An Illustrated Guide To Gastrointestinal Motility

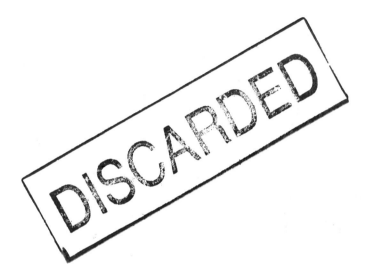

An Illustrated Guide To Gastrointestinal Motility

Edited by

Devinder Kumar

Senior Lecturer in Surgery,
The Queen Elizabeth Hospital,
Birmingham, UK

David Wingate

Professor of Gastrointestinal Science
The London Hospital Medical College,
London, UK

SECOND EDITION

CHURCHILL LIVINGSTONE
EDINBURGH LONDON MADRID MELBOURNE NEW YORK AND TOKYO 1993

Contents

Preface   vii

Acknowledgements   viii

Contributors   ix

SECTION 1
Morphology of the gastrointestinal motor system

1. Gross morphology   3
   D. Kumar

2. The enteric nervous system   10
   J. Christensen

3. Structure of smooth muscle   32
   G. Gabella

SECTION 2
Regulation of gastrointestinal motility

4. The ontogeny of intestinal motor activity   51
   P. J. Milla

5. Intrinsic and extrinsic neural control   64
   D. L. Wingate

6. Motility and regulatory peptides   78
   J. E. T. Fox-Threlkeld

SECTION 3
Modulating factors

7. Modulation of motor activity by sleep   95
   D. Kumar

8. Stress and gastrointestinal motility   104
   F. Musial, P. Enck

9. The immune system   118
   S. M. Collins

10. Food and gastrointestinal motility   130
    L. Bueno, J. Fioramonti

11. Actions of pharmacological agents on gastrointestinal function   144
    T. F. Burks

SECTION 4
The measurement of motility

12. Radiology   165
    E. Corazziari, A. Torsoli

13. Perfused tube manometry   183
    M. Camilleri

14. Ambulant manometry   200
    E. E. Soffer, R. W. Summers

15. Radiotelemetry   211
    D. F. Evans

16. Radioscintigraphy   228
    K. Harding, A. Notghi

17. Ultrasonography   242
    N. K. Ahluwalia, D. G. Thompson

18. Electromyography   256
    G. Coremans

19. Electrical impedance measurements   276
    N. M. Spyrou, F. D. Castillo

20. Electrogastrography   290
    K. L. Koch, R. M. Stern

21. Chemical detection of transit   308
    R. C. Spiller

22. Computerized data analysis   319
    R. B. Hanson

SECTION 5

Normal gastrointestinal motility

23. The oesophagus   337
    G. Vantrappen, J. Janssens

24. The proximal sphincters   357
    J. A. Wilson, R. C. Heading

25. The stomach, pylorus and duodenum   373
    S. S. C. Rao, K. Schulze-Delrieu

26. Biliary tract   393
    J. Toouli

27. The small intestine and the ileocaecal
    region   410
    G. Basilisco, S. F. Phillips

28. Colonic motility   427
    J. Frexinos, M. Delvaux

29. The anorectum   449
    R. Farouk, D. C. C. Bartolo

SECTION 6

Disorders of gastrointestinal motility

30. Motor disorders of the oesophagus   473
    C. E. Pope II

31. Gastro-oesophageal reflux disease   496
    J. E. Richter

32. Motor disorders of the stomach and
    duodenum   522
    G. Stacher

33. Motor disorders of the biliary tract   538
    J. Toouli

34. Ileus and mechanical obstruction   547
    M. J. Benson, D. L. Wingate

35. Chronic pseudo-obstruction   567
    J. Christensen, K. Orvar

36. The irritable bowel syndrome   583
    D. L. Wingate

37. Constipation   595
    G. Devroede

38. Abnormalities of anorectal function   655
    R. L. Grotz, J. H. Pemberton

SECTION 7

Effects of surgery

39. Post-surgical motility disorders   673
    F. Moody, N. Weisbrodt

40. The effects of resection, restorative procedures
    and transplantation on intestinal motility   691
    E. M. M. Quigley

Index   717

Preface

Increasing interest in the subject of the motor function of the gastrointestinal tract is evident both among basic scientists and clinicians. From the former, there are growing volumes of research papers and dedicated symposia; among the latter, gastrointestinal motility disorders are no longer seen merely as obscure rarities. Some techniques for the evaluation of motor function are now widely accepted and used in clinical practice, while new methods promise to unravel many of the 'functional disorders' that form a large part of clinical practice in gastroenterology. New information is accumulating, but much of it is not readily accessible to the clinician or the research worker, and this second edition of *An Illustrated Guide To Gastrointestinal Motility* is intended to remedy this situation.

The aim of this edition remains as before, which is to provide a concise, practical and fully illustrated account, by acknowledged experts, of not only the motor physiology and pathophysiology of the gut, but also of the methods by which it may be studied. The book is divided into sections that reflect the changes that have occurred since the first edition was written. Following the first section on morphology, which is updated but otherwise largely unchanged, new sections deal with the systems that regulate and modulate gastrointestinal motility. In the section on measurement of motility, all the chapters have been rewritten to take account of recent advances; in particular, new techniques of imaging with radioisotopes are described, and

there are now separate chapters on stationary and ambulant manometry. The sections on normal motility and on disorders have been brought up to date by authors who are, with few exceptions, new to the book.

We have been fortunate in assembling a galaxy of talent, and we are deeply grateful to our contributors for the efforts that they have made to create a book intended, above all, to be useful and readable. Readers may notice that there is some repetition between chapters; we have deliberately allowed this because we consider that, whenever possible, a chapter should cover a topic without the constant need for cross-reference to another chapter. This is a large book, and we recognize that only a proportion of readers will set out to read it from cover to cover.

The subject of gastrointestinal motility embraces many different disciplines, from anatomy through electrophysiology to engineering and physics; all those working in these different aspects of motility share a common aim with this book, which is to enable clinicians to provide treatment that is both rational and effective for patients whose digestive tracts move material at the wrong speed, or in the wrong direction, or even not at all.

Birmingham and London, 1993

D.K.
D.L.W.

Acknowledgements

In its finished form, this book has become more encyclopaedic in content and detail than we had imagined at the outset. For this, we are deeply indebted to our contributors for their enthusiasm and to the staff of Churchill Livingstone, in particular Tara Mistry, for their tolerance, ingenuity and constant support.

Contributors

N.K. Ahluwalia
Department of Medicine, Hope Hospital, Salford, UK

David C.C. Bartolo
Department of Surgery, Edinburgh Royal Infirmary, Edinburgh, UK

Guido Basilisco
Cattedra di Gastroenterologia, Padiglione Granelli, Milano, Italy

M.J. Benson
Gastrointestinal Science Research Unit, The London Hospital Medical College, London, UK

L. Bueno
Department of Pharmacology, INRA, Toulouse, France

Thomas F. Burks
The University of Texas, Office of Research and Academic Affairs, Houston, Texas, USA

Michael Camilleri
Professor of Medicine and Consultant in Gastroenterology and Physiology, Mayo Medical School and Mayo Clinic, Rochester, Minnesota, USA

Fortunato D. Castillo
Research Fellow, Gastrointestinal Science Research Unit, The London Hospital Medical College, London, UK

James Christensen
Division of Gastroenterology and Hepatology, The University of Iowa, Iowa City, Iowa, USA

Stephen M. Collins
Intestinal Disease Research Unit, Department of Gastroenterology, McMaster University, Hamilton, Ontario, Canada

Enrico Corazziari
Cattedra di Gastroenterologia I, II Clinica Medica, Policlinico Umberto I, Rome, Italy

G. Coremans
Professor of Medicine, Department of Gastroenterology, University Hospital of Gasthuisberg, University of Leuven, Leuven, Belgium

Michel Delvaux
Department of Gastroenterology and Laboratory of Digestive Motility, Centre Hospitalier Regional, Hôpital de Rangueil, Toulouse Cedex, France

Ghislain Devroede
Department de Chirugie, Centre Hospitalier Universitaire de Sherbrooke, Sherbrooke, Quebec, Canada

Paul Enck
Department of Gastroenterology, Heinrich Heine University Hospitals, Düsseldorf, Germany

D.F. Evans
Senior Lecturer, Gastrointestinal Science Research Unit, The London Hospital Medical College, London, UK

Ridzuan Farouk
Department of Surgery, Royal Infirmary of Edinburgh, Edinburgh, UK

J. Fioramonti
Department of Pharmacology, INRA, Toulouse, France

Jo-ann E.T. Fox-Threlkeld
Professor, School of Nursing, Faculty of Health Sciences, McMaster University, Hamilton, Ontario, Canada

Jacques Frexinos
Department of Gastroenterology and Laboratory of

Digestive Motility, Centre Hospitalier Regional, Hôpital de Rangueil, Toulouse Cedex, France

Giorgio Gabella
Department of Anatomy and Developmental Biology, University College London, London, UK

Richard L. Grotz
Fellow in Colon and Rectal Surgery, Mayo Graduate School of Medicine, Rochester, Minnesota, USA

Russell B. Hanson
Gastroenterology Unit, Mayo Clinic, Rochester, Minnesota, USA

L. Keith Harding
Consultant in Nuclear Medicine, Birmingham Regional Radioisotope Centre, Department of Physics and Nuclear Medicine, Dudley Road Hospital, Birmingham, UK

Robert C. Heading
Department of Medicine, University of Edinburgh, Edinburgh, UK

J. Janssens
Department of Internal Medicine, Division of Gastroenterology, University Hospital Gasthuisberg, University of Leuven, Leuven, Belgium

Kenneth L. Koch
Professor of Medicine, Department of Medicine, Gastroenterology Division, University Hospital, The Milton S. Hershey Medical Centre, The Pennsylvania State University, Hershey, Pennsylvania, USA

Devinder Kumar
Consultant Senior Lecturer, The University of Birmingham, Department of Surgery, Queen Elizabeth Hospital, Birmingham, UK

Peter J. Milla
Senior Lecturer, Gastroenterology Unit, Institute of Child Health, University of London, London, UK

F.G. Moody
Denton A. Cooley Professor and Chairman, Department of Surgery, The University of Texas Medical School, Houston, Texas, USA

Frauke Musial
Department of Biological Cybernetics and Psychobiology, Heinrich-Heine-University, Düsseldorf, Germany

Alp Notghi
Senior Registrar in Nuclear Medicine, Dudley Road Hospital, Birmingham, UK

Kjartan Orvar
Division of Gastroenterology–Hepatology, University of Iowa, Iowa City, Iowa, USA

John H. Pemberton
Associate Professor of Surgery, Mayo Medical School, Clinic and Foundation, Rochester, Minnesota, USA

Sidney F. Phillips
Professor of Medicine, Gastroenterology Research Unit, Mayo Foundation, Rochester, Minnesota, USA

Charles E. Pope II
Department of Veterans Affairs Medical Center, Seattle, Washington, USA

Eamonn M.M. Quigley
Department of Internal Medicine, Section of Digestive Diseases and Nutrition, University of Nebraska, Omaha, Nebraska, USA

Satish S.C. Rao
Assistant Professor of Medicine, Division of Gastroenterology–Hepatology, Department of Internal Medicine, University of Iowa College of Medicine, Iowa City, Iowa, USA

Joel E. Richter
Professor of Medicine, Director of Clinical Research, Division of Gastroenterology, University of Alabama at Birmingham, Birmingham, Alabama, USA

Konrad Schulze-Delrieu
Professor of Medicine, Division of Gastroenterology–Hepatology, Department of Internal Medicine, University of Iowa College of Medicine, Iowa City, Iowa, USA

Edy E. Soffer
Division of Gastroenterology–Hepatology, Department of Internal Medicine, University of Iowa College of Medicine, Iowa City, Iowa, USA

R.C. Spiller
Consultant Physician, University Hospital, Queen's Medical Centre, Nottingham, UK

Nicholas M. Spyrou
Reader in the Department of Physics, Surrey University, Guildford, UK

Georg Stacher
Professor, Psychophysiology Unit, University of Vienna, Vienna, Austria

Robert M. Stern
Professor of Psychology, Psychology Department, The Pennsylvania State University, University Park, Pennsylvania, USA

Robert W. Summers
Division of Gastroenterology–Hepatology,
Department of Internal Medicine, University of Iowa
College of Medicine, and Department of Veterans
Affairs Medical Center, Iowa City, Iowa, USA

D.G. Thompson
Department of Medicine, Hope Hospital, Salford,
UK

James Toouli
Professor and Head of Unit, Gastrointestinal Surgical
and Liver Transplant Unit, Flinders Medical Centre,
Bedford Park, South Australia, Australia

Aldo Torsoli
Cattedra di Gastroenterologia I, II Clinica Medica,
Policlinico Umberto I, Rome, Italy

G. Vantrappen
Department of Internal Medicine, Division of
Gastroenterology, University Hospital Gasthuisberg,
University of Leuven, Leuven, Belgium

N. Weisbrodt
Professor, Department of Physiology and Cell Biology,
The University of Texas Medical School, Houston,
Texas, USA

Janet A. Wilson
Royal Infirmary, Glasgow, UK

David L. Wingate
Gastrointestinal Science Research Unit, The London
Hospital Medical College, London, UK

Morphology of the gastrointestinal motor system

1. Gross morphology of the gastrointestinal tract

D. Kumar

The alimentary tract is a muscular tube extending from the mouth to the anus. It shows a similar structure throughout its entire length, consisting of serosa, muscle layer, submucosa and mucosa. The muscle layer consists of an inner circular and outer longitudinal layer of smooth muscle. The upper third of the oesophagus consists of striated muscle. There are striated muscle sphincters at either end; the upper oesophageal sphincter above and the anal sphincter below. An adequate knowlege of morphology of the gastrointestinal tract is necessary for the successful planning and performance of motility studies.

INNERVATION OF THE GUT

Detailed morphophysiology of the enteric nervous system will be discussed in Chapter 2. Broadly speaking, the nerve supply of the gastrointestinal tract comprises extrinsic and intrinsic components. The extrinsic component is provided by the autonomic nervous system (parasympathetic and sympathetic). The oesophagus, stomach, small intestine and the proximal colon derive their parasympathetic supply from the vagus nerve. The colon is also innervated by the sacral spinal nerves. The sympathetic supply to the gut is through the lower thoracic and lumbar spinal nerves. The intrinsic innervation, now frequently known as the enteric nervous system, is through the submucosal and myenteric plexuses which contain intercommunicating ganglia (Fig. 1.1).

OESOPHAGUS

The oesophagus is a muscular tube extending from the cricoid cartilage to the cardia of the stomach. It descends through the posterior mediasternum and joins the stomach opposite the ninth dorsal vertebra. It is the narrowest part of the alimentary canal.

In the adult, the oesophagus measures approximately 25 cm, the oesophagogastric junction being 40 cm

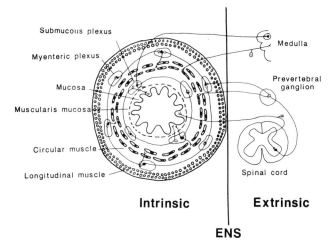

Fig. 1.1 Transverse section of the gut showing the intrinsic plexuses, the extrinsic enteric nervous system (ENS), and some intrinsic and extrinsic interconnections.

from the incisor teeth. In the supine posture with the head fully extended, the distance between the lower incisors and the xiphisternum provides a fairly accurate estimate of the length of the oesophagus. This may be important in studies that require accurate location of the lower oesophageal sphincter.

Structurally, the oesophagus has three layers: an internal or mucosa; a middle or submucosa; and an external or muscular. The external coat consists of an outer longitudinal muscle and inner circular muscle layer. The fibres of the longitudinal layer are in continuity with the inferior constrictor muscle fibres. The fibres of the circular layer are also in continuity with the inferior constrictor muscle fibres above and run transversely in the upper and lower oesophagus. In the central part, they run obliquely. The oesophagus consists of striped muscle in the upper part and involuntary smooth muscle below.

The lower oesophagus and the diaphragmatic hiatus have intrigued investigators for many years and it is, therefore, not surprising that many terminologies and subdivisions of this region are encountered. Figure 1.2 shows a schematic representation of the lower oesophagus and surrounding structures. The oesophagus passes from a low pressure area (thoracic cavity) to a high pressure area (abdominal cavity). The pressure differential between the two cavities is maintained by loose areolar tissue which fills the hiatus around the oesophagus. This is further helped by the presence of the phreno-oesophageal ligament which is inserted into the oesophagus approximately 3 cm above the diaphragmatic opening.

The presence of an anatomical equivalent of the lower oesophageal sphincter has been disputed by most workers. Liebermann-Meffert et al (1979) demonstrated the presence of an asymmetrical thickening of the circular muscle just above the angle of His in the lower oesophagus (Fig. 1.3). It is not certain whether this area of asymmetrical thickening coincides precisely with the lower oesophageal sphincter but the highest pressure is found in the area of greatest muscle thickening (Waldeck et al 1973). It is therefore possible that both anatomical as well as sphincteric factors contribute towards maintaining competence at the gastro-oesophageal junction.

The oesphagus derives its motor nerve supply from the dorsal motor nucleus of the vagus nerve and the nucleus of the spinal accessory nerve which supplies the cervical portion of the oesophagus. The vagus nerve also carries afferent fibres; however, precise details of the afferent supply of the oesophagus are not known. The sympathetic innervation of the oesophagus is derived from the cervical sympathetic ganglia and the thoracic sympathetic chain.

STOMACH

The stomach is the most dilated portion of the gastrointestinal tract. It is J-shaped (Fig. 1.4) in most individuals and has a capacity of approximately 1500 ml in adults. It is located in the upper part of the abdomen and is relatively fixed at its upper and lower ends where it joins the oesophagus and the duodenum respectively. However, its shape and position vary with degree of distension and body pressure. This is important, particularly when carrying out non-invasive studies of gastric emptying, for example epigastric impedance, as change in position during the test can give rise to erroneous results.

The stomach has been divided into various anatomical regions (Fig. 1.4). It consists of the cardia, fundus,

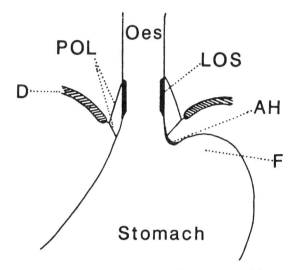

Fig. 1.2 Schematic representation of the anatomy of the lower oesophagus. D = diaphragm; POL = phreno-oesophageal ligament; LOS = lower oesophageal sphincter; AH = angle of His; F = fundus; Oes = oesophagus. (Adapted from Liebermann–Meffert et al 1979)

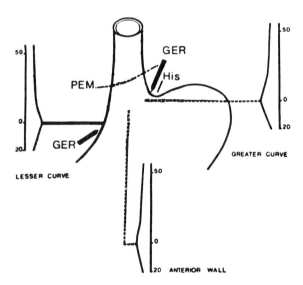

Fig. 1.3 Diagram showing the site of muscular thickness in the lower oesophagus. His = angle of His; GER = gastro-oesophageal ring; PEM = phreno-oesophageal membrane. (Adapted from Liebermann-Meffert et al 1979)

body, antrum and the pylorus. There is a notch-like indentation, known as the incisura angularis, on the lesser curve. The portion of the stomach distal to the incisura angularis is the antrum. Structurally the stomach consists of serosa, a muscular layer, submucosal

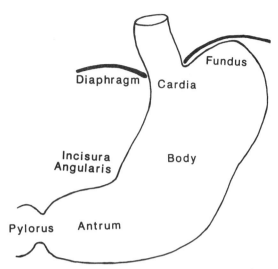

Fig. 1.4 Diagrammatic sketch showing anatomic regions of the stomach.

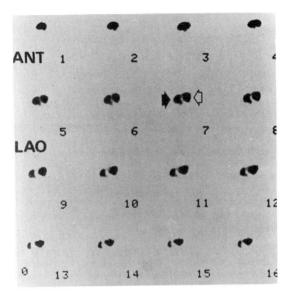

Fig. 1.5 Single photon computed tomography images of the stomach in a healthy subject after ingesting an unhomogenized 900 g meal labelled with ^{99m}Tc-chicken liver. Each 60 s image is acquired every 5.6° throughout 360° rotation of the scintillation camera around the abdomen with the subject in the supine position. Only the first 16 images of a total 64 are shown, representing the anterior (ANT) and left anterior oblique (LAO) positions, or through 90° of rotation counter-clockwise around the abdomen. Note the persistence of the transverse band in frames 5–15. As illustrated here, the band is observed most clearly in the LAO position and is poorly defined in the anterior–posterior position (frames 1–4). The gastric body lies to the right (open arrow, frame 7) and the gastric antrum to the left (closed arrow, frame 7) of the radio-penic region representing the band. (Reproduced with permission from Moore et al, 1986)

layer and mucosa which is the innermost layer. The serosa is derived from the peritoneum and covers the entire surface of the organ except at the points of attachment of the greater and lesser omentum. The muscle coat consists of longitudinal, circular and oblique fibres. The longitudinal fibres are in continuity with the longitudinal muscle of the oesophagus and radiate downwards from the cardia. At the pylorus, they are continuous with the longitudinal fibres of the duodenum. The circular fibres form a uniform layer throughout and lie beneath the longitudinal fibres. At the pylorus, these fibres form a circular ring which projects into the cavity. The oblique fibres are mainly confined to the greater end of the stomach where they descend upon its anterior and posterior surface (Gray 1991). The submucosal coat consists of loose areolar tissue, blood vessels and nerves. The mucosa of the stomach is thrown into folds called rugae which run longitudinally. The rugae become obliterated when the stomach is distended.

Moore et al (1986) have demonstrated the presence of a gastric transverse band representing an anatomical separation between the body and the antrum (Figs 1.5 and 1.6). It has been suggested that this band of separation may play a role in the regulation of emptying from the gastric body into the antrum. Manometrically, the antrum is the most commonly studied part of the stomach as the majority of contractions in this region tend to be occlusive in nature. In contrast, contractions in the body and the fundus of the stomach tend to be non-occlusive and therefore not detected

by intraluminal manometry. The pylorus is the most distal part of the stomach and has a thick muscular wall (Fig. 1.7). It is approximately 1 in long and is usually located 1 in to the right of the midline at the level of the first lumbar vertebra. It is an important landmark as it helps in the placement of the manometric assemblies at or across the pylorus. It can also be identified on manometric tracings because it shows a dual frequency of contractions.

The parasympathetic nerve supply of the stomach is from the right and left vagus nerves. The sympathetic innervation is derived from the coeliac plexus and contains the afferent pain transmitting nerve fibres.

SMALL INTESTINE

The adult human small intestine measures 4–6 m in length. The length seems to vary both with the tone of

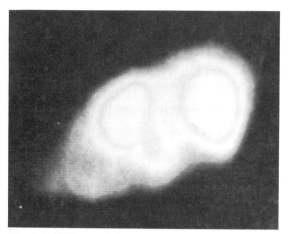

Fig. 1.6 ^{99m}Tc gastric images in a human following solid labelled meal. The scintiphoto was taken 10 min after ingestion of the meal. Gastric antrum lies to the left and gastric body-fundus to the right of the midgastric band. (Reproduced with permission from Moore et al 1986)

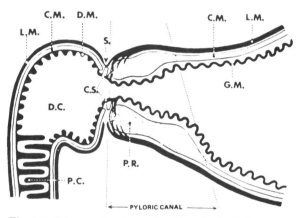

Fig. 1.7 Diagram of gastroduodenal junction in the human being. LM = longitudinal muscle; CM = circular muscle; DM = duodenal mucosa; S = sphincter; DC = duodenal cavity; PC = plicae circulare; PR = pyloric ring; GM = gastric mucosa. (Reproduced with permission from Edwards & Rowlands, 1968)

tion of the duodenum and jejunum, known as the duodenojejunal flexure. It is a useful anatomical landmark in the investigation of the upper small intestine; it helps to anchor manometric assemblies and prevent retraction into the stomach. The diameter of the proximal jejunum is approximately twice that of the distal ileum. The wall of the jejunum is considerably thicker than that of the ileum. The division of the small bowel into jejunum and ileum is somewhat arbitrary; since there is no anatomical landmark but merely a gradual change in size; the proximal two-fifths is generally referred to as the jejunum and the distal three-fifths is called the ileum. The ileum occupies the lower abdomen and a portion of the pelvis.

The food is mixed with the bile and pancreatic secretions and absorption of various nutrients takes place in the small intestine. It is surrounded by the large intestine at the sides and above. The wall of the small intestine consists of four coats; the outer serosa, the muscularis propria, submucosa and the innermost mucosa. The muscular coat consists of an outer longitudinal and inner circular muscle layer. The longitudinal layer is a thin coat of muscle fibres whereas the circular muscle layer forms a thick uniform layer. The muscular coat of the small intestine is thicker in the upper part than in the lower part of the small intestine.

The mucosa of the small intestine is thrown into folds forming valvulae conniventes. They extend across for approximately half to three-quarters of the circumference of the small intestine. These are absent in the ileum. The function of valvulae conniventes is to slow down the passage of food through the small intestine and thus provide an opportunity for the food to be absorbed. The valvulae conniventes also effectively increase the absorptive surface area.

The small intestinal muscosa is marked by the presence of villi. These are longest and most numerous in the duodenum and jejunum. The ileum is characterized by the presence of Peyer's patches which are formed by a group of small round vessicles covered with mucous membrane.

The distal few inches of the terminal ileum are closely applied to the caecum by the superior and inferior ileocaecal ligaments (Fig. 1.8) (Kumar & Phillips 1987) and is therefore the least mobile. The mesentery of the ileum is thicker and contains more fat. This feature may be important in identification of the ileum on fluoroscopy or X-ray films during the placement of tubes in the distal small bowel.

The ileocaecal junction has generally been thought to be a sphincter. Anatomically, it consists of an upper and lower lip. There is no easily identifiable anatomical equivalent of a sphincter at the ileocaecal junction. In

the muscle wall and the method of measurement. This can be important when placing electrodes on the surface of the intestine under general anaesthetic because the actual distance between electrodes may be totally different when the effect of the anaesthetic has worn off and the muscles have regained their normal tone. Therefore, the data obtained from such studies have to be interpreted with caution especially with regard to propagation velocity of various motor events. Except for the duodenum, the small intestine is suspended by a mesentery and has considerable mobility within the abdominal cavity. There is an acute bend at the junc-

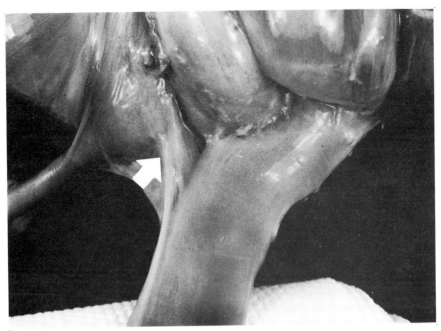

Fig. 1.8 Close-up of the ileocaecal junction showing the superior and inferior ileocaecal ligaments (arrow). (Reproduced with permission from Kumar & Phillips 1987)

fact, the ileal and caecal circular muscle is separated by loose areolar tissue (Fig. 1.9) and the apparent thickening at the junction is due to the superimposition of the ileal muscle on the caecal circular muscle. Kumar and Phillips (1987) have shown that continence at the ileocaecal junction is maintained at least in part of the anatomical configuration of the junction. Division of the ileocaecal ligaments renders the junction incompetent.

LARGE INTESTINE

The large intestine extends from the caecum to the anus and measures approximately 5 feet (1.5 m) in length. It is divided into the caecum, ascending colon, transverse, descending, sigmoid colon and rectum. The caecum is the widest part of the large intestine and the lumen gradually diminishes as far as the rectum where there is a considerable increase in size. In contrast to the small intestine, the large intestine is more fixed in position and has sacculations. The sacculations represent morphological adaptation to the significant amount of non-absorbed fibre reaching the colon, and is related to the occurrence of bacterial fermentation that reduces the fibre to small molecules. The large intestine surrounds the convolutions of the small intestine and forms an arch. The right side ascends from

the caecum to the under surface of the liver forming the hepatic flexure and passes transversely across to the left hypochondriac region in relation to the lower pole of the spleen, forming the splenic flexure, and then descends through the left lumbar region to the left iliac fossa where it forms the sigmoid flexure. It enters the pelvis at the pelvic brim where the rectosigmoid junction lies. The rectum is the most distal and dilated part of the large intestine. It follows the curve of the sacrum and is relatively fixed so that it does not have a great degree of mobility. The rectum passes obliquely downwards from left to right to the midline of the sacrum. It forms a gentle curve to the right side and then comes into the midline to descend further in front of the sacrum and coccyx where it joins the anal canal. The anal canal is a short segment, 3–4 cm long and lies encased in the pelvic floor and the external anal sphincter.

The caecum is the widest part of the large intestine (Fig. 1.10). The rest of the colon is divided into ascending, transverse, descending and sigmoid colon segments. The bulk of the longitudinal muscle in the colon is arranged in three longitudinal bundles called taeniae. The thin layer of intertaeniae longitudinal muscle surrounds the colonic circular muscle layer. The taeniae extend from the base of the appendix to the rectosigmoid junction where they blend with the longitudinal muscle of the rectum. Unlike the ascending

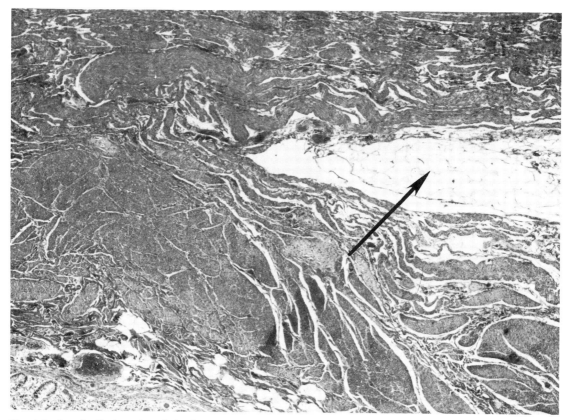

Fig. 1.9 Longitudinal section of the ileocaecal junction showing separation of the ileal and caecal muscle by loose areolar tissue (arrow).

and descending colon, the transverse and sigmoid colon have a mesentery and are therefore mobile. In between the taeniae, the colon forms haustra that allow segmental movements. Different regions of the large intestine have different functions and it is therefore important that data obtained from one segment of the large intestine should be considered with respect to that individual segment and not taken to be representative of the entire colon.

The rectum is the most distal part of the large intestine. It follows the curve of the sacrum and does not have a great degree of mobility. The terminal 3–4 cm form the anal canal. The internal anal sphincter is part of the smooth muscle of the rectum and should be studied in combination with the rectum.

ANORECTUM

The pelvic floor and the anorectum have a complex anatomical structure. The pelvic floor consists of paired striated muscles known as the levator ani. Levator ani muscle is largely composed of the pubococcygeus and the ileococcygeus muscles with some contribution from

the coccygeus muscles close to it. The puborectalis muscle is closely related to and forms an integral part of the levator ani and the external anal sphincter muscle. It helps to angulate the anorectal junction anteriorly. The puborectalis loops around the rectum to form a U-shaped sling and together with the upper part of the internal and external sphincters it forms the anorectal ring which separates the anal canal from the rectum. The levator ani has a dual nerve supply; the pelvic surface is innovated from branches of the fourth sacral nerve and the perineal surface via the perineal branch of the pudenal nerve. The puborectalis muscle is innovated from the inferior rectal nerve.

The upper two-thirds of the rectum is covered by the peritoneum on its anterior surface and only the upper third on its lateral surfaces. The lower third of the rectum is below the peritoneal reflection. The rectum is supported by the lateral ligaments on each side and the anterior extraperitoneal part of the rectum is covered by Denonvilliers fascia which run between the rectum and prostate or vagina. At the level of the anorectal ring the rectum continues downwards as the

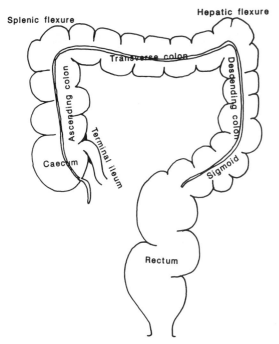

Fig. 1.10 Diagram showing anatomical regions of the large bowel.

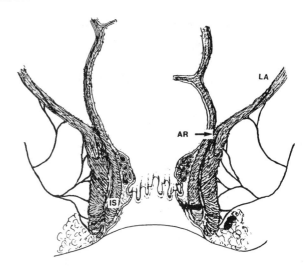

Fig. 1.11 Diagrammatic sketch of the anal canal and lower rectum. AR – anorectal junction; IS – internal sphincter; LA – Levator ani muscle.

anal canal (Fig. 1.11). At this point the lumen of the rectum forms an anteroposterior slit which is closed at all times and helps to maintain continence. The circular smooth muscle of the rectum continues downwards and forms the internal anal sphincter beginning at the level of the anorectal ring. The rounded edge of the internal sphincter can often be palpated 1–2 cm below the dentate line. The involuntary internal sphincter muscle is tonically contracted at rest and provides the resting tone in the anal canal. The longitudinal muscle fibres of the rectum join the medial fibres of the pubococcygeus and puborectalis and travel downwards along the intersphincteric plane, fan out through the subcutaneous portion of the external sphincter and become inserted into the anoderm and perianal skin.

The external anal sphincter is composed of striated muscle and surrounds the internal sphincter. It has a deep part which is closely related to the puborectalis muscle, a superficial part which forms the middle loop of the external anal sphincter and a subcutaneous part which is the lowermost part of the external sphincter.

The mucosa of the anal canal is lined by columnar epithelium in the upper part and stratified squamous epithelium from the dentate line to the anal verge. In between the stratified squamous epithelium and the columnar epithelium there is a band of cuboidal epithelium known as the transitional zone. This transitional zone is only present in approximately 50% of subjects (Chattopadhyay et al 1993). The anoderm has a rich innervation with cutaneous sensory nerve endings whereas the proximal anal canal lacks somatic innervation. The upper anal canal, the rectum, the bladder and genitals are innervated by the autonomic nervous system whereas the external sphincter has a somatic nerve supply.

REFERENCES

Chattopadhyay G, Newbold M, Kumar D 1993 Anal transition zone (ATZ) and the distribution of neuroendocrine cells in the anorectum. Dig Surg 449.

Edwards D A W, Rowlands E N 1968 Physiology of the gastroduodenal junction, in: Code CF, Heidel W (eds) Handbook of Physiology Section 6, Volume 4: 1985–2000

Gray H 1991 Anatomy: descriptive and surgical. Royal Society of Medicine Services Ltd

Kumar D, Phillips S F 1987 The contribution of external ligamentous attachments to function of the ileocaecal junction. Dis Colon Rectum 30: 410–416

Liebermann-Meffert D, Allgower M, Schmid P, Blum A L 1979 Muscular equivalent of the lower oesophageal sphincter. Gastroenterology 76: 31

Moore J G, Dubois A, Christian P E, Elgin D, Alazraki N 1986 Evidence for a midgastric transverse band in humans. Gastroenterology 91: 540–545

Waldeck F, Jennewein H M, Siewert R 1973 The continous withdrawal method for the quantitative analysis of the lower oesophageal sphincter (LES) in humans. Eur J Chir Invest 3: 331–337

2. The enteric nervous system

J. Christensen

INTRODUCTION (Furness & Costa 1987)

The apparent self-determination of the motor behaviour of the gut arises partly from the autonomy of the smooth muscle and partly from the autonomy of the nerves which supply it. The nerves and nerve-associated cells that lie within the walls of the gut and its appendages, called the enteric nervous system (ENS), make up a functional unit capable of such versatility, variety, complexity, and apparent independence in operation that it now receives consideration as an independent control system. Indeed, the original conception of the autonomic nervous system designated three parts, the sympathetic, parasympathetic, and enteric nervous systems. Components of the sympathetic and parasympathetic systems join the ENS to the central nervous system, so that the ENS is not functionally and structurally separated.

The operation of the gut receives constant modulation in normal function. The fact that the gut is never in a steady state requires such modulation. Some of this input is central, though independent of the consciousness. Most of the input, however, comes from sensory nerves in the ENS. Some sensory inputs to motor nerves of the ENS prompt widespread effects, while others produce local responses. Thus, the sensory inputs occur at various levels in the nervous system. Figure 2.1 shows the hierarchy of the extrinsic enteric nerves. Sensory-motor integration occurs in the CNS, in the prevertebral ganglia, and in the intramural plexuses.

THE EXTRINSIC NERVES TO THE GUT: GROSS ARRANGEMENT (DAVISON 1983)

General arrangement

The nerves that pass from the CNS to the gut depart at many levels from the hindbrain and the spinal

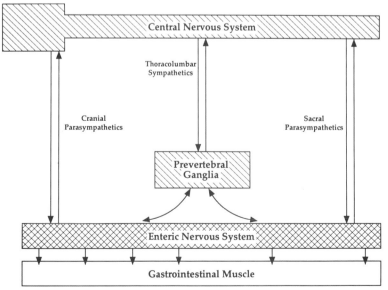

Fig. 2.1 A diagram of the relationship of the ENS to the CNS. Sensory motor integration through reflexes can occur within the ENS, through the prevertebral ganglia, or through the CNS. (From Christensen 1991, with permission.)

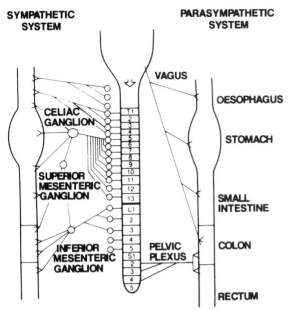

SYMPATHETIC SYSTEM

PARASYMPATHETIC SYSTEM

Fig. 2.2 A diagram of the extrinsic innervation of the gut. CNS structures are not shown. (From Davison 1983, with permission.)

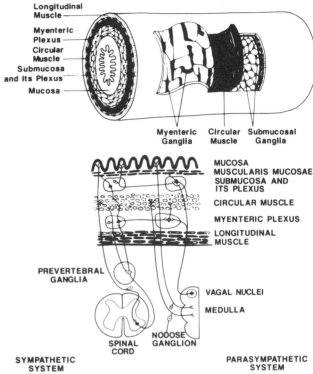

Fig. 2.3 The intramural nerves of the gut. (From Davison 1983, with permission.)

cord. They constitute two principal groups, the thoracolumbar and craniosacral systems, referring to the segments which give them origin. The nerves from the cranial and sacral cord regions resemble one another physiologically, while those from the thoracic and lumbar segments of the cord also resemble one another physiologically, but differ from the craniosacral nerves. The thoracolumbar nerves are commonly called sympathetic, and the craniosacral nerves parasympathetic. These divisions are shown in Figures 2.1 and 2.2.

Craniosacral pathways (Fig. 2.2)

The cranial pathways are the ninth (glossopharyngeal) and tenth (vagus) cranial nerves. The ninth nerve is distributed along the gut as far as the upper oesophageal sphincter. The domain of the tenth nerve extends to the right colon. These cranial nerves arise from nuclei in the region of the fourth ventricle. Each tenth nerve contains a ganglion just beneath the skull, the nodose ganglion, which contains sensory nerve cell bodies. The tenth nerves form a plexus about the distal oesophagus, the oesophageal plexus, branches from which supply the oesophagus. The bundles of the oesophageal plexus fuse above the diaphragm to form the vagal trunks which supply the abdominal gastrointestinal viscera.

The sacral pathways arise from sacral segments 1 to

4 to form the pelvic nerves and the pudendal nerves. The pelvic nerves contribute to the pelvic plexus. The colonic nerves pass from the pelvic plexus to the upper rectum where they penetrate the longitudinal muscle layer to continue within the plane of the myenteric plexus all along the colon. The pudendal nerves supply the striated muscle of the pelvic floor and, to some extent, the colon.

Thoracolumbar pathways (Fig. 2.2)

The thoracolumbar pathways arise from the thoracic and lumbar segments of the cord, traverse the paravertebral ganglia, and pass through the splanchnic nerves to the prevertebral ganglia, the coeliac, superior mesenteric and inferior mesenteric ganglia. From these ganglia, nerves pass alongside mesenteric vessels to reach the gut.

Thoracolumbar pathways entering into craniosacral pathways

The previous paragraphs imply that craniosacral and

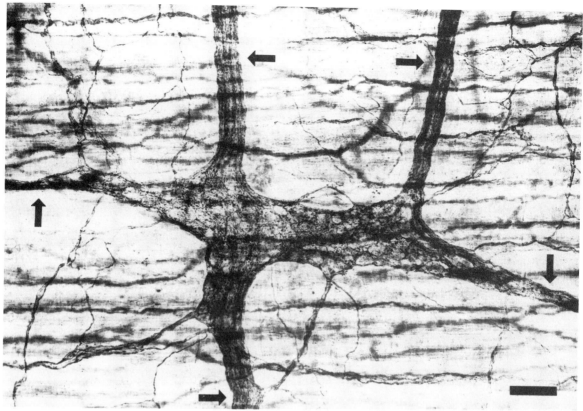

Fig. 2.4   A ganglion of the myenteric plexus of the cat intestine. Neurites, linear black beaded structures fill the ganglion, the interganglionic bundles (➡), and their branches. Cell bodies of ganglion cells appear as open spaces because they do not stain. The secondary plexus lies in the spaces between interganglionic bundles. The tertiary plexus cannot be seen. ▬▬▬ indicates 200 μm. Osmic acid–zinc iodide stain. (From Christensen 1988b, with permission.)

thoracolumbar outflows from the CNS to the CNS remain entirely separate. In fact, however, some admixture occurs in that some thoracolumbar components find their way into craniosacral structures to be distributed along with their branches. The major such mixture occurs in the vagi where, in some species, a large branch departs from a cervical sympathetic ganglion, enters the vagus and decussates with the vagus. Similarly, one or more large branches from the inferior mesenteric ganglion enters into the pelvic plexus to decussate with the branches of that plexus.

THE INTRAMURAL NERVES OF THE GUT: MORPHOLOGY (Gabella 1979, 1987)

General arrangement

Intramural nerve cell bodies are located in ganglia in two planes in the gut wall, the submucosa and the intermuscular plane between the two major muscle layers. These layers of ganglia are the submucous and myenteric plexuses (Fig. 2.3). Other less complex nerve plexuses that contain no ganglia lie just beneath the serosa, deep within the circular muscle layer (only in the intestine), between the circular and oblique muscle layers (only in the stomach), at the interface between circular muscle layer and submucosa (only in the colon), and in the lamina propria throughout the gut.

Histology

Within the collagen sheath of a ganglion, the nerve cell bodies lie in a stroma of glial cells and convoluted neurites (the neuropil). The neurites form synaptic arrangements ('baskets') around ganglion cell bodies. The neuropil and glial cells constitute about half of the mass of a ganglion. Bundles of neurites, which may contain occasional isolated nerve cell bodies, connect adjacent ganglia. These are the interganglionic fascicles. A 'typical' ganglion is shown in Figure 2.4.

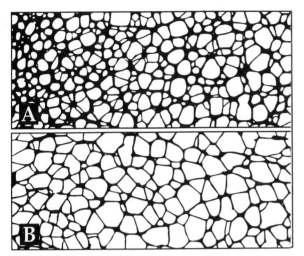

The network formed by the ganglia and interganglionic fascicles of the myenteric plexus is called the primary plexus (Fig. 2.5). Small branches from the interganglionic fascicles form a secondary plexus, devoid of ganglia, that fills the spaces in the primary plexus. In turn, the spaces of the secondary plexus are filled with still smaller fascicles and single neurites that branch from the secondary plexus. This is the tertiary plexus (Fig. 2.6). The secondary and tertiary plexuses are fully formed only in the gastric antrum, the small intestine and the abdominal colon. They are rudimentary or absent in the oesophagus, gastric fundus and pelvic parts of the colon.

The submucous plexus consists of a primary plexus only. It varies greatly in its structure among organs.

The interstitial cells of Cajal (Thuneberg 1982, Rumessen & Thuneberg 1982, Rumessen et al 1982, Christensen 1992)

Ramon y Cajal popularized the idea that certain small

Fig. 2.5 Silhouette drawings of the primary plexus of the colon (**A**) and rectum (**B**) of the guinea pig to illustrate the regularity of the pattern of ganglia connected by interganglionic fascicles. (From Gabella 1987, with permission.)

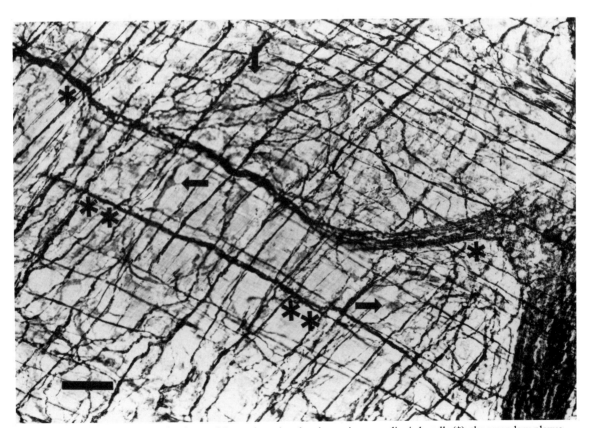

Fig. 2.6 An area of the myenteric plexus of the cat intestine showing an interganglionic bundle (★), the secondary plexus (★★) and the finest bundles which make up the tertiary plexus. Polymorphic cells (➡) are interstitial cells of Cajal. ▬▬▬ indicates 100 μm. Osmic acid–zinc iodide stain. (From Christensen 1988b, with permission.)

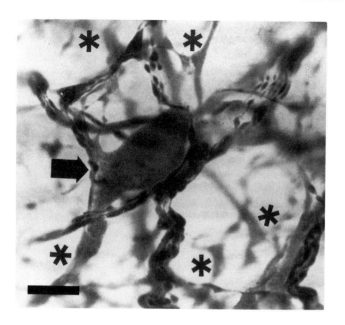

Fig. 2.7   The soma of an interstitial cell of Cajal (➡) surrounded by varicose neurites, black beaded structures, from the cat stomach. The flat, broad, branching processes (*) of this and adjacent interstitial cells appear throughout the field. ▬▬▬ indicates 10 μm. Osmic acid–zinc iodide stain. (From Christensen 1988b, with permission.)

cells, which he called interstitial cells, found in close relationship to networks of axons in the gut wall constitute a structural and functional linkage between axons and muscle or gland cells. These mononuclear polymorphic cells branch profusely, the branches intersecting to form a network throughout which the axons extend (Fig. 2.7). The branches of the interstitial cells form specialized junctions with one another and with smooth muscle cells.

The distribution of these interstitial cells of Cajal differs from one organ to another. In the oesophagus they lie uniformly distributed throughout the circular muscle layer, being absent from the longitudinal muscle layer and sparse in the myenteric plexus. The stomach, where they are distributed in the circular muscle layer and in the plane of the myenteric plexus, contains many fewer interstitial cells in the fundus than in the antrum. Interstitial cells in the small intestine are particularly concentrated in a plane within the circular muscle layer, the deep muscular plexus, and in the plane of the myenteric plexus. In the colon the interstitial cells are most dense on the submucosal surface of the circular muscle layer and in the plane of the myenteric plexus. Figure 2.8 summarizes these distributions.

Interstitial cells possess ultrastructural features which suggest that they have a mesenchymal origin, for they bear certain resemblances to both smooth

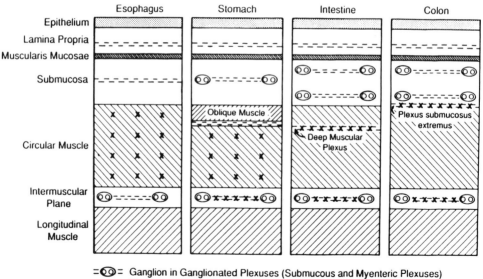

Fig. 2.8   Diagram to compare the distribution of interstitial cells of Cajal in the various regions. (From Christensen 1991, with permission.)

THE ENTERIC NERVOUS SYSTEM

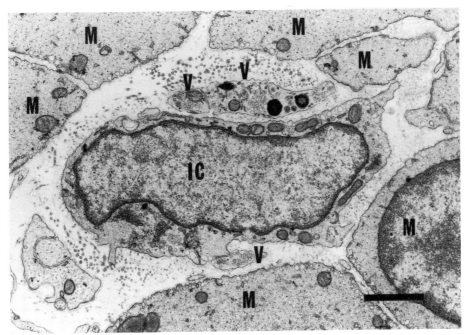

Fig. 2.9 Electron photomicrograph of an interstitial cell of Cajal in the opossum oesophagus. The interstitial cell (**IC**) is surrounded by smooth muscle cells (**M**). Axonal varicosities (**V**) are adjacent. The interstitial cell possesses many mitochondria, caveolae, and an incomplete basal lamina. ▄▄▄▄▄ indicates 1 μm (From Christensen 1988b, with permission.)

muscle cells and fibroblasts (Fig. 2.9), but some observers suggest also that they may be neural or glial in nature.

The idea that interstitial cells may constitute a pacemaker system, generating the electrical slow waves that pace rhythmic peristalsis, has received support from the study of the colon, and is probably true in the small intestine and stomach as well. The cells may also be involved in nerve-to-muscle communication or in providing for electrotonic linkage between muscle cells.

The intramural nerves of the oesophagus
(Christensen & Robison 1982)

The submucous plexus of the oesophagus is nearly devoid of ganglia constituting only a sparse network of axons in most species (Fig. 2.10). For that reason, ganglion cells of the myenteric plexus are probably the source of the abundant nerves found in the relatively thick muscularis mucosae of the oseophagus, and of the sensory nerves in the squamous epithelium (Rodrigo et al 1975).

The myenteric plexus of the oesophagus contains comparatively few ganglion cells (Fig. 2.10). It consists mainly of thick fascicles of neurites running cephalo-caudad and connected by thinner lateral bundles. Secondary and tertiary plexuses are not distinguishable. Ganglia are highly variable in size and shape. Many fascicle branchpoints are devoid of ganglia. Many oesophageal ganglia lie a little away from major fascicles (Fig. 2.11), the so-called parafascicular ganglia. The density of ganglion cells declines along the smooth muscle segment, to reach a nadir at the oesophagogastric sphincter. The myenteric plexus of the striated muscle part of the oesophagus also contains ganglia. Their function there is not clear.

In the oesophageal muscularis mucosae and in the longitudinal muscle layer, the terminal innervation consists of small bundles of neurites and single neurites lying between the muscle bundles. In the circular muscle layer the neurites branch and spread more widely because they must supply the intramuscular interstitial cells which lie in the circular muscle layer (Christensen et al 1987, Daniel & Posey-Daniel 1984). These abundant cells have a sparse cytoplasm surrounding an elliptical nucleus. Broad processes extend from the poles of the elliptical somas of these cells to branch and extend between muscle bundles (Fig. 2.12). The cells lie in chains with their processes entangled.

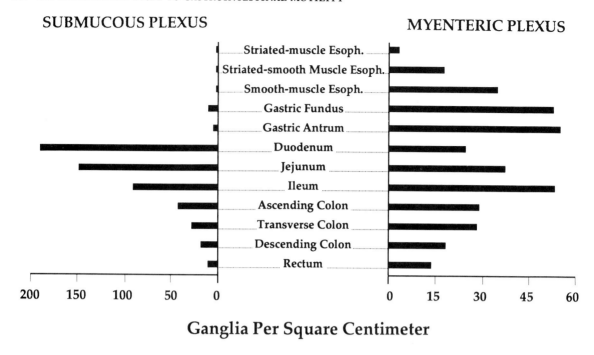

Fig. 2.10 Diagram of the comparative distribution densities of ganglia throughout the submucous and myenteric plexus throughout the gut. The submucous plexus ganglia are much smaller than those of the myenteric plexus, and so this graph does not demonstrate differences in distribution density of neurons. (From Christensen 1991, with permission.)

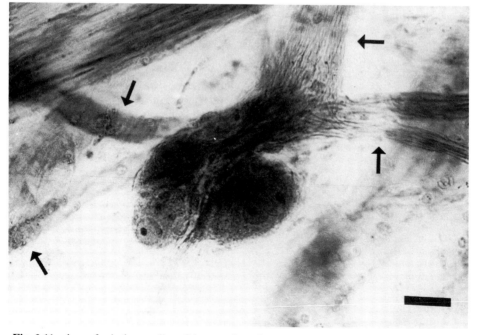

Fig. 2.11 A parafascicular ganglion of the oesophageal myenteric plexus of the opossum. ▬ indicates 25 μm. ➡ indicates the major nerve bundles of the myenteric plexus; note that the nerve cell bodies lie outside the major nerve bundles. Silver stain. (From Christensen 1988b, with permission.)

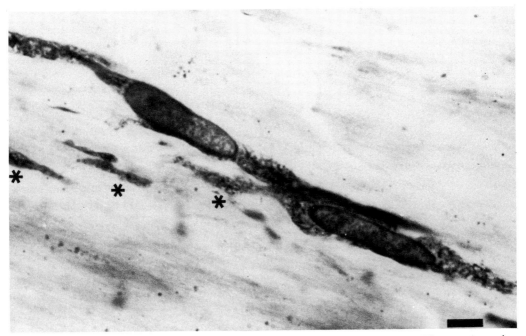

Fig. 2.12 Interstitial cells of Cajal in the circular muscle layer of the opossum oesophagus. There are two oval nuclei with rims of cytoplasm which give off broad flat branches at the poles. Sections pass through processes marked with *. ■■■■ indicates 5 μm. Osmic acid–zinc iodide stain. (From Christensen 1988b, with permission.)

Neurites run along these chains of cells, contacting the processes and somas of the cells. The interstitial cells form gap junctions with the smooth muscle cells. They contain many mitochondria, an extensive endoplasmic reticulum, a conspicuous Golgi apparatus, and many caveolae, suggesting that they are metabolically active (Daniel & Posey-Daniel 1984).

The intramural nerves of the stomach
(Christensen & Rick 1985a, 1985b)

The submucous plexus of the stomach is comparatively sparse, the distribution density of ganglion cells being considerably less than that in the small intestine (Fig. 2.10).

In the fundus, the myenteric plexus ganglia are comparatively sparse, and the secondary and tertiary plexuses are not well developed. In the antrum, the ganglia are larger and more closely spaced and the secondary and tertiary plexuses are dense. The tertiary plexus contains many interstitial cells, each such cell having long processes branching from a small soma about a round or ovoid nucleus. The processes intersect to form a mat, over and within which the neurites lie. Interstitial cells are more prominent in the myenteric plexus of the antrum than they are in that of the fundus (Christensen et al 1992).

The myenteric plexus of the stomach contains coarse nerve bundles, called shunt fascicles, that enter from the oesophagus and branch extensively to spread towards the greater curvature (Fig. 2.13). They give off branches to ganglia (Fig. 2.14), but they do not enter into or pass through ganglia. They disappear into the ganglionated plexus in the distal stomach and along the greater curvature. These shunt fascicles have the structure of extramural autonomic nerves, with a perineurium, a collagen stroma and, a central capillary. They contain myelinated fibres. They may provide a second pathway for vagal fibres to the stomach, parallel to the direct gastric innervation of the stomach from the gastric branches of the vagus.

In the proximal part of the stomach, there is a third layer of muscle (the oblique layer) between the circular muscle layer and the submucosa. The space between the oblique and circular layers contains an aganglionic plexus of branching and intersecting nerve bundles, probably derived from the myenteric plexus. There are no secondary or tertiary plexuses, and interstitial cells are sparse in this space.

The intramural nerves of the small intestine
(Gabella 1987)

The submucous plexus in the small intestine is denser

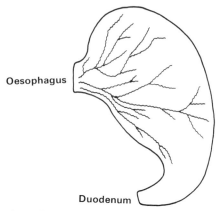

Oesophagus

Duodenum

Fig. 2.13   The distribution of extrinsic nerves ('shunt fascicles') within the plane of the myenteric plexus in the cat stomach. (From Christensen and Rick 1985a, with permission.)

than it is in the other viscera (Fig. 2.10). The ganglia are arranged in two strata, one just beneath the muscularis mucosae (Meissner's plexus) and the other adjacent to the circular muscle layer (Henle's or Schabadasch's plexus). The term 'Meissner's plexus' is also used for the whole of the submucous plexus. To avoid the obvious ambiguity, the more luminal plane

of ganglia is also called the plexus internus, and the more serosal plane the plexus externus (Stach 1972). The ganglia are small, densely distributed and interconnected by interganglionic fascicles.

The myenteric plexus in the small intestine is dense (Fig. 2.10). It contains large and uniformly spaced ganglia with well-developed secondary and tertiary plexuses. The tertiary plexus contains many interstitial cells, like those of the gastric antrum. The plexus shows little variation along the small intestine.

Nonganglionated plexuses of neurite bundles lie in planes beneath the serosa, in the lamina propria, and deep in the circular muscle layer (the plexus muscularis profundus). This latter plexus lies closer to the luminal border of the circular muscle layer than to the serosal border. It constitutes a dense network of neurites with abundant interstitial cells.

The intramural nerves of the colon
(Christensen et al 1984, Christensen & Rick 1987b, Stach 1972)

The submucous plexus, less dense than that of the intestine (Fig. 2.10), constitutes two strata of ganglia,

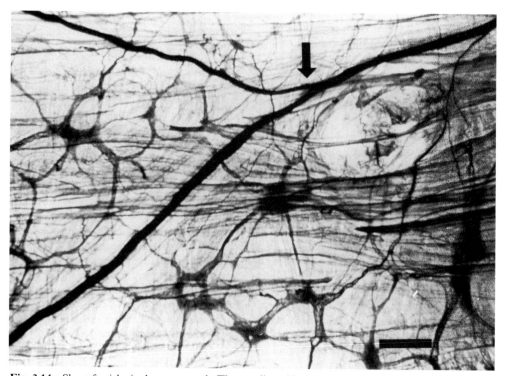

Fig. 2.14   Shunt fascicles in the cat stomach. The ganglia and interganglionic fascicles are overlaid by a thick branching fascicle (➡) which gives off branches to ganglia. ▬▬▬ indicates 1 μm. Silver stain. (From Christensen 1988b, with permission.)

as in the intestine, the plexus internus (Meissner's plexus) and the plexus externus (Henle's or Schabadasch's plexus). The submucous plexus of the colon also contains a unique feature, a dense nonganglionated bed of neurites and interstitial cells on the submucosal surface of the circular muscle layer (Fig. 2.15, 2.16). This, the plexus externus extremus (Stach 1972), has also been called Stach's plexus.

The myenteric plexus in the colon resembles that of the small intestine, with large uniformly-spaced ganglia and well-developed secondary and tertiary plexuses. Interstitial cells abound in the tertiary plexus. In the distal colon, many shunt fascicles (the ascending nerves of the colon) lie among the ganglia (Fig. 2.17). These intramural extensions of the colonic nerves from the pelvic plexus have the structure of peripheral nerves with a perineurium and a dedicated blood supply (Fig. 2.18). They contain myelinated nerve fibres. They give branches to ganglia, disappearing into the ganglionated plexus about half-way up the colon. Ganglion cell density in the myenteric plexus declines along the colon to reach a nadir in the rectum (Fig. 2.10). The rectal plexus consists of coarse nerve bundles with small and sparse ganglia and poorly-developed secondary and tertiary plexuses. This rectal plexus closely resembles that of the smooth-muscled part of the oesophagus.

The intramural nerves of the biliary tract

The biliary tract and gallbladder are relatively sparsely innervated. The innervation is a scanty plexus of small ganglia with a loose net of nerve fascicles that lies mostly on the outer surfaces of the walls.

SENSORY FUNCTIONS IN THE GUT (Wood 1987)

The only established sensory structures in the gut are the intraganglionic laminar endings found in certain ganglia of the myenteric plexus of the oesophagus and stomach (Rodrigo et al 1982). They have not been seen in ganglia of the myenteric plexus elsewhere. These leafy structures usually lie in a part of a ganglion that is devoid of nerve cell bodies (Fig. 2.19).

The morphologically undifferentiated neurites in the gut wall presumably can respond to local stimuli that can excite both pain and reflexes. Undifferentiated neurites abound in the lamina propria of the glandular epithelia as well as in the other layers of the wall.

Reflex motor responses can be demonstrated in response to both mechanical and chemical stimuli. Some of the best known of these reflexes are the following:

Reflex oesophageal peristalsis after oesophageal distension

Localized distension of the distal oesophagus evokes peristalsis in the oesophagus and relaxation of the lower oesophageal sphincter. These responses can be excited both in vitro and in situ. Both central and local pathways mediate the responses.

Reflex relaxation of the stomach in response to an increase in gastric volume

The expansion of the stomach in eating to accommodate the ingested volume represents reflex neurogenic inhibition of the proximal stomach. Both vago-vagal and intramural pathways mediate this reflex.

Reflex control of gastric emptying

Acids, fats, and hypertonic solutions in the duodenum all slow gastric emptying, constituting the major mechanism for the regulation of the delivery of gastric contents to the intestine. The effect is so profound, so sensitive, and so finely modulated that it seems likely to be a reflex. The pathways are unknown.

The peristaltic reflex of the intestine

Distension of the intestine enhances contractions above the distension and inhibits contractions below. The reflex pathways are intramural.

Reflex relaxation of the internal anal sphincter by rectal distension

Distension of the rectum relaxes the internal anal sphincter. The response can be elicited by distension of the descending colon in unanaesthetized humans. The pathways of the reflex are presumably intramural.

THE MORPHOLOGY OF ENTERIC NEURONS AND THEIR PROCESSES

Rapid long-distance transmission in nerves requires them to have long cell processes, axons, which transmit away from the cell soma, and dendrites, which transmit towards the soma. Axons are relatively thick and long and usually arise from a swelling in the soma, the axon hillock, while dendrites are relatively thin and short and lack a swelling at their somal attachments.

Neurons in the intramural plexuses of the intestine have been divided into five classes on the basis of axon and dendrite morphology, the classification of Dogiel (1899) as extended by Stach (1980, 1981, 1982a, 1982b, 1985). This classification has so far found use only in description, not in function. The variety of cell shapes

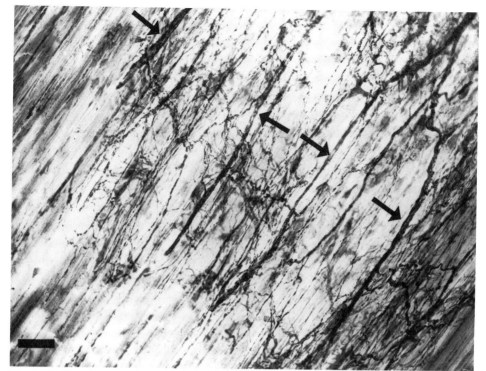

Fig. 2.15 The plexus externus extremus of the cat colon. The plane of section passes deep into the circular muscle layer to the left, but to the right and centre it lies at the submucosal surface of the circular muscle layer. A plexus on this surface constitutes thick bundles of axons (➡) from which small branches ramify over the surface. Interstitial cells of Cajal lie among these branches. ▬▬ indicates 50 μm. Osmic acid–zinc iodide stain. (From Christensen 1988b, with permission.)

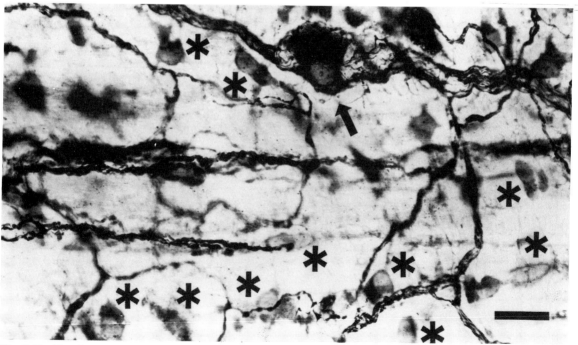

Fig. 2.16 The plexus externus extremus of the cat colon. A single ganglion cell (➡) lies in a thick bundle of neurites, and other such bundles are present in the field. Interstitial cells of Cajal (*) are just out of the focal plane, which was set on the neurites. They lie on the surface of the circular muscle layer. ▬▬ indicates 25 μm. Osmic acid–zinc iodide stain. (From Christensen 1988b, with permission.)

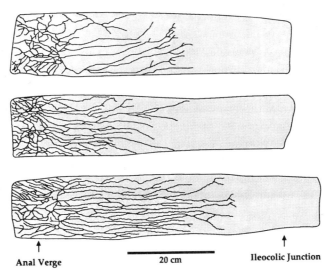

Anal Verge   20 cm   **Ileocolic Junction**

Fig. 2.17 The distribution of the ascending nerves of the colon as traced from three cat colons. (Redrawn from Christensen & Rick 1987)

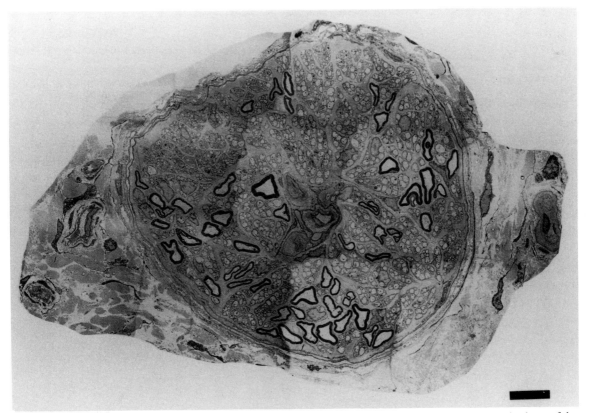

Fig. 2.18 Electron microscopic cross-section of an ascending colonic nerve ('shunt fascicle') from the myenteric plexus of the cat colon. It has the structure of a peripheral nerve, with a perineurium and a central vessel, and it contains many myelin sheaths. Shunt fascicles of the stomach have the same structure. ▬▬ indicates 200 μm.

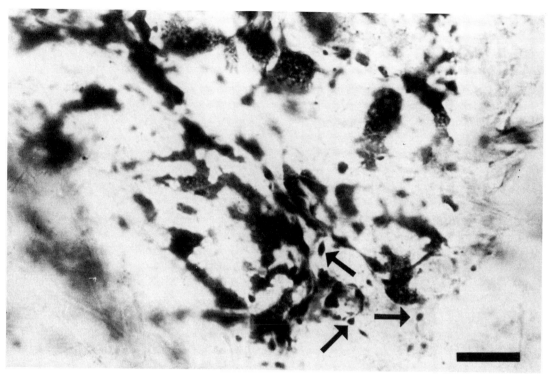

Fig. 2.19   Intraganglionic laminar endings from a ganglion of the opossum oesophagus. This is only the edge of the ganglion and no nerve cell bodies lie in this field. The endings are flat, black, leafy structures with spike-like projections. Such structures occur only in ganglia of the myenteric plexus of the oesophagus and cardia.
▅▅▅▅ indicates 10 μm. ➡ indicates varicosites of axons. Osmic acid–zinc iodide stain. (From Christensen 1988b, with permission.)

is striking. One common form lacks dendrites but has multiple (usually two to four) axons. This, Dogiel's Type II cell, supplies both of the main muscle layers. The other four types of cells have many dendrites and only one axon. They are distinguished on the basis of dendrite length, breadth or shape, and position on the cell soma. The different types of cells occupy different positions in the ganglion. The features of these five types of neurons (as described by Stach) are listed in Table 2.1. These descriptions come from study of the myenteric plexus of the intestine of rodents and the pig.

Table 2.1   The morphological features of the five types of neurons in the myenteric plexus (descriptions from Stach 1980, 1981, 1982a, 1982b, 1985).

Type of cell	Number of dendrites	Shape of dendrites	Position of dendrites	Number of axons	Destination of axons	Position in ganglion
Type I	Many	Short, flat, broad	Radiating from whole cell soma	1	Mostly orad in the plexus	Orad and peripheral parts
Type II	None	–	–	2–5	Muscle layers	Peripheral parts
Type III	Many	Long, thin tapering	Radiating from whole cell soma	1	Mostly aborad in the plexus	Central and aborad parts
Type IV	Many	Long, thin, tapering	Mainly at only one pole or part of soma	1	Submucosal plexus	Not specific
Type V	Many	Short to very long, thin, tapering	Radiating from whole cell soma	1	Mostly aborad in the plexus	In aggregates in central and aborad parts

Table 2.2 Types of vesicles found in autonomic neuromuscular junctions of nerve–nerve synapses. (From Davison 1983, with permission.)

Transmitter	Size of vesicles	Appearances
Cholinergic	35–60 nm 80–110 nm	Small agranular vesicles and some large granular vesicles
Adrenergic	50–90 nm 90–130 nm	Small vesicles with intensely osmiophilic granules, mixed with small agranular and large granular vesicles
Unknown	80–200 nm	Large opaque vesicles (medium electron-dense granule not clearly separated from vesicle membrane) and some small agranular vesicles

New evidence indicates that the forms of ganglion cells differ enormously from one organ to another. Ganglion cells throughout the gastrointestinal tract in a single species, the American opossum, were classified by form and the proportions of the various forms were then calculated from all regions. This study established that the proportions of the various forms are highly organ specific (Christensen 1988a). This finding makes it difficult to understand the functional significance of form in ganglion cells in the myenteric plexus.

Axon terminals have a varicose appearance. The varicosities are nodules containing packets of neural transmitters, stored in the varicosities as vesicles. Vesicles can be classified according to size and to the appearance of their core material in electron microscopy. Cholinergic nerves generally contain small agranular and large granular vesicles. Adrenergic nerves generally contain small vesicles with very dense granules, some small agranular and some large granular vesicles. Other nerves of unknown nature contain large opaque vesicles mixed with small agranular vesicles (Table 2.2).

The fact that varicosities contain several types of vesicles may only mean that vesicles have a different appearance at different stages of filling. It could also mean that a single axon may synthesize several transmitters simultaneously. The old idea of 'one nerve, one transmitter' has been abandoned as not consistent with modern evidence. In fact, the axonal co-localization of neurohormonal transmitters and other substances, mostly peptides, that may be co-transmitters or may also have other functions, provides a 'fingerprinting' method that has permitted a new functional classification of enteric neurons (Furness et al 1992).

Terminal nerve fibres wander among muscle bundles, approaching the muscle cells closely at points. The axons extend a long way among muscle bundles, releasing transmitters over their whole length. Transmitters are released so as to reach the muscle cells as a whole tissue, and they affect a single muscle cell over its whole surface, not through specialized synaptic structures.

NEURONAL PHYSIOLOGY OF THE INTRAMURAL NERVES OF THE GUT (Wood 1987)

Introduction

There are, conceptually, three functional classes of intramural neurons: sensory neurons, internuncial neurons (those which communicate among neurons within the plexuses) and motor neurons. All three classes are presumed to be present in both submucous and myenteric plexuses.

Various functional classifications of intramural neurons exist which are based upon electrophysiological methods. One classification rests on evidence gained from intramural enteric nerves as studied with intracellular microelectrodes inserted into ganglia exposed *in vitro*. Another classification rests on studies made with extracellular electrodes. No full correlations are yet possible either between these electrophysiological classifications, or between them and the morphological classification.

The two classes of enteric nerves found with intracellular recordings

Electrophysiological studies reveal two classes of enteric neurons, called Type 1 and Type 2 neurons, distinguished on the basis of six electrophysiological features (Table 2.3). About one-third of myenteric plexus neurons in the intestine are Type 2, while only a very small fraction of submucous plexus neurons are Type 2.

The classes of enteric nerves found with extracellular electrodes

Another functional classification of enteric neurons is based on their patterns of discharge in spontaneous and evoked activity. These patterns are burst patterns, mechanically-induced patterns and single-spike patterns.

Table 2.3 Electrophysical characteristics of myenteric plexus neurons. (From Davison 1983, with permission.)

Type 1	Type 2
Low resting membrane potential relative to Type 2	High resting membrane potential relative to Type 1
High input resistance relative to Type 2	Low input resistance relative to Type 1
Discharge spikes continuously in response to depolarization by intracellular injection of a current pulse-discharge frequency proportional to current intensity	Discharge one or two spikes only at the onset of injection of a depolarizing current pulse
Excitation at the termination of intracellular injection of a hyperpolarizing current pulse	No excitation at the termination of intracellular injection of a hyperpolarizing current pulse
No hyperpolarizing after-potential	Hyperpolarizing after-potential associated with action potential discharge
Tetrodotoxin-sensitive action potentials	Tetrodotoxin-resistant action potentials

Burst pattern neurons discharge action potentials in bursts. Action potentials occur in short bursts with interspersed long periods of electrical silence. Some neurons, called 'steady burst neurons', discharge this way constantly. Others, called 'erratic burst neurons', do so intermittently, reverting at times to the continuous discharge of action potentials (Fig. 2.20).

Mechanically-induced pattern neurons are silent at rest but discharge action potentials in response to mechanical deformation of the intestinal wall. There are three kinds of patterns (Fig. 2.21). In the 'on' or 'on-off response' pattern, the neuron discharges with a brief burst of spikes at the onset of the deformation of the intestinal wall and, occasionally, at the offset of the deformation. This is the pattern that would be expected from the excitation of a rapidly adapting mechanoreceptor. In the 'sustained response' pattern, the discharge of action potentials begins at the onset of the wall deformation and continues to the end of the deformation. This is the pattern that would be expected from the excitation of a slowly adapting mechanoreceptor. In the 'tonic response' pattern, the discharge of neuronal action potential begins at the onset of the wall deformation and continues for up to 40 s after the offset.

Single-spike pattern neurons discharge single spike action potentials continuously at a low frequency.

These patterns of discharge imply a further way to group enteric neurons into classes. 'Steady burst neurons' are considered to be spontaneous pacemakers. The neurons showing an 'on' or 'on–off response' to mechanical stimulation are probably sensory neurons connected to rapidly adapting mechanoreceptors. Those with the 'sustained response' are thought to be sensory neurons connected to slowly adapting mechanoreceptors. Those with the 'tonic response' may be internuncial neurons, communicating between sensory and motor neurons.

Functional specialization within a neuron

A neuron is not necessarily a single functional unit, always transmitting every stimulus that it receives from its dendrites to its axon. Instead, the membranes of the different parts of a neuron (dendrites, soma, axon hillock and axon) seem to have different electrophysiological properties. A neuron may thus be able to isolate activity in one process, or preferentially to select or to direct the transmission of activity along selected processes. This capacity would allow a single neuron to be a multifunctional unit. If this idea is true, it vastly enhances the versatility and flexibility of the ENS.

Synaptic transmission in intramural enteric nerves

When one nerve cell transmits a signal to another, the membrane of the receiving cell (the postsynaptic cell) shows an immediate small change in membrane potential. This 'pre-potential' may or may not lead to the discharge of a full action potential by the receiving neuron. A fall in resting membrane potential is called an excitatory postsynaptic potential (EPSP), while an increase in resting membrane potential is called an inhibitory postsynaptic potential (IPSP). These are shown in Figure 2.22. EPSPs can be 'fast' (less than 50 ms long) or 'slow' (more than 50 ms long), while IPSPs are always 'slow'.

Fast EPSPs occur in nerve cells of both submucous and myenteric plexuses, in both Type 1 and Type 2 cells. They are mediated by acetylcholine. Slow EPSPs occur only in Type 2 cells. IPSPs occur in Type 1 cells.

Transmitter substances of enteric neurons

Many substances seem to be at least candidates as neurohumoral transmitters in the nerves of the gut. A proposal for a candidate transmitter must satisfy two criteria: it must prove its presence in nerve terminals and its ability to act on muscle or nerve at low ('physiological') concentrations. A proposal for an established transmitter must satisfy further criteria: evidence of its release on nerve stimulation, a full description of mechanisms for its synthesis, release, degradation and/or re-uptake into nerve terminals, and evidence that it acts through a specific receptor in the cell membrane. These latter criteria are not so easily satisfied.

Many nerves contain several candidate transmitters. Some of these substances may act in usual or 'normal' circumstances, while others may be released only in special or 'abnormal' circumstances. Also, transmission could, in some instances perhaps, be electrotonic, mediated by local electrical current flow rather than by neurohumoral transmitters. The best established neurohumoral transmitters are acetylcholine (ACh), noradrenaline (NA), serotonin, substance P, gamma-aminobutyric acid, and the adenine nucleotides. The candidate transmitters include the many recently studied peptides such as vasoactive intestinal polypeptide (VIP), and nitric oxide, previously identified as the endothelium-derived relaxing factor in blood vessels.

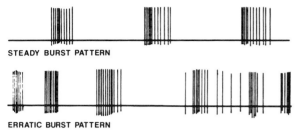

STEADY BURST PATTERN

ERRATIC BURST PATTERN

Fig. 2.20 A diagram of burst patterns of spike discharges from myenteric plexus neurons. (From Davison 1983, with permission.)

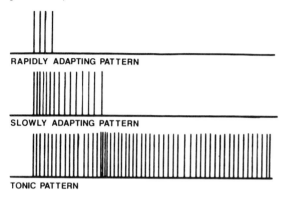

RAPIDLY ADAPTING PATTERN

SLOWLY ADAPTING PATTERN

TONIC PATTERN

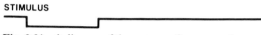

STIMULUS

Fig. 2.21 A diagram of the patterns of response of mechanoreceptive neurons in the myenteric plexus. (From Davison 1983, with permission.)

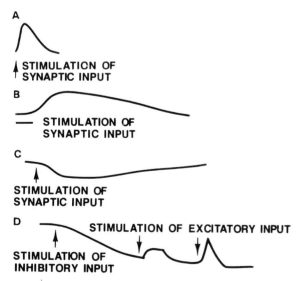

A

STIMULATION OF SYNAPTIC INPUT

B

STIMULATION OF SYNAPTIC INPUT

C

STIMULATION OF SYNAPTIC INPUT

D

STIMULATION OF EXCITATORY INPUT

STIMULATION OF INHIBITORY INPUT

Fig. 2.22 Diagrams of excitatory postsynaptic potentials (EPSPs) and inhibitory postsynaptic potentials (IPSPs). **A** shows fast and **B** slow EPSPs. **C** is an IPSP. **D** shows fast EPSPs superimposed on an IPSP. (From Davison 1983, with permission.)

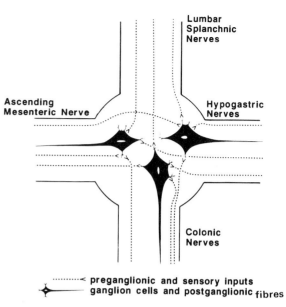

Lumbar Splanchnic Nerves

Ascending Mesenteric Nerve

Hypogastric Nerves

Colonic Nerves

·········< preganglionic and sensory inputs
——← ganglion cells and postganglionic fibres

Fig. 2.23 Pathways through the inferior mesenteric ganglion. Note that every ganglion cell receives inputs from all four groups of nerves, and that postganglionic axons pass to all except the lumbar splanchnic nerves. Some fibres pass through the ganglion without making synapse. (From Davison 1983, with permission.)

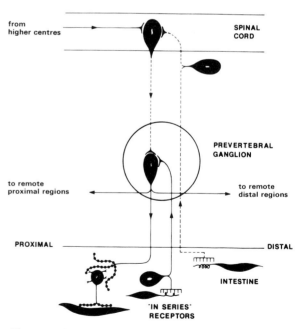

from higher centres

SPINAL CORD

PREVERTEBRAL GANGLION

to remote proximal regions

to remote distal regions

PROXIMAL

DISTAL

INTESTINE

'IN SERIES' RECEPTORS

Fig. 2.24 Pathways for peripheral sympathetic reflexes (——▶——). The long reflex pathway (– – ▶ – –) through the spinal cord which reinforces the peripheral reflex pathway is shown. The long pathway is shown as a monosynaptic path, but polysynaptic pathways could be involved. (From Davison 1983, with permission.)

THE PHYSIOLOGY OF SYMPATHETIC INTEGRATION – THE PREVERTEBRAL GANGLIA (Wood 1987)

Introduction

The prevertebral ganglia of the sympathetic system have several functions. They provide the means to suppress gastrointestinal motility during generalized sympathetic arousal. They constitute stations for the relay of afferent information from the gut to the CNS. And they integrate sensory information and relay it back to the gut over motor pathways to influence motility.

Functional organization of the prevertebral ganglia

Each prevertebral ganglion cell receives synaptic inputs from all fibres that enter the ganglion. Thus, every such cell can integrate information both from the gut and from the CNS. The axons from these cells pass to the gut and to the other prevertebral ganglia. Thus, the three prevertebral ganglia provide for interactions among all parts of the gut, and between the gut and the CNS (Figs 2.23, 2.24). Some entero-enteric reflex interactions take place only through the prevertebral ganglia, independent of the CNS. Such 'local' pathways may be duplicated by longer pathways through the CNS.

Although the nerve cells in these ganglia are thought to be functionally homogeneous, they are not morphologically homogeneous. A small proportion of cells is found to be especially intensely stained by catecholamine fluorescence. No special function of these small intensely fluorescent (SIF) cells is known.

Transmission in the prevertebral ganglia

The prevertebral ganglion cells seem to be physiologically homogeneous. Nerve stimulation of these cells evokes both 'fast' and 'slow' EPSPs, but no IPSPs. That is, all inputs to these nerve cells are excitatory, both those from the preganglionic fibres of CNS origin, and those from the walls of the viscera. A postspike hyperpolarization, like that of the Type 2 cells of the myenteric plexus, terminates the evoked discharge in these cells.

The efferent projections of the prevertebral ganglion cells

The ganglion cell axons pass to the other prevertebral ganglia and to the gut. Those to the gut terminate mainly in relation to enteric ganglion cells and blood vessels. The transmitters of these efferent fibres are catecholamines.

THE PHYSIOLOGY OF PARASYMPATHETIC INTEGRATION (Wood 1987)

Introduction

The long extrinsic pathways of the craniosacral system have been examined almost entirely in the cranial system. The sacral component is relatively neglected.

Sensory functions in the vagi

Vagal sensory endings detect both mechanical and chemical stimulation of the gut through two types of sensory endings. The mucosal ending acts both as a sensitive and rapidly-adapting mechanoreceptor and as a slowly-adapting chemoreceptor, responsive to a variety of substances. The intramuscular ending acts as a slowly-adapting mechanoreceptor, behaving as though arranged in series with the muscle bundles. It is therefore called an 'in-series tension receptor'. These receptors can follow gut volume as well as contractile force. For example, they probably monitor gastric volume in the regulation of gastric emptying.

Vagal sensory fibres emanate from the bipolar ganglion cells of the nodose ganglion. These cells have a somatotopic organization in that ganglion. That is, discrete regions of the nodose ganglion receive separate inputs from the separate organs. This somatotopy probably projects forward into the vagal nuclei in the CNS.

Motor functions in the vagi

The vagus contains both sensory fibres and motor fibres of several kinds. One set of these motor fibres, somatic fibres, innervates the striated muscle of the proximal oesophagus. Autonomic motor fibres include sympathetic postganglionic fibres that enter the vagus from the superior cervical ganglion, and parasympathetic preganglionic fibres that arise in the vagal nuclei. The parasympathetic fibres serve the long reflex pathways that modulate contractions of gut muscle.

Vago-vagal reflexes

The stimulation of the intramuscular in-series tension receptors generally initiates vago-vagal reflexes. The responding vagal motor fibres discharge continuously for a long time, well beyond the duration of the stimulus. The cells of the vagal nuclei possess both excitatory and inhibitory inputs, so that vago-vagal reflexes may involve either or both excitation and inhibition of either or both excitatory and inhibitory motor fibres. Some of these reflex responses reverse when the intensity of stimulation of the sensory limb of the reflex increases. That is, a stimulus that *excites* activity at a low intensity may inhibit activity at a greater intensity. Also, as one group of nerve cells in the vagal nuclei is excited, another group is inhibited. Thus, a high degree of plasticity is possible in the long parasympathetic reflexes.

THE CENTRAL CENTRES INVOLVED IN GUT MOTILITY

Three general methods exist to identify the CNS structures that influence gut motility. First, the use of intracellular dyes permits the tracing of extrinsic nerve trunks back into the CNS. Second, one can observe changes in motility after the stimulation or destruction of central structures. Third, the existence of organizing 'centres' can be inferred from observations of motility itself.

Each method has limitations. Dye tracing methods identify only the immediate central projections of the stained peripheral nerves. The stimulation or destruction of specific central structures may stimulate or destroy not only the nerve cell bodies of that structure but also fibre tracts that pass through the structure without actually involving the function of the structure. And 'centres' are only physiological abstractions, integrators or organizers whose existence must be postulated in order to explain the observed integration of the motor behaviour of the gut.

Some generally accepted 'facts' about some CNS structures involved in the control of motility are presented in Table 2.4.

METHODS TO STUDY THE MORPHOLOGY OF THE NERVES OF THE GUT (Costa et al 1987)

Introduction

Many metachromatic stains stain nervous tissue non-specifically, but the non-selectivity of such stains limits their usefulness. Some methods, like silver impregnation, are only a little more selective for nervous tissue. Other more specific stains are based on the biochemical features of nerves and their associated structures. These include immunohistochemical stains which depend upon the binding of antibodies to proteins or polypeptides located on or in nerve cells. The immunohistochemical methods find use especially in the demonstration of the polypeptides that are candidate neurohumoral transmitters.

General stains

Silver impregnation

The affinity of silver for nerves forms the basis for many methods still used. The many techniques differ only in details, but the most devoted students of one or another structure tend to use one or another of these techniques selectively. All modern methods use a two-stage impregnation. The formalin-fixed tissue is exposed to silver salts in two steps, the first a solution of silver nitrate and the second a solution of ammoniacal silver nitrate, with the ultimate reduction of the silver in a reducing solution. Some methods are capricious, with the quality of staining varying a great deal from tissue to tissue for no apparent reason. The technique of Richardson (1960) is notably reliable, controllable, and predictable.

Supravital methylene blue

Most living cells take up methylene blue, but nerve cells show somewhat greater avidity for the dye than most other cells of the gut wall. The fresh tissue is exposed under standard conditions in vivo or in vitro to a low concentration of the dye. Different workers use slightly different conditions of exposure. The method stains nerve cell bodies well, but it shows their processes poorly. The stain reveals little of the structural details of nerves.

The osmic acid–zinc iodide stain (Maillet 1959)

This simple method reveals a wealth of detail. One immerses fresh tissue in a fresh mixture of osmic acid and zinc iodide for 20–24 h, and then makes sections. The method stains nerves black and it colours other tissues grey, brown, or yellow. It stains varicose nerve processes in fine detail, but it stains nerve cell bodies rather poorly. It also stains the interstitial cells of Cajal with clarity. The density of staining is not fully predictable. The staining reaction probably involves sulphydryl groups in membrane proteins.

Stains for nerve components that are not transmitters

The nissl stains

Basic dyes, like toluidine blue and thionin, stain the acidic proteins of the endoplasmic reticulum and the

Table 2.4 Motility responses evoked by stimulating some CNS areas. (From Davison 1983, with permission.)

Area	Motility responses	Peripheral nerve pathways
Cortex	Excitatory and inhibitory responses from stomach, small intestine, and colon, depending on precise area stimulated	Excitatory effects are mediated through parasympathetic nerves, inhibitory effects through parasympathetic and sympathetic nerves Vagal fibres project to somatosensory cortex and orbital gyrus
Thalamus	Excitatory gastric responses to stimulation of reticular nucleus, anterior nucleus ventralis, lateral pulvinar, and endopeduncular nuclei Inhibitory gastric responses to stimulation of ventral nucleus and antero-medial nucleus	Excitatory and inhibitory pathways are parasympathetic
Amygdaloid complex nuclei	Defaecation, including postural responses	Pelvic nerves and spinal motor neurons
Hypothalamus	Excitatory and inhibitory responses affecting the entire gut	Excitatory effects involve parasympathetic pathways Inhibition involves excitation of nonadrenergic, noncholinergic inhibitory pathways, inhibition of cholinergic pathways (both parasympathetic) and excitation of sympathetic pathways
Mesencephalon and pons	Stimulation of superior colliculi, fasciculus longitudinalis, and reticular substance of pons excites the stomach Stimulation of dorsal tegmentum, medial lemniscus, and reticular substance of pons inhibits the stomach	Excitatory effects are parasympathetic Inhibitory effects are sympathetic
Cerebellum	Increased gastric, intestinal and colonic motility	Sympathetic, probably due to suppression of sympathetic inhibitory tone
Medulla	Excitatory and inhibitory effects on the entire gut	Excitation and inhibition are mediated by parasympathetic pathways; a splanchnic motor area has also been identified

nucleic acids. Because these structures abound in nerve cell bodies, the stain colours neuronal perikarya well. It does not stain nerve processes well.

The NADH stain

The NADH stain is more specific for nerve cell bodies than the Nissl stain. The reaction depends upon the relatively dense distribution of mitochondria, the source of NADH reductase, in nerve cell bodies. The tissue is quick-frozen and thawed and then incubated in nitro-BT with NADH. The resulting dark blue stain demonstrates mainly the nerve cell bodies. It does not colour nerve processes well. The method also stains interstitial cells of Cajal distinctly.

Quinacrine fluorescence

Under suitable conditions of incubation, quinacrine accumulates selectively in enteric neurons, and it can be visualized there by fluorescence microscopy. The stain may be related to the binding of quinacrine to nucleic acids. It stains only some, not all neurons, and only some, not all processes.

Stains for the enzymes related to established neurohumoral transmitters

Acetylcholinesterase stains

The enzyme that degrades ACh should abound in those regions where ACh is produced. Several stains for the localization of this enzyme, using various substrates and inhibitors (to inhibit non-specific cholinesterases), demonstrate nerve cell bodies and processes very strongly. Unfortunately, such stains are not selective for cholinergic neurons.

Catecholamine fluorescence

Catecholamines produce fluorescent compounds when reacted with aldehydes. This reaction allows the use of fluorescence microscopy to localize catecholamines in the enteric nerves. It shows the localization of catecholamine-containing (sympathetic) terminal nerves in the plexuses and around blood vessels.

Immunohistochemical demonstration of peptides

The use of antibodies raised to enteric peptides allows the localization of these peptides in enteric nerves. Several techniques exist, all relying on the specific binding of labelled antibody to the peptide in fresh tissue. By these techniques, one can discover the localization of any peptide for which an antibody exists. In this way, nerves reactive to many peptides, candidate transmitters, have been discovered.

ACKNOWLEDGEMENT

This work was supported by Grant DK 11242 from the National Institutes of Health.

REFERENCES

Christensen J 1988a The forms of argyrophilic ganglion cells in the myenteric plexus throughout the gastrointestinal tract of the opossum. J Auton Nerv Syst 2: 251–260

Christensen J 1988b The enteric nervous system in: Kumar D, Gustavssen S (eds) An Illustrated guide to gastrointestinal motility (lst edn) Wiley, Chichester, pp 9–32

Christensen J 1991 Gastrointestinal motility in: West, J B (ed.) Best and Taylor's physiological basis of medical practice 12th edn,. Williams and Wilkins, Baltimore, MD pp 614–644

Christensen J 1992 Commentary on the morphological identification of the interstitial cells of Cajal. J Auton Nerv Syst 37: 75–88

Christensen J, Rick G A 1985a Shunt fascicles in the gastric myenteric plexus in five monogastric species. Gastroenterology 88: 1020–1025

Christensen J, Rick G A 1985b Nerve cell density in submucous plexus throughout the gut of cat and opossum. Gastroenterology 89: 1064–1069

Christensen J, Rick G A 1987a Intrinsic nerves in the mammalian colon: confirmation of a plexus at the circular muscle–submucosal interface. J Auton Nerv Syst 21: 223–231

Christensen J, Rick G A 1987b The distribution of myelinated nerves in the ascending nerves and myenteric plexus of the cat colon. Am J Anat 178: 250–258

Christensen J, Robison B A 1982 Anatomy of the myenteric plexus of the opossum esophagus. Gastroenterology 83: 1033–1042

Christensen J, Rick G A, Robison B A, Stiles M J, Wix M A 1983 The arrangement of the myenteric plexus throughout the gastrointestinal tract of the opossum. Gastroenterology 85: 890–899

Christensen J, Stiles M J, Rick G A, Sutherland J 1984 Comparative anatomy of the myenteric plexus of the distal colon in eight mammals. Gastroenterology 86: 706–713

Christensen J, Rick G A, Soll D J 1987 Intramural nerves and interstitial cells revealed by the Champy–Maillet stain in the opossum esophagus. J Auton Nerv Syst 19: 137–151

Christensen J, Rick G A, Lowe L S 1992 Distributions of interstitial cells of Cajal in stomach and colon of cat, dog, ferret, opossum, rat, guinea pig and rabbit. J Auton Nerv Syst 37: 47–56

Costa M, Furness J B, Llewellyn-Smith I J 1987 Histochemistry of the enteric nervous system in: Johnson L R, Christensen J, Jackson M J, Jacobson E D, Walsh J H (eds) Physiology of the gastrointestinal tract 2nd edn, vol, 1, Raven Press, New York pp 1–40

Daniel E E, Posey-Daniel V 1984 Neuromuscular structures in opossum esophagus: role of interstitial cells of Cajal. Am J Physiol 246: G305–G315

Davison JS 1983 Innervation of the gastrointestinal tract in: Christensen J, Wingate D L (eds) A guide to gastrointestinal motility Ch. 1 Wright-PSG, Bristol pp 1–47

Dogiel A S 1899 Ueber den Bau der Ganglien in den geflechten des Darmes und der Gallenblase des Menschen und der Säugetiere. Arch Anat Physiol Anat Abt 130–158

Furness J B, Costa M 1987 The enteric nervous system. Churchill Livingstone, Edinburgh

Furness J B, Bornstein J C, Murphy R, Pompolo S 1992 Roles of peptides in transmission in the enteric nervous system. TINS 15: 66–71

Gabella G 1979 Innervation of the gastrointestinal tract. Int Rev Cytol 59: 129–193

Gabella G 1987 Structure of muscles and nerves in the gastrointestinal tract in: Johnson L R, Christensen J, Jackson M J, Jacobson E D, Walsh J H (eds) Physiology of the gastrointestinal tract 2nd edn, Vol. 1 Raven Press, New York pp 335–382

Maillet M 1959 Modifications de la technique de Champy au tetraoxyde d'osmium-iodure de potassium. Resultats de son application à l'étude des fibres nerveuses. C R Soc Biol 153: 939–941

Richardson K C 1960 Studies on the structure of autonomic nerves in the small intestine, correlating the silver-impregnated image in light microscopy with the permanganate-fixed ultrastructure in electron-microscopy. J Anat 94: 457–472

Rodrigo J, Hernandez C J, Vidal M A, Pedrosa J A 1975 Vegetative innervation of the esophagus. III. Intraepithelial endings. Acta Anat 92: 242–258

Rodrigo J, de Filipe J, Robles-Chillida E M, Perez Anton J A, Mayo I, Gomez A 1982 Sensory vagal nature and anatomical access paths to esophageal laminar nerve endings in myenteric ganglia. Determination by surgical degeneration methods. Acta Anat 112: 47–57

Rumessen J J, Thuneberg L 1982 Plexus muscularis profundus and associated interstitial cells. I. Light microscopical studies of mouse small intestine. Anat Rec 203: 115–127

Rumessen J J, Thuneberg L, Mikkelsen H B 1982 Plexus muscularis profundus and associated interstitial cells. II. Ultrastructural studies of mouse small intestine. Anat Rec 203: 129–146

Stach W 1972 Der plexus entericus extremus des Dickdarmes und seine Beziehungen zu den interstitiellen Zellen (Cajal). Z Mikrosk-anat Forsch 85: 245–272

Stach W 1980 Zur neuronalen organisation des plexus myentericus (Auerbach) im Schweinedünndarm. I. Typ I-neurone. Z Mikrosk-anat Forsch 94: 833–849

Stach W 1981 Zur neuronalen organisation des plexus myentericus (Auerbach) im Schweinedünndarm. II. Typ II-neurone. Z Mikrosk-anat Forsch 96: 161–182

Stach W 1982a Zur neuronalen organisation des plexus myentericus (Auerbach) im Schweinedünndarm. III. Typ III-neurone. Z Mikrosk-anat Forsch 96: 497–516

Stach W 1982b Zur neuronalen organisation des plexus myentericus (Auerbach) im Schweinedünndarm. IV. Typ IV-neurone. Z Mikrosk-anat Forsch 96: 972–994

Stach W 1985 Zur neuronalen organisation des plexus myentericus (Auerbach) im Schweinedünndarm. V. Typ V-neurone. Z Mikrosk-anat Forsch 99: 562–582

Thuneberg L 1982 Interstitial cells of Cajal: intestinal pacemaker cells. Adv Anat Embryol Cell Biol 71: 1–130

Wood J D 1987 Physiology of the enteric nervous system in: Johnson L R, Christensen J, Jackson M J, Jacobson E D, Walsh J H (eds) Physiology of the gastrointestinal tract 2nd edn. Vol. 1 Raven Press, New York. pp 67–110

3. Structure of smooth muscle

G. Gabella

The chief muscular component of the wall of the stomach and intestine of vertebrates is the muscle coat or muscularis externa, which ranges in thickness from 50 μm or less in the mouse to 1 mm or more in man. The muscle coat is compact, has well-defined boundaries and has no perimysium. It is crossed by laminae of connective tissue, the intramuscular septa, anchored to the submucosa. Additional musculature forms the muscularis mucosae and the media of intramural blood vessels.

The muscle coat is usually made of two layers of musculature, the longitudinal (outer) layer and the circular (inner) layer (Fig. 3.1); it is not uncommon to find bundles of muscle cells that pass from one layer to the other. The muscle cells lie on planes that are parallel to the serosal surface, but they run orthogonal

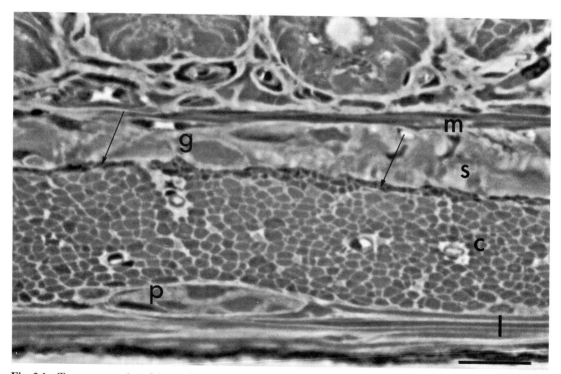

Fig. 3.1 Transverse section of the rat ileum photographed unstained in phase contrast microscopy. The mucosa is at the top, the serosa at the bottom. **c**, circular muscle layer; **l**, longitudinal muscle layer; **m**, muscularis mucosae; **s**, submucosa. Between the two muscle layers is a ganglion of the myenteric plexus (**p**) and in the submucosa there is a ganglion of the submucosal plexus (**g**). At the innermost part of the circular muscle, note a thin layer of small and dark muscle cells (arrows). (Reproduced from Gabella, 1987.) Calibration bar; 30 μm.

to one another in the two layers. Longitudinal and circular muscle layers are firmly anchored to each other; in the interstice between them, one also finds the myenteric plexus, connective tissue, blood vessels and lymphatic vessels. In the innermost part of the circular layer of the small intestine there are special muscle cells that are smaller and denser (s.a.d. cells) than those of the main circular layer (Fig. 3.1) and can be distinguished without difficulty by their characteristic ultrastructure and by the features of the connective tissue surrounding them (Gabella 1987). They usually form a layer that is one or two cells thick and extends over the entire small intestine but it is not found in the large intestine.

In the caecum (of mammals) and in parts of the colon the longitudinal musculature is condensed into cords, or taeniae. Between the taeniae the wall bulges outward forming numerous regular evaginations (haustrations) where the muscle coat is made almost exclusively of circular muscle: the lumen has a profile that ranges from an equilateral triangle (where the circular muscle is fully contracted and runs in straight segments between any two taeniae) to a clover leaf (where the circular muscle is relaxed and bulges out under the pressure of the luminal contents). The taeniae act as longitudinal pillars over which the transverse (circular) musculature hinges inward and outward. This architecture gives a certain rigidity to the organ, despite its bulk, and it allows great, although localized, variations in luminal size to take place.

The intestinal musculature is more than just an assembly of muscle cells. Smooth muscle is a complex tissue; in addition to the principal cell type, smooth muscle cells (which are packed to a density of 190 000/mm^3), there are nerve fibres, Schwann cells, interstitial cells, fibroblasts and cells of lymphatic and blood vessels, mainly endothelial cells (Fig. 3.2). The extracellular space amounts to 20–30%, of the tissue volume, and has a fluid component, the rest being occupied mainly by collagen fibrils and elastic fibres. The collagen fibrils form networks close to the surface of muscle cells and link the cells to one another and to larger arrays of collagen, such as the intramuscular septa or the submucosa or, in some cases, the serosa. The collagen concentration in intestinal muscles is generally higher than that of skeletal and cardiac muscles. The materials of the extracellular space, collagen included, are probably synthesized and secreted, for the most part, by the muscle cells themselves.

SMOOTH MUSCLE CELLS

Muscle cells of the gastrointestinal tract are uninucle-

ated and approximately spindle-shaped; they are 400–600 μm long and measure about 2000 to 4000 μm^3 in volume. The maximum diameter of a muscle cell at rest does not exceed 4 or 5 μm, so that no part of the sarcoplasm is further away from the cell membrane than about 2.5 μm (Fig. 3.3). The surface to volume ratio is relatively high, as there are usually about 1.5 μm^2 of cell surface for every cubic micron of cell volume. The surface of the cells at rest is smooth and regular, except for occasional cell processes. However, when the muscle is fully stretched the cell surface develops shallow longitudinal grooves, whereas in isotonically contracted muscle cells the membrane is thrown into many lamellar evaginations which interdigitate with those from adjacent cells.

CAVEOLAE

Caveolae, cell-to-cell junctions, cell-to-stroma junctions, and dense bands are the main structural specializations found at the cell membrane. Caveolae are stable flask-like invaginations of the cell membrane, about 120 nm long and 70 nm wide; they open into the extracellular space through a neck measuring about 35 nm across. Caveolae are often associated with flattened sacs or with tubules of sarcoplasmic reticulum, although there are no obvious structural links between the two components. Caveolae are mostly grouped into bands, one to four caveolae across, which run parallel to the cell length (Fig. 3.4). There are between 20 and 35 caveolae per square micron of cell surface, and their number does not seem to be affected by stretch or contraction of the muscle. On the whole the caveolae increase the amount of cell membrane by about 70% over the area of the cell surface proper.

DENSE BANDS

Dense bands are patches of electron-dense material, measuring 0.2–0.4 μm in width and 1 or 2 micron long, bound to the cell membrane and located between rows of caveolae; the felt of electron-dense material measures 30 nm or more in thickness. Dense bands are spread over the entire surface of a muscle cell and they occupy between 30 and 50% of the cell profile; towards the tapering ends of the cell this percentage increases and in some small profiles the entire cell membrane is encrusted by dense bands.

A compact bundle of actin filaments penetrates into

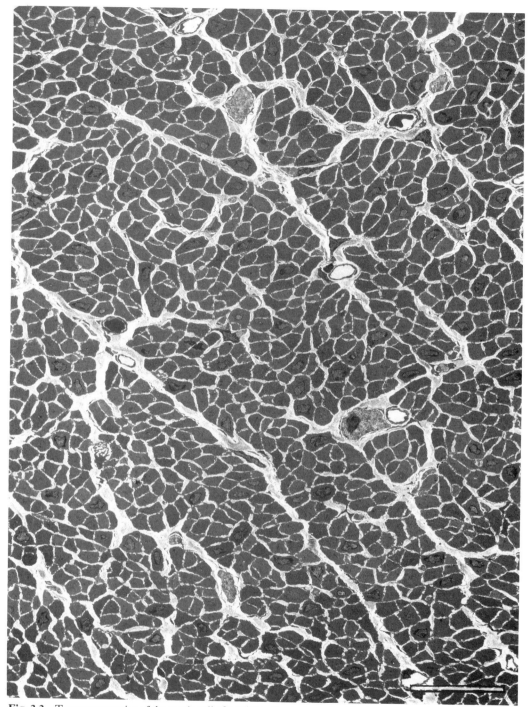

Fig. 3.2   Transverse section of the taenia coli of a guinea-pig photographed in the electron microscope. In addition to smooth muscle cell profiles, one can recognize capillaries, small nerve bundles, interstitial cells, fibroblasts and intramuscular septa. Calibration bar: 20 μm.

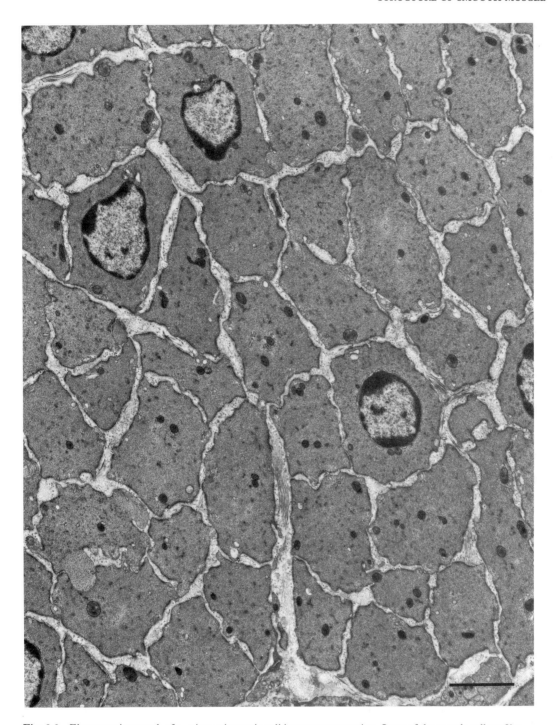

Fig. 3.3 Electron micrograph of a guinea-pig taenia coli in transverse section. Some of the muscle cell profiles display the nucleus; the dark particles are mitochondria. The cells are surrounded by collagen fibrils (small dots in the extracellular space). Calibration bar: 2 μm.

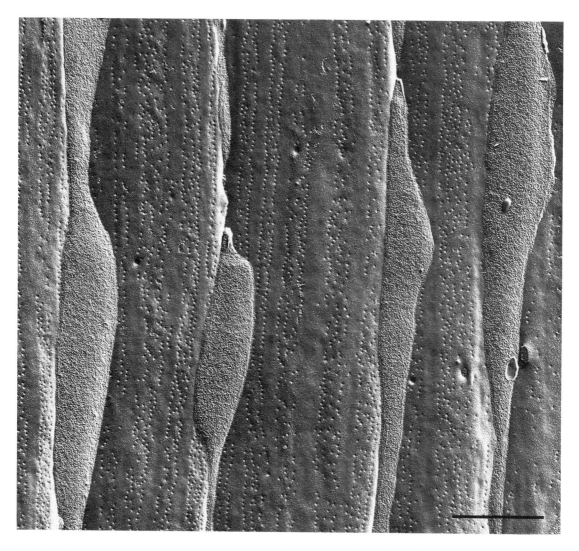

Fig. 3.4 Freeze-fracture preparation of circular muscle of the guinea-pig ileum. The cell membrane shows rows of caveolae arranged longitidinally. Calibration bar: 2 μm.

the felt of electron-dense material, and the contractile apparatus is thus linked to the cell membrane. The actin filaments approach the cell membrane at a very small angle, but the link with the membrane is probably a flexible one that can change during muscle contraction. Also some intermediate filaments reach the dense bands, independently of the actin filaments. Alpha-actinin (Bagby 1980) and vinculin (Geiger et al 1981), two proteins that have been localized at the dense bands by immunocytochemistry, are probably involved in linking actin filaments and cell membrane.

INTERMEDIATE JUNCTIONS

One type of cell-to-cell junction found in intestinal muscles involves the apposition of two dense bands in adjacent cells (Fig. 3.5A). These junctions (intermediate junctions) are of the adherens type, they are elongated (fasciae) and provide mechanical coupling between the two cells. The intercellular gap measures up to 60 nm and is occupied by a layer of electron-dense material that is continuous with the basal laminae investing the two cells and often shows ill-defined periodic densities.

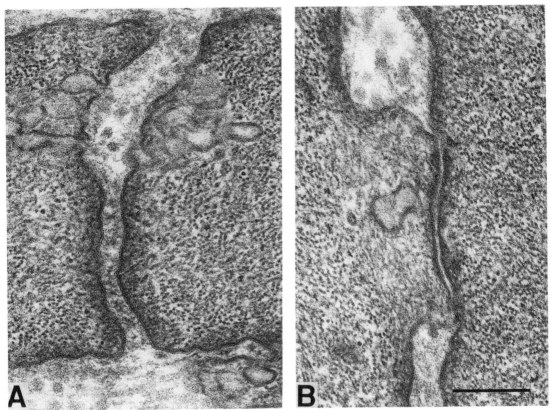

Fig. 3.5 Transverse section of the taenia coli of a guinea-pig. **A** Intermediate junction between two muscle cells. The intercellular gap measures about 50 nm and is occupied by electron-dense material with a faint periodic appearance. Actin filaments and intermediate filaments are associated with the dense bands on either side of the junction. **B** Another type of junction with an intercellular gap of only about 15 nm. Calibration bar (for both micrographs): 0.2 μm.

Other junctions, which may constitute a separate type of junction, are small and patch-like (maculae), have an intercellular gap of about 15 nm, and do not have a clear association with bundles of intracellular filaments (Fig. 3.5B). This type of junction is also occasionally observed between a muscle cell and a Schwann cell or an interstitial cell; on rare occasions it is found between a muscle cell and a varicose axon.

GAP JUNCTIONS

In many intestinal muscles muscle cells are linked by gap junctions (nexuses). These are symmetrical patches (maculae) of the membrane of two cells, occupied by special channels that permit a private exchange of ions and small molecules between two cells and hence provide ionic and metabolic coupling. Their ultrastructure (Fig. 3.6) is identical to that analysed in detail in hepatocytes and cardiac muscle cells. Connexin-43,

the protein of the connexons of heart gap junctions, has also been localized in intestinal gap junctions (Beyer et al 1989). The ultrastructural units of the nexus (connexons bridge the 2–3 nm gap between membranes; in freeze-fracture preparations the connexons appear as intramembrane particles of 8–10 nm diameter and they remain invariably attached to the cytoplasmic (P) leaflet of the membrane (Fig. 3.7A). The packing density of connexons in a junction is about $7000/\mu m^2$. The area of the junction rarely exceeds 0.2 μm, and some junctions are made of only a few connexons (Fig. 3.7B).

Gap junctions are not present uniformly in the various intestinal muscles. In the circular muscle of the small intestine they are abundant in all the species studied. In the circular muscle of the caecum gap junctions are less numerous than in the ileum, and in the colon there are very few (Fig. 3.7B). In many animal species the longitudinal musculature of small and large intestine is virtually devoid of gap junctions.

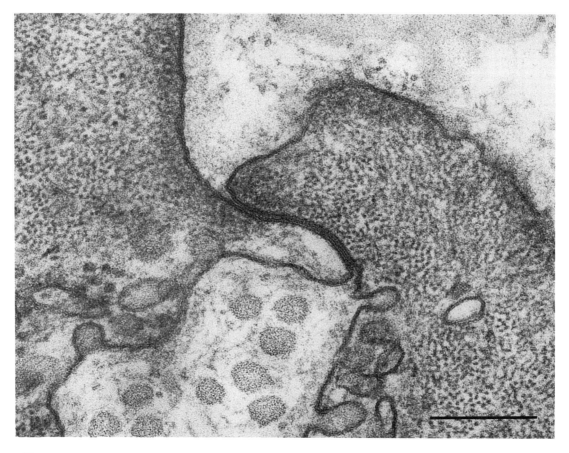

Fig. 3.6 Transverse section of rabbit taenia coli. The two muscle cells are connected by a gap junction. Microfibrils and transversely sectioned collagen fibrils are present in the extracellular space. Calibration bar: 0.2 μm.

In species where gap junctions are also found in the longitudinal musculature, they are rare and exceedingly small. The great variability in the extent of gap junctions in different muscles and their absence in some muscles is difficult to reconcile with the electrophysiological evidence of electrical coupling.

CELL-TO-STROMA JUNCTIONS

Except at the level of specialized junctions the cell membrane is lined by a basal lamina. This has a fuzzy appearance that in certain preparations can be resolved into a fine fibrillar texture. Microfibrils of 11 nm diameter and amorphous materials link the basal lamina, especially where it lies over a dense band, and collagen fibrils and elastic fibres. Junctions between the contractile apparatus of the cell and the stroma of the muscle are thus produced, and these provide a crucial mechanical link for force transference.

SARCOPLASMIC RETICULUM

The sarcoplasmic reticulum is well represented in intestinal muscle cells and constitutes about 2% of the cell volume. Flat and broad cisternae, tubules, networks of tubules and concave sacs are some of the most common forms of smooth sarcoplasmic reticulum. Some cisternae of sarcoplasmic reticulum lie parallel to the cell membrane, and the 10–20 nm gap between the two structures is bridged by dense periodic structures 20–25 nm apart, an arrangement similar to the peripheral coupling between cell membrane and sarcoplasmic reticulum in cardiac muscle cells. The sarcoplasmic reticulum of smooth muscles can accumulate calcium ions and participates in the regulation of calcium concentration in the sarcoplasm (Bond et al 1984). However, the muscles have only a very limited ability of contracting in the absence of extracellular calcium (Casteels and Raeymaekers 1979).

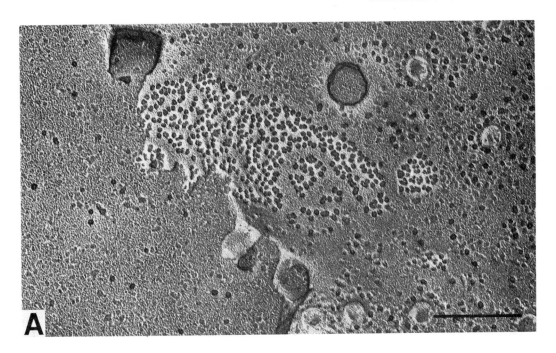

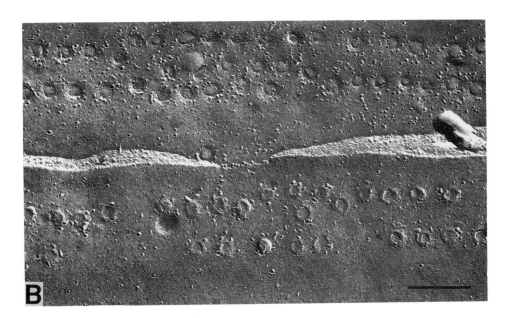

Fig. 3.7 **A** Freeze-fracture preparation of the circular muscle of the guinea-pig jejunum. On the P-face (cell on the right) are the opening of several caveolae, surrounded by a ring of intramembrane particles. In the centre a gap junction is recognizable as a loose aggregation of particles. The adjacent cell (on the left) shows its E-face. **B** Freeze-fracture preparation of the guinea-pig distal colon. The two muscle cells are joined by a very small gap junction, made of only few connexons. Caveolae are seen on the P-face (cell on top) and on the E-face (cell at bottom). The light band across the micrograph is the extracellular space. Calibration bars: 0.2 μm.

MYOSIN FILAMENTS

Up to 90% of the cell volume is occupied by filaments, of which there are three main classes: thick filaments of myosin, thin filaments of actin, and intermediate filaments (Bagby 1983) (Fig. 3.8). Myosin filaments measure 15–17 nm in diameter and have a rather irregular profile. They are labile structures and are easily altered or disrupted by preparative procedures. Myosin molecules isolated from smooth muscles are identical in appearance to those obtained from striated muscles (Elliott et al 1976), but they are chemically distinguishable (Small and Sobieszek 1980). There are also major differences in the way the molecules are packed into filaments, although the exact packing is not yet known. According to one model, myosin molecules are assembled into side-polar filaments having cross-bridges with the same polarity along the entire length of one side of the filaments and the opposite polarity along the other side (Craig and Megerman 1977). The concentration of myosin in smooth muscle (about 16 mg/kg) is about a quarter of that found in skeletal muscle (Murphy et al 1977). Despite the relatively low myosin content, intestinal smooth muscle can generate an amount of force per unit sectional area that is comparable to that of skeletal muscle.

ACTIN FILAMENTS

Actin filaments measure about 7 nm in diameter and are readily preserved in most preparations. They are often arranged in bundles or cables of 10–20 with a square lattice. The bundles split and merge with each other, rather than forming discrete entities, and because of this arrangement many actin filaments do not interact with a myosin filament, at least over part of their length. In a muscle cell in transverse section the apparent ratio of actin filaments to myosin filaments is approximately 12:1 (Bois 1973). The weight ratio of actin to myosin ranges between two and four, and these values are six to 10 times higher than those found in skeletal muscles. Actin filaments penetrate into the dense bodies attached to the cell membrane and into dense bodies (Ashton et al 1975). The latter are electron-dense structures scattered through the sarcoplasm, elongated and extremely variable in size and appearance: a bundle of actin filaments penetrates into each end of a dense body. The polarity of the actin filaments inserted into dense bodies or into dense bands is fixed: the arrowheads formed by decoration of the filaments with the fragment S-1 of myosin always point away from the point of insertion (Bond and Somlyo 1982). The polarity of the actin filaments

is therefore opposite at either side of a dense body, an arrangement similar to that found in actin filaments inserted into Z lines in skeletal muscles.

INTERMEDIATE FILAMENTS

Intermediate filaments measure 10 nm in diameter and in intestinal muscles cells are made of a fibrous protein called desmin or skeletin. They are often closely associated with the amorphous material of dense bands and surround some of the dense bodies, and probably form a mechanical link with them.

OTHER CELL TYPES

Non-muscle cells found in intestinal muscles include fibroblasts and interstitial cells of Cajal. Most intestinal muscles are well vascularized, an exception being the taenia coli of the rabbit, an elastic smooth muscle in which blood vessels are rare. The intramuscular vessels are usually capillaries, most of which run along the muscle length. Large blood vessels traverse the muscle coat obliquely, running within large intramuscular septa. Large lymphatic vessels, which mainly drain lymph from the mucosa, are often seen traversing the circular muscle layer of the intestine; they then travel for considerable distances circumferentially within the interstice between the two muscle layers. The lymphatic vessels, easily recognized through their content, are very thin-walled, have no musculature but do have valves. Their extensive association with the muscle coat of the intestine probably assists lymph transport.

Nerve fibres and Schwann cells form nerve bundles that run between the muscle cells (Fig. 3.9). Vesicle-containing varicosities are found within bundles of all sizes, but they are more frequent in the small ones (Fig. 3.9A). Varicose axons running singly are less common than in other smooth muscles (e.g. vas deferens or iris), but they do occur in intestinal muscles too. Various configurations of intramuscular nerves can be observed, even within the same muscle: they range from isolated varicosities lying very close to, or partly embedded into, a muscle cell, to bundles containing varicosities, located at various distances from muscle cells and interstitial cells.

STROMA

This includes collagen, mostly in the form of fibrils, elastic fibres, microfibrils and amorphous materials. There is evidence that at least part of the stroma is synthesized and secreted by the muscle cells themselves. Collagen concentration in mammalian smooth

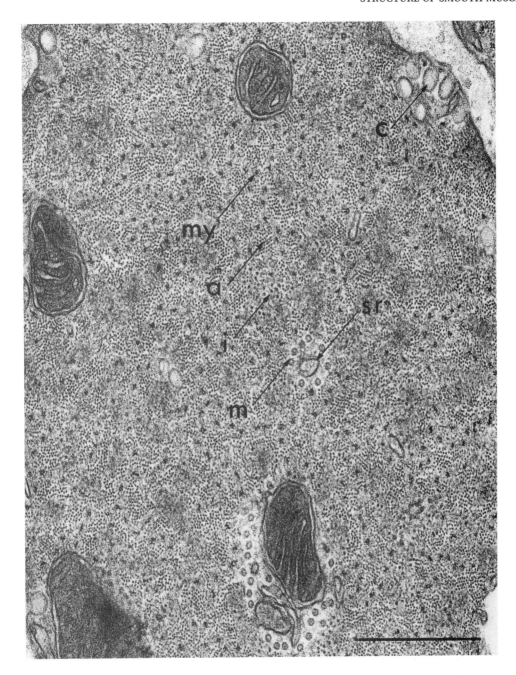

Fig. 3.8 Cytoplasm of a muscle cell of the guinea-pig taenia coli showing mitochondria, microtubules (**m**), sacs of sarcoplasmic reticulum (**sr**) and caveolae (**c**). **a**, actin filaments; **i**, intermediate filaments; **my**, myosin filaments. Calibration bar: 0.5 μm.

muscles is markedly higher than in striated muscles. The high collagen content of intestinal muscles supports the idea that their stroma serves a mechanical role in the transmission of force, and it has been

suggested that it could be regarded as a kind of intramuscular microtendons. Large assemblies of collagen fibrils (collagen fibres) in intramuscular septa and in the submucosa exchange fibrils with each other and

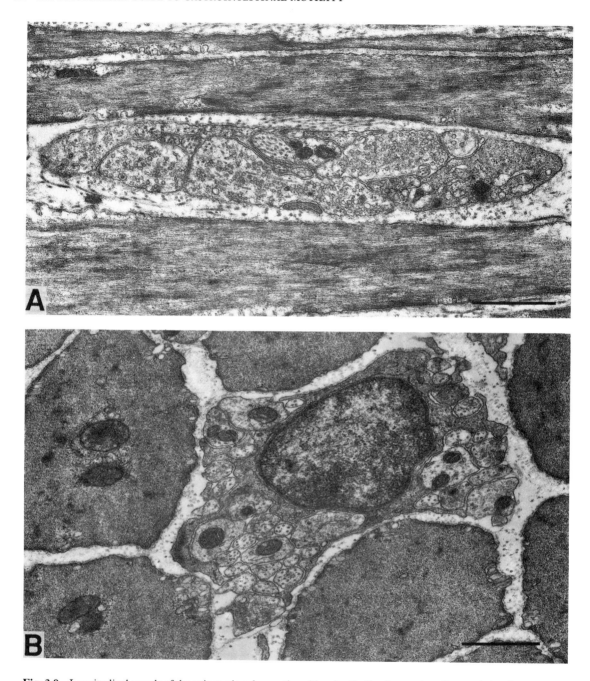

Fig. 3.9 Longitudinal muscle of the guinea-pig colon sectioned longitudinally. A nerve bundle containing three axons (varicosities) packed with synaptic vesicles runs between the muscle cells. **B** Taenia coli of a guinea-pig, in transverse section. A nerve bundle containing several axons runs between the muscle cells. The Schwann cell is sectioned at the level of its nucleus. Calibration bars: 1 μm.

are continuous with individual fibrils running close to the muscle cells. The fibrils are anchored to the muscle cell membrane, especially at the level of dense bands, via fibronectin fibrils, basal lamina and membrane receptors. Most smooth muscles have no tendons and they are not sheathed by a perimysium; tendons are, however, found in the avian gizzard and in smooth muscles inserted to the skeleton, such as the ano-coccygeus and the suspensor duodeni.

Elastic fibres have an indefinite length and anastomose with each other. They are recognized by their amorphous electron-dense core surrounded by microfibrils of 10 nm diameter. The number of elastic fibres in the large intestine is usually modest. An exception are the taeniae of the rabbit colon (and possibly some other intestinal muscles) which are so rich in elastic fibres as to resemble the media of elastic arteries.

MUSCLE AS AN INDEPENDENT EFFECTOR

Although conventionally we talk of a chain of events leading from the CNS, through autonomic ganglia to intramuscular nerve fibres and nerve endings (varicosities) and to smooth muscle cells, the diagram of connections is so complex that only the muscle cell itself can be considered the common final pathway. The muscle cell is an independent effector, which may be influenced, in so far as it has a variety of receptors, by different nerves and by hormones; it is sensitive to temperature and metabolic conditions, and sometimes even to light, it responds to stretch and maybe other mechanical conditions, and it is affected by the degree of coupling with adjacent cells. All these influences are integrated, or computed, to determine whether contraction takes place.

Mechanism of contraction

Intestinal smooth muscles are able to generate a stress comparable to that produced by a skeletal muscle of the same cross-sectional area (Gabella, 1983), in spite of the fact that skeletal muscles have a much higher myosin content (hence a larger number of potential cross-bridges) (Murphy et al 1977). In response to muscle excitation (stimulation of membrane receptors) there is increase in cytoplasmic concentration of calcium ions, released from an intracellular store (such as sarcoplasmic reticulum) or flowing into the cell from the extracellular fluid through opened channels. A myosin light chain kinase is activated and there is phosphorylation of a light chain subunit of myosin; phosphorylated myosin interacts with actin with the formation of cross-bridges which produce contraction (generation of force, shortening). During prolonged contraction of smooth muscle, while force is maintained, phosphorylation decreases, calcium concentration falls, and expenditure of energy decreases; the cross-bridges are then said to be in a condition of latch (latch bridges) (Dillon & Murphy 1982).

Isometric contraction

In isometric contraction a muscle does not change in length: within the muscle there are structural changes, including small variations in length of the cells, to take up any slack in the contractile elements or in the cytoskeleton or in the stroma. A distinctive structural feature of isometrically contracted muscle cells is the chequered appearance of the cell profiles due to areas (or domains) of the cytoplasm that are devoid of myofilaments and are therefore of lighter appearance than areas occupied by myofilaments. Myofilaments are longitudinally arranged and have a higher packing density than in the cells at rest (Gabella 1983, Gillis et al 1988). The force generated isometrically is of the order of 400–500 mN per mm² (or about 5 kg.cm^{-2}) of muscle transverse sectional area, as determined in the taenia coli of the guinea pig; a muscle the size of a pencil (8 mm diameter) should be able to lift about 2 kg.

Isotonic contraction

In isotonic contraction, visceral smooth muscles can shorten to as little as one-fifth of the resting length, and the process is accompanied by vast structural rearrangements. In the intestine, however, the actual amount of shortening is limited by geometrical constraint within the wall. For example, in a full contraction of the circular muscle of the rat distal colon, the muscle thickness is trebled and the mucosa is thrown into tall folds that practically occlude the lumen; therefore, although the muscle has shortened by only about 50%, no further shortening is possible.

The shortening of a smooth muscle in isotonic contraction is accompanied by a lateral expansion of the muscle, such that the increase in sectional area of muscle is about equal to the decrease in muscle length. The structural changes of the contracting muscle are mirrored by changes in the individual muscle cells. Therefore, cells in contracted muscles are shorter and fatter than those of resting muscles. With extensive shortening the cell axis is no longer parallel to the length of the muscle, instead it deviates appreciably, a change particularly apparent in muscles, such as the taeniae, containing many intramuscular septa. While in visceral muscles at rest the cells are straight and virtually parallel to each other, in isotonic contraction they are somewhat contorted; some torsion accompanies their shortening so that they acquire the shape of irregular and long-pitched helices. This change in shape is partly imposed by the connective tissue surrounding each cell and by the adjacent muscle cells and partly due to rearrangement of the contractile units; corkscrew-like shortening is also observed in isolated muscle cells and this suggests a helical arrangement of the cytoskeleton and of the contractile apparatus (Warshaw et al 1987). The cell surface is thrown into myriad laminar projections, which interdigitate with those from adjacent cells and are oriented at an angle to the cell length, forming again a helicoidal system. Cells in isotonic contraction can therefore be recognized (and distinguished from cells at rest) by the size of the profiles, and by the highly corrugated outline of the cells and by their interdigitations. The nucleus is much shortened and fatter, and displays deep crenations. While in the muscle at rest the collagen fibrils surrounding the muscle cells run mainly longitudinally or at a small angle with the cell length, in the shortened muscle the fibrils are wound around the cell and run obliquely or almost transversely, often embedded in the grooves between lamellar projections of the muscle cells.

Passive contraction

There are many passive structural changes in visceral muscle, viz. changes that are imposed by the contraction of adjacent muscle cells or muscle layers. For example, a contraction of the longitudinal muscle shortens the gut and compresses sideways the muscle cells of the circular layer, which thus acquire an elliptic profile; when the circular muscle contracts, the shortening and fattening of the muscle cells produces not only a decrease of the intestine circumference but also a lateral expansion of the muscle so that the gut elongates and the longitudinal muscle cells become longer and thinner.

HYDROSTATS

The helicoidal projections of the cell surface, the grooves housing collagen fibrils, the increase in cell girth, the reorientation of collagen fibrils, suggest that smooth muscle contraction is not well explained as a simple process of shortening (unlike skeletal muscle contraction). The notion of contraction as a change in shape provides a better account of how smooth muscle works. In this context, a comparison is proposed with mechanical structures known as hydrostats, i.e. those muscle that work without the support of a skeleton, such as the tongue of mammals, or the arms of an octopus, or the trunk of an elephant. In order to explain the variety of movements obtained with smooth muscles, and the fact that they contract without the support of a skeleton, and the fact that organs such as

the intestine do elongate, even if actively the muscle can only contract; to explain all this we consider two factors. First, the geometry of the muscle, as exemplified by the very large variety of spatial arrangements of the musculature in different organs, including synergistic or antagonistic combinations of muscles; and, second, the fact that the muscle is chiefly composed of a liquid and is therefore incompressible and of constant volume. Not only the muscle tissue, but also the muscle cells themselves are incompressible. In spite of their different appearance in histological sections, the volume of contracted and relaxed muscle cells is approximately the same. It is therefore correct to regard the contraction of a smooth muscle cell as a change in shape rather than a simple shortening. Fattening of the cells is as effective as their shortening. Collagen tightly wrapped around muscle cells ensures that the changes in shape in every cell and in any direction are added together and contribute to the contraction. The force generated and transmitted is eventually discharged through septa of connective tissue to the submucosa.

SUBMUCOSA

The submucosa of the mammalian intestine is a layer of connective tissue, permeated by numerous arteries, veins, lymphatic vessels and a ganglionated plexus (the submucosal plexus). The most abundant component of the submucosa is collagen, and most of the collagen of the intestinal wall is found in the submucosa. This collagen is connected to the intramuscular septa, and by this means the pull of the muscle bundles is discharged into the submucosa, rather than being transmitted entirely within the muscle over a long distance, for example over the entire circumference of the intestine. In this respect the submucosa acts as the 'skeleton' of the intestine and it also offers a strong resistance to excessive distension. The collagen fibrils of the submucosa are grouped in large bundles (collagen fibres) measuring up to 6 μm in diameter and of indefinite length. These collagen fibres run helicoidally down the length of the intestine forming two intertwined systems, one clockwise the other counterclockwise. This criss-cross arrangement resembles that found in the so-called cross-ply tyres (as opposed to radial tyres), and the angle between the helices (which is 50–55 degrees in the fully distended intestine) varies depending on the amount of longitudinal and radial distension of the gut. The intestinal wall offers, therefore, a strong resistance to excessive distension, while it remains deformable during contractile activity.

DEVELOPMENT OF VISCERAL MUSCULATURE

Smooth muscle cells develop from mesenchymal cells in the wall of the anlagen of viscera and around the endothelium of blood vessels. The precursor cells become elongated, approximately parallel to each other, and myofilaments appear in the deep parts of the cytoplasm. For example, in the primordium of the gizzard muscle of the chick, actin immunofluorescence is detected at 5 days in ovo, myosin is detected a day or two later, filaments can be seen at 10 days, and well formed smooth muscle cells are found from the eleventh day. Subsequently, they gradually acquire membrane specializations, with a specific temporal pattern (Gabella 1989). Caveolae appear at about the thirteenth day and become common at the end of the embryonic life, but they continue to increase in relative frequency after hatching. Gap junctions appear around the sixteenth day as minute aggregates of connexons, which then grow in size, probably by addition of new connexons. In contrast mitochondria and sarcoplasmic reticulum are more abundant in immature muscle cells than in fully differentiated ones.

In a developing smooth muscle all the cells are at the same stage of differentiation and there are no undifferentiated cells kept for development at a later stage. From its early appearance to maturity a smooth muscle increases hundreds of times in mass, by a 2–4-fold increase in cell size and by a very large increase in cell number. Mitoses occur when the cells are already well differentiated: mitosis in a smooth muscle cell occurs at a time when there is already full expression of myofilament proteins and there are membrane specializations (Fig. 3.10). Mitotic muscle cells are found throughout life but are most common at a time before birth (which varies between different muscles) and become rare in the adult unless the tissue is stimulated to hypertrophy. Dividing muscle cells can appear in any part of the muscle. This type of growth is termed intussusceptive as it involves addition of new cells within the texture itself of the muscle rather than at its surface or its ends.

Developing smooth muscles are able to contract from the time the first filaments appear. In addition to synthesizing its contractile apparatus, the developing muscle cell produces a large part of the extracellular components of the tissue, such as collagen, while at the same time already performing some mechanical activity and responding to mechanical influences from its environment.

HYPERTROPHY OF VISCERAL MUSCULATURE

Intestinal smooth muscles undergo a large increase in volume as a consequence of a chronic, partial obstruction impairing the flow of luminal contents. Numerous examples of intestinal muscle hypertrophy are encountered in human medicine, for example in segments of the gut orad to a partial obstruction (aganglionosis, either congenital, as in Hirschprung's disease, or acquired, as in Chagas disease, and ensuing spasm and obstruction; congenital strictures; malformation of sphincters; luminal obstructions by tumoral growths). Intestinal hypertrophy is produced in laboratory animals by experimental stenosis, especially in the small intestine. The partial obstruction of a short segment of the gut slows down the transit of ingesta, causes their accumulation on the oral side, followed by gradual distension of the lumen and hypertrophy of all the coats including the musculature. In contrast, complete occlusion leads to rapid distension followed by necrosis and perforation before there is a growth response in the wall. Hypertrophy of the caecum (enlargement of the organ and thickening of the wall) is observed in animals reared in germ-free conditions, in diabetic animals, and in animals fed with a diet rich in fibre or pectin. Mice with congenital absence of ganglion neurons in the distal colon (lethal spotted mice, Ls/Ls) develop a local obstruction which is followed by an enlargement of the colon and a thickening of the wall on the oral side. In every case, hypertrophy is not an acute process, but requires a stimulus that is persistent and intense, but not such as to cause acute organ failure. Hypertrophy is a response of the muscle or an adaptation to an increase in the functional load on the muscle. There is always a distension of the lumen and an increase not only in thickness but also in extent of the wall: the intestine increases in circumference and in wall thickness, but there is usually no change in length.

In hypertrophy the intestinal musculature can increase 15 times in volume and both layers are affected (Gabella 1990) (Fig. 3.11). In experimental conditions this growth occurs in rats and guinea pigs in 2–5 weeks. The most obvious aspect of muscle hypertrophy is the increase in cell size (cell hypertrophy). In the intestine, muscle cell volume increase by up to about four times. There is also hyperplasia, that is mitosis and increase in muscle cell number: the mitoses occur in fully differentiated muscle cells and are found in both muscle layers. The muscle cells are not only enlarged but acquire a more irregular shape. Their surface is more convoluted, and has deep finger-like or

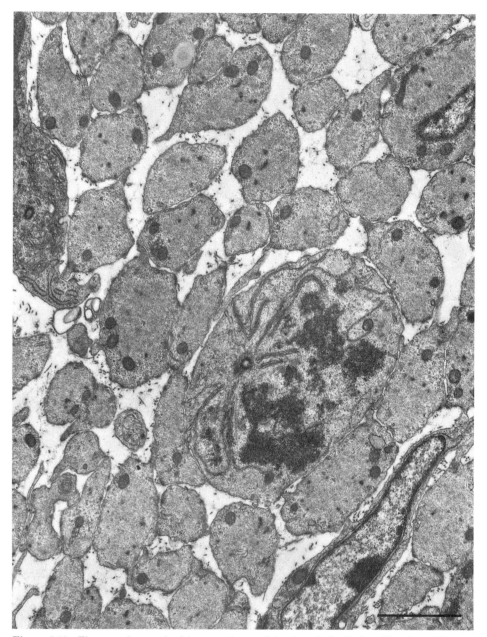

Figure 3.10   Electron micrograph of the musculature of the gizzard of a 20-day-old embryo. The large cell profile in the centre is a muscle cell undergoing mitosis and showing chromosomes, paired cisternae of endoplasmic reticulum and a centriole; at the periphery of the profile there are bundles of myofilaments and other organelles. Calibration bar: 2 μm.

laminar invaginations, covered by a basal lamina and bearing caveolae and dense bands. In spite of the presence of these invaginations, the surface to volume ratio falls from 1.4 to 0.8. All types of filament, thin, thick and intermediate filaments, increase in number, on account of the large increase in cell size. However,

in intestinal hypertrophic muscle cells, actin filaments increase more than myosin filaments and intermediate filaments increase substantially more than either type of myofilament and the cells display large bundles of them. Mitochondria usually increase less than the cell and their spatial density falls, whereas sarcoplasmic

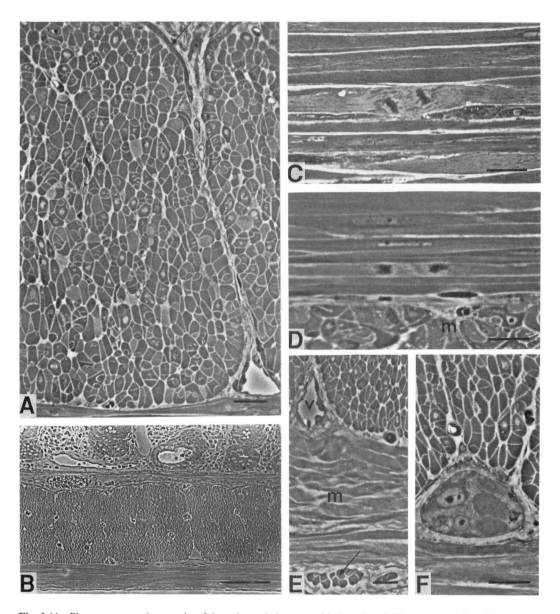

Fig. 3.11 Phase contrast micrographs of the guinea-pig hypertrophic intestine. **A** Transverse section of the circular muscle layer. The enlarged muscle cells have an irregular shape, and their tapering ends are often split into 2–3 processes. The arrow points to a layer of small and dark muscle cells which lines the submucosal surface of the circular muscle and penetrates for some distance along an intramuscular septum. **B** Transverse section of the wall, about 15 cm oral to the obstruction, showing the regular architecture of the muscle and the increase in thickness (cfr. Fig. 3.1). Both muscle layers are hypertrophic. **C** Muscle cell in late anaphase in the circular layer. **D** Muscle cell undergoing mitosis in the circular layer. The circular muscle layer is shown at the bottom. **E** A newly-formed bundle of musculature (arrow), oriented circularly, is seen in the serosa, **m** longitudinal muscle layer. **F** A ganglion of the myenteric plexus surrounded by hypertrophic musculature of the circular (top) and longitudinal (bottom) layer. The small black dots around the ganglion are elastic fibres. Calibration bars: A, C, D, E and F: 20 μm; B: 100 μm.

reticulum is better represented than in control cells. Intramuscular blood vessels, which are mainly capillaries, increase in length and number, and the hypertrophic musculature remains well supplied with blood. The density of innervation of the hypertrophic intestinal musculature is greatly decreased, mainly because the intramuscular nerves are diluted in a much expanded musculature. Characteristically, there is a marked expansion of enteric ganglia and an enlargement of both myenteric and submucosal neurons. In these experimental conditions, neuronal hypertrophy is also found among prevertebral ganglion neurons and dorsal root ganglion neurons.

REFERENCES

Ashton F T, Somlyo A V, Somlyo A P, 1975 The contractile apparatus of vascular smooth muscle: Intermediate high voltage stereo electron microscopy. J Mol Biol 98: 17–29

Bagby R M 1980 Double immunofluorescent staining of isolated smooth muscle cells. I. Preparation of anti-chicken gizzard alpha actinin and its use with anti-chicken gizzard myosin for co-localization of alpha actinin and myosin in chicken gizzard cells. Histochemistry 69: 113–130

Bagby R M 1983 Organization of contractile/cytoskeletal elements in: Stephens N L (ed) Biochemistry of Smooth Muscle, pp 1–84, CRC Press, Boca Raton

Beyer E C, Kistler J, Paul D L, Goodenough D A 1989 Antisera directed against connexin 43 peptides react with a 43-kD protein localized to gap junctions in myocardium and other tissues. J Cell Biol 108: 595–605

Bois R M 1973 The organization or the contractile apparatus of vertebrate smooth muscle. Anat Rec 93: 138–149

Bond M, Kitizawa T, Somlyo A P, Somlyo A V 1984 Release and recycling of calcium by the sarcoplasmic reticulum in guinea-pig portal vein smooth muscle. J Physiol (Lond) 355: 677–695

Bond M, Somlyo A V 1982 Dense bodies and actin polarity in vertebrate smooth muscle. J Cell Biol 95: 403–413

Casteels R, Raeymaekers L 1979 The action of acetylcholine and catecholamines on an intracellular calcium store in the smooth muscle cells of the guinea-pig taenia coli. J Physiol (Lond) 294: 51–68

Craig R, Megerman J 1977 Assembly of smooth muscle myosin into side-polar filaments. J Cell Biol 75(3): 990–996

Dillon P F, Murphy R A 1982 Tonic force maintenance with reduced shortening velocity in arterial smooth muscle. Am J Physiol 242: C102–C108

Elliott A, Offer G, Burridge K 1976 Electron microscopy of myosin molecules from muscle and non-muscle sources. Proc Roy Soc Lond Series B 193: 45–53

Gabella G 1983 Structural apparatus for force transmission in smooth muscles. Physiol Rev 64: 455–477

Gabella G 1987 Structure of muscles and nerves in the gastrointestinal tract in: Johnson L R (ed.) Physiology of the gastrointestinal tract, pp 335–381. Raven Press, New York

Gabella G 1988 Structure of smooth muscle in: Kumar D, Gustavsson S (eds), An illustrated guide to gastrointestinal motility (1st edn), pp 33–45. Wiley, Chichester

Gabella G 1989 Development of smooth muscle: ultrastructural study of the chick embryo gizzard. Anatomy & Embryology 180: 213–226

Gabella G 1990 Hypertrophy of visceral smooth muscle. Anatomy & Embryology 182: 409–424

Geiger B, Dutton A H, Tokuashi K T, Singer S J 1981 Immunoelectron microscope studies of membrane-microfilament interactions: distributions of a-actinin, tropomyosin, and vinculin in intestinal epithelial brush border and chicken gizzard smooth muscle cells. J Cell Biol 91: 614–628

Gillis J M, Cao M L, Godfraind-De Becker A 1988 Density of myosin filaments in the rat anococcygeus muscle, at rest and in contraction. II. J Muscle Research Cell Motil 9: 18–28

Murphy R A, Driska S P, Cohen D M 1977 Variations in actin to myosin ratios and cellular force generation in vertebrate smooth muscles in: Casteels R (ed) Excitation–contraction coupling in smooth muscle, pp 417–424, Elsevier/North-Holland, Amsterdam

Small V J, Sobieszek A 1980 The contractile apparatus of smooth muscle. Int Rev Cytol 64: 241–306

Warshaw D M, McBride W J, Work S S 1987 Corkscrew-like shortening in single smooth muscle cells. Science 236: 1457–1459

Regulation of gastrointestinal motility

4. The ontogeny of intestinal motor activity

P. J. Milla

MORPHOLOGY AND DIFFERENTIATION

The gross morphology of the adult gastrointestinal tract is described in Chapter 1. The complex anatomy of the gut is developed from an initial simple tube.

About 4 weeks after conception the primitive gut consists of a hollow tube from mouth to cloaca suspended dorsally and ventrally by mesenteries. The proximal part of the tube forms the foregut with the oesophagus at the cranial end and a fusiform dilatation, the stomach, appearing at the caudal end of the foregut at about 5 weeks' gestation. The middle portion of the primitive tube forms the midgut – eventually duodenum, small intestine and proximal third of the colon – and the distal portion, the hindgut. The midgut grows rapidly and soon exceeds the capacity of the fetal abdomen, and a loop of gut herniates through the abdominal wall. Between 10 and 12 weeks of gestation the loop returns to the abdominal cavity undergoing a 270° counter-clockwise rotation during the process (Arey 1974). Thus by the end of the first trimester, the layout of the gastrointestinal tract is identical to that found in the newborn infant.

The tissues of the gastrointestinal tract differentiate and mature in a species-dependent pattern which is determined by genetic, environmental and species-specific endogenous regulatory mechanisms. The sequence of development is well established; initially there is primordial differentiation of ecto-, meso- and endoderm followed by interaction of these three layers as anatomical specialization proceeds.

The primitive intestine consists of a single layer of cells arranged radially. Initially the epithelium develops with a change from stratified to columnar cells at about 8 weeks' gestation in a cranio-caudal direction and the development of specialized junctional complexes and secondary lumina. This is followed by remodelling of the mucosa with villi being formed by the fusion of the secondary and primary lumina. Crypts are apparent by 12–13 weeks' gestation (Moxey & Trier 1978). At this same period of time the innervation of

the fetal gut and the muscle coats also develop. In the small intestine the myenteric plexus is visible by 9 weeks' gestation and the submucous plexus by 13 weeks (Hart & Mir 1971). The outer circular muscle is present by 12 weeks, but the longitudinal muscle is not present until 14 weeks, and the inner circular muscle not until 22 weeks of gestation.

A large body of evidence shows that digestive, absorptive and secretory mechanisms are well developed in the alimentary tract by the end of the second trimester.

MOTOR CONTROL SYSTEMS AND THEIR DEVELOPMENT

SMOOTH MUSCLE

There is limited knowledge regarding the morphogenesis and differentiation of smooth muscle cells in the human fetus and infant. Smooth muscle first appears at about 12 weeks of gestation in the outer circular muscular layer and some 2–3 weeks later the longitudinal coat is laid down. The layers adjacent to the submucous plexus, the muscularis mucosae and the inner circular muscle layer however do not occur until later in gestation. The muscularis mucosae is evident at about 22–23 weeks' gestation but it is uncertain when the inner circular muscle layer appears in the human. In the rat it is clear that it does not develop until after birth (Kedinger et al 1990).

In mature smooth muscle cells inherent excitability is shown by rhythmic cyclical depolarization and repolarization of the plasma cell membrane. Studies in the human preterm infant have shown that the frequency of this electrical slow wave increases with increasing post-conceptional age, reflecting developmental changes in the activity of membrane ion pumps and channels or in their modulation (Bisset et al 1988a).

Along the length of the gut there are marked differences in the musculature in both structure and function. Each muscle coat is laid down at specific periods of time during gestation. The contractile proteins of the smooth muscle cells also appear in a hierarchical manner (Kedinger et al 1990), at least in the rat, but there is no information regarding such proteins in the human.

The detection of fibroblastic-like cells in the muscle coats, interstitial cells of Cajal (see Ch. 3), has led to the speculation that these cells may be acting as pacemakers and a body of evidence is assembling which would support this view (Daniel & Berezin 1992). As yet, there is little information regarding their ontogeny; however, from a study of the developing opossum it is clear that interstitial cells are present, but immature with no gap junctions with muscle cells, from very early in development. Gap junctions only become discernible with full maturity (Christensen & Rick 1992).

ENTERIC NERVOUS SYSTEM (ENS)

Information regarding the ontogeny of the enteric innervation in the human is scanty. However the pattern of development of motor activity in the small intestine in all mammals so far studied has been remarkably similar though there are obvious differences in timing (Ruckebusch 1986; Bisset et al 1988a). Thus the body of evidence from the experimental animal is likely to show the general pattern of ontogeny which occurs in the human.

Intrinsic neural elements appear in the fetal gut at a very early stage – first the myenteric plexus followed a week or so later by the submucous plexus. The enteric neurones are generally believed to have migrated to the gut from the neural crest.

Recent studies suggest that this process is closely controlled by the homeobox group of genes that have recently been shown to control segmentation in *Drosophila* (Levine and Harding 1989). Overexpression of the gene Hox 1.4 in transgenic mice has led to the development of a megacolon (Wohlgemuth et al 1989).

Following colonization of the gut there is a prolonged period of maturation during which time many changes occur in the microenvironment of the gut. An increasing body of evidence shows that the microenvironment in which the migrating neural crest cells ultimately find themselves may be critical in their development and may determine the final neurotransmitters expressed by the neurones (Le Dourin 1980, Patterson 1978). Many of the neurones will transiently express catecholamines, but this appears to be an initial phenomenon and is followed by a carefully controlled ontogenic timetable in which cholinergic and serotoninergic neurones develop first, followed by adrenergic and then peptidergic neurones (Gershon et al 1983).

Recent studies in the human fetal oesophagus suggest that peptidergic innervation develops towards the end of the first trimester (Hitchcock et al 1992). The developmental path of the neural precursor cells, however, is open to environmental influences until a very late stage in their maturation. This 'plasticity' of the enteric neurones may therefore be very important in the development of dysmotile states in the infant and child and be of relevance to the functional bowel disorders in the adult. Examples of the environment influencing the development of enteric neurones are the altered expression of extracellular matrix proteins in animals such as the lethal spotted mouse with dysganglionosis of the hind gut (Payette et al 1988).

A number of observations suggest that development of the ENS continues through pregnancy and for at least the first year of life. First, it is a consistent feature of fasting small intestinal motor activity in all mammals that it is cyclical in nature and that when cyclical activity first appears the periodicity is short and this lengthens as the animal matures. In the sheep, the periodicity increases from 30–40 min to 90–120 min between 120 days' gestation and term (Bueno & Ruckebusch 1979). In the premature human neonate there is similarly an increase in periodicity from 10–13 min at 30 weeks' gestation to 40–45 min at term (Wozniak et al 1984; Bisset et al 1988a). It has been suggested that the increase in cycle length is mediated by either an increase in 5-hydroxytryptamine (5HT)-secreting neurones or activation of neurones with 5HT receptors. Such an effect is supported by the presence of large numbers of 5HT receptors within the duodenum (Branchek et al 1984) and the observation that 5HT antagonists in adult sheep reduce the cycle length to that seen in fetal sheep (Ruckebusch 1986). Second, study of argyrophilic neurones in the sigmoid colon of the human neonate show that prior to term no argyrophilic nerves are present, and during the first 6 months of life neurones in the myenteric plexus gradually assume the ability to take up silver (Smith 1993). Third, in the first month of life, neurones of both the submucous and myenteric plexuses of the rectum and sigmoid colon are hyperplastic and may be mistaken for changes of intestinal dysplasia (Smith 1993).

CENTRAL NERVOUS SYSTEM (CNS)

Changes in fasting cycle length are paralleled by changes in electroencephalographic activity. The development of alpha cortical rhythms correlated well with the appearance of organized propagated fasting small intestinal motor activity in the month prior to term in the sheep and to 2 weeks after birth in the dog

(Ruckebusch 1986). A similar increase in sleep cycle occurs at the same time as the increasing fasting cycle length.

It seems clear that the combined maturation of both ENS and CNS together with their interconnections are responsible for many of the major ontogenic changes observed in intestinal motor activity before and after birth (Wozniak et al 1984, Bisset et al 1988, Berseth 1989). The nature of these maturational changes is, however, largely unexplored.

HUMORAL SYSTEM

As the villi and crypts are beginning to form, endocrine cells are first seen in the human fetal small intestine. Initially, the fetal endocrine cells contain two types of secretory granules, one typical of adult-type endocrine cells, and the other characteristic of a very early precursor cell. As gestation increases, these latter cells are lost, leaving a population of the adult-type endocrine cells.

The response of gastrointestinal polypeptide hormones to enteral nutrition has been intensively studied during the preterm period, but very few studies have been conducted later in the first year of life. In those infants born before 33 weeks' gestation, the first feed, whether it is given as a bolus or an infusion, does not produce a significant change in levels of insulin, growth hormone or enteroglucagon, or in glycolytic metabolites compared to the first feed of infants born at term (Lucas et al 1978). If enteral feeding is continued in such preterm infants over the next few weeks a marked postprandial rise in motilin, enteroglucagon and neurotensin is observed (Lucas et al 1980). If however, the infants are fed parenterally and do not receive any enteral nutrition then the basal plasma levels of these hormones is significantly reduced until such time as enteral feeding is introduced. A further series of studies also shows that significant increases in the secretion of polypeptide hormones may be induced by rather limited amounts of enteral nutrition (Lucas et al 1986). These studies show that early enteral nutrition triggers the release of gut hormones and that they may play an important role both in the development of intestinal motility and also in the physiological adaptation to extra-uterine life.

There is little information regarding the effects of weaning from milk feeds, but animal studies suggest that of cholecystokinin, vasoactive intestinal polypeptide and somatostatin rise to significantly greater levels in animals that have been weaned than in those that have been milk fed (Guilloteau 1986). The release of these hormones following feeds may be important in the adaptation of intestinal function to weaning, particularly changes in motor activity.

GASTROINTESTINAL MOTOR ACTIVITY IN THE HUMAN INFANT

It is clear from the above discussion of the control systems of intestinal motor activity that there is a timetable of motor activity development in the gastrointestinal tract, and this may be useful in planning the nutritional care of infants born prematurely.

FETAL AND NEONATAL MOTOR ACTIVITY

Sucking and swallowing

It is well recognized that the human infant in utero swallows amniotic fluid and this has been observed as early as 16 weeks' gestation. By injecting radio-labelled red blood cells into the amniotic fluid, the volume of fluid swallowed has been shown to increase from 2–7 ml/day to about 16 ml/day at around 20 weeks' gestation and to 450 ml/day by term (Pritchard 1966). It is thought that fetal swallowing of amniotic fluid is an important mechanism in the maintenance of amniotic fluid volume late in pregnancy, and conditions in which the foregut is atretic, such as oesophageal and duodenal atresia, are frequently associated with polyhydramnios. However, it is also possible that there are trophic factors in the amniotic fluid that are important in the development of both gut structure and function.

While the infant in utero is able to swallow amniotic fluid, when born prematurely, the infant is unfortunately not able to suck effectively to obtain milk until about 34 weeks' gestation. This is a result of ineffective sucking and an inability to coordinate the oral, pharyngeal and oesophageal phases of swallowing. Attempts to initiate oral feeding in infants born before this time result both in exhaustion of the infant and uncoordinated swallowing and aspiration. As a result, premature infants born before 34 weeks' gestation will require tube feeding. The early feeble and ineffective sucking movements that very premature infants make have been termed 'non-nutritive sucking' to differentiate them from the much more effective nutritive sucking mechanism which develops at about 34–35 weeks of gestation (Herbst 1981, Casaer et al 1982). As the sucking mechanism develops, the premature infant develops short sucking bursts of 5–7 sucks in length at a frequency of approximately 1 Hz. These periods are either preceded or followed by a swallow. Eventually, the infant will develop a more mature pattern of sucking

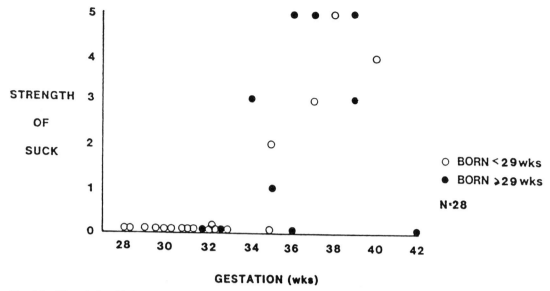

Fig. 4.1   The relationship between nutritive sucking and gestational age.

with prolonged bursts up to 30 sucks long and a frequency double that previously seen. The bursts of sucking are associated with a single swallow towards the end of the burst. Both nutritive and non-nutritive sucking in the infant is a reflex behaviour and, not surprisingly, most studies have shown that its development is related to gestational age. However, a number of other factors have also been shown to affect sucking and these include maternal sedation (Casaer et al 1982), the presence of a nipple and the flow rate of milk (Peiper 1963), length of feeding experience (Crump et al 1958, Casaer et al 1982), taste of the fluid (Maller & Turner 1973) and even visual stimuli (Milewski & Siqueland 1975). It is, however, gestational age and neurological development of both the CNS and ENS that are the strongest determinants of the type and efficiency of sucking, and effective nutritive sucking does not develop until 34–35 weeks' gestation. A study of the ontogeny of small intestinal motor activity (Wozniak et al 1984) showed clearly that the onset of such sucking behaviour parallels the acquisition of mature (cyclical fasting migrating motor complexes (MMCs) and continuous postprandial pattern) patterns of gastric antral and small intestinal motor activity, as shown in Figure 4.1. This pattern of development represents an exception to the usual cranio-caudal gradient, but ensures that the ability to transport food along the gut accompanies the ability to ingest large amounts of food.

Stimulation of non-nutritive sucking has been shown to accelerate the maturation of the sucking reflex, and also to improve enteral feed tolerance and to shorten intestinal transit time. The improved nutrition results in increased infant weight gain when compared to matched infants in whom sucking was not stimulated (Bernbaum et al 1983). It would appear, therefore, that sucking is a conditioned reflex which can be reinforced by learned experience.

SUCKING AND SWALLOWING AFTER BIRTH

The mechanisms of sucking and swallowing

Although sucking and swallowing movements are established before birth, they do not develop fully until a variable period of time after birth. The details of the feeding mechanism in normal infants (Logan & Bosma 1967), full-term neonates (Gryboski 1965) and preterm infants (Gryboski 1969; Daniels et al 1986) have been described in detail. Sucking movements precede swallowing which, in turn, inhibits respiration and is closely coordinated with relaxation of the lower oesophageal sphincter (LOS) and receptive relaxation of the fundus of the stomach. In older infants the first stage of swallowing is voluntary in character but at term or preterm is an involuntary reflex.

Oropharyngeal phase

A bolus of fluid is delivered to the pharynx initially by suction to the nipple and then by tongue action against the palate. A series of coordinated contractions of muscles of the pharynx, soft palate and larynx then pushes the bolus towards the oesophagus without entering the larynx or nasopharynx.

Oesophageal phase

The last stage of swallowing is effected by the inferior constrictor which consists of two parts, the thyropharyngeal muscle above, which is propulsive, and the cricopharyngeal below, which is sphincteric in function and is otherwise known as the superior oesophageal sphincter. Once in the oesophagus, food is propelled by a sequence of peristaltic contractions, initiated by the pharyngeal phases of swallowing through an open and relaxed LOS into the stomach.

THE LOWER OESOPHAGEAL SPHINCTER

Despite the large body of information regarding motor activity of the oesophagus of the older infant, child and adult, knowledge regarding its development is fragmentary, especially in the human. The majority of studies have centred around the gastro-oesophageal junction and the LOS. Recent studies of the LOS in the preterm infant provide evidence that, just as in other parts of the gastrointestinal tract, a developmental timetable is followed and that, initially, sphincter pressures are extremely low. In addition to developmental changes of oesophageal function, there are also changes in the anatomy of the hiatus and of the lower oesophagus.

Anatomy

The anatomy of the gastro-oesophageal junction differs in infants from children and adults. In infants, although the precise anatomy may vary, in general, the crural muscles are thick and relatively well developed, providing an oblique hiatal tunnel which grips the lower oesophagus. The fundus of the stomach and the lower oesophagus are then held in place by a prominent phreno-oesophageal membrane, a tough fibro-elastic layer attached to the thoracic and abdominal aspects of the diaphragm and to the oesophagus within the hiatus. These features differ from the normal anatomy in the adult and both the hiatal tunnel and the membrane are less evident in the older child, suggesting a maturational defect (Eliska 1973). During gestation, the intra-abdominal oesophagus shows a number of developmental changes. At about 8 weeks' gestation, the abdominal oesophagus is as wide and as large as the stomach. Throughout intra-uterine life it becomes gradually less marked and shortens so that by term it is only a few millimetres in length. In postnatal life it again extends over a few years to be 5–15 mm long. The angle between the stomach and the oesophagus is very variable and occasionally longitudinal mucosal folds, as seen in the adult, are present. In infants studied at postmortem, however, there is no evidence of a flap valve although, in a few, thickening of the circular muscle layer has been found.

Some features of the 'anatomical sphincter' are shared by both adults and the newborn infant. The main difference is the prominence in the infant of the diaphragm and the phreno-oesophageal membrane which results in an area of relative constriction of the lower oesophagus and stabilization of the gastro-oesophageal region. Thus, the anatomy of the lower oesophagus in the small infant provides some compensation for the lack of function of the LOS in the very small infant.

Function

Early studies suggested that the human infant has low sphincter pressure at birth (Euler & Ament 1977, Kenigsberg et al 1981) and that in the premature infant there is absence of an anti-reflux barrier for the first few weeks after birth (Boix-Ochoa & Canals 1976). However, the post-conceptional age of the infants studied is not always clear and in few cases were any longitudinal studies made. A more recent study using modern perfused catheter technology overcame most of these objections (Newell 1988). 25 infants of weight range 690–3300 g and mean gestational age 27–41 weeks were studied between 1 day and 9 weeks of age. Using a pull-through technique, fundal pressure, effective sphincter pressure and oesophageal pressure were measured. Fundal pressure was higher than the resting oesophageal pressure in all infants, but all were able to produce a LOS pressure higher than the fundal pressure. Even the smallest most premature infants were found to have a small but effective sphincter pressure. When the data was analysed cross-sectionally, it was shown that sphincter pressure rose with post-conceptional age (Figure 4.2a). However, seven infants studied longitudinally show that there is also a steady rise in pressure with increasing post-conceptual age (Figure 4.2b).

The mechanisms of sphincter maturation are, however, poorly understood. A few studies in the

A

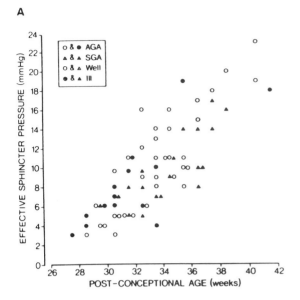

B

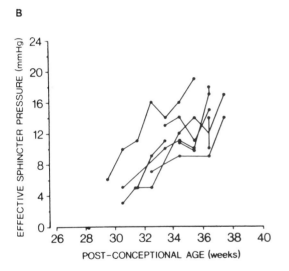

Fig. 4.2 **A** Effective lower oesophageal sphincter pressure and post-conceptional age in infants studied cross-sectionally. **B** Longitudinal studies of effective sphincter pressure in 7 infants born prematurely (adapted fron Newell 1988).

experimental animal have suggested that changes occur in both muscle mass and in sensitivity to neurohumoral agents. In the opossum (Cohen 1974), beagle puppy (Spedale et al 1982) and kitten (Hillemeier et al 1985) muscle mass of the LOS increases with increasing gestation, as does sensitivity to gastrin. This process

continues postnatally. Hillemeier also showed that muscle from the kitten LOS was capable of generating greater forces per unit mass than in the adult cat. Thus, there appears to be a clear pattern of development of at least the LOS smooth muscle with initially small amounts of muscle present capable of generating high forces, which, with increasing age, increases in mass and acquires increasing sensitivity to neurohumoral factors.

Preliminary studies of the body of the oesophagus and sphincter show that tone of both upper and lower sphincters developed before coordinated peristaltic sequences in the body (Ropert et al 1992). Recently the innervation of the oesophagus and the LOS has been studied (Hitchcock et al 1992) and increases in cell size and a reduction in cell and fibre density have been shown, with maturation that continues after the onset of coordinated muscle activity.

THE STOMACH

Studies of motor activity of the stomach are restricted to the measurement of gastric emptying of liquids, usually milk. To date, there have been no systematic observations of either proximal receptive relaxation of the stomach or of contractile activity in the antrum and pylorus of infants born prematurely and at term. It is not clear whether overall there is any effect of gestation on gastric emptying (Siegal et al 1984a), but clinical observation of the extremely premature infant would suggest that emptying is slower than in older infants. However, such infants are particularly prone to a number of extragastrointestinal pathological conditions such as respiratory distress syndrome (Yu 1975) in which delayed gastric emptying has been clearly documented. It is difficult to know therefore whether delayed emptying is a consequence of immaturity, or of the effects of other disease processes.

Although the emptying of a liquid may only require the generation of a pressure gradient between stomach and duodenum, such studies of emptying that have been carried out indicate that a receptor system in the duodenum regulates emptying and operates in a manner qualitatively similar to that in the adult which is described in Chapter 25. Food in the duodenum modulates emptying and composition, digestion and calorie density seem important (Husband & Husband 1969, Siegal et al 1984b). Siegal et al showed that altering the fat content (long chain and medium chain triglyceride – LCT and MCT) altered rates of emptying – inhibition produced by LCTs was much greater than that produced by MCTs. In contrast, alterations in emptying produced by altering the carbohydrate source (glucose, lactose, glucose polymer) were minimal. Changes in the nature of the protein content may also be important. In healthy premature infants, human milk emptied faster than an adapted infant cow's milk based formula of the same calorie density (Cavell 1979).

THE SMALL INTESTINE

There is more information on development of motor activity in the small intestine than for more proximal or distal parts of the gut. Using amniography McLain (1963) showed that there was little or no movement of contrast along the fetal gut before 30 weeks' gestation and, thereafter, there was increasing aboral transit as pregnancy proceeded. Information on the motor activity that underlies such transit was first derived from studies in the experimental animal. Electrodes were surgically implanted in the serosa and muscularis propria of the small intestine of fetal sheep and dogs (Bueno & Ruckebusch 1979). Myoelectric activity was measured in utero and after birth and showed quite clearly that transit in utero was due to fasting motor activity and that there was a species-specific, gestationally-dependent pattern of development. There was a disorganized initial phase with random spiking activity followed by a period of regular spiking activity, and eventually a MMC pattern occurred some days before term in the sheep and about 2 weeks postpartum in the dog. The MMC pattern was qualitatively similar to that found in adult animals, and consisted of periods of regular phasic propagated activity (phase III) followed by periods of quiescence (phase I) and preceded by irregular activity (phase II). Quantitatively, however, the MMC was different with a much shorter cycle length than in the adult animal. The adult patterns of small intestinal motor activity are described in detail in Chapter 27.

Fasting activity

The first direct studies in the human utilized nasojejunal feeding tubes in infants born prematurely (Milla & Fenton 1983). While technically unsophisticated, these human studies showed a similar gestationally-dependent pattern of development of fasting motor activity to that described in the sheep and the dog.

Following these initial studies, the author's laboratory developed a low-compliance, continuous-perfusion manometry system suitable for use in preterm infants as small as 800 g (Bisset et al 1988b). The manometric catheter was constructed from very soft polyvinyl chloride, triple-lumen extrusions (o.d. 1.5 mm; i.d. 0.5 mm) (Dural Plastics Pty, NSW, Australia) with distal perfusion ports 2.5 cm apart. The catheter was perfused at a rate of 0.4 ml per channel per hour using a syringe pump system with an individual syringe for each channel. The catheter and its response characteristics are shown in Figure 4.3. Pressure changes were measured by external Luerlock Mk 3 pressure transducers (Gaeltec, Dunvegan, Isle of Skye, Scotland) and the signal displayed on a multichannel oscillographic chart recorder. Simultaneously the pressure signals were digitized and the data captured on a floppy disk for subsequent display and off-line analysis. The normal methods of placement of the manometric catheter under fluoroscopic control are usually not available in the neonatal nursery and a system of blind placement was devised utilizing the characteristic change in frequency of motor activity from 0.05 Hz (3 cpm) in the stomach to 0.2 Hz (12 cpm) in the duodenum.

Patterns of fasting activity

Despite the narrow catheters used there was no attenuation of the manometric recordings. Artefacts due to body movements, arousals, startles and crying were frequently present but, in spite of this, we (Bisset et al 1988a) and others (Berseth 1989) using a similar recording system were able to show differing patterns of motor activity at differing gestational ages with four stages of development easily discernible (Table 4.1, Fig. 4.4).

Before 31 weeks' gestation low amplitude random contractions without obvious organization or propagation were seen. Some organization of muscle contraction began to appear around 31–34 weeks' gestation and very occasionally as early as 28 weeks with the development of clustered phasic contractions. This activity lasted between 1–20 min and occurred every 4–35 min with a frequency of 0.175–0.19 Hz (10.5–11.5 cpm). This pattern of clustered phasic activity appeared similar to the fetal pattern described in sheep and dogs by Bueno and Ruckebusch (1979). Initially, about half of the clusters of contractions were propagated aborally, but by 34 weeks at least 90% were propagated. As post-conceptional age increased, the clusters of phasic activity became longer and the frequency increased. This prolonged phasic activity was seen variably between 34–36 weeks' gestation. Its nature and cyclical character were, however, poorly developed with very variable intervals between complexes whose length varied between 5–40 min (Table 4.1), but all prolonged phasic activity recorded was propagated aborally. Similar characteristics of clus-

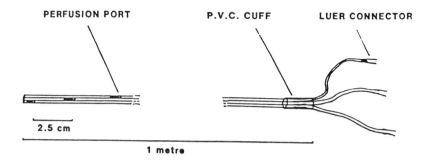

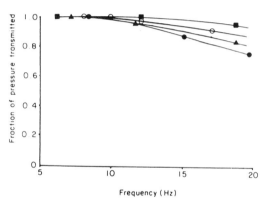

Fig. 4.3   Dimensions and constructional details of miniaturized triple lumen manometric catheter and its pressure response characteristics at different frequencies.

Table 4.1   Stages of fasting small intestinal motor development with corresponding gestational ages and variables of motor activity

Stage	Pattern	Gestational age (wks)	Complex length (min)	Complex interval (min)	Propagation velocity (cm/min)	Frequency (cpm)
1	Random	28–32 (29.5)	[0]	[0]	[0]	10.5–11.5 (11.0)
2	Clustered phasic	28–35 (31)	1–20 (4)	4–35 (12)	0–5 (2.5)	10.5–12.0 (11.0)
3	Prolonged phasic	34–36 (35)	5–40 (12)	4–30 (12)	1–5 (1.4)	11.5–12.5 (11.7)
4	Migrating motor complex	37–42 (39)	3–7 (4)	18–45 (25)	0.7–7.5 (2.5)	11.0–12.5 (12.0)

Data shown as range (median)

tered activity were noted in the studies reported by Berseth (1989). By term, well-defined fasting motor activity was present with distinct phase I, II and III activity. The length of phase III activity and the intervals between phase III were by now much less

variable. These data are summarized in Table 4.1.

If a development motor score is allotted to each pattern then, as shown in Figure 4.5, in subjects studied on repeated occasions, there is an obvious rise in developmental motor score with increasing post-

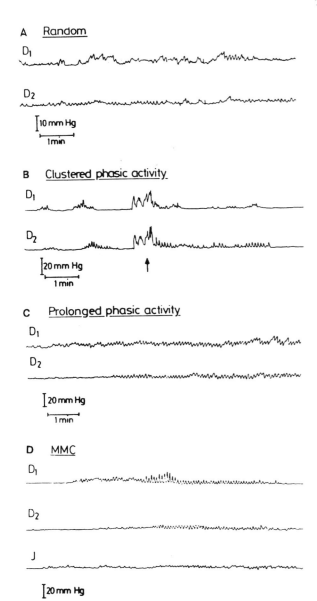

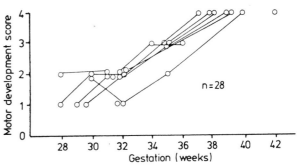

Fig. 4.5 Changes in motor development score as defined in Table 4.1 and Fig. 4.4 with increasing gestational age.

Fig. 4.4 Small intestinal pressure recordings showing: (**A**) random; (**B**) clustered phasic activity; (**C**) prolonged phasic activity, (**D**) MMC activity. (↑) Body arousals frequently occurred during phasic activity. D_1 and D_2 are proximal and distal duodenal ports. J = jejunal port.

Propagation and the subsequent shortening of the duration of prolonged phasic contractions with emergence of MMC activity is, however, much more likely to be caused by the development of inhibitory networks in the ENS and their interface with the CNS. The immaturity of both the ENS and humoral control system is the most likely explanation of the great variability of the phase intermediate between the period of clustered phasic activity and the MMC pattern. In the sheep there is evidence that with increasing gestation there is a threefold increase in the cycle length of the MMC, and that these changes have been associated with the development of serotonergic neurones in the proximal small intestine (Branchek et al 1984, Ruckebusch 1986). There are, however, similarities between these gestationally determined changes in small intestinal motor activity and the effects that total vagotomy has on adult patterns of fasting activity (Diamant et al 1981). This, together with observations of the timing of maturation events determined by the CNS, (Wozniak et al 1984) and the correlation between cyclical timing of electrical activity in the ENS and CNS of cows, sheep and dogs (Ruckebusch 1986) suggest that not only do events in the ENS determine the nature of the pattern of motor activity but also that central control systems that may modulate enteric activity are developing in parallel.

Normal small intestinal motor function was assessed by measuring contractility according to the pressure generated in the gastric antrum and duodenum, degree of propagative activity and frequency of slow wave activity, respectively. The data obtained are shown in Figure 4.6. A significant relationship is evident between each variable and gestation.

The relative development of fasting small intestinal motor activity in man, sheep and dog is shown in Figure 4.7. There is clearly a predetermined timetable of development in each species, with birth having little

conceptional age. The initiation of clustered phasic activity which then becomes more prolonged may be humorally mediated since the secretion of a number of polypeptide hormones involved in motor activity occurs at this gestational age (Aynsley Green 1982).

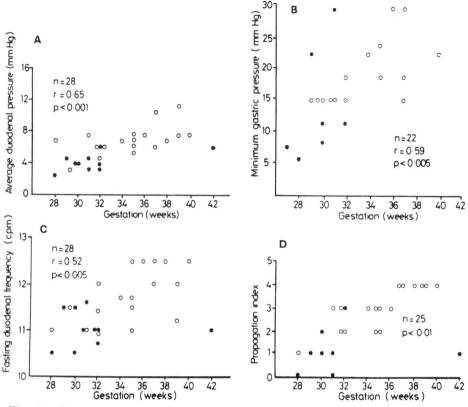

Fig. 4.6 Changes in: (**A**) duodenal pressure; (**B**) gastric antral pressure; (**C**) fasting duodenal frequency and (**D**) propagative activity with increasing gestational age. ○ 'well' infants, ● 'ill' infants.

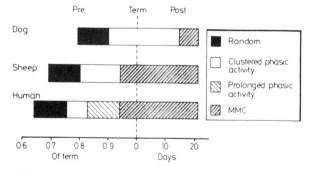

Fig. 4.7 Relative maturation of patterns of small intestinal motor activity in man, sheep and dog.

effect. It should be noted that, although there are many differences in the motor activity of the adult sheep and dog compared with man, studies by both Bisset et al (1988a) and Berseth (1989) support the presence of an inherent programme of development in man which is similar to that in a number of experimental animal species.

Postprandial Activity

In the older child and adult, cyclical fasting or interdigestive motor activity is disrupted after a meal and replaced by continuous activity that promotes mixing and segmentation of the luminal contents. There is, however, little information regarding the development of the motor response to food in the human infant or in the experimental animal but, as the motor response to food varies with the nature of the food and the ability of the gut to respond to that stimulus, it is likely to be different in the preterm infant. Using the same recording system as described above, Bisset et al (1989) studied intestinal motor activity following a bolus feed. One of three responses occurred and these are shown in Figure 4.8:

1. In the smallest infants before 31 weeks' post-conceptional age, who were usually receiving low volumes of continuous enteral feed, postprandial activity did not occur, and if a fasting pattern was seen this was not disrupted by either the bolus or the continuous enteral feed.

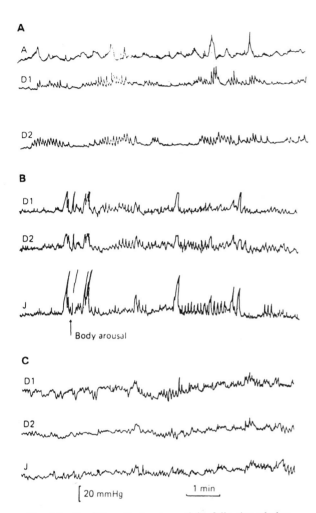

Fig. 4.8 Small intestinal motor activity following a bolus feed in infants of **A** 30 weeks' post-conceptional age **B** 35 weeks; **C** full term. (GA = gastric antrum, D = duodenum, J = jejunum.)

2. Between 31–35 weeks' post-conceptional age, the infants received a larger volume of feed which induced a degree of postprandial activity, but frequently the underlying fasting pattern remained, as shown in Figure 4.8b where clustered phasic activity is superimposed on a background of more random postprandial activity.

3. In infants over 35 weeks' post-conceptional age who were receiving large volumes of bolus feed, there was disruption of the cyclical fasting activity and replacement with continuous activity; towards the end of the postprandial period fasting activity returned giving a pattern similar to that seen in Figure 4.8b.

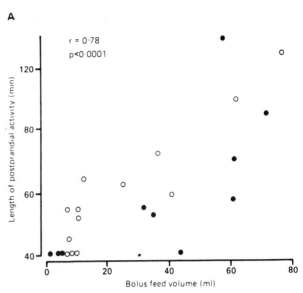

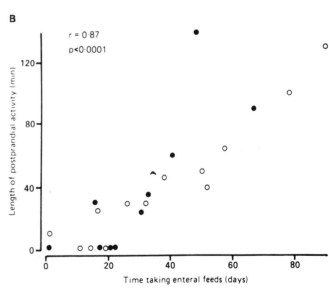

Fig. 4.9 Length of postprandial activity plotted against **A** volume of bolus feed and **B** length of time on enteral feeds. ○ = born 29 weeks' gestation, ● = born > 29 weeks gestation.

Recently, Berseth & Nordye (1992) have also shown that tolerance of enteral feeds is closely correlated with the development of a continuous pattern of activity in response to food and a more clearly apparent cyclical pattern of fasting activity.

Table 4.2   Correlation of variables with length of postprandial activity

Variable	Correlation coefficient
Post-conceptional age	0.66
Increasing feed interval	0.66
Postnatal age	0.78
Volume of bolus feed	0.78
Volume of daily feed	0.80
Time receiving enteral feeds	0.87
$P < 0.005$ in all cases	

A multiple regression model with the length of postprandial activity as the dependent variable and post-conceptional age, bolus feed volume and time fed enterally as independent variables showed that the length of time which the infant had spent taking feeds was the most important determinant, with the feed volume being of lesser importance (Fig. 4.9). These factors are shown in Table 4.2.

COLON

While there is limited information regarding colonic motor activity in the adult human, there is no information regarding the ontogeny of such activity in either the human or the experimental animal.

CONCLUSIONS

From the fragmentary studies performed so far, it seems clear that the development of motor activity – primarily dependent on neuronal activity such as sucking, swallow-induced peristalsis in the oesophagus, and fasting small intestinal activity – occurs according to a timetable which is similar in all species studied and is gestationally dependent, but the timing of it during gestation is species specific. Although these activities are primarily determined by neural development there is a very limited amount of information to suggest that cortisol may advance the timing and rate of development of at least duodenal motor activity (Morriss et al 1986). Postprandial events including gastric emptying and continous postprandial motor activity in the small intestine, however, appear to be dependent on the nature of the humoral response to food, provided that the muscle coats of the gut and enteric nerves are able to respond. The nature of the maturational changes described in this chapter are, however, almost totally unexplored.

REFERENCES

Arey L B 1974 Developmental anatomy. W B Saunders, Philadelphia

Aynsley Green A 1982 The control of the adaptation to postnatal nutrition in: Monographs in paediatrics, Karger Basel. pp 59–87

Bernbaum J C, Gilberto R P, Watkins J B, Peckham G J 1983 Non nutritive sucking during gavage feeding enhances growth and maturation in premature infants. Pediatrics 71: 41–45

Berseth C L 1989 Gestational evolution of small intestinal motility in preterm and term infants. J Pediatr 115: 646–651

Berseth C L, Nordye C K 1992 Manometry can predict feeding readiness in preterm infants. Gastroenterology 103: 1523–1528

Bisset W M, Watt J B, Rivers R P A, Milla P J 1988a Ontogeny of fasting small intestinal motor activity in the human infant. Gut 29: 483–488

Bisset W M, Watt J B, Rivers R P A, Milla P J 1988b The measurement of small intestinal motor activity in the preterm infant. J Biomed Eng 10: 155–158

Bisset W M, Watt J B, Rivers R P A, Milla P J 1989 Postprandial motor response of the small intestine to enteral feeds in preterm infants. Arch Dis Child 64: 1356–1361

Boix-Ochoa J, Canals J 1976 Maturation of the lower oesophagus. J Pediatr Surg 11: 749–756

Branchek T, Kates M, Gershon M D 1984 Enteric receptors for 5 hydroxytryptamine. Brain Res 324: 107–118

Bueno L, Ruckebusch Y 1979 Prenatal development of intestinal myeloelectric activity in dogs and sheep. Am J Physiol 237: E61–E67

Casaer P, Daniels H, Devlieger H, DeCock P, Eggermont E 1982 Feeding behaviour in preterm neonates. Early Human Dev 7: 331–346

Cavell B 1979 Gastric emptying in preterm infants. Acta Paediatr Scand 68: 725–730

Christensen J, Rick G A 1992 The development of esophageal interstitial cells in the opossum. Gastroenterology 102: A437

Cohen S 1974 Developmental characteristics of lower esophageal sphincter function: a possible mechanism for infantile chalasia. Gastroenterology 67: 252–258

Crump E P, Gore P M, Morton C 1958 The sucking behaviour in premature infants. Hum Biol 30: 334–340

Daniel E E, Berezin I 1992 Interstitial cells of Cajal: are they major players in control of gastrointestinal motility. J Gastrointest Motil 4: 1–24

Daniels H, Casaer P, Devlieger H, Eggermont E 1986 Mechanisms of feeding efficiency in preterm infants. J Pediatr Gastrointest Nutr 5: 593–596

Diamant N E, Hall K, Mui H, El Sharkowy T Y 1980 Vagal control of the feeding motor pattern in the lower esophageal sphincter, stomach, and upper small intestine of the dog. Proc 7th Int Symp G I Motility, Raven Press, New York pp 365–378

Eliska O 1973 Phreno-oesophageal membrane and its role in the development of hiatal hernia. Acta Anat 86: 137–150

Euler A R, Ament M E 1977 Value of oesophageal manometric studies in gastroesophageal reflux of infancy. Pediatrics 59: 58–61

Gershon M D, Payette R F, Rothman T P 1983 Development of the enteric nervous system. Fed Proc 42: 1620–1625

Gryboski J D 1965 The swallowing mechanism of the neonate: I Esophageal and gastric motility. Pediatrics 35: 445–452

Gryboski J D 1969 Suck and swallow in the premature infant. Pediatrics 43: 96–101

Guilloteau P 1986 Digestion des proteines chez le jeune ruminant. Doctoral thesis, University of Paris

Hart S L, Mir M S 1971 Adrenoreceptors in the human foetal small intestine. Br J Pharmacol 41: 567–569

Herbst J J 1981 Development of suck and swallow. J Paediatr Gastroenterol Nutr 2: S131–S135

Hillemeier C, Gryboski J, McCallum R, Biancani P 1985 Developmental characteristics of the lower esophageal sphincter in the kitten. Gastroenterology 89: 760–766

Husband J, Husband P 1969 Gastric emptying of water and glucose solutions in the newborn. Lancet ii: 409–411

Hitchcock R J I, Pemble M J, Bishop A E, Spitzz L, Polak J M 1992 The ontogeny and distribution of neuropeptides in the human fetal and infant oesophagus. Gastroenterology 102: 840–849

Kedinger M, Simon-Assmann P, Bouziges F, Arnold C, Alexandre E, Haffen K 1990 Smooth muscle actin expression during rat gut development and induction in fetal skin fibroblastic cells associated with intestinal embryonic epithelium. Differentiation 43: 87–97

Kenigsberg K, Aiges H, Alperstein G 1981 A unique device to measure lower oesophageal sphincter pressure in unsedated infants. J Pediatr Surg 16: 370–373

Le Dourin N M 1980 The ontogeny of the neural crest in avian embryo chimeras. Nature 286: 663–669

Levine M S, Harding K W 1989 Drosophila: the zygotic contribution in: Glover D M, Harnes B D (eds) Genes and embryos. IRL Press, London pp 39–94

Logan W J, Bosma J F 1967 Oral and pharyngeal dysphagia in infancy. Pediatr Clin N Am 14: 47–54

Lucas A, Bloom S R, Aynsley Green A 1978 Metabolic and endocrine events at the time of the first feed of human milk in preterm and term infants. Arch Dis Child 53: 731–736

Lucas A, Adrian T E, Christofides N, Bloom S R, Aynsley Green A 1980 Plasma motilin, gastrin and enteroglucagon and enteral feeding in the human newborn. Arch Dis Child 55: 673–677

Lucas A, Bloom S R, Aynsley Green A 1986 Gut hormones and 'minimal enteral feeding'. Acta Paediatr Scand 75: 719–723

McLain C R 1963 Amniography studies of the gastrointestinal motility of the human fetus. Am J Obstet Gynecol 86: 1079–1087

Maller O, Turner R E 1973 Taste in acceptance of sugars in human infants. J Comp Physiol 84: 496–502

Milewski A K, Siqueland E R 1975 Discrimination of color and pattern novelty in one month old infants. J Exp Child Psychol 19: 122–136

Milla P J, Fenton T R 1983 Small intestinal motility patterns in the perinatal period. J Pediatr Gastroenterol Nutr 2: S141–S144

Morriss F H, Moore M, Weisbrodt N W, West M 1986 Ontogenic development of gastrointestinal motility. IV. Duodenal contractions in preterm infants. Pediatrics 78: 1106–1113

Moxey P C, Trier J S 1978 Specialized cell types in the human fetal small intestine. Anat Rec 191: 269–286

Newell S J 1988 The lower oesophageal sphincter in the preterm infant in: Milla P J (ed.) Disorders of gastrointestinal motility in childhood. Wiley, Chichester pp 39–50

Patterson P M 1978 Environmental determination of autonomic neurotransmitter ferreteon. Ann Rev Neurosci 1: 1–17

Payette R F, Tennyson V M, Pomeranz H D, Pham T D, Rothman T P, Gershon M D 1988 Accumulation of components of basal laminae: association with the failure of neural crest cells to colonize the presumptive aganglionic bowel of ls/ls mutant mice. Dev Biol 125: 341–360

Peiper A 1963 Cerebral functioning in infancy and childhood. Consultants Bureau, New York

Pritchard J A 1966 Fetal swallowing and amniotic fluid volume. Obstet Gynecol 28: 606–610

Ropert A, Schwartz I, Defawe G, Reaper A, Dabadie A, Lebar R, Le Marec B 1992 Prospective study of esophageal motor disorders in premature infants. Gastroenterology 102: A507

Ruckebusch Y 1986 Development of digestive motor patterns during perinatal life: mechanisms and significance. J Pediatr Gastroenterol Nutr 5: 523–536

Siegal M, Krantz B, Lebenthal E 1984a The effect on gastric emptying of isocaloric feedings in premature infants. Pediatr Res 18: 212A

Siegal M, Lebenthal E, Krantz B 1984b Effect of caloric density on gastric emptying in premature infants. J Pediatr 104: 118–122

Smith V V 1993 Chronic intestinal pseudo-obstruction. PhD thesis, University of London

Spedale S B, Weisbrodt N W, Morriss J R 1982 Ontogenic studies of gastrointestinal function. II. Lower esophageal sphincter maturation in neonatal beagle puppies. Pediatr Res 16: 851–855

Wohlgemuth D J, Behringer R R, Mostoller M P, Brinsten R L, Palmiter R D 1989 Transgenic mice overexpressing the mouse homeobox gene Hox 1.4 exhibit abnormal gut development. Nature 337: 464–467

Wozniak E R, Fenton T R, Milla P J 1984 The development of fasting small intestinal motor activity in the human neonate in: Roman C E (ed.) Gastrointestinal motility. MTP Press, Lancaster pp 265–270

Yu V Y H 1975 Effect of body position on gastric emptying in the neonate. Arch Dis Child 50: 500–504

5. Intrinsic and extrinsic neural control

D. L. Wingate

INTRODUCTION AND HISTORICAL PERSPECTIVE

The anatomy of the innervation of the gut is described in the first two chapters of this volume. In this chapter, the allocation of the control of motor function between the different elements of the nervous system is reviewed.

For much of the twentieth century, physiologists and pharmacologists have believed and taught that the motor control of the gut was a function of the central nervous system (CNS) mediated by two opposing components of the autonomic nervous system (ANS), these being two of the three divisions of the ANS originally postulated by Langley. The parasympathetic system was held to be excitatory and the sympathetic system inhibitory, with acetylcholine and noradrenaline as the respective neurotransmitters (Fig. 5.1). Even at the end of the century, this is what many practising physicians believe – because knowledge imparted at university tends to remain ingrained – and, in the author's experience, these beliefs are shared by many who work in medicinal pharmacy and are responsible for designing remedies for motor disorders.

At the beginning of the century Bayliss and Starling had expressed the opinion that the peristaltic reflex was mediated through the intrinsic nerves of the gut; it was these nerves that were classified as the third, or enteric division of the ANS by Langley, and which are now collectively known as the enteric nervous system (ENS). Because they seemed to have no obvious function, the ganglia of the intrinsic plexuses were not central to the 'classical' concept of motor control, but in the 1960s, this concept began to fall apart. The discovery by Burnstock that post-ganglionic neurones in the gut, that utilized neurotransmitters that were not acetylcholine or noradrenaline (non-adrenergic non-cholinergic – NANC) and appeared to have an inhibitory function introduced a new element into the model.

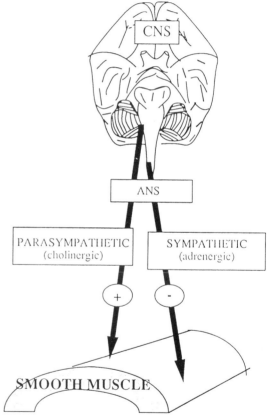

Fig. 5.1 'Classical' concept of extrinsic neural control of the gut.

Subsequently it became clear that the extrinsic nerves of the gut do not directly innervate the smooth muscle fibres of the gut, from which it followed that both inhibitory and excitatory functions are mediated by post-ganglionic neurones of the ENS (Fig. 5.2).

The impact of these discoveries was at first obscured by the excitement generated by the discovery of numerous putative 'gut hormones', unveiled in a seemingly

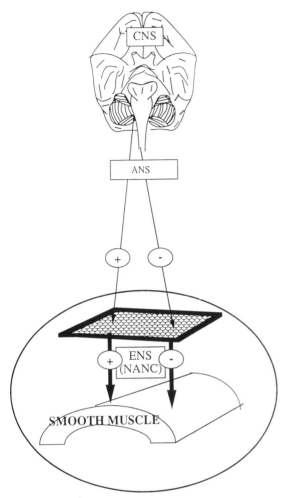

Fig. 5.2 Modification of the 'classical' concept following the discovery of NANC nerves (the hatched plane represents, in this and some subsequent figures, the ganglionic layer of the myenteric plexus). The NANC innervation that was originally postulated was post-ganglionic.

endless sequence in the 1970s from the laboratories of V Mutt, S R Bloom, J C Brown, and others. For a time it seemed as though the control of all gut functions (including motility) should be attributed to hormones, and it is therefore important to understand why it has subsequently become clear that this is not the case.

INTRINSIC INNERVATION (ENS)

Much of the evidence for the control of motility by the

ENS has been derived from the study of periodic motor activity, first observed during the nineteenth century, but not studied experimentally until the work of V N Boldyreff in 1902–5. He established that the motor and secretory activity of the fasting canine stomach and duodenum, in conscious animals, alternates between prolonged (> 70 min) 'rest' and brief (5 min) episodes of work marked by high amplitude contractions (Fig. 5.3), and, furthermore, that this pattern is abolished by feeding. This work attracted much attention at the time, but was subsequently largely forgotten (Wingate 1981) until Szurszewski (1969) not only confirmed similar periodicity in the small intestine, but showed that periodic motor complexes, subsequently known as migrating myoelectric (or motor) complexes (MMCs) migrate slowly along the length of the small intestine. Code and Marlett (1975) extended these observations, identifying four phases of the fasting cycle and showing that the interruption of the MMC cycle by food is not only a gastric phenomenon (as shown by Boldyreff), but also occurs in the small intestine. Vantrappen et al (1977) confirmed the migration of MMCs in man, but the periodicity in man was subsequently shown to be much more variable than in the trained laboratory dog.

In relation to the function of the ENS, the significance of periodicity resides in the fact that all evidence (Wingate 1983, Sarna 1985) points to the fact that it is a biorhythm generated within the ENS; it is not dependent upon extrinsic innervation, but is a phenomenon that survives even in extrinsically denervated and transplanted bowel. It is a programme of motor activity present in virtually all mammalian and avian species so far studied. In terms of motor function, therefore, it is clear that the different programmes of motor activity that prevail according to physiological conditions are resident within the intrinsic neuronal circuitry of the bowel (Fig. 5.4).

In functional terms, there are close parallels between CNS and ENS (Fig. 5.4). Just as the spinal reflex is the integrated building block of programmed locomotor movement, so the peristaltic reflex is the building block of the motor programmes of the gut, and it is not merely coincidental that the architecture of the myenteric plexus shows structural homologies with cerebral cortex. Wood (1984) drew attention to the brain-like function of the ENS, and it has become known colloquially as 'the little brain in the gut'.

The 'little brain' shows one important difference from the 'big brain'; whereas the cerebral brain has a complex but characteristic morphology, with different areas specialized for particular functions, the ENS is arranged in

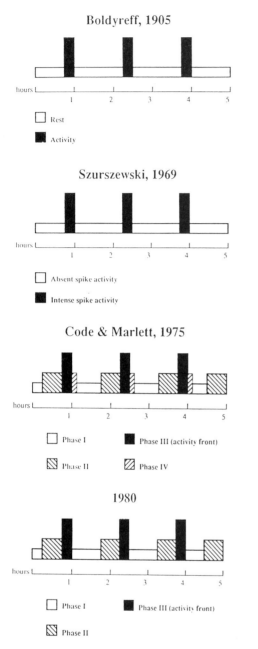

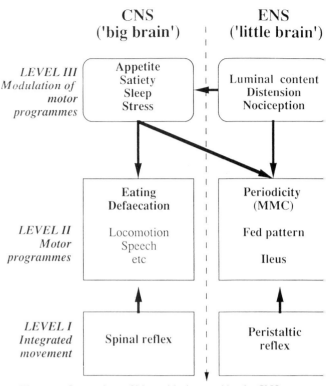

Fig. 5.4 Comparison of hierarchical control by the CNS and ENS.

Fig. 5.3 Evolution of the nomenclature of periodic activity. Note that there was little change between 1905–69. Code and Marlett defined phase II and phase IV in 1975 but, subsequently (circa 1980), the concept of phase IV was largely abandoned as it is only occasionally identifiable.

layers that completely invest the gut tube but has no identified areas of specialized structure or function. The circuitry for peristalsis is contained in a sequence of overlapping segments that are replicated along the length of the gut tube. Coordination between these segments is achieved not so much by neurones that run both orad and caudad within the plexus as by the prevertebral ganglia; information can be rapidly transferred between distant regions of the gut (for example, ileum and duodenum) through the prevertebral ganglia, and it is through these ganglia that entero–enteric inhibitory reflexes are mediated. Reflex pathways through the prevertebral ganglia are oligosynaptic, whereas in the myenteric neurons, axial neurones are short requiring information transmitted over a distance to cross many synapses (Fig. 5.5).

Variations in the period of the MMC cycle have attracted much attention from investigators, and have provided important evidence on the contribution of the different levels of the nervous system to the control of bowel motility. Phase III of the MMC is invariably followed by a period of motor quiescence (phase I), and it has been postulated by Sarna (1985) that the first part of phase I represents a 'refractory phase', during which fasting contractions cannot occur (Fig. 5.6). This concept is supported by the observation that

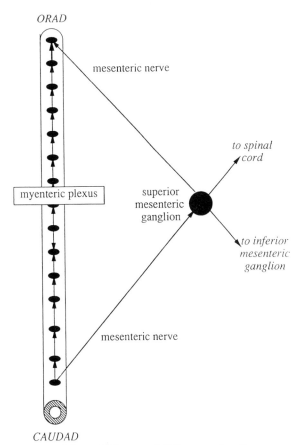

ORAD

mesenteric nerve

myenteric plexus

superior mesenteric ganglion

to spinal cord

to inferior mesenteric ganglion

mesenteric nerve

CAUDAD

Fig. 5.5 Schematic diagram of different modes of communication between remote regions of the bowel. Transmission through the essentially monosynaptic prevertebral ganglion is more rapid and of higher fidelity than along the synaptic chain of the myenteric plexus.

Refractory Phase (R)

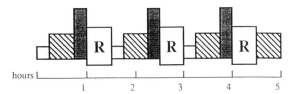

hours

Post-surgical ileus

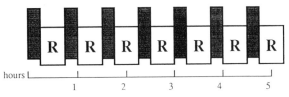

hours

Fig. 5.6 Concept of the refractory phase of the MMC (upper panel) and refractory phase (R) is a period in which phase II and phase III of the MMC cannot occur. The interval between the end of the refractory phase and the occurrence of phase II and phase III is variable and modulated by multiple factors. When the cycling frequency of the MMC is rapid, as in post-surgical ileus (lower panel), a phase III episode is seen at the end of each refractory phase.

during early phase I, the bowel is refractory to exogenous motilin or erythromycin, which in other parts of the cycle will stimulate a premature phase III episode. It might be reasonable to speculate that if the period of the cycle could be shortened to be approximately equal to the refractory phase, phase III episodes would occur in rapid succession without an intervening phase II, and this is in fact what happens in the proximal small bowel during the first few hours of post-surgical ileus (Fig. 5.6). However, it seems that the stimulus of food can overcome the refractory phase; irrespective of the phase of the cycle in which it occurs, ingestion of a meal stimulates an almost immediate transition to the non-periodic and apparently chaotic motor pattern – the 'fed' pattern – that characterizes the post-prandial phase (Fig. 5.7).

The periodic MMC cycle, the 'fed' pattern, and the

paralytic response of ileus to a noxious stimulus all appear to be programmes that are resident within the ENS, which thus appears to be self-sufficient in terms of the control of motility (Fig. 5.8). It is now clear that the extrinsic innervation of the gut is predominantly sensory, or afferent with respect to the CNS (Fig. 5.9). Within a relatively short space of time, starting from the concept that gut motility is 'controlled' by two divisions of the ANS, it now seems permissible to question whether the extrinsic innervation of the gut is important in the control of motility; this question will be considered below.

'GUT HORMONES'

The discovery of numerous gut hormones, with the rediscovery of periodic activity, has already been pointed out and it was less than surprising that, in the mid 1970s, eminent investigators proposed that changes in gut motility due to feeding were true hormonal effects, caused by the postprandial release of gastrin and CCK. While these did not account for the phenomenon of periodic activity, but only for its abolition by

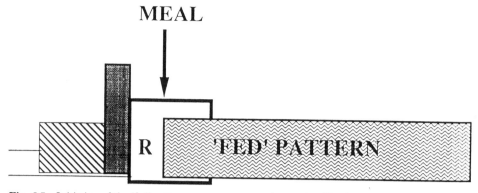

Fig. 5.7   Initiation of the 'fed' pattern can occur at any time and unlike the resumption of the MMC cycle, there does not appear to be a refractory phase.

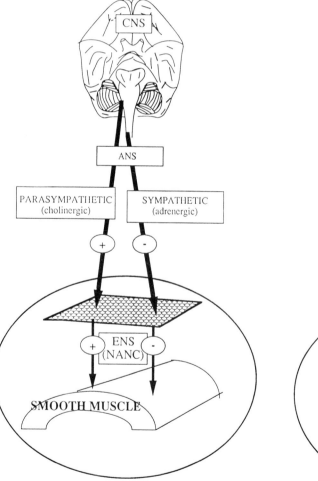

Fig. 5.8   Autonomy of the ENS in the control of motility. Motor programmes are generated within the ENS and the contribution of extrinsic innervation is limited to modulation.

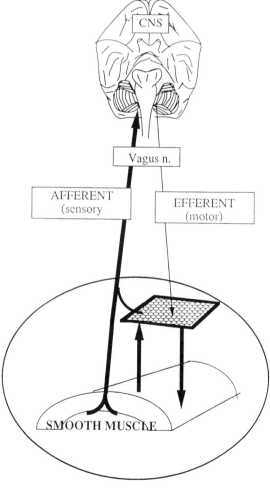

Fig. 5.9   The majority of vagal fibres are afferent and the vagus should be regarded as, above all, a sensory nerve.

food, apparently stronger evidence was to come. In 1976, two groups of investigators (Itoh et al 1976, Wingate et al 1976) proposed that phase III of the MMC was the result of a peak of plasma motilin, since a premature MMC could be elicited by the administration of exogenous synthetic motilin. For a time, it seemed as though all the patterns of bowel motility could be explained as humoral effects due to the release of 'hormones', but this is no longer believed to be the case.

There are several reasons for disenchantment with the hormonal hypothesis (Wingate 1976):

1. Although there are changes in plasma levels of 'hormones', these are very variable within and between different individuals; there is no predictable relation between plasma level and response.
2. In marked contrast to the endocrine glands, clinical syndromes arising from excess or deficient humoral concentrations are largely absent.
3. Although many experiments have shown functional changes in response to infusion of 'hormones', the plasma levels required to achieve these changes are pharmacological rather than physiological.

4. Attempts to simulate physiological changes in plasma levels do not produce appropriate physiological changes in motor activity.
5. In contrast with the frustrating struggle to validate the hormonal hypothesis, neurophysiologists have convincingly demonstrated the primacy of neural control in the regulation of motility.

Above all, it has become clear that the major function of the peptides that were considered, two decades ago, to be true 'hormones', is as regulatory peptides acting as neuromodulators and neurotransmitters not only in the gut, but elsewhere in the body, and above all within the CNS. Even CCK, originally postulated as the humoral agent responsible for gallbladder contraction, is now regarded primarily as both a peripheral and central neuropeptide, while the question of its physiological action on the gallbladder still remains a matter of controversy. Even the role of motilin remains in doubt; while it is clear that motilin release and the occurrence of a gastroduodenal phase III are associated phenomena, it is not clear which is cause and which is effect (Sarna 1985).

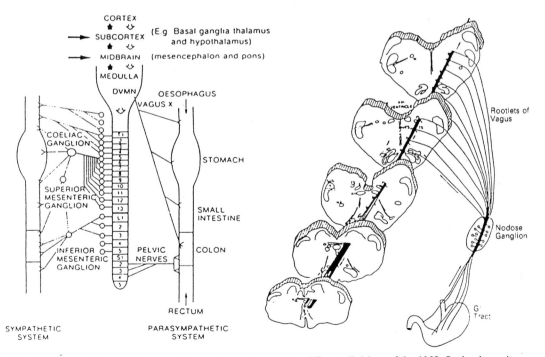

Fig. 5.10 Left: schematic diagram of the territory subserved by different divisions of the ANS. Such schematic diagrams oversimplified the complexity of neural connections. The vagal nuclei are not a single point in the brain stem but longitudinal structures as illustrated in the exploded view of the brain stem (right). Vagal afferent fibres are inserted over a considerable distance of the nuclei of the solitary tract rather than at a single point.

As is discussed in the next chapter, there is no question that there are important actions of regulatory peptides in relation to motility, but the bulk of evidence suggests that these effects are neurally rather than humorally mediated.

EXTRINSIC INNERVATION (ANS and CNS)

The extrinsic innervation of the gut is provided by sympathetic and parasympathetic nerves that transfer information between the ganglionic networks of the ENS and CNS (Fig. 5.10). As pointed out above, they were originally visualized as pathways for the transmission of commands from the CNS to effector systems in the gut, but in terms of motor control, it is likely that their function is predominantly sensory. The best

studied of these elements are the vagus nerves, because it is possible, at least in experimental animals, to track nerve impulses from the abdomen up to the brain; since there are no synapses between the vagal receptors in the gut wall and the vagal nuclei in the brain stem, information is not dissipated en route, although convergence takes place within the dorsal vagal complex in the brain stem.

Much of the information passed from the gut to the spinal cord and brain stem is destined for onward transmission, but the extrinsic nerves also form reflex arcs between sensory receptors in the gut and motor neurones in the ENS. The vagovagal reflex arc is the best understood of these and can serve as a paradigm for other similar but less accessible reflex arcs. In such a reflex arc, it is important to remember that the efferent segment between the CNS and the myenteric plexus is in terms of function, sensory rather than motor (Fig. 5.11), since the circuitry for the motor programmes of the gut is located not in the brain stem, but in the ENS.

Sensory receptors in the gut are sensitive to various sensory modalities; in the mucosa there are receptors that respond to touch, and also to chemical change, whereas in the muscle layers, there are tension receptors. The pattern of nerve impulses from these receptors indicates both static and dynamic (rate of change) changes in luminal conditions, and in wall tension (Fig. 5.12). Recordings from single vagal afferents in anaesthetized laboratory animals demonstrate sensory responses to acute changes (Fig. 5.13). Subtler techniques are required to demonstrate vagovagal activity in conscious animals. In sheep, Miolan and Roman (1978) divided one vagus nerve, and implanted the rostral cut end into an isolated portion of the diaphragm. Following complete recovery from surgery, electromyography of the re-innervated muscle in the conscious animals revealed patterns of discharge that closely tracked the motor activity of the stomach, reaching a crescendo during phase III of the gastric motor complex.

The function of the vagovagal arc that has been most clearly demonstrated is the initiation of the enteric response to a meal. Although there are direct sensory afferents from the gut mucosa to the myenteric plexus, the receptors that detect the arrival of a meal are vagal receptors that relay directly to the brain stem. The interruption of periodic activity and the initiation of the postprandial pattern of motility is dependent upon the integrity of the vagovagal pathway; acute blockade of this pathway during the postprandial phase produces a premature, and physiologically inappropriate, resumption of periodic activity (Hall et al 1982). Other meal-initiated functions, such

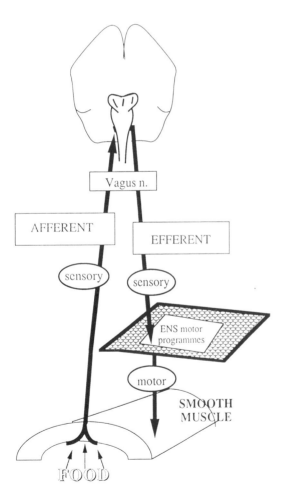

Fig. 5.11   The vagovagal reflex arc. Since the motor programmes are contained within the ENS, the efferent vagus is in functional terms an afferent or sensory limb of the arc.

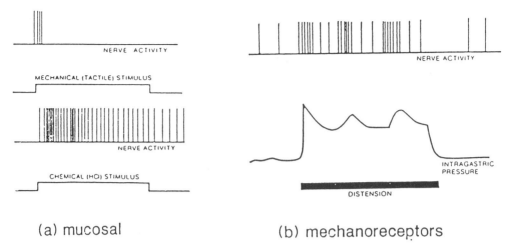

Fig. 5.12 Schematic representation of different patterns of discharge from two types of vagal afferent receptors. On the left, two different types of mucosal receptors are shown: the upper receptor is an 'on' receptor that responds to application of a tactile stimulus whereas the lower receptor responds to chemical stimulus with a sustained discharge.

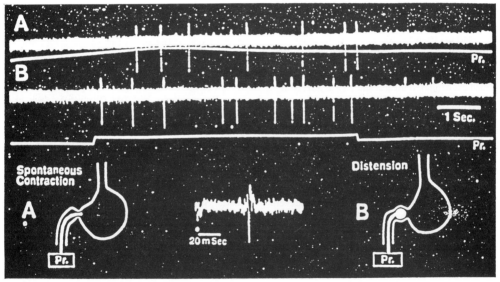

Fig. 5.13 Recording from vagal afferent receptor in pyloric smooth muscle. **A** shows firing in a single afferent fibre in response to a spontaneous phasic contraction. Note that the discharge starts near the peak of the pressure wave and continues until the pressure returns to the baseline. **B** shows firing in the same fibre in response to passive distension of the pylorus by a balloon. These recordings were obtained in an anaesthetized animal.

as acid secretion and receptive accommodation in the gastric fundus are also vagovagally mediated. Clinically, this is utilized therapeutically in the reduction of acid secretion by vagotomy, but, depending upon the extent of vagotomy, this beneficial effect is accompanied by other predictable but unwanted side-effects

such as early satiety (due to failure of receptive accommodation) and diarrhoea that may be associated with an impaired postprandial motor response in the small bowel (Thompson et al 1982).

The vagovagal pathway, however, is more than a simple reflex arc (Fig. 5.14). Information from the

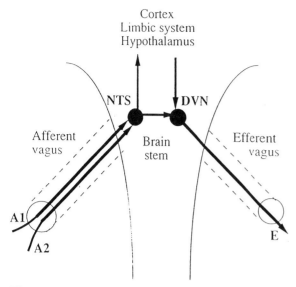

Cortex
Limbic system
Hypothalamus

NTS   DVN

Afferent   Brain   Efferent
vagus   stem   vagus

A1

A2

E

Fig. 5.14 Schematic representation of traffic through the dorsal vagal complex. A nerve cell body in the nucleus of the solitary tract (NTS) is depicted as receiving inputs from two vagal afferents (A1, A2). The NTS neurone projects in two directions, rostrally to higher brain centres and locally to a neurone in the dorsal vagal nucleus (DVN). The DVN neurone receives inputs from NTS and also from higher centres and projects its output as a vagal efferent fibre. Even in this simplified diagram, it can be seen that information from the gut can be utilized in two ways, to keep higher centres informed of changes in the gut and also as a relay in the vagovagal arc. The vagovagal information can also be modified in the DVN by commands from higher CNS centres.

afferent vagus arrives in the afferent nucleus of the tractus solitarius (NTS) within the dorsal vagal complex (DVC). It can then be passed to the efferent dorsal nucleus of the vagus nerve (DVN), but it is also transmitted rostrally towards the hypothalamus and cortex; by this means, the presence of ingesta in the gut influences appetite and satiety which are regulated in the hypothalamus. The interconnections between NTS and DVN may be a single interneuron, or several interneurons. Finally, output from the efferent nerve cell body in the DVN may be modulated by descending impulses from higher brain centres. This modulation may be mediated within the DVN by the local release of neuropeptides, which can attenuate (Ewart & Wingate 1983a) or amplify (Ewart & Wingate 1983b) changes in firing patterns of DVC neurones evoked by the stimulation of vagal sensory receptors in the gut.

Neuronal recordings from the vagus nerves and brain stem are only possible in experimental animals, but these have revealed that the brain stem is kept

fully informed at all times of motor events in the foregut and of the presence of different nutrients within the gut lumen. One experimental approach is illustrated in Figs 5.15–5.18, in which the firing pattern of single nerve cells in the DVC is recorded during physiological stimulation of the foregut (Ewart & Wingate 1984). The experimental set-up is illustrated in Fig. 5.15. These experiments are far from simple, since they involve stereotactic positioning of a micro-electrode with a 6-μ tip in the DVC in an anaesthetized rat that has been previously prepared with an intragastric balloon inserted through a gastrostomy, and a cannulated segment of duodenum that can be perfused with saline or nutrient solutions. Different cells show different patterns of response, most responding to one or other rather than both stimuli; when a response is obtained it may be an 'on' response (increased firing rate in response to a stimulus) or an 'off' response (stimulus-induced inhibition of firing).

Direct study of the vagovagal arc is possible because of the relative simplicity of the neuronal circuitry. It has to be assumed that similar reflex arcs operate through the sympathetic and pelvic nerve afferents and the spinal cord, but these remain to be clearly demonstrated because of the complexity and inaccessibility of the neuronal pathways, which also include the prevertebral ganglia. Such a reflex arc has been illustrated (Fig. 5.19) in an ex vivo preparation by Kreulen and Szurszewski (1979). But while this experiment yields an apparently clear-cut result, in vivo there is a potential reflex arc between colonic segments through the spinal cord, and at this end of the bowel, it becomes difficult to determine the hierarchical level through which such reflexes operate, and the influence of descending modulation from efferent tracts in the spinal cord. Similar entero-enteric inhibitory mechanisms have been demonstrated in vivo in animals (Da Cunha Melo et al 1981) and in man (Kellow et al 1987), but it remains to be determined whether these reflexes operate solely through the prevertebral ganglia or whether the pathway involves the spinal cord.

Nonetheless, assuming similarity of structure and function between man and animals used in experimental studies, it seems clear that the brain receives continuous and detailed information on the digestive system – but little or none of this sensory information is normally projected into consciousness. A good meal is appreciated through the special senses of taste and smell, but not through visceral sensation. The central need for this information is not hedonistic, but for the modification of behaviour, and in particular ingestive and excretory activity.

Apart from reflex arcs through the vagus and brain

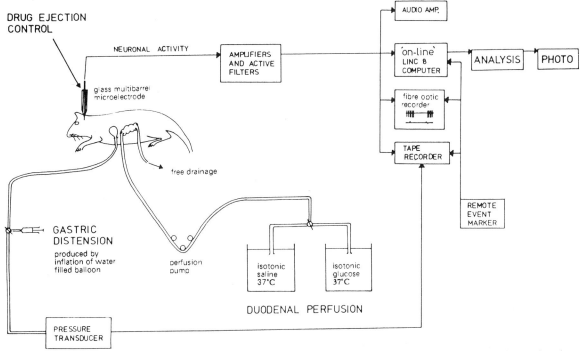

Fig. 5.15 Block diagram of experiment to record input from vagal afferents in the brain stem. See text for further explanation. (Adapted with kind permission from Ewart and Wingate 1984.)

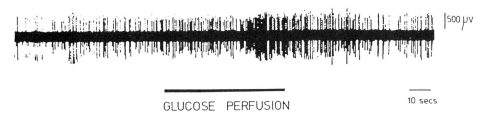

Fig. 5.16 Recording from dorsal vagal complex (DVC). Cell showing 'on' response to duodenal glucose perfusion. (Adapted with kind permission from Ewart and Wingate 1984.)

stem, and through the spinal nerves and the spinal cord, the functional role of extrinsic *motor* innervation of the gut remains to be clarified. Many experiments in animals have been done in which electrical or chemical stimulation of the brain or spinal cord alters motor function, but often these changes duplicate control mechanisms that are now known to exist within the ENS, and it is uncertain whether these evoked responses simulate physiological actions. In man, neurological diseases that are known to cause dysfunction of the digestive tract offer useful potential models, but interpretation of changes is not simple. Parkinson's disease, for example, is associated with disturbances of gastrointestinal motor function, but it is not clear

whether this is due to lesions within the CNS, or due to the histopathological changes that have been reported within the intrinsic innervation of the gut.

THE BRAIN–GUT AXIS

The term 'brain–gut axis' has no precise scientific meaning, but is a convenient phrase for the description of the static (morphological) and dynamic (functional) relationship between the digestive tract – and, in particular, the ENS – and the CNS. During recent years, improved techniques in neuroscience have considerably enlarged our knowledge of the morphology and neurochemistry of brain–gut interaction (Singer &

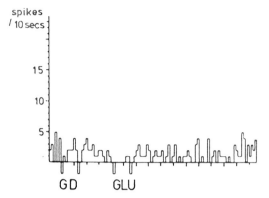

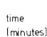

Fig. 5.17 Recording from a DVC cell showing no response to gastric distension (GD) but 'off' response to duodenal glucose perfusion (GLU)

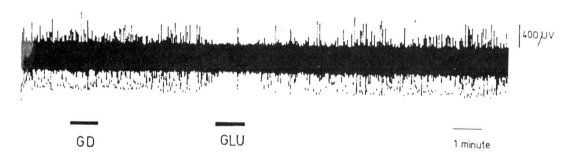

Goebell 1989, Tache & Wingate 1991), but the accumulation of detailed information tends to obscure the broad concepts that have emerged. Numerous pathways between brain and gut have been demonstrated, but the extent to which these are utilized in the normal physiology of the gut is much less certain. Just as road maps give no clues to the volume and nature of the vehicles that use the roads, the demonstration of neural pathways does not provide information on their physiological usage. This presents particular problems in the unravelling of brain–gut communication, since there are many different routes in parallel from CNS to ENS. An attempt to summarize the neurobiology of the system is thus as likely to be misleading as informative; it is perhaps more useful to provide an overview of the functional relationships between brain and gut.

Through the process of swallowing, the digestive tract receives, digests, and assimilates nutrients. This involves not only the mechanical breakdown of ingesta, but also chemical breakdown through the action of digestive secretions. Salvage of the secreted fluid and solutes leaves only indigestible material as a semi-solid residue to be excreted in the act of defaecation. Ingestion and excretion involve behavioural activities by the whole organism, and are thus under the control of the CNS.

Thus, it is no more than logical that each end of the digestive tract is guarded by sphincteric mechanisms (the upper oesophageal sphincter and the external anal sphincter) that consist of striated muscle under the direct control of the CNS. On the enteric side of each of these sphincters is a second sphincter (the lower oesophageal sphincter and the internal anal sphincter) that is a smooth muscle sphincter under the control of enteric neurones. In the long length of digestive tube between these barriers, it is the ENS that governs propulsion.

The motor programme of swallowing is initiated by the act of eating or drinking; the programme involves not only the motor function of the oropharynx, but also initiates an automatic motor sequence in the oesophagus that is mediated through enteric (post-ganglionic) neurones. The central control of this process – the decision to swallow – is modulated by feedback to the brain from the gut. The sensation of satiety, which provides a negative feedback to the process of ingestion appears to be mediated through vagal sensory receptors in the gut that monitor the volume and chemical content of the stomach and proximal bowel. The situation at the distal end of the gut is a mirror image; the stimulus for excretion is provided by rectal filling that

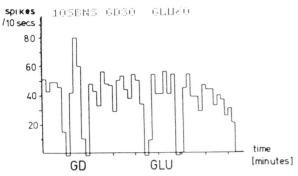

Fig. 5.18 The lower trace shows the pattern of spike discharge; the upper histogram shows the same events as a spike frequency histogram. (Reproduced by kind permission from Ewart and Wingate 1984.)

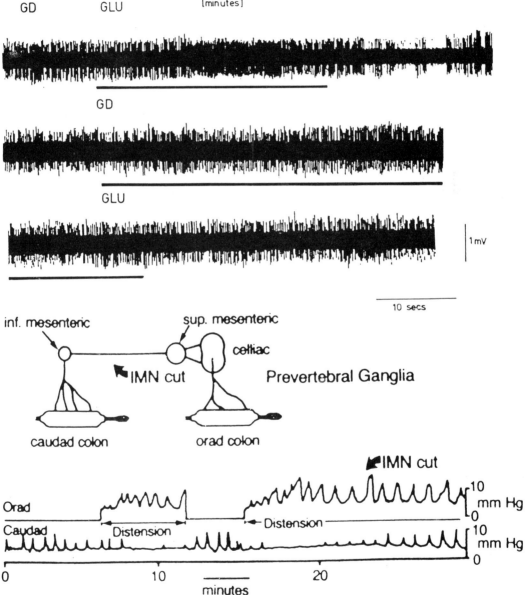

Fig. 5.19 A distal reflex arc through prevertebral ganglia is illustrated by this preparation, which consists of two segments of isolated guinea pig colon, connected only by the intermesenteric nerve (IMN) between the superior and inferior mesenteric ganglia. When the orad segment is distended, spontaneous contractile activity in the caudad section is inhibited, but returns when the distention is removed. When the IMN is severed during a second period of distension of the orad segment, the inhibition is abolished. (Adapted with kind permission from Wood and Wingate 1988.)

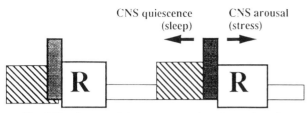

CNS quiescence (sleep)   CNS arousal (stress)

Fig. 5.20 Stress and sleep representative of opposite poles of activity.

is under enteric and not central control; whether or not this stimulus is followed by defaecation is determined by the CNS; it is a behaviour that is, in many species, dependent upon social context.

Interactions between the brain and gut that are relevant to the motor function of the gut may be grouped under three headings:

1. Gut functions initiated by CNS
   a. Input (swallowing)
   b. Output (defaecation)
2. CNS states that modulate gut motor function
   a. Arousal
      – *sleep/wake*
   b. Negative affect (nociception)
      – *stress, nausea*
   c. Positive affect (hedonistic)
      – *pleasure, contentment*

3. CNS functions modulated by gut
   a. Appetite
   b. Satiety
   c. Visceral nociception
   d. Other

The first group of functions are covered in other chapters of this volume, as are, to some extent, the second group. As an example of the latter, it is known that the state of the brain (arousal vs quiescence) is an important factor (Fig. 5.20) in determining the periodicity of the MMC cycle (Valori et al 1986, Kellow et al 1990). It is perhaps important to point out that the experimental protocols for studying affective influences on motor function are unipolar, with negative affect being the test condition. The effect of positive affect (pleasure, contentment, satisfaction) on the gut remains formally unexplored, but is perhaps embodied in the experience of everyday life.

Likewise, the third group in the list remains unexplored and largely disregarded. Interdisciplinary collaboration, so far lacking, is required, for example between those who study motor activity and those who study ingestive behaviour. It remains only to be pointed out that the brain–gut axis is also the gut–brain axis.

REFERENCES

Code C F, Marlett J A 1975 The interdigestive myoelectric complex of the stomach and small bowel of dogs. J Physiol (Lond) 246: 298–309

Da Cunha Melo J, Summers R W, Thompson H H, Wingate D L, Yanda R 1981 Effects of intestinal secretagogues and distension on small bowel motility in fasted and fed conscious dogs. J Physiol 321: 483–494

Ewart W R, Wingate D L 1983a Central representation and opioid modulation of gastric mechanoreceptor activity in the rat. Am J Physiol 244: G27–G32

Ewart W R, Wingate D L 1983b Cholecystokinin octapeptide and central representation of gastric mechanoreceptor activity in the rat. Am J Physiol 244: G613–G617.

Ewart W R, Wingate D L 1984 Central representation of arrival of nutrient in the duodenum. Am J Physiol 246: G750–G756

Hall K E, El-Sharkawy T Y, Diamant N E, 1982 Vagal control of migrating motor complex in the dog. Am J Physiol 243: G276–G284.

Itoh Z, Honda R, Hiwatashi K, Takeuchi S, Aizawa I, Takanayagi R, Couch E F 1976 Motilin-induced mechanical activity in the canine alimentary tract. Scand J Gastroenterol Suppl 39: 83–110

Kellow J E, Gill R C, Wingate D L 1987 Modulation of human upper gastrointestinal motility by rectal distension. Gut 28: 864–868

Kellow J E, Gill R C, Wingate D L 1990 Prolonged ambulant recordings of small bowel motility demonstrate abnormalities in the irritable bowel syndrome. Gastroenterology 98: 1208–1218

Kreulen D L, Szurszewski J H 1979 Reflex pathways in the abdominal prevertebral ganglia: evidence for a colo-colonic inhibitory reflex. J Physiol Lond 295: 21–32

Miolan J P, Roman C 1978 Discharge of efferent vagal fibers supplying gastric antrum: indirect study by nerve suture technique. Am J Physiol 235: E366–E373

Sarna S K 1985 Cyclic motor activity; migrating motor complex: 1985. Gastroenterology 89: 894–913

Singer M V, Goebell H (eds) 1989 Nerves and the Gastrointestinal Tract. MTP Press, Lancaster.

Szurszewski J H 1969 A migrating electric complex of the canine small intestine. Am J Physiol 217: 1757–1763

Tache Y, Wingate D L (eds) 1991 Brain-Gut Interactions. CRC Press, Boca Raton

Thompson D G, Ritchie H D, Wingate D L 1982 Patterns of small intestinal motility in duodenal ulcer patients before and after vagotomy. Gut 23: 517–523

Valori R M, Kumar D, Wingate D L 1986 Effects of different types of stress and of 'prokinetic' drugs on the control of the fasting motor complex in humans. Gastroenterology 90: 1890–1900

Vantrappen G, Janssens J, Hellemans J, Ghoos Y 1977 The interdigestive motor complex of normal subjects and patients with bacterial overgrowth of the small intestine. J Clin Invest 59: 1186–1196

Wingate D L 1976 The eupeptide system: a general theory

of gastrointestinal hormones. Lancet i: 529–532

Wingate D L 1981 Backwards and forwards with the migrating motor complex. Dig Dis Sci 26: 641–666

Wingate D L 1983 Complex clocks. Dig Dis Sci 28: 1133–1140

Wingate D L, Ruppin H, Green W E R et al 1976 Motilin-induced electrical activity in the canine gastrointestinal tract. Scand J Gastroenterol, 11 (Suppl 39): 111–118

Wood J D 1984 Enteric neurophysiology. Am J Physiol 247: G585–G598

Wood J D, Wingate D L 1988 Gastrointestinal Neurophysiology, American Gastroenterological Association Undergraduate Teaching Project Unit 20, Milner-Fenwick, Timonium

FURTHER READING

Readers interested in more detailed information on this topic are referred to:

Wood J D (ed) 1989 Motility & Circulation. Vol 1, The Gastrointestinal System, Section 6, Handbook of Physiology, American Physiological Society, Bethesda.

6. Motility and regulatory peptides

J. E. T. Fox-Threlkeld

INTRODUCTION

The advent of immunohistochemistry, radioimmuno-assays, microanalytic, synthetic and molecular biological techniques has increased the number of biologically active peptides with gut motor activity on exogenous administration, but understanding the endogenous role of these requires appropriate potent selective non-peptide antagonists, few of which are available. The following reviews are recommended Furness & Costa 1987, Daniel et al 1989a,b, Daniel et al 1992a,b, Ekblad et al 1990.

PEPTIDE FAMILIES AND MODES OF ACTION

Table 6.1 gives the most common peptides/peptide families with gastrointestinal motor functions. Most peptides are not exclusive to the gut but are found peripherally in the lungs, the heart and cardiovascular system, the genitourinary tract and in the central nervous system (CNS).

A peptide or family member may be exclusive to endocrine cells, released extracellularly, with action at an adjacent cell termed paracrine, while delivery via the circulation is termed endocrine. A peptide exclusive to nerves and delivered via the circulation is termed neuroendocrine (e.g. oxytocin or vasopressin), none of which have been identified for the gut, but if delivered locally the action is termed neuromodulator or neurotransmitter.

True nerve–nerve synapses are present in enteric nerves. Motor end plates are present only in the striated muscle segments of the gut. The smooth muscle of the gut does not have neuromuscular junctions. Peptides released from nerve endings or varicosities must diffuse 5–100 times the distance of the motor end plate, a condition which leads to delay of onset or prolongation of the activity of the peptide.

NEUROMODULATORS, RATE OF DEGRADATION (Checler 1990)

The action of neurotransmitters such as acetylcholine (ACh), although longer in smooth muscle than in striated muscle, is completed within milliseconds. However, the action of most neuropeptides lasts for seconds to minutes, thus setting the conditions for the action of the neurotransmitter and fulfilling a neuromodulator role.

Differences in duration of action may reflect deactivation time. Thus, high acetylcholinesterase levels rapidly terminate the action of ACh, but peptides are hydrolysed by local concentrations of peptidases which are bond-specific rather than compound-specific. Bond specificity of the peptidases has prevented development of drugs such as cholinesterase inhibitors, since the antagonism of one peptidase increases all peptide levels, but has led to the synthesis of degradation-resistant peptides with prolonged actions. Some peptides are inactivated by the endocytotic incorporation of the receptor-bound molecule into the cell.

CO-LOCALIZATION, SYNTHESIS, STORAGE AND RELEASE

With the advent of immunohistochemistry, 'Dale's principle' (popularized by Eccles) of one nerve, one transmitter has been disproved. Sequential and simultaneous immunostaining techniques have found up to five different transmitters/modulators in the same nerve. This may be a mix of peptides or peptides and transmitters, such as ACh or nitric oxide (NO). Control of the release of multiple transmitters from a single nerve type by differing firing patterns is just beginning to be studied (Hokfelt 1991, Kupfferman 1991). Co-released peptides, hydrolysed by the

Table 6.1 Peptides of the gastrointestinal tract

Family	Mammalian	Non-mammalian
VIP/GIP/secretin/ glucagon	Vasoactive intestinal peptide (VIP) Peptides histidine, isoleucine & methionine (PHI/PHM) Gastric inhibitory peptide (GIP) Secretin Glucagon/glicentin/oxyntomodulin/glucagon-like peptides 1 & 2 Growth hormone releasing factor (GRF)	Helospectins Helodermins
Neurokinin/ tachykinin	Substance P Neurokinin A/Substance K Neurokinin B	Uperolein/Physalaemin/Scyliorhinin I Kassinin/Eledoisin/Scyliorhinin II
Opiates	Met/Leu enkephalin Dynorphin β-endorphin (+ multiple extended forms of the above) Morphiceptins (milk-derived)	Casamorphins Dermorphins Kytorphins
Bombesin/GRP	Gastrin releasing peptide (GRP) Neuromedin B	Bombesin/Alytesin Ranatensin/Litorin Phyllolitorin
PP/NPY/PYY	Peptide proline proline (PP) Peptide tyrosine tyrosine (PYY) Neuropeptide tyrosine (NPY)	
Neurotensin	Neuromedin N Neurotensin Kinetensin	LANT-6 Xenopsin
Gastrin/CCK	Cholecystokinin CCK 8, 22, 33, 39, & 58 Gastrin 4, 5, 6, 14, 17, & 34	Caerulein
Calcitonin	Calcitonin Calcitonin gene related peptide (CGRP) α & β	
Others (unrelated)	Galanin Motilin Somatostatin	

(Fox 1989a,b, McDonald 1990a,b, Dockray 1992)

same enzyme may alter the others' hydrolysis and action.

Neuropeptides are synthesized as large precursors on the ribosomes in the nerve soma. Cleavage from the precursor involves removal of the signal peptide in the endoplasmic reticulum. Post-translational processing of further cleavage, amidation, phosphorylation, sulphation and glycosylation occurs in the Golgi apparatus. The secretory granules are transported down the axon to the nerve terminals and varicosities and stored in large, dense-cored vesicles. A single precursor can be cleaved to varying lengths, e.g. the gastrin family (Table 6.1), or may contain several peptide family members, e.g. vasoactive intestinal peptide (VIP) and peptide HI (PHI) or peptide HM (PHM) found at different loci in the same gene. There may be more than one gene coding for different precursors, e.g. three genes code for opiate peptide precursors, all containing the active enkephalin sequence.

Peptide release from neural or endocrine granules is calcium dependent. Studies on control of release, using radioimmunoassay for detection, may apply electrical field stimulation or add depolarizing concentrations of potassium in the presence of tetrodotoxin to block sodium channels or scorpion venom to open sodium channels.

Table 6.2   Possible sites and mechanisms of motor actions of peptides

| Action | Prejunctional | | Postjunctional | |
	Stimulation of	Inhibition of	Muscles	Other cell types
Excitation	Excitatory post-junctional nerves	Inhibitory post-junctional nerves	Contract	Release excitants
Inhibition	Inhibitory post-junctional nerves	Excitatory post-junctional nerves	Relax	Release inhibitors

RECEPTORS AND SECOND MESSENGERS
(Ahmad et al 1990, Vincent & Kitabgi 1990)

Radioligand binding techniques, used initially in the CNS and on cultured cells, and highly selective peptide and non-peptide agonists and antagonists have shown that many of the peptide families act at different receptor subtypes, and these can be isolated, synthesized and characterized. After receptor binding, adenylate cyclase and/or guanylate cyclase levels may be altered resulting in changes in cyclic adenosine monophosphate (cAMP or guanosine monophosphate (cGMP), G proteins activated, ion channels gated, and phospholipase C and the phosphatidyl inositol pathways activated. The action of a peptide will depend upon the type of second messenger present in the cell.

SITES AND MECHANISM OF ACTION (Fox-Threlkeld 1990, Fox et al 1985, Daniel et al 1989b)

The overall action of a peptide is the algebraic sum of all its excitatory and inhibitory actions at many cell types within the system, as detailed in Table 6.2. Many peptides have both excitatory and inhibitory actions in the same tissue. Furthermore, expression of the action of a peptide may depend upon the mode of delivery of the peptide, the experimental conditions and the presuppositions. In man, with a peptide given intravenously and motor activity monitored by serosal electrodes or intraluminal apparatus, resulting activity may depend on release of compounds from the vascular endothelium, immune cells, systemic nerves (peptides rarely cross the blood–brain barrier), enteric nerves, or a direct muscle action, or all of the above.

Although use of some antagonists is possible in man, determination of sites of action may require in vitro and animal in vivo studies. Species differences are understandable. However, differing responses depending on the experimental preparation are not well recognized. For example, gastrin contracts the isolated gastric muscle cell at 10^{-13}M, the muscle cell of the isolated strip at 10^{-8}M, but muscle cell activation is absent when examined in situ, suggesting that the isolation procedures upregulate receptor population, begging the question of the functional receptor in situ in conscious man. Thus studies of intravenous peptides allow little physiological interpretation and studies in isolated cells exaggerated interpretations. Study of physiological significance requires potent, highly selective non-peptide antagonists; peptide based antagonists are expensive and have low potency. Many long-held beliefs based on pharmacological actions of peptides, such as the role of cholecystokinin (CCK) in the gastrocolic reflex (Niederau et al 1992), may disappear once appropriate antagonists are available for these endogenous peptides (Hokfelt 1991).

THE OPIATES

Tincture of opium was used to treat diarrhoea in prehistory. Endogenous mammalian opioids were discovered in the 1970s, and the exorphins, or casomorphins, of milk and the dermorphams and kytorphans of frog skins have been discovered since then.

Peptide structure, precursors and localization
(Daniel et al 1989b, Allescher & Ahmad 1990, Furness & Costa 1987, Furness et al 1992)

The enkephalin structure R-Tyr-Gly-Gly-Phe-Met (Met enkephalin) or R-Tyr-Gly-Gly-Phe-Leu (Leu enkephalin) is common to three precursors: pro-opiomelanocortin expressed mainly in the pituitary and CNS contains, adrenocorticotrophic hormone (ACTH) besides the C-terminally extended Met enkephalin which is known as β endorphin and is co-released as a hormone with ACTH; proenkephalin A, expressed in central and peripheral nerves and in the adrenal medulla, contains four Met enkephalins, one Leu enkephalin and several C-terminally extended Met enkephalins; and prodynorphin expressed in nerves has the Leu enkephalin backbone and contains several lengths of dynorphin, α and β neoendorphin, and rimorphin.

In the myenteric plexus of the guinea pig ileum, neural soma containing dynorphin and enkephalins project:

a. to sympathetic ganglia;
b. orally to the circular muscle (co-localized with ACh and tachykinins;
c. directly to the circular muscle (enkephalins co-localized with ACh and tachykinins),
d. anally to the circular muscle with both short and long projections (dynorphin co-localized with NO and VIP).

In the submucous plexus, dynorphin can be found in nerves with projections:

a. to villi and myenteric plexus co-localized with ACh, tachykinins and neuromedin U (sensory);
b. to the villi co-localized with VIP, galanin and neuromedin U (secretomotor);
c. in the plexus co-localized with ACh (interneurones);
d. to villi co-localized with ACh, CCK, calcitonin gene-related peptides (CGRP), neuromedin U, neuropeptide Y (NPY) somatostatin and sometimes galanin (secretomotor).

Opiate receptor subtypes (Goldstein & Naidu 1989, Ahmad et al 1990)

Opiate receptors concerned with gastrointestinal motility are found in the CNS, the spinal cord, and peripheral and enteric nerves. Five opiate receptor subtypes have been identified: μ (classic agonist morphine); δ (recognizing the enkephalins, particularly Leu); κ (recognizing the endogenous dynorphin); ε (recognizing β endorphin); and σ found only in the CNS. The gut has μ, δ and κ receptor subtypes as determined by selective agonists and antagonists. In the canine small intestine, binding studies indicate the presence of opiate receptors only on neural membranes, with a μ:δ:κ ratio of 40:40:15 for the deep muscular plexus and the myenteric plexus, and 64:24:12 for the submucous plexus. In the guinea pig ileum, activation of μ receptors in the myenteric plexus, and δ receptors in the submucous plexus inhibits excitatory nerves by hyperpolarization of the membrane and prolongation of the duration of the after-hyperpolarization by increasing potassium conductance dependent on release of stored intracellular calcium, similar to the adrenergic receptor (North et al 1987). Activation of κ receptors decreased the inward calcium conductance and had no effect on the potassium conductance. Both μ and κ receptors could be demonstrated on the same cell (North 1986).

Sites and mechanisms of enteric actions along the gut (Manara and Biachetti 1985, Daniel et al 1989a,b, Fox 1989b, Allescher & Ahmad 1990)

The existence of functional opiate receptors on smooth muscle cells is controversial. In the dog, although opiates contract isolated cells, only inhibition of nerve stimulated motility occurs in vitro in strips, and binding is only to nerve membranes. In vivo, exogenous opiates excite by inhibiting tonic release of the inhibitory transmitter NO and inhibit by inhibiting release of excitatory transmitters (Daniel & Fox-Threlkeld 1992). In contrast the rat colon appears to have excitatory smooth muscle receptors for opioids.

In the guinea pig myenteric plexus longitudinal muscle, the standard bioassay preparation, opiates inhibit spontaneous and nerve-stimulated contractions by inhibiting release of the excitatory neurotransmitters such as ACh and substance P at μ and κ receptors.

The role of *endogenous* opiates in control of motility is less clear, although delivery of an opiate antagonist to the tolerant gastrointestinal tract of the opiate abuser causes dramatic gut effects. At the level of the enteric nervous system (ENS), endogenous opiates appear to be involved in the proximal excitation of the enteric reflex and in the noncholinergic component of excitation induced by motilin. Endogenous opiates are also involved in the reduction of VIP-dependent secretion.

Table 6.3 gives an overview of the actions of exogenous opiates and, where studied by use of antagonists, the actions of endogenous opiates along the gastrointestinal tract in man. Central sites of action were distinguished from peripheral sites of action when the agonist or antagonist given did not cross the blood–brain barrier. When opiates are given for analgesia the actions on gastrointestinal motility often become troublesome side-effects, particularly in the gallbladder (Humphries & Flemming 1992). Also, although the action of opiates on absorption is not examined in this chapter, any slowing of transit will increase absorption by prolonging the exposure of the contents to the absorptive surface.

The opiates are involved in complex actions controlling motility in the gastrointestinal tract. Although the resulting action of an opiate administered systemically may be excitation, in sites where detailed studies have been carried out, excitation results from inhibition of inhibition. This is best borne out by studies of the actions of opiates on neural receptors where μ and δ receptor activation result in hyperpolarization and κ activation reduces calcium entry into the cell. Both of these actions reduce release of transmitter from nerve, but the resulting action depends on whether the

Table 6.3 Opiate actions along the gastrointestinal tract in man

Organ	Compound	Exogenous action	Site of action	Endogenous action	Site of action
Oesophagus	FK33-824	Increase peristaltic amplitude and contraction	Peripheral	?	
LOS	Morphine	Decrease resting tone and relaxation	Central or peripheral	Modulates tone and relaxation	?
Antrum	β endorphin	Inhibited contractions	Peripheral	Stress-induced inhibition of activity	Peripheral, central in sheep
Gastric emptying	Morphine	Delayed	Central or peripheral	No effect with naloxone	
Pylorus	β endorphin	Increased activity	Peripheral	No effect with naloxone	
Small intestine	β endorphin Loperamide Morphine	Induce phase III of MMC during fed or fasting state	Peripheral Peripheral Peripheral or central	Abolished phase III	Peripheral or central
Small intestinal transit	Loperamide Codeine	Inhibition	Peripheral Central or peripheral	?	
Gall bladder	Morphine	Increases biliary pressure	Peripheral	?	
Ileocaecal sphincter	Morphine	No effect	?	?	
Colon	Morphine	Increase in non-propulsive contractions	Central or peripheral	Inhibition of transit	Central or peripheral
Anal sphincter	Morphine	Increased tone	Central or peripheral	?	

Manara 1985

neurotransmitter was excitatory or inhibitory to the target organ. Reduction of excitation leads to inhibition, while reduction of inhibition leads to excitation.

MOTILIN AND THE ERYTHROMYCIN BASED MOTILIDES (Itoh 1989, McIntosh & Brown 1990)

Motilin (22 amino acids) is found exclusively in gastrointestinal M and enterochromaffin endocrine cells of the duodenum and upper jejunal mucosa and acts in an endocrine or possibly a paracrine fashion.

Peptide structure, precursors, localization and receptors

Motilin was isolated from the porcine gut by Brown on the basis of its ability to increase motor activity of the canine upper gut. The 115 amino acid prepromotilin is processed to motilin 22 by removal of the N-terminal 25 amino acid signal peptide and the 68 amino acid C-terminal peptide. Human and porcine motilin are identical, but dog motilin has five different amino acids at positions 7, 6, 12, 13 and 14. Biological activity appears to reside in the 1–15 sequence. Erythromycin was found to have similar motor actions as motilin in man and dog given either orally or intravenously, and erythromycin and the structurally-related motilides, of which EM-536 (8,9-anhydroerythromycin A 6,9-hemiketal-propagyl-bromide) is the most potent, bind to the motilin receptor and displace [^{125}I]motilin with an IC_{50} of 40 nM. This property of erythromycin is now being exploited to increase gastric emptying in patients suffering from diabetic gastroparesis (Janssens et al 1990). However the propensity of the motilin receptor to become downregulated upon continued exposure to either motilin or erythromycin (tachyphylaxis) limits its long-term administration and efficacy as a prokinetic agent.

Motilin receptors as determined by physiological studies are located on the upper gastrointestinal smooth muscle in man and rabbits, and exclusively on nerves in dogs, opossums, guinea pigs and pigs. Isolated muscle cells prepared from the guinea pig stomach and the dog stomach and small intestine contract to motilin, but, since the isolated strip does not contract to motilin in the absence of nerves and binding cannot be demonstrated, isolation of the cells may induce a function not found in situ. There are no studies to confirm or deny the presence of motilin receptors on nerves in man or rabbit. In the rabbit, both porcine and canine motilin had similar potencies in functional and binding studies (K_δ = 1 nM, B_{MAX} = 40 fmol/mg protein). Erythromycin and motilin 1–14 also bind to these receptors.

Enteric actions, mode of delivery and release, sites and mechanisms (Allescher et al 1990, Daniel et al 1989b, Fox 1989a)

Although motilin may have undocumented local paracrine actions, its function is presumed to be one of a true hormone delivered to the site of action through the circulation. Intraduodenal acid, fat, bile salts, gastric distention and phase III of the migrating motor complex (MMC) commencing in the stomach are potent stimuli for release in man. In dogs, intraduodenal alkali, electrical stimulation of the vagus or intrinsic enteric nerves, and antral and duodenal intra-arterial ACh infusions release motilin, and neural stimuli are blocked by either hexamethonium or atropine, suggesting that the motilin cell receives cholinergic neural input and has muscarinic receptors.

In the rabbit, the action of motilin on the smooth muscle cell depends upon entry of calcium through verapamil-sensitive channels. Electrophysiological studies found that motilin depolarized the membrane, reduced membrane resistance and reduced the electrical control activity from 18 cycles per min (cpm) to 1 cpm. Trains of spike potentials occurred on these slow oscillations accompanied by muscle contractions.

In vivo in the dog, which has only neural receptors, motilin releases ACh to act at both muscarinic and nicotinic sites. There is a decreasing gradient of sensitivity along the gut to motilin. The stomach which has only muscarinic receptors responds to the lowest concentrations of motilin. The cholinergic component decreases in sensitivity along the small intestine and the noncholinergic component, which results from release of endogenous opiates, is constant along the small intestine. Since in the dog small intestine, opiates produce excitation by inhibiting release of the nonadrenergic noncholinergic (NANC) inhibitory transmitter NO, one would expect that motilin acts to inhibit NO as well. Motilin also inhibits release of VIP but this inhibition may not influence motility.

The sequence of events at the neural receptors for motilin then is:

1. Motilin → postjunctional cholinergic nerves → release of acetylcholine → stimulation of muscarinic receptors on smooth muscle → increased motility.
2. Motilin → prejunctional cholinergic nerves → release of acetylcholine → stimulation of nicotinic receptors → release of endogenous opiates → inhibition of NO release → disinhibition of smooth muscle → increased motility.

Intravenous infusions of motilin excite the upper gastrointestinal tract in the conscious dog, man and opossum (and pig after prolonged fasting). During fasting, low concentrations induce premature phase III contractions of the MMC. These commence in the oesophagus and sweep through to the ileum and involve a contraction and emptying of the gallbladder. At least in the dog (not tested in man) these motilin-induced phase are blocked by atropine. When motilin is infused in the fed state in dogs, much higher concentrations are required to induce an amplification of the fed pattern (not phase III type contractions) during feeding.

Peripheral immunoreactive motilin levels cycle in some association with the MMC. Motilin levels peak in dogs as the cycle passes through the upper duodenum, and motilin and motor activity have been shown to increase motilin levels in the dog. When motilin was immunoneutralized in dogs using anti-rabbit motilin serum, the MMC was abolished in the antrum and duodenum concomitant with abolition of the motilin cycles, but the distal jejunum and ileum continued MMC-like activity suggesting a causative action in the upper gut only. However, when motor cycles were interrupted by intravenous gastrin or CCK, or intracerebral CRF, the motilin cycles continued. Thus endogenous motilin release may not be sufficient to produce the phase III activity in all circumstances but may be involved in the amplification of the stimuli and coordination of the activity. In man, motilin cycles only coincided with the passage of phase IIIs through the duodenum if the MMC commenced in the stomach. In both man and dog erythromycins have similar actions to motilin.

The ability of erythromycin (acting at motilin receptors) has been exploited to increase gastric emptying in gastroparetic patients. In this case intravenous erythromycin is more effective than oral erythromycin. In normal man, intravenous erythromycin can overcome the inhibition of gastric emptying induced by intraduodenal fat. The mechanism of this acceleration appears to be an inhibition of pyloric contractions accompanying the strong gastric contractions (Fraser et al 1992).

Coincident with the initiation of contractions by motilin or phase III of the intestinal MMC, the gallbladder contracts. That this is part of the integrated cycle rather than a direct action of motilin on the gallbladder, is suggested by the finding that neither the rabbit or human gallbladder contract in vitro to motilin (Pomeranz et al 1983). Erythromycin given orally reduces the gallbladder volume in normal subjects and in patients with gallstones, and reverses the gallbladder motility defect found in some patients with gallstones (Catnach et al 1992).

TACHYKININS (Leeman et al 1991, Fox 1989b, Allescher & Ahmad 1990)

Substance P (SP), the initial enteric neuropeptide to be biologically identified, was extracted from equine intestines and brains by von Euler and Gaddum in 1931, recognized as a sensory transmitter by Lembeck in 1953, and sequenced, purified and synthesized by Leeman and coworkers in 1970. SP is extensively distributed in secretmotor and sensory nerves in the gut and virtually all other organs. Neurokinins A (NKA) and B (NKB), and neuropeptide K have been identified as the mammalian relatives of SP; the precursor proteins have been identified and the related genes sequenced. The capacity of capsaicin, the active ingredient in hot peppers, to selectively deplete or degenerate sensory fibres is a useful tool for studying sensory tachykinins. Other members of the tachykinin family have been identified in species as diverse as molluscs and amphibians, suggesting that the tachykinins appeared early in evolution. Although not proven, Lembeck suggested that they serve the function of amplification of a peripheral injury signal in lower species.

Peptide structure, precursors, localization and receptor subtypes (Allescher & Ahmad 1990, Furness & Costa 1987, Sternini 1991, Ekblad et al 1991, Burcher et al 1991)

The mammalian tachykinins (SP, NKA, NKB and neuropeptide K) and their molluscan, fish and amphibian relatives (Table 6.1) have in common the C-terminal pentapeptide -Phe-X-Gly-Leu-Met-NH_2, where X is either the aromatic or branched chain amino acid Phe, Val, Ile or Tyr.

Two preprotachykinin (PPT) genes have been identified. PPT-A encodes for SP and NKA and its extended form neuropeptide K, and PPT-B encodes for NKB. However PPT-A may be processed to give only SP (α-PPT-A), or from two slightly different processing paths, SP and NKA (β-PPT-A) and SP and the extended NKA neuropeptide K (γ-PPT-A).

Using highly selective antisera, no NKB has been found in enteric nerves and no studies distinguish NKA from SP nerves. In the guinea pig enteric nerve cell bodies in the myenteric plexus containing immunoreactive SP have projections:

a. to the circular muscle and its deep muscular plexus;
b. to the submucous plexus;
c. in both anal and oral directions in the myenteric plexus;
d. to the mucosa.

A further population of enteric nerve cell bodies in the submucous plexus has projections to the mucosa. Cell bodies of sensory afferents in the dorsal root ganglia have projections to the submucosa and blood vessels. Some sensory afferent fibres also travel in the vagus. Some populations of tachykinin afferent nerves, but not enteric nerves, also contain CGRP.

Three subtypes of tachykinin receptors (NK_1, NK_2 and NK_3) have been defined using highly selective agonists and specific arteries containing only one receptor type. These receptor subtypes have been sequenced, cloned and expressed in Xenopus oocytes. However, there may be at least two subtypes each of NK_1 and NK_2 receptors. The endogenous tachykinins show the following relative potency orders for the three subtypes: NK_1 – SP > NKA > NKB; NK_2 – NKA > NKB > SP; and NK_3 – NKB > NKA > SP.

In the gastrointestinal tract NK_1 or SP-preferring receptors are found both pre- and postfunctionally, NK_2 receptors post-junctionally and NK_3 receptors prejunctionally. These three receptor subtypes depend upon the C-terminus of the tachykinins. There are other processes which depend upon the N-terminus of SP, which may be important in gastrointestinal function, for example, release of histamine and prostanoids upon the degranulation of mast cells.

Sites and mechanisms of action along the gut

Tachykinins are stimulants. They excite smooth muscle directly and they release neurotransmitters, the contents of mast cells and mediators from the vascular endothelium. The motor action found on application of a tachykinin will therefore depend on the experimental preparation used and the presence or absence of these components. Tachykinins contract isolated smooth muscle cells by increasing the calcium available to the contractile mechanism by a number of processes, including decreasing K^+ conductance, opening depolarization-evoked Ca^{2+} channels and stimulating phosphatidyl inositol turnover. Electrophysiological studies have shown that stimulation of ACh release results from Ca^{2+}-dependent inhibition of K^+ conductance with stimulation in some cells of adenylate cyclase as the second messenger. Inhibition of acetylcholine release probably results from release of the inhibitory NO from nerves or the endothelium.

Antidromic release of SP in the skin, from afferent sensory nerves, degranulates mast cells causing release of histamine which in turn increases the permeability of local capillaries (the classic triple response). This may also happen in the gut as SP-containing nerves are found in close proximity to mast cells and Swain et

Table 6.4 Motor actions of endogenous tachykinins

Site	Species	Muscle	Action	Stimulus
Oesophagus	Opossum	M mucosa	Contraction	HF field
		longitudinal	Contraction	HF field
LOS	Cat	Circular	Contraction	Luminal acid
Stomach	Cat	Circular	Contraction	Mucosal heating, bradykinin
	Rat	Circular	Spasm	Ulcer induction (ethanol)
Pylorus	Cat	Circular	Contraction	HF splanchnic
Small intestine	Rat	Blood vesels	Vasodilatation	Mucosal/serosal warming
	Guinea pig	Segment	Peristalsis	Local distention
Colon	Dog	M mucosa	Contraction	HF field
	Cat	Circular	Contraction	HF sympathetic

HF = High frequency electrical stimulation
Fox 1989b

al (1992) have found sensory nerve SP content increased in the inflamed gut.

The profound vasodilation induced by intravenous infusions of tachykinin and the paucity of highly potent selective antagonists prohibit human studies using intravenous tachykinins, so data must be obtained from in vitro and animal studies.

Endogenous tachykinins appear to be involved in proximal excitation in the peristaltic reflex by increasing excitability of other neurons. Endogenous tachykinins appear to interact with the release of a number of noncholinergic enteric transmitters. Serotonin and neurotensin release SP, opiate and α adrenergic tolerance appear to have a tachykinin component and, as described above, release of NO may contribute to motility changes. Table 6.4 gives the excitatory responses which have an identified role for local release of endogenous tachykinins. In man, increases in plasma immunoreactive tachykinins as well as other peptides have been found to be associated with carcinoid syndrome and may account for the altered gastrointestinal motility seen with the syndrome.

A major role has been established in other organs for tachykinins in inflammation and mucosal oedema but, other than studies on ulcerogenesis, this function has not been examined for the gut.

VASOACTIVE INTESTINAL POLYPEPTIDE
(VIP) FAMILY (McDonald 1990, Allescher & Ahmad 1990, Daniel et al 1989b, Fox 1989b, Dockray 1992)

The endocrine members of this family are secretin, the glucagons and gastric inhibitory polypeptide (GIP), while VIP and PHI (porcine)/PHM (human) and the hypothalamic peptide growth hormone-releasing factor (GHRF or somatocrinin) are found in nerves. Three selective receptor groups recognize:

a. the glucagons;
b. VIP, PHI/PHM, secretin and GHRF;
c. GIP, but not members of the other group.

Activation of VIP receptors stimulates adenylate cyclase and the increase in cAMP results in a cell-specific action (i.e. a muscle cell relaxes, an enterocyte secretes chloride).

Peptide structure, precursors, localization and receptors

VIP and PHI/PHM require the full 28/27 amino acids for full binding and function with certain internal amino acids substitutions maintaining potency. Aminopeptidase removal of the N-terminal residue follows receptor binding and allows internalization of the VIP/receptor complex where degradation is completed.

VIP and PHI/PHM share the same gene, and the precursor preproVIP is post-translationally processed to VIP and PHI/PHM and three other extended peptides. These neuropeptides are abundant in intrinsic and extrinsic gastrointestinal nerves. In the guinea pig myenteric plexus, separate populations of VIP nerves project to sympathetic ganglia, the circular muscle and deep muscular plexus in short and long distal projections, the submucous plexus distally and the myenteric plexus distally. Nerve cell bodies in the submucous plexus have projections to the mucosa. Nerves of unidentified origins terminate on blood vessels. VIP and ACh are co-localized in many postganglionic parasympathetic nerves and at least in the pancreas and salivary glands potentiate secretion. In the guinea pig ileum VIP co-localizes with galanin, opioids, NPY, CCK and gastrin releasing peptide (GRP).

The VIP group of receptors recognizes secretin, VIP/PHI and GHRF, and subtypes have differing affinities for the preferred peptide. Radioligand binding studies in the canine gut (Mao et al 1991) find VIP receptors on enterocytes, synaptosomes from the myenteric, submucous and deep muscular plexus, and purified plasma membranes from the longitudinal muscle and sphincter circular muscle membranes but not on plasma membranes of the intestinal circular muscle.

Enteric actions, sites and mechanisms (Daniel et al 1989b, Allescher & Ahmad 1990, Dockray 1992)

VIP relaxes those smooth muscle cells (isolated or in situ) which have receptors for VIP and respond to increases in adenylate cyclase and thus cAMP, with a reduction in intracellular Ca^{2+} concentration. However, stimulation of VIP receptors on nerves releases ACh in the guinea pig ileum, and on the interstitial cells of Cajal hyperpolarizes these cells influencing the contraction frequency. Thus the responses to VIP are complex and may vary from tissue to tissue. For example, in the opossum lower oesophageal sphincter (LOS), VIP moderately hyperpolarizes the membrane and relaxes the LOS (a direct muscle action), while in the oesophageal body moderate hyperpolarization is followed by depolarization, spikes and phasic contractions (catecholamines appeared to release VIP in this case). Because VIP relaxes sphincters (nerve-induced relaxation reduced by VIP antiserum) and certain isolated smooth muscle cells, VIP was considered the most likely candidate for the elusive nonadrenergic noncholinergic (NANC) inhibitory neurotransmitter. However, NO (Moncada 1992, Stark & Szurszewski 1992) has been shown to be the NANC transmitter primarily responsible for the inhibitory junction potential (IJP), while VIP has little or no effect on the membrane potential or the IJP in some tissues. Thus, study of the interactions and relative contributions of VIP, NO and the initial NANC candidates, the purines, to inhibition of motility is important. Since VIP and NO synthase are co-localized in guinea pig enteric nerves – blockade of NO synthase reduces VIP output and the NO donor, Na nitroprusside, stimulates VIP release – VIP may be an important neuromodulator. Detailed analysis awaits appropriate antagonists.

Endogenous release of VIP participates in, but is not completely responsible for, nerve-induced relaxation of: the LOS of opossum, cat, pig, and dog and man; the circular muscles of stomach of the dog, ferret and guinea pig; the canine pylorus; and the human ileum. Endogenous release of VIP appears to be responsible for inhibition of the muscularis mucosa of the canine antrum and colon. The relaxation of colon and

internal anal sphincter of the opossum and man, and descending inhibition in the guinea pig colon has a VIP component. However the role of VIP in the small intestine is unclear. VIP levels are tonically elevated and additional VIP has mixed effects, but inhibition of tonic levels is not always associated with excitation. When inhibition of tonic VIP release is dissociated from inhibition of tonic NO release, NO not VIP appears to be responsible for tonic suppression of motility (Fox-Threlkeld et al 1991), correlating with the lack of VIP binding sites on intestinal circular muscle plasma membranes. PHI/PHM produce similar responses to VIP.

GALANIN (Hokfelt et al 1991)

Galanin is a neuropeptide widely distributed throughout the central, peripheral and enteric nervous system in afferent and efferent nerves.

Peptide structure, precursors, localization

Porcine, rat and bovine galanins have 29 amino acids; human galanin has 30 amino acids with the N-terminal 1–15 amino acids being identical in each species and fully functional at the single receptor so far identified. Porcine, rat and bovine preprogalanins have 123 amino acids and the genes have been cloned (Rokaeus & Waschek 1991).

Galanin-containing nerve cell bodies originating in the myenteric plexus project distally. Galanin is most frequently found co-localized with VIP (Ekblad et al 1991).

Galanin inhibits adenylate cyclase in pancreatic β cells where it also activates ATP-sensitive and G-protein-regulated K^+ channels leading to closure of Ca^{2+} channels. Galanin binds to both nerve and muscle membranes in the canine ileum.

Enteric actions, sites and mechanisms
(Fox-Threlkeld 1991)

Except for the sphincters, galanin excites longitudinal muscles by a direct muscle action while circular muscles are inhibited either by a direct action or inhibition of excitatory transmitters. If release of inhibitory neural transmitters is inhibited excitation may occur. In sphincters, galanin may either excite or inhibit depending on the sphincter. Microelectrode studies in the guinea pig enteric nerves demonstrated that galanin increased K^+ conductance and blocked voltage-sensitive Ca^{2+} channels. There is no information available on the role of endogenous galanin in control of gastrointestinal motility.

NEUROTENSIN FAMILY (Daniel et al 1989b)

Neurotensin (13 amino acids), named for its ability to reduce blood pressure, was isolated originally from the hypothalamus. Subsequently identified members of this family, including the co-localized neuromedin N (6 amino acids), are widely distributed in central and peripheral nerves in mammals, birds, fish and amphibians, as well as ileal endocrine cells. The most potent stimulus for endocrine release of neurotensin is luminal fat but, since no non-peptide selective antagonist is available, its participation in the integrated motor responses is unknown, although neurotensin receptors are present on gastrointestinal muscles and nerves.

Peptide structure, precursors, localization and receptors (McDonald 1990b, Ahmad et al 1990, Vincent & Kitabgi 1990, Kostka 1990)

The neurotensin family share the biologically active C-terminal tetrapeptide -Pro-Tyr-Ile-Leu-OH, except in amphibians where Trp is substituted for Tyr with a shortened or substituted N-terminal portion. Preproneurotensin contains both neurotensin and two copies of neuromedin N. Neurotensin appears to be contained in cultured but not in situ nerves and antisera do not distinguish neurotensin from neuromedin N.

Enzymes which inactivate neurotensin in the C-terminal producing the inactive neurotensin$_{1-8}$ and neurotensin$_{1-11}$ are present in the gastrointestinal tract (Checler 1990). The very rapid degradation of neurotensin$_{9-13}$ ($t_{1/2}$ = 0.5 min) in the gut suggests a paracrine action. Neuromedin N is rapidly degraded by aminopeptidases.

Neurotensin binds to receptors on circular, but not longitudinal, muscle plasma membranes and on deep muscular plexus and submucous plexus, but not myenteric plexus synaptosomes. There is no evidence for specific subtypes of neurotensin receptors.

Receptors in the CNS are coupled to G proteins and stimulate phospholipase C and inositol phospholipids while inhibiting adenylate cyclase. In gut muscles, neurotensin receptors inducing excitation open L-type Ca^{2+} channels while those inducing inhibition open apamin-sensitive K^+ channels which depend upon entry of extracellular Ca^{2+}.

Sites and mechanisms of actions (Daniel et al 1989b, Allescher & Ahmad 1990

Neurotensin produces complex actions at multiple receptor sites in a single tissue segment. As an example,

the canine ileal circular muscle is excited by neurotensin by a direct smooth muscle action, release of excitatory neurotransmitters and excitatory agents from mast cells, and is inhibited by neurotensin by a direct smooth muscle action and release of norepinephrine. Also, neurotensin and neuromedin are potent stimulators of VIP secretion.

Intravenous infusions of (Gln^4)-neurotensin reduced the cholinergic component of resting LOS pressure, and decreased antral contraction frequency while increasing duodenal contraction frequency. Gastric emptying was delayed after neurotensin infusion. If infused during fasting, neurotensin converted the fasting pattern of small intestinal motility into the irregular pattern of fed motility. In the colon there was increased motor activity with an increased faecal volume and induction of defaecation with neurotensin infusion. The human gallbladder dilated during neurotensin infusion. Given that fat induces release of neurotensin it has been tempting to speculate that the above responses, which are all (except for the gallbladder) responses to fat, are actions of endogenous release of neurotensin. Until antagonists are available this is truly speculation.

BOMBESIN/GASTRIN RELEASING PEPTIDE (GRP)

The mammalian (GRP and neuromedin B) family members are found in the central, peripheral and enteric nerves, and have actions at multiple sites. Only peptide antagonists are available, so limiting understanding of endogenous actions (Houben & Denef 1991). No receptor subtypes have been identified.

Peptide structure, precursors and localization (McDonald 1990b)

The bombesin/GRP family has been divided into three subgroups on the basis of final seven amino acids in the biologically active C terminal. Bombesin, alytesin and the GRPs share a -Trp-Ala-Val-Gly-His-Leu-Met-NH$_2$ terminus; the neuromedin B group of neuromedin B, ranatensin R, ranatensin and litorin have substitutions at Val and Leu, and the phyllolitorin subgroup (no mammalian counterpart) has substitutions at His.

The GRP gene is found on human chromosome 18 while that for neuromedin B on chromosome 15.

In the guinea pig ileum (Furness & Costa 1987) sparse populations of nerve cell bodies in the myenteric plexus project:

a. to the sympathetic ganglia,
b. distally within the myenteric plexus;
c. to the deep muscular plexus;
d. to the submucous plexus co-localized with CCK, dynorphin, enkephalin and VIP.

Mucosal fibres are frequent in the stomach and large intestine but sparse in the small intestine (Ekblad et al 1990).

Sites and mechanisms of enteric actions (Daniel et al 1989b, Fox-Threlkeld 1990)

GRP often acts as an interneuronal transmitter, is involved in several reflexes and rarely acts directly on smooth muscle in vivo. However, isolated strips and cells contract to GRP and bombesin suggesting that smooth muscle receptors are downregulated in vivo.

Exogenous GRP stimulates LOS contractions by releasing SP and ACh, and endogenous GRP may participate in the LOS response to distal oesophageal acidification. In the canine stomach circular muscle, GRP releases ACh in vivo, while in the muscularis mucosa it releases SP. In the canine small intestine, GRP appeared to release ACh to activate inhibitory muscarinic autoreceptors which may be the mechanism by which intravenous bombesin interrupts phase of the MMC in man. Except in rodents where a smooth muscle action may occur, bombesin-induced gallbladder contractions depend on release of ACh. Release of excitatory neurotransmitters, ACh for the muscularis externa and SP for the muscularis mucosa, appears to account for the excitatory action of bombesin in the colon.

NPY/PYY/PP

Pancreatic polypeptide (PP) is found in pancreatic endocrine cells, neuropeptide Y (NPY) is exclusive to nerves both centrally and peripherally (frequently in sympathetic nerves) and peptide YY (PYY) is found in both enteric endocrine cells and nerves.

Peptide structure, precursors, localization and receptors (McDonald 1990b, Dockray 1992, Sheikh 1991)

Each of these three peptides is 36 amino acids in length, with 8 amino acids different between porcine NPY and PYY, and 15 amino acids different between PYY and PP. The genes encoding the precursors have been identified as well as the preproprotein precursors.

In the guinea pig, sympathetic nerve cell bodies containing NPY and noradrenaline (NA) project to the blood vessels, while populations of nerve cell bodies in the myenteric plexus project:

a. to the circular muscle and deep muscular plexus;
b. distally in the plexus;
c. to the mucosa.

These nerves also may contain dynorphin, enkephalin, VIP or GRP. Submucous plexus nerve cell bodies, containing CCK, CGRP, somatostatin and ACh, have projections to the mucosa (Furness & Costa 1987). In the rat submucosal neurons, NPY and VIP are co-localized and project orally to the villi (Ekblad et al 1990).

At least two receptor subtypes have been distinguished for NPY – Y_1 and Y_2. Y_1 receptors appear to correspond to functional prejunctional receptors, requiring whole NPY. Y_2 receptors bind the C-terminal fragments of NPY and appear to be localized postjunctionally. A further receptor type may recognize PYY preferentially. NPY receptors appear to be linked to a pertussis-sensitive G protein and activation inhibits adenylate cyclase.

Enteric actions, sites and mechanisms and actions along the gastrointestinal tract (Fox 1989a, Dockray 1992)

In the guinea pig and cat small intestine and colon, NPY and PYY inhibit contractions by releasing NA to α_2 adrenoceptors on cholinergic nerves. In the dog ileum, NPY and PYY excite the circular muscle in vivo and ex vivo by inhibiting release of NO. The concomitant inhibition of VIP may be important in the potent inhibition of intestinal secretion by PYY and NPY.

PYY inhibits gastric emptying in man. Since in the dog infusions of PYY matching endogenously released PYY after oleic acid intraduodenal infusion also inhibited gastric emptying, PYY was suggested as candidate for the ileal brake hormone (Sheikh 1991).

SOMATOSTATIN

Somatostatin is widely distributed throughout the gastrointestinal tract in both endocrine cells and nerves. Endocrine cells in the stomach have long processes terminating on adjacent cells suggesting a paracrine action. Only one receptor type has been described.

Peptide structure, precursors and localization
(Dockray 1992, Furness & Costa 1987, Ekblad et al 1990)

Somatostatin 14 (the neural peptide) is N-terminally extended to somatostatin 28 (the endocrine peptide) which retards degradation and prolongs action. The somatostatin 14 structure is conserved across birds, fishes and mammals, with structural variations in the lower vertebrate somatostatins. Preprosomatostatin has a single copy of somatostatin 28 and post-translates into 28 or 14 depending on the cell type. Mucosal endocrine cells produce mainly somatostatin 28 while enteric nerves predominately produce somatostatin 14. Somatostatin nerve cell bodies in the guinea pig sympathetic ganglia project to the submucous plexus and the villi. Populations of cell bodies in the myenteric plexus project:

a. distally in the plexus;
b. downward to the submucous plexus;
c. downward to the villi;
d. within the same myenteric ganglia.

Cell bodies in the submucous plexus have projections, also containing choline acyl transferase, CCK, CGRP and NPY, extending to the villi. In the rat myenteric plexus somatostatin containing nerves have short distal projections, while those in the dog are longer.

Sites and mechanisms of enteric actions (Dockray 1992, Daniel et al 1989b, Ekblad et al 1990)

Somatostatin acts mainly as an inhibitory interneuronal transmitter in controlling motility. Hypopolarization to somatostatin results from an increase in an inwardly rectifying K^+ conductance in guinea pig submucous plexus nerves, depolarization results from an inactivation of a resting K^+ conductance in myenteric plexus neurons while inhibition of cAMP occurs elsewhere.

Intravenous somatostatin reduces gastric emptying, initiates fasting jejunal phase III of the MMC in man during fasting and in dogs during fasting and in the fed state. Intra-arterial somatostatin stimulates canine ileal motility concomitant with inhibition of tonic VIP levels, by a direct smooth muscle action and by inhibiting NO and VIP release which may explain phase III generation. In the rat, intracerbroventricular somatostatin increased the frequency of phase III activity. In the rat colon, somatostatin enhanced VIP release and descending relaxation. Somatostatin had no effect on neurally-stimulated contractions of the isolated human appendix.

CALCITONIN GENE RELATED PEPTIDE
(CGRP) (Fox 1989b, Ekblad et al 1990, McDonald 1990b, Dockray 1992)

CGRP is a neuropeptide with potent vasodilatory actions when co-released with SP from peripheral sensory nerves, where it increases vasodilation but not vasopermeability in the triple response.

Peptide structure, precursors, localization and receptor subtypes

CGRPα, co-expressed in sensory nerves with SP, results from alternate mRNA processing of the precursors from the calcitonin gene and CGRP β, expressed in enteric nerves from a gene not encoding for calcitonin.

In the guinea pig and rat CGRP/SP-containing capsaicin afferent nerves have their cell bodies in the dorsal root ganglia and project to the submucosa and the blood vessels. Intrinsic nerves in the guinea pig myenteric and submucous plexus contain, as well choline acyl transferase, CCK, NPY and somatostatin and project to the mucosa. In the rat small and large intestine myenteric plexus, cell bodies have projections to the muscle. Myenteric plexus neurons also project orally and anally in the small intestine, but only anally in the large intestine.

No CGRP-receptor subtypes have been identified, but with amino acid differences between human α and β CGRP and the finding that β but not α human CGRP stimulates acid secretion in man this suggests multiple receptor types.

Enteric actions, sites and mechanisms of actions along the gastrointestinal tract

Low concentrations of CGRP relax rat and guinea pig ileal longitudinal muscle, an action mimicked by capsaicin treatment, suggesting sensory release of CGRP, since co-released SP contracts. CGRP relaxed the precontracted isolated guinea pig ileal cells by increasing cAMP, and excited strips of muscle by releasing ACh and histamine. CGRP depolarized AH/type 2 neurons mimicking slow synaptic depolarization. The interactions between endogenous release of CGRP and SP in inflamed enteric tissues have not been studied.

GASTRIN/CHOLYCYSTOKININ (CCK)

The mammalian members of this family of peptides (Table 6.1) are found in both nerves and endocrine cells.

Peptide structure, precursors, localization and receptor subtypes (Dockray 1992, Daniel et al 1989b, Allescher & Ahmad 1990, Furness et al 1992)

Gastrin, CCK and caerulein share the biologically active C-terminal pentapeptide, R-Gly-Trp-Met-Asp-Phe-NH$_2$, which has the Tyr sulphated. Gastrin is exclusive to gut endocrine cells, while CCK is found in endocrine cells and enteric nerves. Some gastrin and CCK nerves of the CNS project to the gut. Gastrin and CCK genes have been cloned and precursor proteins identified.

In the guinea pig ileum, sparse separate populations of CCK nerve cell bodies have projections:

a. to the sympathetic ganglia;
b. distal in the plexus;
c. deep in the circular muscle;
d. deep in the villi.

CCK-containing cells in the submucosa project to the mucosa and these also contain ACh, CGRP, dynorphin, NPY, somatostatin, neuromedin U and sometimes galanin, and may affect water and electrolyte secretion.

Receptor subtypes have the following differences: CCK-A receptors have an agonist preference of CCK-8 > > > gastrin, and the modified benzodiazopine L-364,718 antagonist has a 55-fold higher affinity for CCK-A receptors than CCK-B receptors; CCK-B receptors have a preference of CCK (10X) > gastrin, and the antagonist L-365, 260 has a 90-fold higher affinity for CCK-B receptors than CCK-A receptors. Gastrin receptors supposedly recognize CCK and gastrin equally, but since the CCK-B antagonist has the same affinity for gastrin as CCK-8, the gastrin and CCK-B receptor may be the same.

Sites and mechanisms of enteric actions (Daniel et al 1989b, Fox-Threlkeld 1990, Allescher & Ahmad 1990, Dockray 1992)

Exogenous CCK or gastrin stimulate motor activity by direct action on smooth muscle and release of excitatory transmitters. Inhibitory responses result from release of inhibitory transmitters. The well-documented receptors on isolated smooth muscle cells of the stomach and gallbladder appear to be downregulated in vivo and excitation results from cholinergic nerve stimulation. Occupation of CCK-A receptors releases ACh to produce phasic activity, while occupation of CCK-B receptors releases SP to produce a tonic response in the guinea pig ileum (Forno et al 1992).

Excitation of isolated circular muscle cells appears to be only partially dependent on entrance of extracellular Ca^{2+} and may mobilize inositol trisphosphate as a second messenger.

Exogenous gastrin and CCK in the cat and man decreased LOS resting tone by releasing inhibitory transmitters. In the cat, after neural blockade, direct muscle excitation occurred. The upper stomach was excited and the antrum inhibited by exogenous gastrin and CCK in vivo, in most species tested, while excitation occurs in vitro. The pylorus was also contracted in man and dog but relaxed in the cat. Direct smooth muscle effects were excitatory in the dog. The potent inhibition of gastric emptying by CCK was attributed to the decrease in antral contractions coupled with a decreased pyloric opening and decreased duodenal contractions. Exogenous CCK or gastrin convert the fasted pattern to the fed pattern. Colonic motility is increased by CCK in vivo and in vitro. CCK gets its name from its ability to contract the gallbladder and concomitantly relax the sphincter of Oddi so increasing gallbladder emptying.

The endogenous effects attributed to CCK and gastrin, listed in Table 6.5, can only be demonstrated with CCK-A antagonists. The action of CCK-B antagonists, originally presumed to act preferentially on central receptors requires examination, since there is increasing evidence for peripheral CCK-B receptors. The following exogenous actions of CCK or gastrin could not be confirmed by, primarily, CCK-A antagonists: a role in LOS tone; decreased gastric emptying of saline, acid or osmotic agents in the rat, and de-

Table 6.5 Endogenous effects of CCK/gastrin demonstrated by antagonists

Site	Species	Action	Antagonist
Stomach	Rat, Cat, Man	Increased gastric emptying	CCK-A
Small intestine	Dog	Reduced postprandial activity	CCK-A
Colon	Man	Reduced transit time	CCK-A
Gallbladder	Man	Maintains resting tone	CCK-A
		Meal induced contractions	

Dockray 1992

creased emptying of peptones in the cat; a role in acid-induced pyloric sphincter contractions in the dog; a role in a small intestinal transit, and a role in the gastrocolic reflex.

CONCLUSION

Since the explosive increase in the number of known peptides in the early 1970s a great deal has been learned about their location, what controls their release, what types of receptors they stimulate, what the intracellular second mechanisms of their actions are, and what addition of these peptides do to many experimental preparations ranging from intact man to isolated cell. However, information about what these peptides actually do when they are released locally is lacking. This will only come with the advent of the potent non-peptide antagonists, some of which are becoming available.

REFERENCES

Ahmad S, Allescher H-D, Kwan C-Y 1990 Receptors for neuropeptides: ligand binding studies in: Daniel E E (ed.) Neuropeptide function in the gastrointestinal tract. CRC Press, Baton Rouge, FL, pp 209–230

Allescher H-D, Ahmad S 1990 Postulated physiological and pathophysiological roles on motility in: Daniel E E (ed.) Neuropeptide function in the gastrointestinal tract. CRC Press, Baton Rouge, FL, pp 309–400

Burcher E, Mussap C J, Geraghty D P, McLure-Sharp J M, Watkins D J 1991 Concepts in characterization of tachykinin receptors. Ann N Y Acad Sci 632: 123–136

Catnach S M, Fairclough P D, Trembath R C et al 1992 Effect of oral erythromycin on gallbladder motility in normal subjects and subjects with gallstones. Gastroenterology 102: 2071–2076

Checler F 1990 Peptidases and neuropeptide-inactivating mechanisms in the circulation and in the gastrointestinal tract in: Daniel E E (ed.) Neuropeptide function in the gastrointestinal tract. CRC Press, Baton Rouge, FL, pp 273–308

Daniel E E, Collins S M, Fox J E T, Huizinga J D 1989a Pharmacology of drugs acting on gastrointestinal motility in: Schultz S G, Wood J D, Rauner B B (eds) Handbook of Physiology, Section 6 The Gastrointestinal System American Physiological Society, Bethesda, MD pp 715–758

Daniel E E, Collins S M, Fox J E T, Huizinga J D 1989b Pharmacology of neuroendocrine peptides in: Schultz S G, Wood J D, Rauner B B (eds) Handbook of Physiology, Section 6 The Gastrointestinal System. American Physiological Society, Bethesda, MD pp 759–816

Daniel E E, Fox-Threlkeld J E T 1992 Role of opioid receptor subtypes in control of gastrointestinal motility in: Holle G E Advances in the innervation of the gastrointestinal tract. Demeter Verlag Grafelfing pp 341–356

Daniel E E, Tomita T, Tsuchida S, Wanatabe M (eds) 1992 Sphincters: normal function – changes in diseases. CRC Press Boca Racon, FL.

Dockray G J 1992 Transmission: peptides 2 in: Burnstock G, Hoyle C H V (eds) Autonomic neuroeffector mechanisms. Harwood Academic Publishers, Chur, Switzerland pp 409–464

Ekblad E, Hakanson R, Sundler F 1990 Microantomy and chemical coding of peptide containing neurons in the digestive tract in: Daniel E E (ed.) Neuropeptide function in the gastrointestinal tract. CRC Press, Baton Rouge, FL, pp 131–179

Ekblad E, Hakanson R, Sundler F 1991 Galanin in enteric nerves in: Hokfelt T, Bartfai T, Jackobitwitz D, Ottoson D (eds) Galanin a multifunctional peptide in the neuro-endocrine system. Macmillan Press, Hampshire pp 135–147

Forno G D, Pierta C, Uriciuoli M, Van Amsterdam F T M et al 1992 Evidence for two cholecystokinin receptors mediating the contraction of the guinea pig isolated ileum longitudinal muscle myenteric plexus. J Pharm Exp Ther 261: 1056–1063

Fox J E T 1989a Mechanisms of motilin excitation as determined by in situ and in vitro studies in Itoh Z (ed.) Motilin. Academic Press, Maebashi, Japan pp 73–89

Fox J E T 1989b Control of gastrointestinal motility by peptides: old peptides, new tricks – new peptides, old tricks. Gastroenterol Clin N Am 18: 163–177

Fox J E T, Collins S M, Daniel E E 1985 Expression of peptide responses depends upon study environment in: Lewin M J M, Bonfils S (eds) Regulatory peptides in digestive, nervous and endocrine systems. INSERM Symposium 25, Elsevier Science Publishers pp 265–268

Fox-Threlkeld J E T 1990 Neuropeptide motor actions vary between in vivo and in vitro experimental conditions in: Daniel E E (ed.) Neuropeptide function in the gastrointestinal tract. CRC Press, Baton Rouge, FL, pp 181–191

Fox-Threlkeld J E T 1991 Galanin and gastrointestinal function in: Hokfelt T, Bartfai T, Jackobitwitz D, Ottoson D (eds) Galanin a multifunctional peptide in the neuro-endocrine system. Macmillan Press, Hampshire, pp 275–286

Fox-Threlkeld J E T, Manaka H, Manaka Y, Cipris S, Daniel E E 1991 Stimulation of circular muscle motility of the isolated perfused canine ileum: relationship to VIP output. Peptides 12: 1039–1045

Fraser R, Shearer T, Fuller J, Horowitz M, Dent J 1992 Intravenous erythromycin overcomes small intestinal feedback on antral, pyloric and duodenal motility. Gastroenterology 103: 114–119

Furness J B & Costa M 1987 The enteric nervous system. Churchill Livingstone, Edinburgh

Furness J B, Bornstein J C, Murphy R, Pompolo S 1992 Roles of peptides in transmission in the enteric nervous system. TINS 15: 66–71

Goldstein A, Naidu A 1989 Multiple opioid receptors: ligand

selectivity profiles and binding site signatures. Mol Pharmacol 36: 265–272

Hokfelt T 1991 Neuropeptides in perspective: the last 10 years. Neuron 7: 867–879

Hokfelt T, Bartfai T, Jackobitwitz D, Ottoson (eds) 1991 Galanin a new multifunctional peptide in the neuro-endocrine system. Werner-Gren International Symposium Series 58, Macmillan Press, Hampshire

Houben H, Denef C 1991 Bombesin receptor antagonists and their use in the evaluation of paracrine and autocrine intercellular communication in: Agarwal M K (ed.) Antihormones in health and disease. Front Horm Res, Basel Karger, Basel pp 176–195

Humphries H K, Flemming N W 1992 Opioid induced spasm of the sphincter of Oddi apparently reversed by nalbuphine. Anesth Analg 74: 308–310

Itoh Z 1989 Motilin. Academic Press, Maebashi, Japan

Janssens J, Peeters T L, Vantrappen G et al 1990 Improvement of gastric emptying in diabetic emptying by erythromycin–preliminary studies. N Engl J Med 322: 1028–1031

Kostka P 1990 Gastrointestinal neuropeptides and second messenger systems in: Daniel E E (ed) Neuropeptide function in the gastrointestinal tract. CRC Press, Baton Rouge, FL, pp 249–272

Kupfferman I 1991 Functional studies of cotransmission. Physiol Rev 71: 683–732

Leeman S E, Krause J E, Lembeck F (eds) 1991 Substance P and related peptides. Ann NY Acad Med

Manara L, Biachetti A 1985 The central and peripheral influences of opioids on gastrointestinal propulsion Annu Rev Pharmacol Toxicol 25: 249–273

Mao Y K, Burnett W, Coy D H, Tougas G, Daniel E E 1991 Distribution of vasoactive intestinal polypeptide (VIP)-binding in circular muscle and characterization of VIP-binding in canine small intestinal mucosa. J Pharmacol Exp Therap 258: 986–991

McDonald T J 1990a A historical overview of the gastroenteropancreatic regulatory peptides in: Daniel E E (ed.) Neuropeptide function in the gastrointestinal tract. CRC Press, Baton Rouge, FL, pp 1–18

McDonald T J 1990b Gastroenteropancreatic regulatory peptide structures: an overview in: Daniel E E (ed.)

Neuropeptide function in the gastrointestinal tract. CRC Press, Baton Rouge, FL, pp 19–86

McIntosh C H S, Brown J C 1990 Motilin: isolation, secretion, actions and pathophysiology in: Scarpingnato C, Bianchi Porro G (eds) Clinical investigation of gastric function. Front Gastrointest Res 17: 307–352

Moncada S 1992 The L-arginine: nitric oxide pathway. Acta Physiol Scand 145: 201–227

Niderau C, Faber S, Karaus M 1992 Cholecystokin's role in regulation of colonic motility in health and in irritable bowel syndrome. Gastroenterology 102: 1889–1898

North R A 1986 Opioid receptor types and membrane ion channels. TINS 7: 114–117

North R A, Williams J T, Supernant A M, Christie M J 1987 μ and δ receptors belong to a family of receptors that are coupled to potassium channels. Proc Natl Acad Sci USA 84: 5487–5491

Pomeranz I S, Davison J S, Shaffer E A 1983 In vitro effects of pancreatic polypetide and motilin on contractility of human gallbladde. Dig Dis Sci 28: 539–544

Rokaeus A, Waschek J A 1991 Cloning and expression of porcine and bovine galanin in: Hokfelt T, Bartfai T, Jackobitwitz D, Ottoson D (eds) Galanin a multifunctional peptide in the neuro-endocrine system. Macmillan Press, Hampshire, pp 27–36

Sheikh S 1991 Neuropeptide Y and peptide YY: major modulators of gastrointestinal blood flow and function. Am J Physiol 261: G701–G715

Stark M E, Szurszewski J H 1992 Role of nitric oxide in gastrointestinal and hepatic function and disease. Gastroenterology 102: 1928–1949

Sternini C 1991 Tachykinin and calcitonin gene-related peptide immunoreactivities and MRNA's in the mammalian enteric nervous system and sensory ganglia in: Costa M (ed.) Sensory nerves and neuropeptides in gastroenterology. Plenum Press, New York, pp 39–51

Swain M G, Agro A, Blennerhassett P, Stanisz A, Collins S M 1992 Increased levels of substance P in the myenteric plexus of trichinella infected rats. Gastroenterology 102: 1913–1919

Vincent J-P, Kitabgi P 1990 Receptors for neuropeptides: receptor isolation studies and molecular biology in: Daniel E E (ed.) Neuropeptide function in the gastrointestinal tract. CRC Press, Baton Rouge, FL, pp 231–248

Modulating factors

7. Modulation of motor activity by sleep

D. Kumar

INTRODUCTION

The human gastrointestinal tract exhibits phasic and period motor activity comprised of three phases; phase I of motor quiesence, phase II of irregular activity and phase III of regular sustained contractions at a frequency of 9–12 per min. This periodic activity has been described as a motor complex which travels down the intestine with a periodicity of 90–120 min. The interdigestive motor activity is disrupted by food. Ingestion of a meal produces intense irregular activity that lasts for 3–4 h. The CNS is functionally characterized by the rapid eye movement (REM) and non-REM sleep cycle. Both of these biorhythms are marked by repetitive brief phases of maximal activity. In humans, the periodicity of these activities is similar; this similarity raises the possibility that they are driven by the same oscillator and indeed this has been suggested by a previous report (Finch et al 1982). This hypothesis has profound physiological implications in that if there is a common oscillator then either the brain controls the gut or the gut controls the brain, or both are under the control of some other as yet unidentified oscillator. It seems improbable that the brain is under the dominance of the gut; the opposing proposition suggests that gut function is subservient to the brain. This is indirectly supported by the observations that the motor activity of gastrointestinal tract in man is modified during sleep. During wakefulness, the effect of stimuli such as stress and meals is superimposed on the basal activity and reflects the effect of these stimuli on what can be regarded as normal human intestinal motility. The motor rhythm in the gut is more regular at night and this suggests possible interactions between sleep and gastrointestinal motor activity. This interaction between sleep and gastrointestinal motility can take place in three different states:

1. Fasting state
2. Postprandial state
3. Interaction between the two biorhythms.

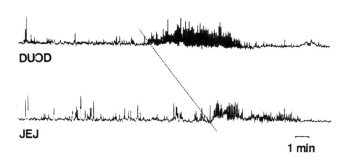

DIURNAL MMC (AWAKE)

DUOD

JEJ

1 min

NOCTURNAL MMC (ASLEEP)

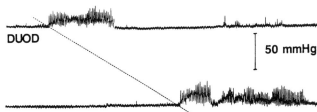

DUOD

50 mmHg

JEJ

Fig. 7.1 Examples of diurnal and nocturnal MMC in the proximal small bowel. Diagonal lines, marking onset of phase III in each example illustrate circadian variation in migration velocity of phase III. Vigorous irregular contractile activity (phase II) precedes phase III in the waking record but is absent in the sleeping record.

FASTING STATE

Phase II activity

During sleep, phase II of the migrating motor complex (MMC) cycle is virtually absent (Gill et al 1987). The duration of phase II activity is significantly reduced both during diurnal and nocturnal sleep (Table 7.1) (Kumar et al 1990a). During sleep, it is often impossible to differentiate between phase I and phase II

Table 7.1 Characteristics of MMC during 24-hour recording that included either regular or reversed sleep cycle

	MMC period [min]	Phase II duration [min]
Regular sleep cycle		
Awake	141 ± 60	123 ± 62
Asleep	105 ± 39	3 + 6
Significance	P < 0.02	P < 0.009
Reversed sleep cycle		
Awake	109 ± 30	81 ± 32
Asleep	76 ± 12	25 ± 22
Significance	P < 0.03	P < 0.02

Values are means ± SE

activity because the majority of phase III fronts are preceded by motor quiesence (Fig. 7.1). This suggests a CNS modulation for phase II activity. Phase II activity is absent during sleep when CNS function is diminished, and present during waking when there is CNS arousal. Other factors such as psychological stress and the presence of luminal contents that is sufficient to sustain the post prandial response may also be implicated in the longer duration of phase II activity seen during the day.

In a 24-h manometric recording of colonic motor activity in healthy man, Narducci et al (1987) showed that the motility index decreased significantly during sleep; phases of motor quiescence lasted up to 2 h (Fig. 7.2) and were interrupted by little motor activity during the night, when the subjects slept. Similar findings have been reported by Frexinos et al (1985) in the myoelectric spiking activity of the human colon.

Phase III activity

Phase III fronts occur more regularly during sleep and the MMC cycle length is significantly shorter when compared to that seen during wakefulness (Kumar et al 1990a). These differences are maintained when the sleep cycle is reversed and the subjects are sleeping during the day (Table 7.1).

In addition to variations in cycle length, the human MMC exhibits a significant variation in propagation velocities between wakefulness and sleep (Kumar et al 1986). Similar observations were made for MMCs in healthy sheep and pigs supplied with adlibitum rations each morning and adapted to a 12-light, 12-dark schedule. In all species, the nocturnal velocity of MMC propagation in the proximal small bowel was lower than the diurnal velocity. In man, diurnal velocity was more than double nocturnal velocity (Fig. 7.1), whereas in the ruminants the ratio of diurnal to nocturnal

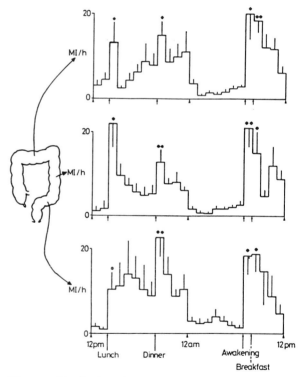

Fig. 7.2 Motility index/hour of the colon during the 24-h recording period. Asterisks indicate significant differences (*p < 0.05, **p < 0.01) in respect to the fasting and pre-waking values. (From Narducci et al 1987 with permission.)

velocity was 1.5:1. When the distribution of MMCs was plotted in relation to time, it was obvious that the velocities varied in an approximately sinosoidal form (Fig. 7.3a,b). These data support the concept of a circadian variation in mammalian MMC propagation

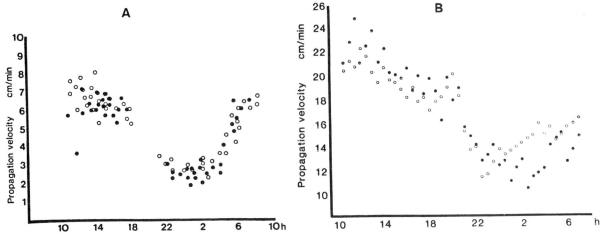

Fig. 7.3 A Propagation velocity of human MMCs in relation to time. Filled circles represent patients with IBS and open circles represent normal subjects. From Kumar et al (1986) with permission. **B** Propagation velocity of porcine MMCs in relation to time. Filled circles denote pigs fed at 8 a.m. and open circles fed at 8 p.m.

velocity rather than the function of variation in intraluminal content.

POSTPRANDIAL STATE

Ingestion of a meal disrupts fasting periodic motor activity in humans and other mammalian species by inducing a postprandial pattern of recurrent but irregular contractions (Code & Marlett 1975, Vantrappen et al 1977). It has been shown in a canine model that the initiation and maintenance of a postprandial pattern is dependent on vagal integrity (Hall et al 1986) and that acute vagal blockade abolishes postprandial motor activity (Chung & Diamant 1987). In humans, vagotomy delays the onset of postprandial activity and shortens its duration (Thompson et al 1982). Other factors such as extrinsic nerves, luminal stimuli and humoral factors have also been implicated in the modulation of postprandial activity. The duration of the postprandial pattern also appears to depend on the volume, caloric content and the distribution of calories in the ingested food (Schang et al 1978, Wingate et al 1979). Recently, the role of sleep in the modulation of the duration of human postprandial motor activity has been reported (Kumar et al 1989). The effect of the presence of food in the gastrointestinal tract on proximal small bowel motility during sleep was measured in eight healthy ambulant subjects. The subjects ate a standard 540 kcal evening meal on the first day. On the following day they ate a similar meal at lunchtime and then another standard meal late in the evening 15 min before going to bed. In this study, the duration of

postprandial activity was significantly (p < 0.001) shortened after a late meal, but there was no difference in the postprandial activity after lunch and an evening meal. At the end of the postprandial pattern, the subsequent fasting pattern following the three meals did not show any differences in the MMC characteristics. MMC cycle lengths were similar as was the duration of phase II of the MMC cycle. These data showed that in healthy subjects postprandial activity was diminished during sleep whereas the consumption of a late meal restored the phase II activity usually absent during sleep (Fig. 7.4). This altered postprandial response during sleep may have important clinical implications. This may be particularly relevant in night shift workers and people travelling across several time zones. It is possible that in our study the onset of sleep immediately after the ingestion of a meal suppressed vagal activity thereby reducing the motor response to food. The other intriguing observation from this study was the persistence of phase II activity after the onset of sleep after a late meal. It would appear that in addition to CNS arousal there are other factors modulating phase II activity of the MMC cycle. Slow gastric emptying during sleep may have contributed to the prolongation of phase II activity in that the amount of nutrient stimulus received by the upper small intestine was not enough to disrupt the fasting MMC cycle but was enough to contribute a regular phasic activity preceding each MMC cycle. Food in the gastrointestinal tract during sleep appears to be received as in the vagally denervated gut. Postprandial motor activity in the small bowel is modulated both by CNS arousal

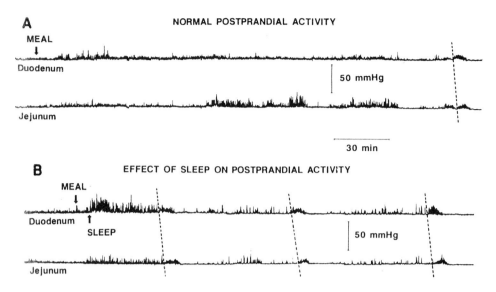

Fig. 7.4 **A** Normal response to a meal in a healthy subject. **B** Effect of sleep on postprandial activity after a late meal. Phase III activity is indicated by broken lines showing onset of phase III at each of the two sensors. Note return of phase III activity fronts approximately 40 min after subject went to bed. Also note the presence of phase II activity preceding nocturnal phase IIIs.

and by nutrients stimulation of receptors in the small bowel. These changes may be relevant to the patho-physiology and management of gastrointestinal dysfunction and disease.

RELATIONSHIP BETWEEN TWO BIORHYTHMS

Several studies on the relationship between the two biorhythms have produced contradictory results (Helm et al 1948, Lavie et al 1978, Yaruyra-Tobias et al 1970). Since the two biorhythms, MMC cycle and the REM–non-REM sleep cycle, have similar periodicities, it is tempting to hypothesize that the two rhythms are interrelated. In a recent study Kumar et al (1990a) tested the validity of this hypothesis by creating experimental conditions where the sleep cycle was acutely reversed. If there was a true relationship between the two biorhythms, it would become apparent by maintaining that relationship when the sleep cycle is reversed. Kumar et al (1990a) did not report either a modulatory relationship or an association between the two major biorhythms. The absence of such a correlation between the two biorhythms both during a regular sleep cycle and a reversed sleep cycle strongly suggested that the two cycles are independent of each other. The distribution of the various sleep stages and MMCs is shown in Fig. 7.5 and the proportion of

REM and non-REM sleep for day and night time sleep and the total number of MMCs occuring in REM and non-REM sleep is shown in Fig. 7.6. The number of MMCs in any given sleep stage was directly proportional to the percentage of total sleep time occupied by that sleep stage (Fig. 7.7). This distribution was maintained during diurnal sleep. These data support the lack of association between human MMCs and REM episodes.

Periodic motor activity has also been described in the human rectum (Kumar et al 1990c). This periodic activity occurs in the form of rectal motor complexes (RMCs) which are seen as bursts of powerful contractions resembling phase III of the small bowel MMC. The RMCs also occur more regularly during sleep and the cycle length is shorter. Since the MMC cycle and the RMCs are more regular during sleep and exhibit periodic activity, we tested the hypothesis of a common control mechanism for the two rhythms by prolonged simultaneous recording of small bowel and rectal motor activity in eight healthy adults. The number of RMCs and MMCs was identical in two subjects and differed by only one in five other subjects (Fig. 7.8). Both RMCs and MMCs were less frequent in the first 12 h in which the subjects were awake and consumed main meals. There was no obvious relationship between the timing of RMCs and MMCs. The association of the RMC cycle with the REM and non-REM brain cycle

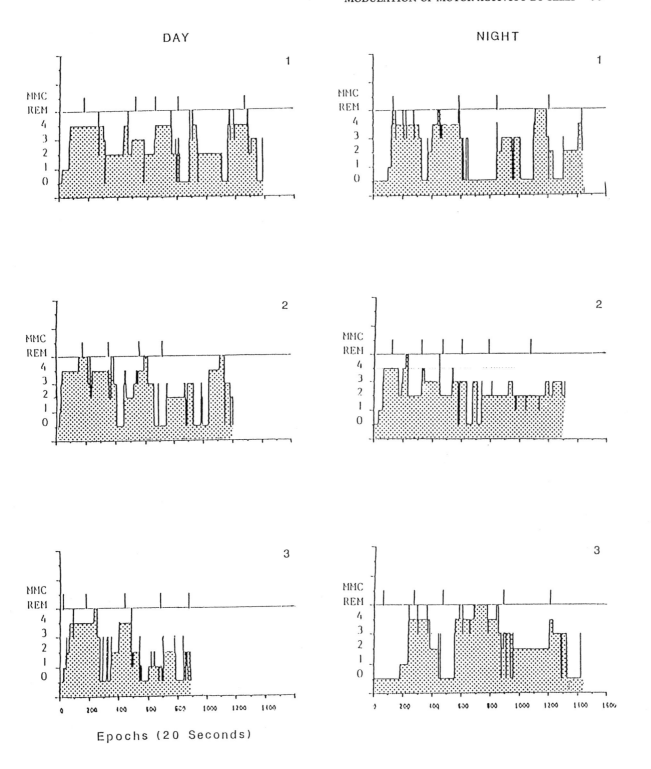

Fig. 7.5 Distribution of MMCs in real time (20-s epox on X axis for different sleep stages in three healthy subjects during normal (right) and reversed (left) sleep. Upper vertical bars indicate timing of duodenojejunal phase III of MMCs.

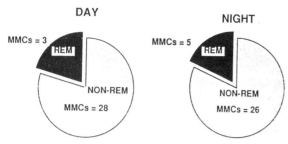

Fig. 7.6 Proportions of REM and non-REM sleep for day and night time sleep and total number of MMCs occurring in REM and non-REM sleep.

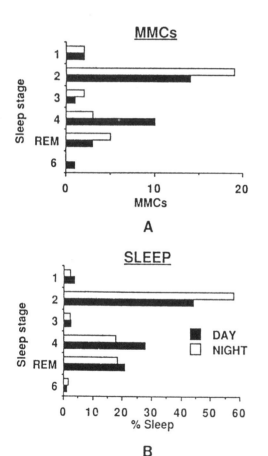

Fig. 7.7 **A** Total number of MMCs in various sleep stages for diurnal and nocturnal sleep. **B** Percentage of total sleep time occupied by various sleep stages during diurnal and nocturnal sleep.

remains to be formally tested, but the occurrence of RMCs in the waking state when the REM and non-REM cycle is abolished is against this possibility.

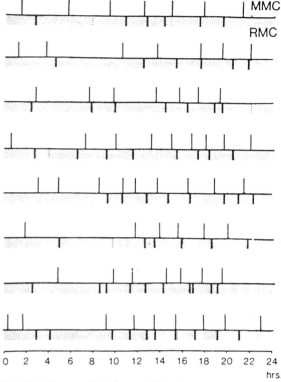

Fig. 7.8 Temporal incidence of MMCs and RMCs. Each line represents a single subject; timing of onset in duodenum of phase III of MMC is indicated by vertical bar above the line and of RMC by vertical bar below the line. Horizontal scale shows time elapsed (in hours) from onset of recording.

Effect of a late meal on REM–non-REM sleep

The modulation of the duration of human postprandial motor activity by sleep has been documented (Kumar et al 1989). Whether the presence of food in the gastrointestinal tract during sleep had any modulatory effect on the REM–non REM sleep activity was recently investigated in eight healthy subjects (Kumar et al 1991). The subjects ate a standard 600 kcal meal at 6 p.m. on the first day and 15 min before going to bed on the second day. The percentage of total sleep time occupied by REM sleep was similar for the two nights. However, REM latency after a late meal was significantly shorter ($p < 0.01$) whereas stage 2 and 3/4 did not differ significantly between the two nights. A late meal followed by sleep appears to modify the REM–non-REM sleep cycle. These data strongly suggest that the interaction between the CNS and enteric nervous system (ENS) not only takes place during wakefulness but also during sleep.

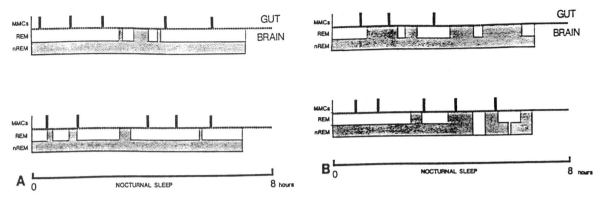

Fig. 7.9 Schematic representation of incidence of MMCs and REM sleep in **A** two healthy controls and **B** two patients with IBS. The incidence of MMC phase III is indicated by vertical black bars above the broken line; the shaded areas below the line indicate sleep. Zero time is the onset of sleep in all subjects. The duration of sleep is similar in all four subjects; in one of the patients with IBS, two episodes of waking occurred during the night. Both show increased duration of REM sleep episodes as compared with the controls.

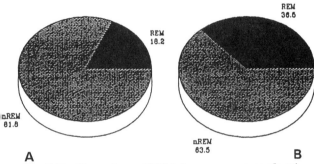

Fig. 7.10 Comparisons of REM sleep as percentage of total sleep in controls (**A**) and patients with IBS (**B**).

Sleep and the irritable bowel syndrome

An intermittent small bowel dysrhythmia has recently been described in the irritable bowel syndrome (IBS) (Kumar & Wingate 1985, Kellow & Phillips 1987, Kellow et al 1990). A feature of this abnormality is that it is absent during sleep; this suggests that although enteric motility is programmed at the level of the ENS, CNS arousal is a required element in the expression of the disorder. In health, the intestinal (MMC) and sleep (REM–non-REM) biorhythms have been shown to be asynchronous (Kumar et al 1990a). Perturbation of enteric motor activity has been shown in the IBS; comparable data for the CNS are lacking. In a recent study, the hypothesis that CNS arousal is a necessary condition for expression of the IBS and that it may reflect inappropriate brain gut interaction was tested further by synchronous sleep and upper small bowel motility measurements in six healthy subjects and six patients with IBS (Kumar et al 1992). During sleep, there was no difference in intestinal motility between the two groups. As previously discussed, there

was no temporal relationship between phase III activity and REM sleep in either group (Fig. 7.9). The total duration of sleep was similar between the two groups, but in five of the six IBS patients, REM sleep occupied more than 25% of the total sleep time. This is above the generally accepted upper limit of the normal range (Jouvet 1969). The difference in REM sleep between control and IBS subjects (Fig. 7.10) was statistically significant ($p < 0.01$). The increase in REM sleep was a result of longer periods of REM sleep; the number of REM episodes and the REM latency did not differ significantly between the two groups, nor did the number of MMCs during sleep. These data raise the question of whether IBS is a result of abnormal CNS function rather than a disorder of gut function. The demonstration of abnormal CNS function in IBS is consistent with the clinical impression of psychopathology in IBS, supported by a detailed study of this subject (Hislop 1971). However, one recent study showed that the incidence of psychoneurosis is similar in patients with abdominal pain and altered bowel habit irrespective of the organic or functional relation of these symptoms (Smith et al 1990) whereas another study of patients in whom small bowel motor abnormalities have been documented showed only an excessive level of anxiety but not depression as compared with patients with organic gut disorders (Kumar et al 1990b).

Thus, it appears that patients with IBS have CNS dysfunction. Motor abnormalities disappear during sleep in the absence of CNS arousal as does sensory perception whereas perturbation of the CNS by mental stress potentiates motor abnormalities and symptoms. The hypothesis that the CNS dysfunction is secondary to a primary gut abnormality, however, unlikely it may seem, can only be tested by a formal study of sleep in other enteric disorders.

IS IT IMPORTANT TO RECORD MOTILITY DURING SLEEP?

One of the most important aims of measuring gastrointestinal motor activity is to be able to distinguish between normal and abnormal motor activity. The 'normal range' for motor activity in the gastrointestinal tract is constantly challenged as more studies are carried out in different parts of the world under different circumstances. Most of the observed variation in the so-called normal activity is seen during waking hours.

Even with the advent of newer techniques that allow prolonged and ambulant monitoring (Gill et al 1990), very few studies report data that include a period of normal sleep. It is now well documented that CNS arousal and factors such as psychological stress can modify fasting and possibly even postprandial motor activity resulting in a paroxysmal abnormality of motor function (Kumar & Wingate 1985, Valori et al 1986). Since we know that during sleep in the absence of CNS arousal, paroxysmal abnormalities of motor activity are absent, motility measurements during sleep may be the most reliable way (Fig. 7.11) of differentiating between normal motor activity, paroxysmal disorders and organic pathology such as neuropathies and myopathies.

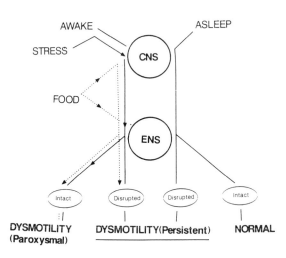

Fig. 7.11   A schematic diagram showing how sleep recordings can help to differentiate between normal and abnormal motility.

REFERENCES

Chung S A, Diamant N E 1987 Small intestinal motility in fasted and post prandial states; effect of transient vagosympathetic blockade. Am J Physiol 252: G301–G308

Code C F, Marlett J A 1975 The interdigestive myoelectric complex of the stomach and small bowel of dogs. J Physiol Lond 246: 289–309

Finch P M, Ingram D M, Henstridge J D, Catchpole B N 1982 Relationship of fasting gastroduodenal motility to the sleep cycle. Gastroenterology 83: 605–612

Frexinos J, Bueno L, Fioramonti J 1985 Diurnal changes in myoelectric spiking activity of human colon. Gastroenterology 88: 1104–1110

Gill R C, Kellow J E, Wingate D L 1987 The migrating motor complex (MMC) at home. Gastroenterology 92: 1405

Gill R C, Kellow J E, Browning C, Wingate D L 1990 The use of intraluminal strain-gauges for recording ambulant small bowel manometry. Am J Physiol 258: G610–G615

Hall K E, El-Sharkawy T Y, Diamant N E 1986 Vagal control of canine postprandial upper gastrointestinal motility. Am J Physiol (Gastrointest Liver Physiol 13) G501–G510

Helm J D, Kramer D P, MacDonald R M, Ingelfinger F J 1948 Changes in motility of the human small intestine during sleep. Gastroenterology 10: 135–137

Hislop I G 1971 Psychological significance of the irritable bowel syndrome. Gut 12: 452–457

Jouvet M 1969 Biogenic amines and the states of sleep. Science 163: 32–41

Kellow J E, Phillips S F 1987 Altered small bowel motility in irritable bowel syndrome is correlated with symptoms.

Gastroenterology 92: 1885–1893

Kellow J E, Gill R C, Wingate D L 1990 Prolonged ambulant manometry of small bowel motility demonstrates abnormalities in irritable bowel syndrome. Gastroenterology 98: 1208–1218

Kumar D, Wingate D L 1985 The irritable bowel syndrome: a paroxysmal motor disorder. Lancet 2: 973–977

Kumar D, Wingate D, Ruckebusch Y 1986 Circadian variation in the propagation velocity of the migrating motor complex. Gastroenterology 91: 926–930

Kumar D, Soffer E E, Wingate D L, Britto J, Das-Gupta A, Mridha K 1989 Modulation of the duration of human prostprandial motor activity by sleep. Am J Physiol 256: G851–G855

Kumar D, Idzikowski C, Wingate D L, Soffer E E, Thompson P, Siderfin C 1990a Relationship between enteric migrating motor complex and the sleep cycle. Am J Physiol 259, G983–G990

Kumar D, Pfeffer J, Wingate D L 1990b Role of psychological factors in the irritable bowel syndrome. Digestion 45: 80–87

Kumar D, Thompson P D, Wingate D L 1990c Absence of synchrony between human small intestinal migrating motor complex and rectal complex. Am J Physiol 258 (Gastrointest. Liver Physiol 21): G171–G172

Kumar D, Thompson P D, Wingate D L, Vesselinova-Jenkins C K, Libby G 1992 Abnormal REM sleep in the irritable bowel syndrome. Gastroenterology 103: 12–17

Kumar D, Tsang G, James R 1991 Impact of a late meal on rapid eye movement/non-rapid eye movement sleep activity. Gut 32: A1248

Lavie P, Kripke D F, Hiatt J F, Harrison J 1978 Gastric rhythms during sleep. Behav Biol 23: 526–530

Narducci F, Bassoti G, Gaburri M, Morelli A 1987 Twenty four hours manometric recording of colonic motor activity in healthy man. Gut 28: 17–25

Schang J C, Dauchel J, Sava P, Angel F, Grenier J F 1978 Specific effects of different food components on intestinal motility: electromyographic study in dogs. Eur Surg Res 10: 425–432

Smith R C, Greenbaum D S, Vancouver J B et al 1990 Psychosocial factors are associated with health care seeking rather than diagnosis in irritable bowel syndrome. Gastroenterology 98: 293–301

Thompson D G, Ritchie H D, Wingate D L 1982 Patterns of small intestinal motility in duodenal ulcer patients before and after vagotomy. Gut 23: 517–523

Valori R M, Kumar D, Wingate D L 1986 Effects of different types of stress and of prokinetic drugs on control of the fasting motor complex in humans. Gastroenterology 90: 1890–1900

Vantrappen G, Janssens J, Ghoos Y 1977 The interdigestive motor complex of normal subjects and patients with bacterial overgrowth of the small intestine. J Clin Invest 59: 1158–1166

Wingate D L, Pearce E, Ling A, Boucher B, Thompson H, Hutton M 1979 Quantitative effect of oral feeding on gastrointestinal myoelectric activity in the conscious dog. Dig Dis Sci 24: 417–423

Yaruyra-Tobias J A, Hutcheson J S, White L 1970 Relationship between stages of sleep and gastric motility. Behav Neuropsychiatry 2: 22–24

8. Stress and gastrointestinal motility

F. Musial   P. Enck

INTRODUCTION

The term 'stress' in everyday life is often used in situations of challenge or exhaustion associated with feelings of agression or depression. In a psychobiological approach, stress is an intrinsic part of the life of every organism. It is experienced in situations of confrontation with an enemy or a rival in the competition for resources, territories and mates. In this sense, stress is a useful biological instrument which enables the individual to cope with environmental challenges.

The clinician is most likely to be confronted with stress in the form of maladaptive reactions to environmental challenges. Therefore, stress in a clinical setting may be seen as one factor in the aetiology of a disease or a symptom, or as a concommitant factor of disease that affects its course and severity. Furthermore, disease itself has to be considered as a physiological, social and psychological stressor to the individual.

'Functional disorders' – abnormal organ function in the absence of an identified pathological cause – include psychosomatic disorders, and are generally accepted as common manifestations of dysfunction due to stress. Functional disorders are common in the gastroenterology clinic, and frequently the symptoms suggest disordered motility; thus, a link between stress and disturbances in motility seems highly probable. The reality is less certain, because the topic is more complex than it seems at first sight. As will be seen from the first part of this chapter, attempts to validate the relationship using experimental stress paradigms have produced results that appear to be inconsistent. In the subsequent section, we have attempted to show that a more rigorous approach to measuring stress and its effects shows the problem to be complex, and we conclude by considering some aspects that should be considered, but have too often been ignored, in the design of experimental and clinical studies.

EXPERIMENTAL INVESTIGATIONS OF STRESS ON MOTILITY IN HUMANS AND ANIMALS

Oesophagus

Probably the first to describe stress effects on oesophageal motility were Wolf & Almy (1949), who discussed unpleasant life situations with dysphagic patients during fluoroscopy and found non-propulsive contractions. A more recent study by Ayres et al (1989) in healthy volunteers and patients with irritable bowel syndrome compared a psychological stressor (dichotomous listening) to a physical stressor (cold pressor test). The results showed that stress increased the amplitude of contractions and the number of simultaneous contractions. A recent study by Zacchi et al (1992) demonstrated an inhibitory effect of physical but not of mental stress on the lower oesophageal sphincter pressure in healthy humans implying that stress may be associated with an increase in oesophageal reflux. According to Penagini et al (1992), however, the rate of transient lower oesophageal sphincter relaxations was markedly inhibited during the cold pressor test, associated with a decrease in reflux episodes.

Table 8.1 summarizes human research data so far. It becomes evident that stress has a predominantly excitatory effect on the oesophagus. No results of animal studies have been reported.

Stomach

Animal studies

As recently reviewed by Enck & Holtmann (1992), a variety of species (rat, monkey, dog, mouse) and stressors (restraint, foot shock, cold, noise, fear) have been used in animal experiments; 'psychological' components of stress were exhibited only in a minority of studies (Gué et al 1991, Enck et al 1989, Enck & Wienbeck 1989) (Fig. 8.1), but a consistent inhibitory effect of stress on gastric motility and emptying was

Table 8.1   Stress effects on oesophageal motility – human studies

Author, Year	Cont./Pat.*		Stressor applied	Effect observed
Wolf 1949		14	Stress interview	↓ motility: oesophageal body
Rubin 1962	5		Stress interview	↑ non-propulsive contractions
Stacher 1979 (a)	16		Acoustic stimuli	↑ non-propulsive contractions
Stacher 1979 (b)	22		Acoustic stimuli	↑ non-propulsive contractions
Cook 1987	13		Dichotic listening	↑ upper sphincter pressure
Young 1987	14		White noise/CPT	↑ amplitude/velocity of contractions
Soffer 1988	8	8	CPT, delayed AF, VG	No effects, no differences
Anderson 1989	20	19	Noise/cognitive tasks	↑ amplitude of contractions
Cook 1989	13	8	Dichotic listening	↑ upper sphincter pressure
Ayres 1989	17	12	Dichotic listening/CPT	↑ amplitude/simultaneous contraction
Zacchi 1992	10		Dichotic listening/CPT	↓ LOS pressure only with CPT
Penagini 1992	9		CPT	↓ No LOS relaxations, reflux

CPT: cold pressor test; AF: audio feedback; VG: video games; LOS: lower oesophageal sphincter;
*Cont./Pat.: Number of controls and patients studied

Table 8.2   Stress effects of stomach emptying – animal studies

Author/Year	Species	Stressor applied	Effects observed
Glavin 1977	Rat	Restraint, foot shock	↑ (48 h), ↓ (96 h)
Dubois 1978	Monkey	Avoidance	↓
Galligan 1983	Rat	Foot shock	No effect
Costall 1983	Guinea pig	Handling, noise	↓↓
Koo 1985	Rat	Cold	↑ (< 1 h), ↓ (>2 h)
Gué 1987a	Mouse, rat	Cold, noise	↑, ↑
Williams 1988	Rat	Wrap restraint	No effect
Lenz 1988	Rat	Restraint	↓
Taché 1988	Rat	Tail shock	↓
Enck 1988	Rat	Passive avoidance	↓
Gué 1989	Dog	Noise	↓
Gué 1990	Mouse, rat	Noise/cold/restraint	↑ (non-caloric) ↓ (else)

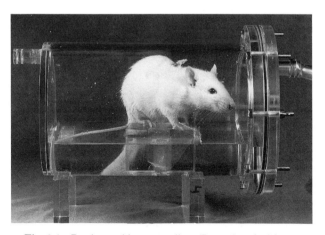

Fig. 8.1   Passive avoidance paradigm (Reproduced with permission from Enck & Wienbeck 1989.)

demonstrated (Fig. 8.2, Table 8.2). As a variety of biochemical studies data have shown, these effects are most likely to be mediated by CNS release of coricotrophin releasing factor (CRF) (Taché et al 1990).

A recent study in dogs showed that 1 h acoustic stress led to an inhibition of the gastric migrating motor complex (MMC) as well as to an increase in plasma cortisol (Fig. 8.3) (Gué et al 1987). In a later study, similar stress effects were inhibited by fedotozine, an opioid agonist (Fig. 8.4) (Gué et al 1990). The authors suggest that the blocking effect may be mediated through κ receptors in the gut wall that activate vagal afferent fibres (Gué et al 1988).

Human studies

In their classical experiment on the fistulated patient

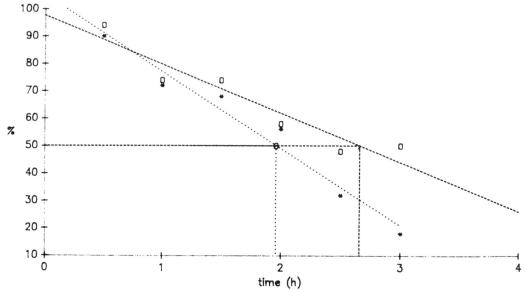

Fig. 8.2 Delayed gastric emptying after passive avoidance in rats. The graph shows the percent of actual food intake of 5 g which remained in the stomach after rest (. . . . . .) and after stress (- - - - - -). A linear regression provided best fit to the data. $T\frac{1}{2}$ was calculated on these functions: 1.97 h after rest and 2.66 h after stress. (Reproduced with permission from Enck et al 1989.)

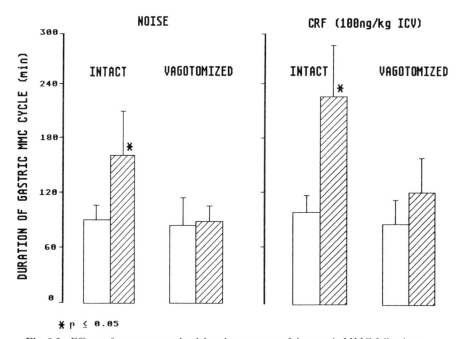

Fig. 8.3 Effects of vagotomy on the delayed occurrence of the gastric MMC following acoustic stress by noise and intracerebroventricular (ICV) injection of CRF (100 ng/kg). The duration of the gastric MMC cycle before (□) and after (■) acoustic stress or ICV administration of CRF (mean ± SD) is indicated. (Reproduced with permission from Gué et al 1987.)

Table 8.3   Stress effects on gastroduodenal motility – human studies

Author/Year	C/P	Technique	Stressor applied	Effect observed
Wittkower 1931	17	Aspiration for GE	Hypnotic emotions	No response
Jungmann 1952	55	Fluoroscope for GM	Noise	↑ No/ampl of C
Davis 1969	19	EGG	Mental arithmetic	↑ ampl. of C
Cann 1983	8	Scintigraphy for GT	CPT, CLS	No change of GE
Stanghellini 1983	6	Manometry for GM	CPT, CLS	↓ antral motility
Camilleri 1984	8	Manometry for GM	TENS	↓ antral motility
Fone 1990		Manometry, GE	CPT	↓ GM, GE

C/P: number of controls, patients studied
GE: gastric emptying; GM: gastric motility; GT: gastric transit; C: contractions; CPT: cold
pressor test; CLS: cold labyrinthine stimulation; TENS: transcutaneous nerve stimulation

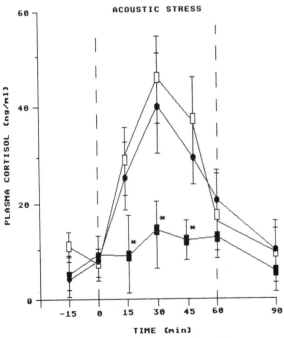

Fig. 8.4   Influence of acoustic stress with or without previous oral (PO) or intravenous (IV) administration of fedotozine on plasma cortisol level in dogs ($n = 4$). ✱ = significantly different ($p < 0.05$) from corresponding control values. (Reproduced with permission from Gué et al 1990.)

Tom, Wolf & Wolff (1943) suggested that gastric motility decreased when the subject was fearful, but increased with anger. This early work showed that the effects might depend on the kind of stressor used in the experiment. A traditional paradigm to induce different emotions is the variation of 'controllability' of the experimental situation. In a study by Davies et al (1969) using the electrogastrogram (EGG) as a non-invasive measurement of gastrointestinal motility, healthy young volunteers were randomly assigned to two different groups. The 'executives' were able to avoid unpleasant noise whereas the controls received the same amount of noise as the 'executives', but were not able to avoid the aversive stimulation. Subjects in the executive group showed more and prolonged EGG responses. Furthermore, Fedor and Russel (1965) found that the unsuccessful avoidance of noise was associated with a greater amplitude of 3 cpm waves in the EGG.

Camilleri et al (1984) showed that transcutaneous electrical nerve stimulation inhibited the postcibal increase in in antral motility in healthy volunteers. In a later study (Camilleri et al 1986) in patients with idiopathic dyspepsia, only patients with normal antral motility prior to stress application showed a regular reduction in antral pressure in response to stress, while in patients with postprandial hypomotility, stress tended to increase antral motility (Fig. 8.5). The results of human studies are summarized in Table 8.3.

Both animal and human studies of the effects of stress on upper gastointestinal functions indicate a predominant inhibition in all species. However, with certain techniques, a dual response – an initial increase and a subsequent delay of emptying – has been observed (Glavin et al 1977, Koo et al 1985). This emphasizes the importance of studying the kinetics of gastric emptying rather than using a single determination of the state of gastric filling, as has been done in most of the animal studies.

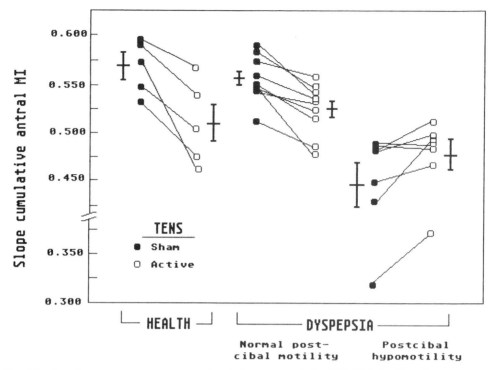

Fig. 8.5 Antral response to transcutaneous electrical nerve stimulation (TENS) in health and functional dyspepsia. Data shown as the slopes of cumulative antral motility indices. Bars refer to mean ± SEM. (Reproduced with permission from Camilleri et al 1986.)

Table 8.4 Stress effects on small bowel transit – animal studies

Author/Year	Species	Stressor	Effect	T[1]	GE[2]
Brown 1966	Rat	Restraint	↓	F	Yes
Galligan 1983	Rat	Foot shock	No effect	C	Yes
Appelbaum 1985	Rat	Restraint	↓	F	Yes
Gué 1987	Mouse, rat	Cold, noise	↑, no effect	C	Yes
Williams 1988	Rat	Restraint	↓	C	No
Lenz 1988	Rat	Restraint	↓	C	No
Enck 1989	Rat	Avoidance	↑	F	Yes
Barone 1990	Rat	Cold restraint	No effect	C	Yes

1. T: Technique to assess transit: marker front (F) or geometric centre (C)
2. GE: confounding gastric emptying (GE) and small bowel transit

Small bowel

Animal studies

One of the major problems of studying the effect of stress on small bowel transit time, is to differentiate between gastric and intestinal effects. Most of the techniques that have been used are not able to do this, (Table 8.4) but confound, for example, a gastric delay with an acceleration in the small bowel, resulting in a net 'zero' effect.

There are few published studies in which canine small bowel motility has been recorded directly in the fasted state (Gué et al 1987, 1988, 1990). The results showed that while stress inhibited the occurrence of gastric phase III, it had no effects on duodenal motility. In the fed state, stress delayed the recovery of the MMC by extending the period of the jejunal postprandial motor activity. There was no change in the amplitude but the frequency of contractions increased.

Table 8.5 Stress effects on small bowel motility – human studies

Author/Year	C/P	Technique	Stressor applied	Effect observed
McRae 1982	7	Manometry	Dichotic listening	↓ No. phase III
Valori 1986	37	Radiotelemetry	DAF, video games	↓ No. phase III
Barcley 1987	15/37	Perfusion for transit	Dichotic listening, CPT	↑ transit time
Holtmann 1989	14	Manometry	Mental arithmetics	↓ No. phase III
Kellow 1992	10/10	Manometry	'Stroop test', problem solving	↓ phase II

C/P: controls, patients studied; DAF: delayed auditory feedback; CPT: cold pressor test

Table 8.6 Stress effects on large bowel transit – animal studies

Author/Year	Species	Technique[1]	Stressor	Effects
Bindra 1953	Rat	Pellets	Foot shock	No effect
Broadhurst 1957	Rat	Pellets	Restraint	↑
Roth 1979	Rat	Pellets	Light/noise	↑
Ossenkopp 1982	Rat	Pellets	Rotation	↑
Galligan 1983	Rat	Transit	Foot shock	No effect
Williams 1988	Rat	Pellets, transit	Restraint	↑
Lenz 1988	Rat	Transit	Restraint	↑
Enck 1989	Rat	Transit	Avoidance	↑
Barone 1990	Rat	Pellets, transit	Restraint	↑

[1] Technique to assess colonic transit: pellet excretion or transit measurement

Human studies

In humans, small bowel transit time is mostly assessed using the hydrogen breath test. But again, this method reflects oro-caecal transit time and is, therefore, confounded by gastric emptying. Intraluminal manometry does not measure transit, but can be used to study patterns of motor activity. A variety of mental stressors have been shown to disturb interdigestive small bowel motility in healthy volunteers, resulting in a decreased number of observed MMCs. Such stressors were dichotomous listening (McRae et al 1982), delayed auditory feedback and video games (Valori et al 1986), and mental arithmetic (Holtmann et al 1989). O'Brien et al (1987) compared the cold pressor test to dichotomous listening in normal volunteers and found that the physical stressor significantly delayed oro-caecal transit time whereas mental stimulation did not. Furthermore, the autonomic responses of the subjects to the stressor adapted in dichotomous listening but not in the cold pressor test. In concordance with such inhibition of transit, Kellow and colleagues (1992) found a sustained suppression of phase II motility of the MMC in the duodenum and jejunum in healthy subjects following various psychological stressors. The results of studies are listed in Table 8.5.

The delay of oro-caecal transit in response to stress observed by Cann et al 1983) (Fig. 8.6A) was comparable to that of rats under stress (Enck et al 1989) (Fig. 8.6B), measured with a similar technique, the breath hydrogen test (Enck & Wienbeck 1989). Overall, the inhibitory effect observed in most human studies supports the notion that where the opposite has been found in animals, this may be due to technical problems in measuring such effects rather than to true differences in stress response.

Large Bowel

Animal studies

A classical measure of stress in animals is faecal pellet output (Hall 1934). The number of stools and their consistency have been used as a measure of 'emotionality' in animals. In contrast to other digestive organs there is general agreement that stress accelerates colonic transit (Table 8.6) even though the underlying motor events are still a matter of controversy (Enck & Holtmann 1992).

There have been relatively few studies measuring the effects of stress on colonic activity directly. Conditioned responses to a previously fearful experience have been shown to increase colonic spike bursts in the caecal and proximal colon (Gué et al 1991). The effect can be modified by the nature of the stressor (Primi & Wingate 1990). The most likely mediator of reduced colonic transit time during stress exposure is again CRF (Mönnikes et al 1991, Lenz et al 1988).

Human studies

The first studies dealing with stress and colonic motility in man by Almy et al (1947, 1950), showed that different emotional states like anger, anxiety, or hostility had differential effects on colonic motility.

The 'irritable bowel syndrome' (IBS) is probably the functional disease that has most often been associated with stress. Welgan and coworkers (1985, 1988) have shown that psychological stressors designed to

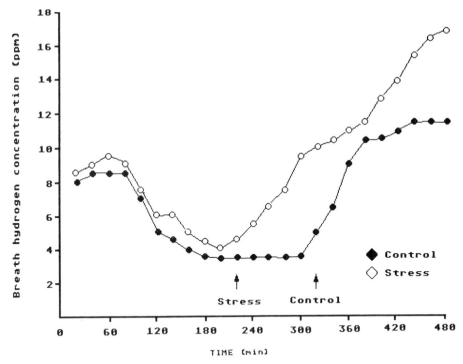

Fig. 8.6A   Mean breath hydrogen levels for subjects during control and stress studies respectively. Note similarity in profile of curves, but also there was a 'shift to the left' during stress studies with rise in breath hydrogen level occurring well before rise during control studies. (Reproduced with permission from Cann et al 1983.)

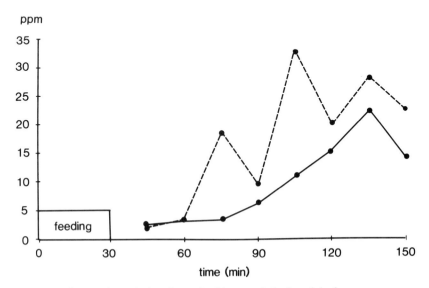

Fig. 8.6B   Orocaecal transit time determined by cumulative breath hydrogen concentration of exhaled air after rest (solid line) and after passive avoidance stress (dashed line) in rats. (Reproduced with permission from Enck et al 1989.)

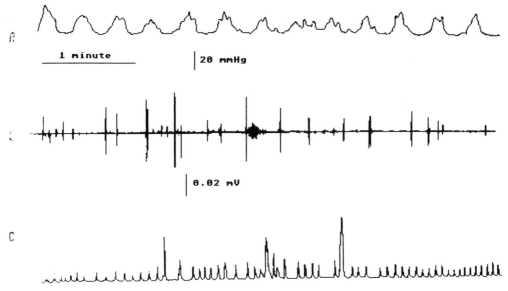

Fig. 8.7A The colonic motor and spike potential activity during mental stress in a patient with IBS. (**A**) Colonic motor activity, (**B**) spike potential activities, and (**C**) pneumogram. (Reproduced with permission from Welgan et al 1988.)

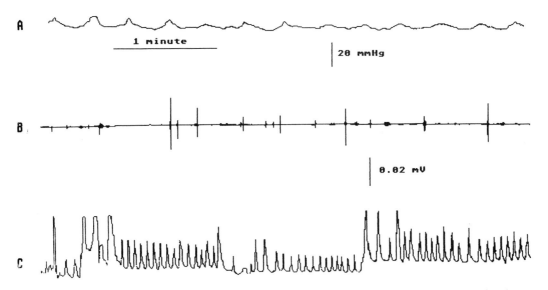

Fig. 8.7B The colonic motor and spike potential activity from the same patient depicted in Figure 7A after the stressor was eliminated. (**A**) Colonic motor activity, (**B**) spike potential activities, and (**C**) pneumogram. (Reproduced with permission from Welgan et al 1988.)

produce anger (criticism of the subject's performance in an intelligence test) and anxiety (threat of a health hazard) were effective in increasing colonic motor and spiking activity in normal healthy volunteers and in patients with IBS (Fig 8.7A,B), with the response in the IBS patients being more pronounced. However, subjective anger ratings were increased in the IBS group as compared to controls so that the result may

Table 8.7   Stress effects on large bowel motility – human studies

Author/Year	Cont./Pat.	Technique	Stressor applied	Effect observed
Almy 1949	7	Proctoscope	CPT, headache	↑ contractile activity
Chaudhary 1961	16/32, 38	Manometry	Stress interview	↑ motility
Sarna 1982	17/16	Colon EMG	Stress interview	No effect
Narducci 1985	6/11	Colon EMG	CPT, Stroop test	↑ motility and EMG
Welgan 1985	10/12	Manometry	CPT, arithmetics	↑ motility
Welgan 1988	10/12	Colon EMG	Induced anger	↑ No. of spikes (IBS)
Frexinos 1989	12	Colon EMG	CPT	No effect

CPT: cold pressor test; EMG: electromyography; IBS: irritable bowel syndrome; Cont./Pat.: numbers of controls and patients studied

reflect no more than a stronger affective response to the stressor in the patient group.

Narducci et al (1985) found similar increases in colonic motility in response to cold pressor test and cognitive stressful tasks in patients with IBS and normal healthy volunteers. Another psychological stressor, the mirror drawing test, increased the colonic motility index in patients with IBS but not in healthy controls; this effect was accompanied by an increase in plasma motilin and heart rate variability (Fukudo & Suzuki 1987). Table 8.7 lists the human studies of stress effects on large bowel motility.

CONCEPTS OF STRESS

Because of the many diferential effects that stress may have on intestinal and extraintestinal functions, a unifying concept is required to integrate these observations. We will briefly discuss three such theories which have been used to explain consistent and inconsistent results in experimental stress research.

Stress as a physiological response

Hans Selye was the first to describe the physiological reaction in experimental animals that has become known as the 'stress response' (Seyle 1950). He defined stress as a stereotypic set of physiological reactions in response to a noxious stimulus, known as the 'general adaptation syndrome'.

Two physiological systems are involved in the general adaptation syndrome:

1. The pitutary adrenal–cortical system
2. The sympathetic adrenal–medullary system.

During the first stage of the syndrome, the alarm reaction, adrenocorticotrophin hormone is released from the pituitary gland and leads to the adrenal excre-

tion of cortisol and corticosterone. Sympathetic nerves stimulate the medullary adrenals to release adrenaline and noradrenaline. The result is an increase in heart rate and blood pressure, deeper and more rapid respiration, and increased circulation in the skeletal muscle. At the same the time blood circulation in the renal and gastrointestinal system is decreased. The increased demand for glucose is covered by the reduction of glycogen in the liver and the transformation of protein into glucose. Immune and inflammatory responses are reduced. The whole reaction prepares the animal for a 'fight or flight' response. If the stressor continues, the animal can adapt to the situation for some time, with the immune and reproductive functions reduced. But if the stressor continues without the opportunity for recovery, the eventual consequence will be the death of the animal.

With increasing interest in the concept of stress and its application to humans, this definition had to be modified. The role of subjective factors, e.g. emotions (Mason 1968), had to be taken into account. Furthermore, the stress reaction not only differs between individuals and but also between different types of stressors. The concept of the specify of the stimulus or situation and the individual, or reaction has been proposed by Engel (1972).

Environment and the individual

In psychophysiological research, a variety of stimulus categories are used to classify stimuli as 'stressors':
1. External stressors
   - change of sensory input, either as an excess or deprivation of sensory information (e.g. light, noise)
   - pain stimuli (e.g. electrical, mechanical, thermic stimulation or lesions) or real or simulated situations of danger (e.g. accidents, surgery, fight–flight situations)

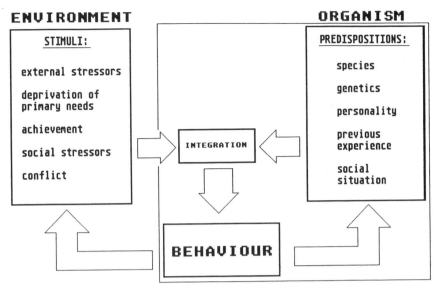

Fig. 8.8 Summary of organic and environmental aspects of stress research.

2. Deprivation of primary needs
   - water, sleep, food, temperature
3. Achievement
   - failure, overtaxation (e.g. time pressure, distraction), Undertaxation (monotony)
4. Social stressors
   - social isolation, interpersonal conflicts, bereavement
5. Conflict
   - decision between different alternatives, uncertainty and unpredictability of future events.

Obviously, not all of these stressors can be applied to every experimental subject, or in every laboratory situation. Certain categories of stressors, such as achievement, are only applicable to human subjects. Others, like external stressors or even social stressors, can be used in a wide variety of species and laboratory settings. Examples of social stressors in animals are early maternal separation and crowding.

Not only may the characteristics of stressors lead to differences in the physiological stress response, but also the differences between the individuals, depending on genetic predispositions, previous experience or personality differences, can change the subjects' ability to cope with a stressor. Therefore, stress can also be seen as a relational or transactional concept, describing the interactions of a person or any other biological system with the environment. According to Lazarus and Launier (1978), the three major stress relevant relationships between an individual and its environment are: harm–loss, threat and challenge. The new aspect in their approach is, to not define stress in variables like 'person' or 'stimulus', but to appreciate stress as a permanent flow process of interactions between a particular person and an environment of specific characteristics.

Figure 8.8 attempts a summary of different aspects of stress research that one has to be aware of in the discussion of experimental findings.

Stress and disease: reaction stereotypes and maladaptation

In most cases, the stress response is limited in time and extend. Nevertheless, in some individuals the response may not attenuate but persist, due to genetical predisposition, previous experiences, or other factors. This could lead to an overstimulation of certain organ systems and may result in persistent symptoms. Henry and Stephens (1977) suggested a two-dimensional concept to explain disease generation from the dysregulation of two different behavioural systems. They suggest, that a psychosocial stimulus perceived by an organism, that is not inhibited at higher cortical levels through coping patterns or social assets, leads to an activation of the limbic system. Such a psychosocial stimulus can be the failure to control territory, failure to achieve desired goals, or the anticipated loss of attachments. If the consequence of this behavioural

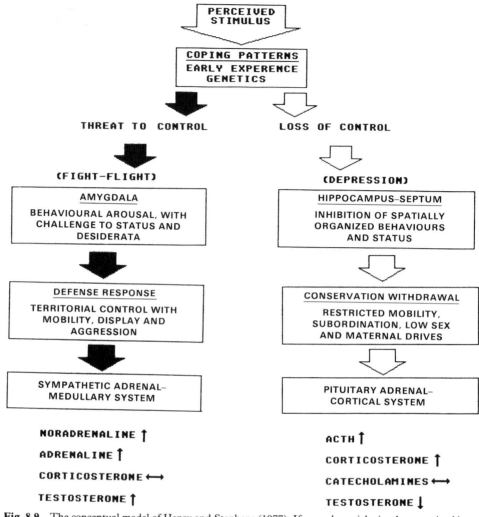

Fig. 8.9 The conceptual model of Henry and Stephens (1977). If a psychosocial stimulus perceived by an organism is not inhibited at higher levels by interaction with coping patterns and social assets, then a response of the limbic system will ensue. The amygdala and the sympathetic adrenal-medullary are activated when the organism is challenged in its control of the environment. By contrast, when there is loss of territorial control and failure to meet expectations, the hippocampal pituitary adrenal–cortical system becomes more involved as the conservation–withdrawal response is aroused. The physiologic consequences of these two response patterns differ as shown; ↔ indicates no change. (Reproduced with permission fron Henry & Stephens 1977.)

incompetence is *threat* of territorial control, the outcome will be a stimulation of the amygdala and the sympathetic adrenal–medullary system, which prepares for a fight–flight response and may be associated with feelings of aggression in humans. If the consequence is the *definite loss* of territorial control or a vital expectation, the outcome will be a stimulation of the hippocampus–septum region together with the pituitary adrenal–cortical system. This response is assumed

to be associated with feelings of depression and helplessness. Figure 8.9 summarizes the possible physiological consequences of the two response patterns.

The outcome of the individual's evaluation of potential loss or threat of control is dependent on its perception of self being dominant or subordinate. This implies that the social position determines the organism's perception of dominance and may, therefore, contribute to the frequency of occurrence of one or the other response patterns. As a stereotypic stress response, the overstimulation of one system does not necessarily lead to manifest disease, but such stereotypic stress responses may, in combination with other factors, contribute to the aetiology of disease.

RESEARCH PERSPECTIVES

Published data provide overwhelming evidence for the effects of experimental stress on gastrointestinal motility. Beyond this basic agreement, however, it is necessary to identify the factors affecting stress responses, both in their degree as well as in their direction, in different digestive organs. This may help clarify why, in most studies in which patients were included, no difference in their stress responses compared to healthy controls was found (see Tables 8.1, 8.3, 8.5, 8.7).

It has yet to be determined whether acute (experimental) stress as used in most experimental studies elicits similar responses to the long-term 'chronic' stress of which patients usually complain. It was shown recently that long-term exposure to a stressor elicits remarkably different responses in the gastrointestinal tract of the rat as compared to short-term stress. Specifically the colon appears to respond to restraint with delayed but excessive activity even when the stressor is removed (Wittmann et al 1990). Such effects have also been observed in in vitro preparations of colonic segments of pre-stressed animals (Collins et al 1989). Experimental ulcer research has shown that repetitive exposure to a severe stressor may result in enhanced susceptibility and vulnerability to subsequent 'minor' stressors (Murison et al 1986, 1989, Overmier et al 1987), while chronic mild restraint may even have a protective effect on gastric mucosal injury induced by restraint (Wallace et al 1983, Overmier et al 1985).

With respect to clinical research, similar questions arise: what are the effects of long-term stress in humans? Does habituation of gastrointestinal motility responses occur? Is the response of patients with functional gastrointestinal disorders due to both acute and chronic stress different to that of healthy volunteers? Which pathways are involved in the motility responses to acute and chronic stress? Does repeated (or chronic) stress result in alterations of motility patterns which persist even during absence of stress? Are stress-induced changes of gastrointestinal motility associated with the occurrence of symptoms in patients with functional gastrointestinal disorders?

It is therefore clear that the design and conduct of stress studies on the motor activity of the gut require careful thought, and assumptions that the chosen stressor can be easily equated with other stressors and with life stress are wrong. Expert psychophysiological and statistical input are required preconditions for the development of experimental protocols, and thus a multidisciplinary approach is mandatory. In an area where imprecision has too often been the rule, the aims of research or clinical study should be precisely focused. For studies on patients, the problems are even more daunting because of the difficulty of selecting appropriate controls; it may be convenient to assume that hospital patients and paid healthy volunteers will have similar affective responses to stressors, but it is unlikely to be true. Nonetheless, this is a research field that deserves support because of its relevance to actual clinical problems, and the real possibility that research outcomes will have a positive impact on clinical practice.

REFERENCES

Almy T P, Tulin M 1947 Alterations in colonic functions in man under stress: experimental production of changes simulating the 'irritable' colon. Gastroenterology 8: 616–626

Almy T P, Abbott F K K, Hinkle L E 1950 Alterations in colonic function in man under stress. IV. Hypomotility of the sigmoid colon, and its relationship to the mechanisms of functional diarrhoea. Gastroenterology 15: 95–103

Anderson K O, Dalton C B, Bradley L A, Richter J E 1989 Stress induced alterations of esophageal pressure in healthy volunteers and non-cardiac chest pain patients. Dig Dis Sci 34: 83–91

Appelbaum B D, Hotzmann S G 1985 Restraint stress has no effect on morphine-induced inhibition of gastrointestinal transit in the rat. Physiol Behav 34: 995–997

Ayres R C S, Robertson D A F, Naylor K, Smith C L 1989 Stress and esophageal motility in normal subjects and patients with the irritable bowel syndrome. Gut 30: 1540–1543

Barcley G R, Turnberg L A 1987 Effect of psychological stress on salt and water transport in the human jejunum. Gastroenterology 93: 91–97

Barone F C, Deegan J F, Price W J et al 1990 Cold-restraint stress increases rat fecal pellet output and colonic transit. Am J Physiol 258: G329–G337

Bindra D, Thompson W R 1953 An evaluation of defecation and urination as measures of individual differences in emotionality. J Comp Physiol Psychol 46: 43–45

Broadhurst P L 1957 Determinants of emotionality in the rat. Br J Psychol 48: 1–12

Brown M S, Groves W G 1966 Intestinal propulsion in restrained and unrestrained rats. Proc Soc Exp Biol Med 121: 989–995

Camilleri M, Malagelada J-R, Kao P C, Zinsmeister A R 1984 Effect of somatovisceral reflexes and selective dermatomal stimulation on postcibal antral pressure activity. Am J Physiol 247: G703–G708

Camilleri M, Malagelada J-R, Kao P C, Zinsmeister A R 1986 Gastric and autonomic responses to stress in functional dyspepsia. Dig Dis Sci 31: 1169–1177

Cann P A, Read N W, Cammack J et al 1983 Psychological stress and the passage of a standard meal through the stomach and small intestine in man. Gut 24: 236–240

Collins S, Vermillion D, Blennerhassett P, Randall B 1990 The effects of repeated acoustic or hypothermic stress on smooth muscle and enteric nerve function in vitro in the rat in: Bueno L, Collins S, Junien J L (eds) Stress in digestive motility. Libbey Press, London, pp 151–155

Cook I J, Dent J, Shannon S, Collins S M 1987 Measurement of upper esophageal sphincter pressure. Effects of acute mental stress. Gastroenterology 93: 526–532

Cook I J, Dent J, Collins S M 1989 Upper esophageal sphincter tone and reactivity to stress in patients with a history of globus sensation. Dig Dis Sci 34: 672–676

Costall B, Cummings S J, Nayor R J, Simpson K H 1983 A central site of action for benzamide facilitation of gastric emptying. Eur J Pharmacol 91: 197–205

Davis R C, Berry F, Paden A 1969 The effect of certain tasks and conditions on gastrointestinal activity. Indiana University, Bloomington, Indiana (Technical Report). Cited by Stern R, 1983 Responsiveness of the stomach to environmental events. In: Hölzl R, Whitehead, W E (eds), Psychophysiology of the gastrointestinal tract. Plenum Press, New York

Davison J S 1983 Innervation of the gastrointestinal tract in: Christensen J, Wingate D L (eds) A guide to gastrointestinal motility. Ch 1, Wright-PSG, Bristol, pp 1–47

Dubois A, Natelson B H 1978 Habituation of gastric function suppression in monkeys after repeated free-operant avoidance session. Physiol Psychol 6: 524–528

Enck P, Wienbeck M 1989 Repeated noninvasive measurement of gastrointestinal transit in rats. Physiol & Behav 46: 633–637

Enck P, Holtmann G 1992 Stress and gastrointestinal motility in animals: a review of the literature. J Gastrointest Mot 4: 83–90

Enck P, Merlin V, Erckenbrecht J F, Wienbeck M 1989 Stress effects on gastrointestinal transit in the rat. Gut 30: 455–459

Engel B T 1972 Response specificity in: Greenfield N S, Sternbach R A (eds) Handbook of psychophysiology. Holt, Rhinehart & Winston, New York, pp 571–575

Fedor J H, Russel R W 1965 Gastrointestinal reactions to response-contingent stimulation. Psychol Rep 16: 95–113

Fone D R, Horowitz M, Maddox A, Akkermans L M, Read N W, Dent J 1990 Gastroduodenal motility during the delayed gastric emptying induced by cold stress. Gastroenterology 98: 1155–1161

Fukudo S, Suzuki J 1987 Colonic motility, autonomic function, and gastrointestinal hormones under psychological stress on irritable bowel syndrome. Tokohu J Exp Med 151: 373–385

Galligan J J, Porreca F, Burks T F 1983 Footshock produces analgesia but no gastrointestinal motility effects in the rat. Life Sci 33: 473–475

Glavin G B, Mikhail A A 1977 Stress duration, gastric emptying, and ulcer development in three strains of rats. Biochem Med 18: 58–63

Gué M, Fioramonti J L, Bueno L 1987a Comparative influence of acoustic and cold stress on gastrointestinal transit in mice. Am J Physiol 253: G124–G128

Gué M, Fioramonti J L, Bueno L 1987b Influence of acoustic stress by noise on gastrointestinal motility in dogs. Dig Dis Sci 32: 1411–1417

Gué M, Honde C, Pascaud X et al 1988 CNS blockade of acoustic stress-induced gastric motor inhibition by κ-opiate antagonist in dogs. Am J Physiol 254: G802–G807

Gué M, Peeters T, Depoortere I, Vantrappen G, Bueno L 1989 Stress-induced changes in gastric emptying, postprandial motility, and plasma gut hormone levels in dogs. Gastroenterology 97: 1101–1107

Gué M, Junien J L, Pascaud X, Bueno L 1990 Antagonism of stress-induced gastric motor alteration and plasma cortisol release by fedotozine (JO 1196) in dogs. J Gastrointestinal Motility 2: 258–264

Gué M, Junien J L, Bueno L, 1991 Conditioned emotional response in rats enhances colonic motility through the central release of corticotrophin-releasing factor. Gastroenterology 100: 964–970

Hall C S 1934 Emotional behaviour in the rats: 1. Defecation and urination as measures of individual differences in emotionality. J Comp Psychol 18: 385–403

Henry J, Stephens P 1977 Stress, health and social environment: a sociobiologic approach to medicine. Springer, New York.

Holtmann G, Enck P 1991 Stress and gastrointestinal motility in humans: a review of the literature. J Gastrointest Mot 3: 245–254

Holtmann G, Singer M V, Kriebel R et al 1989 Differential effects of acute mental stress on gastric acid, pancreatic enzyme secretion and gastroduodenal motility. Dig Dis Sci 34: 1701–1707

Jungmann H, Venning P 1952 Radiological investigation of stomach following a loud auditory stimulus. Br J Radiol 25: 201–208

Kellow J E, Langeluddecke P M, Eckersley G M, Jones M P 1992 Effects of acute psychologic stress on small-intestinal motility in health and the irritable bowel syndrome. Scand J Gastroenterol 27: 53–58

Koo M W L, Ogle C W, Cho C H 1985 The effects of cold-restraint stress on gastric emptying in rats. Pharmacol Biochem Behav 23: 969–972

Lazarus R S, Launier R 1978 Stress-related transactions between person and environment in: Pervin L A (ed.) Perspectives in interactional psychology. Plenum Press, New York. pp 287–327

Lenz H J, Raedler A, Greten H et al 1988 Stress induced gastrointestinal motility and secretory responses in rats are mediated by endogenous corticotropin-releasing factor. Gastroenterology 95: 1510–1517

McRae S, Younger K, Thompson D G, Wingate D L 1982 Sustained mental stress alters human jejunal motor activity. Gut 23: 404–409

Mason J W 1968 A review of pschoendocrine research on the pituitary-adrenocortical system. Psychosom med 30: 576–607

Mönnikes H, Schmidt B G, Taché Y 1991 CRF in the paraventricular nucleus (PVN) is involved in mediating psychological stress-induced stimulation of colonic transit in the conscious rat. Gastroenterology 100: A656 (abstract)

Murison R, Overmier J B, Skoglund E J 1986 Serial stressors: prior exposure to a stressor modulates its later effectiveness on gastric ulcerations and corticosterone release. Behav Neural Biology 45: 246–253

Murison R, Overmier B J, Glavin G B 1989 Stress-rest cyclicity in the pathogenesis of restraint-induced stress gastric ulcers in rats. Physiol Behav 45: 809–813

Narducci F, Snape W J, Battle W M et al 1985 Increased colonic motility during exposure to a stressful situation. Dig Dis Sci 30: 40–44

O'Brien J D, Thompson D G, Burnham W R et al 1987 Action of centrally mediated autonomic stimulation on human upper gastrointestinal transit: a comparative study of two stimuli. Gut 28: 960–968

Ossenkopp K P, Frisken N L 1982 Defaecation as an index of motion sickness in the rat. Physiol Psychol 10: 355–360

Overmier J B, Murison R, Skoglund E J, Ursin H 1985 Safety signals can mimic responses in reducing the ulcerogenic effects of prior shock. Physiol Behav 13: 243–247

Overmier J B, Murison R, Ursin H, Skoglund E J 1987 Quality of post-stressor rest influences the ulcerative process. Behav Neurosci 101: 246–253

Penagini R, Bartesaghi B, Biachi P A 1992 Effects of cold stress on lower esophageal sphincter competences and gastroesophageal reflux in healthy subjects. Dig Dis Sci 37: 1200–1205

Primi M P, Wingate D L, 1990 Stress and gut motor functions in the rat? It depends on what you measure. J Gastrointest Motility 2: 156 (abstract)

Roth K A, Katz R J 1979 Stress, behavioral arousal, and open field activity – a reexamination of emotionality in the rat. Neurosci Biobehav Rev 3: 247–263

Rubin J, Nagler R, Spiro H M, Pilot L M 1962 Measuring the effect of emotions on esophageal motility. Psychosom Med 90: 170–176

Seyle H 1950 The physiology and pathology of exposure to stress. ACTA INC. Medical Publishers, Montreal

Soffer E E, Scalabrini P, Pope C E, Wingate D L 1988 Effects of stress on oesophageal motor function in normal subjects and in patients with irritable bowel syndrome. Gut 29: 1591–1594

Stacher G, Steinringer H, Landgraf M 1979 Acoustically evoked esophageal contractions and defense reaction. Psychophysiology 16: 234–241

Stacher G, Steinringer H, Landgraf M 1979 Tertiary esophageal contractions evoked by acoustical stimuli. Gastroenterology 77: 49–54

Stanghellini V, Malagelada J-R, Zinsmeister A R, Go V L W, Kao P C 1983 Stress-induced gastroduodenal motor disturbances in humans: possible humoral mechanisms. Gastroenterology 85: 83–91

Taché Y, Ishikawa T, Stephens R, Hagiwara M 1988 Stressor specific alterations of gastric function in the rat: role of brain TRH and CRF. Gastroenterology 94: A452 (abstract)

Taché Y, Garrick T, Raybould H 1990 Central nervous system action of peptides to influence gastrointestinal motor function. Gastroenterology 98: 517–528

Valori R M, Kumar D, Wingate D L 1986 Effects of different types of stress and of 'prokinetic' drugs on the control of the fasting motor complex in humans. Gastroenterology 90: 1890–1900

Wallace J L, Track N S, Cohen M 1983 Chronic mild restraint protects the rat gastric mucosa from injury by ethanol or cold restraint. Gastroenterology 85: 370–375

Welgan P, Meshkinpour H, Hoehler F 1985 The effect of stress on colon motor and electrical activity in irritable bowel syndrome. Psychosom Med 47: 139–149

Welgan P, Meshkinpour H, Beeler M 1988 Effect of anger on colon motor and myoelectric activity in irritable bowel syndrome. Gastroenterology 94: 1050–1056

Wittkower E 1931 Zur affektiven Beeinflussung der Magensekretion. Klin Wochenschr 10: 1811–1813

Wittmann T, Crenner F, Angel F et al 1990 Long-duration stress. Immediate and late effects on small and large bowel motility. Dig Dis Sci 35: 495–500

Wolf S, Wolff H 1943 Human gastric function. Oxford University Press, New York.

Wolf S, Almy T P 1949 Experimental observations on cardiospasm in man. Gastroenterology 13: 401–421

Young L D, Richter J E, Anderson K O et al 1987 The effect of psychological and environmental stressors on peristaltic oesophageal contractions in healthy volunteers. Psychophysiology 24: 132–141

Zacchi P, Falchini M, Rossi C et al 1992 Lower esophageal sphincter but not esophageal body responds to stress. Gastroenterology 102: A538 (abstract)

9. The immune system

S. M. Collins

INTRODUCTION

There is increasing awareness of the ability of the immune system to influence physiological activity in the gut. Since the immune system in the gut is located within or is adjacent to the mucosa, it is not surprising to find that most of the work on immunophysiological interactions has addressed interactions between the immune system and epithelial cells as a basis for symptom development in the inflamed gut (Fig. 9.1). A large part of this work has been performed using nematode infections in small mammals as a model (Russell & Castro 1987).

More recent work has addressed the possibility that deeper layers of the gut wall, namely the neuromuscular tissues, may also be influenced by the immune system. The rationale for studying this interaction is derived not only from the example set by previous work on immunophysiological interactions in the mucosa, but also on clinical demonstrations of altered motility in the context of inflammation or immune activation in the gut caused by the following:

- IBD
- Acid peptic disease
- Scleroderma
- Coeliac dosease
- Enteric infections
- Pseudo-obstruction
- Food allergy
- IBS

At present, information regarding the influence of the immune system on neuromotor function is restricted to pathological conditions. There is, as yet, little information regarding the role of the resident immune or inflammatory cell population in modulating gastrointestinal physiology under normal conditions, although observations in germ-free animals suggest that this may be an interesting field of study (Thompson & Trexler 1971, Abrams & Bishop 1967).

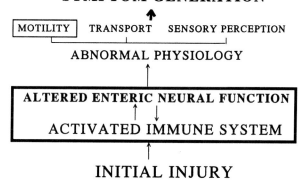

Fig. 9.1 Interactions between the immune and physiological systems produce widespread disturbances in gut function that are the basis for symptom generation in the inflamed bowel.

DEMONSTRATIONS OF ALTERED MOTILITY IN THE INFLAMED OR SENSITIZED GUT

Altered motility in peptic oesophagitis

Peptic oesophagitis is perhaps the most common example of altered motility associated with inflammation. Changes include a reduction in lower oesophageal sphincter (LOS) pressure, as well as changes in the motor activity in the distal oesophagus with a reduction in the clearance of acid (Kahrilas et al 1986). While some of these changes may precede and predispose to acid reflux, studies in the cat provide clear evidence that they may also occur as a result of acid-induced oesophagitis (Eastwood et al 1975). Intermittent perfusion of acid into the oesophagus over 4 days induced severe oesophagitis accompanied by a substantial fall in LOS pressure that recovered in 3–4 weeks.

Altered motility in the context of acid-peptic disease

Motility disturbances have been described in patients with peptic ulceration (Garrett et al 1966, Malagelada et al 1977), although the topic has yielded conflicting results (Holt et al 1986). Changes in the structure of the muscularis externa have also been described in ulcer patients; hypertrophy of muscle and structural alterations in enteric nerves have been described in specimens resected from patients with gastric ulcer (Lieberman-Meffert & Allgower 1977). In addition, others have shown increased numbers of mast cells in the muscle layers below gastric ulcer craters (Hiatt & Katz 1962). A more recent study (Moore et al 1986)) demonstrated an inverse correlation between the degree of gastritis and postprandial motor activity recorded manometrically from the antrum. These findings raise the possibility that the presence of inflammation in the gastric mucosa is accompanied by alterations in gastric motility.

Altered motility in disorders of the small intestine

Alterations in motility have also been described in other conditions associated with inflammation or sensitization of the gut. Liu et al (1975) provided radiological evidence of rapid gastrointestinal transit of barium in patients with allergy to milk protein following antigen challenge. Transit abnormalities have also been demonstrated in the small intestine of patients with untreated coeliac disease (Spiller et al 1987). Taken together, these findings raise the possibility that antigen-driven changes in the mucosal immune system result in changes in gastrointestinal motility.

There may also be an immunological basis for the severe disturbance of motility observed in certain cases of intestinal pseudo-obstruction. Histological evaluation of full-thickness gut biopsies have identified lymphoid infiltration of smooth muscle or the myenteric plexus in patients with pseudo-obstruction as part of a para-neoplastic syndrome (Krishnamurthy et al 1986, Chinn & Schuffler 1988).

Another clinical observation supporting the concept of immune activation of motility comes from side-effects of treatment with immune mediators. Gamma interferon treatment of hepatitis, for example, is associated with gastrointestinal symptoms, such as vomiting and altered bowel habit, suggestive of altered motility. The use of interleukin-2 (IL-2) in the treatment of cancer is also associated with similar side-effects and a report of megacolon with subsequent perforation has been described as a complication of IL-2 therapy (Schwartzenruber et al 1988).

Altered motility in the context of idiopathic inflammatory bowel disease (IBD)

The strongest body of evidence that inflammation in the gastrointestinal tract is associated with altered motility comes from structural and functional studies on patients with IBD.

Initial studies of motility patterns in IBD described a marked reduction in the basal contractile activity in the sigmoid colon of patients with ulcerative colitis (Kern et al 1951, Spriggs et al 1951). Since the dominant motor pattern in this region is that of segmental contractions, which serve to retard the faecal stream, the marked diminution in activity observed in IBD patients promotes accelerated colonic transit which, in turn, results in diarhoea (Chaudhary & Truelove 1961, Connell 1962, Almy 1961).

Garrett et al (1967) demonstrated that small concentrations of opiate that had no effect in normal subjects caused substantial increases in contractile activity in the sigmoid colon of patients with active colitis. Opiate administration produced large-amplitude segmental contractions which may predispose to the development of megacolon (McInerney et al 1962). The reflex increase in colonic motility that follows the ingestion of a meal was substantially decreased in patients with ulcerative colitis (Snape et al 1980, Loening-Baucke et al 1989), suggesting that motility apparatus of the inflamed gut exhibits altered responsiveness not only to pharmacologic stimuli, but also to endogenous stimuli.

The observation that the changes in motor activity seemed to return to normal following remission of IBD (Kern et al 1951) suggested that altered motility occurred as a consequence of the inflammatory process. Altered motility in IBD may occur not only as a result of changes in smooth muscle and enteric effector nerve function, but also as a result of changes in afferent nerve activity. This concept is supported by the clinical observations of increased sensitivity of the rectum to distension in patients with colitis (Farthing & Lennard-Jones 1978, Rao et al 1988). This could result from increased sensitivity of sensory nerves, and/or a decrease in the elastic properties of the gut wall subsequent to chronic inflammation (Denis et al 1979).

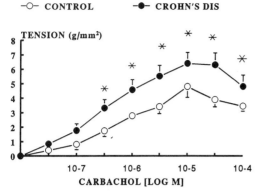

Fig. 9.2   Isometric tension development by human longitudinal muscle from patients with and without Crohn's disease, following stimulation by carbachol. (Adapted from Vermillion et al 1991b.)

STUDIES ON ENTERIC NERVES AND SMOOTH MUSCLE FROM THE INFLAMED HUMAN GUT

Thickening of the muscularis interna and externa is a well recognized phenomenon in IBD (Morson & Dawson 1979) and may reflect inflammation-induced hypertrophy and/or hyperplasia of muscle cells. Muscle, rather than fibrosis, accounts for the benign strictures that occur in ulcerative colitis (Goulston & McGovern 1969). It has also been shown that hyperplasia of smooth muscle in the muscularis mucosae contributes to intestinal strictures in Crohn's disease (Lee et al 1991, Graham et al 1988). In addition to muscle cell proliferation, fibrosis also contributes to strictures in Crohn's disease and is due, in large part, to the production of type V collagen by smooth muscle cells.

A recent study has demonstrated changes in the contractility of muscle from the inflamed small intestine of patients with Crohn's disease, compared to responses in muscle from patients without IBD (Vermillion et al 1991b). In longitudinal muscle from Crohn's disease patients there was a significant increase in the maximum contraction induced by carbachol but not histamine, but there was no change in the ED_{50} values for these agonists (Fig. 9.2). In contrast, in circular muscle from Crohn's disease patients there was a sevenfold decrease in the ED_{50} value for carbachol but no change in maximum contraction induced by carbachol. Since no differences were observed between the two groups when muscle was stimulated with depolarizing concentrations of KCl, these data suggest that the altered contractility of muscle from Crohn's disease patients is due to changes at the recep-

tor level, either in the ligand-recognition properties of the receptor, or in its coupling to second messenger systems in the muscle cell.

In contrast to the increased contractility of muscle from the inflamed small intestine, colitis appears to be associated with a decrease in muscle contractility. Although earlier reports yielded equivocal results regarding the excitability of colonic muscle from patients with ulcerative colitis (Koch et al 1988, Huizinga et al 1991), a more recent report has described a significant reduction in tension development by circular muscle from patients with ulcerative colitis (Snape et al 1991). Furthermore, and in further contrast to findings in the small intestine, reduced tension was observed following KCl stimulation, indicating a post-receptor change in excitation–contraction coupling in the muscle.

There have been a large number of studies describing structural changes in enteric nerves in IBD. Early studies described significant increases in the number of ganglion cells in the myenteric plexus of patients with Crohn's disease (Storsteen et al 1953) or ulcerative colitis (Davis et al 1953). Interestingly, increased numbers of ganglion cells were observed in non-inflamed regions. Later studies described damaged to myenteric nerves in IBD, particularly in severe or chronic IBD (McInerney et al 1962, Okamoto et al 1964, Siemers et al 1974, Oehmichen & Reifferscheid 1977). Electron microscopy of tissue from Crohn's disease has demonstrated axonal degeneration in the submucous and myenteric plexuses.

The enteric plexuses in Crohn's disease are infiltrated by a number of different types of inflammatory cells, including plasma cells, lymphocytes and mast cells (Dvorak et al 1979, 1980). In addition, there is expression of Class II major histocompatibility complex on Schwann cells in the myenteric plexus of patients with Crohn's disease, a finding that suggests that damage to the enteric nerves is immunologically mediated (Geboes et al 1992).

Inflammation is associated with changes not only in the structure of enteric nerves, but also in neurotransmitter content and receptors. For example, there have been reports of increased substance P (SP) concentrations in the gut in IBD (Koch et al 1987) as well as an increase in SP receptors (Mantyh et al 1988). Since SP is present in sensory nerve fibres in the gut, increases in SP and its receptor have implications for the increased sensory perception in the gut of patients with active IBD (Mantyh et al 1989). An increase in biologically active amines, together with prominence of catecholamine-containing nerves has also been described in patients with active colitis (Penttila et al 1975, Kyosola et al 1977). There are, however, conflicting reports of changes in vasoactive intestinal peptide (VIP) containing nerves (Bishop et al 1980, Sjolund et al 1983, O'Morain et al 1984, Koch et al 1987). There have been few in vitro studies on enteric neural function in IBD. Koch et al (1990) associated a reduction in inhibitory junction potential in circular muscle of Crohn's colitis with a decrease in the VIP content of the tissue.

MECHANISTIC INSIGHTS DERIVED FROM ANIMAL STUDIES

Conceptual approach

The immune system may alter gastrointestinal motility by influencing the contractility, coupling and mass of smooth muscle, by influencing the excitability, distribution and content of intrinsic and extrinsic nerves, or by influencing hormone synthesis and release by endocrine cells of the gut. With respect to the changes in neuromodulation of motility, this may occur via an effect on efferent or afferent nerve function.

We have investigated the immonomodulation of smooth muscle and myenteric nerve function in the rat during acute inflammation resulting from primary infection with the nematode parasite *Trichinella spiralis*. During infection, the parasite invades the epithelium of the jejunum where it causes an acute inflammatory reaction that is largely limited to the mucosa and lamina propria. The inflammation is maximal between days 5–7 post-infection; the organism is either expelled in the faeces after 21 days, or gains access to the circulation and migrates to skeletal muscle where it encysts. The parasite does not penetrate the gut wall beyond the epithelium.

Primary infection with *Trichinella spiralis* produces an increase in spiking activity in the small intestine (Palmer et al 1984), and this is accompanied by changes in transit (Castro et al 1977). Subsequent exposure to the parasite produces an increase in myoelectrical activity in the small intestine within 15 min (Palmer & Castro 1986). In both cases, the infection-associated motility changes have been shown to occur in extrinsically denervated segments of intestine, indicating that they are likely mediated by altered function in smooth muscle and intrinsic nerves (Alizadeh et al 1987, 1989).

Mechanisms underlying altered smooth muscle function in the inflamed intestine

Initial experiments demonstrated that primary nematode infection was associated with increased isometric force generation by longitudinal muscle from the inflamed jejunum (Vermillion & Collins 1988a, Fox-Robichaud & Collins 1986, Farmer 1981). Circular muscle behaves quite differently, exhibiting a decrease in tension generation following nematode infection (Crosthwaite et al 1990). The two to threefold increased tension development by longitudinal muscle was expressed per unit cross-sectional area of muscle; the actual increase in tension development in situ would be substantially higher as infection also results in a twofold increase in muscle mass due to a combination of hypertrophy and hyperplasia (Blennerhassett et al 1992).

Increase tension development in longitudinal muscle was not due to a change in the number or affinity of muscarinic cholinergic receptors, and was not restricted to stimulation by muscarinic agonists (Fox-Robichaud & Collins 1986, Muller et al 1989). These findings prompted an examination of receptor-independent changes in excitation–contraction coupling as a basis for the increased tension development. Others have showed an increase in the actin and myosin content of muscle in this model (Bowers et al 1986). In addition, there is a marked ($>80\%$) suppression of the Na–K pump in longitudinal muscle from inflamed jejunum of Trichinella-infected rats (Muller et al 1989). Since the pump is electrogenic in this tissue, contributing to membrane polarity, a suppression of pump activity would serve to depolarize the membrane and render the cell more excitable. The suppression of the Na pump was specific for longitudinal muscle and did not occur in circular muscle from the inflamed jejunum (Fig. 9.3). Since mRNA for the Na pump α-1 subunit was also substantially reduced, the findings indicate that the change occurs at the level of the gene, at a pretranslational step (Khan & Collins 1993).

Smooth muscle function in the inflamed intestine may be altered by changes in the biovailability of neurotransmitters and other stimuli. While this may occur as a result of changes in the cellularity of the tissue or in the excitability of nerves, it may also result from alterations in the activity of degradative enzymes. An example is neutral endopeptidase (NEP), a metaloenzyme that degrades SP in the gut. In the inflamed intestine of Trichinella-infected rats, the activity of NEP is reduced $>80\%$ (Hwang et al 1992). This serves to increase the biovailability of SP which in turn causes greater stimulation of muscle cells (Djokic et al 1989). The factors contributing to alter muscle contractility in the inflamed gut are summarized in Figure 9.4.

The relationship between altered contractility of muscle and the inflammatory process has been

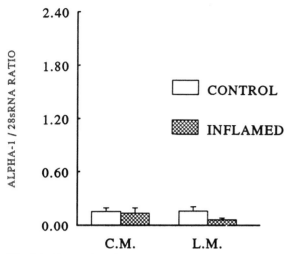

Fig. 9.3 Expression of mRNA for the α-1 isoform of the sodium pump in circular (**CM**) and longitudinal (**LM**) muscle from the inflamed jejunum of Trichinella-infected rats, using quantitative polymerase chain reaction (PCR) with 28s RNA as the co-amplified internal control. (Adapted from Khan and Collins 1993.)

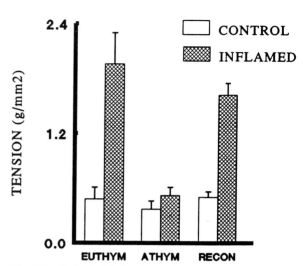

Fig. 9.5 Carbochol-induced muscle contraction from control and inflamed euthymic, athymic and T-cell reconstituted rats, illustrating the T-lymphocyte dependence of contraction in the Trichinella-infected rat model. (Adapted from Vermillion et al 1991a.)

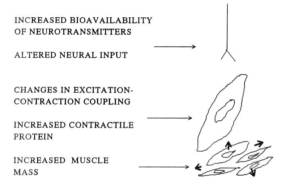

Fig. 9.4 Summary of factors that influence smooth muscle contraction in the inflamed bowel.

investigated. The inflammatory response is monitored by the measurement of the activity of tissue myeloperoxidase (MPO), an enzyme found primarily in polymorphs and the activity of which correlates well with the histological assessment of acute inflammatory infiltrate (Smith & Castro 1978). Trichinella infection produces an increase in MPO activity in the jejunum, and corticosteroid treatment of animals during infection attenuates the acute inflammatory response, as illustrated by a suppression of the increase in MPO activity; attenuation of the inflammatory response in this manner also prevented the changes in smooth muscle contraction (Marzio et al 1990). These findings provide evidence of a *causal* relationship between the inflamma-

tory process and altered muscle function. A similar strategy was used in Trichinella-infected mice to establish that changes in intestinal transit occur as a consequence of inflammation (Sukhdeo & Croll 1981). It should be emphasized, at this point, that MPO activity is being used simply as a *marker* of the inflammation and attenuation of MPO activity per se is not necessarily evidence of the involvement of MPO-producing cells in causing altered muscle function; identification of the cell types involved requires a more selective strategy.

Previous studies have shown that the expulsion of Trichinella larvae from the intestine is markedly delayed in athymic animals, implicating a role for T-lymphocytes. This prompted an evaluation of the T-cell dependence of altered smooth muscle function in this model. Infected congenitally athymic rats develop acute inflammation in the jejunum but this was not accompanied by increased tension development by jejunal longitudinal muscle, suggesting T-cell dependence. As shown in Figure 9.5 this was confirmed by demonstrating that successful reconstitution of T-cell function in congenitally athymic rats by grafting cells from thymus-bearing littermates prior to infection was accompanied by restoration of increased muscle tension (Vermillion et al 1991a).

In addition to inducing changes in muscle contraction, inflammation also produces changes in the growth of muscle. In the Trichinella-infected rat, there is a two to threefold increase in the thickness of the muscularis externa. Morphometric analysis together with

IMMUNOMODULATION OF
SMOOTH MUSCLE FUNCTION

ACUTE INFLAMMATORY RESPONSE

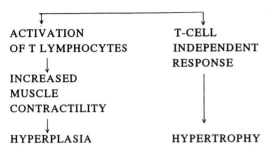

Fig. 9.6 Summary of T-lymphocyte dependent and independent changes in the rat intestine following inflammation with *Trichinella spiralis*.

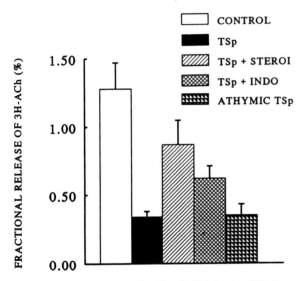

Fig. 9.7 The effect of *Trichinella spiralis* infection (**TSp**) on the release of ³H-acetylcholine from the jejunal myenteric plexus. Illustrated are the effects of corticosteroid treatment (**STEROI**), indomethacin (**INDO**) and the athymic status of infected rats (**ATHYMIC TSp**). Only corticosteroid attenuated the suppression of ACh release.

³H-thymidine incorporation studies have indicated that the increased muscle mass is due to a combination of hypertrophy and hyperplasia (Blennerhassett et al 1992). The increased mitotic rate observed in the Trichinella-infected rat is not seen in infected athymic rats, suggesting that the hyperplasia is dependent on T-lymphocytes. This is in contrast to muscle hypertrophy which is present in infected athymic rats, thus

indicating that inflammation-induced hypertrophy and hyperplasia are due to different components of the inflammatory response (Blennerhassett et al 1990). The extent of T-cell dependent changes in muscle are summarized in Figure 9.6.

Mechanisms underlying altered neural function in the inflamed intestine

We have studied neurotransmitter content and release in myenteric nerves from the jejunum of Trichinella-infected rats. Cholinergic nerves take up less choline than control tissues and release proportionately less acetylcholine (ACh) following electrical or chemical stimulation (Collins et al 1989). As shown in Figure 9.7 the suppression of cholinergic nerve function is attenuated by corticosteroid treatment of infected rats but is present in infected athymic animals, indicating that it is due to the inflammatory response but, in contrast to altered muscle function, is not dependent on the presence of functioning T-lymphocytes (Collins et al 1992a). Similar changes occurred with respect to the release of ³H-noradrenaline (³H-NA) from sympathetic nerves in the myenteric plexus (Swain et al 1991).

Inflammation is known to be associated with increases in SP in joints and in the airways, where it is believed to contribute to the inflammatory process. As shown in Figure 9.8 we found a fivefold increase in the immunoreactive SP content of the myenteric plexus of the inflamed jejunum but not the ileum of Trichinella-infected rats (Swain et al 1992). The SP was believed to be present in nerves as it could be depleted from the tissue after exposure to the neurostimulant scorpion venom in vitro. Treatment of rats with capsaicin prior to infection abrogated the increase in SP, suggesting a sensory or afferent nerve origin. Finally, steroid treatment of infected rats prevented the increase in SP, indicating that this is due to the inflammatory response (Fig. 9.9). However, in contrast to the suppression of cholinergic nerve function, the increase in SP was not evident in infected athymic rats, suggesting T-lymphocyte dependence. The effects of inflammation on neural function are summarized in Figure 9.10.

The mechanics underlying the changes in adrenergic and peptidergic nerves in model have been explored. This was preceded by a characterization of changes in cytokine expression in the region of the myenteric plexus-longitudinal muscle of the Trichinella-infected rat intestine. Interestingly, the study identified constitutive expression of interleukin-1β (IL-1β) in the myenteric plexus of non-infected control rats. There was a substantial increase in mRNA for IL-1β, as well as

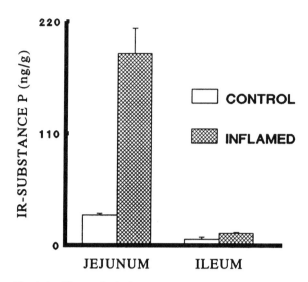

Fig. 9.8 Changes in the immunoreactive (IR) substance P content of the myenteric plexus and longitudinal muscle in the inflamed jejunum and non-inflamed ileum of Trichinella-infected rats.

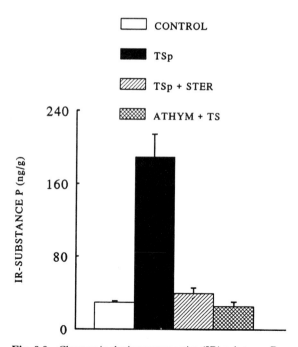

Fig. 9.9 Changes in the immunoreactive (IR) substance P content of the myenteric plexus and longitudinal muscle of the inflamed jejunum of Trichinella-infected (TSp) rats following corticosteroid treatment, and in athymic infected rats. (Adapted from Swain et al 1992.)

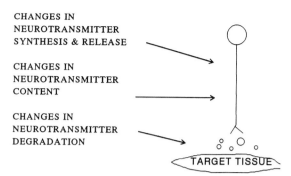

Fig. 9.10 Summary of the changes that lead to altered neural function in the inflamed gut.

IL-1α, commencing within 24 h of infection. This was accompanied by the expression of IL-6 and tumour necrosis factor α (TNFα) (Khan et al 1992). These findings prompted an investigation of the ability of these cytokines to influence function in myenteric nerves of the rat small intestine.

Human recombinant interleukin-1β (hrIL-1β) had no immediate effect on neurotransmitter release from cholinergic or adrenergic nerves in the rat myenteric plexus. However, prolonged exposure of the tissue to hrIL-1β caused a concentration-dependent suppression of ³H-ACH or ³H-NA release (Hurst & Collins 1993, Main et al 1991). In both instances, the effect of hrIL-1β could be prevented by boiling the cytokine for 20 min, thus excluding an effect due to contamination by endotoxin (Stanley et al 1992). Moreover, the effect was blocked either by neutralizing anti-IL-1 antibody or by an IL-1 receptor antagonist (Fig. 9.11). The effect of hrIL-1β was dependent on protein synthesis and involved the release of endogenous IL-1 (Hurst & Collins 1993, Main et al 1991), most likely from macrophage-like cells previously identified in the myenteric plexus by others (Mikkelsen et al 1985). TNFα also caused suppression of ³H-NA release from myenteric nerves, and the effect was mediated, at least in part, by the release of endogenous IL-1 (Hurst & Collins 1992). These findings are summarized in Figure 9.12. Other possible sources of IL-1 are shown in Table 9.1. The site of action of endogenous IL-1 is thought to be on myenteric neurons since suppression of NA release was apparent when the cytokine was exposed to a preparation of varicosities from the myenteric plexus (Hurst & Collins 1990).

IL-1β also causes an increase in immunoreactive SP in the myenteric plexus. The action of IL-1β is concentration and time dependent, and is maximal after 6-h incubation with the tissue (Hurst et al 1992b).

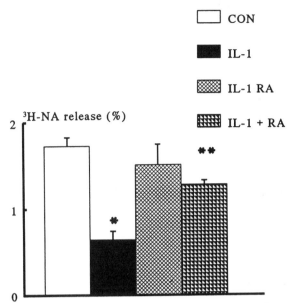

Fig. 9.11 The suppression of ³H-noradrenaline release from longitudinal muscle myenteric plexus preparations of rat intestine, following exposure to hrIL-1β. The data show that the effect can be reversed by an IL-1 receptor antagonist. (Reproduced with permission from Hurst & Collins 1993.)

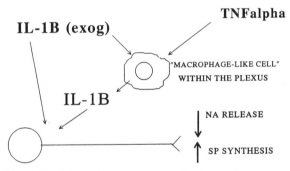

Fig. 9.12 Schematic representation of actions and interactions of cytokines in the rat myenteric plexus.

Table 9.1 Potential sources of IL-1 in the LM-MP preparation

Source	Reference
Macrophages	Mikkelsen et al 1988
Glial or Schwann cells	Giulian et al 1986
Smooth muscle cells	Warner et al 1987

These observations, therefore, demonstrate the ability of IL-1β to produce changes in myenteric nerves similar to those observed in the Trichinella-infected rat model, and suggest the cytokine as a putative mediator of those

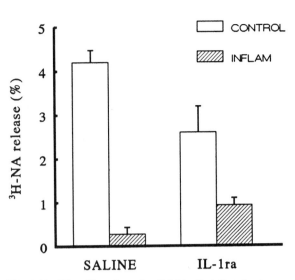

Fig. 9.13 The effect of treating Trichinella-infected rats with an IL-1 receptor antagonist (IL-1ra) versus saline, on the release of ³H-noradrenaline.

changes. To examine this, rats were treated with the IL-1 receptor antagonist delivered by a mini-pump to the peritoneal cavity during Trichinella infection. Tissues were then examined for their SP content and ability to release ³H-NA. Treatment with IL-1 receptor antagonist (IL-1ra) attenuated (by >50%) both the increase in SP and the suppression of NA release (Fig. 9.13) observed in (saline treated) Trichinella-infected rats (Collins et al 1992b). These findings, therefore, are consistent with the hypothesis that IL-1 mediates the changes in adrenergic and peptidergic nerves in the inflamed intestine of Trichinella-infected rats.

Local and systemic effects of inflammation

It is not uncommon for diarrhoea to occur in patients with inflammation restricted to a relatively limited section of the gut. This raises the possibility that inflammation at one site may alter function at another site in the gut. It has been shown that intestinal motility is altered in patients with ulcerative colitis (Manousos & Salem 1965). It is of interest to note the morphological studies in man have, for example, identified ultrastructural changes in enteric nerves in non-inflamed gut segments (Dvorak et al 1980). Results of recent studies in animals provide a functional correlate of these observations. In the Trichinella-infected rat, inflammation of the jejunum also caused changes in smooth muscle contraction in jejunal segments excluded from the gut prior to infection (Marzio et al

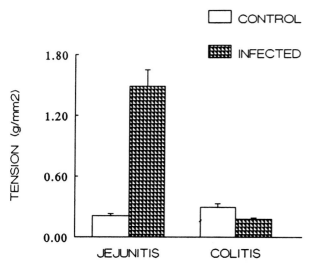

Fig. 9.14 Comparison of changes in carbachol-stimulated tension development following jejunitis or colitis, induced in each case by local application of *Trichinella spiralis* larvae. (Adapted from Vermillion & Collins 1988a and Grossi et al 1993.)

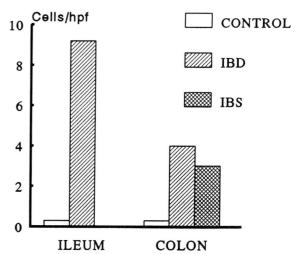

Fig. 9.15 Mast cells per high power field in the muscularis externa from patients with inflammatory bowel disease (IBD) or irritable bowel syndrome (IBS). (Adapted from Hiatt et al 1962.)

1990). In preliminary studies involving rats with colitis induced by intrarectal administration of trinitrobenzene sulphonic acid (TNB) in ethanol (Morris et al 1989), we have observed similar changes in the release of ^{3}H-NA from the myenteric plexus. In this model, inflammation is restricted to the distal colon, yet a marked suppression of ^{3}H-NA release is observed not only in the inflamed region but also in the non-inflamed transverse colon and terminal ileum. The mechanisms underlying the remote effects of inflammation on motility are not presently known.

Regional differences in muscle responses to inflammation

It has long been recognized that inflammatory mediators such as prostaglandins exert different effects on circular and longitudinal muscle within a given region of the gut, as well as in different regions of the gut (Sanger et al 1980, Goldenberg & Subers 1991, Ishizawa & Minowa 1982). It is therefore not surprising to observe qualitative differences in the responses of muscle to inflammation. For example, as shown in Figure 9.14 inflammation induced by Trichinella infection in the jejunum produces increased tension development (Vermillion & Collins 1988a) whereas inflammation induced by *Trichinella spiralis* in the distal colon is associated with a decrease in tension

development (Grossi et al 1993). This trend appears to hold true in man. For example, Crohn's disease produces increased tension development by muscle of the small intestine (Vermillion et al 1991b) whereas colitis is associated with a decrease in tension development (Snape et al 1991).

Muscle responses to different inflammatory stimuli

The question may be raised as to whether inflammation induced by different stimuli produce similar changes in tissue responsiveness? It would seem reasonable to expect similar changes provided comparisons are made within the same species and gut region, and over the same time frame as it is likely that acute and chronic inflammation have different mediator profiles. This question was formally addressed in a recent study in which muscle responses were determined following the induction of distal colitis using four different models. A similar decrease in muscle tension development was observed following the induction of colitis by TNB, ethanol, acetic acid or mitomycin (Grossi et al 1993). Similar data were obtained with respect to the suppression of NA release from the myenteric plexus in distal colitis induced by TNB or *Trichinella spiralis* infection. Taken together, these findings indicate that inflammation-induced changes in enteric nerve and muscle in a given tissue are independent of the manner in which inflammation is induced.

Mast cells and altered motility

Increased numbers of mast cells are found in the gut in a variety of conditions that include ulcerative colitis and Crohn's disease (Hiatt & Katz 1962). In addition mast cells are thought to mediate changes in gut function in food allergy. The demonstration of a close anatomical relationship between mast cells and nerves in the gut (Stead et al 1987), together with the demonstration of Pavlovian conditioning of mast cell degranulation in the gut (MacQueen et al 1989) raises the possibility that mast cells may be involved in other conditions that may include IBS. Indeed, as shown in Figure 9.15, increased mast cell numbers have been reported in the muscle layers of patients with IBS or 'spastic colitis' (Hiatt & Katz 1962).

An animal model of food protein hypersensitivity has yielded new information regarding motor responses to antigen exposure in the gut. Exposure of egg albumen-sensitized rats to the antigen produced propulsive motor changes along the small intestine which were associated with diarrhoea (Scott et al 1988). Studies in vitro indicate that antigen exposure of intestinal muscle from sensitized rats results in contraction that is mediated by 5-hydroxytryptamine, and is likely to be mediated by mast cells (Scott et al 1990). The extent to which enteric nerves are involved in antigen-induced motor changes remains to be elucidated.

Mastocytosis occurs not only as a result of immunologic sensitization, but may also occur as a result of manipulation of the bowel at surgery. Studies in the rat have shown that handling of an intestinal segment at surgery results in the appearance of increased number of mast cells in the subserosal region of the longitudinal muscle evident several weeks later. It is believed that the physical trauma results in mast cell degranulation which serves as a stimulus for mast cell proliferation (Vermillion & Collins 1988b). Regardless of the manner in which mastocytosis is induced, the presence of these cells in the muscle layers provides a potential stimulus for intestinal dysmotility.

REFERENCES

Abrams G D, Bishop J E 1967 Effect of normal microbial flora on gastrointestinal motility. Proc Soc Exp Biol (NY) 126: 301–304

Alizadeh H, Castro G A, Weems W A 1987 Intrinsic jejunal propulsion in the guinea pig during parasitism with *Trichinella spiralis*. Gastroenterology 93: 784–790

Alizadeh H, Weems W A, Castro G A 1989 Long-term influence of enteric infection on jejunal propulsion in guinea pigs. Gastroenterology 97: 1461–1468

Almy T P 1961 Observations on the pathologic physiology of ulcerative colitis. Gastroenterology 40: 299–306

Bishop A E, Polack J M, Bryant M G et al 1980 Abnormalities of vasoactive intestinal polypeptide containing nerves in Crohn's disease. Gastroenterology 79: 853–860

Blennerhassett M G, Vignjevic P, Vermillion D L et al 1990 Intestinal inflammation induces T-lymphocyte dependent hyperplasia of jejunal smooth muscle. Gastroenterology 98: A328 (abstract)

Blennerhassett M G, Vignjevic P, Vermillion D L et al 1992 Inflammation causes hyperplasia and hypertrophy in smooth muscle of the rat small intestine. Am J Physiol 262: G1041–G1046

Bowers R L, Castro G A, Weisbrodt N M 1986 Alterations in intestinal smooth muscle of the rat induced by Trichinella spiralis. Gastroenterology 90: 1353 (abstract)

Castro G A, Post C A, Roy S A 1977 Intestinal motility during the enteric phase of trichinosis in immunized rats. J Parasitol 63: 713–719

Chaudhary N A, Truelove S C 1961 Human colonic motility: a comparative study of normal subjects, patients with ulcerative colitis and patients with irritable bowel syndrome. I. Resting patterns of motility. Gastroenterology 40: 1–17

Chinn J S, Schuffler M D 1988 Paraneoplastic visceral neuropathy as a cause of severe gastrointestinal motor dysfunction. Gastroenterology 95: 1279–1286

Collins S M, Blennerhassett P A, Blennerhassett M G et al 1989 Impaired acetylcholine release from the myenteric plexus of Trichinella-infected rats. Am J Physiol 257: G898–G903

Collins S M, Blennerhassett P, Vermillion D L et al 1992a Impaired acetylcholine release in the inflamed rat intestine is T-cell independent. Am J Physiol 263: G198–G201

Collins S M, Blennerhassett P, Hurst S et al 1992b The role of endogenous interleukin-1B in enteric nerve and muscle changes in the inflamed nematode-infected rat intestine. Gastroenterology 102(4): A608 (abstract)

Connell A M 1962 The motility of the pelvic colon. Part II. Paradoxical motility in diarrhea and constipation. Gut 3: 342–348

Crosthwaite A I P, Huizinga J D, Fox J E T 1990 Jejunal circular muscle motility is decreased in nematode-infected rat. Gastroenterology 98: 59–65

Davis D R, Dockerty M B, Mayo C B 1953 The myenteric plexus in regional enteritis: a study of the number of ganglion cells in the ileum in 24 cases. Surg Gynecol Obstet 101: 208–216

Denis P, Collin R, Galmiche J-P 1979 Elastic properties of the rectal wall in normal adults and in patients with ulcerative colitis. Gastroenterology 77: 45–48

Djokic T D, Sekizawa K, Borson D B et al 1989 Neutral endopeptidase inhibitors potentiate substance P-induced contraction in gut smooth muscle. Am J Physiol 256: G39–G43

Dvorak A M, Connell A B, Dickersin G R 1979 Crohn's disease, a scanning electron microscopic study. Hum Path 10: 165–177

Dvorak A M, Osage J E, Monahan R A et al 1980 Crohn's disease: transmission electron microscopic studies. III Target tissues. Proliferation of an injury to smooth muscle and the autonomic nervous system. Hum Pathol 11: 620–634

Eastwood G L, Castell D O, Higgs R H 1975 Experimental esophagitis in cats lowers esophageal sphincter pressure. Gastroenterology 69: 146–153

Farmer S G 1981 Changes in the responsiveness of intestinal smooth muscle to agonists in rat infected with Nippostrongylus brasiliensis. Br J Pharmacol 74: 199

Farthing M J G, Lennard-Jones J E 1978 Sensitivity of the rectum to distension and the anorectal distension reflex in ulcerative colitis. Gut 19: 64–69

Fox-Robichaud A E, Collins S M 1986 Altered calcium-handling properties of jejunal smooth muscle from the nematode-infected rat. Gastroenterology 91: 1462–1469

Garrett J M, Summerskill W J H, Code C F 1966 Antral motility in patients with gastric ulcer. Am J Dig Dis 11: 780–789

Garrett J M, Sauer W G, Moertel G C 1967 Colonic motility in ulcerative colitis after opiate administration. Gastroenterology 53: 93–100

Geboes K, Rutgeerts P, Ectors N 1992 Major histocompatibility class II expression on the small intestinal nervous system in Crohn's disease. Gastroenterology 103: 2 439–447

Goldenberg M M, Subers E M 1991 The effect of leukotriene D4 on the isolated stomach and colon of the rat. Life Sci 33: 2121–2127

Goulston S J M, McGovern V J 1969 The nature of benign strictures in ulcerative colitis. New Engl J Med 281: 290–295

Graham M F, Diegelmann R F, Elson C O et al 1988 Collagen content and types in the intestinal strictures of Crohn's disease. Gastroenterology 94: 257–265

Grossi L, McHugh K, Collins S M 1993 On the specificity of altered muscle function in experimental colitis in rats. Gastroenterology 104: (in press)

Hiatt R B, Katz J 1962 Mast cells in inflammatory conditions of the gastrointestinal tract. Am J Gastroenterol 37: 541–548

Holt S, Heading R C, Taylor T V et al 1986 Is gastric emptying abnormal in duodenal ulcer? Dig Dis Sci 31: 685–692

Huizinga J D, Vermillion D L, Cuthbert C et al 1991 Smooth muscle function in inflammatory bowel disease in: Snape W J, Collins S M (eds) Effects of immune cells and inflammation on smooth muscle and enteric nerves. CRC Press, Boca Raton, FL pp 109–118

Hurst S M, Collins S M, 1990 The regulation of ³H-noradrenaline release from rat myenteric plexus synaptosomes. Gastroenterology 99: A328 (abstract)

Hurst S, Collins S M 1992 The mechanisms of action of tumour necrosis factor-induced suppression of noradrenaline release from rat myenteric plexus. Gastroenterology 102(4): A460 (abstract)

Hurst S M, Collins S M 1993 Interleukin-1β modulation of noradrenaline release from rat myenteric nerves. Am J Physiol 264: G30–G35

Hurst S, Stepien H, Stanisz A et al 1992 The relationship between the pro-inflammatory peptide interleukin-1β (IL-1β) and substance P in the inflamed rat intestine. Gastroenterology 102(4): A460 (abstract)

Hwang L, Okamoto A, Leichter R et al 1992 Neutral endopeptidase (NEP, EC 3.4.24.11) is down regulated in the intestine by infection with Trichinella spiralis. Gastroenterology 102(4): A927 (abstract)

Ishizawa M, Minowa T 1982 Effects of PGD_2 and PGF_2 alpha on longitudinal and circular muscles of guinea-pig isolated proximal colon. Prostaglandins 24: 843–850

Kahrilas P J, Dodds W J, Hogan W J et al 1986 Esophageal peristaltic dysfunction in peptic esophagitis. Gastroenterology 91(4): 897–904

Kern F J, Almy T P, Abbot F K et al 1951 Motility of the distal colon in nonspecific ulcerative colitis. Gastroenterology 19: 492–503

Khan I, Blennerhassett P, Gauldie J et al 1992 Cytokine mRNA profile in smooth muscle from the inflamed intestine of the nematode-infected rat. Gastroenterology 102(4): A645 (abstract)

Khan I, Collins S M 1993 Altered sodium pump gene expression in the inflamed intestine of the nematode infected rat. Am J Physiol (in press)

Koch T R, Carney A, Go V L W 1987 Distribution and quantification of gut neuropeptides in normal intestine and inflammatory bowel diseases. Dig Dis Sci 32: 369–376

Koch T R, Carney J A, Go V L W et al 1988 Spontaneous contractions and some electrophysiological properties of circular muscle from normal sigmoid colon and ulcerative colitis. Gastroenterology 95: 77–84

Koch T R, Carney J A, Go V L W et al 1990 Altered inhibitory innervation of circular smooth muscle in Crohn's colitis. Association with decreased vasoactive intestinal polypeptide levels [published erratum appears in Gastroenterology 1990 (Oct) 99(4): 1199]. Gastroenterology 98: 1437–1444

Krisnamurthy S, Schuffler M D, Belic L et al 1986 An inflammatory axonopathy of the myenteric plexus producing a rapidly progressive intestinal pseudo-obstruction. Gastroenterology 90: 754–758

Kyosola K, Penttila O, Salaspuro M 1977 Rectal mucosal adrenergic innervation and enterochromaffin cells in ulcerative colitis and irritable colon. Scand J Gastroenterol 12: 363–367

Lee E Y, Stenson W F, Deschryver-Kecskemeti K 1991 Thickening of muscularis mucosae in Crohn's disease. Mod Pathol 4: 87–90

Lieberman-Meffert D, Allgower M 1977 The morphology of antrum-pylorusin gastric ulcer disease. Prog Surg 15: 109–139

Liu H Y, Whitehouse W M, Giday Z 1975 Proximal small bowel transit pattern in patients with malabsorption induced by bovine milk protein ingestion. Radiology 115: 415–420

Loening-Baucke V, Metcalf A M, Shirazi S 1989 Rectosigmoid motility in patients with quiescent and active ulcerative colitis. Am J Gastroenterol 84: 34–39

McInerney G T, Sauer W G, Baggenstoss A H et al 1962 Fulminating ulcerative colitis with marked colonic dilation: a clinicopathologic study. Gastroenterology 42: 244–257

MacQueen G, Marshall J, Perdue M et al 1989 Pavlovian conditioning of rat mucosal mast cells to secrete rat mast cell protease II. Science 243: 83–85

Main C, Blennerhassett P, Collins S M 1991 Human recombinant interleukin-1 beta (HrIL-β) suppresses the release of ³H acetylcholine (³H-ACh) from rat myenteric plexus. Gastroenterology 100: A833 (abstract)

Malagelada J-R, Longstreth G R, Deering T B et al 1977 Gastric secretion and emptying after ordinary meals in duodenal ulcer. Gastroenterology 73: 989–994

Manousos O N, Salem S N 1965 Abnormal motility of the

small intestine in ulcerative colitis. Gastroenterologica 1044: 249–257

Mantyh C R, Gates T S, Zimmerman R P et al 1988 Receptor binding sites for substance P, but not substance K or neuromedin K, are expressed in high concentrations by arterioles, venules, and lymph nodules in surgical specimens obtained from patients with ulcerative colitis and Crohn's disease. Proc Natl Acad Sci USA 85: 3235–3239

Mantyh P W, Catton M D, Boehmer C G et al 1989 Receptors for sensory neuropeptides in human inflammatory diseases: implications for the effector role of sensory neurons. Peptides 10: 627–645

Marzio L, Blennerhassett P, Chiverton S et al 1990 Altered smooth muscle function in worm-free gut regions of Trichinella-infected rats. Am J Physiol 259: G306–G313

Mikkelsen H B, Thuneberg L, Rumessen J J et al 1985 Macrophage-like cells in the muscularis externa of the mouse small intestine. Anat Rec 213: 77–86

Moore S C, Malagelada J R, Shorter R G et al 1986 Interrelationships among gastric mucosal morphology, secretion and motility in peptic ulcer disease. Dig Dis Sci 31: 673–684

Morris G P, Beck P L, Herridge M S et al 1989 Hapten-induced model of chronic inflammation and ulceration in the rat colon. Gastroenterology 96: 795–803

Morson B, Dawson IMP 1979 Gastrointestinal pathology. 2nd edn. Blackwell Scientific, Oxford

Muller M J, Huizinga J D, Collins S M 1989 Altered smooth muscle contraction and sodium pump activity in the inflamed rat intestine. Am J Physiol 257: G570–G577

Oehmichen M, Reifferscheid P 1977 Intramural ganglion cell degeneration in inflammatory bowel disease. Digestion 15: 482–496

Okamoto E, Kakutani T, Iwasaki T et al 1964 Morphological studies on the myenteric plexus of the colon in chronic ulcerative colitis. Med J Osaka Univ 15: 85–105

O'Morain C, Bishop A E, McGregor G P et al 1984 Vasoactive intestinal peptide concentrations and immunocytochemical studies in rectal biopsies from patients with inflammatory bowel disease. Gut 25: 56–61

Palmer J M Castro G A 1986 Anamnestic stimulus-specific myoelectric responses associated with intestinal immunity in the rat. Am J Physiol 250: G266–G273

Palmer J M, Weisbrodt N M, Castro G A 1984 Trichinella spiralis: intestinal myoelectrical activity during enteric infusion in the rat. Exp Parasitol 57: 132–141

Penttila O, Kyosola K, Klinge E et al 1975 Studies on rectal mucosal catecholamines in ulcerative colitis. Ann Clin Res 7: 32–36

Rao S S C, Read N W, Stobart J A H et al 1988 Anorectal contractility under basal conditions and during rectal infusion of saline in ulcerative colitis. Gut 29: 769–777

Russell D A, Castro G A 1987 Physiology of the gastrointestinal tract in the parasitized host in: Johnson L R (ed.) Physiology of the gastrointestinal tract. Raven, New York pp 1749–1780

Sanger G J, Bennett A 1980 Regional differences in the responses to prostanoids of circular muscle from guinea-pig isolated intestine. J Pharm Pharmacol 32: 705–708

Schwartzenruber D, Lotze M T, Rosenberg S A 1988 Colonic perforation. An unusual complication of therapy with high dose interleukin-2. Cancer 62: 2350–2353

Scott R B, Diamant S C, Gall G A 1988 Motility effects of intestinal anaphylaxis in the rat. Am J Physiol 255: G505–G511

Scott R B, Gall D G, Maric M 1990 Mediation of food protein-induced jejunal smooth muscle contraction in sensitized rats. Am J Physiol 259: G6–G14

Siemers P T, Dobbins W O 3rd 1974 The Meissner plexus in Crohn's disease of the colon. Surg Gynecol Obstet 138: 39–42

Sjolund K, Schaffalitzky O B, Muckadell D E et al 1983 Peptide-containing nerve fibres in the gut wall in Crohn's disease. Gut 24: 724–733

Smith J W, Castro G A 1978 Relation of peroxidase activity in gut mucosa to inflammation. Am J Physiol 235: R72–R79

Snape W J, Matarazzo S A, Cohen S 1980 Abnormal gastrocolonic response in patients with ulcerative colitis. Gut 21: 392–396

Snape W J, Williams R, Hyman P E 1991 Defect in colonic muscle contraction in patients with ulcerative colitis. Am J Physiol 261: G987–G991

Spiller R C, Lee Y C, Edge C et al 1987 Delayed mouth–caecum transit of a lactulose labelled liquid test meal in patients with steatorrhoea caused by partially treated coeliac disease. Gut 28: 1275–1282

Spriggs E A, Code C F, Bargen J A et al 1951 Motility of the pelvic colon and rectum of normal persons and patients with ulcerative colitis. Gastroenterology 19: 480–491

Stanley E, Stead R, Collins S M 1992 E. coli endotoxi exerts a biphasic effect on acetylcholine release from rat myenteric plexus. Gastroenterology 102(4): A700 (abstract)

Stead R H, Tomioka M, Quinonez G et al 1987 Intestinal mucosal mast cells in normal and nematode infected rat intestines are in intimate contact with peptidergic nerves. Proc Natl Acad Sci USA 84: 2975–2979

Storsteen K A, Kernohan J W, Bargen J A 1953 The myenteric plexus in chronic ulcerative colitis. Surg Gynecol Obstet 97: 335–343

Sukhdeo M V K, Croll N A 1981 Gut propulsion in mice infected with Trichinella spiralis. J Parasitol 67: 906–910

Swain M G, Blennerhassett P A, Collins S M 1991 Impaired sympathetic nerve function in the inflamed rat intestine. Gastroenterology 100: 675–682

Swain M G, Agro A, Blennerhassett P et al 1992 Increased levels of substance P in the myenteric plexus of Trichinella-infected rats. Gastroenterology 102: 1913–1919

Thompson G R, Trexler P C 1971 Gastrointestinal structure and function in germ-free or gnotobiotic animals. Gut 12: 230–235

Vermillion D L, Collins S M 1988a Increased responsiveness of jejunal longitudinal muscle in Trichinella-infected rats. Am J Physiol 254: G124–G129

Vermillion D L, Collins S M 1988b Nonspecific induction of mast cell hyperplasia in intestinal smooth muscle. Gastroenterology 94: A479 (abstract)

Vermillion D L, Ernst P B, Collins S M 1991a T-lymphocyte modulation of intestinal muscle function in the Trichinella-infected rat. Gastroenterology 101: 31–38

Vermillion D L, Huizinga J D, Collins S M 1991b Altered smooth muscle function in Crohn's disease. FASEB J 5(5) Part II: A1062 (abstract)

10. Food and gastrointestinal motility

L. Bueno   J. Fioramonti

INTRODUCTION

The major function of the digestive tract is to digest food, assimilate nutrients and expel non-digestible residues. These functions are directly related to the motility of the digestive tract which is responsible for the intestinal delivery and transport of digesta.

The fact that feeding affects gastrointestinal and colonic motility has been known since the last century when Beaumont (1833) described the changes in amplitude and frequency of gastric contractions asociated with feeding. Recently it has been shown that these changes are related to the nature of food and caloric intake.

PATTERNS OF GASTROINTESTINAL MOTILITY AND DIGESTIVE STATUS

Stomach

In many species manometric recordings of antral motility during fasting or interdigestive period exhibit a cyclic pattern of high-amplitude contractions grouped in phases separated by periods of quiescence and appearing at 90–120 min intervals (Fig. 10.1). The fundamental characteristic of fundic motility is the presence of a steady resting potential of the smooth muscle cells with no regular fluctuations (slow waves) at least in dog and man (Kelly et al 1969, Hinder & Kelly 1977). The other important property of the proximal stomach is receptive relaxation, mediated by inhibitory neurons in vagal nerves (Abrahamsson 1973), which enables it to accommodate food delivered by the oesophagus. The contractions of the corpus and the antrum are coordinated; in the dog a slow contraction of the corpus lasting approximately 30 s is associated with 3–5 more rapid contractions of the antrum (Gill et al 1985). After a meal, the digestive pattern is characterized by steady low-amplitude contractions (4–5 per min) in the gastric antrum with no significant motor activity in the gastric body. Motor patterns of the fasting stomach have been described in Chapter 4.

A cyclic pattern of gastric motility has been found in the dog (Itoh et al 1977) and in man (Rees et al 1982). In the rat (Bueno et al 1982a) and the rabbit (Deloof & Rousseau 1985) there is no cyclic organization of the gastric motility, and feeding induces an increase of both amplitude and frequency of the contractions.

Small intestine

The basic motor pattern of many animal species investigated consists of migrating motor (or myoelectric) complexes (MMCs), first identified as 'a caudad band of large-amplitude action potentials starting in the duodenum and traversing the small bowel' (Szurszewski 1969). Each MMC corresponds to three consecutive phases: phase I has little or no contractile activity (quiescent phase), phase II has intermittent and irregular contractions, while the contractions of phase III occur at their maximal rate, which is determined by the frequency of the slow waves. The duration of phase III activity is relatively constant, but that of other phases varies from cycle to cycle depending on the flow of digesta (Ruckebusch & Bueno 1977). Depending on the animal species, the MMC cycle length varies between 60 and 120 min (Bueno & Ruckebusch 1978) except in rats in which MMCs recur at 15–20 min intervals (Ruckebusch & Fioramonti 1975). The human MMC is described in greater detail in Chapter 4.

Feeding is accompanied by a disruption of the intestinal MMC to give a 'postprandial' pattern characterized by the irregular occurrence of contractions similar to those observed during phase II of the MMC (Bueno et al 1975, Code & Marlett 1975) (Fig. 10.2).

This disruption of the MMC pattern and its replacement by a 'fed' pattern is related to multiple factors, including the energy content of the meal, the nature of nutrients and the frequency of meals and is mediated through mixed neural and humoral factors. In dogs (Fig. 10.3), it has been established that there is a linear

Proximal stomach

50 g

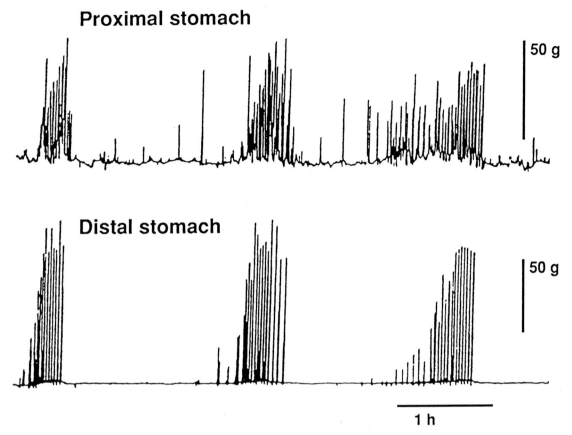

Distal stomach

50 g

1 h

Fig. 10.1 Cyclic patterns of contractions recorded in conscious dogs during fasting with strain gauges sutured on the proximal and distal stomach. (From Gill et al 1985.)

relationship between the duration of the postprandial state of gut motility and the energy content of a meal (De Wever et al 1978). However, non-nutrient factors are also involved in the postprandial disruption of the MMC pattern, since sham-feeding significantly delays the next phase III in man (Defilippi & Valenzuela 1981). On the other hand, meal frequency modulates the effects of feeding on small intestinal motility. For example, in pigs (Ruckebusch & Bueno 1976) and in rats (Ruckebusch & Ferre 1973), ingestion of a daily large meal disrupts the MMC for several hours while under *ad lib* feeding the MMC frequency is similar to that observed in the fasted state. However, in adult as well as in neonatal pigs, feeding a standard meal only induces a 1-h delay in the onset of the next phase III (Burrows et al 1986, Rayner & Wenham 1986).

Large intestine

A universal pattern analogous to that observed for the

small intestine has not been found for the large bowel. A common feature of the colon in all mammalian species investigated is a duality of the contractile activity: tonic contractions corresponding to myoelectrical events characterized by short spike bursts and phasic contractions corresponding to long spike bursts. However, the spatial and temporal organization of these two kinds of contractions which form the colonic motor pattern is specific to each mammalian species so far investigated. This pattern is independent of colonic anatomy and of the traditional regimen of the animal species, but gross similarities exist within species producing moulded faeces such as the pig, the dog or man, and within species that form faeces in pellets such as the rabbit or the sheep (Fioramonti 1981).

In dogs high-amplitude colonic contractions are grouped in phases lasting 4–6 min and appearing at a rate of 2–3 per h in the fasted state with an increase in frequency (4–5 per h) during the 10 h after a daily meal (Fioramonti & Bueno 1983a). In man the most

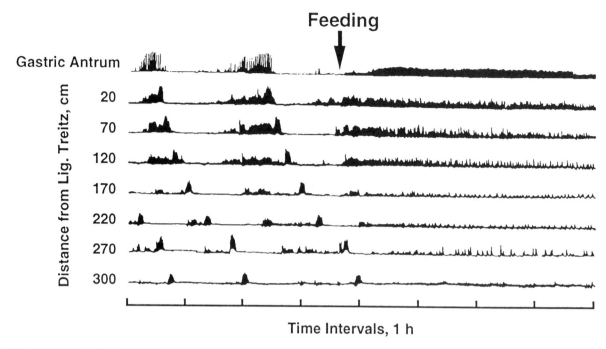

Fig. 10.2 Disruption of MMCs on the stomach and small intestine after feeding in a conscious dog chronically fitted with strain gauge transducers. (From Itoh & Sekiguchi 1984.)

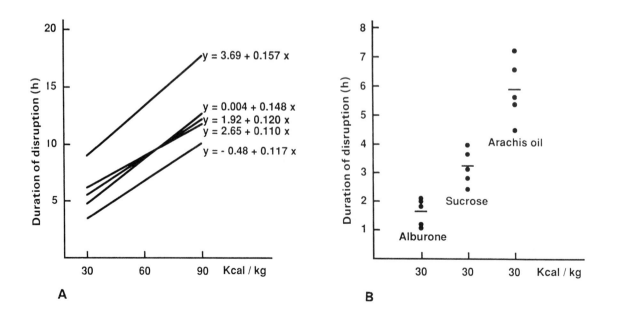

Fig. 10.3 Duration of the postprandial disruption of MMCs on the jejunum after feeding three different quantities of the same meal (**A**) or equicaloric amounts of three food components **B** in five dogs. (From De Wever et al 1978.)

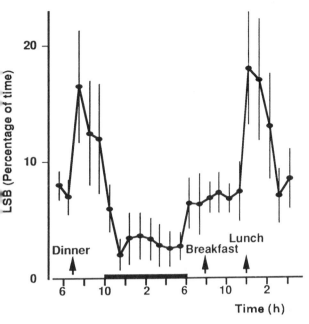

Fig. 10.4   Hourly variation of the LSB activity of the transverse colon in 10 healthy subjects, showing an inhibition during the night time (▬▬▬) and an increased activity for the 3 hours following a 1000 Kcal dinner and lunch. (From Frexinos et al 1985.)

typical characteristic of colonic motility, not seen in animals, consists of a very low activity during the night (Frexinos et al 1985). After a 3000–4000 kJ meal the frequency of colonic contractions is increased for 2–3 h. Such an increase in colonic motility after a meal seems to be a common feature (Fig. 10.4).

RELATIONSHIPS BETWEEN MOTILITY AND FLOW OF DIGESTA

Stomach

In terms of transit of digesta the three major functions of the stomach are the receipt of food, the storage of ingested food and the emptying of liquids and solids.

The entry of a large amount of food into the stomach leads to adaptive (or receptive) relaxation of the muscle wall and permits the fundus and the upper body to act as a reservoir (Jahnberg 1977). The rhythmic contractions of the distal stomach are thought to control the trituration and emptying of solids, whereas the tonic contractions of the proximal stomach govern the rate of emptying of liquids. The pylorus prevents duodenogastric reflux, but is also a true sphincter that controls the emptying of food from the stomach.

Small intestine

The greatest flow of digesta occurs generally during the postprandial disruption of the MMC pattern, but the role of MMCs in the propulsion of digesta is not negligible since, at least in dogs, gastric emptying is not terminated when the MMCs reappear on the jejunum (Banta et al 1979). However the propulsive role of each phase of the MMC still remains controversial depending on the experimental model: the maximal transit rate of a marker has been found associated with phase III using a jejunal isolated loop (Sarr et al 1980) or with phase II when experiments were performed on an intact intestine in the same species.

Using an electromagnetic flowmeter to measure digesta flow continuously and electromyography to record intestinal motility, it has been observed in sheep that the majority of intestinal contents flowed intermittently for periods of 10–15 min at the same frequency as the MMC (Fig. 10.5.). Two-thirds of this flow occurred in the 4–6 min immediately preceding the periods of phase III migration (Bueno et al 1975).

Postprandial contractile patterns and transit and the distance over which the contractions are propagated vary according to the nature of the ingesta (Fig. 10.6) (Schemann & Ehrlein 1986).

Large intestine

The two kinds of colonic contractile activity have opposite effects on the propulsion of digesta. Phasic contractions ensure the mixing and the aboral progression of colonic contents while the tonic activity acts as a brake.

In dogs the spontaneous fluctuations of the phasic activity are positively correlated with the spontaneous changes in the velocity of transit of a marker introduced in the proximal colon (Fioramonti et al 1980). Similarly in pigs, a low-residue diet induces a threefold increase in colonic mean retention time which was related to a decrease in phasic activity and an increase in tonic activity (Fioramonti & Bueno 1980) (Fig. 10.7).

However, in humans, despite the many studies of colonic motility or colonic transit time, relations between muscle activities and digesta movement have not been fully elucidated.

HORMONAL CONTROL OF THE POSTPRANDIAL PATTERN

A hormone may be implicated in the change from the fasted to the fed motor pattern if its release occurs after a meal and if its infusion, at physiological doses,

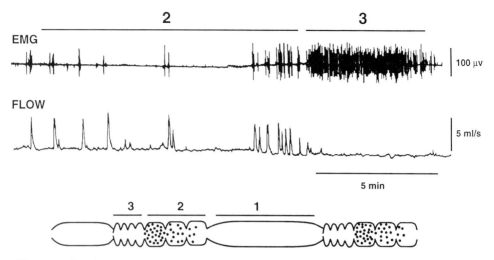

Fig. 10.5 Simultaneous recording of spiking myoelectrical activity and flow of digesta in the jejunum in the sheep. The greatest flow occurs at the end of phase II. No flow was observed during phase III and phase I. (Adapted from Bueno et al 1975.)

in fasted subjects induces a motor pattern typical of the fed state. Summaries of studies showing some effects of infused hormones on motor or myoelectric patterns in different species are represented in Table 10.1.

Hormones involved

Among the hormones released by a meal, gastrin (Weisbrodt et al 1974, Marik & Code 1975, Wingate et al 1978a), insulin (Bueno & Ruckebusch 1976), cholecystokinin (CCK) (Mukhopadhyay et al 1977, Wingate et al 1978a), secretin, glucagon (Wingate et al 1978b), and neurotensin (Al Saffar & Rosell 1981; Thor et al 1982) alter the cyclic pattern of the MMC when infused intravenously (Table 10.2). This suggests that these substances may play a role in the change of the motility pattern after feeding. However, it is unlikely that a single hormone is responsible for the postprandial change of the gastrointestinal motor pattern since for each hormone there are arguments against a physiological motor action. For example, in dogs a long-lasting disruption of the MMC occurs after fat ingestion, but with no significant increase in plasma gastrin and insulin (Eeckhout et al 1978). Indeed significant increases in gastrin and insulin concentrations in blood induced by glucose ingestion or intravenous infusion are not associated with a disruption of the MMC pattern (Eeckhout et al 1978). Similarly the disruptive effect on MMCs of insulin infusion is abolished in pigs when a normal blood glucose level is maintained

by a concomitant glucose infusion (Rayner et al 1981). On the other hand, infusions of CCK or gastrin, or both, disrupt the duodenal MMC in dogs, but the cyclic peaks of motilin concentrations in blood persist, while in the same animals plasma motilin is reduced after a meal (Lee et al 1980). Moreover, analysis of intestinal myoelectric activity in dogs indicates that the pattern of contractions induced by CCK, secretin or gastrin infusion is different from that observed after a meal (Wingate et al 1978a).

In rats as well as in humans neurotensin infusion induces a pattern of intestinal contractions very similar to that observed after feeding (Al Saffar & Rosell 1981, Thor et al 1982). In rats intestinal neurotensin exhibits circadian variations, with a maximum during the nighttime which corresponds to a period of intense ingestive behaviour associated with the disruption of MMCs (Ferris et al 1986). However, in man the plasma concentration of neurotensin induced by an infusion that is able to disrupt the MMC pattern is much greater than the plasma concentration observed after a meal (Shaw & Buchanan, 1983).

Regulation by hormones of the postprandial pattern of gastrointestinal motility is a very attractive hypothesis and hormones are undoubtedly involved in the disruption of the MMC, at least in the stomach, since feeding abolishes the MMC in an autotransplanted fundic pouch (Thomas & Kelly 1979). However, nervous factors are also of importance since vagotomy delays the onset of the fed pattern (Ruckebusch & Bueno 1977) and the MMCs occurring in an

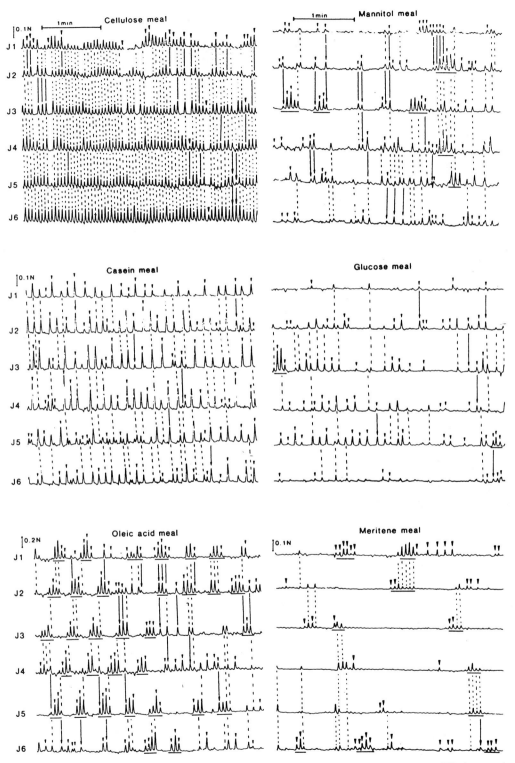

Fig. 10.6 Variations in postprandial contractile patterns, transit and distance of propagation differing according to nature of ingesta (Schemann & Ehrlein 1986).

Table 10.1 Comparative effects of the systemic infusion of gastrointestinal hormones on cyclical variations in the fasted state in human and animal species.

	Induction of phase III	Increase in MMC frequency	Suppression of fed pattern	Species	References
Motilin	G + + D + +	–	°	Dog	Wingate et al (1976) Thomas et al (1979) Itoh et al (1978) Poitras et al (1980) Chey et al (1978)
	G + + D + +	°/ +	ND	Man	Lux et al (1980) Vantrappen et al (1979) Peeters et al (1980)
	G° D°	°	°	Pig	Borody et al (1981) Bueno et al (1982b)
	G° D + /°	°	°	Sheep	Bueno et al (1977)
Somatostatin	G° D + +	+ +	+	Dog	Bueno et al (1982b) Poitras et al (1980)
	G° D + +	–	ND	Pig	Bueno et al (1982b)
	G° D°	+ +	ND	Man	Peeters et al (1983)
Pancreatic polypeptide	G° D°	+ + +	°	Dog	Bueno et al (1982b)
	G° D + +	+ + +	ND	Pig	Bueno et al (1982b)
	G – D°	°	°	Man	Janssens et al (1982)

+ increase; ° no effect; – decrease; G gastric; D duodenal; ND not determined

Table 10.2 Comparative effects of systemic infusion of gastrointestinal (GI) and pancreatic hormones released after feeding on the GI motor pattern in human and animal species.

	Disruption of MMC pattern	Initiation of fed pattern	Duration of fed pattern	Species	References
Pancreatic hormones					
Insulin	+ + +	+ +	+ +	Dog, sheep	Bueno et al (1977)
				Rat	Pascaud et al (1982)
Pancreatic polypeptide	°	°	–	Dog, pig	Bueno et al (1982b)
	+	+	°	Man	Peeters et al (1983)
Somatostatin	+ (GD)	°	°	Dog, pig	Poitras et al (1980) Bueno et al (1982b)
				Man	Peeters et al (1983)
Glucagon	+	0	0	Dog	Wingate et al (1978b)
Secretin	+	0	+	Dog	Wingate et al (1978a)
GI hormones					
Motilin	°			Dog	Itoh et al (1975) Wingate et al (1976)
				Man	Rees et al (1982)
Gastrin	+ +	+	°	Dog	Eeckhout et al (1978) Marik & Code (1975) Weisbrodt et al (1974)
				Cow	Wingate et al (1978a)
CCK₃₃, CCK₈	+ +	+ + +	+ +	Dog	Weisbrodt et al (1976) Mukhopadhyay et al (1977) Wingate et al (1978a)
				Rat	Bueno & Ferre (1982)
				Sheep	Bueno & Fioramonti (1980)
Neurotensin	+ +	+ +	+ / –	Rat	Al Saffar & Rosell (1981) Thor et al (1982)

+ increase: ° no effect; – decrease; GD gastroduodenal; CCK cholecystokinin

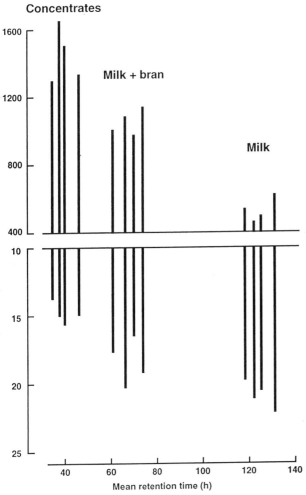

Fig. 10.7 Relationship between colonic transit time and colonic spiking activity in four pigs on three different diets. The lowest LSB activity and the highest SSB activity was associated with a prolonged transit time on a fibre free diet (milk). (From Fioramonti & Bueno 1980.)

Central versus peripheral site of action

Numerous findings indicate a link between the brain and the digestive tract in both physiological and pathological states. Smith et al (1977) showed that the thyrotropin-releasing hormone, administered into the lateral ventricle of the brain (intracerebroventricular [i.c.v.] administration) stimulated colonic motility in anaesthetized rabbits. Bueno & Ferre (1982) showed that central administration of somatostatin at a picomolar dose (inactive by the systemic route) increases the frequency of jejunal MMC in the rat while, in contrast, i.c.v.-administered CCK disrupts the MMC pattern. Since then, increasing evidence has accumulated that several neuropeptides may affect the pattern of gastrointestinal motility when centrally administered. These peptides may be divided into two groups according to the digestive state and the corresponding motor profile under consideration.

The first group includes peptides, CCK being an important example, which disrupt the MMC pattern after central administration. After feeding, CCK-like immunoreactivity has been found to increase in the primate hypothalamus (Schick et al 1987). Central administration of CCK disrupts the jejunal MMC and induced a fed pattern in both rats (Bueno & Ferre 1982) and dogs (Karmeli et al 1987). More recently, it was shown that central administration of antiserum against CCK or the CCK-receptor antagonist asperlicin after a meal restored the MMC pattern in rats (Duc 1988). These results support a physiological role of CCK at the central level in the postprandial disruption of the MMC pattern but this is likely to be mediated by neuronal rather than circulating CCK.

At the peripheral level the postprandial role of CCK in the control of the gastrointestinal motor pattern may also be neuronal since CCK_8 immunoreactivity has been demonstrated in axons and nerve cell bodies of the enteric nervous system (Larsson & Rehfeld 1979). Moreover, one of the main mechanisms involved in the effects of CCK is an indirect action resulting in an increase in acetylcholine release from intramural cholinergic nerves (Gerner & Haffner 1977). Circulating CCK may alter the motor activity directly by binding to specific receptors located on the smooth-muscle-cell membrane (Morgan et al 1978) but a central component connot be excluded since intravenous administration of CCK_8, which does not cross the blood–brain barrier (Zhu et al 1986), has been found to activate hypothalamic neurons (Renaud et al 1987) and to increase CCK concentrations in the lateral hypothalamus (McLaughlin et al 1986).

In agreement with the concept of a physiological

autotransplanted segment of dog jejunum are not disrupted by feeding (Sarr & Kelly 1981).

The motility of the colon is stimulated after feeding. Intravenous infusion of postprandially-released hormones such as gastrin (Snape et al 1978), CCK (Renny et al 1983) or neurotensin (Thor & Rosell 1986) stimulate colonic motility. However, no information is available to confirm a physiological role for these hormones in the control of the colonic motor response to eating for which a neural mechanism (Snape et al 1979), associated in dogs with the entry of digesta into the colon (Fioramonti & Bueno 1983a), seems probable.

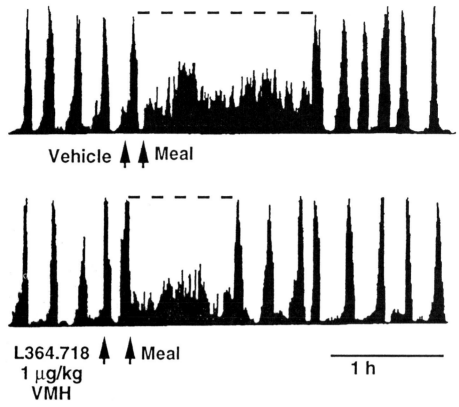

Fig. 10.8 Reduction of the duration of postprandial disruption of duodenal MMCs after a microinjection of L 364 718, A CCK$_A$ antagonist, into the ventromedial hypothalamus (VMH) nucleus in the rat. (From Liberge et al 1990.)

role for CCK released in the central nervous system CNS in response to feeding, it has been recently shown in rats that the CCK$_A$ receptor antagonist devazepide injected bilaterally into the ventromedial nucleus of the hypothalamus (VMH) greatly reduces the duration of the postprandial pattern after a given meal (Fig. 10.8), an effect not reproduced by similar administration into the lateral hypothalamus (Liberge et al 1990). In addition while CCK$_8$ microinjected into the VMH mimics the increase in colonic motility observed after a meal, devazepide injected in the same brain nucleus just prior to feeding abolishes the colonic response to the meal in rats. This result supports the hypothesis that CCK$_8$ released in the CNS mediates, in rats, the motor adaptation of the small intestine and the proximal colon to the postprandial state (Liberge et al 1991).

In agreement with such a hypothesis, it was recently shown that addition of fat to a standard meal in dogs dose-dependently inhibits the postprandial increase in pyloric contractions and slows gastric emptying (Fig. 10.9). However not only CCK$_8$ but also endogenous opioids and prostaglandins are involved in the mediation of these effects (Lopez et al 1991a,b).

Another peptide with a potent central action which disrupts the MMC pattern is corticotropin-releasing factor (CRF) but the effects of i.c.v. administration are limited to the stomach (Bueno & Fioramonti 1986). This action which suppresses gastric MMC does not involve a peripheral release of corticotropin and cortisol. In addition, acoustic stress in dogs reproduces the central effect of CRF on gastric motility (Gué et al 1987). Since CRF is known to be released by stress (Rivier et al 1982), this peptide may be responsible at the central level for the digestive motor disturbances observed in stressful conditions. This hypothesis is supported by observations in mice showing that the acceleration of gastric emptying of nutritive meals induced by acoustic or cold stress is blocked by i.c.v. administration of an antiserum against CRF (Bueno & Gué 1988).

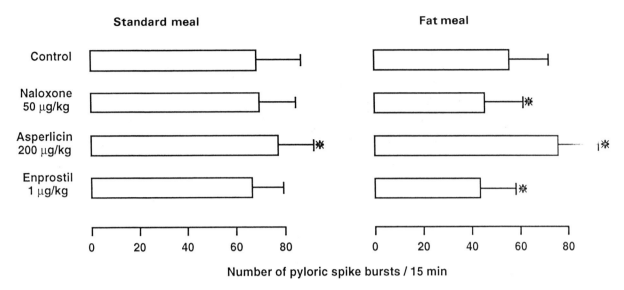

Fig. 10.9 Frequency of spike bursts corresponding to pyloric contractions after a standard or a fat enriched meal in dogs. The opiate antagonist naloxone and the prostaglandin E_2 analogue emprostil inhibit pyloric motility after a fat meal only. The CCK antagonist asperlicin increases the number of pyloric contractions after both meals. (Adapted from Lopez et al 1991a,b.)

The second group of peptides with a central site of action on digestive motility are those that restore a MMC pattern in the jejunum when given i.c.v. after a meal. Such an effect is not sufficient to prove a central physiological action, but it suggests that the CNS is involved in the normal postprandial disruption of the intestinal MMC pattern. For example, MMC disruption can be blocked by i.c.v. administration of calcitonin, neurotensin or growth-hormone-releasing factor (Bueno et al 1985a) as well as interleukin (IL) β at doses ineffective by the systemic route.

The mechanisms involved in the central action of these peptides are different. The central effect of calcitonin, neurotensin and IL1 involves a release of prostaglandins since it is blocked by indomethacin (Bueno et al 1985a), while that of GHRF is mediated through dopaminergic receptors since it is blocked by dopamine antagonists (Bueno et al 1985b).

The disruptive effects of centrally-administered CRF on the gastroduodenal MMC pattern in the fasted state, as well as the action of centrally administered calcitonin in restoring the MMC pattern at the jejuno-ileal level in the fed state, are blocked by vagotomy (Bueno et al 1985a, Gué et al 1987). This is consistent with the neural inhibition of phase III activity by food which has been shown to be mediated by extrinsic nerves (Ruckebusch & Bueno 1977, Diamant et al 1980).

NUTRITIONAL IMPLICATIONS

Intestinal motility, digestive secretions and intestinal absorption are closely-related processes that control nutrient absorption and the digestion of food. Thus, the influence of food components on the release of gastrointestinal hormones may be considered a link between nutrition and digestive motility.

Hormonal influence of food components on digestive motility

The duration of the MMC disruption after a meal depends much more on the physico-chemical composition of the food than on its volume or its energy content. For example, ingestion of 125 kJ/kg in the form of arachis oil in dogs disrupts the MMC pattern for 6 h while an isoenergetic meal of milk protein induces a MMC disruption for only 2 h (De Wever et al 1978). However, the effect of fats cannot be related to circulating levels of insulin or gastrin since their plasma concentration remains unchanged after the ingestion of arachis oil (Eeckhout et al 1978). The digestive motor responses to fat in a meal may be mediated by circulating CCK which is mainly released after the ingestion of fat, at least in humans (Liddle et al 1985), and which is considered to have a physiological effect on gastric emptying (Debas et al 1975). However, a role for gastrin in the postprandial MMC disruption

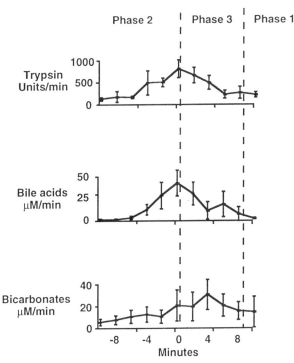

Fig. 10.10 Relationships among duodenal MMC and pancreatic and biliary flow in dogs. The maximal output of trypsin, bile acids and bicarbonates appears at the onset of phase III. (From Keane et al 1980.)

cannot be excluded, since during total parenteral nutrition in dogs the MMC pattern persists in association with depressed concentrations of serum and antral gastrin (Weisbrodt et al 1976).

Similarly at colonic level the fat component of the diet has been found to be the predominant stimulus of colonic motor activity in response to eating (Wright et al 1980). However, CCK, which also stimulates colonic motility, cannot be considered as the major mediator of the colonic response to fat ingestion since stimulation of muscarinic receptors is required in the fat response but not in the CCK-induced colonic stimulation (Renny et al 1983).

Hormonal control of digestive motility and nutrient absorption

Exocrine secretion and mucosal absorption vary synchronously with patterns of motor activity and may also be affected by peptides that alter motility.

Pancreatic and biliary flow are associated with duodenal MMC. In dogs, maximal outputs of lipase (EC 3.1.1.3) and bilirubin appear during the duodenal propagation of phase III activity (Dimagno et al 1979). Similarly bile acids, trypsin and bicarbonate outputs are maximal during phase III activity (Keane et al 1980) (Fig. 10.10). However, the amount of pancreatic enzymes secreted during phase III activity was found

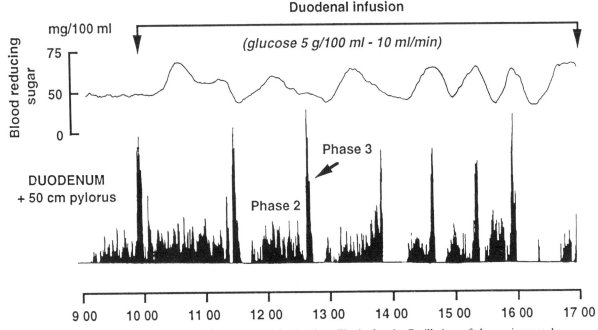

Fig. 10.11 Relationships between glucose absorption and duodenal motility in the pig. Oscillations of glycaemia are at the same frequency than duodenal MMC during continuous infusion of glucose into the duodenum. (From Fioramonti et al 1982.)

to be 50% of that secreted during a similar time following ingestion of a meal.

Studies of absorption in animals prepared with isolated intestinal loops indicate that the rate of digesta passage affects the uptake of nutrients (Sarr et al 1980). In experiments with intact animals the maximal absorption of glucose occured during the later stages of phase II activity of the MMC (Fig. 10.11), when the rate of transit was fastest compared with other phases of the intestinal motor complex (Fioramonti & Bueno 1983). These relationships between intestinal motility and absorption have been indirectly confirmed by the presence of the highest values of potential difference across the mucosa during phase III activity in dogs as well as in humans (Read 1980). Moreover,

mesenteric arterial blood flow, which controls passive paracellular absorption but also active transcellular transport through the oxygen supply, exhibits cyclic variations at the same frequency as recurrent MMC (Fig. 10.10). Minimal blood flow occurs during the periods of intestinal motor quiescence (Fioramonti & Bueno 1983b) and maximal mesenteric blood flow has been observed after a meal (Vatner et al 1970). Digestive hormones act on smooth muscles of both arteries and small intestine, but their effects can be similar or opposite. For example, gastrin and CCK increase and somatostatin decreases both blood flow and intestinal motility, while glucagon inhibits motility and increases blood flow (Fondacaro 1984).

REFERENCES

Abrahamsson H 1973 Studies on the inhibitory nervous control of gastric motility. Acta Physiol Scand 390 suppl: 1–38

Al Saffar A, Rosell S 1981 Effects of neurotensin and neurotensin analogues on the migrating myoelectrical complexes in the small intestine of rats. Acta Physiol Scand 112: 203–208

Banta C A, Clemens E T, Krinsky M M et al 1979 Sites of organic acid production and patterns of digesta movements in the gastrointestinal tract of dogs. J Nutrition 109: 1592–1600

Beaumont W 1833 Experiments and observation on the gastric juice and the physiology of the digestion. F P Allen, Plattsburgh

Borody T J, Byrnes D J, Slowiaczek J G et al 1981 Motilin and migrating myoelectric complexes in pigs. J Physiol 310: 37P–38P

Bueno L, Ferre J P 1982 Central regulation of intestinal motility by somatostatin and cholecystokinin octapeptide. Science 216: 1427–1429

Bueno L, Fioramonti J 1980 Rhythms of abomaso-intestinal motility in: Ruckebusch Y, P Thivend P, (eds) Digestive physiology and metabolism in ruminants. MTP Press, Lancaster, pp 53–80

Bueno L, Fioramonti J 1986 Effects of corticotropin-releasing factor, corticotropin and cortisol on gastrointestinal motility in dogs. Peptides 7: 73–77

Bueno L, Gué M 1988 Evidence for the involvement of corticotropin-releasing factor in the gastrointestinal disturbances induced by acoustic and cold stress in mice. Br Res 441: 1–4

Bueno L, Ruckebusch M 1976 Insulin release and jejunal electrical activity in dogs and sheep. Am J Physiol 230: 1538–1544

Bueno L, Ruckebusch Y 1978 Migrating myoelectrical complexes. Disruption, enhancement and disorganisation in: Duthie H L (ed.) Proceedings of the 6th International Symposium on Gastrointestinal Motility, Edinburgh, 1977 MTP Press, Lancaster, pp 83–90

Bueno L, Fioramonti J, Ruckebusch Y 1975 Rate of flow of digesta and electrical activity of the small intestine in dogs and sheep. J Physiol 249: 69–85

Bueno L, Weekes T E C, Ruckebusch Y 1977 Effects of diet on the motility of the small intestine and plasma insulin levels in sheep. Annales de Recherches Vétérinaires 8: 95–104

Bueno L, Ferre J P, Fioramonti J et al 1982a Control of the antral motor response to feeding by gastric acid secretion in rats. J Physiology 325: 43–50

Bueno L, Fioramonti J, Rayner V et al 1982b Effects of motilin, somatostatin and pancreatic polypeptide on the migrating myoelectric complex in pigs and dogs. Gastroenterology 44: 1395–1402

Bueno L, Fargeas M J, Fioramonti J et al 1985a Central control of intestinal motility by prostaglandins: a mediator of the action of several peptides in rats and dogs. Gastroenterology 88: 1888–1894

Bueno L, Fioramonti J, Primi M P 1985b Central effects of growth hormone-releasing factor (GRF) on intestinal motility in dogs: involvement of dopaminergic receptors. Peptides 6: 403–407

Burrows C F, Meritt A M, Tash J 1986 Jejunal myoelectrical activity in the conscious neonatal pig. J Physiol 374: 349–357

Chey W Y, Lee K Y, Tai H H 1978 Endogenous plasma motilin concentration and interdigestive myoelectric activity of the canine duodenum in: Bloom S R (ed.) Gut hormones. Churchill Livingstone, Edinburgh, pp 355–358

Code C F, Marlett J A 1975 The interdigestive myoelectric complex of the stomach and the small bowel of dogs. J Physiol 246: 298–309

De Wever I, Eeckhout C, Vantrappen G et al 1978 Disruptive effect on test meals on interdigestive motor complex in dogs. Am J Physiol 235: E661–E665

Debas H T, Farooq O, Grossman M I 1975 Inhibition of gastric emptying is a physiological action of cholecystokinin. Gastroenterology 68: 1211–1217

Defilippi C, Valenzuela J E 1981 Sham feeding disrupts the interdigestive motility complex in man. Scand J Gastroenterol 16: 977–979

Deloof S, Rousseau J P 1985 Specific effects of thoracic vagotomy on the electrical activity of the gastric antrum and pylorus in rabbits. Quarterly J Exp Physiol 70: 491–501

Diamant N E, Hall K, Mui H et al 1980 Vagal control of the feeding motor pattern in the lower oesophageal sphincter, stomach and small intestines of dog in: Christensen J (ed.) Gastrointestinal motility. Raven Press, New York, pp 365–370

Dimagno E P, Hendricks J C, Go V L W et al 1979 Relationships among canine fasting pancreatic and biliary secretions, pancreatic duct pressure, and duodenal phase III motor activity. Boldyreff revisited. Dig Dis Sci 24: 689–693

Duc F 1988 Contribution à l'étude du contrôle hormonal sur la motricité duodénale chez le rat. Rôle privilégié de la cholecystokinin (Hormonal control of duodenal motility in the rat. Role of cholecystokinin). Doctoral thesis, University of Lyon

Eeckhout C, De Wever I, Peeters I et al 1978 Role of gastrin and insulin in postprandial disruption of migrating complex in dog. Am J Physiol 235: E666–E669

Ferris C F, George J K, Alberts H E 1986 Circadian rhythm of neurotensin levels in rat small intestine. Reg Pept 15: 285–292

Fioramonti J 1981 Etude comparée des fonctions motrices du gros intestin (A comparative study of large intestine motor functions). Doctoral thesis, University of Toulouse

Fioramonti J, Bueno L 1980 Motor activity in the large intestine of the pig related to dietary fibre and retention time. Br J Nutr 43: 155–162

Fioramonti J, Bueno L, Ruckebusch Y 1982 Blood sugar oscillations and duodenal migrating myoelectric complexes. Am J Physiol 242: G15–G20

Fioramonti J, Bueno L 1983a Diurnal changes in colonic motor profile in conscious dogs. Dig Dis Sci 28: 257–264

Fioramonti J, Bueno L 1983b Relationship between intestinal motility and mesenteric blood flow in the conscious dog. Am J Physiol 246: G108–G113

Fioramonti J, Garcia-Villar R, Bueno L et al 1980 Colonic myoelectrical activity and propulsion in the dog. Dig Dis Sci 25: 641–646

Fondacaro J D 1984 Intestinal blood flow and motility in: Shepherd A P, Granger N (eds) Physiology of the intestinal circulation. Raven Press, New York, pp 120–170

Frexinos J, Bueno L, Fioramonti J 1985 Diurnal changes in myoelectric spiking activity of the human colon. Gastroenterology 88: 1104–1110

Gerner T, Haffner J F W 1977 The role of local cholinergic pathways in the motor responses to cholecystokinin and gastrin in isolated guinea-pig fundus and antrum. Scand J Gastroenterol 12: 7571–7578

Gill R C, Pilot M A, Thomas P A et al 1985 Organization of fasting and postprandial myoelectric activity in stomach and duodenum of conscious dogs. Am J Physiol 249: G655–G661

Gué M, Fioramonti J, Frexinos J et al 1987 Influence of acoustic stress by noise on gastrointestinal motility in dogs. Dig Dis Sci 32: 1411–1471

Hinder R A, Kelly K A 1977 Human gastric pacesetter potential. Site of origin, spread, and response to gastric transection and proximal gastric vagotomy. Am J Surgery 133: 29–33

Itoh Z, Sekiguchi T 1984 Interdigestive motor activity in health and disease in: Polak J M, Bloom S R, Wright N A, Butler A G (eds) Physiology of the gut. Glaxo Group Research, Ware, UK, pp 121–134

Itoh Z, Aizawa I, Takeuchi S et al 1975 Hunger contractions and motilin in: Vantrappen, G (ed.) Proceedings of the 5th International Symposium on G I Motilin. Typoff, Herentals pp 48–55

Itoh Z, Aizawa I, Takeuchi S et al 1977 Diurnal changes in gastric motor activity in conscious dogs. Dig Dis Sci 22: 929–935

Itoh Z, Takeuchi S, Aizawa I et al 1978 Changes in plasma motilin concentration and gastrointestinal contractile activity in the conscious dog. Am J Dig Dis 23: 929–935

Jahnberg T 1977 Gastric adaptative relaxation. Scand J Gastroenterol 12, Suppl: 1–32

Janssens J, Hellemans J, Adrian T E et al 1982 Pancreatic polypeptide is not involved in the regulation of the migrating motor complex in man. Reg Pept 3: 41–49

Karmeli R, Kamei C, Schamlz P et al 1987 The effect of intracerebroventricular perfusion with CCK-OP on gastrointestinal myoelectric activity in the dog. Dig Dis Sci 32: 916

Keane F B, DiMagno E P, Dozois R R et al 1980 Relationships among canine interdigestive exocrine pancreatic and biliary flow, duodenal motor activity, plasma pancreatic polypeptide and motilin. Gastroenterology 78: 310–316

Kelly K A, Code C F, Elveback LR 1969 Patterns of canine gastric electrical activity. Am J Physiol 217: 461–470

Larsson L I, Rehfeld U R 1979 Localization and molecular heterogeneity of cholecystokinin in the central and peripheral nervous system. Br Res 165: 201–218

Lee K Y, Kim P S, Chey W Y 1980 Effects of a meal and gut hormones on plasma motility and duodenal motility in dog. Am J Physiol 238: G280–G283

Liberge M, Arruebo P, Bueno L 1990 CCK8 neurons of the ventromedial (VMH) hypothalamus mediate the upper gut motor changes associated with feeding in rats. Br Res 508: 118–123

Liberge M, Arruebo P, Bueno L 1991 Role of hypothalamic cholecytstokinin octapeptide in the colonic motor response to a meal in rats. Gastroenterology 100: 441–449

Liddle R A, Goldfine I D, Rosen M S et al 1985 Cholecystokinin bioactivity in human plasma: molecular forms, responses to feeding and relationship to gallbladder contraction. J Clin Invest 75: 1144–1152

Lopez Y, Fioramonti J, Bueno L 1991a Action of endogenous prostaglandins on postprandial pyloric motility: a possible modulation by fats. Prostaglandins 42: 313–320

Lopez Y, Fioramonti J, Bueno L 1991b Central and peripheral control of postprandial pyloric motility by endogenous opiates and cholecystokinin in dogs. Gastroenterology 101: 1249–1255

Lux G, Femppel J, Lederer P et al 1980 Somatostatin induces interdigestive intestinal motor and secretory complex-like activity in man. Gastroenterology 78: 1212

McLaughlin C L, Baile C A, Della-Fera MA 1986 Changes in brain CCK concentrations with peripheral CCK injections in Zucker rats. Physiol and Behav 36: 477–482

Marik F, Code C F 1975 Control of the interdigestive myoelectric activity in dogs by the vagus nerves and pentagastrin. Gastroenterology 69: 387–395

Morgan K G, Schmalz P F, Go V L W et al 1978 Electrical and mechanical effects of molecular variants of CCK on antral smooth muscle. Am J Physiol 235: E324–E239

Mukhopadhyay A K, Thor P J, Copeland E M et al 1977 Effect of cholecystokinin on myoelectric activity of small bowel of the dog. Am J Physiol 232: E44–E47

Pascaud X, Ferre J P, Genton M et al 1982 Intestinal motility response to insulin and glucagon in streptozotocin diabetic rats. Can J Physiol Pharmacol 60: 960–967

Peeters T L, Janssens J, Vantrappen G R 1983 Somatostatin and the interdigestive migrating motor complex in man. Reg Pept 5: 209–217

Peeters T L, Vantrappen G, Janssens J 1980 Fasting plasma motilin levels are related to the interdigestive motility complex. Gastroenterology 79: 716–719

Poitras P, Steinbach J H, Van Devenier G 1980 Motilin-independent ectopic fronts of the interdigestive myoelectric complex in dogs. Am J Physiol 239: G125-G220

Rayner V, Wenham G 1986 Small intestinal motility and transit by electromyography and radiology in the fasted and fed pig. J Physiol 379: 245–256

Rayner V, Weekes T E C, Bruce J B 1981 Insulin and myoelectric activity of the small intestine of the pig. Dig Dis Sci 26: 33–41

Read N W 1980 The migrating motor complex and spontaneous fluctuations of transmural potential difference in the human small intestine in Christensen J (ed.) Gastrointestinal motility. Raven Press, New York, pp 299–306

Rees W C W, Malagelada J R, Miller L J et al 1982 Human interdigestive and postprandial gastrointestinal motor and gastrointestinal hormone patterns. Dig Dis Sci 527: 321–329

Renaud L P, Tang M, McCann M J et al 1987 Cholecystokinin and gastric distension activate oxytocinergic cells in rat hypothalamus. Am J Physiol 253: R661–R665

Renny A, Snape W J, Sun E A et al 1983 Role of cholecystokinin in the gastrocolonic response to a fat meal. Gastroenterology 85: 17–21

Rivier C, Rivier J, Vale W 1982 Inhibition of adrenocorticotropic hormone secretion in the rat by immunoneutralisation of corticotropin releasing factor. Science 218: 377–378

Ruckebusch Y 1971 The effect of pentagastrin on the motility of ruminant stomach. Experientia 24: 1185–1186

Ruckebusch Y, Bueno L 1976 The effect of feeding on the motility of the stomach and small intestine in the pig. Br J Nutr 35: 397–405

Ruckebusch Y, Bueno L 1977 Migrating myoelectrical complex of the small intestine. An intrinsic activity mediated by the vagus. Gastroenterology 73: 1309–1314

Ruckebusch M, Ferre J P 1973 Origine alimentaire des variations nycthémérales de l'activité électrique de l'intestin grêle chez le rat (Alimentary origin of the nycthemeral variations of intestinal activity in the rat). Comptes Rendus de la Société de Biologie 167: 2005–2009

Ruckebusch M, Fioramonti J 1975 Electrical spiking activity and propulsion in small intestine in fed and fasted rats. Gastroenterology 68: 1500–1508

Sarr M G, Kelly K A 1981 Myoelectric activity of the autotransplanted canine jejuno ileum. Gastroenterology 81: 303–310

Sarr M G, Kelly K A, Phillips S F 1980 Canine jejunal absorption and transit during interdigestive and digestive motor states. Am J Physiol 239: G167–G172

Schemann M, Ehrlein H -J 1986 Postprandial patterns of canine jujunal motility and transit of luminal content. Gastroenterology 90: 991–1000

Schick R F, Reilly W M, Roddy D R et al 1987 Neuronal

cholecystokinin-like immunoreactivity is postprandially released from primate hypothalamus. Br Res 418: 20–26

Schippers E, Janssens J, Vantrappen G et al 1986 Somatostatin induces ectopic activity fronts via a local intestinal mechanism during fed state or pentagastrin infusion. Am J Physiol 250: G149–G154

Shaw C, Buchanan K D 1983 Intact neurotensin (NT) in human plasma: response to oral feeding. Regulatory Peptides 7: 145–153

Smith J R, Lahann T R, Chesnut R M et al 1977 Thyrotropin releasing hormone: stimulation of colonic activity following intracerebroventricular administration. Science 196: 660–662

Snape W J, Matarazzo A, Cohen S 1978 Effect of eating and gastrointestinal hormones on human colonic myoelectrical and motor activity. Gastroenterology 75: 373–378

Snape W J, Wright S H, Battle W M et al 1979 The gastrocolic response: evidence for a neural mechanism. Gastroenterology 77: 1235–1340

Szurszewski J H 1969 A migrating electric complex of the canine small intestine. Am J Physiol 217: 1757–1763

Thomas P A, Kelly K A 1979 Hormonal control of interdigestive motor cycles of canine proximal stomach. Am J Physiol 237: E192–E197

Thomas P A, Kelly K A, Go V L W 1979 Does motilin regulate canine interdigestive gastric motility? Dig Dis Sci 24: 577–582

Thor K, Rosell S 1986 Neurotensin increases colonic motility. Gastroenterology 90: 27–31

Thor K, Rosell S, Rokaeus A et al 1982 (GIn⁴)-neurotensin changes the motility pattern of the duodenum and proximal jejunum from a fasting-type to fed-type. Gastroenterology 83: 569–574

Vantrappen G, Janssens J, Peeters T L et al 1979 Motilin and the interdigestive migrating motor complex in man. Dig Dis Sci 24: 497–500

Vatner S F, Franklin D, Van Citters R L 1970 Mesenteric vasoactivity associated with eating and digestion in the conscious dog. Am J Physiol 219: 170–174

Weisbrodt N W, Copeland E M, Kearley R W et al 1974 Effects of pentagastrin on electrical activity of small intestine of the dog. Am J Physiol 277: 425–429

Weisbrodt N W, Copeland E M, Thor P J et al 1976 The myoelectric activity of the small intestine of the dog during total parenteral nutrition. Proceedings of the Society for Experimental Biology and Medicine 153: 121–124

Wingate D L, Ruppin H, Green W E R et al 1976 Motilin-induced electrical activity in the canine gastrointestinal tract. Scand J Gastroenterol 11, suppl 39: 111–118

Wingate D L, Pearce E A, Hutton M et al 1978a Quantitative comparison of the effects of cholecystokinin, secretin and pentagastrin on gastrointestinal myoelectric activity in the conscious fasted dog. Gut 19: 593–601

Wingate D L, Pearce E A, Thomas P A et al 1978b Glucagon stimulates intestinal myoelectric activity. Gastroenterology 74: 1152

Wright S H, Snape W J, Battle W et al 1980 Effect of dietary components on gastrocolonic response. Am J Physiol 238: G228–G232

Zhu X G, Greeley G H, Lewis B G et al 1986 Blood–CSF barrier to CCK and effect of centrally administered bombesin on release of brain CCK. J Neurosci Res 15: 393–403

11. Actions of pharmacological agents on gastrointestinal function

T. F. Burks

Drugs that affect gastrointestinal motility have become valuable in the management of a number of diseases. In particular, newer drugs that possess novel mechanisms of action and that act with greater specificity than older drugs are proving their therapeutic worth. The importance of several recent entries into therapeutics has been twofold: the drugs produce beneficial changes in motility and they have revealed the presence of motility components of disease pathophysiology. As understanding of motility control mechanisms has improved, new uses of established drugs have found application in sometimes unexpected ways. We can anticipate rapid progress in the area of pharmacotherapy of disorders of gastrointestinal motility.

Diverse types of drugs are capable of causing changes in patterns of contraction of gastrointestinal smooth muscle (Table 11.1). Often, a change in gastrointestinal motility is the intended effect of the drug.

However, in many cases changes in gastrointestinal motility are undesired side-effects of drug therapy. For example, tricyclic antidepressant drugs used for therapy of affective disorders or histamine H_1 antagonists given for relief of allergic symptoms may induce undesired changes in motility because of intrinsic anticholinergic actions of these classes of drugs. Whether drugs are considered as therapeutic agents intended to bring about relief from a disease process, as experimental tools to probe gastrointestinal biology, or simply as sources of annoying side-effects, it is essential to consider their cellular mechanisms of action to utilize their therapeutic or experimental value optimally or to minimize their gastrointestinal side-effects. Drug actions are generally explicable in terms of increasing or decreasing functions of one or more specific influences that regulate smooth muscle excitability or contractility. In most cases, the actions of the drugs may be relatively simple and straightforward. The complexity encountered in their actions results from the confusing array of multiple systems that regulate smooth muscle contractions.

Table 11.1 General classification of drugs that increase gastrointestinal contractions ('stimulatory') or inhibit contractions ('inhibitory')

Stimulatory	Inhibitory
Cholinergic agonists	Adrenergic agonists
Acetylcholinesterase inhibitors	Dopamine ‡
Prokinetic agents	Anticholinergics†
Opioid agonists *	Phenothiazines
Adrenergic blockers	Tricyclic antidepressants
Ergotamine	Histamine H_1 antagonists
Vasopressin	Calcium blockers
Cholecystokinin	Progestins
Gastrin	Oestrogens
Bile salts	Xanthines
	Papaverine
	Glucagon
	Nitrates
	Iron

* Decrease contractions of antrum; † Includes both muscarinic and nicotinic antagonists; ‡ Increases contractions of colon

MECHANISMS OF DRUG ACTIONS

Sites of action

The usual first step in defining the mechanism of motility action of a particular drug requires identification of the site(s) of action. Established sites of action of drugs that affect gastrointestinal motility include gastrointestinal smooth muscle, intrinsic nerves of the gut, autonomic ganglia, the spinal cord, and the brain (Fig. 11.1).

A number of drugs, hormones and neurotransmitter chemicals act directly upon smooth muscle. In the laboratory, drugs that act directly on gastrointestinal smooth muscle can be studied by a variety of techniques, such as use of tetrodotoxin or by use of dispersed smooth muscle cells. These and other types of

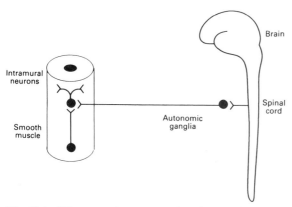

Fig. 11.1 Diagrammatic representation of potential sites of actions of drugs that influence gastrointestinal motility. Drugs may act in the brain, spinal cord, at autonomic ganglia, gut intramural neurons, or upon gut smooth muscle.

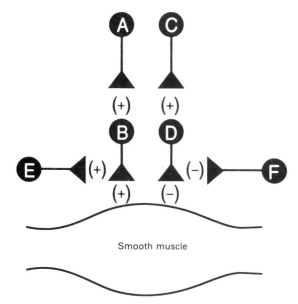

Fig. 11.2 Diagrammatic representation of neural control systems that regulate gastrointestinal smooth muscle. Neural pathway A-B represents an excitatory (+) neural system. Pathway C-D represents an inhibitory (−) neural system. Neuron E can produce an excitatory effect by facilitation of pathway A-B. Neuron F can produce excitation by inhibition of pathway C-D (disinhibition). The excitability of the smooth muscle at any moment will be influenced by the net excitatory or inhibitory effects of these nerve pathways.

preparations have been employed to demonstrate that gastrointestinal smooth muscle cells can respond directly to a large number of chemicals.

Many drugs can exert their pharmacological actions within the wall of the bowel by effects on the enteric

nervous system (ENS) rather than by, or in addition to, direct actions on the smooth muscle. The ENS, containing two ganglionated plexuses (myenteric plexus and submucous plexus), is a complex neuronal network embedded in the wall of the digestive tube (Costa et al 1987). It contains a number of neurons approximately equal to the number in the spinal cord and may be considered to represent a third component of the autonomic nervous system (ANS), along with the sympathetic and parasympathetic divisions. The ENS contains both afferent and efferent neurons and is responsible for coordination of motility to bring about carefully controlled transit of luminal contents through the digestive tract. The rich network of nerve cell bodies and fibres offers an array of possibilities for drug action that can increase or decrease release of excitatory or inhibitory neurotransmitters in the smooth muscle layers (Fig. 11.2).

The ganglia of the sympathetic division of the ANS provide an extramural target of drug, hormone and neurotransmitter action. It is becoming increasingly apparent that both paravertebral and prevertebral sympathetic ganglia are important information integration processing stations that participate in regulation of gastrointestinal motility. The ganglia receive sensory information from the digestive organs and motor (efferent) signals from the spinal cord; this information is processed through local neural circuits and is relayed to the enteric nerves by postganglionic sympathetic fibres.

The spinal cord was only fairly recently identified as a site of drug action of importance in regulation of gastrointestinal motility (Porreca et al 1983; Porreca & Burks 1983). Drugs and neurotransmitter substances can act within the spinal cord both in ascending (afferent) and descending (efferent) pathways to alter autonomic outflow to the gastrointestinal tract.

It has been known for many years that the brain can influence gastrointestinal motility. Even the ancients recognized the connection between strong emotions and bowel function. However, recognition that drugs can act in the brain to influence gastrointestinal motility has come more recently (Burks 1978). It is now evident that the brain is an important site of action for several types of drugs that influence gastrointestinal motility.

It is often difficult to determine the relative importance of individual sites of drug action when the drug in question acts at multiple sites. However, understanding of its action at each site contributes greatly to overall understanding of the drug's mechanism of action.

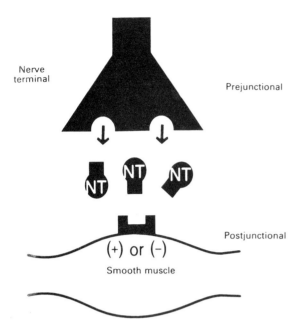

Fig. 11.3 Diagrammatic representation of neuro-effector communication between a nerve terminal and gastrointestinal smooth muscle. Neurotransmitter molecules released from the prejunctional nerve terminal act at postjunctional smooth muscle receptors to produce excitation (+) or inhibition (−), depending on the type of receptor.

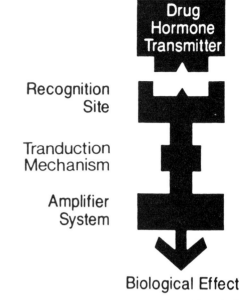

Fig. 11.4 Diagrammatic representation of the principal elements of drug receptor systems. The receptor consists of a recognition site coupled by means of a transduction mechanism to an intracellular amplifier system. The drug, hormone or neurotransmitter molecule combines with the recognition site to activate the transduction mechanism and produce a biological effect by means of the amplifier system.

Receptors

Most drugs that affect gastrointestinal motility do so by means of actions at specific cellular receptors. The receptors may exist physiologically for the purpose of receiving messages from endogenous neurotransmitters, hormones, paracrine and autocrine chemicals (Fig. 11.3). Most neural and smooth muscle receptors of importance in gastrointestinal motility occur on the outer side of the cell's plasma membrane and penetrate through the membrane to the interior of the cell. Great progress has occurred recently in understanding the structure and functions of membrane receptors. Chemically, receptors that have been characterized consist of complex proteins or glycoproteins.

Each receptor consists of three major components (Fig. 11.4): a recognition site, a transduction mechanism, and an amplifier system. The recognition site is that component of the transmembrane receptor that resides on the extracellular surface of the cell and binds to the drug, hormone or neurotransmitter molecules it recognizes. The receptor recognition site presents a specific array of physical and chemical features complementary to those of the messenger molecules it binds. There is thus a mutual chemical

attraction between the messenger molecule and the corresponding receptor recognition site. Once binding between the drug, hormone or neurotransmitter molecule and the receptor recognition site has occurred, the binding may lead to activation of the transduction mechanism. It is the ability to activate the transduction mechanism that separates agonists from antagonists. The best characterized of the transducer systems involves proteins that bind guanosine triphosphate (GTP), and the proteins are thus called 'G proteins'. The importance of the transducer G proteins is the interesting way they are connected to the amplification system to provide either positive or negative regulatory influences (Fig. 11.5).

Three major types of receptor-coupled cellular amplification systems have been identified: ion channels, cyclic nucleotides, and phosphoinositide metabolites. Some receptors, such as the nicotinic cholinergic receptor, are coupled directly to membrane ion channels. Other membrane receptors may be coupled to adenylate cyclase, which generates cyclic adenosine monophosphate (cAMP), or to guanylate cyclase, which generates cyclic guanosine monophosphate (cGMP). Receptors that are positively coupled to adenylate

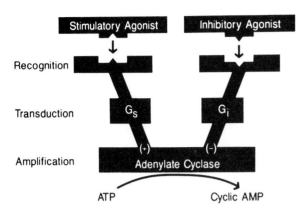

Fig. 11.5 Diagrammatic representation of coupling of diffent receptors to a single intracellular amplifier system. The recognition site for the cellular receptor for the stimulatory agonist is coupled by means of a G_s protein to the intracellular enzyme, adenylate cyclase. The recognition site of the cellular receptor for the inhibitory agonist is coupled by means of a G_i protein to intracellular adenylate cyclase. Binding of the stimulatory agonist to its receptor activates G_s, which in turn activates adenylate cyclase and results in production of cyclic AMP. Binding of the inhibitory agonist activates G_i, which in turn inhibits adenylate cyclase activity and decreases production of cyclic AMP.

cyclase, such as β-adrenergic receptors, are linked to a stimulatory G protein (G_s) which is, in turn, linked to the cyclase. Binding of agonist drugs to the β-adrenergic receptor activates the stimulatory G protein, which increases adenylate cyclase activity. As a result, more adenosine triphosphate (ATP) is converted by the cyclase to cAMP. Through a series of chemical steps, the cAMP results in activation of intracellular protein kinase. Other receptors, such as δ opioid receptors and some muscarinic cholinergic receptors, may be negatively coupled to adenylate cyclase by means of an inhibitory G protein (G_i). In this case, binding of the agonist to the recognition site activates the inhibitory G protein, which inhibits enzymic activity of the coupled adenylate cyclase and decreases the amount of cAMP generated. The third major type of amplification system of importance in gastrointestinal smooth muscle is inositol trisphosphate (IP_3). Membrane receptors, such as those for cholecystokinin and some muscarinic cholinergic receptors, are coupled through a regulatory G protein to phospholipase C, which mobilizes the membrane lipid, phosphatidylinositol 4,5-biphosphate, which is hydrolysed to yield inositol-1,4,5-trisphosphate and diacylglycerol. In terms of contraction of gastrointestinal smooth muscle, all three types of amplifier systems act to increase or decrease availability of calcium to the

contractile proteins (Hartshorne 1987). the practical significance of the transducer and amplification systems is the potential ability to develop totally new drugs that influence motility by acting on these mechanisms. For example, calcium entry blocking drugs alter motility by decreasing the influx of calcium required by many agents for generation of contractions.

Characteristics of drugs

Drugs that act as smooth muscle or neural membrane receptors may be classified as 'agonists' or 'antagonists'. Agonists are molecules that bind to receptors (possess 'affinity') and, once bound, can activate the transducer mechanism to which the receptor is coupled (possess 'efficacy'). Thus, interaction of an agonist with its corresponding cellular receptors will bring about a change in cellular function. The specific change, an increase or a decrease in function, depends on the type of tranducer mechanism and amplifier system coupled to the receptor. For example, activation of an intestinal smooth muscle muscarinic cholinergic receptor leads to contraction of the muscle cell. Conversely, activation of a smooth muscle β-adrenergic receptor leads to relaxation of the smooth muscle cell. In both cases, the respective receptors were activated by agonist molecules. However, the amplifier system connected to the smooth muscle muscarinic cholinergic receptor (IP_3) increases availability of calcium to smooth muscle and generates contraction. Activation of the β-adrenergic receptor increases production of intracellular cAMP and decreases availability of calcium to the contractile proteins, thus causing relaxation. Most smooth muscle cells contain many individual types of receptors. For example, an individual gastrointestinal smooth muscle cell may possess receptors for acetylcholine, 5-hydroxytrytamine (5-HT), histamine, cholecystokinin, substance P, and angiotensin, each of which leads to smooth muscle contraction, and receptors for noradrenaline (NA), nitric oxide, and glucagon, which generally cause relaxation. Multiple receptors coupled by different mechanisms to the contractile machinery provide both a large number of mechanisms for physiological regulation of contractile activity and potential sites of drug action.

Antagonists are drugs that have affinity for receptor recognition sites, but lack the ability to activate the transduction mechanism. Thus, antagonists are molecules lacking in efficacy. Because they do not activate receptor-linked transduction mechanisms, pure antagonists cannot directly influence cellular function. Their effect is to block actions of agonists. When

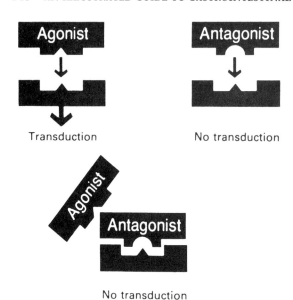

Fig. 11.6 Diagrammatic representation of cellular actions of receptor agonists and antagonists. Binding of the agonist to the receptor recognition sites activates the transduction mechanism leading to a biological response. Binding of an antagonist to the receptor recognition sites does not bring about transduction. The antagonist occupies the recognition site and competes with agonist molecules for binding.

administration of an antagonist results in a change in contractile activity, it is because the antagonist blocked receptor activity of an agonist (Fig. 11.6).

Antagonists are generally classified according to whether they act through competitive or non-competitive mechanisms. Competitive antagonists bind reversibly to receptors and thereby compete with agonist molecules for occupancy of the recognition site. The antagonism produced by competitive antagonists can be overcome by the addition of more agonist (Fig. 11.7), that is, the effect of a competitive antagonist is surmountable. Non-competitive antagonists, on the other hand, do not simply compete with agonist molecules for the receptor recognition site. Some, such as phenoxybenzamine or chlornaltrexamine, produce essentially permanent alkylation of the receptor recognition site. This type of blockade cannot be overcome by the addition of more agonist. Typically, competitive antagonists cause a shift in the agonist dose-response curve parallel to the right (Fig. 11.7). When sufficient amounts of agonist are added in the presence of the competitive antagonist, a full response to the agonist can be achieved. It is characteristic that the dose of agonist required for a half-maximal response (D_{50}) is increased in the presence of a competitive antagonist.

By contrast, non-competitive antagonists generally reduce the maximum response that can be produced by the agonist with relatively little change in the agonist D_{50} values.

Indirectly acting drugs

Some drugs can produce biological effects indirectly by promoting release of neurotransmitter or neurohormone that in turn interacts with the cellular receptor. For example, tyramine can release NA from the terminals of adrenergic nerves. The NA released by tyramine can then interact with neural or smooth muscle receptors. Actions of tyramine may be blocked pharmacologically in two ways. A treatment may be given that blocks ability of tyramine to release NA. For example, treatment of the preparation with cocaine prevents neural uptake of tyramine and thus blocks its ability to release NA. Another approach is to block NA receptors by use of α- or β-adrenergic antagonists.

In vivo, drugs may act at remote sites to promote release of an intermediate mediator. For example, drugs may release catecholamines from the adrenal medulla or promote formation of antiotensin. These effects may be brought about by direct drug action or can be secondary to an unrelated pharmacological action, such as drug-induced decreases in blood pressure.

Another indirect way that drugs can act is by altering catabolism of neurotransmitter chemicals. For example, acetylcholinesterase inhibitors may produce indirect cholinergic actions by preventing enzymatic hydrolysis of neurally secreted acetylcholine. Uptake inhibitors, such as cocaine, desipramine or fluoxetine, can prevent inactivation of NA and 5-HT that occurs by neural uptake.

DRUG ACTIONS

Cholinergic drugs

Acetylcholine (ACh) has been recognized as an important neurotransmitter since the early years of this century (Dale 1914). In the digestive tract, ACh generally induces smooth muscle contraction by direct actions at smooth muscle muscarinic receptors or at neural nicotinic cholinergic receptors. The excitatory response to activation of smooth muscle muscarinic receptors is thought to arise from activation of phospholipase C, resulting in intracellular formation of IP_3, which causes release of calcium ions that activate contractile proteins (Harden et al 1986). ACh is rarely used for therapeutic

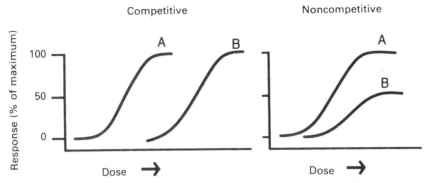

Fig. 11.7   Conceptual dose-response curves illustrating actions of competitive and non-competitive antagonists. In both panels, curve A shows the response to the agonist alone. Curve B shows the response to the same agonist in the presence of an antagonist. A competitive antagonist shifts the agonist dose-response curve parallel to the right with the same maximal response attained even in the presence of the antagonist. A non-competitive antagonist displaces the agonist dose-response curve downward, decreasing the maximum response to the agonist that can be attained.

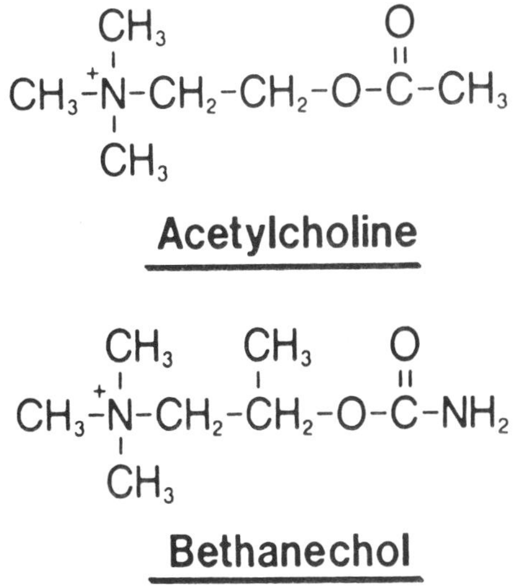

$$CH_3\overset{\overset{\displaystyle CH_3}{|}}{\underset{\underset{\displaystyle CH_3}{|}}{N}}-CH_2-CH_2-O-\overset{\overset{\displaystyle O}{\|}}{C}-CH_3$$

Acetylcholine

$$CH_3\overset{\overset{\displaystyle CH_3}{|}}{\underset{\underset{\displaystyle CH_3}{|}}{N}}-CH_2-\overset{\overset{\displaystyle CH_3}{|}}{CH_2}-O-\overset{\overset{\displaystyle O}{\|}}{C}-NH_2$$

Bethanechol

Fig. 11.8   Chemical structures of acetylcholine and bethanechol.

purposes because of its lack of receptor selectivity and its rapid hydrolysis by acetylcholinesterase and plasma cholinesterase. Many synthetic analogues of ACh have been synthesized that exhibit selectivity for muscarinic cholinergic receptors and resistance to hydrolysis by acetylcholinesterase and plasma cholinesterase. The best known of the directly acting selective ACh-like drugs is bethanechol (Fig. 11.8). While both are choline esters, bethanechol differs chemically from ACh in two important ways. In bethanechol, a methyl

group is substituted in the β position relative to the ammonium function. The β-methyl substitution confers selectivity for muscarinic cholinergic receptors. Also, an amide group is substituted for the methyl function of the acetate portion of the molecule. The resulting carbamyl ester of choline is resistant to hydrolysis by both acetylcholinesterase and plasma cholinesterase. Bethanechol is thus a selective muscarinic receptor agonist with a relatively long duration of action. It is related chemically and pharmacologically to carbachol, which also possesses the carbamyl ester function, and to methacholine, which contains a β-methyl function. Because of its muscarinic selectivity and resistance to enzymatic hydrolysis, bethanechol is the directly acting cholinergic agonist most often used in gastroenterology and serves as the prototype of this class of drugs.

Bethanechol and other muscarinic cholinergic agonists produce contractions of gastrointestinal smooth muscle. The excitatory effects of muscarinic agonists on isolated muscle cells from longitudinal and circular muscle layers of the small intestine of various species, including the human, have been demonstrated (Bitar et al 1982, Makhlouf 1987). In in vitro preparations of gastrointestinal smooth muscle, muscarinic cholinergic agonists produce increases in smooth muscle tone and amplitude of contractions. In animals and humans, ongoing cholinergic neurotransmission to gastrointestinal smooth muscle is of importance in maintaining normal contractility and propulsion of intestinal contents (Galligan & Burks 1986, Nowak et al 1986, Borody et al 1985). Subcutaneous administration of

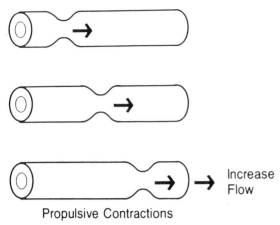

Propulsive Contractions

Fig. 11.9 Diagrammatic representation of propulsive intestinal contractions typical of those induced by cholinergic agonists.

bethanechol induces contractions of smooth muscle in the body of the oesophagus, lower oesophageal sphincter, stomach, small intestine, large intestine, and the internal anal sphincter (Nostrant et al 1986, Burks 1987, Burleigh & D'Mello 1983, Roman & Gonella 1987). Coordination of contractile activity is important in gastric emptying and propulsion of contents through the small intestine (Camilleri et al 1986a, Meyer 1987). Bethanechol and related muscarinic cholinergic agonists produce aborally moving contractions that increase intestinal propulsion (Fig. 11.9). For this reason, bethanechol is often listed as a prokinetic drug (see below), even though it is often less effective than other drugs in the prokinetic category.

Bethanechol can be of limited clinical utility in the treatment of certain cases of gastroparesis and post-operative abdominal distension (Taylor 1990a). Careful use of bethanechol can increase gastric emptying and promote intestinal propulsion. Because it can increase oesophageal motility and lower oesophageal sphincter pressure, bethanechol can decrease gastro-oesophageal reflux (Thanik et al 1982). Bethanechol causes contractions of the human gallbladder and promotes gallbladder emptying (Fisher et al 1985).

Bethanechol and other cholinergic agonists can produce a wide variety of distressing and serious side-effects that effectively limit their therapeutic use. In the gastrointestinal tract, muscarinic cholinergic agonists stimulate gastric and pancreatic secretion, and can produce abdominal cramps and watery diarrhoea. These drugs also slow the heart and can produce vasodilatation and hypotension. Because of the possibility of serious adverse cardiovascular effects, bethane-

chol should not be administered intravenously. The muscarinic agonists produce contraction of the urinary bladder and induce urination. They also act at the sweat glands to induce sweating. Bethanechol and other muscarinic agonists can produce bronchial constriction, especially in patients with asthma. Contraindications of the use of muscarinic agonists include peptic ulcer disease, heart block, and reactive or obstructive pulmonary disease. Whenever bethanechol is given by injection, atropine should be available as an antidote in the event of serious adverse effects.

Experimental evidence has recently been provided for at least three subtypes of muscarinic receptor, termed M_1, M_2 and M_3. The muscarinic receptor subtypes are differentiated primarily by the actions of antagonists (Watson et al 1986). Gastrointestinal smooth muscle receptors contain primarily the M_2 subtype of receptors, whereas gastric acid secretion is stimulated both by the M_1 and M_3 subtypes of muscarinic receptors. Agonist and antagonist drugs selective for each subtype of muscarinic receptor should eventually become available.

Nicotinic cholinergic receptors

Nicotinic cholinergic receptors of importance to gastrointestinal motility are located primarily on autonomic ganglion cells in the wall of the bowel or in sympathetic ganglia. Sympathetic ganglionic transmission is much more complex than is generally appreciated. Recording of ganglionic electrical potential during stimulation of preganglionic fibres yields a complex wave form characterized by a rapid depolarization, a slow hyperpolarization, and a late depolarization (Fig. 11.10). The initial depolarization results from actions of neurally secreted ACh at ganglion cell nicotinic cholinergic receptors. The slow hyperpolarization is mediated by catecholamines released from small ganglionic interneurons that are activated by the neurally secreted ACh acting at muscarinic cholinergic receptors (Libet 1970). The late depolarization results from actions of neurally secreted ACh at ganglion cell muscarinic cholinergic receptors. Nerve impulses are initiated in the ganglion cells and postganglionic fibres by the nicotinic receptor-mediated rapid depolarization. The actions of ACh at the ganglionic nicotinic receptors can be mimicked by other chemicals, including nicotine. As illustrated in Figure 11.11, nicotine can combine with the ENS ganglion cell nicotine cholinergic receptor to generate a nerve action potential and release of ACh from the terminals of the postganglionic fibres. In the gastrointestinal tract, many postganglionic cholinergic fibres terminate near the smooth muscle layers and the

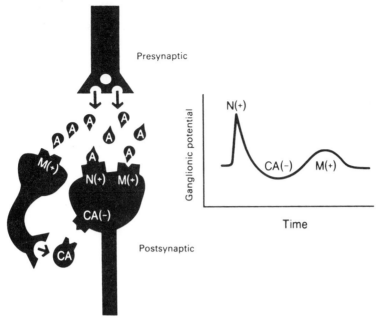

Fig. 11.10 Diagrammatic representation of the components of sympathetic ganglionic neurotransmission. Acetylcholine (A) released from the presynaptic nerve terminal interacts with principal ganglion cell nicotinic (N) excitatory receptors (+) and with muscarinic (M) excitatory receptors. Acetylcholine also interacts with excitatory muscarinic receptors in ganglionic interneurons that release catecholamines (CA). The catecholamine released from the ganglionic interneuron interacts with inhibitory (−) receptors (CA) on the principal ganglion cell. The panel on the right illustrates the ganglionic electrical potentials generated by each component of the transmission process. Acetylcholine activation of nicotinic receptors causes a rapid depolarization, activation of catecholamine receptors causes a late hyperpolarization, and activation of ganglion cell muscarinic receptors causes late depolarization.

neurally secreted ACh acts at smooth muscle muscarinic cholinergic receptors to cause contractions. Thus, nicotine and other ganglionic nicotinic agonists can produce contraction of smooth muscle by activating cholinergic neurons in the wall of the gut. In some species, stimulation of nicotinic cholinergic receptors results in intestinal inhibition, presumably as a result of activating inhibitory neural pathways (Burks et al 1974).

Ganglionic stimulants are not employed as therapeutic agents.

Acetylcholinesterase inhibitors

Acetylcholinesterase is the enzyme responsible for terminating synaptic and neuro-effector actions of ACh. Drugs that inhibit actions of acetylcholinesterase allow a local accumulation of ACh that can act at postsynaptic acetylcholine receptors. Acetylcholinesterase inhibi-

tors are examples of indirectly acting cholinergic drugs.

The classical acetylcholinesterase inhibitor is physostigmine, also known as eserine. However, physostigmine can cross the blood–brain barrier and produce undesired effects in the CNS. For this reason, neostigmine (Fig. 11.12) is more useful therapeutically. Neostigmine is a quarternary amine and does not effectively cross the blood–brain barrier. Edrophonium is related chemically to neostigmine, but exhibits a shorter duration of action. The organophosphate drugs, insecticides and nerve gases, such as diisopropylfluorophosphate, malathion and tabun, are extremely potent, irreversible acetylcholinesterase inhibitors. Organophosphate acetylcholinesterase inhibitors are rarely used in gastroenterology.

Neostigmine and other reversible acetylcholinesterase inhibitors increase the motor activity of the stomach, small intestine, and large intestine. Muscle tone,

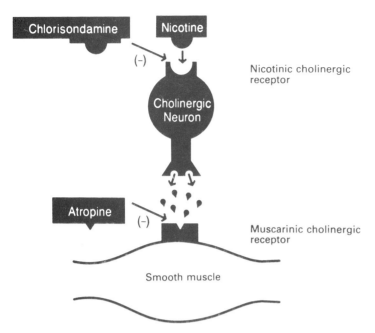

Fig. 11.11 Diagrammatic representation of excitatory actions of nicotine on gastrointestinal smooth muscle. Nicotine acts at ganglionic nicotinic receptors of cholinergic neurons, causing the neuron to release acetylcholine from their nerve terminals. The acetylcholine interacts with smooth muscle muscarinic cholinergic receptors. The interaction of nicotine with the nicotinic receptor can be blocked by ganglion blocking drugs, such as chlorisondamine. Acetylcholine actions on smooth muscle can be blocked by the muscarinic antagonist, atropine.

amplitude of phasic contractions, and gastrointestinal propulsion are stimulated. The overall stimulatory effect of acetylcholinesterase inhibitors on gastrointestinal motility represents a combination of actions within the myenteric plexus and in the muscle layers. Cholinesterase inhibitors can be useful for management of abdominal distention and paralytic ileus (Taylor 1990b).

The major shortcoming of acetylcholinesterase inhibitors as therapeutic agents is their relative lack of selectivity in that they indirectly activate both nicotinic and muscarinic cholinergic receptors at all sites of cholinergic neurotransmission. Gastrointestinal symptoms of side-effects may include nausea and vomiting, abdominal cramps, and diarrhoea. Other side-effects can include excess salivation, hypotension, sweating, urination, and lacrimation. Atropine is an effective antidote.

Cholinergic antagonists

Atropine is the prototype of the selective muscarinic cholinergic receptor antagonists. Atropine and scopolamine, which are pharmacologically similar, are natural plant alkaloids. A number of synthetic congeners of atropine have been prepared. The synthetic muscarinic receptor antagonists include methantheline (Fig. 11.13), propantheline, tridihexethyl, anisotropine, clidinium, and numerous others. In general, the synthetic

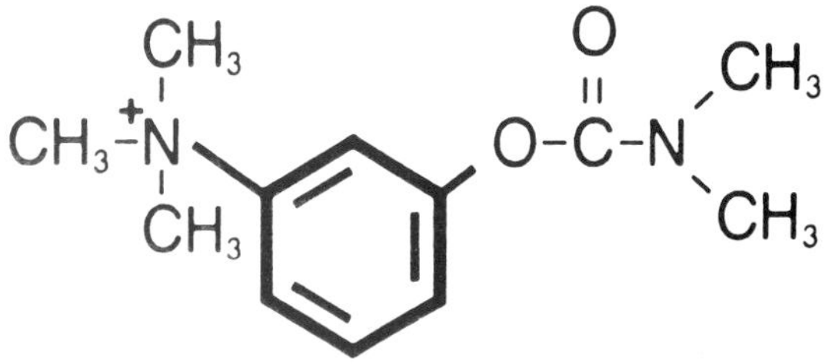

Fig. 11.12   Structure of neostigmine.

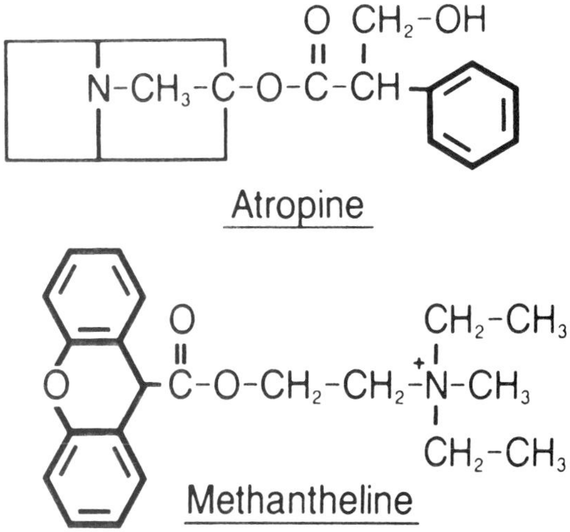

Fig. 11.13   Structures of atropine and methantheline.

Table 11.2 Receptor preferences for selected adrenergic and DA agonists

Drugs	Receptor types				
	α_1	α_2	β_1	β_2	DA
Natural					
Adrenaline	+	+	+	+	
Noradrenaline	+	+	+		
Dopamine	+		+		+
Synthetic					
Phenylephrine	+				
Clonidine		+			
Isoproterenol			+	+	
Dobutamine			+		
Metaproterenol				+	

+ = Significant agonist activity

drugs possess quarternary ammonium structures and are somewhat more specific than the natural compounds for the gastrointestinal tract. Atropine and related compounds are competitive antagonists at muscarinic cholinergic receptors. That is, they compete with ACh for the receptor recognition site, but, lacking ability to activate the transducer mechanism, simply occupy the binding site to prevent access of acetylcholine to the receptor. Because of the importance of ongoing cholinergic neurotransmission in regulation of gastrointestinal contractions and propulsion, the muscarinic receptor antagonists can significantly reduce the incidence and amplitudes of contractions and inhibit gastrointestinal propulsion (Borody et al 1985, Nowak et al 1986).

While muscarinic receptor antagonists can decrease gastrointestinal motility and transit, their use is generally associated with uncomfortable side-effects such as dry mouth, difficulty in urination, and constipation. In sufficient doses, atropine and other antimuscarinic drugs can decrease gastric acid secretion and pancreatic secretion. Pirenzepine, an antagonist at the M_1 subtype of muscarinic receptors, can decrease gastric secretion with minimal effects on smooth muscle (Watson et al 1986). Pirenzepine has been used on a limited basis as an antisecretory drug in the management of peptic ulcer disease. An experimental drug, AF-DX 116, is a selective antagonist at the M_2 subtype of muscarinic receptors. It is probable that new drugs with selectivity for individual subtypes of muscarinic cholinergic receptors will become useful therapeutic agents in the future.

Ganglion blocking drugs are neural nicotinic receptor antagonists. High (toxic) doses of nicotine alone can cause varying degrees of ganglionic blockade.

Drugs that act selectively as ganglion blockers include chlorisondamine, hexamethonium, mecamylamine, and trimethaphan. These drugs are all competitive antagonists at ganglionic nicotinic receptors. Ganglionic blocking drugs decrease gastrointestinal contractions and transit, mainly by actions at ganglion cells of the myenteric plexus. The ganglion blocking drugs are rarely used in modern medicine. Because they block both sympathetic and parasympathetic ganglionic transmission (Fig. 11.11), these drugs are non-specific and produce many troublesome side-effects. In particular, they lower blood pressure and frequently cause postural hypotension.

It should be noted that certain neuromuscular blocking agents, such as d-tubocurarine, can also block ganglionic neurotransmission.

Adrenergic and anti-adrenergic drugs

Adrenergic receptor agonists and antagonists are seldom used at present in therapy of motility gastrointestinal disorders, but can produce profound motility effects. Actions of this class of drug are complex because of multiple types of adrenergic receptors (adrenoceptors). Adrenergic receptors were originally divided into two types, alpha and beta (Ahlquist 1948). Subsequently, subtypes were identified (Lands et al 1967, Langer 1974). Postsynaptic (postjunctional) NAα receptors are mainly classified as the α_1 subtype. α_2 receptors are mainly located at presynaptic (prejunctional) neural sites and are responsible for negative feedback inhibition of neurotransmitter release. Postjunctional α_2 receptors have been identified in vascular smooth muscle and in intestinal epithelial cells. β_1 adrenergic receptors occur primarily in the heart, whereas β_2 adrenergic receptors occur in smooth muscle of the gastrointestinal tract, bronchi, and blood vessels. β_3 receptors occur in the gastrointestinal tract and on some fat cells. Dopamine (DA) receptors occur on neurons and in some vascular smooth muscle. In the gastrointestinal tract, the wall of the stomach, small intestine, and large intestine is relaxed by activation of α and β receptors. Activation of DA receptors generally causes relaxation in the small intestine, and contraction in the large intestine. Activation of α_1 adrenergic receptors causes contraction of the ileocaecal junction. The inhibitory effects of α_1 and β_1 receptors result primarily from neural actions in the myenteric plexus. Activation of α_2 prejunctional receptors can also cause inhibition of the intestine by decreasing release of excitatory neural transmitter. Activation of smooth muscle β-adrenergic receptors causes smooth muscle relaxation (Makhlouf 1987). The smooth

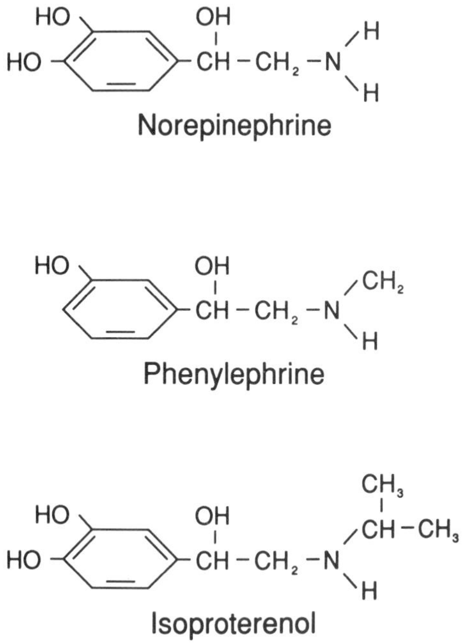

Fig. 11.14   Structures of norepinephrine (noradrenaline), phenylephrine and isoproterenol (isoprenaline).

Table 11.3   Receptor preferences of selected adrenergic and DA antagonists

Drugs	\(\alpha_1\)	\(\alpha_2\)	\(\beta_1\)	\(\beta_2\)	DA
	\multicolumn{5}{c}{Receptor types}				
Phenoxybenzamine	+	+			
Phentolamine	+	+			
Prazosin		+			
Labetalol	+		+	+	
Propanolol			+	+	
Nadolol			+	+	
Metoprolol			+		
Atenolol			+		
Tolamolol			+		
Butoxamine*				+	
Droperidol	+				+
Haloperidol					+

+ = Significant antagonist activity; * = Experimental compound

Table 11.4   Mechanisms of action of prokinetic drugs

Prokinetic drug	Proposed mechanism
Bethanechol	Stimulation of muscarinic receptors
Metoclopramide	Blockade of D$_2$ receptors
Domperidone	Blockade of peripheral D$_2$ receptors
Cisapride	Stimulation of 5-HT$_4$ receptors
Erythromycin	Stimulation of motilin receptors

muscle component of the relaxation may occur primarily from activation of β_2- and β_3-adrenergic receptors (Ek et al 1986).

The receptor types and subtypes activated by natural and synthetic adrenergic agonists are shown in Table 11.2. Most of the agonists decrease gastrointestinal motility. The structures of NA, phenylephrine and isoproterenol are given in Fig. 11.14. The gastrointestinal actions of the adrenergic agonists tend to be transient and gastrointestinal side-effects, other than nausea and vomiting, are rare.

The α_2 agonist, clonidine, has been employed therapeutically as an antidiarrhoeal drug. While α_2 agonists can decrease gastrointestinal motility, the principal antidiarrhoeal effect of clonidine is attributable to its effect on mucosal transport of fluid and electrolytes. Clonidine acts prejunctionally at secretomotor neurons in the submucosal plexus to decrease release of secretory neurotransmitters and also acts directly at mucosal crypt cell α_2 receptors to inhibit secretion. Clonidine thereby reduces secretion of fluid into the intestinal lumen and tends to restore net absorptive functions to the intestinal mucosa. Lidamidine, also an α_2 agonist, appears to produce its antidiarrhoeal effect by a similar mechanism. The major side-effect of clonidine is hypotension.

Some adrenergic drugs can act indirectly by promoting release of NA from its storage sites in adrenergic nerve terminals. The prototype indirectly acting adrenergic drug is tyramine. Tyramine acts almost exclusively by release of endogenous NA. Ephedrine and amphetamine produce their adrenergic actions partly by release of neural NA. NA uptake inhibitors, such as cocaine and desipramine, can produce NA-like effects by preventing neural uptake of NA.

Adrenergic receptor antagonists are slightly less complex than the agonists. The receptor selectivities of prototypic adrenergic and DA receptor antagonists are given in Table 11.3.

Under certain circumstances, administration of α- and β-adrenergic receptor antagonists may be associated with increased gastrointestinal motility and transit. Because adrenergic agonists generally inhibit gastrointestinal motility, it is assumed that blockade of endogenous catecholamines is responsible for the intestinal stimulation that can occur after α or β blockade. However, certain adrenergic antagonists, such as phentolamine, may possess intrinsic intestinal stimulatory activity.

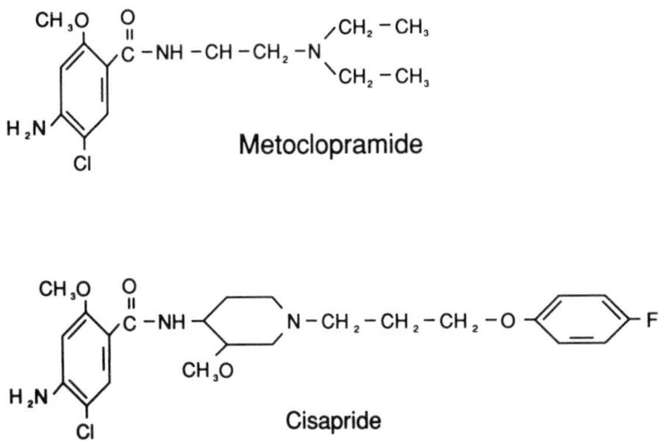

Fig. 11.15 Structures of metoclopramide and cisapride.

Prokinetic drugs

The prokinetic drugs can be divided by pharmacological mechanism into four general categories (Table 11.4): (1) drugs with direct cholinergic receptor agonist properties (e.g. bethanechol) or inhibitors of acetylcholinesterase (e.g. neostigmine), (2) those with pronounced dopamine (D_2) receptor antagonist properties (e.g. metoclopramide and domperidone), (3) drugs that act as agonists at 5-hydroxytryptamine 5-HT$_4$ receptors (e.g. cisapride), and (4) those that probably act as agonists at gastrointestinal motilin receptors (e.g. erythromycin). Each category has distinct advantages in certain situations, but those with primary actions at 5-HT$_4$ or motilin receptors generally display the most favourable therapeutic profiles for clinical use.

Cholinergic agents

It has been known for years that bethanechol and similar muscarinic agonists, as well as acetylcholinesterase inhibitors, increase the incidence and amplitudes of contractions of gastrointestinal smooth muscle. These cholinergic agonists also improve coupling of contractions in local areas to generate propulsive waves that increase flow through the intestinal lumen. Unfortunately, the cholinergic agonists fail to improve antro-duodenal coordination necessary for effective gastric emptying and they can increase gastric and intestinal secretions, leading to acid hypersecretion and luminal accumulation of fluid, and even to diarrhoea. For these reasons, the cholinergic agonist drugs have not been employed extensively as prokinetic agents.

Dopamine antagonists

DA receptor antagonist drugs, such as metoclopramide, are much more selective in their actions than bethanechol or neostigmine, even though the smooth muscle muscarinic M_2 receptor is the final cellular link in the prokinetic effects of both dopamine antagonist and direct cholinergic drugs. It was initially difficult to establish DA receptor antagonism as the fundamental basis of metoclopramide actions because the role of DA dopamine as a regulator of motility was uncertain and because different types of DA receptors may mediate qualitatively different gastrointestinal responses (Lombardi et al 1986, Burks 1987, Wiley & Owyang 1987). However, it is now clear that DA acting at neural D_2 receptors is an important inhibitory regulator of motility because activation of D_2 receptors reduces release of ACh from cholinergic motor neurons that innervate gastrointestinal smooth muscle (Schuurkes & VanNeuten 1981, Kurosawa et al 1991). Metoclopramide and domperidone act as antagonists at the inhibitory neural D_2 receptors and, by removing DA-mediated inhibition, increase the release of ACh from the excitatory motor neurons (Takahashi et al 1991). Thus, the final mediator of the stimulatory effect is ACh, which acts at smooth muscle M_2 receptors to bring about contraction (Hay & Man 1979). A major advantage of the DA antagonist drugs, metoclopramide and domperidone, over direct cholinergic agents, such as bethanechol, is that the DA antagonists do not create sustained increase in ACh activation of smooth muscle M_2 receptors, but only intensify the pulsatile release of ACh resulting from normal discharge of the cholinergic motor neurons. Intensification and amplification of ACh release maintains normal patterns of coordinated motor activity. Indeed, one of the striking properties of DA antagonist prokinetic drugs is improvement of the antro-duodenal coordination necessary for optimal gastric emptying. In addition, metoclopramide and domperidone increase the amplitude and force of antral contractions.

Metoclopramide (Fig. 11.15) and domperidone increase gastric motility and gastric emptying (Schulze-Delrieu 1981). The effect of these prokinetic drugs on gastric emptying is of therapeutic value in the treatment of diabetic gastroparesis and dystophia myotonia (Snape et al 1982, Horowitz et al 1987). Metoclopramide, in particular, is also an effective antiemetic drug. Because of differing pharmacokinetic properties, metoclopramide crosses the blood–brain barrier more effectively than domperidone and metoclopramide produces much more profound CNS effects than domperidone. While improved gastric emptying may contribute to antinausea and antiemetic effects, the central DA receptor antagonist actions of metoclopramide provide the major basis of its antiemetic effects. D_2 receptors are located in the brainstem area postrema and the

Table 11.5 5-HT receptor mechanisms and preferences of selected drugs

Receptor types	Mechanisms*	Agonists	Antagonists
5-HT$_{1A}$	↓cAMP		Methysergide
			Methiothepin
5-HT$_{1C}$	IP$_3$		Ritanserin
5-HT$_{1D}$	↓cAMP	Sumatriptan	
5-HT$_2$	IP$_3$		Ketanserin
5-HT$_3$	Cation channel		Ondansetron
			Granisetron
5-HT$_4$	↑cAMP	Cisapride	
		Renzapride	

* Cellular mechanisms associated with receptor activation

nearby vomiting centres. These receptors can be activated by DA and DA analogues, such as apomorphine, to induce emesis. Emesis produced by DA or apomorphine is inhibited by metoclopramide. It is used therapeutically to treat non-specific emesis and to reduce nausea and vomiting associated with cancer chemotherapy.

The CNS action of metoclopramide to block DA receptors figures prominently in the adverse effects of metoclopramide: hyperprolactinaemia, galactorrhoea, breast tenderness, extrapyramidal symptoms and sedation.

Domperidone rarely causes extrapyramidal symptoms, but can cause hyperprolactinaemia and associated side-effects.

Because the DA antagonist drugs increase motility and propulsion by increasing release of neural ACh in the upper gut, their motility effects can often be blocked by atropine and other drugs with M$_2$ receptor antagonist activity, including some H$_1$ histamine antagonists. Domperidone is less affected by antimuscarinic drugs than metoclopramide (Reynolds 1989).

5-Hydroxytryptamine agonists and antagonists

5-HT has pronounced effects on gastrointestinal motility and tone. Its effects are mediated by multiple types and subtypes of 5-HT receptors in the central and peripheral nervous systems and on smooth muscle (Table 11.5). The neural and smooth muscle actions of 5-HT are associated with three distinct cellular amplifications systems: increases or decreases in production of cAMP, increase in formation of diacylglycerol and IP$_3$, or opening of membrane channels for sodium and potassium (Table 11.5).

Some recently introduced antiemetic drugs, such as ondansetron, produce their antiemetic effects by block-

ade of 5-HT$_3$ receptors on vagal afferent nerves and in the CNS. These drugs have shown clinical utility in management of nausea and vomiting, especially the symptoms associated with emetogenic cancer chemotherapeutic drugs, such as cisplatin. However, 5-HT$_3$ receptor antagonists have relatively little effect on motility or propulsion in the gastrointestinal tract (Gullikson et al 1991).

Cisapride (Fig. 11.15) and some related prokinetic drugs are agonists at neural 5-HT$_4$ receptors in cholinergic motor pathways that provide excitatory innervation to gastrointestinal smooth muscle (Nemeth et al 1985, Dumuis et al 1989, Linnik et al 1991). Activation of 5-HT$_4$ receptors by agonist drugs results in increased release of neural ACh and stimulation of the smooth muscle. Cisapride thus increases the incidence and force of gastric and intestinal contractions, and improves antro-duodenal coordination to enhance gastric emptying (McCallum et al 1988). Cisapride also increases tone of the lower oesophageal sphincter and can increase intestinal propulsion. Because ACh is the final mediator of its stimulatory actions, the effects of cisapride can be blocked by atropine and other antimuscarinic drugs.

Cisapride appears to improve gastric emptying of solids and liquids in patients with diabetic gastroparesis and other disorders of gastric emptying (Stacher et al 1987, Feldman & Smith 1987). Cisapride has been shown effective in reducing delayed intestinal transit in some patients with chronic intestinal pseudo-obstruction (Camilleri et al 1986b). Cisapride does not block DA receptors and thus does not produce extrapyramidal symptoms or release prolactin. The most common side-effect associated with cisapride therapy is an increase in the number of bowel movements.

Motilin agonists

Erythromycin has recently been shown to exert pronounced prokinetic actions, possibly as a result of agonist actions at gastrointestinal motilin receptors (Itoh et al 1984, Peeters et al 1989). Erythomycin and several structurally related analogues, many of which do not possession antibacterial activity, mimic the gastrointestinal stimulatory properties of motilin in dogs and humans (Inatomi et al 1989). However, it is not totally clear that all prokinetic effects of erythromycin can be attributed to actions at motilin receptors because erythromycin also produces some motility changes that differ from those of motilin (Otterson & Sarna 1990, Minocha & Galligan 1991). However, erythromycin binds to motilin receptors and, like motilin, it induces migrating motor complexes in the small intestine.

Table 11.6 Receptor preferences of selected opioid agonists

Ligands	Receptor types		
	μ	δ	κ
Nonpeptides			
Morphine	+ +	+	+
Sufentanyl	+ +		
U-50 488			+ +
Peptides			
Pro-opiomelanocortin family			
β-Endorphin	+ +	+	
Proenkephalin family			
[Met⁵]enkephalin	+	+ +	
[Leu⁵]enkephalin	+	+ +	
Peptide E	+ +	+	
Prodynorphin family			
Dynorphin-(1-17)	+		+ +
α-Neoendorphin	+	+	+ +
Synthetic peptides			
DAGO	+ +		
PLO17	+ +		
DPDPE		+ +	

+ + = Preferred receptor type; + = Significant agonist activity

Erythromycin accelerates gastric emptying and intestinal propulsion. Experimental studies have indicated a profound effect of erythromycin on gastric emptying rates in patients with diabetic gastroparesis (Janssens et al 1990).

Opioid drugs

Opium and opium-derived drugs have been used in medicine for literally thousands of years, mainly for their effects on gastrointestinal function and as analgesics. The motility effects of opioids have been studied extensively in modern times (Burks et al 1982, Kromer 1988). One of the most striking pharmacological features of opioid drugs is their ability to produce constipation. The mechanism of the constipating action of opioids has been explored in detail.

It has been evident since the 1960s that morphine and other opioid drugs must act at specific pharmacological receptors to produce their biological effects (Martin 1967). Saturable, stereospecific opioid binding sites in brain and intestine were described in 1973 (Pert & Snyder 1973). Within 2 years, endogenous opioid peptides, [Met⁵]enkephalin and [Leu⁵]enkephalin, were discovered (Hughes 1975). Discovery of other brain, pituitary, gut and adrenal opioid peptides followed. It is now apparent that the endogenous opioid peptides are derived from three families of precursor peptides: pro-opiomelanocortin, proenkephalin, and prodynorphin (Table 11.6). As studies of the endogenous opioid peptides progressed, the concept of mul-

[Met⁵]enkephalin

    Try-Gly-Gly-Phe-Met

DAGO

    Tyr-D-Ala-Gly-N-MePhe-Gly-ol

PLO17

    Tyr-Pro-MePhe-D-Pro-NH₂

DPDPE

    Tyr-D-Pen-Gly-Phe-D-Pen

Fig. 11.16 Amino acid sequences of [Met⁵]enkephalin, DAGO, PLO17 and DPDPE.

tiple types of opioid receptors was reinforced. Three major types of opioid receptors can be demonstrated in a variety of mammalian tissues: μ, δ and κ. Morphine, methadone, meperidine (pethidine), codeine and other opioid drugs produce their effects by means of agonist actions at receptors for the endogenous opioids. Different opioid ligands display different preferences for the multiple types of opioid receptors (Table 11.6). For example, morphine is μ-receptor preferring but can act also at δ and κ opioid receptors. Sufentanyl and the experimental peptides, DAGO and PLO17 (Fig. 11.16), act almost exclusively at μ opioid receptors (James & Goldstein 1984). The experimental peptide, DPDPE (Figure 11.16), acts selectively at δ opioid receptors (Mosberg et al 1983). U-50488 acts selectively at κ opioid receptors (Von Voigtlander et al 1983). However, most peptide and non-peptide ligands interact with more than one type of receptor. The gastrointestinal functional significance of multiple types of opioid receptors has revealed a rich complexity. Opioid drugs can affect gastrointestinal motility by actions in the brain, spinal cord, intrinsic neurons, and directly on smooth muscle (Stewart et al 1977, 1978). The different anatomical sites of action often involve different types of optoid receptors (Burks et al 1987). Motility responses to opioid agonists appear to involve primarily μ and δ opioid receptors (Hirning et al 1985, Vaught et al 1985).

Systematic administration of morphine results in characteristic changes in gastrointestinal motility. Typically, gastric emptying is inhibited, small bowel transit is delayed, and colonic transit is prolonged. When contractile activity is measured, morphine is generally found to increase the incidence and amplitudes of randomly distributed segmenting contractions similar

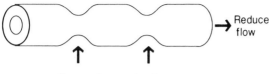

Segmenting contractions

Fig. 11.17 Diagrammatic representation of the effects of opioids on intestinal motility. Opioids increase segmenting contractions that increase intraluminal pressure and thereby increase resistance to flow. Intestinal flow is thereby decreased.

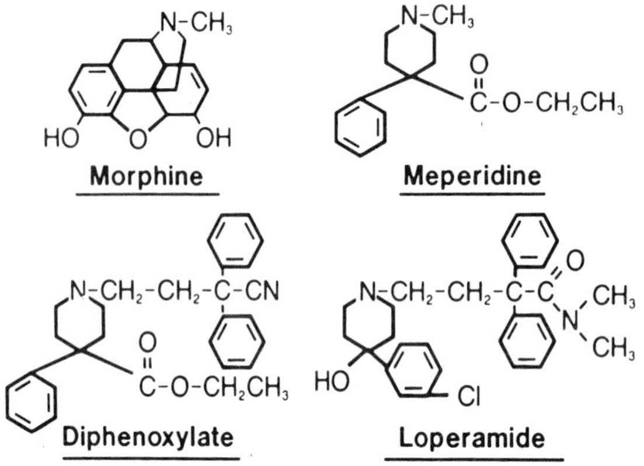

Fig. 11.18 Structures of morphine, meperidine, diphenoxylate and loperamide.

to phase III of the migrating myoelectric complex. The segmenting, non-propulsive contractions increase resistance to flow and decrease the transit of intestinal contents (Fig. 11.17). Morphine has also been found to initiate 'premature' phase III migrating complex activity (Borody et al 1985, Matsumoto et al 1986). Like synthetic opioids, human β-endorphin decreases antral contractions and delays gastric emptying (Camilleri et al 1986c).

Presently available opioid agonist drugs, such as morphine (Fig. 11.18), produce changes in gastrointestinal motility and contractions of the sphincter of Oddi, inhibit outflow of bile, promote intestinal absorption of fluid and electrolytes, and induce constipation. Several synthetic opioids related chemically to meperidine (pethidine) are employed in therapeutics primarily as antidiarrhoeal drugs. The two best known synthetic antidiarrhoeal opioids are diphenoxylate and loperamide (Fig. 11.18). These drugs produce naloxone-reversible changes in gastrointestinal motility and delay of intestinal transit (Basilisco et al 1987, Kachel et al 1986). While diphenoxylate and loperamide resemble meperidine chemically, meperidine itself (Fig.

CCK-8

Asp-Tyr-Met-Gly-Trp-Met-Asp-Phe-NH₂
SO₃

Substance P

Arg-Pro-Lys-Pro-Gln-Gln-Phe-Phe-Gly-Leu-Met-NH₂

Bombesin

Glp-Gln-Arg-Leu-Gly-Asn-Gln-Trp-Ala-Val-Gly-His-Leu-Met-NH₂

Fig. 11.19 Amino acid sequences of cholecystokinin octapeptide (CCK-8), substance P and bombesin.

11.18) is relatively non-constipating. The antidiarrhoeal properties of loperamide may result in part from non-opioid mechanisms (Reynolds et al 1984).

Special care must be taken in use of opioids as non-specific antidiarrhoeal drugs, since opioids may exacerbate enteric infections by invasive organisms (DuPont & Hornick 1973). Opioids are generally considered only for short-term use, as tolerance to the motility effects can occur (Burks & Long 1967) and opioids that cross the blood–brain barrier (morphine, codeine and other alkaloid-type opioids) can induce dependence. The major hazard associated with acute medical use of opioids is respiratory depression. Naloxone is an effective antagonist.

Peptides

Cholecystokinin (CCK) is a brain-gut peptide that serves both neurotransmitter and hormonal functions. It is released after meals from endocrine cells in the mucosa of the upper small intestine. CCK exists in multiple molecular forms, but the principal smaller form is the carboxyl-terminal octapeptide known as CCK-8 (Fig. 11.19). CCK is a potent stimulant of gallbladder contraction and of sphincter of Oddi relaxation (Walsh 1987). CCK induces contractions of gallbladder both by direct actions on smooth muscle CCK receptors and indirectly by increasing neural release of ACh (Behar & Biancani 1987, Harada et al 1986). CCK also induces contractions of intestinal smooth muscle, both by direct actions at smooth muscle CCK receptors and indirectly by release of ACh (Stewart & Burks 1977, Grider & Makhlouf 1987). Pharmacological doses of CCK inhibit gastric emptying and postprandial delay of gastric emptying has often been ascribed to physiological actions of CCK (Liddle et al 1986). However, potent and selective CCK antagonists, such as L-364718 or devazepide (Pendleton et al 1987), fail to block postprandial inhibition of gastric emptying and call into question a physiological role of CCK in regulation of gastric emptying. CCK may serve as a sensory neurotransmitter in ganglionic reflex pathways regulating gastrointestinal motility (Schumann & Kreulen 1986).

The tachykinins, also known as neurokinins, are neurotransmitters in peripheral sensory pathways (Buck & Burks 1986). Substance P (Fig. 11.19) and substance K (also known as neurokinin alpha and neuromedin L) and neurokinin beta (also known as neuromedin K) occur in neurons associated with both sensory and motor function (Mantyh et al 1984). Multiple types of tachykinin receptors occur in gastrointestinal nerves and smooth muscle (Mantyh et al 1984, Burcher et al 1986). Evidence has been put forward that substance P or a related tachykinin is responsible for initiation of intestinal reflexes responsible for postoperative ileus and ileus produced by peritoneal irritation (Holzer et al 1986).

A number of other gastrointestinal hormones produce motility effects when administered exogenously (Walsh 1987). Somatostatin, gastrin, motilin, and other hormones produce changes in motility that may eventu-

ally be of therapeutic value. Gastrin-releasing peptide, the mammalian equivalent of bombesin, produces striking changes in gastrointestinal motility and transit after peripheral or central administration in animals (Koslo et al 1986). Interestingly, the actions of bombesin may result primarily from effects in sensory neural pathways.

CONCLUSIONS

A great deal has been learned about the motility effects of drugs in the past few years. With increasing recognition of the importance of disorders of gastrointestinal motility in a number of disease states, additional new drugs will be introduced for therapeutic use in regulation of motility. Likewise, new approaches will be available to eliminate or combat the motility side-effects of drugs directed at other therapeutic endpoints.

Acknowledgements

Supported by US Public Health Service grant DA02163. The assistance of Ms Susan Fernandez is gratefully acknowledged.

REFERENCES

Ahlquist R P 1948 A study of the adrenotropic receptors. Am J Physiol 153: 586–600

Basilisco G, Camboni G, Bozzani, A, Paravincini M, Bianchi P A 1987 Oral naloxone antagonizes loperamide-induced delay of orocecal transit. Dig Dis Sci 32: 829–832

Behar J, Biancani P 1987 Pharmacologic characterization of excitatory and inhibitory cholecystokinin receptors of the cat gallbladder and sphincter of Oddi. Gastroenterology 92: 764–770

Bitar K N, Saffouri B, Makhlouf G M 1982 Cholinergic and peptidergic receptors on isolated human antral smooth muscle cells. Gastroenterology 82: 832–837

Borody T J, Quigley, E M M, Phillips S F, Wienbeck M, Tucker R L, Haddad A, Zinsmeister A R 1985 Effects of morphine and atropine on motility and transit in the human ileum. Gastroenterology, 89: 562–570

Buck S H, Bucks T F, 1986 The neuropharmacology of capsaicin: review of some recent observations. Pharmacol Rev 38: 179–226

Burcher E, Buck S H, Lovenberg W, O'Donohue T L 1986 Characterization and autoradiographic localization of multiple tachykinin binding sites in gastrointestinal tract and bladder. J Pharmacol Exp Ther 238: 819–831

Burks T F 1978 Central sites of action of gastrointestinal drugs. Gastroenterology 74: 322–324

Burks, T F 1987 Actions of drugs on gastrointestinal motility in: Johnson L R (ed.) Physiology of the gastrointestinal tract, 2nd edn, Raven Press, New York pp 723–724

Burks, T F, Galligan J J, Hirning L D, Porreca F 1987 Brain, spinal cord and peripheral sites of action of enkephalins and other endogenous opioids on

gastrointestinal motility. Gastroenterol Clin Biol 11: 44B–51B

Burks T F, Hirning L D, Galligan J J, Davis TP 1982, Motility effects of opioid peptides in dog intestine. Life Sci 31: 2237–2240

Burks T F, Jacquette D L, Grubb M N 1974 Motility responses of dog and monkey isolated perfused intestine to morphine, 5-hydroxytryptamine and cholinergic stimulants. Gen Pharmacol 5: 213–216

Burks T F, Long J P 1967 Responses of isolated dog small intestine to analgesic agents. J Pharmacol Exp Ther 158: 264–271

Burleigh D E, D'Mello A 1983 Neural and pharmacologic factors affecting motility of the internal anal sphincter. Gastroenterology 84: 409–417

Camilleri M, Brown M L, and Malagelada J-R 1986a Relationship between impaired gastric emptying and abnormal gastrointestinal motility. Gastroenterology 91: 94–99

Camilleri M., Brown, M L Malagelada J-R 1986b, Impaired transit of chyme in chronic intestinal pseudoobstruction-correction by cisapride. Gastroenterology 91: 619–626

Camilleri M, Malagelada J-R, Stanghellini V, Zinsmeister A R, Kao P C, Li C H 1986c Dose-related effects of synthetic human β-endorphin and naloxone on fed gastrointestinal motility. Am J Physiol 251: G147–G154

Costa M, Furness J B, Llewellyn-Smith I J 1987 Histochemistry of the enteric nervous system in: Johnson L R (ed.) Physiology of the gastrointestinal tract, 2nd edn, Raven Press, New York pp. 1–40

Dale H H 1914 The actions of certain esters and ethers of choline, and their relation to muscarine. J Pharmacol Exp Ther 6: 147–190

Dumuis A, Sebben M, Bockaert J 1989 The gastrointestinal prokinetic benzamide derivatives are agonists at the non-classical 5-HT receptor (5-HT$_4$) positively coupled to adenylate cyclase in neurons. Naunyn-Schmiedeberg's Arch Pharmacol 340: 403–410

DuPont H L, Hornick R B 1973 Adverse effects of Lomotil therapy in shigellosis. J Am Med Assoc 226: 1525–1528

Ek B A, Bjellin L A C, Lundgren B T 1986 β-Adrenergic control of motility in the rat colon. I. Evidence for functional separation of the β_1- and β_2 -adrenoceptor-mediated inhibition of colon activity. Gastroenterology 90: 400–407

Feldman M, Smith H J 1987 Effect of cisapride on gastric emptying of indigestible solids in patients with gastroparesis diabeticorum–a comparison with metoclopramide and placebo. Gastroenterology 92: 171–174

Fisher R S, Rock E, Malmud L S 1985 Cholinergic effects on gallbladder emptying in humans. Gastroenterology 89: 716–722

Galligan J J, Burks T F 1986 Cholinergic neurons mediate intestinal propulsion in the rat. J Pharmacol Exp Ther 283: 594–598

Grider J R, Makhlouf G M 1987 Regional and cellular heterogeneity of cholecystokinin receptors mediating muscle contraction in the gut. Gastroenterology 92: 175–180

Gullikson G W, Loefler R F, Virina M A 1991 Relationship of serotonin-3 receptor antagonist activity to gastric emptying and motor-stimulating actions of prokinetic drugs in dogs. J Pharmacol Exp Ther 258: 103–110

Harada T, Katsuragi T, Furukawa T 1986 Release of acetylcholine mediated by cholecystokinin receptors from the guinea pig sphincter of Oddi. J Pharmacol Exp Ther 239: 554–558

Harden T K, Tanner L I, Martin M W et al, 1986 Characteristics of two biochemical responses to stimulation of muscarinic cholinergic receptors in: Levine R R, Birdrall N J M, Giachetti A, Hammer R, Iverson L L, Jenden D J, North R A, (eds) Subtypes of muscarinic receptors II. Elsevier, Amsterdam pp 14–18

Hartshorne D J 1987 Biochemistry of the contractile process in smooth muscle in: Johnson L R (ed.) Physiology of the gastrointestinal tract, 2nd edn, Raven Press, New York pp 432–482

Hay A M, Man W K 1979 Effect of metoclopramide on guinea pig stomach. Gastroenterology 76: 492–496

Hirning L D, Porreca F, Burks T F 1985 Mu, but not kappa, opioid agonists induce contractions of the canine small intestine, ex vivo. Eur J Pharmacol 109: 49–54

Holzer P, Lippe I T, Holzer-Petsche U 1986 Inhibition of gastrointestinal transit due to surgical trauma or peritoneal irritation is reduced in capsaicin-treated rats. Gastroenterology 91: 360–363

Horowitz M, Maddox A, Maddern G J, Wishart J, Collins P J, Shearman J C 1987 Gastric and esophageal emptying in dystrophia myotonica–effect of metoclopramide. Gastroenterology 92: 570–577

Hughes J 1975 Isolation of an endogenous compound from the brain with pharmacological properties similar to morphine. Brain Res 88: 295–308

Inatomi N, Satoh H, Maki Y, Hashimoto N, Itoh Z, Omura S 1989, An erythromycin derivative, EM-523, induces motilin-like gastrointestinal motility in dogs. J Pharmacol Exp Ther 251: 707–712

Itoh Z, Nakaya M, Suzuki T, Arai H, Wakabayashi K 1984 Erythromycin mimics exogenous motilin in gastrointestinal contractile activity in the dog. Am J Physiol 247: G688–G694

James I F, Goldstein A 1984 Site-directed alkylation of multiple opioid receptors. I. Binding selectivity. Mol Pharmacol 25: 337–342

Janssens J, Peeters T L, Vantrappen G et al 1990 Improvement of gastric emptying in diabetic gastroparesis by erythromycin. New Eng J Med 322: 1028–1031

Kachel G, Ruppin H, Hagel J, Barina W, Meinhardt M, Domschke W 1986 Human intestinal motor activity and transport: effect of a synthetic opiate. Gastroenterology 90: 85–93

Koslo R J, Burks T F, Porreca F 1986 Centrally administered bombesin affects gastrointestinal transit and colonic bead expulsion through supra-spinal mechanisms. J Pharmacol Exp Ther 238: 62–67

Kromer W 1988 Endogenous and exogenous opioids in the control of gastrointestinal motility and secretion. Pharmacol Rev 40: 121–162

Kurosawa S, Hasler W L, Owyang C 1991 Characterization of dopamine receptors in guinea pig stomach: dopaminergic vs adrenergic receptors. Gastroenterology 100: 1224–1231

Lands A M, Luduena F P, Buzzo H J 1967 Differentiation of receptors responsive to isoproterenol. Life Sci 6: 2241–2249

Langer S Z (1974) Presynaptic regulation of catecholamine release. Biochem Pharmacol 23: 1793–1800

Libet B 1970 Generation of slow inhibitory and excitatory postsynaptic potentials. Fed Proc 29: 1945–1956

Liddle R, Morit E, Conrad C, Williams J 1986 Regulation of gastric emptying in humans by cholecystokinin. J Clin Invest 77: 992–996

Linnik M D, Butler B T, Gaddis R R, Ahmed N K 1991 Analysis of serotonergic mechanisms underlying benzamide-induced gastroprokinesis. J Pharmacol Exp Ther 259: 501–507

Lombardi D M, Grous M, Fine C F et al 1986 DA, Receptor mediates dopamine-induced relaxation of opossum lower esophageal sphincter in vitro. Gastroenterology 91: 533–539

McCallum R W, Prakash C, Campoli-Richards D M, Goa K L 1988 Cisapride: a preliminary review of its pharmacodynamic and pharmacokinetic properties, and therapeutic use as a prokinetic agent in gastrointestinal motility disorders. Drugs 36: 652–681

Makhlouf, G M 1987 Isolated smooth muscle cells of the gut in Johson L R (ed.) Physiology of the gastrointestinal tract, 2nd edn. Raven Press, New York pp 555–569

Mantyh P W, Goedert M, Hunt S P 1984 Autoradiographic visualization of receptor binding sites for substance P in the gastrointestinal tract of the guinea pig. Eur J Pharmacol 100: 133–134

Martin W R 1967 Opiod antagonists. Pharmacol Rev 19: 463–521

Matsumoto T, Sarna S K, Condon R E, Cowles V E, Frantzides C 1986 Differential sensitivities of morphine and motilin to initiate migrating motor complex in isolated intestinal segments. Gastroenterology 90: 61–67

Meyer J H 1987 Motility of the stomach and gastroduodenal junction in: Johnson L R (ed.) Physiology of the gastrointestinal tract, 2nd edn. Raven Press, New York pp 613–629

Minocha A, Galligan J J 1991 Erythromycin inhibits contractions of nerve-muscle preparations of the guinea pig small intestine. J Pharmacol Exp Ther 257: 1248–1252

Mosberg H I, Hurst R, Hruby V J, Gee K, Yamamura H I, Galligan J J, Burks T F 1983 Bis-penicillamine enkephalins possess highly improved specificity towards delta opioid receptors. Proc Natl. Acad Sci USA 80: 5871–5874

Nemeth P R, Ort C A, Zafirov D H, Wood J D 1985 Interactions between serotonin and cisapride on myenteric neurons. Eur J Pharmacol 108: 77–83

Nostrant T T, Sams J, Huber T 1986 Bethanechol increases the diagnostic yield in patients with esophageal chest pain. Gastroenterology 91: 1141–1146

Nowak T V, Harrington B, Karlbfleisch J H, Amatruda J M 1986 Evidence for abnormal cholinergic neuromuscular transmission in diabetic rat small intestine. Gastroenterology 91: 124–132

Otterson M F, Sarna S K 1990 Gastrointestinal motor effects of erythromycin. Am J Physiol 259: G355–G363

Peeters T G, Matthijs G, Depoortere I, Cachet T, Hoogmartens J, Vantrappen G 1989 Erythromycin is a motilin receptor agonist. Am J Physiol 257: G470–G474

Pendleton R G, Bendesky R J, Schaffer L, Nolan T E, Gould R J, Clineschmidt B V 1987 Roles of endogenous cholecystokinin in biliary, pancreatic and gastric function: studies with L-364, 718, a specific cholecystokinin receptor antagonist. J Pharmacol Exp Ther 241: 110–116

Pert C B, Snyder S H 1973 Opiate receptor: demonstration in nervous tissue. Science (Washington) 179: 1011–1014

Porreca F, Burks T F 1983 The spinal cord as a site of opioid effects on gastrointestinal transit in the mouse. J Pharmacol Exp Ther 227: 22–27

Porreca F, Filla A, Burks T F 1983 Spinal cord-mediated opiate effects on gastrointestinal transit in mice. Eur J Pharmacol 86: 135–136

Reynolds J C 1989 Prokinetic agents: a key in the future of gastroenterology. Gastroenterol Clin No Amer 18: 437–457

Reynolds I J, Gould R J, Snyder S H 1984 Loperamide: blockade of calcium channels as a mechanism for antidiarrheal effects. J Pharmacol Exp Ther 231: 628–632

Roman C, Gonella J 1987 Extrinsic control of digestive tract motility in: Johnson L R (ed) Physiology of the gastrointestinal tract, 2nd edn., pp 507–53, Raven Press, New York.

Schulze-Delrieu K 1981 Metoclopramide. N Engl J Med 305: 28–33

Schumann M A, Kreulen D L 1986 Action of cholecystokinin octapeptide and CCK-related peptides on neurons in inferior mesenteric ganglion of guinea pig. J Pharmacol Exp Ther 239: 618–625

Schuurkes J A J, Van Neuten J M 1981 Is dopamine an inhibitory modulator of gastrointestinal motility? Scand J Gastroenterol 67: 33–36

Snape W J, Battle W M, Schwartz S S, Braunstein S N, Goldstein H A, Alavi A 1982 Metoclopramide to treat gasroparesis due to diabetes mellitus. Ann Int Med 96: 444–446

Stacher G, Bergmann H, Wiesnagrotzki S, Kiss A, Schneider C, Mittelback G, Gaupmann G, Hobart J 1987 Intravenous cisapride accelerates delayed gastric emptying and increases antral contraction amplitude in patients with primary anorexia nervosa. Gastroenterology 92: 1000–1006

Stewart J J, Burks T F 1977 Actions of cholecystokinin octapeptide on smooth muscle of isolated dog intestine. Am J Physiol 232: E306–E310

Stewart J J, Weisbrodt N W, Burks T F 1977 Centrally mediated intestinal stimulation by morphine. J Pharmacol Exp Ther 202: 174–181

Stewart J J, Weisbrodt N W, Burks T F 1978 Central and peripheral actions of morphine on intestinal transit. J Pharmacol Exp Ther 205: 547–555

Takahashi T, Kurosawa S, Wiley J W, Owyang C 1991 Mechanism for the gastrokinetic action of domperidone. Gastroenterology 101: 703–710

Taylor P 1990a Cholinergic agonists in Gilman A G, Rall T W, Nies A S, Taylor P (eds) Goodman and Gilman's the pharmacological basis of therapeutics, 7th edn. Macmillan, New York pp 122–130

Taylor P 1990b Anticholinesterase agents in Gilman A G, Rall T W, Nies A S, Taylor P (eds) Goodman and Gilman's the pharmacological basis of therapeutics, 7th edn. Macmillan, New York pp 131–149

Thanik K, Chey W K, Shak A, Hamilton D, Nadelson N 1982 Bethanechol or cimetidine in the treatment of symptomatic reflux esophagitis. Arch Intern Med 142: 1479–1481

Vaught J L, Cowan A, Jacoby H I 1985, μ and δ, but not κ, opioid agonists induce contractions of the canine small intestine in vivo. Eur J Pharmacol 109: 43–48

Von Voigtlander P F, Lahti R A, Ludens J H 1983 U-50, 488H: a selective and structurally novel non-mu (kappa) opioid agonist. J Pharmacol Exp Ther 24: 7–12

Walsh J H 1987 Gastrointestinal hormones in Johnson L R (ed.) Physiology of the gastrointestinal tract, 2nd edn. Raven Press, New York pp 181–253

Watson M, Roeske W R, Vickroy T W et al 1986 Biochemical and functional basis of putative muscarinic receptor subtypes and its implications in: Levine R R, Birdsall N J M, Giachietti A et al (eds) Subtypes of muscarinic receptors II, Elsevier, Amsterdam pp 46–55

Wiley J, Owyang C 1987 Dopaminergic modulation of rectosigmoid motility: action of domperidone. J Pharmacol Exp Ther 242: 548–551

The measurement of motility

12. Radiology

E. Corazziari   A. Torsoli

Radiology offers qualitative or semi-quantitative information on the motor behaviour of the alimentary canal. Following the administration of a carefully selected material, X-rays can indirectly reveal wall contractions, as well as displacement of contents. The degree of luminal distension can provide some information on tonicity and/or capacitance of the viscus.

RADIOLOGICAL TECHNIQUES

Fluoroscopic observation is the most valuable radiological test for the investigation of motor activity of the gastrointestinal tract. Image intensifier systems (Wolf & Khilnani 1966) offer a better resolution of the images, significantly reduce radiation, and make telefluorography, photofluorography, cinefluorography and magnetic tape recording possible (Gebauer et al 1967).

Cinefluorography enables the evaluation of rapid motor sequences by slow motion or still picture analysis (Cohen & Wolf 1968).

Fluoroscopic images converted into video signals and recorded on magnetic tape or disk can be immediately displayed by playback. Adequate radiological evaluation of rapid motor sequences can thus be obtained by spot-camera imaging.

LIMITATIONS OF RADIOLOGICAL TECHNIQUE

Radiology carries the risk of radiation exposure and, therefore, only few and short-lasting motor events can be observed. With the exception of the colon, radiological description concerns motor events, elicited by intraluminal distension due to contrast medium, which are not physically and chemically comparable to those induced by food.

Radiology detects wall movement caused by contraction of the circular muscle layer but it is inadequate in the investigation of motor events of the longitudinal layer. Finally, radiological observations are essentially qualitative in nature and, with a few exceptions, do not allow quantification of the data.

RADIOLOGICAL EVALUATION OF DEGLUTITION AND DEFAECATION

Deglutition and defaecation are functions controlled at a conscious level and performed by integrated actions of several striated muscles. These events are rapid and can only be evaluated by means of slow motion or frame-by-frame analysis of cinefluorographic or videotape recordings.

Deglutition

The mechanism of normal deglutition is shown in Figure 12.1 (Montesi et al 1987).

The main indication for the radiologic investigation of deglutition is oropharyngeal dysphagia. Major structural abnormalities which may affect the swallowing act are webs, rings and diverticula. Deranged function of deglutition may affect the oral, pharyngeal and pharyngo-oesophageal phases. Defective mastication and tongue contractility, as well as that of buccal, masticatory and glossal coordination, may impair oral clearance and bolus transport to the pharynx. Regurgitation of the ingesta into the rhynopharynx may occur when the closure of the velopharynx is absent or delayed. Failure of the pharyngeal constrictor to produce coordinated peristaltic activity leads to retention of the bolus within the pharynx (Fig. 12.2). Defective closure of the laryngeal vestibule is visualized by entrance of contrast medium into the upper airways; and defective movement of the epiglottis becomes apparent as partial mobility or immobility (Fig. 12.3). Dysfunction of the cricopharyngeus may be apparent as a failure to relax, thus obstructing, totally or partially, the passage of the pharyngeal contents into the oesophagus (Fig. 12.4); relative to the time period of deglutition, the dysfunc-

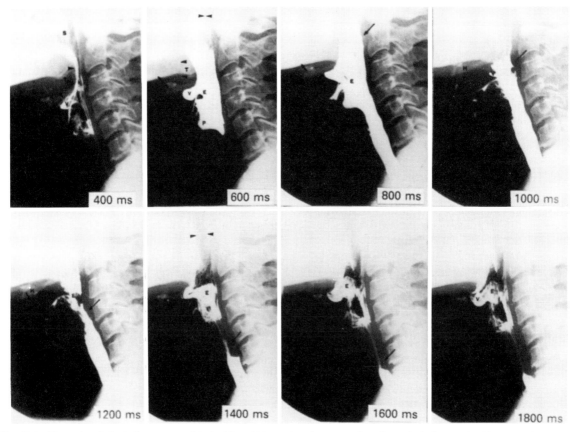

Fig. 12.1 Normal radiological sequence of deglutition. 400 ms after the onset of swallow, the bolus, pushed into the pharynx by the tongue, is displaced posteriorly (arrows) and the valleculae (V) become evident. The tongue and the hyoid bone move slightly forward. After 600 ms the bolus is filling the pharynx, the base of the tongue moves forward, the valleculae and the pyriform recesses (P) are distended; the palatopharyngeal isthmus (facing arrows) is closed; the hyoid bone moves upward and forward; the epiglottis (E) is in a horizontal position. After 800 ms, the bolus has reached the cervical oesophagus; concomitantly the cricopharyngeal muscle relaxes and the peristaltic contraction of the superior pharyngeal constrictor occurs (long arrow); a small amount of barium can be detected in the subepiglottic space. After 1000 ms the bolus is pushed by the peristaltic contraction of the medial pharyngeal constrictor (long arrow), the hyoid bone (H) has reached its highest level close to the mandible and the thyroid cartilage; the epiglottis is almost completely inverted, the valleculae and the pyriform sinuses are no longer outpouching. After 1200 ms the bolus is pushed distally by the peristaltic contraction. After 1400 ms the palotopharyngeal isthmus opens, the hyoid bone and the larynx move downward, the epiglottis moves upright and air fills the larynx. After 1600–1800 ms the pharyngolaryngeal structures are back to the resting position and the primary peristaltic contraction of the cervical oesophagus (arrow) pushes the bolus into the thoracic oesophagus. (From Montesi et al 1987 with permission.)

tion may occur in the early, late or during the entire phase of cricopharyngeal relaxation (Curtis et al 1991).

Any of the above-mentioned abnormalities may be present alone, but the concomitant presence of two or more abnormalities may frequently occur in the same patient (Ekberg & Nylander 1982a,b).

Defaecation

Following the rectal injection of a contrast medium, carefully prepared to simulate physical characteristics of faeces, the dynamic events during straining and defaecation can be visualized. The radiological examination is performed by taking the lateral pelvic view at rest, and during straining and defaecation with the patient sitting on a radiolucent commode (Mahieu et al 1984a,b, Ekberg et al 1990). At rest, the anorectal angle is about 90° and the anorectal junction which identifies the level of the pelvic floor is located less than 2 cm below the pubococcygeal line. During straining, the pelvic floor descends by no more than 2 cm and as tone of the puborectalis decreases, the anorectal angle straightens out to about 137°.

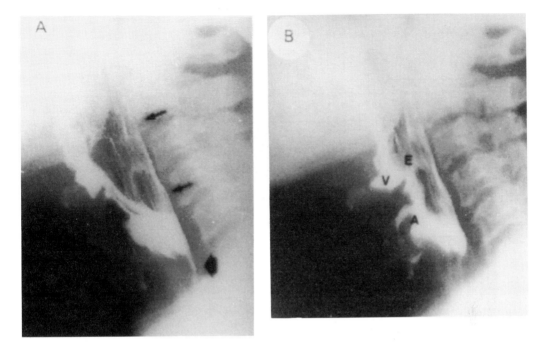

Fig. 12.2 Paresis of the pharyngeal constrictors. Retention of the bolus in the oro- and hypopharynx due to lack of contraction of the pharyngeal constrictors. **A** Failure of elevation of the hyoid bone and larynx. **B** Aspiration of contrast into the larynx. **A**, arytenoid cartilage; **V**, ventricle; **E**, epiglottis. (By courtesy of A. Montesi.)

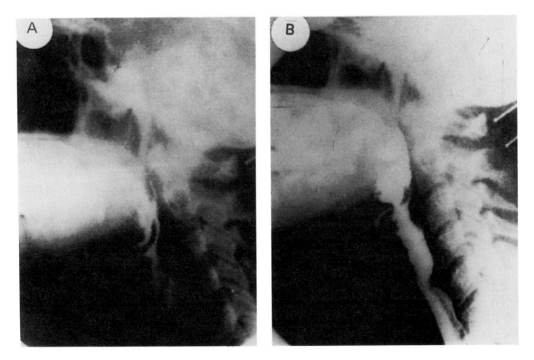

Fig. 12.3 Immobile epiglottis. During the passage of the bolus through the (**A**) oro- and (**B**) hypopharynx the epiglottis remains still. (By courtesy of A. Montesi.)

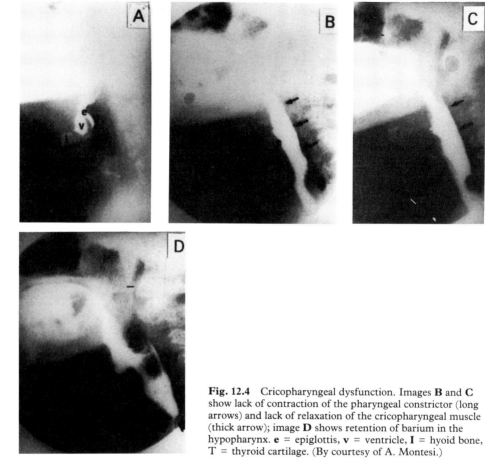

Fig. 12.4   Cricopharyngeal dysfunction. Images **B** and **C** show lack of contraction of the pharyngeal constrictor (long arrows) and lack of relaxation of the cricopharyngeal muscle (thick arrow); image **D** shows retention of barium in the hypopharynx. **e** = epiglottis, **v** = ventricle, **I** = hyoid bone, T = thyroid cartilage. (By courtesy of A. Montesi.)

During defaecation, as the pelvic floor descends the distal rectum and the anal canal open up and are progressively filled by contrast medium. At the end of defaecation the lumen of the anal canal and distal rectum close, the pelvic floor rises, and the anorectal angle is restored (Fig. 12.5).

Defaecography is usually performed in patients with:

1. Dyschezia (feeling of difficult and/or incomplete rectal emptying);
2. Faecal incontinence other than that caused by rectal impaction;
3. Anal or perianal pain syndrome;
4. Solitary rectal ulcer syndrome;
5. Rectal intussusception and prolapse.

An open anal canal and a wide anorectal angle at rest and/or the inability to retain contrast medium on request is indicative of sphincter insufficiency in faecal incontinence. Common findings, during evacuation, in dyschezia patients are failure of the anorectal angle to widen (Fig. 12.6), anal canal to open (Fig. 12.7) and high-frequency alternating contraction/relaxation pattern of the puborectalis, and a rectal emptying time over 30 s; these findings appear to be the radiologic counterpart of pelvic floor dyssynergia (Badiali et al 1991).

Abnormalities of the smooth outline of the rectum may be apparent as irregularity of the mucosa and/or infoldings of the mucosa and the rectal wall. When these infoldings become thicker and descend during straining, they may give rise to internal intussusception and/or external prolapse. Such defaecographic findings are relatively common in the solitary rectal ulcer syndrome, rectal prolapse and anal/perianal pain syndrome.

The location of the pelvic floor may be abnormally low at rest or during evacuation. In females, the degree of perianal descent is age related, and an abnormal

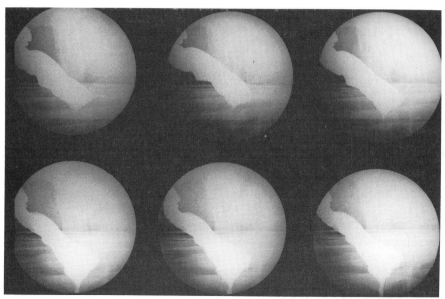

Fig. 12.5 Normal radiological sequence of defaecation. Defaecography in latero-lateral view. To be read from left to right. Resting condition (first image) followed by straining with progressive lowering of the pelvic floor, relaxation of the puborectalis sling (visible as widening of the rectoanal angle) and opening of the distal rectum and anal canal (subsequent two images); evacuation (images of the bottom line). (By courtesy of F I Habib.)

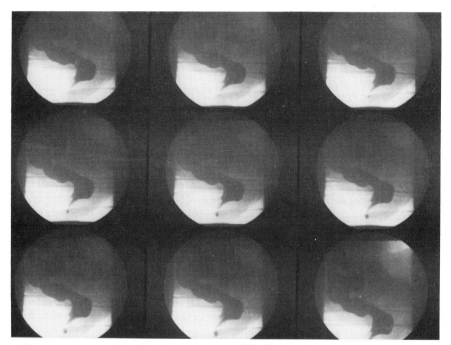

Fig. 12.6 Rectoanal discordination. Defaecography in latero-lateral view. To be read from left to right. During evacuation the puborectalis sling does not relax and there is inadequate opening of the anal canal. (By courtesy of F I Habib.)

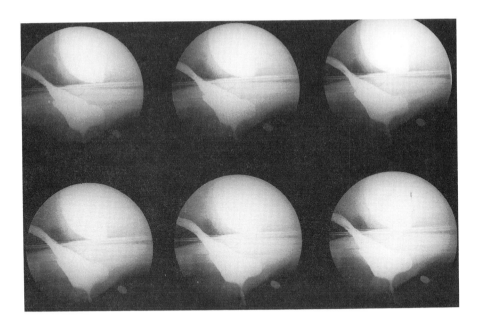

Fig. 12.7   Rectonal discordination. Cysto-defaecography in latero-lateral view. To be read from left to right. Resting condition (first image); straining and evacuation (last five images). During evacuation normal relaxation of the puborectalis sling is not accompanied by adequate opening of the anal canal. A small rectocele is also visible. (By courtesy of F I Habib.)

descent of the perineum is frequently found in association with one or more of the previously described abnormalities (Habib et al 1992). Rectocele is also a frequent finding in females at defaecography (Fig. 12.8).

The clinical value of proctography is still under scrutiny since (1) some findings such as rectocele and intussusception are commonly present in asymptomatic control subjects, and (2) the size of the anorectal angle and the depth of the puborectalis indentation are difficult to measure reproducibly.

Examination of the recto-anal tract can also be performed by using a barium-filled balloon (balloon proctography) instead of a semi-solid bolus. There is, however, loss of information concerning details of the rectal mucosa and overall emptying of the rectum (Preston et al 1984).

Since radiologic investigation of defaecation involves a substantial amount of radiation exposure it has been recommended that this investigation is performed only when other investigations fail to provide a diagnosis (Whitehead et al 1992).

WALL MOVEMENTS

Segmenting stationary contractions

Segmenting contractions appear radiologically as stationary non-propagating ring-like indentations of the wall, which totally or partially occlude the lumen, dividing the viscus into segments. These contractions may, however, give rise to pressure gradients determining displacement of contents in either direction.

In the oesophagus, local intermittent contractions (tertiary contractions) may appear isolated or simultaneously at different levels (Fig. 12.9). Their infrequent occurrence is compatible with a normal oesophageal function. Their frequent and/or simultaneous occurrence at multiple levels, sometimes associated with curling of the oesophagus, is suggestive of an oesophageal motor abnormality (Fig. 12.10).

In the stomach, stationary wall movements do not present the characteristic segmentary ring-like contractions, but rather appear as slow tonic variation. This type of motor activity, which takes place in the fundus and upper two-thirds of the corpus, is difficult to

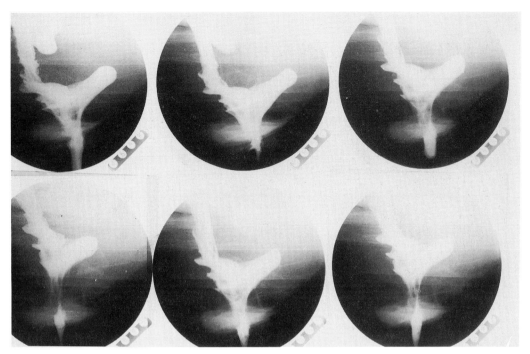

Fig. 12.8 Intussusception and rectocele. Defaecography in latero-lateral view – to be read from left to right: during the evacuation phase a large rectocele is visible. An intrarecto-anal intussusception is also visible. (By courtesy of F I Habib.)

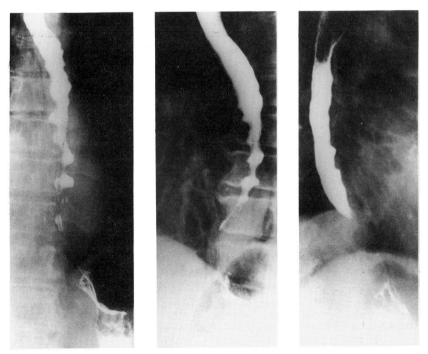

Fig. 12.9 Segmenting contractions of the oesophagus. Three oesophagograms of the same patient showing segmenting contractions and their variability during a short observation period.

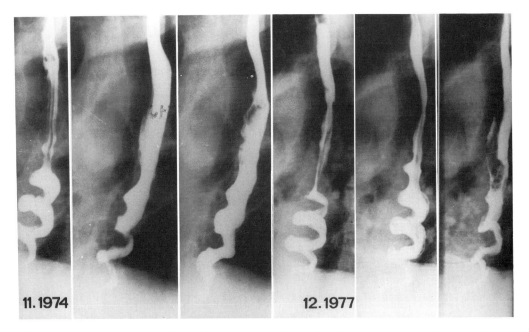

Fig. 12.10 Segmenting contractions of the oesophagus. Two series of oesophagograms performed at 3 year intervals in the same patient with diffuse oesophageal spasm. The two series are strikingly similar and show a corkscrew appearance of the oesophageal body despite the absence of any symptoms during the radiological examinations.

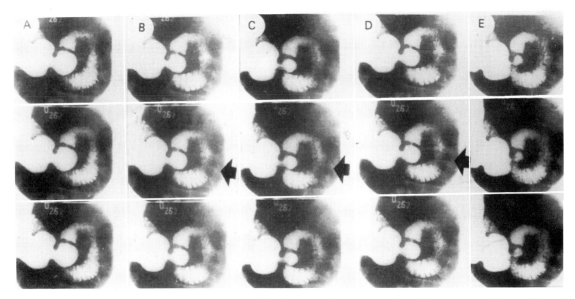

Fig. 12.11 Segmenting contraction of the duodenum. Cinefluorographic sequence taken in the prone position – to be read from top to bottom: **A** Duodenum filled with barium; **B**, **C** Ring-like constriction as indicated by arrows; **D** Duodenal wall starts relaxing without forward progression of either constriction or barium; **E** Duodenal wall fully relaxed and distribution of barium similar to that seen in **A**. (From Torsoli et al 1971 with kind permission.)

investigate radiologically as no critical or well-identifiable changes of the wall profile can be detected.

At the level of the small intestine, segmenting activity appears as 1–2 cm long annular contractions occurring at intervals of 3–4 cm. They are usually isolated (Fig. 12.11) and sometimes simultaneous at different

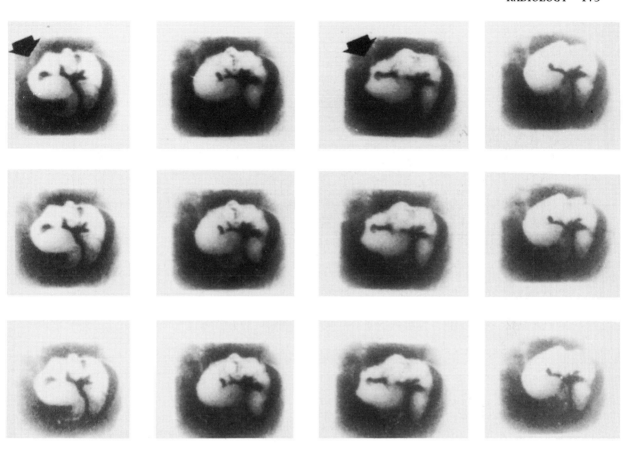

Fig. 12.12   Segmenting contraction of the colon. Cinefluorographic sequence of the sigmoid colon contrasted with barium sulphate administered per os. To be read from top to bottom and from left to right: annular segmenting contraction occurs twice in the sequence on the left side of the sigmoid (arrows).

levels. Annular contractions may sometimes occur for short periods in adjacent intestinal tracts causing bi-directional displacement of contents ('to and fro' or 'pendular' movements) (Hertz 1907).

At the level of the large intestine, segmenting activity is characterized by localized wall contractions which, partly or completely, involve the circumference of the colon (Ritchie 1968). They represent more than 90% of the entire colonic motor activity (Fig. 12.12) and originate, for the major part, at the level of the stable interhaustral folds (Torsoli et al 1971b).

Peristalsis

The peristaltic motor event is visualized as an aborally directed ring-like contraction, which, at least in the oesophagus and small and large intestine, appears to follow a circumscribed dilatation of the walls.

In the oesophagus primary peristalsis follows an act of swallowing and it is seen to progress from the pharynx to the oesophagogastric junction. Secondary peristalsis is not preceded by the oropharyngeal phase of deglutition and usually originates in the middle-distal part of the oesophagus (Turano 1957).

In the distal stomach, circular ring-like indentations which start in the corpus and move slowly towards the pylorus are visible on contrast examination (Smith et al 1957). In some instances, the indentations are shallow and fade out at the antrum, do not reach the pylorus, or do not produce any substantial movement of the contents. In other instances, the indentations deepen as they move distally, occluding the lumen as they reach the incisura angularis; at 3–4 cm from the pylorus the antrum appears to contract simultaneously (antral systole). This type of contraction causes displacement of contents towards the pylorus and, as the terminal antral contraction takes place, barium may be either pushed forward into the duodenum if the

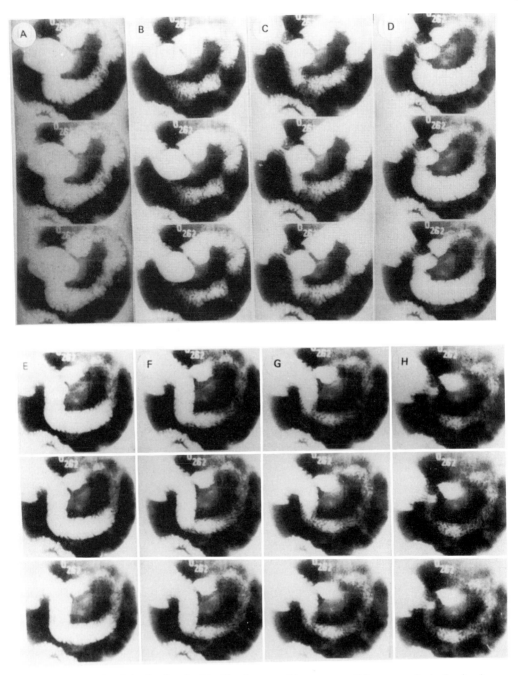

Fig. 12.13 Antral and duodenal peristalsis. Cinefluorographic sequence of the antro-pyloric-duodenal tract taken in prone position – To be read from top to bottom: **A** Annular contraction of the antrum moving distally (**B, C** and **D**) propelling barium into the duodenum, (**B, C**); **D** constriction appearing just beyond the duodenal bulb and propelling barium into the ascending duodenum (**E** and **F**) and beyond the duodeno-jejunal flexure (**G** and **H**).

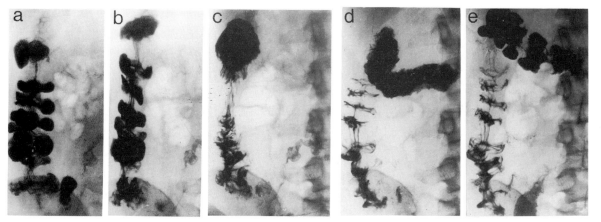

Fig. 12.14 Lower gastrointestinal series showing a peristaltic movement (right colon). Haustra modify orientation (**b**) and then disappear (**c**) as contents are displaced distally (**c** and **d**). Haustra are present again in the segment proximal to the displaced contents (**d**) and then at the level of contents (**e**) after termination of the motor event. (From Torsoli et al 1966 with permission.)

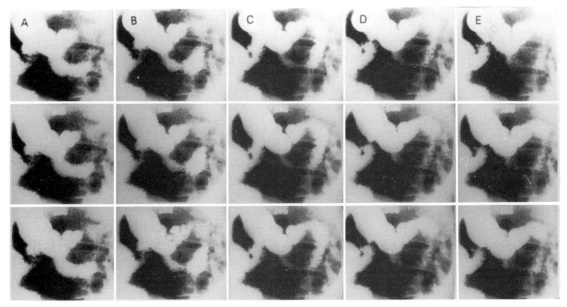

Fig. 12.15 Retrograde duodenal contractions. Cinefluorographic sequences of the antro-pyloric-duodenal tract taken in prone position. **A** Barium contrast in the stomach and the ascending part of the duodenum. **B** A duodenal constriction appears just before the ascending duodenal loop and moving backward propels barium into the descending duodenal loop (**C** and **D**) and then into the duodenal bulb and the stomach (**D** and **E**).

pylorus is open (Fig. 12.13), or propelled backwards into the stomach if the pylorus is closed (Smith et al 1957, Carlson et al 1966).

At the level of the small bowel, peristaltic movements displace contrast medium for short distances (4–5 cm). In the duodenum, however, movement of contents over longer distances (up to and beyond the ligament of Treitz) may be seen (Fig. 12.13) (Torsoli et al 1971a).

At the level of the colon, peristalsis begins with a progressive change in the spatial orientation of the colonic folds, which rapidly disappear. Then a concentric contraction starts at the cranial end of the unsegmented tract and moves distally, preceded by dilatation of the lumen. Subsequently, haustrations reappear first in the segment proximal to the displaced contents and then at the level of the segment where contents have been displaced (Fig. 12.14) (Torsoli et al 1971b).

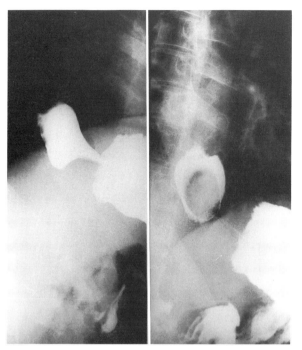

Fig. 12.16 Oesophagograms in a patient with dysphagia and recurrent episodes of chest pain after a Nissen fundoplication for reflux oesophagitis. Liquid barium is emptied from the oesophagus into the stomach; conversely (on the right) a solid bolus (marshmallow) is retained above the fundoplication. (By courtesy of F I Habib.)

Retrograde motor activity

Retrograde displacement of contents for short distances can be detected occasionally in the small bowel, but a sequential orally directed wall contraction has only been described in the duodenum (Fig. 12.15) (Borgstrom & Arborelius 1971, Torsoli et al 1971a). Retrograde displacement of contents for medium and large distances occurs in the colon, but the underlying motor mechanism is not clear.

TRANSIT

Depending upon the anatomic structure, the specific motor pattern of each segment and the physical characteristics of the contents, the transit rate varies in different parts of the gastrointestinal tract. Since its earliest clinical application radiology has been used to evaluate the progression of a radio-opaque bolus. This approach has the advantage of simplicity but only gives a semi-quantitative evaluation as it detects the head and, less precisely, the body and tail of the radio-opaque bolus. Furthermore, the great variability in viscosity and stability of the barium sulphate suspension may affect the final interpretation, even when the technique is standardized (Miller 1967).

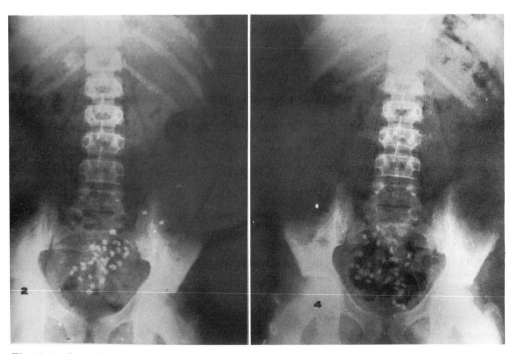

Fig. 12.17 Large bowel segmental transit time. Chronic non-organic constipation with rectal slowing of transit (dyschezia). On days 2 and 4 after ingestion, radio-opaque markers are retaind in the rectal ampulla.

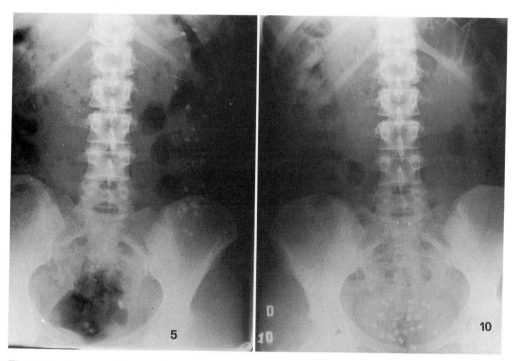

Fig. 12.18   Large bowel segmental transit time. Chronic non-organic constipation with colonic and rectal slowing of transit. On day 5 after ingestion, radio-opaque markers are retained in the left colon in the presence of an empty rectum; on day 10 markers are retained in the rectal ampulla.

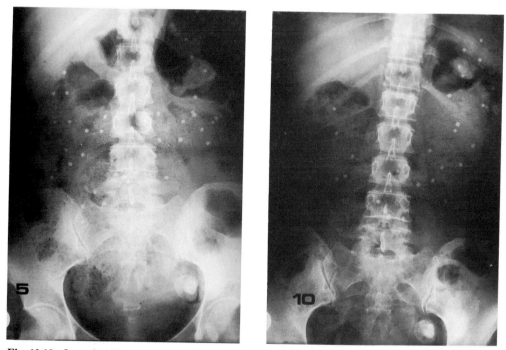

Fig. 12.19   Large bowel segmental transit time. Chronic non-organic constipation with colonic slowing of transit in a patient with colostomy performed at the level of the distal left colon after a stercoral perforation. On days 5 and 10 after ingestion, markers are retained in the colon proximal to the colostomy.

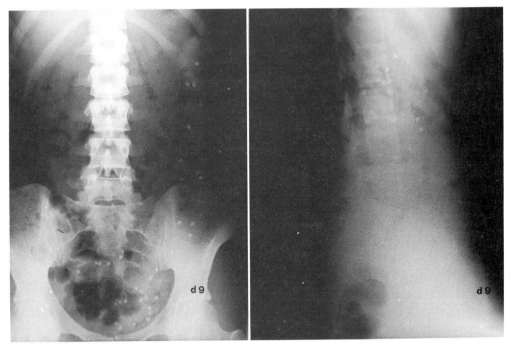

Fig. 12.20 Large bowel segmental transit time. Chronic non-organic constipation with colonic slowing of transit. X-ray discrimination between sigmoid and rectal location of the markers by means of a radiogram performed in lateral view. On day 9 after ingestion, an anteroposterior view of the abdomen depicts markers scattered along the descending colon and within the pelvis (in the rectum?); a lateral view shows an empty rectum indicating that markers are retained in the descending colon and sigmoid only.

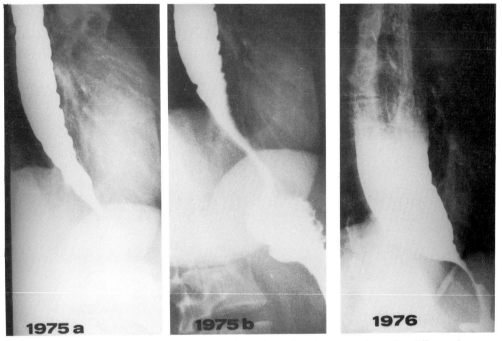

Fig. 12.21 Mega-oesophagus. Oesophagograms of a patient with achalasia, performed at different times. Note progressive dilatation of the oesophageal body.

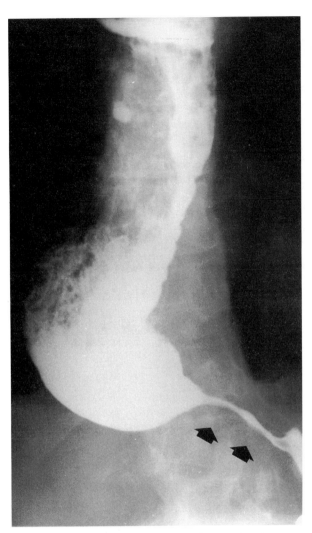

Fig. 12.22   Mega-oesophagus. Oesophagogram showing dilated oesophageal body with retention of barium and ingesta secondary to leiomyoma (arrows) located at the oesophagogastric junction.

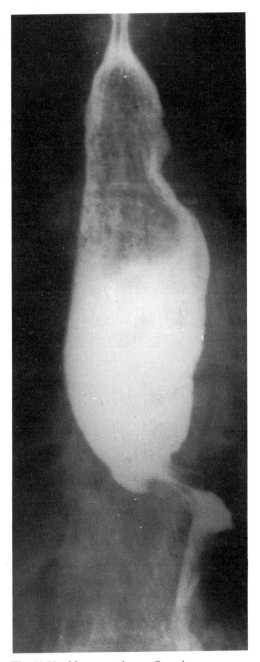

Fig. 12.23   Mega-oesophagus. Oesophagogram showing dilated oesophageal body with retention of barium and air level in a patient with scleroderma.

Oesophageal transit depends on gravity, consistency of the bolus and oesophageal motor activity. In the erect position, non-viscous boluses reach the oesophagogastric junction with the aid of oropharyngeal pressure and gravity. Peristaltic contractions occur after the passage of the bolus and empty the oesophageal body of any residual contents. Conversely, in the supine position oesophageal transit of a viscous bolus depends entirely upon pressure gradients caused by propulsive motor activity. To detect subtle changes in oesophageal transit, it is necessary to challenge the oesophagus with a solid radio-opaque bolus swallowed in the supine position (Fig. 12.16).

The radiological demonstration of the passage of

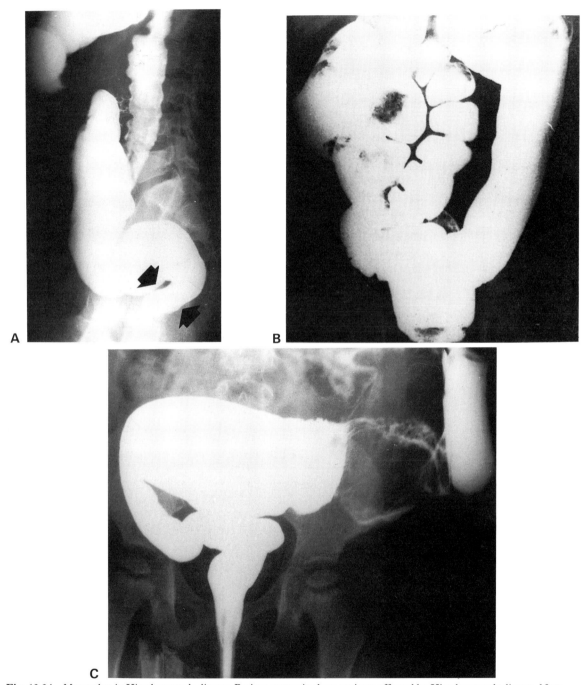

Fig. 12.24   Megacolon in Hirschsprung's disease. Barium enema in three patients affected by Hirschsprung's disease. Note different length of the aganglionic segment and large bowel distension proximal to it. **A** shows involvement of the distal part of the rectum, **B** shows involvement of the entire rectum, **C** shows involvement of the rectum and sigmoid. Transition zone is better appreciated in the lateral view (arrows) of a barium enema performed without previous large bowel preparation. Transition zone cannot be detected in patients with ultra-short Hirschsprung's disease.

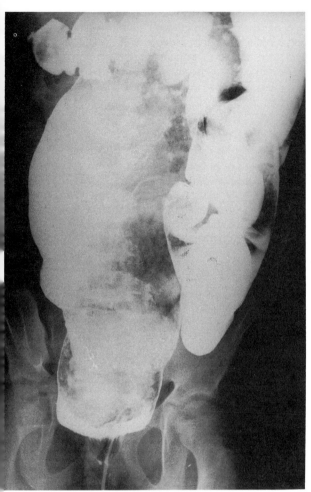

Fig. 12.25 Megarectum and megacolon in chronic idiopathic constipation. Barium enema shows extremely distended rectum and colon in the absence of any transition zone.

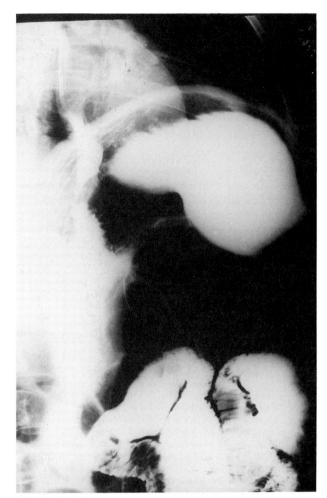

Fig. 12.26 Megastomach and mega-small bowel in chronic idiopathic intestinal pseudo-obstruction. Upper gastrointestinal series of a patient with recurrent episodes of intestinal obstruction who has been previously submitted to total colectomy and a negative laparotomy. Note gaseous distension of the stomach and the small bowel.

barium from the stomach into the oesophagus in the supine position, and in the absence of physical efforts which may increase the abdominothoracic pressure gradient, is a definitive diagnostic sign of gastro-oesophageal reflux.

The gastric emptying of a barium meal cannot be considered an accurate method to evaluate transit of food through the stomach; however, the retention of barium contrast in the stomach of fasting patients for several hours suggests an abnormally prolonged gastric emptying time. In the evaluation of patients with slow gastric emptying it might be useful to perform a radiological investigation with solid food impregnated with barium or with corpuscular radio-opaque markers to detect delayed gastric emptying of solid components

(Bertrand et al 1980), in the presence of normal liquid emptying.

Detection of contrast medium in the stomach subsequent to its introduction directly into the duodenum via a fine catheter has been used to detect duodenogastric reflux. Evaluation of the small bowel transit by means of a barium meal is inaccurate (Thompson & Saunders 1972).

Particulate radio-opaque markers (3 × 5 mm, polyethylene and 20% w/w barium sulphate) are more suitable for measuring transit of semi-solid/solid contents through the large bowel. Following the ingestion of markers, X-ray films or fluoroscopic observation of the abdomen at regular time intervals (Hinton et al 1969, Chaussade et al 1986) can be used to detect their location within the large bowel. The distribution of markers in various segments of the colon and rectum can provide valuable information on transit in patients with constipation (Corazziari et al 1975) (Figs. 12.17–12.20).

DILATATION OF THE LUMEN

Capacitance and tone of the alimentary canal may vary widely and cannot be measured accurately. Nonetheless, abnormal dilatation of the lumen, 'megalumen', is easily detected radiologically and indicates the presence of either a functional or mechanical obstruction distally or the loss of tone in the dilated viscus. Accordingly, mega-oesophagus (Figs. 12.21–12.23), megastomach, megacolon and megarectum (Figs. 12.24, 12.25) are common findings in the presence of ineffective relaxation of the lower oesophageal sphincter, the pylorus and the anal canal, respectively. Less commonly, however, one or more segments of the alimentary tract appear dilated in the presence of wall hypotonicity secondary to either myopathies or neuropathies (Fig. 12.26).

CONCLUSION

In conclusion, radiology is still the most reliable method to evaluate motor function of the striated muscles at the level of the oropharynx and the anorectum and to measure transit through the large bowel. In other areas, it should be used to complement methods that offer quantitative measurements.

REFERENCES

Badiali D, Habib F I, Corazziari E et al 1991 Manometric and dafaecographic patterns of straining. J Gastrointestinal Motil 3: 171

Bertrand J, Metman E H, Dorval E D, Rouleau P H, D'Hueppe A, Philippe L 1980 Etude du temps d'évacuation gastrique de repas normaux au moyens de granules radio-opaque. Applications cliniques et validation. Gastroenterol Clin Biol 4: 770–776

Borgstrom S, Arborelius M 1971 A technique for studying propulsion and the displacement of contents in the duodenum and proximal jejunum. Rendic R. Gastroenterol 3: 174–177

Carlson H C, Code C F Nelson R A 1966 Motor action of canine gastroduodenal junction: a cineradiographic, pressure and electric study. Am J Dig Dis 11: 155–172

Chaussade S, Roche H, Khyara A, Couterier D, Guerre J 1986 Mesure du temps de transit colique (TTC): description et validation d'une nouvelle technique. Gastroenterol Clin Biol 10: 385–389

Cohen B R, Wolf B S 1968 Cineradiographic and intraluminal pressure correlations in the pharynx and oesophagus in: Code C F (ed.) Alimentary canal. American Physiological Society, Washington, DC pp 1841–1860

Corazziari E, Dani S, Pozzessere C, Anzini F, Torsoli A 1975 Colonic segmental transit times in chronic nonorganic constipation. Rendic Gastroenterol 7: 67–69

Curtis D J, Ekberg O, Montesi A 1991 Swallowing: a radiologic perspective. Gastroenterol Int 4: 47–54

Ekberg O, Nylander G 1982a Cineradiography of the pharyngeal stage of deglutition in 150 individuals without dysphagia. Br J Rad 55: 253–257

Ekberg O, Nylander G 1982b Cineradiography of the pharyngeal stage of deglutition in 250 dysphageal patients. Br J Rad 55: 258–262

Ekberg O, Mahieu P H G, Bartram C I, Piloni V 1990 Defaecography: dynamic radiologic imaging in proctology. Gastroenterol Int 3: 57–62

Gebauer A, Lissner J, Schott O 1967 Roentgen television. Grune & Stratton, New York

Habib F I, Corazziari E, Viscardi A, Badiali D, Torsoli A 1992 Role of body position, gender and age on pelvic floor location and mobility. Dig Dis Sci 37: 500–505

Hertz A F 1907 The passage of food along the alimentary canal. Guy Hosp Rep 61: 389–427

Hinton J M, Lennard-Jones J E, Young A C 1969 A new method for studying gut transit times using radioopaque markers. Gut 10: 842–847

Mahieu P, Pringot J, Bodart P 1984a Defecography: I. Description of a new procedure and results in normal patients. Gastrointest Radio 9: 247–251

Mahieu P, Pringot J, Bodart P 1984b Defecography: II. Contribution to the diagnosis of defecation disorders. Gastrointest Radio 9: 253–261

Miller R E 1967 Barium sulphate as a contrast medium in: Margulis A R, Burheune H J (eds) Alimentary tract roentgenology. Mosby, Saint Louis pp 25–36

Montesi A, Piloni V, Pesaresi A, Antico E, Blasetti R 1987 Le tube digestif. Approche radiologique fonctionelle. Radiology in mobile organs: the gastrointestinal tract. Radiologie du Cepur 9: 95–103

Preston D M, Lennard-Jones J E, Thomas B M 1984 The balloon proctogram. Br J Surg 71: 29–32

Ritchie J A 1968 Colonic motor activity and bowel function. Part I. Normal movement of contents. Gut 9: 442–456

Smith A W M, Code C F, Schlegel J F 1957 Simultaneous cineradiographic and kimographic studies of human gastric antral motility. J Appl Physiol 11: 12–16

Thompson, J R, Sanders I 1972 Lactose barium small bowel study. Efficacy of a screening method. Am J Roentgen 116: 276–278

Torsoli A, Corazziari E, Waller S L, Anzini F 1971a Duodenal peristalsis in man. Rendic Gastroenterol 3: 168–173

Torsoli A, Ramorino M L, Ammaturo M V, Capurso L, Arcangeli G, Paoluzi P 1971b Mass movements and intracolonic pressures. Am J Dig Dis 16: 693–696

Turano L 1957 Malattie non neoplastiche dell'esofago in: Pozzi L (ed.) Atti Congr. Ital. Med. Intern. Pozzi, Rome pp 1–72

Whitehead W E, Devroede G, Habib F I, Meunier P, Wald A 1992 Functional disorders of the anorectum. Gastroenterol Int 5: 92–108

Wolf B S, Khilnani M T 1966 Progress in gastroenterological radiology. Gastroenterology 51: 542–559

13. Perfused tube manometry

M. Camilleri

INTRODUCTION

The greatest assets of perfused tube manometry in the investigation of the motor function of the alimentary tract are its simplicity, the robust nature of its components, and the general applicability of the method to several regions. By merely modifying the distribution of the manometric side-holes, the investigator is able to evaluate a variety of regions. The method is thus versatile and can be adapted to achieve the desired amount of detail in examining the pressure profile throughout the digestive tract. This simplicity, relatively low running costs, and the extensive experience of several laboratories has rendered manometry an integral part of the diagnostic armamentarium in many gastroenterology clinics. Manometry of the oesophagus and anorectal region will be covered in other chapters of this volume.

This chapter will focus on the methodology and application of perfused tube manometry to evaluate motor function of the stomach, small bowel, and colon, with particular emphasis on the technical details involved in the use of manometric studies in the clinical arena.

It is almost a decade since gastroduodenojejunal manometry was moved from the physiology-oriented laboratory and applied in the investigation of patients with unexplained upper gastrointestinal symptoms at tertiary referral centres. At our institution, a standardized laboratory-based test was started in 1982. This test is performed at least 48 h after cessation of all medications that may affect motility. In our laboratory, a multilumen manometric assembly with five or six sensors across the antropyloroduodenal segment is placed into the proximal digestive tract without sedation; recordings are obtained for 3 h during fasting and for 2 h after ingestion of a standardized 535 kcal solid-liquid meal (Malagelada et al 1986). To date, we have employed the simple, cheap, pneumohydraulic perfusion manometry; in recent years, other laboratories have successfully used microtransducer systems (Mathias et al 1985b) particularly in ambulatory studies (Kellow et al 1990), which are discussed in a separate chapter.

EQUIPMENT FOR MANOMETRIC RECORDINGS

The equipment required for manometric recordings (Arndorfer et al 1977) consists of a low compliance, pneumohydraulic perfusion system that is linked to a multilumen assembly of manometric catheters via interposed strain gauges. The hydraulic capillary infusion system achieves high fidelity recording of intraluminal pressure at an infusion rate (0.1–0.3 ml/min) that is quite low so as to interfere as little as possible with motor function. Pneumohydraulic perfusion is achieved by use of degassed water in a reservoir that is maintained at a high constant pressure (1000 mm Hg or 15 p.s.i.); the latter pressure is reduced to atmospheric level before entering the manometric assembly by capillary tubing which provides a high resistance to flow (Fig. 13.1).

Two theories are provided to explain how manometric recordings are obtained. First, the constant flow of a low (0.1–0.3 ml/min) volume of degassed water through the manometric catheters is simply impeded by a contraction that coincides in location with the position of the catheter side-hole. This resistance to water flow depends on the amplitude and duration of the contraction within the viscus, and the degree to which the lumen is occluded; thus, the pressure which is transmitted to the strain gauge by the constant perfusion system reflects the pressure within the lumen and can be recorded on a paper chart or electronic recorder. The second explanation is that the water-filled column within the perfused tube acts as a manometer. Thus, pressure events in the gastrointestinal tract have little effect on the flow rate of water through the tube because the pressure within the manometric catheter is low in comparison with the pressure in the

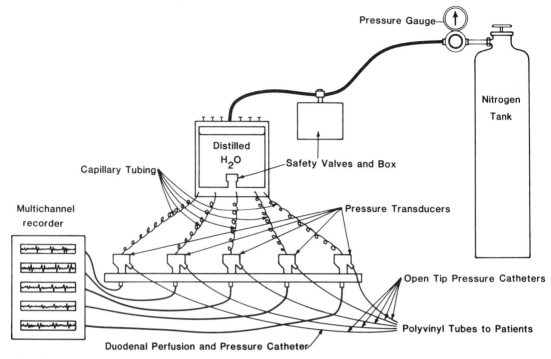

Fig. 13.1   Diagram of low-compliance pneumohydraulic system of perfusion manometry. Reproduced by permission of Mayo Foundation. (From Malagelada J-R et al 1986.)

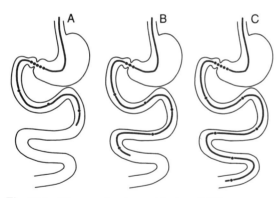

Fig. 13.2   Diagram showing positioning of different manometric assemblies in the upper gastrointestinal tract. The manometric sites across the antroduodenal junction should be closely spaced, e.g. 1 cm apart. (Reproduced by permission of Mayo Foundation from Malagelada et al 1986.)

the pressure gradient created by increased pressure within a sealed compartment around the side-hole within the hollow organ and is recorded by the strain gauge.

Irrespective of which explanation is correct, phasic pressure activity is easily recorded, provided the catheter is positioned in a part of the viscus where a critical degree of luminal conclusion occurs, such as in the small intestine and in the distal 3–5 cm of gastric antrum. In contrast, luminal occlusion is rare or infrequent in some regions of the digestive tract, such as the fundus of the stomach or colon, and perfusion manometry is of limited value in those regions.

A large variety of systems incorporate perfusion devices, strain gauges and recording appliances. Those used in the oesophagus also incorporate a sleeve device (Dent 1976). The investigator's choice of the location of manometric side-holes is probably the most important factor in establishing reliable recordings that provide worthwhile information for the practising clinical gastroenterologist.

Figure 13.2 shows the three standard tubes available in our gastroduodenojejunal manometry laboratory.

water reservoir. With the compliance of the infusion system minimized, the manometric catheter itself becomes the major source of compliance in the recording system; fluid flows within the manometer along

The two tubes that are most extensively used have five or six side-holes, 1 cm apart; these side-holes straddle the antroduodenal junction; three to six other side-holes, each 10 cm apart, are located in the small bowel. The tube with three closely-spaced side-holes is usually used to assess phasic pressure activity in the gastric remnant of patients with partial gastrectomy. Colonic manometric catheters are typically constructed with evenly-spaced ports in most laboratories.

GASTRODUODENOJEJUNAL MANOMETRY

Placement of manometric tubes into the upper digestive tract

The traditional way to place decompression, aspiration, or perfusion tubes into the small intestine has utilized a mercury-weighted bag at the end of the tube. This method is certainly applicable in the research laboratory when healthy subjects are studied; however, in patients with motility disorders of the upper gastrointestinal tract, such systems are generally ineffective; transport of the tubes far enough to precisely locate the manometric ports at desired sites cannot be achieved with a mercury-weighted tube. Failure rates of almost 40% have been recorded using this method (Quigley et al 1992). Since 1982, we have adopted two other approaches to placement of manometric tubes.

The first approach involves the use of a steerable Teflon catheter which is passed through the mouth and positioned with the aid of fluoroscopy into the proximal jejunum. A 3–4 m guide wire is then passed through the centre of the Teflon catheter and positioned securely with the tip advanced well into the jejunum. The Teflon catheter is then withdrawn leaving the guide wire in place, and a multilumen manometric assembly with a central channel is threaded slowly along the guide wire. Fluoroscopy is used to monitor the position of the catheter and to advance the guide wire if it slips back during the process of advancing the manometric tube. In our experience, it is useful to have one assistant hold the guide wire taut while the operator slides the manometric assembly over it. Prior to doing so, the central channel of the manometric assembly is lubricated with a low-fat aerosolized 'frying oil'.

The second approach for manometric tube placement in our laboratory utilizes a preliminary upper gastrointestinal endoscopy. A 9–11 mm outside diameter endoscope is used. The throat is sprayed with local anesthetic, and no intravenous sedation is used. This approach has the added advantage of directly excluding mechanical obstructions or significant mucosal disease and permits biopsy or aspiration of fluid from the distal duodenum in patients with suspected scleroderma or amyloidosis. The endoscope is passed into the descending or third portion of the duodenum, and a 3–4 m guide wire is then introduced through the biopsy channel and advanced over the angle of Treitz into the proximal jejunum under fluoroscopic control. The upper digestive tract is deflated, and after withdrawing the endoscope, the manometric assembly is passed over the guide wire as described above.

For recordings of the more distal small bowel, most investigators utilize an inflatable balloon at the tip of a mercury-weighted assembly. This allows for more rapid distal migration of the manometric assembly (Kerlin et al 1983).

Practical clues for optimal recording of gastroduodenojejunal manometry

The precise positioning of manometric side-holes in the small bowel is not crucial since lumen-occluding contractions are reliably detected at all levels. In contrast, the positioning of manometric side-holes across the antroduodenal junction is of critical importance if any valuable information about antral motility is to be acquired. At least five manometric side-holes, spaced by 0.3–2 cm (e.g. in Dent's laboratory) or 1 cm (in our laboratory and others') are essential since lumen-occluding contractions are only detected in the terminal 3–5 cm of antrum (Fig. 13.3). For purposes of standardization within and between individuals, we have assessed antral motility in the manometric recording corresponding to a position 1 cm proximal to the pyloric tracing. Hence, it is crucial to accurately localize the pyloric tracing throughout these studies. The human pylorus can be identified manometrically (Camilleri et al 1986b), by one of three patterns (Fig. 13.4):

1. A combination of antral (broad, high amplitude pressure waves, typically associated with similar waves at a rate of up to 3 per min in more proximal sites) and duodenal (lower amplitude, shorter duration, higher frequency) pressure activity;
2. Antral pressure activity associated with tonic elevation of baseline pressure;
3. Antral pressure activity with duodenal pressure activity 1 cm distally.

When typical antral pressure activity is associated with duodenal bulb pressure activity 1 cm distally, the pyloric profile lies between the sensors. Although this profile does not precisely localize the pylorus, identifying

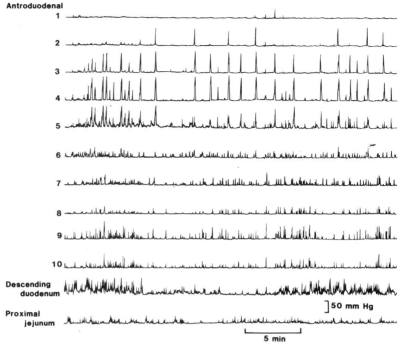

Fig. 13.3A Postprandial gastrointestinal pressure activity in a healthy volunteer, using 10 antroduodenal recording sites each separated by 1 cm. Pyloric activity is identified in lane 5, antral contractions in lanes 2–4; note the paucity of contractions in lane 1, which is 4 cm proximal to the pylorus. (Reproduced by permission of Mayo Foundation from Malagelada J-R et al 1986.)

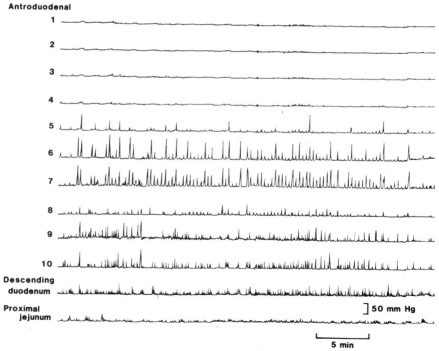

Fig. 13.3B A tracing similar to that shown in Figure 13.3A. In the healthy control, lane 4 (3 cm proximal to the pyloric tracing shown in lane 7) demonstrates virtually no antral contraction. Note also the greater sensitivity of recording of antral contractions in lane 6 (1 cm from the pylorus) than lane 5 (2 cm from pylorus). (Reproduced by permission of Mayo Foundation from Malagelada J-R et al 1986.)

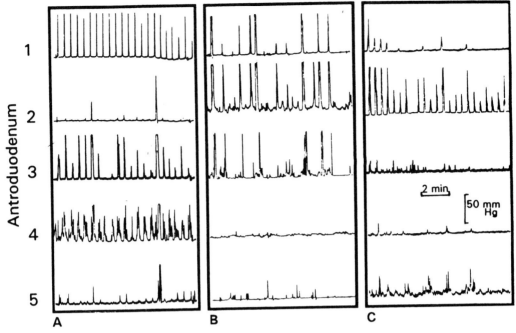

Fig. 13.4 Manometric patterns of postprandial pyloric pressure activity. In **A**, pyloric activity in lead 4 shows a combination of antral and duodenal waves; note the high amplitude regular activity in antrum in leads 1 and 3, with *apparent* reduction in frequency in lead 2 due to failed luminal occlusion. In the **B**, pyloric activity in lead 2 is characterized by antral-type waves associated with tonic elevation of baseline pressure; some pyloric activity is also detected in lead 3 by the contraction of antral and duodenal waves. Note duodenal bulb (lead 4) is relatively quiescent. In **C**, lead 2 shows antral-type waves and lead 3 duodenal-type waves; the pyloric pressure profile is missed, but the position of the tube is appropriate to record distal antral motility.

this sequence of profiles is useful since it reassures the operator that the tube is in the correct position.

Thus, the aim of the assistant monitoring the acquisition of manometric data is to keep the pyloric recording in the middle of the multiple tracings recorded from the antroduodenal junction, typically in lead 3 or 4. This goal can be achieved quite easily, even during the fasting period (Fig. 13.5), after a short period of training. Only minor adjustments of tube position are necessary during the fasting observation period.

Just prior to ingestion of the test meal, in anticipation of the gastric accommodation response, the catheter assembly should be advanced 3–5 cm. Once the meal is ingested, the pressure profile of the antroduodenal junction should be continually assessed (Fig. 13.5), and the tube may be introduced or withdrawn to keep the pyloric tracing in lead 3 or 4. During the second postprandial hour, recovery of gastric tone compensates for the initial relaxation or accommodation response and results in relative caudad movement of the manometric assembly; hence, some withdrawal of the tube is sometimes necessary usually at 1–2 cm steps.

Practical advantages of manometry over other investigations of motor function in the upper digestive tract

There are several clinically-available tests of gastric motor function which are discussed elsewhere in this book, including impedance, scintigraphy, ultrasonography, and electrogastrography. Manometry provides a more detailed profile of motor function of the antropyloroduodenal region and of the small intestine. The propagation and the contractile amplitude of pressure activity of long lengths of small bowel can be assessed with only a minor increase in the calibre of the manometric assemblies.

After the initial costs necessary to purchase the equipment, manometric studies can be performed safely and efficiently by trained paramedical staff under supervision of the gastroenterologist. The training period can be as short as 1 month in a centre with high volume use of manometry. The equipment is generally robust, and repairs and maintenance are far less frequent or costly than applies to other clinical

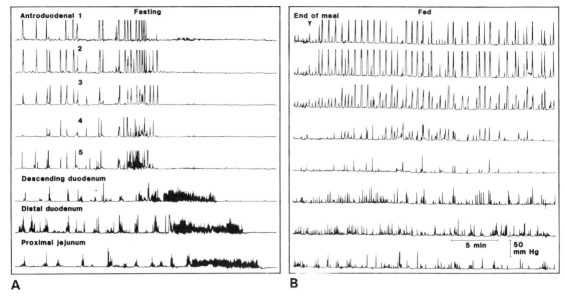

Fig. 13.5   Normal gastric duodenal and jejunal pressure activity. **A** (fasting) shows an interdigestive migrating motor complex, and **B**, the small, irregular, but persistent phasic pressure activity in the antrum and proximal small bowel. (Reproduced by permission of Mayo Foundation from Malagelada et al 1986.)

tests that assess motility of the stomach, such as a gamma camera.

The physiologic significance of the manometric pressure profile is discussed below. Differentiation from normal patterns of motor function (Fig. 13.5) can be achieved by manometry and several other modalities of investigation. However, there are two specific, clinically-relevant questions regarding upper gastro-intestinal motor function that are, at present, exclusively addressed by manometry: first, is the pathophysiologic process (Camilleri 1990) suggestive of a neuropathy or a myopathy? (Fig. 13.6); and second, does the motility disorder affect the stomach or small bowel, or both? These two points are discussed further below. Despite these practical advantages, it is also clear that manometry has its limitations; hence, a balanced approach to its use and the information it provides is still warranted.

What disease or pathophysiologic processes can be identified?

Studies of gastrointestinal pressure activity provide evidence of a pathophysiologic process (Malagelada et al 1986, Camilleri 1990) and, hence, are not diagnostic of any specific disease per se. However, they provide strong corroborative evidence of abnormal motility, generally imply an associated neuropathic, myopathic or obstructive process, and provide a lead to the diagnosis.

We have performed over 2000 gastroduodenojejunal manometric tracings at the Mayo Clinic GI Motility Laboratory; five types of pathophysiologic abnormalities are easily recognized in patients with motility disorders (Camilleri 1993). These are reviewed extensively in other chapters and are summarized below.

(1) Patterns suggestive of mechanical obstruction

Two patterns have been reported: first, a sustained (typically for more than 30 min postprandial pattern of 'minute' clustered contractions (Fig. 13.7) separated by gaps or periods of motor quiescence of variable duration (Summers et al 1983, Camilleri 1989); second, repetitive, simultaneous, prolonged contractions (Fig. 13.8) in the proximal small bowel (Camilleri 1989).

(2) Low amplitude contractions usually at several levels, which are typical of a myopathic process

These are found in patients with progressive systemic sclerosis or hollow visceral myopathy (Fig. 13.6).

(3) Normal amplitude, but abnormally propagated ('uncoordinated') phasic pressure profiles in the stomach and small bowel, suggestive of a neuropathic process

These features are often identifiable during phase II and during the activity front or phase III of the

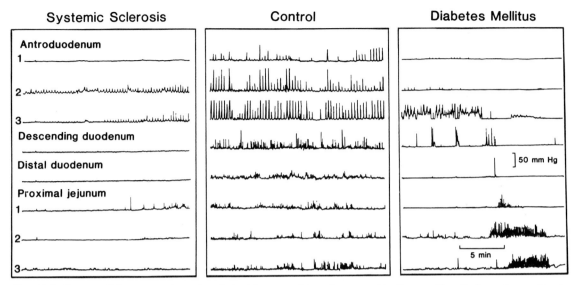

Fig. 13.6 Postprandial manometric tracings in health, myopathic and neuropathic diseases. Note the irregular persistent normal amplitude pressure activity in health, the low amplitude normal frequency antral activity in systemic sclerosis, and lack of antral contractions (leads 1 and 2), prominent pyloric tonic and phasic pressure activity, and the persistence of activity fronts postprandially. (Reproduced with permission from Camilleri M 1991.)

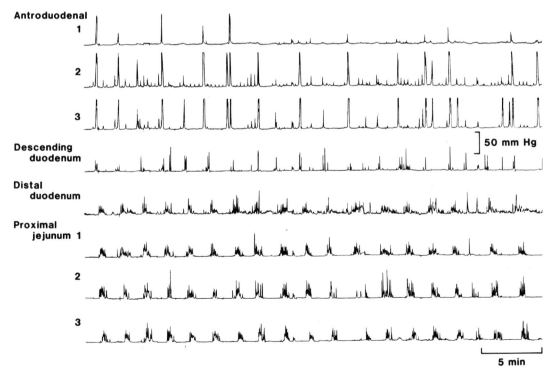

Fig. 13.7 Regular small intestinal clustered contractions separated by quiescence in a patient with mechanical obstruction. (Reproduced by permission of Mayo Foundation from Malagelada J-R et al 1986.)

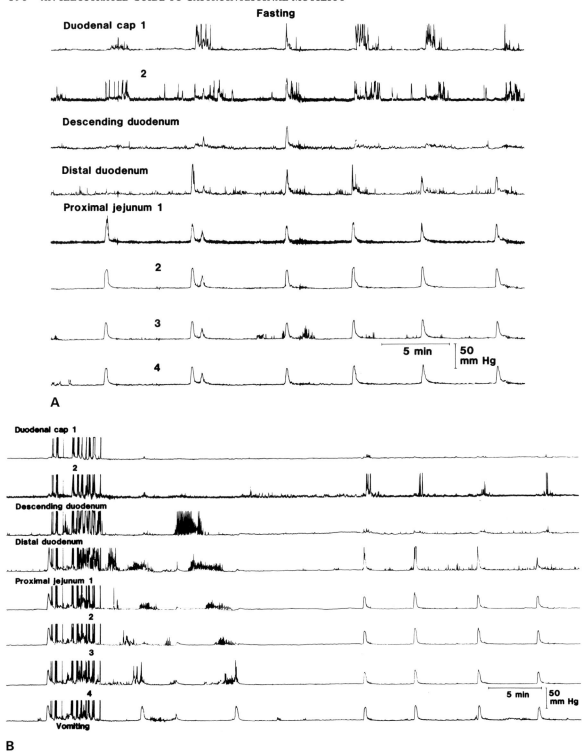

Fig. 13.8   Prolonged high amplitude contractions in the small intestine of a patient with mechanical obstruction. Note these contractions are observed fasting (**A**) and postprandially (**B**). (Reproduced by permission of Mayo Foundation from Malagelada J-R et al 1986.)

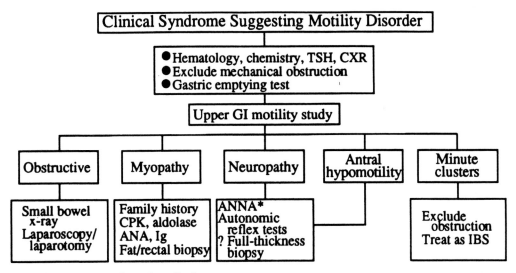

Fig. 13.9   Algorithm for evaluation of patients with suspected gastrointestinal motility disorders. (Reproduced with permission from Camilleri M (in press).)

digestive migrating motor complex (MMC). The persistence of fasting patterns after ingestion of a moderate sized meal (> 400 kcal) is also suggestive of a neuropathic process (Fig. 13.6).

(4) Postprandial antral hypomotility characterized by normal amplitude but infrequent contractions

The latter can be quantitated and compared with data from normal subjects (Malagelada et al 1986), and is typically found in association with diabetes mellitus, vagotomy, and postviral or idiopathic gastroparesis.

(5) A pattern of minute clustered contractions coincident with abdominal pain has been described in patients with irritable bowel syndrome

However, this pattern (Kellow & Phillips 1987) may be unassociated with pain and is also observed in healthy controls.

Strictly speaking, these abnormal pressure profiles have not been validated in man; thus, histologic correlates of these profiles are only rarely unavailable. However, the profiles and their pathophysiologic significance are based on a large body of literature on damage to the enteric nervous system (ENS) or experimental extrinsic denervation (e.g. vagotomy, splanchnicectomy) in animals. The basis for these manometric criteria is beyond the scope of this chapter.

These pressure profiles lead to further investigations (Camilleri 1990) to firmly establish the diagnosis (see Fig. 13.9). An abnormal autonomic reflex test leads to a search of diseases affecting the CNS (e.g. brainstem tumor (Wood et al 1985)) or peripheral neuropathy (e.g. heavy metal poisoning, porphyria, paraneoplastic syndrome (Sodhi et al 1989, Lennon et al 1991). In the absence of an associated autonomic neuropathy, it is assumed that the 'neuropathic' dysmotility identified by manometry represents a disorder of the ENS. Thus, on the basis of clinical and manometric criteria, the condition chronic idiopathic intestinal pseudo-obstruction (CIIP) is diagnosed (Stanghellini et al 1987). Some of the pressure profiles originally described in CIIP (such as nonpropagated bursts of phasic pressure activity (Stanghellini et al 1987)) have been reported in patients with the clinical diagnosis of irritable bowel syndrome (IBS) (Kellow et al 1990). Since there are no clinically-applicable methods to prove the diagnosis of CIIP, it is virtually impossible to absolutely differentiate these two conditions solely by manometry (Read 1987). Morphologic studies on full-thickness biopsies of intestine may increase the diagnostic rate (Krishnamurthy & Schuffler 1987) but do not significantly alter the management of these CIIP patients. These findings in adult patients have been largely confirmed in the paediatric age group (Hyman et al 1990).

When should gastroduodenal manometry be performed?

Studies of motility should follow *careful* exclusion of mucosal, structural or metabolic disorders and mechanical obstruction (see Fig. 13.9) by endoscopy and radiologic studies. A common indication for manometry is to confirm the presence of an 'organic' disorder of function in patients with a known underlying disease process, such as diabetes mellitus or progressive systemic sclerosis, that may affect digestive motor function (Fig. 13.9). A careful gastric and small bowel transit test by scintigraphy, using a radiolabel linked to a non-digestible solid, may be an alternative approach (Camilleri et al 1991b). In a tertiary referral practice, these tests are usually performed after a therapeutic trial has failed.

Upper gastrointestinal manometry is also commonly performed in patients with unexplained nausea, vomiting, abdominal pain and distension, or those with an abnormal gastric emptying test in the absence of an etiologic diagnosis. In a tertiary referral practice, the diagnostic algorithm outlined in Figure 13.9 and reviewed in detail elsewhere (Camilleri 1990) leads to the new diagnosis of organic diseases, such as brain tumours, paraneoplastic neuropathy or sporadic hollow visceral myopathy, or the identification of an undiagnosed mechanical obstruction.

In the presence of abnormal gastric emptying, manometry is useful to determine whether the abnormal motility of the upper gastrointestinal tract is generalized or restricted to the stomach (Camilleri et al 1986a). This information permits a logical choice of patients with isolated motor dysfunction of the stomach in whom enteral nutrition via a jejunal feeding tube is a viable option. The manometric profile is also of prognostic value; it identifies those patients with a myopathic process in whom prokinetic agents are less likely to be efficacious, and in whom parenteral nutrition is frequently necessary.

Is there a role for manometric studies following gastric surgery?

The patient with post-vagotomy antral hypomotility can be easily identified; this antral hypomotility was the most clearly recognizable motor dysfunction among 60 patients with post-surgical gastric stasis seen in our laboratory (Fich et al 1990). Although a few patients have very abnormal motility in the jejunal limb after Roux gastrectomy (Mathias et al 1985a), the most characteristic 'abnormalities' found in symptomatic post-gastric surgery patients (Fich et al 1990) are also

found in asymptomatic patients (Miedema et al 1992). The lack of propulsion of food from the denervated fundus may be as important as the jejunal loop dysmotility in the Roux stasis syndrome; this part of the stomach cannot be adequately assessed by current manometric methods.

In summary, there is little clinically useful information obtained by studying motor function of the gastric remnant after partial gastrectomy in symptomatic patients. The effects of vagotomy without gastric resection are easily identified manometrically (Fich et al 1990), but these effects are just as easily identified by the clinical history, and endoscopy or a gastric emptying test.

Practical significance of the upper gastrointestinal pressure profile

Apart from the pathophysiologic significance discussed above, gastroduodenojejunal manometry has provided some information regarding the mechanical properties of the stomach and small bowel in health (Camilleri et al 1985, Houghton et al 1988) and disease (Camilleri et al 1986a, Greydanus et al 1990). Thus myopathic and neuropathic processes result in delayed gastric and small bowel transit (Greydanus et al 1990); and postprandial antral hypomotility is associated with prolonged gastric emptying of solids (longer lag time, slower post-lag rate of emptying (Camilleri et al 1986a)).

The manometric pressure profile also provides information that leads to more logical therapeutic approaches. As stated above, patients with selective antral hypomotility may be efficiently supported by enteral feeding; in our practice, a nasoenteric tube is placed, and enteral formula is infused at rates of up to 80 ml/h; if tolerated, it is likely that chronic feeding by means of a percutaneous enteral tube would be a viable, longer-term approach to nutrition. In patients with a myopathic process, prolonged trials with prokinetic agents and enteral nutrition are avoided, and treatment is based on parenteral feeding, oral supplements as tolerated, and suppression of bacterial overgrowth in the small bowel.

Few studies have attempted to use the digestive tract's pressure profile as a predictor of the therapeutic response. The persistence of fasting MMCs may indicate a greater likelihood to respond to prokinetic agents (Hyman et al 1991). Gastric emptying and small bowel transit studies may provide an alternative approach with possible advantages: they are non-invasive, easily repeatable, and provide a clearer, functional interpretation of the response to therapy (Camilleri et al 1989).

However, if there is no identified underlying disease, it may be impossible to predict whether the pathophysiologic process is neuropathic or myopathic solely by measuring transit and, hence, decisions regarding use of prokinetics or choice of nutritional support may still necessitate manometry.

Pitfalls in the application of gastroduodenojejunal manometry

Caution is necessary in the interpretation of motility tracings; there are several pitfalls during acquisition of the pressure profile, and precautions are necessary to achieve a technically-satisfactory recording. First, it must be emphasized that the human interdigestive motility is extremely variable (Kellow et al 1986) and that the absence of a phase III of the MMC during a 3-h fasting period is not per se abnormal, except in systemic sclerosis (Rees et al 1982, Greydanus & Camilleri 1989). About 60% of patients have at least one interdigestive MMC during a 3-h fasting period. Thus, in a series of 114 consecutive patients (Bharucha et al 1993), the number of MMCs in 3-h was 1.15 ± 0.12 (range: 0–5). The distribution of the number of MMCs in the 3-h fasting period in this cohort of patients was: 0 in 47, 1 in 34, 2 in 13, 3 in 10, 4 in 9, and 5 in 1 patient. Thus, the amplitude, frequency of contractions, velocity of propagation, and characteristics of propagation of the phase III can be examined in many patients in a 3-h tracing; however, more prolonged studies are needed to thoroughly evaluate the MMCs, and this is discussed in the chapter on ambulant manometry.

Second, assessment of the amplitudes of pressure profiles necessitates: careful calibration before and after each study; assessment of the response profile and fidelity of the recording device; use of degassed water for perfusion at a constant pressure; and flushing each manometer when shifts in baseline pressure occur, or when low amplitude pressures are recorded.

Third, assessment of distal antral motility necessitates the use of a multilumen (five or six) catheter assembly and a well-trained assistant who is able to identify the manometric pressure profiles of the pylorus and duodenal bulb. The golden rule in our practice is to maintain the 'pyloric tracing' in the middle of the five or six antroduodenal pressure profiles by advancing or withdrawing the manometric catheter assembly.

Finally, manometric tracings, like X-rays and other investigations, should be interpreted cautiously, with knowledge of the other information regarding each patient. One must also acknowledge that, as with oesophageal manometry, certain manometric criteria are more reliable than others. Thus, abnormal propagation of phase III of the MMC, sustained incoordinated pressure activity, quantitated antral hypomotility and an early return to MMC activity within 2 h of the ingestion of the 530 kcal meal (Stanghellini et al 1987) are easily interpreted. By way of contrast, it is more difficult to interpret the significance of 'bursts' (Malagelada et al 1986, Summers et al 1983) and 'clusters' (Kellow et al 1990, Summers et al 1983, Kellow & Phillips 1987). By following these simple principles, manometry provides a useful assessment of pathophysiology that complements clinical, transit (Camilleri et al 1989), and pathologic (Camilleri et al 1991a) criteria.

Future refinements in gastroduodenojejunal manometry

Several novel research approaches may be applied in the clinical motility laboratory in the future.

The 'sleeve'

Addition of a sleeve to measure pyloric contractility has the attraction of assessing, in detail, the function of the sphincter per se (Dent 1976). The sleeve is claimed to be superior to manometry in detection of pyloric motility (Heddle et al 1988). Although there have been a large number of studies in health (reviewed in Horowitz & Dent 1991), this sleeve methodology has not been evaluated as extensively in disease states. The pylorus typically functions as an integral part of the antropyloroduodenal segment in the postprandial period (Camilleri et al 1985, Horowitz & Dent 1991). Its function can usually be consistently monitored postprandially using standard manometry provided manometric ports are not spaced more than 1 cm apart (Fig. 13.10). In disease states such as diabetic autonomic neuropathy (Mearin et al 1986), or following pharmacologic perturbations with intravenous β-endorphin (Camilleri et al 1986b) or intraduodenal lipid (Horowitz & Dent 1991), pylorospasm or isolated pyloric pressure waves are not the only abnormalities. The changes in pyloric motor function with intraduodenal lipid are associated with significant inhibition of distal antral and duodenal contractility as well as inhibition of proximal antral and probably corpus motility (Prather et al 1992b). Hence, the impaired gastric emptying in these circumstances is likely to be multifactorial, rather than being specifically due to pylorospasm. At present, it is unclear whether the detailed sleeve assessment of the pylorus is essential in patients

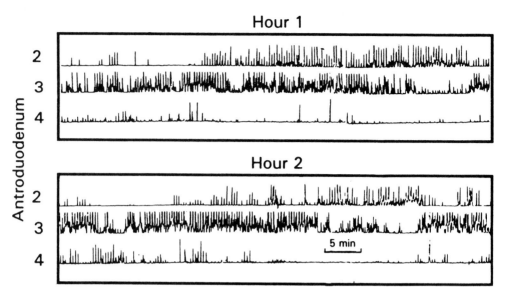

Fig. 13.10 Two-hour postprandial tracing of antropyloric region in a patient with diabetes mellitus. Note the consistent recording of pyloric motility, characterized by combined antral and duodenal waves sometimes associated with baseline elevation.

seen in the clinical gastrointestinal motility laboratory. In fact, a preliminary report suggests that among 16 patients with gastroparesis, the number of localized pyloric contractions that are unassociated with antral waves is not different from health (Fraser et al 1992).

From a technical standpoint, if a 4–5 cm long sleeve is added to the manometric assembly, it is important to fashion several manometric side-holes (e.g. 1 cm apart) spanning the assembly in the region of the sleeve. This is necessary to ensure that distal antral contractions can be detected as separate events from the sleeve-recorded 'pyloric' waves since the sleeve would record any occluding events occurring over its length (4–5 cm), which is far in excess of the anatomical length of the pylorus.

The barostat

The barostat provides an excellent method to study reflex motor function of the proximal stomach in health (Rouillon et al 1991) and following gastrectomy (Azpiroz & Malagelada 1987). Whereas the barostat or a latex balloon may be useful to identify the visceral hypersensitivity of dyspeptic patients (Mearin et al 1991, Lémann et al 1991a), its role in the evaluation of postprandial gastric *motor* function is unclear, especially in the absence of previous partial gastric resection.

Ambulatory recordings

Will ambulatory pressure recordings using solid state transducers mounted on a nasojejunal tube become a routine test in the gastrointestinal motility laboratory? This is addressed further in Chapter 15. The impressive technologic advances that led to the ambulatory recordings have also provided important descriptive observations, chiefly on the timing, periodicity and characteristics of the MMC (Kellow et al 1990). Previous limitations regarding the number of recording sites will likely be overcome. For postprandial recordings, it will be particularly important to have a sufficient number of transducers in the antropyloro-duodenal junction, since movements of the catheter by 2–3 cm may preclude any measurement of distal antral pressure activity. As further studies may show other advantages of prolonged recordings, the place of ambulant pressure measurement will be clearer.

Computerization

This is discussed in Chapter 22.

COLONIC MANOMETRY

A handful of laboratories have applied manometric measurements to the evaluation of colonic motor function in health and disease. Our group's experience is restricted to observations in the research laboratory. However, other groups (Soffer et al 1989, Narducci et al 1987, Bassotti & Gaburri 1988, Bazzocchi et al 1990, Moreno-Osset et al 1989, Reddy et al 1991) have pioneered the use of colonic manometry for diagnostic purposes. Following the lead of the Adelaide group in the upper digestive tract (Horowitz & Dent 1991), the combination of manometry and scintigraphy by Snape's group (Bazzocchi et al 1990, Moreno-Osset et al 1989, Reddy et al 1991) has provided a powerful combination that assesses pressure profile patterns in the colon and their functional significance.

Placement of manometric tubes into the lower digestive tract

Placement of colonic manometric catheters is usually achieved by a retrograde approach. In our laboratory, this involves colonoscopy, placement of a guide wire through the biopsy channel of the endoscope and allowing it to coil in the ascending colon to facilitate its anchoring. After withdrawing the colonoscope, the manometric assembly is threaded over the guide wire under fluoroscopic control. Other groups pass a smaller manometric catheter through the biopsy channel of the colonoscope for studies of the left colon's motility; a third approach is to drag the motility tube along the colonoscope by means of a silk thread tied to the tip of the manometric assembly; the thread is passed retrogradely up the biopsy channel of the colonoscope. In my experience, the latter method is technically the most difficult; hence, I routinely use the guide wire method. Finally, a French group (Lémann et al 1992) first pass an orally-ingested, weighted string through to the anal canal, and then attach and drag a manometric assembly of catheters to the desired position in the lower digestive tract.

Clues for optimal recording of colonic manometry

As with any intraluminal pressure recording, pressure changes are not necessarily generated from motor activity at the recording site; when a segment is filled with a continuous column of content, it acts as a common cavity which may be pressurized by a contraction anywhere along its length. Hence the colon needs to be thoroughly cleansed, and preferably emptied, at the time of manometric recordings. We routinely prepare the colon with large volumes of an osmotic laxative, and stop high residue foods for at least 24 h prior to colonoscopy. During the latter, we deliberately aspirate

all pools of liquid content prior to placing the guide wire. Gas used to inflate the colon during examination and guide wire placement is aspirated prior to removal of the endoscope. This is important since fidelity of colonic manometry depends on the diameter of the lumen (von der Ohe et al 1992).

Manometry compared to other methods in evaluating colonic motility

The relative roles of manometry, myoelectric studies, and transit measurements in the assessment of colonic motility remain unclear. Transit measurements (e.g. radiopaque markers, scintigraphy) appear to provide an overall functional assessment of the colon, and, if sufficiently detailed, can be useful to define regional colonic function (Proano et al 1990, Stivland et al 1991, Vassallo et al 1992). Manometric patterns in health are being extensively studied, and their alteration by disease processes are clearer. For example, high amplitude propagated waves in the colon appear to play an important role in normal defecation, including mass movements; they are deficient in patients with idiopathic constipation, and are frequent in patients with functional diarrhoea (Narducci et al 1987, Bassotti & Gaburri 1988, Bazzocchi et al 1990, Moreno-Osset et al 1989, Reddy et al 1991).

Recent advances with a delayed-release capsule have facilitated detailed measurements of regional transit without the need for intubation (Proano et al 1990, Stivland et al 1991, Vassallo et al 1992). Future research will shed light on the relative indications for each method in assessing colonic motor function.

At present, it is not clear whether or when colonic manometry should be performed in the diagnostic process. Certain pitfalls in colonic manometry are worth mentioning: first, the degree of colonic cleansing may influence the pressure profile (Lémann et al 1991b, 1992); the colonic diameter influences quantitation of intraluminal pressure (von der Ohe et al 1992); finally, the 'diagnostic' validity of colonic pressure profiles requires confirmation by larger studies.

Future refinements of colonic manometry

Novel approaches that are currently being applied in the research laboratory may be used in the colonic motility laboratory in the future.

The barostat

By conforming to the internal outline of the colonic segment, the barostat (Azpiroz & Malagelada 1987)

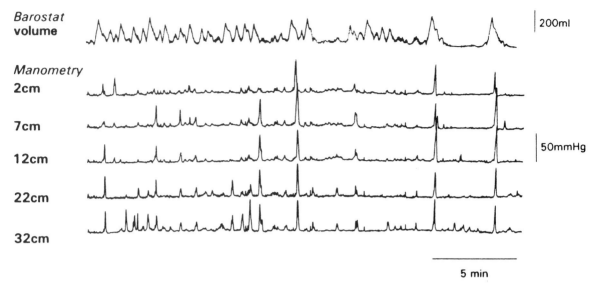

Fig. 13.11 Combined manometric and barostat tracing during fasting from the transverse colon of a healthy volunteer. Distances of manometric side-holes from the barostat bag are shown at left. Note the intermittent phasic pressure activity measured by manometry and the phasic volume waves measured by means of a 10-cm long barostat bag.

provides a means to overcome difficulties in recording phasic and tonic pressure activity in the colon. Work from the laboratory of Phillips (Steadman et al 1991, 1992) has validated the use of the barostat in the colon. Our group has recently shown (Fig 13.11) that the volume tracing obtained with the barostat can be resolved into two components: a baseline volume, which reflects colonic tone; and phasic volume events, which coincide with manometrically-recorded phasic pressure activity. Moreover, the barostat detects about 50% more waves than simultaneous manometry when the colonic diameter exceeds 5 cm (von der Ohe et al 1992).

Ambulatory recordings

These are discussed in Chapter 14. They are technically feasible (Soffer et al 1989); however, initial results in health show that motor activity in the large bowel is characterized by scant, irregular contractions, with infrequent bursts that do not conform to any pattern. No motor coordination (Soffer et al 1989) is apparent using recording sites 45 cm apart. With this background of 'normal' colonic motility patterns, it remains to be seen whether colonic motility recorded either manometrically or by ambulatory recordings with microtransducers can be used to identify disease states.

SUMMARY AND A LOOK AT THE FUTURE

Gastroduodenojejunal pressure measurements have proved their value as adjuncts in the clinical diagnosis of upper gastrointestinal motility disorders (Malagelada et al 1986, Camilleri 1990) in the past decade. They are an integral part of studies in the diagnostic units of several tertiary referral centres. The future will likely clarify their role further. In particular, it is expected that less costly but accurate, non-invasive measurements of gastric, small bowel, and colonic transit will be performed routinely (Camilleri et al 1991b, Camilleri & Zinsmeister 1992) prior to intubated studies of the pressure profiles of those regions. The application of scintigraphy to assess antral wall motion (Urbain et al 1990) appears a particularly exciting development that may replace the need to measure antral pressure activity by an intraluminal sensor. Other radiologic techniques are being studied. Magnetic resonance imaging (MRI) has been reported in preliminary studies (Schwizer et al 1990) of gastric emptying, and ultra-fast computer tomography (CT), or the dynamic spatial reconstructor (Kumar et al 1987) has been used to evaluate emptying across the canine gastric outflow tract. These studies appear to bring the assessment of gastric motility to the threshold of the diagnostic imaging unit. However, radiation exposure, high costs, lack of availability of instruments, and the relatively prolonged observations necessary to assess gastrointestinal motor function suggest that the application of MRI and ultra fast CT will lag behind their use in cardiac and haemodynamic studies. At present, novel research studies are describing other methods to measure gastroduodenal flow (Malbert & Ruckebusche 1991) and the longitudinal vector of forces in the distal stomach (Vassallo et al 1992, Prather et al 1992a, Prather et al 1992b).

The roles of these new methods in the diagnostic laboratory are still unclear; however, the fact that so much research continues in the evaluation of motor function of the digestive tract testifies to the need to understand the motor function of this region better, and to develop methods that may be applied in future clinical practice. Meanwhile, manometry or solid state transducer measurements of the stomach and small bowel have proven their clinical usefulness and will continue to be applied in the diagnostic and research laboratories.

The precise place of manometry in the diagnosis of colonic motility disorders requires further research. For several decades, it has been shown that such studies are technically possible; what is required is a clearer understanding of the value of the information obtained with pressure profiles relative to some of the more sophisticated colonic transit measurements (Camilleri & Zinsmeister 1992) that are now available. Future research should also clarify this question.

ACKNOWLEDGEMENTS

I wish to thank the assistants in the Clinical GI Motility Laboratory at Mayo Clinic for their challenging comments and excellent monitoring of manometric studies 1982–1992. I also thank Cindy Stanislav for typing and preparing the manuscript of this chapter.

REFERENCES

Arndorfer R C, Stef J J, Dodds W J et al 1977 Improved infusion system for intraluminal esophageal manometry. Gastroenterology 73: 23–27

Azpiroz F, Malagelada J R 1987 Gastric tone measured by an electronic barostat in health and postsugical gastroparesis. Gastroenterology 92: 934–943

Bassotti G, Gaburri M 1988 Manometric investigation of high-amplitude propagated contractile activity of the human colon. Am J Physiol 255: G660–G664

Bazzocchi G, Ellis J, Villaneuva-Meyer J et al 1990 Postprandial colonic transit and motor activity in chronic constipation. Gastroenterology 98: 686–693

Bharucha A E, Camilleri M, Low P A et al 1993 Autonomic dysfunction in gastrointestinal motility disorders. Gut 34: 397–401

Camilleri M 1989 Jejunal manometry in distal subacute mechanical obstruction: significance of prolonged simultaneous contractions. Gut 30: 468–475

Camilleri M 1990 Disorders of gastrointestinal motility in neurologic diseases. Mayo Clin Proc 65: 825–846

Camilleri M 1991 Medical treatment of chronic intestinal pseudoobstruction. Practical gastroenterology 15: 10–22

Camilleri M 1993 Study of human gastroduodenojejunal motility: applied physiology in clinical practice. Dig Dis Sci 38: 785–794

Camilleri M, Zinsmeister A R 1992 Towards a relatively inexpensive, noninvasive, accurate test for colonic motility disorders. Gastroenterology 103: 36–42

Camilleri M, Malagelada J-R, Brown M L et al 1985 Relation between antral motility and gastric emptying of solids and liquids in humans. Am J Physiol 249: G580–G585

Camilleri M, Brown M L, Malagelada J-R 1986a Relationship between impaired gastric emptying and abnormal gastrointestinal motility. Gastroenterology 91: 94–99

Camilleri M, Malagelada J-R, Stanghellini V et al 1986b Dose-related effects of synthetic human β-endorphin and naloxone on fed upper gastrointestinal motility. Am J Physiol 251: G147–G154

Camilleri M, Malagelada J-R, Abell T L et al 1989 Effect of six weeks of treatment with cisapride in gastroparesis and intestinal pseudoobstruction. Gastroenterology 96: 704–712

Camilleri M, Carbone L D, Schuffler M D 1991a Familial enteric neuropathy with pseudo-obstruction. Dig Dis Sci 36: 1168–1171

Camilleri M, Zinsmeister A R, Greydanus M P et al 1991b Towards a less costly but accurate test of gastric emptying and small bowel transit. Dig Dis Sci 36: 609–615

Dent J 1976 A new technique for continuous sphincter pressure measurement. Gastroenterology 71: 263–266

Fich A, Neri M, Camilleri M et al 1990 Stasis syndromes following gastric surgery: clinical and motility features of sixty symptomatic patients. J Clin Gastroenterol 12: 505–512

Fraser R, Horowitz M, Maddox A, Dent J 1992 Gastroparesis is not associated with increased localized pyloric contractions. Gastroenterology 102: A449

Greydanus M P, Camilleri M 1989 Abnormal postcibal antral and small bowel motility due to neuropathy or myopathy in systemic sclerosis. Gastroenterology 96: 110–115

Greydanus M P, Camilleri M, Colemont L J et al 1990 Ileocolonic transfer of solid chyme in small intestinal neuropathies and myopathies. Gastroenterology 99: 158–164

Heddle R, Dent J, Tooulli J et al 1988 Topography and

measurement of pyloric pressure waves and tone in humans. Am J Physiol 255: G490–G497

Horowitz M, Dent J 1991 Disordered gastric emptying: mechanical basis, assessment and treatment in: Dent J (ed.) Baillière's clinical gastroenterology: practical issues in gastrointestinal motor disorders, Vol 5. Baillière Tindall, London pp 371–407

Houghton L A, Read N W, Heddle R et al 1988 Relationship of the motor activity of the antrum, pylorus, and duodenum to gastric emptying of a solid-liquid mixed meal. Gastroenterology 94: 1285–1291

Hyman P E, Napolitano J A, Diego A et al 1990 Antroduodenal manometry in the evaluation of chronic functional gastrointestinal symptoms. Pediatrics 86: 39–44

Hyman P E, DiLorenzo C, Flores A F et al 1991 Antroduodenal manometry predicts response to cisapride in children with chronic intestinal pseudoobstruction (abstract). Gastroenterology 100: A452

Kellow J E, Borody T J, Philips S F et al 1986 Human interdigestive motility: variations in patterns from esophagus to colon. Gastroenterology 91: 386–395

Kellow J E, Phillips S F 1987 Altered small bowel motility in irritable bowel syndrome is correlated with symptoms. Gastroenterology 92: 1885–1893

Kellow J E, Gill R C, Wingate D L 1990 Prolonged ambulant recordings of small bowel motility demonstrate abnormalities in the irritable bowel syndrome. Gastroenterology 98: 1208–1218

Kerlin P, Tucker R, Phillips S F 1983 Rapid intubation of the ileocolonic region of man. Australian N Z J Med 13: 591–593

Krishnamurthy S, Schuffler M D 1987 Pathology of neuromuscular disorders of the small intestine and colon. Gastroenterology 93: 610–639

Kumar D, Ritman E L, Malagelada J-R 1987 Three-dimensional imaging of the stomach: role of pylorus in the emptying of liquids. Am J Physiol 253: G79–G85

Lémann M, Dederding J P, Flouré B et al 1991a Abnormal perception of visceral pain in response to gastric distension in chronic idiopathic dyspepsia: the irritable bowel syndrome. Dig Dis Sci 36: 1249–1254

Lémann M, Flourie B, Picon L et al 1991b Is the motor activity different in the unprepared and prepared human colon? Gastroenterology 100: A462

Lémann M, Picon L, Flourie B et al 1992 Relationship between high amplitude propagated contractions and transit in the unprepared human colon. Gastroenterology 102: A474

Lennon V A, Sas D F, Busk M F et al 1991 Enteric neuronal autoantibodies in pseudoobstruction with small-cell lung carcinoma. Gastroenterology 100: 137–142

Malagelada J-R, Camilleri M, Stanghellini V 1986 Manometric diagnosis of gastrointestinal motility disorders. Thieme, New York

Malbert C H, Ruckebusche Y 1991 Relationship between pressure and flow across the gastroduodenal junction in dogs. Am J Physiol 260: G653–G657

Mathias J R, Fernandez A, Sninsky C A et al 1985a Nausea, vomiting, and abdominal pain after Roux-en-Y anastomosis: motility of the jejunal limb. Gastroenterology 88: 101–107

Mathias J R, Sninsky C A, Millar H D et al 1985b Development of an improved multi-pressure-sensor probe for recording muscle contraction in human intestine. Dig Dis Sci 30: 119–123

Mearin F, Camilleri M, Malagelada J-R 1986 Pyloric dysfunction in diabetics with recurrent nausea and vomiting. Gastroenterology 90: 1919–1925

Mearin F, Cucala M, Azpiroz F, Malagelada J-R 1991 The origin of symptoms on the brain–gut axis in functional dyspepsia. Gastroenterology 101: 999–1006

Miedema B W, Kelly K A, Camilleri M et al 1992 Human gastric and jejunal transit and motility after Roux gastrojejunostomy. Gastroenterology 103: 1133–43

Moreno-Osset E, Bazzocchi G, Lo S et al 1989 Association between postprandial changes in colonic intraluminal pressure and transit. Gastroenterology 96: 1265–1273

Narducci F, Bassotti G, Gaburri M, Morelli A 1987 Twenty-four hour manometric recording of colonic activity in healthy man. Gut 28: 17–25

Prather C M, Camilleri M, Thomforde G M et al 1992a Forces in the distribution and emptying of different solids from the human stomach. Gastroenterology 102: A502

Prather C M, Camilleri M, Thomforde G M, Forstrom L A 1992b Axial forces in an experimental model of gastric stasis in man. Gastroenterology 102: A501

Proano M, Camilleri M, Phillips S F et al 1990 Transit of solids through the human colon: regional quantification in the unprepared bowel. Am J Physiol 258: G856–G862

Quigley E M M, Donor M J P, Lane M J, Gallagher T F 1992 Antroduodenal manometry. Usefulness and limitations as an outpatient study. Dig Dis Sci 37: 20–28

Read N W 1987 Functional gastroenterological disorders: the name's the thing . . . (editorial) Gut 28: 281–284

Reddy S N, Bazzocchi G, Chan S et al 1991 Colonic motility and transit in health and ulcerative colitis. Gastroenterology 101: 1289–1297

Rees W D W, Leigh R J, Christofides N D et al 1982 Interdigestive motor activity in patients with systemic sclerosis. Gastroenterology 83: 575–580

Rouillon J-M, Azpiroz F, Malagelada J-R 1991 Sensorial and gastrointestinal reflex pathways in the human jejunum. Gastroenterology 101: 1606–1612

Schwizer W, Fried M, Siebold K et al 1990 Magnetic resonance imaging (MRI) – a new tool to measure gastric emptying in man. Gastroenterology 98: A389

Sodhi N, Camilleri M, Camoriano J H et al 1989 Autonomic function and motility in intestinal pseudoobstruction caused by paraneoplastic syndrome. Dig Dis Sci 34: 1937–1942

Soffer E E, Scalabrini P, Wingate D L 1989 Prolonged ambulant monitoring of human colonic motility. Am J Physiol 257: G601–G606

Stanghellini V, Camilleri M, Malagelada J-R 1987 Chronic idiopathic intestinal pseudoobstruction: clinical and intestinal manometric findings. Gut 28: 5–12

Steadman C J, Phillips S F, Camilleri M et al 1991 Variation of muscle tone in the human colon. Gastroenterology 101: 373–381

Steadman C J, Phillips S F, Camilleri M et al 1992 Control of muscle tone in the human colon. Gut 33: 541–546

Stivland T, Camilleri M, Vassallo M et al 1991 Scintigraphic measurement of regional gut transit in idiopathic constipation. Gastroenterology 101: 107–115

Summers R W, Anuras S, Green J 1983 Jejunal manometry patterns in health, partial intestinal obstruction, and pseudoobstruction. Gastroenterology 85: 1290–1300

Urbain J-L, Van Cutsem E, Siegel J A et al 1990 Visualization and characterization of gastric contractions using a radionuclide technique. Am J Physiol 259: G1062–G1067

Vassallo M, Camilleri M, Phillips S et al 1992 Transit through the proximal colon influences stool weight in the irritable bowel syndrome. Gastroenterology 102:102–108

Vassallo M, Camilleri M, Hanson R B, Thomforde G M 1992 Axial forces in the emptying of solids and liquids from the human stomach. Am J Physiol 263: G230–G239

von der Ohe M, Hanson R B, Camilleri M 1992 Barostat recordings of intracolonic pressure activity: comparison with manometry in healthy subjects. Gastroenterology – 103:1378

Wood J R, Camilleri M, Low P A, Malagelada J-R 1985 Brainstem tumor presenting as an upper gut motility disorder. Gastroenterology 89: 1411–1414

14. Ambulant manometry

E. E. Soffer   R. W. Summers

BACKGROUND

The ability to record gut motility in ambulant subjects is advantageous for both clinical and research purposes. The earliest attempts used the technique of radiotelemetry, employing radio-pills. These were small capsules, containing a pressure-sensing device and a radio-transmitter. They were first introduced in the late 1950s, but little useful information was gained because they were free-floating and were propelled along the gut without knowledge of their location. They were used more effectively two decades later when miniaturization of equipment made prolonged ambulatory recording feasible and tethering of the capsules demonstrated motor events occurring at fixed loci in the intestine (Thompson et al 1980). However, the restriction posed by the antennae placed on the subject, the signal loss and the peroral insertion of the relatively large sized radio-pill limited the usefulness of this technique. The introduction of multiple miniature strain gauge pressure transducers mounted within thin catheters introduced transnasally, was an important step forward (Mathias et al 1985). Later, a recording technique using a portable tape recorder, sampling analogue signals from catheter-mounted strain gauges, demonstrated for the first time the feasibility of prolonged (up to 72 h) ambulant monitoring of proximal small bowel motility in subjects who were free to conduct their normal activity at home and at work (Kellow et al 1990). In a different approach, an analogue to digital converter was developed so that data could be stored on a portable solid state recorder (Husebye et al 1988). The feasibility of prolonged ambulant monitoring of small bowel motility was later demonstrated using solid state recording techniques (Soffer et al 1991). Solid state recorders are now the state-of-the-art in conducting ambulatory studies.

EQUIPMENT

The intraluminal recording probe has strain gauge pressure transducers incorporated in specially designed catheters. The coating material and flexibility vary among manufacturers, but catheters in general are quite flexible and have a small diameter (approximately 3 mm). Small bowel catheters have a central lumen, allowing for inflation of a small latex balloon which facilitates the progression of the catheter in the intestine. The number of sensors in the probe, and their location, depend on the study design and segment of gut monitored. The more sensors, however, the larger the catheter, making transnasal insertion more difficult, and reducing the tolerance of the subject. With current technology, it is difficult to produce catheters for ambulatory studies with more than six sensors. The addition of each sensor adds to the cost of the catheter, but new transducers are much more durable than early models, thus prolonging the life of the catheter and thereby reducing the cost of individual tests.

Solid state recorders are produced by a number of companies and vary in size and weight, but all are small enough to be easily carried within small shoulder bags. Memory ranges from 1–2 megabytes, but as size and price of memory chips is decreasing, more memory will be available in even smaller recorders. Down-loading to the computer is facilitated by the digital output, and the software usually includes an analysis program. Event markers help to note various physiological (meals, evacuation) or pathological (pain, nausea, etc.) events during the recording. (For commercially available systems see Further information.)

PLACEMENT OF THE CATHETER

The manometry catheter, with a small latex balloon tied to its tip, is inserted intranasally with the subject in the sitting position. We use a local anaesthetic spray for the hypopharynx and a similar spray, or a gel, for the nose to facilitate the passage. After the tube is advanced to a distance of 40–50 cm, the subject is fluoroscoped in the supine position, to verify catheter position. The catheter is then advanced and manipulated toward the pylorus. Once in the antrum, the subject is placed in the right lateral position, and the tube is advanced into the duodenum. There the balloon is inflated using the central lumen and the catheter is allowed to advance by propulsive motor activity. The subject is periodically checked until sensors have reached the desired position. Using catheters with three sensors spaced 10 cm apart, we position the proximal sensor in the mid duodenum and the two distal sensors in the proximal jejunum. In normal subjects, the tube will reach the desired position almost invariably within 2 h, and then the balloon is deflated. Patients with gastroparesis require manual manoeuvring of the catheter through the pylorus. In patients with intestinal dysmotility, e.g. scleroderma, progression of the catheter in the intestine can be slow, and can take up to 12 h before the desired position is reached. The patient, however, does not need to be present in the motility laboratory during this entire period; when we anticipate a serious motor disorder, we often begin the tube placement on the night before the recording is to begin. We are usually successful and have had to employ endoscopy for catheter placement only infrequently. However, if time is a factor, passage can be greatly facilitated by grasping the catheter tip in the stomach with an endoscopically directed snare, manipulating it into the distal duodenum and releasing it there before withdrawing the endoscope.

PROTOCOL FOR THE STUDY

Medications which might affect intestinal motility should be discontinued 24 h before the procedure. If gastroparesis is suspected, solid food should be withheld for at least 24 h. We insert the catheter in the morning, between 07:00–09:00, after an overnight fast. A single 600–700 kcal meal is given at about 15:00 –16:00 (water is allowed ad lib) and the subject is asked to go to sleep at about 23:00 and to return for catheter removal the next morning. Subjects are encouraged to engage in their normal activity at home. This protocol permits a period of 6–8 h of daytime fasting, an equal time after a meal, and about the same recording time during sleep. Allowing subjects to consume the usual three meals a day results in postprandial motor activity constituting most of the waking hours, with only a few migrating motor complexes (MMCs) observed, as has been previously described (Thompson et al 1981). Specific research protocols may require

variations on this theme. Our standard sampling rate is 2 Hz. Using a datalogger with 2 megabytes of memory, and a catheter with three sensors, one can record continuously for at least 72 h, if necessary. Sampling frequency of 2 and 16 Hz detected the same number of phasic events, though amplitude was slightly higher with the higher frequency (Husebye et al 1990), and we consider the lower frequency to be adequate for clinical purposes.

PATTERNS OF SMALL BOWEL MOTILITY

The three phases of the MMC are shown in Figure 14.1. Figure 14.2, taken from a fasting subject, demonstrates the irregular contractile activity during phase II in the awake state. Phase II constitutes the majority of the total cycle length. In contrast, Figure 14.3 demonstrates an equal duration of recording during sleep. Phase II is very short and phase I accounts for most of the cycle length. The cycle length is decreased resulting in an increase in MMC incidence as has been previously described (Thompson et al 1980, Kellow et al 1990). The transition from sleep to the awakened state is usually quite obvious (Figure 14.4), with an instantaneous increase in motor activity, occurring in all channels at the onset of consciousness.

The change in contractile activity induced by food, the so-called fed pattern, is depicted in Figure 14.5. With prolonged recording, the increased activity typical of the fed pattern is sustained in the upper intestine for only part of the duration of the postprandial period, typically 1–2 h. After this the pattern is indistinguishable from phase II, until the appearance of the next activity front. Figures 14.6–14.7 were obtained from patients with scleroderma, showing low amplitude of contractions and lack of fed pattern after a meal. Figure 14.8 is obtained from a sleeping patient with pseudo-obstruction. Although no intestinal tissue was available for histological studies, this pattern is most consistent with visceral neuropathy. It is particularly dramatic when compared to the inactive bowel as seen normally during sleep (Figure 14.3). Figure 14.9 demonstrates intestinal activity during sleep in a patient with diabetes mellitus. Phase II shows marked clustered contractile activity while phase III is normal. In this patient, waking daytime activity was normal, and the abnormal pattern, consistent with visceral neuropathy, was seen only during sleep.

INTESTINAL MANOMETRY – STATIONARY OR AMBULATORY?

With improved technology, stationary recording of

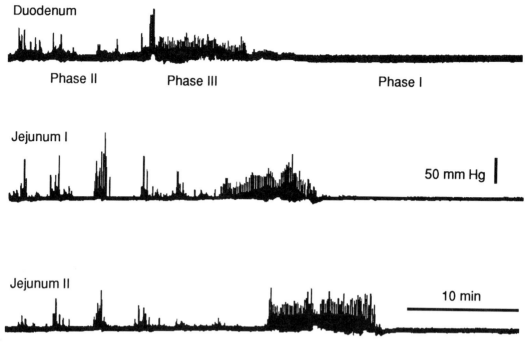

Fig. 14.1   The three phases of the normal MMC. Phase II consists of intermittent activity. Phase III, the most distinct, consists of a short burst of regular pressure waves that migrates aborally, followed by a period of quiescence, which is phase I.

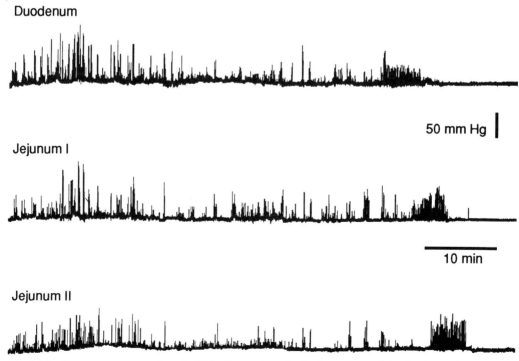

Fig. 14.2   Demonstrates approximately 1.5 h of normal awake, fasting motor activity. In the awake state phase II accounts for most of the MMC cycle.

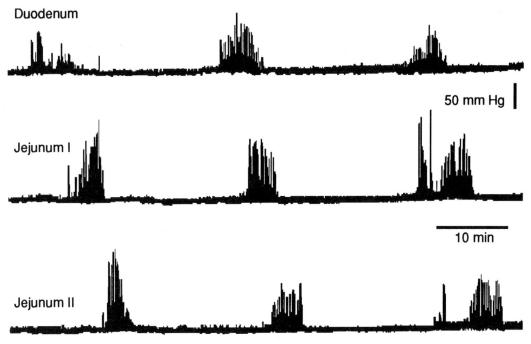

Fig. 14.3   The normal MMC during sleep is characterized by marked hypoactivity, with phase I accounting for most of the cycle length, and by increased cycle frequency.

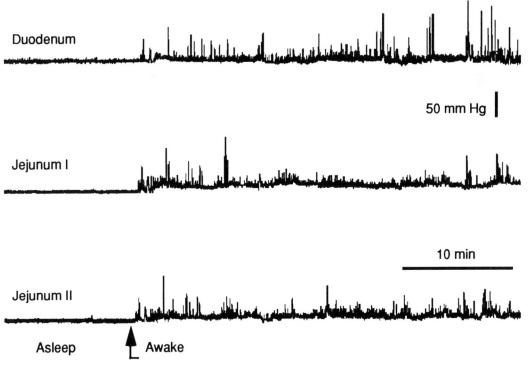

Fig. 14.4   Awakening is recognized by a marked, instantaneous increase in motor activity and is an easily recognized phenomenon on inspection of the tracing.

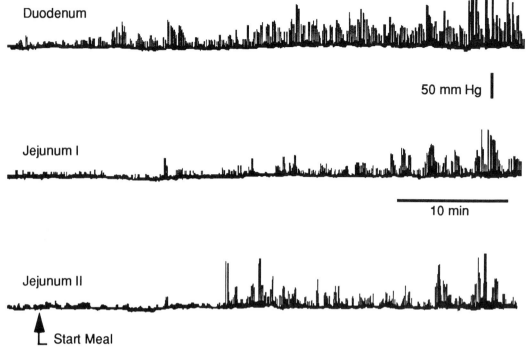

Fig. 14.5 The ingestion of food results, within minutes, in increased rate of contractions which is similar in appearance to an active phase II.

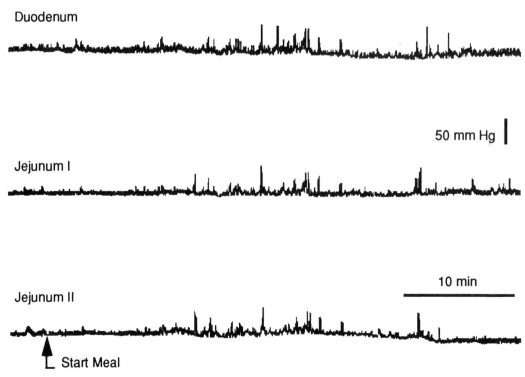

Fig. 14.6 Abnormal hypoactive response to food in a patient with scleroderma. The contractile activity following the meal could not be distinguished from the phase II that preceded it. The pressure waves are infrequent and of low amplitude.

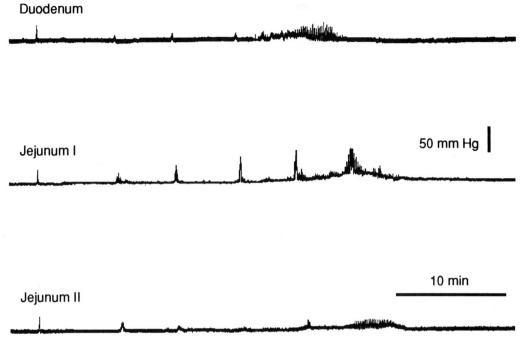

Fig. 14.7   Low amplitude MMC in a patient with scleroderma. Also, this was the only phase III observed in 24 h of recording, another abnormal finding.

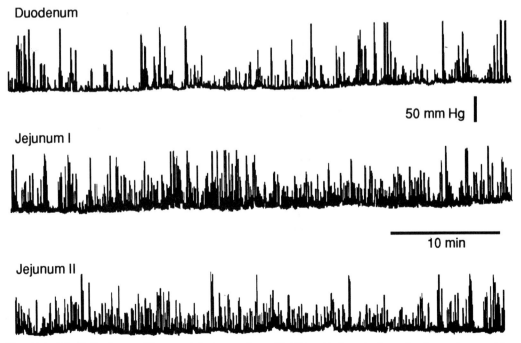

Fig. 14.8   Markedly abnormal hyperactivity in a patient with idiopathic intestinal pseudo-obstruction requiring chronic parenteral nutrition. This pattern was seen throughout the night and the day with hardly any periods of quiescence. No motor complexes were seen. This 'intestinal equivalent' of ventricular fibrillation illustrates the fact that uncoordinated hypermotility, like hypomotility, can result in abnormal function.

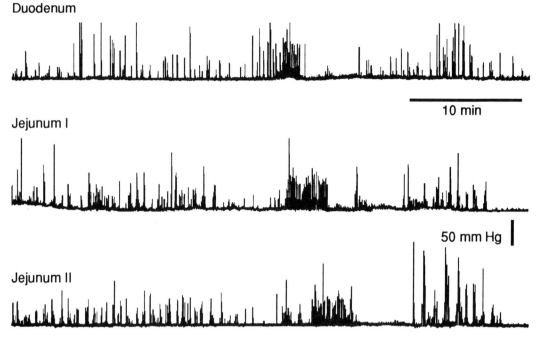

Fig. 14.9 Clustered motor hyperactivity during sleep was the only abnormality detected in this patient with diabetes mellitus. Diurnal motor activity and appearance of phase III during sleep were normal.

intestinal motor activity has been the most widely used technique for more than a decade (Arndorfer et al 1977). Ambulatory recording using radiotelemetry, strain gauge catheters with miniaturized tape recorders, or lately, solid state recorders has been gaining popularity. Which one should be used? We will attempt to answer this question considering all aspects of a motility recording system, from recording fidelity to price and logistics.

Length of recording sessions

The first question, of course, is whether there is any advantage in recording intestinal motility over prolonged periods of time for clinical purposes, or is the standard stationary recording during 3–4 hours of fasting and 1–2 hours postprandially sufficient. Our experience and that of others (Thompson et al 1980, Kellow et al 1986, Quigley et al 1992) has highlighted the marked variability of fasting and fed motor patterns both within and between subjects. In normal fasting individuals, during diurnal recording, we have observed MMC cycle intervals as short as 25 min, while in others, in contrast, only a single activity front was seen during 7 h. The length and configuration of

phase III are also quite variable, all of which make short studies more difficult to interpret. Decisions about what is normal and what is abnormal should be based on recording duration of sufficient length to sample all of the various motility patterns. The motor pattern during sleep is more 'predictable' with long periods of quiescence, more regular, and more frequent MMC cycles (Thompson et al 1980, Kellow et al 1990). For that reason, we believe that most motor abnormalities can be better appreciated during sleep. Figure 14.9 is a case in point. This diabetic patient's daytime motility pattern appeared normal. The abnormality emerged during sleep, demonstrating a markedly active clustered motor pattern. The increased contractile activity in a patient with pseudo-obstruction (Figure 14.8) was observed during the day, but was better highlighted during sleep. A more complete discussion of intestinal motor patterns is to be found in later chapters. We consider three patterns as unequivocal markers of abnormal motility:

1. Deviation from normal fasting sleep pattern, with increased contractile activity and reduction in phase I activity;
2. Failure of the fed pattern to be established after a meal;

3. No evidence of at least a single phase III in 6–7 of recording while fasting.

Retrograde or non-migration of activity fronts (phase III), infrequent, low amplitude pressure waves after a meal, or postprandial clustered contractions alternating with quiescent periods are among other reported abnormal motility patterns. However, development of aetiologic diagnoses requires consideration of all other clinical data.

Equipment fidelity

Tube-mounted strain gauges have been compared with an open-tip perfused-tube system in an animal study, and the authors concluded that strain gauge sensors distorted contractile events (Valori et al 1986). However, in a similar study in humans using a non-compliant catheter referenced to atmospheric pressure, the recordings failed to document such distortions (Gill et al 1990), prompting the authors to speculate that the distortions seen in the animal studies could be caused by deformation of the catheter at sites away from the sensors. Both studies found the in-dwelling strain gauges to be more sensitive in detecting intraluminal pressure changes.

Logistics

Due to its flexibility and small diameter, the strain gauge catheter is very well tolerated. The transnasal insertion is easy, it does not interfere with eating, and sleep is not disturbed. Advancing the strain gauge catheter through the pylorus in patients with gastroparesis can be difficult, as is the case with perfused tube assembly (Quigley et al 1992). Endoscopy may be needed to aid in advancement of both types of catheters into the duodenum. However, given the prolonged period of recording in an ambulatory study, the interpretability of the motility study following endoscopy with sedation and air insufflation is less of a problem than it is with the perfused catheter. With multiple perfused lumens and longer recording sessions the volume of water entering the intestine becomes a significant problem. Absorption of this fluid increases the need for frequent urination, and it is possible that the volume may alter the motor patterns in subtle ways.

With only 2–3 strain gauges in a catheter, the antrum cannot be reliably studied. However, with increasing memory in the solid state dataloggers, catheters with 5–6 strain gauges can be used, allowing for prolonged recording from the antrum as well as the duodeno-jejunum.

A major drawback of stationary recording has been the need for nursing personnel to supervise the patient and care for the equipment throughout the study, which in effect may last a whole day. This is unnecessary with ambulatory recording. A major disadvantage of the ambulatory system is its price and the fragility of the strain gauges which may periodically malfunction. However, these expenses are, to a great extent, offset by saving personnel time, and by the ability to display the analogue form on a printer rather than use an expensive chart recorder. As noted earlier, current strain gauge catheters are much more durable and last longer than early models. Also, with the addition of an isolation device, the system can be used for short-term, on-line recording, comparable to those obtained using existing stationary systems. Such a system, comprised of a solid state recorder, a strain gauge catheter, a personal computer and a printer can serve a dual purpose: a stationary system and an ambulatory one.

The ambulatory systems in research

The impact of ambulatory recording is perhaps better recognized in the area of research. Here, ambulatory systems have allowed investigators to conduct studies which would have been impossible to perform with stationary systems. It has allowed the study of effects of a stressful drive through heavy traffic on intestinal motility (Kumar & Wingate 1985), made possible the study of exercise effects on intestinal and oesophageal motility (Soffer et al 1991, Soffer et al 1993), and another paper initiated a flurry of studies on the relationships between oesophageal motor events, luminal pH and non-cardiac chest pain (Janssens et al 1986). In studies of this nature, the free mobility of the subjects, afforded by an ambulatory system, is essential. Advantage of a different kind is offered in studies which require the repetitive use of variables such as studying the effect of different meals (Soffer & Adrian 1992) or different drug doses on intestinal motility (Soffer & Launspach 1993). An ambulatory system allows a single intubation and prolonged recordings, while a stationary system requires repeated intubation of the same subjects.

At the University of Iowa we have been using an ambulatory recording system, consisting of a strain gauge catheter and a solid state recorder, for the last 4 years. It is used for research, and for clinical purposes, and has completely replaced the previous stationary system which used perfused catheters. Patient compliance has been very good, and the system enthusiastically accepted by the nursing and physician personnel. Clinically, we have found the results of the prolonged recording to be more conclusive, and initially found it necessary, on occasion, to perform an ambulatory test after a perfused tube manometric study yielded equivocal results.

INTESTINAL MOTILITY – IS IT CLINICALLY USEFUL?

This is a key question, whether one employs an ambulatory or a stationary recording technique. Intestinal manometry is useful and important clinically if the limitations of the technique are recognized (Quigley 1992). The information gained must be interpreted in the context of the rest of the clinical data in order to draw the correct conclusions. The symptoms, the concurrent medical problems, the background of operative therapy, the medications, the family history, the physical examination, the plain and contrast radiographic studies, the studies of transit and the histologic examination of the gut are just some of the data that contribute to our understanding of motility disorders. The gut is limited in the ways it can express underlying disease processes, and this is true with regard to manometric findings as well as symptoms. Though 'myopathic' and 'neuropathic' (Camilleri & Malagelada 1984, Camilleri et al 1985, Dooley et al 1988) motility patterns have been described, based on findings in subgroups of patients, it is important to remember that with only few exceptions data are not available correlating manometric and pathologic findings. Different pathologic processes may produce the same abnormal patterns and so manometry cannot diagnose a disease. Manometry can detect, however, deviations from the normal pattern and define those deviations as consistent with visceral myopathy or neuropathy. Also, hardly any correlation is available between manometry and functional studies, such as gastric emptying or intestinal transit. What is one to make of abnormal motor pattern in the presence of normal functional studies or vice versa?

The above limitations notwithstanding, we have found intestinal motility studies helpful in evaluating patients with consistent gastrointestinal symptoms, with no evidence of organic lesions (Malagelada & Stanghellini 1985). In such patients the distinction between 'functional' and organic symptoms can sometimes be quite difficult, and the detection of gut motor abnormalities helps to clarify the picture. We have found motility studies to be helpful in determining the presence and extent of gut motor abnormalities in contemplating surgical interventions in patients with defaecation disorders. If small bowel motility patterns are seriously disturbed, we are reluctant to recommend

subtotal colectomy for severe constipation. This situation suggests a widespread motor disorder which is unlikely to respond to colonic resection.

Assessment of the underlying pathology, based on the manometric findings, can aid in choosing an appropriate drug therapy from the limited menu available for dysmotility syndromes. For instance, cholinergic agents might be expected to be more effective in motor disorders consistent with visceral myopathy rather than neuropathy (Christensen et al 1990). Octreotide, a somatostatin analogue may be expected to be more helpful in patients who do not generate spontaneous MMCs, as suggested by a recent report on the use of the drug in patients with scleroderma (Soudah et al 1991). As stressed before, the marked variability observed in normal subjects needs to be kept in mind in order to avoid labelling variants of normal as pathologic processes.

WHAT IS IN STORE FOR THE FUTURE?

Measurement of gastrointestinal pressure changes is still a relatively young discipline. Significant advances in ambulatory monitoring technology have occurred in the past 10 years and it is anticipated that this will not be a static area of investigation. Smaller, more durable and less expensive strain gauge catheters are likely to be developed so that more sensors can be incorporated into a single catheter. Prototype catheters using fibreoptic bundles have already been developed and the technology appears to hold great promise. It will be important to develop pressure sensors which are capable of reliably detecting pressure changes over longer segments or in sphincters. Again early models have already been developed, but they are not in widespread use. While the oesophagus and small bowel have been the major focus of attention, further studies are likely to concentrate on the stomach and colon.

Catheters will likely be developed which incorporate sensors for detection of other events in addition to pressure. In the oesophagus, detectors of hydrogen ion concentration have been combined with strain gauges yielding important observations correlating pH and motor patterns. It would be useful to add measurements of myoelectric activity from bipolar electrodes. Strain gauges are reliable in detecting phasic activity in the gut, but are of little use in monitoring changes in tone. Two promising techniques have been developed to approach this problem, the barostat and a probe to measure cross-sectional area (Danish device) (Aspiroz & Malagelada 1985, Gregersen et al 1990). Other devices are being studied to measure the force of aborally-moving propulsive contractions. Unfortunately none of these is available in the ambulatory state. Badly needed are simple devices to measure transit. Incorporation of these devices into intraluminal catheters will contribute a great deal to the understanding of the motor function and dysfunction of the gastrointestinal tract.

The use of the computer has greatly facilitated the analysis of large volumes of data. Yet it is likely that current programs are primitive in their development. Pressure changes with respect to time can be analysed with all existing programs, but patterns of contractions are much more important in determining the function of the gut. Thus the use of closely-spaced sensors and the analysis of the relationship between pressure changes from adjacent sensors will aid in the understanding of propulsive forces and transit of intraluminal contents.

Some of the developments which are likely to occur

have been outlined. Some will be important, others will not survive and others not yet anticipated will find their way from the research laboratory into the clinical arena. Ambulatory manometry is an important development which extends our ability to understand gastrointestinal motor function. It is well on its way to replacing short-term stationary recording using perfused catheters.

ACKNOWLEDGEMENTS

The authors gratefully acknowledge the efforts of Ms Jan Launspach in obtaining the recordings and preparing the illustrations. This work was supported in part by research funds from the Department of Veterans Affairs and Janssen Pharmaceutica.

REFERENCES

Arndorfer R C, Stef J J, Dodds W J et al 1977 Improved infusion system for intraluminal esophageal manometry. Gastroenterology 73: 23–27

Azpiroz F, Malagelada J-R 1985 Physiological variations in canine gastric tone measured by an electronic barostat. Am J Physiol 248: G229–G237

Camilleri M, Malagelada J-R 1984 Abnormal intestinal motility in diabetics with the gastroparesis syndrome. Eur J Clin Invest 14: 420–427

Camilleri M, Malagelada J-R, Stanghellini V et al 1985 Gastrointestinal motility disturbances in patients with orthostatic hypotension. Gastroenterology 88: 1852–1859

Christensen J, Dent J, Malagelada J-R et al 1990 Pseudo-obstruction. Gastroenterology International 3: 107–119

Dooley C P, El Newhi H M, Zeidler A et al 1988 Abnormalities of the migrating motor complex in diabetics with autonomic neuropathy and diarrhea. Scand J Gastroenterol 23: 217–233

Gill R C, Kellow J E, Browning C et al 1990 The use of intraluminal strain gauges for recording ambulant small bowel motility. Am J Physiol 258: G610–G615

Gregersen H, Kraglund K, Djurhuus J C 1990 Variation in duodenal cross-sectional area during the interdigestive migrating motility complex. Am J Physiol 259: G26–G31

Husebye E, Skar V, Osmes M 1988 Digital ambulatory registration of small-intestine motility. Scand J Gastroenterol 23 (Suppl 145): 30

Husebye E, Skar V, Aalen O O, Osnes M 1990 Digital ambulatory manometry of the small intestine in healthy adults. Estimates of variation within and between individuals and statistical management of incomplete MMC periods. Dig Dis Sci 35: 1057–1065

Janssens J, Vantrappen G, Ghillebert G 1986 24-hour recording of esophageal pressure and pH in patients with non-cardiac chest pain. Gastroenterology 90: 1978–1984

Kellow J E, Borody T J, Phillips S F et al 1986 Human interdigestive motility: variations in patterns from esophagus to colon. Gastroenterology 91: 386–395

Kellow J E, Gill R C, Wingate D L 1990 Prolonged ambulant

recordings of small bowel motility demonstrated abnormalities in the irritable bowel syndrome. Gastroenterology 98: 1208–1218

Kumar D, Wingate D L 1985 The irritable bowel syndrome: A paroxysmal motor disorder. Lancet 2: 973–977

Malagelada J-R, Stanghellini V 1985 Manometric evaluation of functional upper gut symptoms. Gastroenterology 88: 1223–1231

Mathias J R, Sninsky C A, Millar H D et al 1985 Development of an improved multi-pressure-sensor probe for recording muscle contraction in human intestine. Dig Dis Sci 30: 119–123

Quigley E M M 1992 Intestinal manometry – technical advances, clinical limitations. Dig Dis Sci 37: 10–13

Quigley E M M, Donovan J P, Lane M J et al 1992 Antroduodenal manometry. Usefulness and limitations as an outpatient study. Dig Dis Sci 37: 20–28

Soffer E E, Adrian T E 1992 The effect of meal composition and sham feeding on duodenojejunal motility in humans. Dig Dis Sci 37: 1009–1014

Soffer E E, Launspach J 1993 The effect of misoprostol on postprandial intestinal motility and orocecal transit time in humans. Dig Dis Sci 38: 851–855

Soffer E E, Summers R W, Gisolfi C 1991 The effect of exercise on intestinal motility and transit in trained athletes. Am J Physiol 260: G698–G702

Soffer E E, Merchant R K, Duethman G et al 1993 The effect of graded exercise on esophageal motility and gastroesophageal reflux in trained athletes. Dig Dis Sci 38: 220–224

Soudah H C, Hasler M L, Chung O 1991 Effect of octreotide on intestinal motility and bacterial overgrowth in scleroderma. N Engl J Med 325: 1461–1467

Thompson D G, Wingate D L, Archer L et al 1990 Normal pattern of human upper small bowel motor activity recorded by prolonged radiotelemetry. Gut 21: 500–506

Thompson D G, Archer L, Green W J, et al 1981 Fasting motor activity occurs during a day of normal meals in healthy subjects. Gut 22: 489–492

Valori R M, Collins S M, Daniel E E et al 1986 Comparison of methodologies for the measurement of antroduodenal motor activity in the dog. Gastroenterology 91: 546–553

FURTHER INFORMATION

Strain-gauge catheter suppliers
Gaeltec Ltd
Dunvegan, Isle of Skye
Scotland IV55 8GU
Phone: 047–022385
Fax: 047–202369

Konigsberg Instruments
2000 E Foothills Blvd
Pasadena, CA 91107
Phone: (818) 449–0016

Medical Measurement Inc
(Gaeltec Ltd)
53 Main Street
Hackensack, NJ 07601
Phone: (201) 489–9400
Fax: (800) 833–8031
Telex: 6971380

Millar Instruments Inc
PO Box 18227
6001 Gulf Freeway
Houston, TX 77023–5417
Phone: (713) 923–9171
Telex: 791288

Solid state recorder suppliers
Gaeltec Ltd
Dunvegan, Isle of Skye
Scotland IV55 8GU
Phone: 047–022385
Fax: 047–202369

Medical Measurement Inc
(Gaeltec Ltd)
53 Main Street
Hackensack, NJ 07601
Phone: (201) 489–9400
Fax: (800) 833–8031
Telex: 6971380

Medical Measurement Systems
PO Box 40178
7504 RD Enschede, Holland
Phone: 31–53–308–803
Fax: 31–53–308–801

Sandhill Scientific Inc
1501-N West Campus Drive
Littleton, CO 80120–4535
Phone: (303) 797–6544
          (800) 468–4556
Fax: (303) 795–8587

Synectics Medical Inc
1425 Greenway Dr, Suite 600
Irving, T X 75038–2482
Phone: (214) 518–0518
Fax: (214) 518–0080

Synectics Medical Inc
Renstiernas Gata 12
S-11631
Stockholm, Sweden
Phone: 468–7430850
Fax: 468–405424

15. Radiotelemetry

D. F. Evans

BACKGROUND

The terms endoradiosondes, radiotelemetry capsules (RTCs), radiocapsules and radiopills are all descriptions of ingestible telemetric sensors for measurement of gastrointestinal function. They were first developed over 30 years ago, almost simultaneously on both sides of the Atlantic (Farrar et al 1957, Mackay & Jacobson 1957). Although initially received by the medical and scientific community with much interest, the use of these devices has had a chequered history. Most studies using telemetry were performed in the 1960s and although mainly addressing gastrointestinal function some reports had novel, if not astounding, applications (Fox et al 1970, Worrell et al 1963) investigating areas otherwise impossible with existing technology.

Interest waned in the 1970s, partly because of technical difficulties in measurement, but also because of a lack of knowledge of basic physiology of the gastrointestinal tract. However, in the past 15–20 years there has been a rapid increase in our knowledge of gastrointestinal tract function and a partial resurgence in the use of telemetry capsules for clinical investigation and research. A further important factor affecting the progress of development has been the increase in complexity and size of the electronics industry in such areas as microcircuitry and microelectronics, computer development and signal processing. This chapter will attempt to map the development of radiotelemetry in research and describe the state of the technology, recording equipment and analytical methods to which such devices are currently being put to in gastrointestinal applications.

PRINCIPLES

Ingestible telemetry capsules measure useful parameters from hollow organs within the body using the principle of radiotransmission. The capsules consist of a transducer, which detects the measure, and electronic circuitry to convert the measurements to a radiofrequency, and an aerial to transmit this signal through body tissue. Transmitted radio signals are detected and interpreted by specially designed external radioreceivers remote from the subjects (Wolff 1961). The advantage of these systems is that functional information can be detected without discomfort, pain or hazard to the subject. Of equal importance is the ability to make measurements over long periods, a facility that we now know is essential in the accurate study of gastrointestinal function.

DESCRIPTION

General applications

Radiocapsules can be used to measure physiological parameters in a number of ways. They were originally designed to be ingested orally and to transmit data as they traversed unhindered through the gastrointestinal tract. They have however been used in a variety of other ways, both in the gastrointestinal tract and in other organs. One possibility is temporary attachment or tethering in the gut lumen or other hollow organs. Another is semi-permanent implantation in the lumen or in body tissue.

Radiocapsule types

Currently there are four main types of radiopills available: pH, pressure, temperature and redox potential. All are available commercially (Remote Control Systems, London and Heidelberg, Inc USA) and are used predominantly in research (Fig.15.1a). All capsules use similar principles of transduction but there have been alternative approaches to the design of transmission and demodulation characteristics of the resultant signal.

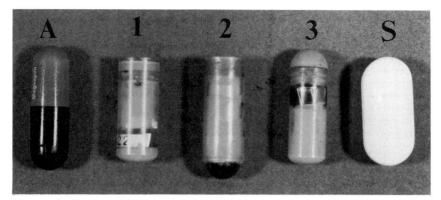

Fig. 15.1A Three types of commercially available radiotelemetry capsules scaled to Magnapen (**A**) and sucralfate (**S**) tablets. From left to right: **1** Pressure-sensitive for implantation, tether or free-fall applications, with integral battery. **2** pH sensitive with integral battery and screw-cap for replaceable reference electrode and tether; also for implantation, tether or free fall applications. **3**. Semi-disposable temperature-sensitive type with replaceable battery.

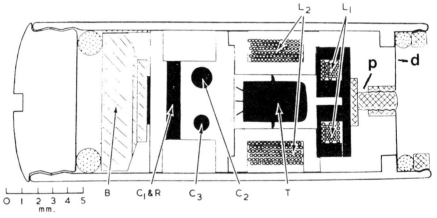

Fig. 15.1B Schematic diagram of principles of operation of inductance type pressure-sensitive radiocapsule. Pressure impinging on diaphragm (**d**), approximates pot core (**p**) to inductance L_1). Oscillator circuit powered by battery (**B**) comprises transistor (**T**) and capacitors and resistors (C_{1-3} and **R**). Radiosignal is transmitted by aerial coil L_2 to remote receiver. (Adapted from Watson et al 1962.)

Pressure

Pressure radiotelemetry capsules are basically miniature cable-free pressure transducers. There are two main types.

Inductance The principle of operation of this type of radiocapsule is shown in Fig. 15.1B. Details of various types can be found elsewhere (Watson et al 1962, Watson 1981, Lambert et al 1982).

The capsule consists of an envelope of perspex, polycarbonate or stainless steel. The dimensions are such that the capsule can be swallowed and will travel through the digestive tract without becoming obstructed. Capsules are, typically, approximately 25–30 mm in length by 6–10 mm in diameter. Power is derived from miniature batteries which are either replaceable or embedded in epoxy resin, in which case the capsule is discarded once the battery is exhausted. Activation of power is achieved either by some form of switch within the battery compartment or by simple removal of the battery. Battery life varies from 60–90 h for the reusable types or 2–3 months for the implantable type.

A gold-plated or stainless steel circular diaphragm

mounted in one end of the pressure capsule acts as the pressure sensor. The capsule operates by deformation of the diapragm (d) by surrounding pressure fluctuations. This alters the inductance (L_1) of a ferrite pot core by the proximity of the ferrite disc mounted on the back of the diaphragm. The inductance change correspondingly alters the frequency of an oscillating transistor circuit (Clapp oscillator) and this signal is transmitted by a small copper coiled aerial (L_2) within the envelope. Transmission frequency is tunable, with a small set screw in the diaphragm, in the range 150–400 kHz, with a net change of approximately 20 kHz per 100 mmHg. The overall pressure range of the capsules is up to 300 mmHg and the transmission distance through body tissue is approximately 0.5–0.75 m.

An improved version of the pressure capsule has recently been introduced (Remote Control Systems, London) with major improvements such as extension of the battery life to over 60 days. The capsule is also smaller than the existing type, has a fixed frequency and an intergral, encapsulated mercury battery. Capsules can be tuned by the manufacturer to different frequencies to facilitate simultaneous, multiple site recordings from within the gut. This is particularly useful if peristalsis is to be measured with tethered or implanted units.

Strain gauge Pressure sensitive capsules have also been manufactured utilizing semiconductor or wire strain gauges as the principle of transduction (Browning et al 1981). Pulsed transmission conserves battery life (5–8 days) and allows for simplified demodulation and receiving equipment (Browning et al 1983). However the unit cost is high (2–3 times the inductance type) and the devices are only available to special order (Gaeltec Ltd, Isle of Skye, Scotland).

pH

pH sensitive radiotelemetry capsules (Jacobson & Mackay 1957, Watson & Paton 1965). have been used extensively to measure gastro-oesophageal reflux and gastric pH (Branicki et al 1982, Cheadle et al 1988) in relation to acid-related disorders in the upper gastrointestinal tract, but have also been used to yield information about intestinal and colorectal pH (Bown et al 1974, Evans et al 1988a).

There are two types of pH-sensitive telemetry capsules. The first, and probably the most common, is the hydrogen ion-sensitive glass electrode. The capsule incorporates a pH-sensitive glass electrode and an inbuilt sodium chloride reference cap (Colson & Watson 1979). The second type of pH-sensitive capsule utilizes

a poly- or monocrystalline antimony sensor, the so called 'Heidelberg capsule' (Noller 1962). Both types of capsules are sensitive to pH but have different operating characteristics. Other principles have been researched (Rawlings & Lucas 1985, Schepel et al 1984) but, to date, glass and antimony remain the primary techniques in general use.

Glass Glass pH-sensitive capsules consist of a cylindrical glass envelope incorporating a pH-sensitive glass electrode and a KCl/NaCl reference electrode. The most widely used capsule (Remote Control Systems, London) contains an inbuilt mercury battery with a useful life of 60–90 days, but with documented life under continuous in vivo conditions of > 150 days (Swain et al 1992). The voltage detected by the hydrogen ion-sensitive glass is transducted and transmitted by the encapsulated electronics using similar principles to the pressure capsule. The transmission centre frequency is 400 ± 50 kHz with a sensitivity of 3.3 kHz per pH unit. Temperature coefficient is 0.03 pH units/°C. pH drift is typically < 0.5 pH units per usage cycle and the capsule is reusable after sterilization. The screw-in reference caps are disposable and must be replaced after every use as they are a major source of contamination.

Antimony The Heidelberg capsule (Heidelberg Inc, New York, USA) has been used for many years for the assessment of gastric pH using the 'Bicarbonate test Zeit'. Battery life (~ 6h), drift and a high temperature coefficient (0.1 pH units/°C) limit its use to short-term experiments.

Temperature and redox potential

Telemetry capsules to detect temperature and redox potential within the gastrointestinal tract are also available (Remote Control Systems, London). Their usage has been limited (Moller & Bojsen 1975, Edholm et al 1973, Stirrup et al 1990, Steele et al 1991) and at present it is difficult to predict their impact on research into gastrointestinal function.

Receiving and recording systems

Display and recording systems for telemetry capsules consist of three major components. An aerial to detect radio transmissions from capsules, a decoding receiver similar to a domestic radio, and a recording medium to display or store data. Figure 15.2 illustrates the basic system requirements of a telemetry system. With the move towards ambulatory monitoring, the use of portable tape or digital data storage devices is becoming more widespread.

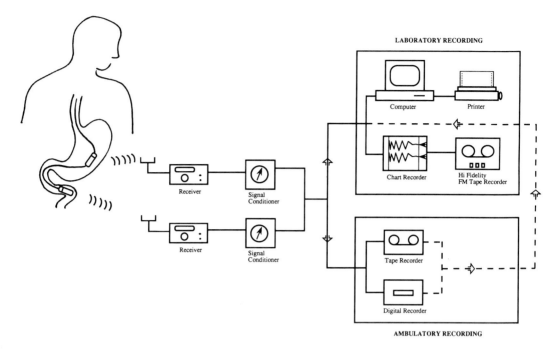

Fig. 15.2   Schematic diagram of data collection and storage equipment for ingested radiotelemetry capsules. Simple systems may have display and hard copy facility only. Ambulatory systems require the recording facility in order to collect data in the field. Data from such systems can be replayed through recorder or computer.

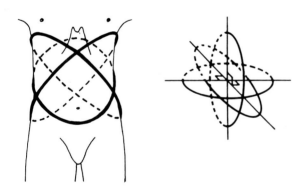

Fig. 15.3   Typical multiple aerial configuration for radio capsules. Orthogonally mounted body-borne aerials capture the strongest signal as the radiopill tumbles through the gastrointestinal tract. (Valori 1988)

Aerials

The aerial detecting system is normally body-borne, i.e. positioned next to the body surface, overlying and surrounding the position of the capsule. In the simplest form the aerial consists of a copper coil, often wound around a ferrite rod to improve reception. The aerial is tuned to radio transmissions to give maximum signal strength. Aerials may be single or multiple, in order to most efficiently detect transmissions from the capsule. Multiple aerial systems reduce the amount of signal loss and may be in the form of circular, flattened discs, or a bandolier which completely encircles the torso. Freely moving capsules tumbling through the gut ideally require a multiple aerial system with selective switching controlled by an electronic switching unit (Jacob 1973). Excessive signal loss is the major cause of poor recordings and this is due to the dipole characteristics of transmissions from the capsule, signals being maximum in the longitudinal axis of the capsule. By arranging three aerials orthogonally around the body, a strong signal will be detected no matter how the pill lies within the gut (Fig. 15.3). With the introduction of microelectronics, it is possible to incorporate automated aerial switching into the receiver.

Receivers and recorders

Radiotelemetry capsule receiving systems consist of radio receivers tuned specifically to the capsule frequen-

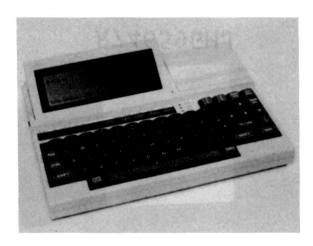

Fig. 15.4 Digitally tuned, computer designed, laboratory type radiotelemetry receiver for pH, pressure and temperature. (Thorburn et al 1989.)

cies with additional filtering to overcome interference from outside sources. Most receivers are frequency modulated (FM) and incorporate a variable tuning control to capture signals from capsules transmitting in the range 250–550 kHz. Other systems use pulsed transmission principles which involve switching the incoming signal to a zero state for part of the time (Browning et al 1983), this helps to conserve capsule battery life. Commercial systems currently available are limited to small companies (Remote Control Systems, London (Thorburn et al 1989) (Fig. 15.4) and some users design and build their own units.

Traditionally, signals derived from the radio receivers were displayed and recorded onto chart recorders and data was stored on FM tape recorders. Recently, the use of digital storage media in the form of computer memory allows for analogue to digital conversion and long-term storage on hard or floppy disk.

Receivers – portable In the past 10 years there has been a move towards monitoring gastrointestinal function in near physiological conditions, as it is now known that many measurements of gut function are altered by physical and psychological state. Previous studies have shown that gastrointestinal motility is modified by ambulatory state and psychological and physical stresses (Evans et al 1984, Kumar et al 1989, Valori et al 1986). Other factors that are influenced by motility are also influenced by ambulation. Gastrooesophageal reflux is more frequent and of greater severity under normal physiological conditions when compared to that seen in bed-bound patients (Branicki et al 1982, Schlesingler 1985). The move towards

ambulatory measurement has required the development of portable recording systems.

The first ambulatory receivers for radiotelemetry capsules were home-built (Slater et al 1982, Browning et al 1983) and were designed to record on to portable battery-powered miniature tape recorders. Figure 15.5 illustrates such a device. Subjects wear an aerial, a receiver and a recorder in a waist belt. Radiocapsules can be tethered or freely moving within the gastrointestinal tract.

Since the advent of high-capacity digital storage media, there has been a change from analogue to digital data storage. With ambulatory devices, both the receiver and the data storage can be conveniently located in one unit. Two such systems are currently available which allow for detection and recording of data from pH or pressure telemetry capsules. The Flexilog 1010 recorder (Oakfield Instruments, Oxon Ltd, Eynsham, Oxford) and the Albyn PH100 recorder (Albyn Medical, Dingwall, Scotland) capture signals from ingested radiopills and store the data in solid-state memory at 0.15 Hz (Fig. 15.6). These devices are primarily designed for pH measurement but, with modifications to the sampling rate, they, and other similar devices with larger memory, could be used to record motility information from pressure-sensitive radiocapsules.

Data handling and analysis

Telemetred signals may be displayed and recorded on chart recorders for on-line, real-time hard copy and stored on magnetic tape in analogue form, or digitally on computer for subsequent analysis.

Analysis of recordings is governed by the type of signal originally recorded and the degree of calculation required from the original data. Signals from pressure capsules depend on the site of recording and resultant traces have been analysed manually or digitized to enable some form of computer scoring. Various groups have devised semi-automated or automated analytical methods of analysis for motility and pH recordings (Reynolds et al 1986, Rogers & Misiewicz 1989, Emde et al 1990, Benson et al 1992).

APPLICATIONS

General considerations

For human studies, telemetry capsules are normally ingested untethered, freely passing through the gastrointestinal tract under normal peristalsis. Alternatively, capsules have been tethered either singly (Watson &

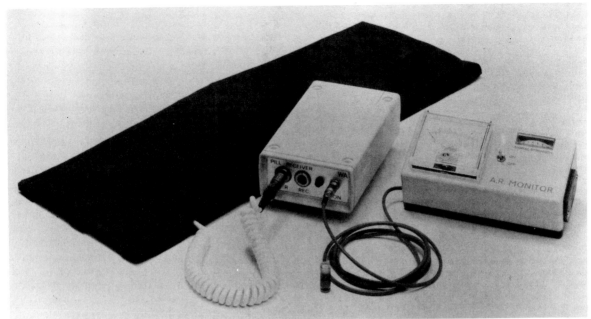

Fig. 15.5 Portable telemetry receiver and monitor unit. The aerial belt contains three aerials and the receiver has automated signal switching to achieve maximum signal capture. (Slater et al 1982)

Paton 1965, Thompson et al 1980, Evans et al 1984, Gilbert et al 1988) or using two or more capsules tied together (Evans et al 1982, Valori et al 1986). In theory, many capsules could be strung together like a 'string of pearls' allowing for multiple measurements along the whole length of the gut. Practically, the maximum number of sensors possible with the transmission characteristics of available capsules is three (Morris et al 1987), numbers being limited by the frequency separation necessary to allow for clear transmission of signals without interference between transducers.

Clearly, the most desirable use of radiopills is in ambulatory subjects. This offers totally non-invasive measurement without tubes or wires. However, interpretation of signals from a freely moving capsule depends on a knowledge of the position of the capsule within the gastrointestinal tract and also assumptions that the freely moving capsule will detect true pressure changes as would be monitored by a stationary device. This is of most relevance to capsules moving rapidly through the gut, as in the oesophagus and the small intestine (Fig. 15.7).

In other parts of the gut, such as the colon, movement of the luminal contents is infrequent due to the high proportion of segmental to peristaltic contractions. Pressure artefacts caused by movement are therefore unlikely to be a major consideration. Reynolds et al (1989) found that free-moving pressure-sensitive capsules remained in the right colon for up to 13 h (mean 8.6 h), demonstrating that movement is infrequent in the large bowel.

The remaining possibility for radiocapsules is to have them permanently or semipermanently implanted. Surgical implantation is possible, but such a procedure negates the attraction of the non-invasive nature of the method. Some studies have been performed in animal models (Dahlgren & Thoren 1967, Lincoln et al 1974) but no surgical implantation of radiopills has so far been reported in man. Our group have been investigating the feasibilty of long-term implantation of radiopills in the gut lumen using endoscopically controlled stapling devices (Swain et al 1989) and have recently reported, successful gastric implantation of a pH-sensitive radiocapsule for 3 months without complication (Swain et al 1992). Over 1000 h of recording were achieved using this technique and it appears feasible to adopt this methodology in other parts of the gastrointestinal tract.

Pressure-sensing applications

Oesophageal pressure

In their present form, pressure-sensitive radiotelemetry capsules are not suitable for oesophageal studies. Firstly, the pressure-sensitive diaphragm is end

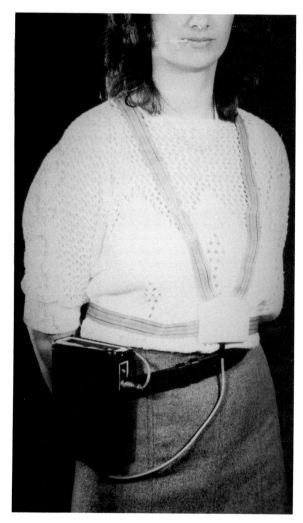

Fig. 15.6   Ambulatory digital storage pH recorder for use with pH telemetry capsule (Flexilog 1010, Oakfield Instruments, Oxon, Eynsham, Oxford). Aerial belts are worn around the chest or abdomen depending on the position of the capsules within the gastrointestinal tract.

poor understanding of the significance of motility patterns (Connell & Rowlands 1960, Misiewicz et al 1966). Classification of motility patterns in the 1970s (Szurszewski 1969, Vantrappen et al 1977) stimulated a new interest in the study of gastrointestinal motility including studies with telemetry.

The telemetry technique was regarded as being less invasive, more comfortable and less stressful than the classical tube methods, and in the 1980s some reports were published using the technique for physiological (Thompson et al 1980, Evans et al 1982) and pathological studies (Thompson et al 1979, Foster et al 1982).

Although the attraction of telemetry capsules was seen to be one of greater subject comfort and ease of positioning of transducers without the need for X-rays, in practice, this technique has all but been abandoned because of major operational difficulties. Problems have been encountered in obtaining sensors and there has been a general lack of the expertise required to operate equipment. The introduction of smaller, comfortable, tube mounted devices, such as multiple strain gauge catheters, and the use of portable digital recorders has largely overcome the need for tethered telemetry capsules for the measurement of gastrointestinal motility. Perhaps, with development of less invasive methods of implantation there may be a further revival of this application in the future.

Colon and rectum

The most attractive measurement modality using pressure radiocapsules in the gastrointestinal tract is in the colon and rectum. Due to general inaccessibility of the colon there have been few studies of motility in this area, especially in the caecum and right side of the colon. Consequently, our understanding of colonic motility remains incomplete. Animal studies have increased our knowledge of the physiology of the colon to some extent (Fioramonti et al 1980), but species differences in morphology and function have limited extrapolation of results to man. Tube-mounted sensors have been adopted by some investigators for studies in man, but the methodology used to place the tubes has limited their usefulness to short-term measurement in the left colon, although, recently, strain-gauge catheters have been used for ambulatory recordings.

A freely moving ingested telemetry capsule offers an attractive option in which pressures in both the right and left side of the colon may be measured as the capsule slowly passes through. If two or more capsules are swallowed 12 h apart, it is possible to measure pressures from the right and left side of the colon simultaneously. The technique is safe and without

mounted and may not accurately detect peristalsis from the circular muscle contractions of the oesophageal body. Secondly, the capsules would require tethering to prevent caudad movement into the stomach and this could cause severe discomfort to the patient, especially during swallows.

Gastric and small intestinal pressure

Telemetry is an attractive alternative to nasogastric intubation with tube-borne measuring devices for motility studies, but early studies were hindered by a

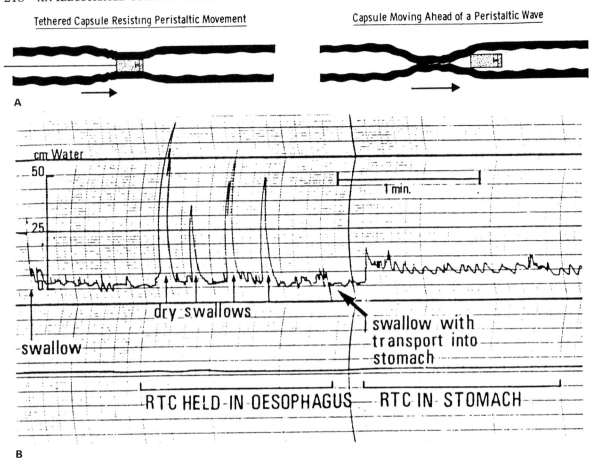

Fig. 15.7   Pressure waves recorded by a stationary tethered radiopill and the same pill moving freely with the oesophagus. **A** shows the difference between the two situations, and **B** illustrates differences in pressures recorded by the capsule when tethered and moving freely.

patient discomfort. The major disadvantages are that only one sensor is ever employed at any one site and capsules are untethered and will move with normal peristalsis. However, these problems have not prevented researchers from using the technique.

Holdstock and Misiewicz in the 1960s and 1970s made extensive measurements in the colon with a single, freely moving radiocapsule (Misiewicz et al 1966, Misiewicz 1968, Holdstock et al 1970). Their work was mainly involved with identification and classification of motility patterns. Wilson in 1975, attempted to examine the effect of surgery and anaesthesia on colonic ileus using a single untethered radiocapsule ingested prior to operation. Others have extended these studies using multiple radiocapsules (Morris et al 1987).

Recently, pressure telemetry has been used to measure colonic motility with conventional receiving equip-

ment and in ambulatory subjects using portable monitoring systems (Lamont et al 1987, Reynolds et al 1988, Jones et al 1989, Thorburn et al 1992). In general, measurements with a single untethered capsule are in agreement with laboratory based studies using standard tube methods. Reynolds described three levels of motility during 24-h periods of measurement. A basal or interdigestive period during daytime recording, a postprandial or meal-stimulated period and a nocturnal period. Figure 15.8 illustrates colonic motility in each of these states in an ambulant subject. Figure 15.9 summarizes levels of activity in a group of normal individuals and these show similar trends to the patterns of activity published by others using perfused tubes. Clearly no information about peristalsis is available using this technique, but as almost all of the contractions are segmental (Connell 1965), the information gathered by the telemetry method is still

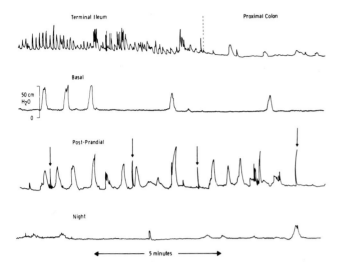

Fig. 15.8 Colonic motility patterns in interdigestive (basal), postprandial and nocturnal state in ambulatory subject using free-moving pressure-sensitive radiocapsule. The transition from ileum to caecum during phase III of migrating motor complex can be clearly seen. Arrows indicate signal loss or pressure artifact caused by gross body movement. (Reynolds et al 1989).

useful in defining colonic motor function. Thorburn and colleagues (1992), using a single untethered pressure radiocapsule, showed differences in motility response between the left and right side of the colon in a study of the effects of isphagula husk on colonic motility in diverticular disease. Measurements were made, without discomfort, in a group of elderly patients with chronic gastrointestinal disorders. It is unlikely that such patients would have been studied with standard tube methods.

With the advent of new technology, especially with the possibility of temporary implantation, improvements in methodology may be introduced in the future and studies may be possible with multiple capsules implanted at colonoscopy.

Rectal motility can be measured by inserting a radiopill into the rectum either with a finger or through a rigid sigmoidoscope (Lord 1963, Chattopadhay et al 1990). The technique has been used by few, as measurements can easily be made using conventional methods, without the complication of the telemetry. The passage of the radiopill through the anal canal at defaecation can also give useful information about straining and peak defaecatory pressures in conditions such as haemorrhoids, but to date this area has not been extensively studied.

Other

Pressure-sensitive radio capsules have been utilized to measure motility and related parameters in other parts of the digestive system. Mitchenere et al (1981)

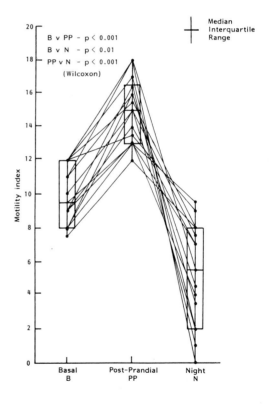

Fig. 15.9 Circadian levels of colonic motility as measured by pressure sensitive radiocapsule in ambulant subjects. Motility indices are from five healthy subjects studied on three occasions. Basal (**B**) is daytime interfood period, postprandial (**PP**) is 2 h after food and night (**N**) is during sleep period. (Reynolds et al 1989)

implanted a pressure sensitive radiopill in the gallbladder of pigs at laparotomy and recorded pressure profiles in the gallbladder lumen in response to drugs and food in the conscious animal.

Other researchers have used free fall pressure radiocapsules to measure intra-abdominal pressure changes as an indirect measure of stresses related to back injuries. Davis and Stubbs (1978) and Davis et al (1977), calculated safe levels of manual forces for various forms of weight lifting in manual workers by measurements of intragastric pressure (and thereby intra-abdominal pressure) induced by lifting. Although not specifically related to gastrointestinal motility, intra-abdominal and intragastric pressures are important as anti-reflux factors related to lower oesophageal sphincter (LOS) function and are therefore of interest to gastroenterologists.

Pressure-sensitive radiopills have also been used to measure contractile or intrinsic pressures in other motile organs. Vaginal (Fox et al 1970), uterine (Persianinov & Davydov 1971), bladder (Gleason et al 1965) and cranial pressures (Currie et al 1971) have all been studied by insertion or implantation of pressure capsules. Other sites are only limited by the ingenuity and imagination of budding telemetrists!

pH sensing applications

Upper gastrointestinal tract

pH-sensitive radiocapsules have been used for many years to investigate upper gastrointestinal pH in relation to acid secretion. As some of the conditions caused by gastric acid factors are thought to be related to or caused by motility disorders, e.g. gastro-oesophageal reflux (GOR) and antroduodenal hypomotility, it is relevant to discuss the technology in this section.

Oesophageal. The idea of a tethered pH-sensitive radiopill is not new. Fehr et al (1966) used a 'Heidelberg' capsule to assess LOS competence in patients with a hiatus hernia by performing a modified 'Tuttle' test. The tethered pH capsule was used to map pH profiles across the LOS as a guide to the severity of the hernia. Interest in oesophageal pH monitoring was revived in the late 1970s and early 1980s by the introduction of the concept of 24-h studies as a diagnostic indicator for gastro-oesophageal reflux disease (GORD) (DeMeester et al 1976). The introduction of ambulatory methods further stimulated the revival and an explosion of interest was evident by the number of research publications over the next 10 years (Evans 1987, Atkinson 1987). Telemetric methods for assess-

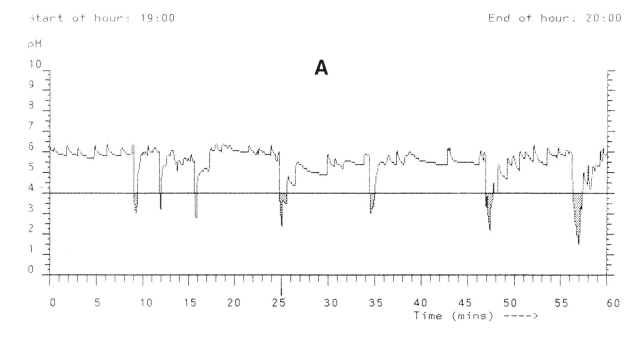

Start of hour: 19:00 End of hour: 20:00

Time (mins) ---->

Number of detected episodes = 5 Exposure time below pH 4.0 is 3 mins 48 secs

ment of GORD were among the first to advocate 24-h outpatient assessment (Branicki et al 1982, Vitale et al 1984). Figure 15.10 shows examples of GOR extracted from 24-h pH traces. Reflux and its correlation with symptoms can be clearly seen.

24-h pH monitoring is now regarded as the 'gold

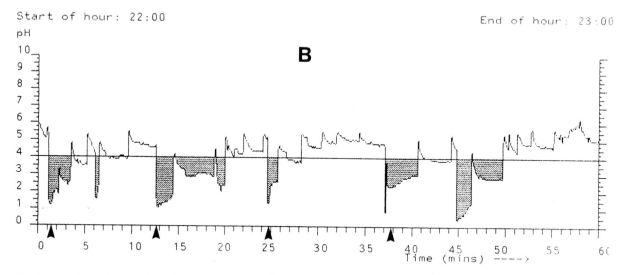

Number of detected episodes = 6 Exposure time below pH 4.0 is 25 mins 18 secs

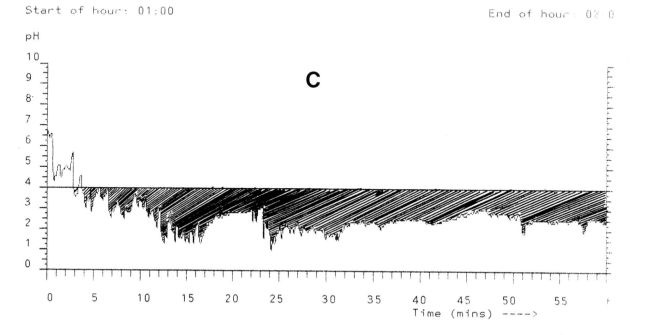

Number of detected episodes = 1 Exposure time below pH 4.0 is 56 mins 24 sec

Fig. 15.10 24-h pH profiles of a normal subject (**A**) and patients with mild (**B**) and severe (**C**) pathological GOR. An event marker (▲) correlates symptoms with reflux.

standard' investigation for the diagnosis and assessment of GORD in both adults and children. Equipment using telemetric methods is commercially available from two companies in the UK (Oakfield Instruments, Oxon, Eynsham, Oxford and Albyn Medical, Ross-shire, Scotland). Although the use of telemetry capsules has been largely superseded by smaller, less-expensive, semi-disposable pH electrodes, telemetry remains an option where electrodes are unsuitable or difficult to use. For example, some patients may not tolerate nasal intubation using an electrode but may find the swallowing of a tethered pH radiocapsule a more attractive alternative.

Gastrointestinal tract

Studies of gastric and duodenal pH using tethered radiocapsules were common in the late 1960s and early 1970s (Watson & Paton 1965, Williamson et al 1969). Capsules were swallowed on a suitable length of tethering material (usually silk or linen thread) and allowed to settle in the liquid pool of the stomach. Some studies used free-fall radiopills, relying on a long gastric residence time, to collect information about gastric acid secretion and duodenal pH (Staveny et al 1966, Yarborough et al 1969, Stack 1969). The major thrust of these early studies was to use the pH capsules as an alternative to gastric acid secretion tests. The technique lost its relevance as gastric secretion tests went out of vogue in the 1970s.

pH radiocapsules continue to be used by some researchers for gastric pH studies, particularly in long-term (24-h) measurements (Reynolds et al 1987, Patel et al 1992). This type of study has been stimulated by the need to have more detailed information about circadian patterns of gastric pH in relationship to acid suppression by acid blocking drugs.

The advantages conferred by telemetry over conventional glass electrodes are, patient acceptability (thin, braided, nylon tethers are more comfortable than electrode cables), cable-free measurement (ability to remove equipment to undress and shower etc.) and possibly more accurate representation of overall pH of the gastric pool. The latter because the radiopill on its flexible tether is more likely to maintain contact with gastric juice and also has a greater surface area of pH-

sensitive glass by comparison with standard pH electrodes and is less likely to become contaminated by food residue.

Small intestinal pH has also been measured with some success. One major advantage over glass electrodes is the ability to place the capsules at any site, without X-ray screening, the position being identified by the length of the tethering thread. Physiological studies have established normal levels in fasting and fed states (Watson & Paton 1965) and measurements have been made in diseases that affect small intestinal function, such as cystic fibrosis (Gilbert et al 1988), and after gastrointestinal surgery (Watson et al 1966).

There have been few studies using tethered pH radiocapsules in the colon due to the length of tether material required if capsules are introduced orally. Chattopadhay et al (1990), inserted a pH capsule into surgically refashioned rectums (ileal pouch) in patients with 'pouchitis' to examine pH profiles in relation to the inflammation in the pouch. Other possibilities exist but as yet have been untried.

Free-fall applications of pH capsules

pH-sensitive radio capsules may also be used as a free-moving pH sensor if allowed to pass unhindered through the gastrointestinal tract. Specific interests have driven researchers to use such a system to investigate total gastrointestinal pH or to concentrate on small areas. A major hurdle was a knowledge of the precise location of a free-fall pill as it tumbled through the gut lumen.

Early studies simply documented a total profile without much consideration of position. Meldrum et al (1972) were the first to document pH profiles along the whole length of the gut using a pH-sensitive radiocapsule. Whole gut pH profiles were measured on two normal controls and seven patients with 'miscellaneous gastrointestinal disorders'. The group extended these studies by investigating the effects of lactulose on ileal and caecal pH in normal subjects (Bown et al 1974). Studies were all performed in the laboratory as recording and receiving equipment at that time did not lend itself to ambulatory monitoring

Ambulatory studies of gastrointestinal pH were de-

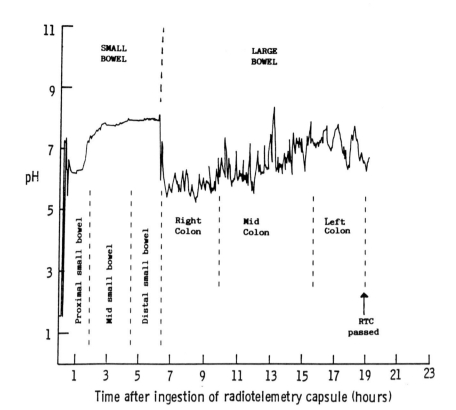

Fig. 15.11 Example of a gastrointestinal pH profile from a control subject. Important landmarks are gastric to duodenal transition (pH 1.5 to pH 6) and ileum to caecum transition (pH 8 to pH 6). (Evans et al 1988a)

veloped to examine the possibility of pH as a marker of colorectal cancer. The system consisted of a modified glass pH-sensitive radiotelemetry capsule (Remote Control Systems, London) (Colson et al 1981) and a commercially developed digital receiver/recorder (Medilog 1000, Oxford Medical Systems/Oakfield Instruments, Oxon, Eynsham, Oxford). The recorder sampled pH from the radiocapsule at 12 s intervals as it tumbled through the gastrointestinal tract. The maximum recording time of 48 h was sufficient for total gastrointestinal transit in most subjects. Capsule location was achieved by intermittent surface localization with a directional aerial connected to a hand-held receiver. Maximum signal strength pinpointed the position of the radiopill in the abdomen and this was documented on a body map divided into nine segments. Additional information was obtained from the recordings. The three important markers were the transition from stomach to duodenum, ileum to caecum and movement of the capsule from the right to the left iliac fossa signifying caecal to rectal movement. Figure 15.11 is an example of a normal pH profiles obtained from a study where over 70 subjects were examined in

an attempt to establish normal ranges. Detailed methodology and normal values can be found elsewhere (Evans et al 1988a,b).

This method has been adopted to examine pH profiles in various gastrointestinal diseases in order to use pH as a possible marker of specific pathology (Gilbert et al 1988, Evans et al 1988a, Pye et al 1990, Raimundo et al 1992).

Gastrointestinal pH profiles are also of growing interest to the pharmaceutical industry in the area of targeting drugs to specific areas of the gastrointestinal tract by the use of pH-dependent polymer coatings.

Implantation

The remaining option in the use of pH-sensitive radiopills is temporary or long-term implantation in the gastrointestinal tact. pH sensors can be implanted at most sites in the gut of animal models at open surgery by suturing them into the gastrointestinal lumen with non-absorbable material. Used in this way capsules will transmit usable data for the duration of the battery life (with modern capsules typically up to 3 months) (Alday & Goldsmith 1975).

In man, implantation of telemetry devices has not been common, but with the introduction of less invasive endoscopically controlled clip fixing devices and stapling machines there may be as yet undiscovered uses for pH telemetry. McLauchlan et al (1989), showed considerable regional variations in gastric body and antral pH by clipping two pH-sensitive electrodes to the gastric mucosa during upper gastrointestinal endoscopy using a commercially available clip fixing device (Olympus HX-2L). Studies such as this may modify the approach to measurement of gastric pH, demonstrating a requirement for more than one sensor to obtain representative values of pH in the stomach.

Swain and colleagues (1992), have recently demonstrated the feasibility of long-term implantation of a pH-sensitive radiopill in the stomach in man. A single pH capsule was implanted in the gastric body of its inventor using an endoscopic transmural 'stapling machine' during upper gastrointestinal endoscopy. The capsule remained in situ for 108 days without complication and was removed endoscopically only after the capsule battery had failed. There was no evidence of inflammation or ulceration at the implantation site and there was no discomfort or pain to the subject. A total of 1200 h of recording were achieved using a portable pH recorder, demonstrating the usefulness of the technique. It remains to be seen whether this technique proves safe and useful and becomes adopted by the medical community.

Transit

Ingested, untethered radiotelemetry capsules in all forms behave like a large undigestible object moving through the gut. Although the transit time of such an object may not be identical to the semi-liquid content of the small intestine or the solid content of the distal colon, this has not deterred researchers from utilizing the technology in this area of study.

Early studies (Waller 1975) used a pressure-sensitive radiocapsule labelled with μCi of ^{51}Cr and plotted gastrointestinal transit with a collimated scintillation counter. Pressure patterns from the capsule aided localization by identification of the different pressure profiles observed in the stomach and small and large intestine. Figure 15.12 shows the different pressure patterns generated by the stomach, small intestine and caecum during fasting and after food. These patterns can be used to identify the transition from one gut compartment to another and, when plotted against time, can also be used as a measure of transit.

Other studies have utilized pH capsules, with or without radiolabels to plot movement of luminal content within the gastrointestinal tract (Mojaverian et al 1989, Hardy et al 1991, Coupe et al 1991). The technique relies on the distinctive and reproducible pH changes seen during transition from stomach to small intestine and terminal ileum to caecum (Bown et al 1974, Evans et al 1988a) which can be easily detected by the pH capsule and used to assess gastric residence time and small intestinal transit (Figure 15.11).

Pharmaceutical scientists have made particular use of this type of information in studies focused on the targeting of drug dosage forms at particular sites in the gut (Hardy et al 1991, Coupe et al 1991). A new approach is to coat tablets with an enteric resistant polymer which dissolves at a specific pH. By using such coatings, drugs can theoretically be delivered to specific distal gastrointestinal sites, for example, the delivery of 5 ASA compounds to the colon in inflammatory bowel conditions. Telemetry is likely to be of continuing interest in the evaluation of novel drug-targeting experiments of this kind.

SUMMARY

The utilization of radiotelemetry technology as a measurement system in the gastrointestinal tract has been a specialized science since its conception in the 1960s. Utilization of the technique for medical and scientific research has waxed and waned, depending to a large degree on the efforts of small groups of enthusiasts, supply of appropriate hardware and an imaginative approach to potential applications. It is unlikely that this technique will ever see widespread use unless good clinical applications are found that are better than, or at least equal to, existing methods for data gathering. The technology should also be less invasive and as technically easy to use as current methods.

If medical telemetry is ever going to advance into the twenty-first century, a number of inputs are essential. Research and development into new devices using 1990s technology will require large sums of money and the committment of large corporate organizations to support such development. The developer would need to have strong links with the end user, who will ultimately determine the direction that the development will follow. New enthusiasm might, perhaps, be generated with the possibility of safe, minimally-invasive endoscopic implantation of radiocapsules. The medical and scientific world awaits this concept with interest. Until this happens, the radiopill is likely to remain a novelty in the hands of a few enthusiasts!

FASTING MOTILITY   POST-PRANDIAL   MOTILITY

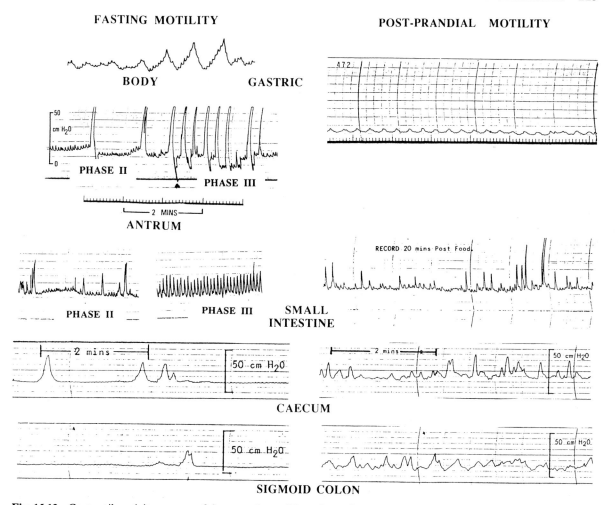

Fig. 15.12 Contractile activity patterns of the stomach, small intestine and caecum. The amplitude, duration and frequency of the pressure waves during fasted and fed state, recorded by a free-fall pressure radiocapsule, can be used to differentiate stomach, small intestine and colon.

REFERENCES

Alday E S, Goldsmith H S 1975 Radiotelemetric monitoring of H ion levels of the small intestine (in dogs). Surg Gynecol Obstet 141: 549–551

Atkinson M 1987 Monitoring oesophageal pH. Gut 28: 509–514

Benson M J, Castillo F D, Demitrakopolous J, Spyro N, Wingate D L 1993 The computer as referee in small bowel motility analysis. Am J Physiol (in press)

Bown R L, Gibson J A, Sladen G E, Hicks B, Dawson A M 1974 Effects of lactulose and other laxatives on ileal and colonic pH as measured by a radiotelemetry device. Gut 15: 999–1004

Branicki F J, Evans D F, Ogilvie A L, Atkinson M, Hardcastle J D 1982 Ambulatory monitoring of oesophageal pH in reflux oesophagitis using a portable radiotelemetry system. Gut 23: 992–998

Browning C, Valori R, Wingate D L, MacLachlan D 1981 A new pressure-sensitive ingestible radiotelemetric capsule. Lancet 2(8245): 504–505

Browning C, Valori R M, Wingate D L 1983 Receiving, decoding and noise limiting systems for a new pressure-sensitive ingestible radio telemetric capsule. J Biomed Eng 5(3): 262–266

Chattopadhay G, Kumar D, Keighley M R B, Oya M 1990 Ileal pouch pH: a regulatory mechanism for evacuation Gut 31: A1171

Cheadle W G, Vitale G C, Sadek S A, Cuschieri A 1988 Computerized ambulatory esophageal pH monitoring in 50 asymptomatic volunteer subjects. Results and clinical implications. Am J Surg 155(3): 503–508

Colson R H, Watson B W, 1979 Improved techniques in the construction of pH sensitive radio pills in: Almaner C J, MacDonald D W (eds) A handbook on biotelemetry and radio tracking. Pergamon Press, Oxford pp 209–227

Colson R H, Watson B W, Fairclough P D et al 1981 An

accurate long-term pH sensitive radio pill for ingestion and implantation. Biotelem Patient Monit 8: 213–217

Connell A M 1965 Significance of the pressure waves of the sigmoid colon. Am J Dig Dis 10: 455–462

Connell A M, Rowlands E N 1960 Wireless telemetry from the digestive tract. Gut 1: 266–272

Coupe A J, Davis S S, Evans D F, Wilding I R 1991 Correlation of the gastrointestinal transit of non-disintegrating tablets with gastrointestinal motility. Pharm Res 8: 1281–1285

Currie J C M, Riddle H C, Watson B W 1971 The use of telemetry to study the physiological and clinical variations in intracranial pressure in man in: Stott F D (ed.) Biotelemetry, (Proc. Int. Symposium on Biotelemetry) Meauder, Nijmegen pp 326–331

Dahlgren S, Thoren L 1967 Intestinal motility in low small bowel obstruction, Acta Chir Scand 133: 417–421

Davis P R, Stubbs D J 1978 Safe levels of manual forces for young males. Applied Ergonomics 9(1): 33–37

Davis P R, Stubbs O A, Ridd J 1977 Radio pills: their use in monitoring back stress. J Med Eng Technol 1: 209–212

DeMeester T R, Johnson L F, Joseph G J, Toscano M S, Hall A W, Skinner D B 1976 Patterns of gastroesophageal reflux in health and disease, Ann Surg, 184: 459–470

Edholm O G, Fox R H, Wolff H S 1973 Body temperature during exercise and rest in cold and hot climates. Arch du Sci Physiol 27: 339–345

Emde C, Armstrong D, Bumm R, Kaufhold H J, Riecken E O, Blum A L 1990 Twenty four hour continuous ambulatory measurement of oesophageal pH and pressure: a digital recording system and computer aided manometry analysis. J Ambul Monit 3: 47–62

Evans D F 1987 Ambulatory oesophageal pH monitoring-an update, Br J Surg 74: 157–161

Evans D F, Foster G E, Hardcastle J D 1982 The motility of the human antrum and jejenum during the day and during sleep. An investigation using a radiotelemetry system in: Wienbeck M (ed.) Motility of the digestive tract. Raven Press, New York pp 185–193

Evans D F, Foster G E, Hardcastle J D 1984 Does exercise affect gastrointestinal motility in man? in: Roman C (ed.) Proc. of IX Int. Symp. on Gastrointestinal Motility. MTP Press, Lancaster pp 272–284

Evans D F, Pye G, Bramley R, Clark A G, Dyson T J, Hardcastle J D 1988 Measurement of gastrointestinal pH in normal ambulant human subjects. Gut 29: 1035–1041

Evans D F, Pye G, Opare-Sem P, Kotoh S, nii-Amon Kotei D 1988 Is colorectal cancer risk increasing in urban Ghanaians? Ghana Med J 22: 8–16

Farrar J T, Zworykin V K, Baum J 1957 Pressure sensitive telemetry for study of gastrointestinal motility. Science 126: 975–976

Fehr H, Staveney L S, Hamilton T, Sircus W, Smith A N 1966 Hiatal hernia investigated by pH telemetry. Am J Dig Dis 10: 747–752

Fioramonti J, Garci-Villar R, Bueno L, Ruckebusch Y 1980 Colonic myoelectrical activity and propulsion in the dog. Dig Dis Sci 25: 641–646

Foster G E, Arden-Jones J R, Beattie A, Evans D F, Hardcastle J D 1982 Abnormal motility and gastrointestinal disease. The 'Q' complex in: Wienbeck M (ed.) Motility of the digestive tract. Raven Press, New York pp 427–433

Fox C A, Wolff H S, Baker J A, 1970 Measurement of intra-vaginal and intrauterine pressures during human coitus

by radiotelemetry. J Reprod Fertil 227: 243–251

Gilbert J, Kelleher J, Littlewood J, Evans D F 1988 Ileal pH in cystic fibrosis. Sc J Gastroenterol 23(suppl): 132–134

Gleason D M, Lattimer J K, Bauxbaum C 1965 Bladder pressure telemetry. J Urology 94: 252–256

Hardy J G, Lamont G L, Evans D F, Haga A K, Gamst O N 1991 Evaluation of an enteric-coated naproxen pellet formulation. Aliment Pharmacol Therap 5: 69–75

Holdstock D J, Misiewicz J J, Smith T, Rowlands E W 1970 Propulsion in the human colon and its relationship to meals and somatic activity. Gut 11: 19–31

Jacob R, Riddle H, Watson B W 1973 Circuit for searching for a signal from a three aerial system during induction loop telemetry. Biomed Eng 8: 292–295

Jacobson B, Mackay R S 1957 A pH endoradiosonde. Lancet 269: 1224

Jones V, Evans D F, Lamont G, Watson R, Macpherson M 1989 The effect of Didrogesterone on colonic motility and transit in women with premenstrual syndrome (PMT). Gut 30: A1464

Kumar D, Soffer E E, Wingate D L, Britto J, Das-Gupta A, Mridha K 1989 Modulation of the duration of human post-prandial motor activity by sleep. Am J Physiol 256: G851–G859

Lambert A, Crenner F, Schang J C, Scmitt S, Grenier J K 1982 A new intraluminal autonomous capsule to be swallowed for recording the electrical and mechanical activity of the intestine in dog and in man in: Wienbeck M (ed.) Motility of the gastrointestinal tract. Raven Press, New York pp 251–255

Lamont G L, Evans D F, Reynolds J R 1987 Symptoms of IBS and objective measurements of large bowel function. Gut 28: 1321

Lincoln D W, Boer K, Swaab D 1974 Measurement of intramammary pressure in rats by a pressure sensitive radio pill. Physiol Behav 12: 289–292

Lord P H 1973 A treatment of third degree haemorrhoids. Br J Hosp Med 6: 347–350

Mackay R S, Jacobson B 1957 Endoradiosonde. Nature 179: 1239–1240

McLauchlan G, Fullarton G M, Grean G P, McCol K E L 1989 Comparison of gastric body and antral pH: a 24 hour ambulatory study in healthy volunteers. Gut 30: 573–578

Meldrum S J, Watson B W, Riddle H C, Sladen G E, Bown R L 1972 pH profile of gut as measured by radiotelemetry capsule. BMJ 2: 104–106

Misiewicz J J 1968 Measurement of intraluminal pressures. Radiotelemetry, design of manometric studies and computer analysis of records. Am J Dig Dis 13: 389–396

Misiewicz J J, Waller S L, Eisner M 1966 Motor responses of the human gastrointestinal tract to 5-HT in vivo and in vitro. Gut 7: 208–217

Mitchenere P, Adrian T E, Hobbs K E F, Bloom S R 1981 The effects of caerulein and a meal stimulation on gallbladder intraluminal pressure and bile flow in pigs. Br J Surg 68: 154–157

Mojaverian P, Chan K, Desai A, John V 1989 gastrointestinal transit of a solid indigestible capsule as measured by radiotelemetry and dual gamma scintigraphy. Pharmaceutical Research 6: 719–724

Moller U, Bojsen J 1975 Temperature and blood flow measurements in and around 7, 12 Dimethylbenz (a) anthracene induced tumours and Walker 256 carcinosarcomas in rats. Canc Res 35: 3116–3121

Morris D L, Clark A G, Evans D F, Hardcastle J D (1987) Triple radiotelemetric pill study of post-operative ileus. Digestive Surgery 4: 160–163

Noller H G 1962 Results of examination of stomach function with the Heidelberg capsule. Fortsch Med 9: 351

Patel N, Ward U, Rogers M J, Primrose J N 1992 Nighttime and morning dosing with H_2-receptor antagonists: studies on acid inhibition in normal subjects. Aliment Pharmacol Ther 6: 381–387

Persianinov L S, Davydov S N 1971 A radiotelemetric study of uterine activity in labour. Act Obstet Gynecol Serd 50: 269–273

Pye G, Evans D F, Ledingham S J, Hardcastle J D 1990 Gastrointestinal intraluminal pH in normal subjects and those with colorectal adenoma or carcinoma. Gut 31: 1355–1358

Raimundo A H, Evans D F, Rogers J, Jameson J, Silk D B A 1992 Intestinal pH in ulcerative colitis: acute (untreated) and in remission on 5 ASA: Gut 33 (supp): S63

Rawlings J M, Lucas M L 1985 Plastic pH electrodes for the measurement of gastrointestinal pH. Gut 26: 203–207

Reynolds J R, Evans D F, Hillier J, Hardcastle J D 1986 Analysis of ambulatory colonic motility records using a BBC (B) microcomputer. J Med Comp 9: 129–134

Reynolds J R, Walt R P, Clarke A G, Hardcastle J D Langman M J S 1987 Intragastric pH monitoring in acute upper GI bleeding and the effects of intravenous cimetidine and ranitidine. Aliment Pharmacol Ther 1: 23–30

Reynolds J R, Evans D F, Clark A G, Hardcastle J D 1988 The effect of mebeverine, isphagula husk and combination therapy on colonic motor activity in healthy men studied using a portable radiotelemetey system. J Amb Monit 1: 223–232

Reynolds J R, Evans D F, Clarke A G, Hardcastle J D 1989 Reproduciblity and variation of 24 hour ambulatory colonic motility in normal subjects. J Amb Monit 2: 303–312

Rogers J R, Misiewicz J J 1989 Fully automated computer analysis of intracolonic pressures. Gut 30: 642–649

Schpel S J, de Rooij N F, Koning G, Oesburg B, Zijlistra W G 1984 In vivo experiments with ISFET electrodes. Med Biol Eng Comput 22: 6–11

Schlesinger P K, Donahue P E, Schmid B, Layden T J 1985 Limitations of 24-hour intraoesophageal pH monitoring in the hospital setting. Gastroenterology 89: 797–804

Slater E J, Evans D F, Foster G E, Hardcastle J D 1982 A portable radiotelemetry receiver for ambulatory monitoring. Biomed Eng 4: 247–251

Stack B H R 1969 Use of the Heidelberg pH capsule in the routine assessment of gastric acid secretion. Gut 10: 245–246

Staveney L S, Hamilton M B, Sircus M D, Smith A N 1966 Evaluation of the pH sensitive telemetering capsule in the estimation of gastric secretory capacity. Am J Dig Dis 11: 753–760

Steele R J C, Ledingham S J, Iftikhar S Y, Hardcastle J D 1991 Redox potential in the lower oesophagus. Gut 32: A585

Stirrup V, Ledingham S J, Thomas M, Pye G, Evans D F 1990 Measurement of redox potentials in the GI tract in man. Gut 31: A1171

Swain C P, Brown G, Mills T N 1989 An endoscopic stapling device: development of a new flexible endoscopically controlled device for placing multiple transmural staples in gastrointestinal tissue. Gastrointest Endosc 35: 338–339

Swain C P, Evans D F, Glynn M, Brown G, Mills T 1992 Endoscopic sewing machine used to achieve continuous non-invasive monitoring of gastric pH for three months in man. Gastrointest Endosc 38: 278

Szurszewski J H 1969 A migrating electric complex of the canine small intestine. Am J Physiol 217: 1757–1763

Thompson D G, Laidlow J M, Wingate D L 1979 Abnormal small bowel motility demonstrated by radiotelemetry in a patient with irritable colon. Lancet 1321–1323

Thompson D G, Wingate D L, Archer L, Benson M J, Green J, Hardy R J 1980 Normal patterns of human upper small bowel motor activity recorded by prolonged radiotelemetry. Gut 21: 500–506

Thorburn H A, Carter K B, Goldberg J A, Findlay I G 1989 Remote control systems radiotelemetry receiver: its use in colonic motility measurement. J Med Eng Technol 15: 252–256

Thorburn H A, Carter K B, Goldberg J A, Findlay I G 1992 Does isphagula husk stimulate the entire colon in diverticular disease? Gut 33: 352–356

Valori R M, Kumar D, Wingate D L 1986 Effects of different types of stress and of prokinetic drugs on the control of the fasting motor complex in humans. Gastroenterology 90: 1890–1900

Valori R M 1988 Radiotelemetry in: Kumar D, Wingate D L (eds) Illustrated guide to gastrointestinal motility, 2nd edn. Wiley, Chichester pp 77–80

Vantrappen G, Janssens J, Peters T L 1977 The interdigestive migrating motor complex of normal subjects and patients with bacterial overgrowth. J Clin Invest 59: 1158–1166

Vitale G C, Cheadle W G, Sadek S A, Michel M E, Cuchieri A 1984 Computerised 24 hour pH monitoring and esophagogastroduodenoscopy in the reflux patient. Ann Surg 200: 724–728

Waller S L 1975 Differential measurement of small and large bowel transit times in constipation and diarrhoea: a new approach. Gut 16: 372–378

Watson B W 1981 Clinical uses of radio pills. Br J Hosp Med 25: 618–624

Watson B W, Ross B, Kay A W 1962 Telemetering from within the body using a pressure sensitive radio pill. Gut 3: 181–186

Watson W C, Paton E 1965 Studies on intestinal pH by radiotelemetry. Gut 6: 606–612

Watson W C, Watt J K, Paton E, Glen A, Lewis G J T 1966 Radiotelemetry studies of jejunal pH before and after vagotomy and gastroenterostomy. Gut 7: 700–705

Williamson J M, Russell R J, Goldberg A 1969 A screening technique for the detection of achlohydria using the Heidelberg capsule. Scand J Gastroenterol 4: 369–375

Wilson J P 1975 Post operative motility of the large intestine in man. Gut 16: 689–692

Wolff H S 1961 The radiopill. New Scientist 261: 419–421

Worrell D W, Watson B W, Shelley T 1963 Intravesical pressure measurement in women during movement using a radio pill and air probe. J Obs & Gyn. 70: 957–967

Yarborough D R, McAlhany J C, Cooper N, Weidner Jr M G 1969 Evaluation of the Heidelberg capsule. Method of tubeless gastric analysis. Am J Surgery 117: 185–192

16. Radioscintigraphy

K. Harding   A. Notghi

INTRODUCTION

Nuclear medicine tests have contributed much to the understanding of gastrointestinal motility (Harding & Robinson 1991). The radiation dose is smaller than for conventional radiology, particularly for prolonged studies, and because gamma cameras are linked to digital computers quantification is relatively easy. However, compared with conventional radiology, computerized tomography, ultrasound or magnetic resonance imaging, the resolution of scintigraphic tests is relatively poor, but this is far outweighed by the functional information which is available. For most tests the patient needs to starve for at least 4 h, but other preparation is minimal, and reactions to radiopharmaceuticals are rare. Intubation is rarely required.

The radioactive tracer moving backwards and forwards in the stomach or in loops of bowel causes problems in quantification because isotope near the camera is detected more efficiently. This complication can largely be overcome by using the geometric mean of an anterior and a posterior detector. Geometric mean is calculated as ($\sqrt{}$(anterior x posterior counts)), and this parameter is virtually depth independent (Hardy & Perkins 1985). Generally, a double-headed camera is not available, so most departments collect alternate anterior and posterior views. It is usual to take both gamma camera pictures and simultaneous digital computer pictures. The gamma camera pictures, which may be analogue or digital, are important for positioning the patient and for checking computer-derived data. More important in motility studies is the data acquired using the computer. Regions of interest (ROI) may be drawn round portions of the gut and their emptying or filling pattern determined.

Choice of radionuclide

Several radionuclides are used in scintigraphy and these are chosen because they have no beta emission, and therefore a low radiation dose. The most readily available and commonly used is ^{99m}Tc, which has a half-life of 6 h. It has a gamma energy of 140 keV, which is particularly suitable for radionuclide imaging. This energy is close to ideal because the gamma rays are not easily absorbed in the patient, but are readily detected using a gamma camera. In many tests of gastrointestinal function a longer half-life radionuclide is required, or a second isotope. In this case it is usual to use ^{111}In, which has a 2.8 day half-life and two gamma energies of 250 and 170 keV. Unfortunately it interferes to some extent with ^{99m}Tc detection because of scatter into the ^{99m}Tc window especially of the 170 keV photons. The extent of this scatter varies with depth within the patient, which changes as the markers travel through the gastrointestinal tract. Yet another radionuclide, ^{113m}In, has been used but is now difficult to obtain. This has a relatively high gamma energy of 390 keV and a short half-life of 1.7 h.

Dosimetry

Dosimetry in scintigraphic procedures is shown in Table 16.1. Effective dose equivalent (EDE) is a whole body dose which takes into account both the radiation dose and the sensitivity of different organs in the body. It allows comparison of nuclear medicine tests with radiological ones, although in the latter case much of the radiation is absorbed by the skin. With many studies the EDE is less than 2 mSv, and comparable to background radiation level. Table 16.2 shows the EDE from a variety of radiological procedures, and it can be seen that these are generally higher than those in Table 16.1, especially for barium studies or computerized tomography. It should also be noted that the figure for screening is the radiation dose per minute and for some studies, for example videoproctography, screening may continue for several minutes.

Comparison with yearly background figures is a difficult concept and an alternative way of looking at the information is in terms of risks. Table 16.3 shows

Table 16.1 Radiation dosimetry for nuclear medicine studies

Radio-nuclide	Study	Administered activity MBq	Radiation dose EDE–mSv
^{99m}Tc	Oesophageal	40	1
^{99m}Tc	Gastric emptying	12	0.3
^{111}In	Gastric emptying	12	3.6
^{99m}Tc	Biliary-HIDA	150	2
^{111}In	Colonic transit	2	0.8
^{99m}Tc	Defaecography	200	0.3

(Source: Department of Health 1992)

Table 16.2 Radiation dose for radiological procedures

Study	Radiation dose EDE–mSv
Abdominal film	1.4
Barium meal	3.8
Barium enema	7.7
Cholecystogram	1.2
CT abdomen	8.8
CT pelvis	9.4
Screening	1.0/min

Shrimpton 1988, Womack & O'Connell 1991, Shrimpton et al 1991

Table 16.3 A comparison of radiation risks with those in everyday life

1–2 mSv	Natural background radiation in a year
2 mSv	Travelling 300 miles by car
5 mSv	Drinking 1 glass of wine a day for 1 year
10 mSv	Travelling 500 miles by motorcycle
10 mSv	Chance of the average person of 30 dying in any 2-month period

Harding & Robinson 1991

some risks taken in everyday life and the equivalent EDE (Shields & Lawson 1987). It is clear that the radiation risk of imaging is small compared with those risks which are accepted by many people, and more important, with the risk of an adult dying from any cause.

OESOPHAGEAL TRANSIT AND REFLUX

Oesophageal disease causes chest pain, and in some patients this may be difficult to differentiate from that of myocardial ischaemia. Barium studies are generally used to show motility or reflux, and on endoscopy the inflammatory response to reflux is evident. These studies are also important to exclude structural changes, especially when the patient also has dysphagia. The test which many believe definitive for reflux is to use ambulatory pH monitoring.

Oesophageal transit

Protocol

Radionuclide oesophageal studies were first described by Katzem (1972), and Kaul et al in 1985 suggested that scintigraphy was more sensitive than radiology or pH monitoring in detecting episodes of reflux. Scintigraphy has the advantage of being physiological, non-invasive, and the equipment required is available in the average district hospital, unlike that used for manometry. For oesophageal transit studies the patient is usually studied in the supine position initially, although if transit is delayed repeat images are taken in the sitting position so that the added effect of gravity can be investigated. A ^{99m}Tc label is used, and this may be attached to diethylene-triamine-pentacetic-acid (DTPA) for a liquid swallow or sulphur colloid in scrambled egg for a semi-solid test medium. The patient is asked to take a swallow of 20–40 MBq in a volume of 10–20 ml and then not swallow for the next 30 s. Subsequently a further swallow of radiopharmaceutical is undertaken followed by a dry swallow at 15 s. This test has poor reproducibility, and some authors recommend that up to six swallows are undertaken in order to assess the patient properly (Bartlett 1986).

Data analysis

The oesophagus is divided into upper, middle and lower thirds, taking care not to involve the stomach in the lower third. The total oesophageal transit time is normally less than 9 s with upper, middle and lower third transit times of 1, 2 and 6 s respectively.

Results

Various patterns of oesophageal motility disorder have been described. In the adynamic oesophagus such as occurs with scleroderma or achalasia there is decreased movement throughout the three regions with an incoordinate fragmentation of the bolus. Achalasia classically shows hold-up in the lower third of the oesophagus. Reflux from the stomach may also be demonstrated. The easiest way to present the images is as a condensed dynamic sequence as described by Svedberg (1982). Essentially each image is compressed along the X axis and presented as a thin vertical strip. This strip is then placed adjacent to the strip for the

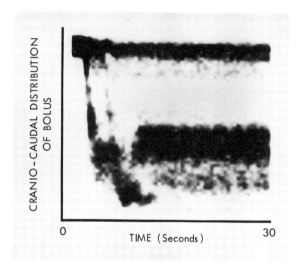

Fig. 16.1 Functional image of a normal swallow. Time scale 30 s, Y-axis corresponds to the length of the oesophagus with the oral cavity at the top and gastric fundus at the bottom (Harding & Robinson 1991).

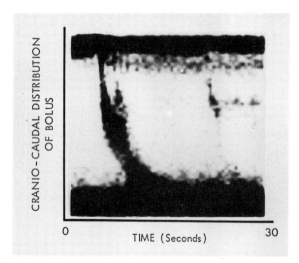

Fig. 16.2 Functional image of a patient with reflux, showing hold up of the swallowed bolus in mid and lower oesophagus after a normal peristaltic wave has passed (Harding & Robinson 1991).

next frame and a composite picture is produced showing the transit of the radiopharmaceutical down the oesophagus. Thus the set of frames acquired during the study is compressed into a single image. An example is shown in Figures 16.1 and 16.2.

GASTRO-OESOPHAGEAL REFLUX

Protocol

Radionuclides can be used to show reflux from the stomach into the oesophagus or indeed into the lung. The radiopharmaceutical is again either sulphur colloid or DTPA labelled with a ^{99m}Tc and the administered activity up to 40 MBq. It is incorporated into acidified orange juice, the acid being present to delay gastric emptying. The patient may be imaged lying or semi-recumbent. In a semi-recumbent position only one episode of reflux, of duration less than 20 s is expected during a 40 min study.

Alternative tests

Alternatively the radiopharmaceutical is given in the evening and the lung imaged the following morning to show gastro-pulmonary reflux. This test is now rarely used. In children a modification of the test has been used where radiolabelled milk is given and the child is imaged the following morning. Thirdly the so-called binder test (Fisher et al 1976) is a modification of the gastro-oesophageal reflux test. Essentially an abdominal binder is applied and the pressure increased in steps of 20 mm from 0–100 mmHg. Most departments consider this test unphysiological, and although the original authors found the test sensitive and accurate, others have not achieved consistently good results.

GASTRIC EMPTYING

Whole stomach emptying

Gastric emptying tests have mainly been used to assess patients after peptic ulcer surgery. Such patients may be difficult to assess from their symptoms and objective measurements of emptying allow gastric stasis or dumping to be proved. Indeed the two conditions may coexist. In addition, gastric emptying has a useful place in children with persistent vomiting or who fail to thrive and have other negative investigations. It has also been used to evaluate the effect of drugs or surgery on emptying, delayed emptying in diabetics and evaluating its treatment with erythromycin, and the result of surgery in patients with obesity having gastric operations to reduce the capacity of the stomach.

Protocol

Patients should be fasted, and alcohol and cigarettes avoided prior to the test. Many different meals incorporating a non-absorbable marker have been used to examine gastric emptying. Meyer et al (1976) injected chickens with colloid, and then subsequently removed their liver, cooked it and used it as a meal for measuring gastric emptying. While this technique is elegant it is quite unnecessary for routine gastric emptying studies. The important points in choosing a meal are that there is both a liquid and solid component and the meal is standardized (Donovan & Harding 1986), as the rate of gastric emptying depends on the volume of the meal, the calorie and fat content and the size of particles. Some centres do liquid and solid meal emptying on separate days, and others use a dual isotope technique usually with ^{99m}Tc and ^{111}In. The most commonly used non-absorbable markers have been DTPA and colloids. Gravity affects gastric emptying, particularly after gastric operations, and it is important that the position in which the patient is studied is also standardized. In the lying position abnormalities may not be detected.

Data acquisition

It is usual to collect computer frames at 1–5 min intervals, and camera pictures of the study are taken every 5 min. With a liquid meal it is only necessary to continue the study for 40 min, whereas with solid meals 90 min is preferable (Harding & Robinson 1991). Data recording should begin as soon as the patient starts the meal because there is often early emptying prior to the peak counts in the stomach being achieved, and early emptying is an important parameter of gastric motility. It is useful to place ^{57}Co markers on the iliac crests so that the patient can be repositioned accurately, particularly when alternate posterior and anterior pictures are taken in order to determine the geometric mean of counts in the stomach. The counts in the whole field of view of the camera are proportional to the meal volume, and this allows the volume of meal remaining in the stomach to be plotted against time (Harding & Donovan 1988). When dual isotopes are used it is important to correct the data for down scatter from the higher energy isotope (usually ^{111}In) into the lower energy window (usually ^{99m}Tc).

In addition, because of scatter, counts from the stomach may be detected outside the stomach ROI, and a correction may need to be applied (Donovan & Harding 1986).

Data analysis

It is conventional to fit a linear or logarithmic line to the emptying data of the stomach. Many departments use a logarithmic curve, but some argue that with liquid meals the curve is more nearly linear. With logarithmic methods, data points at that less than 25% of the peak volume in the stomach should be discarded, because at this stage the counts from the stomach are very low and subject to a number of errors, and in any case the bulk of the meal has by then emptied (Harding & Donovan 1988). Particularly with solid meals a lag phase may be apparent, when no emptying occurs. This is mainly due to meal moving anteriorly from the fundus of the stomach to the antrum where it is detected more efficiently.

In some departments the time for half of the meal to empty is used (T50%). This parameter gives no information about early emptying which is an important consideration in patients with dumping.

Results

The two common disorders detected using this technique are dumping and stasis. Dumping is associated with rapid early emptying and a reduced peak volume in the stomach. With a meal volume of 400 ml, approximately one third of the patients with a peak volume of less than 240 ml would have symptoms of dumping. Surprisingly the other two-thirds seem unaffected by this rapid emptying. With stasis approximately half the patients with a $T\frac{1}{2}$ of 150 min are symptomatic. Those who have had ulcer surgery tend to have abnormal gastric emptying results, with the older Polya operation causing both a reduced peak volume in the stomach and delayed emptying. The more selective operations result in less abnormality of emptying (Donovan & Harding 1986).

Difficulties with the test

The only restriction of the test is in those with large stomachs where the stomach may overlap the bowel. In such patients alternative techniques such as intubation have to be used (Wolverson et al 1982). Other important points which have already been described are relating counts to volume in order to detect early emptying, forward movement of the meal and scatter.

Fundal and antral emptying

This is a variant of the gastric emptying test where fundal and antral emptying are examined separately. In most patients a transverse band is apparent across the stomach in isotope gastric emptying studies, and

Fig. 16.3   Gastric emptying study showing clear distinction of the fundus from the antrum.

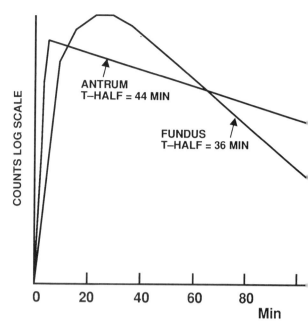

Fig. 16.4   Fundal and antral emptying curves. The fundus fills first and then empties into the antrum. The $T\frac{1}{2}$ of the two curves is indicated.

this is presumed to divide the stomach into fundal and antral sections. Curves can then be obtained for the two parts of the stomach separately, and the patterns of emptying from fundus to antrum, and antrum to the duodenum examined (Figs 16.3 and 16.4). Images are usually collected every 30 s, and time–activity curves derived for the two halves of the stomach.

The fundus fills first and empties in a linear pattern. The fundus initially empties into the antrum; in normal subjects Sheiner et al (1990) found that the counts in the antrum remain more or less constant during the process of emptying. Others have found a reduction in antral activity with time once it has filled from the fundus. Sheiner also investigated patients after peptic ulcer surgery and showed no antral plateau after vagotomy and pyloroplasty, and no delayed antral filling after proximal vagotomy. All forms of vagotomy resulted in slower fundal filling, possibly related to the time taken to eat a solid meal. Collins et al (1991) have shown that the liquid phase of the meal tends to be dispersed throughout the stomach, whereas the solid phase collects in the fundus and gradually enters the antrum (as described by Sheiner).

The role of fundal and antral emptying studies is not yet clear.

BILIARY DYNAMICS

Derivatives of imminodiacetic acid (HIDA), labelled with ^{99m}Tc, allow high-quality images of the biliary system to be obtained. They have been used in a variety of clinical circumstances.

Enterogastric reflux

Enterogastric reflux has been believed for many years to cause symptoms such as nausea and epigastric pain. It has also postulated as an aetiological agent in the production of duodenal and gastric ulcer. However reflux has been shown to occur in normal subjects, with a somewhat higher incidence in duodenal ulcer and higher still in gastric ulcer (Harding 1989). It seems unlikely however that these differences are causative in peptic ulceration. After peptic ulcer surgery some patients complain of persistent bile vomiting, epigastric pain and heartburn. In those where endoscopy has revealed no recurrence of the ulcer, the possibility of bile reflux should be considered. As such patients are difficult to evaluate, it is important to confirm that the patient has bile reflux before Roux-en-Y diversion. This technique can also

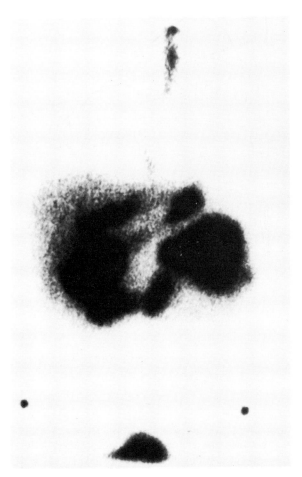

Fig. 16.5 Reflux of bile to the stomach and oesophagus during a HIDA study. There is some activity in the urinary bladder and [57]Co markers on the iliac crests.

be used to evaluate oesophageal reflux in those who have had total gastrectomy. Bile in the oesophagus causes severe symptoms, but again it is necessary to prove that such reflux can be induced before revisional surgery is considered.

Radiopharmaceutical

If the patient is not jaundiced di-ethyl HIDA is a satisfactory radiopharmaceutical. Peak biliary excretion occurs at 45–60 min after injection, and there is a close correlation between the amount of HIDA and bile acid in the stomach (Harding at al 1984). In jaundiced patients other forms of HIDA which are excreted at high bilirubin levels are necessary, for example, tri-bromo-methyl or iodo-HIDA. However,

with these different preparations the time of peak excretion will vary, as will the extent of uptake by the liver and excretion by the kidneys.

Protocol

The patient should starve overnight. Reflux studies are usually undertaken in the lying position, and because the studies take 90 min or more, it is particularly important to use [57]Co markers on the anterior iliac crests so that should the patient move the pictures can be repositioned.

The radiopharmaceutical is given intravenously, and data acquisition begins after injection, with 30 s computer images and 2 min gamma camera pictures. Frequent images are needed because interpretation often depends on a careful examination of the sequence of images. To ensure that the gallbladder contracts, intravenous cholecystokinin (CCK) or a liquid fatty meal are given at 45 min, which corresponds with the peak output of HIDA into the bowel. The incidence of reflux using these two agents varies (Harding 1989). CCK must always be given slowly, over 2 min or more, and may be associated with transient cramping pain, but severe pain is rare.

Results

An example of reflux into the stomach is shown in Figure 16.5. Such reflux can be quantified and related, for instance, to the amount of isotope injected, or to the counts in the liver, but these measurements seem to add little to assessment as to whether reflux is present or not. The test is sensitive to 1% of the administered HIDA in the stomach, but reproducibility is only 75%, (Sorgi et al 1984) due to day-to-day variation in reflux. Oesophageal reflux of bile is readily detected (Fig. 16.5).

Acute cholecystitis

While ultrasound is reliable for the detection of stones in the gallbladder or wall thickening in chronic cholecystitis, diagnosis of acute cholecystitis is rather more difficult. However, in most cases there is blockage of the cystic duct, or stasis of bile in those with acalculus cholecystitis. Diagnosis of cholecystitis can be made using HIDA as described in the previous section. In acute cholecystitis there is failure of the gallbladder to fill within 60 min of the start of the study (Fig. 16.6), although Weismann et al (1981) have shown that in occasional patients the gallbladder does not fill for 4 h. Delayed filling is usually due to chronic cholecystitis,

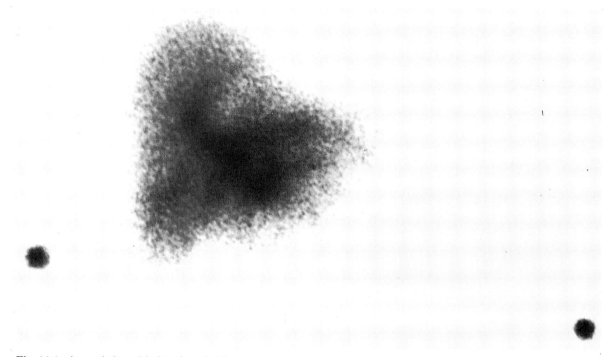

Fig. 16.6　Acute cholecystitis. Intrahepatic bile ducts are visualized but there is no gallbladder filling.

but filling may also be impaired with biliary tract obstruction, hepatocellular disease, after parenteral nutrition and occasionally with acalculous cholecystitis. Johnson and Coleman (1982) have reviewed the reliability of this test from several published papers and find the sensitivity is 95–100% with a specificity of 76–99%.

Chronic cholecystitis

Some patients have symptoms of gallbladder disease, such as right upper quadrant pain and sometimes biliary colic, but ultrasound fails to show any gallstones or other definite evidence of gallbladder disease. There has been much discussion as to whether they have a disorder of gallbladder motility which would be relieved by surgery and HIDA studies are helpful. Preparation of the patient and conduct of the test are as described previously, and the counts are determined in a ROI around the gallbladder, and in a background area within the liver. Krishnamurthy et al (1981) described the concept of radionuclide ejection fraction (EF) of the gallbladder. This is identical to the method used in cardiac studies and requires measurement of counts in the gallbladder before and after contraction.

After subtracting background (B) the EF is the difference between the counts in the uncontracted (GBu) and contracted gallbladder (GBc) divided by those in the uncontracted gallbladder and multiplied by 100.

$$EF = \frac{GBu - GBc}{GBu - B} \times 100\%$$

The normal range depends on the agent used to contract the gallbladder, and the period over which this is given. Some authors use a fatty meal, but most have chosen CCK for gallbladder motility studies. Using CCK the normal subject's EF is approximately 60%. Krishnamurthy described a group of patients with an average EF of 38% and whom he considered had chronic cholecystitis (Krishnamurthy et al 1983). In a subsequent paper Krishnamurthy et al (1984) also proposed measuring the latent period between injection of CCK and the beginning of contraction, the ejection period and the rate of contraction of the gallbladder.

Results

Results using this technique have been variable. In the detection of chronic cholecystitis Middleton and

Williams (1992) have examined 89 patients and used an EF of less than 35% as being indicative of a poorly functioning gallbladder. They found a true positive rate of 94% compared with gallbladder histology. Fink-Bennett et al (1991) examined 374 patients, 124 of whom have had cholecystectomy. Decreased function in the gallbladder was identified in 94% of patients with histopathologically confirmed chronic acalculus cholecystitis or cystic duct syndrome. Both of these authors infused CCK over a 2–3 min period. On the other hand Westlake et al (1990) using an infusion of CCK over 15–20 min concluded that decreased EF does not predict the presence of chronic cholecystitis without gallstones, and that the value of cholescintigraphy in patients with acalculus right upper quadrant pain was low. Raymond et al (1988) also found similarly poor results, but again they used a prolonged infusion of CCK.

Few authors have used the other parameters discussed by Krishnamurthy, but Winslet et al (1990) have shown that cholecystectomy relieves symptoms in patients who often have very longstanding symptoms (median 24 months) when any of the factors described by Krishnamurthy was abnormal.

Difficulties with the test

The main problem with the test relates to the fact that the gallbladder is a small organ, with a large count rate. These counts are therefore scattered into the adjacent liver tissue and it is important to choose a background area away from the gallbladder, and not including one of the major intrahepatic ducts.

Using a 2–3 min injection of CCK the results have been impressive in detecting those with chronic cholecystitis who would be relieved by cholecystectomy. More data are however required before this can be recommended as a routine indication for cholecystectomy.

COLONIC TRANSIT

Chronic constipation is common and in patients where structural changes have been eliminated by barium studies or endoscopy, transit studies of the colon are appropriate. Traditionally these have been undertaken using radio-opaque markers, but as with all radiological techniques the radiation dose depends on the number of films taken and may be large (Krevsky et al 1986). Many techniques have been described, but generally these involve intubation and therefore cannot be considered physiological. Alternatively a non-absorbable (Waller 1975) or slow release capsule (Chacko et al 1990) have been used. Transit studies are particularly important in determining whether one segment of the colon is responsible for the constipation, and therefore whether the disease is amenable to subtotal colectomy.

Protocol

Patients are usually starved overnight and the test begins early the next morning. A non-absorbable tracer is given by mouth and images are taken over 24–48 h. Because of the long transit time ^{111}In is usually used as the marker for DTPA although others have used [131]I (Smart et al 1991). Unfortunately ^{131}I gives a high radiation dose and this obviates the great benefit of the radionuclide test. Because of the varying delay produced by gastric emptying not all the tracer leaves the stomach at the same time after oral administration. However radionuclide usually collects at the ileocaecal region approximately 4 h after administration and then passes into the colon as a bolus. Stivland et al (1991) have however described a more reliable method of delivering the radionuclide into the small bowel. The radioactive tracer is absorbed on to amberlite resin and this is incorporated into a conventional gelatin capsule. The capsule is then coated with a methacrylate polymer which renders it insoluble in the acidic pH of the stomach. As the pH increases in the small bowel, the capsule gradually disintegrates and releases the resin as a bolus so that colonic transit can be examined.

Data acquisition

[57]Co markers are placed on the anterior iliac crests for positioning the patient. Imaging begins 4 h after the capsule has been ingested. The capsule may by then have reached the terminal ileum assuming small bowel transit is normal. The data is also collected on computer, and for accurate quantification the geometric mean is used so alternate anterior and posterior images are required. It is convenient to set the gamma camera so that both the ^{111}In and the [57]Co markers are imaged simultaneously. Sets of images are required at approximately hourly intervals once the meal has entered the caecum, and this continues for the whole of the first day. The patients return on the following day when images are taken every 2–4 h depending on the extent of transit. When there is no detectable activity remaining in the bowel or after 3 days the study is terminated. Recent experience suggests, however, that images at the end of the first day and at any time on the second or third days are sufficient.

Data analysis

The location of the bulk of the meal can be described using the 'geometric centre' (Krevsky et al 1986).

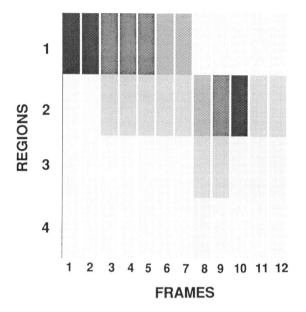

Fig. 16.7 Condensed images of the colon. Frame number is on the X-axis. Retrograde movement of faecal material seen between frames 8 and 9.

From the geometric mean counts the percentage of activity in each of several regions of the colon, from the caecum to the rectum, is calculated and multiplied by the region number. As originally described seven regions were defined between the ileocaecal area, and the faeces. The sum of these figures allows assessment of the transit of the bulk of the meal, but does not indicate any forward or backward spread which tends to occur in normal as well as abnormal subjects. Alternatively the geometric mean data can be presented as a series of curves, with one curve for each region of interest. The interpretation of the multiple curves is difficult, and it is particularly difficult to compare a series of patients. The simplest way of displaying the data is to use a condensed parametric image. This has already been described in the section on oesophageal imaging. However, because the patient goes home at night there is a long gap between the image at the end of one day and at the start of the next day and expressing the results in terms of images is therefore misleading. Notghi et al (1993) have chosen to express the parametric image with time along the X-axis, and a comparison of the image plotted against frame number and against time is shown in Figures 16.7 and 16.8. In these images the counts in each region are presented as shades of grey, and the darker areas representing

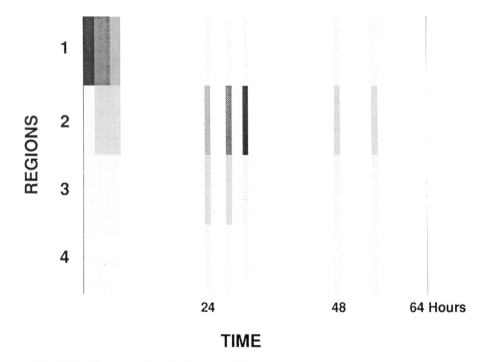

Fig. 16.8 The same patient is shown as in Figure 16.7 but time is on the X-axis rather than frame number.

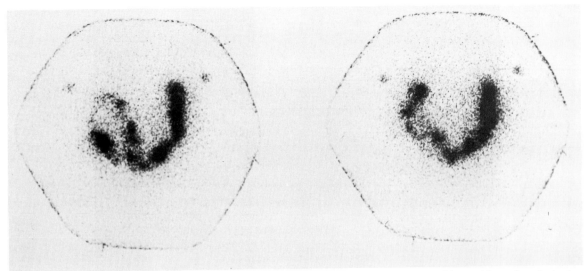

Fig. 16.9 Movement of the colon within the abdomen between successive frames may cause problems with overlap of colonic segments.

higher count rates. A smaller number of regions has been used than those for geometric mean calculations; region 1 is the caecum to hepatic flexure; 2 the transverse colon; 3 the splenic flexure; and 4 the rest of the colon and rectum.

Results

In normal patients Notghi et al (1993) have found small bowel transit varied between 1 and 8 h. For such studies this was considered as time zero. At this time 50% (SD 20%) of the meal was in the colon. By 4 h 46% (SD 18%) was in the caecum and 30% (SD 20%) in the transverse colon. Generally activity has not at that stage reached the left colon as the right colon is the main storage area. By 24 h approximately half of normal subjects will have excreted the activity, and in the remainder the majority of the activity is in the rectum. All normal subjects have generally evacuated the whole of the meal by 48 h.

Difficulties with the test

The main problem with the test is due to the complex three-dimensional structure of the colon and its constant movement in the abdomen. The ⁵⁷Co markers are essential to align the images, since there are no anatomical landmarks available for much of the study. The problem of colonic movement can largely be overcome by using generous regions of interest, but if there are exaggerated movements of the colon, more

than one region of interest may be required for the set of images (Fig. 16.9).

Colon transit studies allow the segmental transit of faecal material to be examined in a physiological manner and the sites of impaired transit to be determined. As experience grows with the technique it may become possible to define the precise place of subtotal colectomy in these patients who often present a difficult management problem.

SCINTIGRAPHIC DEFAECOGRAPHY

The video-proctogram is usually used to examine the process of defaecation in those with normal barium enema and sigmoidoscopy, but who complain of symptoms such as tenesmus, proctalgia, excess straining or incomplete evacuation. It may also be useful in those with constipation or faecal incontinence. While this is useful for functional abnormalities such as rectocele, mucosal prolapse or intussusception, it is not quantitative and has a fairly high radiation dose of 1 mSv/min of screening (Padovani et al 1987). Attempts have been made to assess defaecation by inserting a technetium-filled balloon in the rectum (Barkel et al 1988, O'Connell et al 1986). More recently a technique has been described by Papachrysostomou et al 1992 using an artificial stool of potato mash containing 200 MBq ⁹⁹ᵐTc which is placed into the rectum via a wide bore tube. The volume of artificial stool used depends on the capacity of the rectum which has been previously determined.

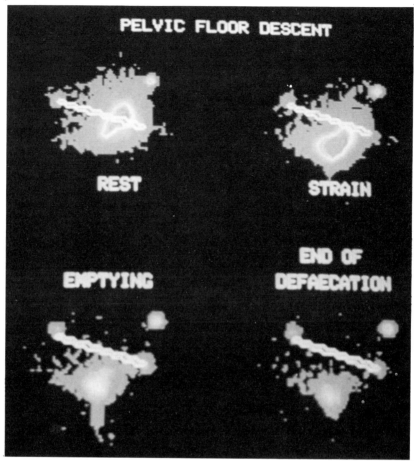

Fig. 16.10 Defaectography showing the images at rest, straining, emptying, and at end of defaecation. Marked pelvic floor descent on straining.

Papachrysostomou used suppositories to prepare the bowel prior to the test. In order to determine the anorectal angle a Foley catheter containing a small amount of ^{99m}Tc was inserted into the rectum. Hutchinson et al (in press) have suggested a technique which is essentially similar, but with 200 ml oat porridge as the artificial stool and 100 MBq ^{99m}Tc as the radioactive label. They have used no prior bowel preparation and have not found a catheter necessary to determine the line of the anal canal.

Protocol

The artificial stool is inserted into the rectum by tube with the patient in the left lateral position and imaging begins immediately. 2–5 images are collected for a total of 5–10 min. It is necessary to have a commode, and for lateral views of the pelvis be be taken. The patient is first asked to hold the artificial stool in the rectum, then to squeeze the anal sphincter, and then to evacuate the stool (Fig. 16.10). The stool is collected into a plastic bag and the activity determined. Hutchinson et al (in press) used radioactive markers on the symphysis pubis, lumbo-sacral junction and on the coccycx in order to determine the precise position of the artificial stool in relation to these anatomical landmarks.

Data analysis These tests provide continuous qualitative information about the process of defaecation. Efficiency of evacuation can be quantified as can the physiological significance of rectocele or prolapse. By determining the reduction of counts in the rectum the efficiency of defaecation can be measured (approximately 60% in normal patients), as can the rate of evacuation. Any activity above the plane of the pubic and coccygeal markers is considered to be in the sig-

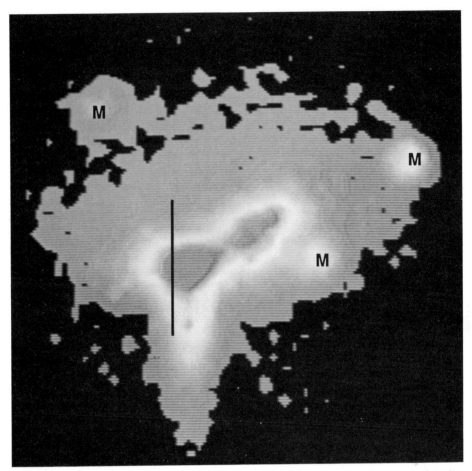

Fig. 16.11 Rectocele is evident as a bulge in front of the anterior rectal canal (in front of the line indicated). The position of marker sources is shown by the letter 'M'.

moid colon. The anorectal angle can be considered either in relation to a catheter inserted into the rectum, or the longitudinal axis of the anal canal. Rectocele can be easily identified (Fig. 16.11) as can descent of the pelvic floor. Hutchinson et al (in press) found that constipated patients evacuated 0.8% per second whereas incontinent patients evacuated 2.7% per second. It seems likely however that these parameters will depend on the amount of stool inserted.

Difficulties with the test

There are no particular problems in doing the test,

data collection is straightforward, and from the patient's point of view it is not as unpleasant as video-proctography. However the test is still embarrassing for the patient and care must be taken to ensure that the patient has a screen put round them and that the room contains the minimum number of people.

Although experience with defaecating proctograph is at present limited it has the advantages of being simpler and giving a lower radiation dose than video proctography. The functional data obtained are currently being evaluated and as more departments use the technique standardization of the protocol may be achieved.

REFERENCES

Barkel D C, Pemberton J H, Kazim L E et al 1988 Scintigraphic assessment of the anorectal angle in health and after ileal pouch – anal anastomosis. Ann Surg 208: 42–49

Bartlett R J V 1986 Scintigraphy of the oesophagus in: Robinson P J A (ed) Nuclear gastroenterology. Churchill Livingstone, Edinburgh pp 1–23

Chacko A, Szaz K F, Howard J, Cummings J H 1990 Non-invasive method for delivery of tracer substances or small quantities of other materials to the colon. Gut 31: 106–110

Collins P J, Houghton L A, Read N W et al 1991 Role of the proximal and distal stomach in mixed solid and liquid emptying. Gut 32: 615–619

Department of Health 1992 Notes for guidance on the administration of radioactive substances to persons for the purposes of diagnosis, treatment or research. Department of Health, London

Donovan I A, Harding L K 1986 Gastric emptying in: Robinson P J A (ed) Nuclear gastroenterology. Churchill Livingstone, Edinburgh pp 24–35

Fink-Bennett D, DeRidder P, Kolozsi W Z et al 1991 Cholecystokinin cholescintigraphy: detection of abnormal gallbladder motor function in patients with chronic acalculus gallbladder disease. J Nucl Med 32: 1695–1699

Fisher R S, Malmud L S, Roberts G S, Lobis I F 1976 Gastro-oesophageal scintigraphy to detect and quantitate G E reflux. Gastroenterology 70: 301–308

Harding L K 1989 Gastrointestinal tract in: Sharp P F, Gemmell H, Smith F W (eds) Practical nuclear medicine. I R L, Oxford pp 193–209

Harding L K, Donovan I A 1988 Gastric emptying: gastro-oesophageal reflux in: Rhys-Davies E, Thomas W E G (eds), Nuclear medicine – applications to surgery. Castle House Publications, Tunbridge Wells pp 42–51

Harding L K, Robinson P J A 1991 Clinician's guide to nuclear medicine – gastroenterology. Churchill Livingstone, Edinburgh pp 22–30

Harding L K, Sorgi M, Wolverson R L, Mosimann F et al 1984 The pharmacokinetics of ^{99m}Tc HIDA in man and its relationship to intragastric bile acids. Scand J Gastroenterol 19 (Suppl 92): 27–29

Hardy J G, Perkins A C 1985 Validity of the geometric mean correction in quantification of whole bowel transit. Nucl Med Commun 6: 217–224

Hutchinson R, Mostafa A B, Deen K I, Grant E A, Smith N D, Harding L K, Kumar D Scintigraphic defaecogram: quantitative and dynamic assessment of anorectal function (in press)

Johnson D G, Coleman R E 1982 New technique in radionuclide imaging of the alimentary system. Radiol Clin N America 20: 635–651

Katzem I 1972 A new scintigraphic technique for the study of the oesophagus. AJR 115: 681–689

Kaul B, Petersen H, Grette K et al 1985 Scintigraphy, pH measurements, and radiography in the evaluation of gastro-oesophageal reflux. Scand J Gastroenterology 20: 289–294

Krevsky B, Malmud L S, D'Ercole F et al 1986 Colonic transit scintigraphy. A physiological approach to the quantitative measurement of colonic transit in humans Gastroenterology 91: 1102–1112

Krishnamurthy G T, Bobba U R, Kingston E 1981 Radionuclide ejection fraction: a technique for quantitative analysis of motor function of the human gallbladder. Gastroenterology 80: 482–490

Krishnamurthy G T, Bobba U R, McConnell D et al 1983 Quantitative biliary dynamics: introduction of a new, non-invasive scintigraphic technique. J Nucl Med 24: 217–223

Krishnamurthy G T, Bobba U R, Langrell K 1984 The gallbladder emptying response to sequential exogenous and endogenous cholecystokinin. Nucl Med Commun 5: 27–33

Meyer A H, MacGregor I L, and Gueller R 1976 ^{99m}Tc tagged chicken liver as a marker of solid food in the human stomach. Am J Dig Dis 21: 296–304

Middleton G W, Williams JH 1992 Is gallbladder ejection fraction a reliable predictor of acalculus gallbladder disease? Nucl Med Commun 13: 894–896

Notghi A, Kumar D, Panagamuwa B et al 1993 Measurement of colonic transit time using radionuclide imaging: analysis by condensed images. Nucl Med Commun 14: 204–211

O'Connell P R, Kelly K A, Brown M L 1986 Scintigraphic assessment of neorectal motor function. J Nucl Med 27: 460–464

Padovani R, Contento G, Fabretto M et al 1987 Patients doses and risks from diagnostic radiology in North East Italy. Br J Radiol 60: 155–165

Papachrysostomou M, Griffin T M J, Ferrington C et al 1992 A method of computerised isotope dynamic proctography. Eur J Nucl Med 19: 431–435

Raymond F, Lepanto L, Rosenthall L, Fried G M 1988 Technetium-99m-IDA gallbladder kinetics and response to CCK in chronic cholecystitis. Eur J Nucl Med 14: 378–381

Sheiner H J, Quinlan M S, Thompson I J 1990 Gastric motility and emptying in normal and post-vagotomy subjects. Gut 21: 753–759

Shields R A, Lawson R S 1987 Effective dose equivalent. Nucl Med Commun 8: 851–855

Shrimpton P C 1988 Are x-rays safe enough? in: Faulkner K, Wall B F (eds) Patient doses and the risks in diagnostic radiology. Institute of Physical Sciences in Medicine, York pp 41–53

Shrimpton P C, Jones D G, Hillier M C, Wall B F, et al 1991 Survey of CT practice in the UK. Part 2: Dosimetric aspects. HMSO, London NRPB-R249

Smart R C, McLean R G, Gaston-Parry D et al 1991 Comparison of oral iodine-131-cellulose and indium-111-DTPA as tracers for colonic transit scintigraphy: analysis by colonic activity profiles. J Nucl Med 32: 1668–1674

Sorgi M, Wolverson R L, Mosimann S, Donovan I A, Alexander-Williams J, Harding L K 1984 Sensitivity and reproducibility of a bile reflux test using ^{99m}Tc HIDA. Scand J Gastroenterol 19 (Suppl 92): 30–32

Stivland T, Camilleri M, Vassallo M et al 1991 Scintigraphic measurement of regional gut transit in idiopathic constipation. Gastroenterology 101: 107–115

Svedberg J B 1982 The bolus transport diagram: a functional display method applied to oesophageal studies. Clin Phys Physiol Meas 3: 267–272

Waller, S L 1975 Differential measurement of small and large bowel transit times in constipation and diarrhoea. Gut 16: 372–378

Weissmann H S, Badia J, Sugarman L A et al 1981 Spectrum of cholescintigraphic patterns in acute cholecystitis. Radiology 138: 167–175

Westlake P J, Hershfield M B, Kelly J K et al 1990 Chronic right upper quadrant pain without gallstones: does HIDA

scan predict outcome after cholecystectomy? Am J
Gastroenterol 85: 986–990

Winslet M, Harding L K, Neoptolemos J P 1990 Biliary
dyskinesia as a cause of upper abdominal pain. Nucl Med
Commun 11: 56 (abstract)

Wolverson R L, Harding L K, Alexander-Williams J et al
1982 Improvement of double-dye dilution technique for
measuring gastric emptying. Gastroenterology 82: 1213

Womack N R, O'Connell P R 1991 Dynamic assessment of
ano-rectal function in: Kumar D, Waldron D J, Williams
N S (eds) Clinical measurement in coloproctology.
Springer, London pp 50–59

17. Ultrasonography

N. K. Ahluwalia   D. G. Thompson

HISTORY OF ULTRASOUND

The quest to detect different fragments of the ill-fated Titanic at the bottom of the sea in 1912 and enemy submarines during World War I led an English physicist, Lord Rayleigh, and a French physicist, Paul Langevin, to describe a method of transmitting ultrasonic waves through water using a quartz crystal to generate the waves (Langevin & Chilowski 1916). The industrial use of diagnostic ultrasound flourished in the 1940s but it was left to Professor Ian Donald at Glasgow University, in the 1950s to discover its diagnostic potential in the field of medicine by generating two-dimensional images (Donald et al 1958). Since the mid-1970s, it has become an indispensable tool of immense diagnostic potential in clinical practice which is still being exploited.

After two-dimensional imaging, the next major step, in medical ultrasonics, was the development of real-time imaging. In real-time ultrasonography, the images are refreshed so rapidly that the eye cannot see the change and thus gives an impression of continuously moving images. However, poor resolution of the images prevented its widespread application until recent improvements in transducer design resulted in high-resolution and acceptable images. The additional introduction of freeze-frame capability has now allowed widespread use of real-time high-resolution ultrasound in studying dynamic imaging of structures such as an active fetus, heart, etc.

In the space of 20 years, ultrasound has undergone dramatic changes, the major part of which has occurred in the latter decade. In recent years, the introduction of transducers, capable of continuously emitting sounds (Evans et al 1989), has added another dimension to studying flow velocity and quantitating magnitude of forward and retrograde flow. Real-time ultrasound and Doppler scanning are used routinely in cardiovascular practice and are now readily available in most X-ray departments (AIUM 1984, Cartwright et al 1984, Kinnear Wilson & Waterhouse 1984).

Early use of gastrointestinal ultrasound was limited to the evaluation of fluid collections, such as ascites and abscess cavities, but as the technology improved it became valuable for defining normal and abnormal solid viscera. Until recently, however, use of ultrasound to study the presence of intraluminal hollow abdominal viscera was unusual, primarily due to gas, which presents a physical barrier to the passage of an ultrasound beam. This problem has now largely been circumvented by careful positioning of the transducer to 'work around' gas, by filling the organ with water (McMahon et al 1979, Warren et al 1978) to displace bowel loops and provide a cystic 'acoustic window' (Fleischer et al 1981). A water-filled stomach thus became useful as an 'acoustic window' for studying the pancreas and its vascular accompaniments during which studies the incidental occurrence of visible contractions of the antral wall was reported as early as 1979 (Weighall et al 1979).

DEVELOPMENT OF ULTRASOUND FOR GASTROINTESTINAL MOTILITY

With advancements in technology and the availability of real-time, high-resolution ultrasonography, it has become possible to reliably study the gastric wall and its motor physiology. Bateman et al (1977) first exploited its potential in measuring the volume of the stomach. In their technique the long axis of the stomach was first identified, using the scanning probe 'free hand' technique followed by the use of a gantry to constrain the plane of the scan to remain perpendicular to the stomach's long axis. Finally, a series of scans for volume measurement were obtained by traversing the scanning probe along the axis of the stomach (Fig. 17.1). They employed this technique to measure gastric emptying of liquids and found the half-time of emptying ($T\frac{1}{2}$) of 500 ml orange cordial to be 22.0 min, which decreased significantly after administration of 10 mg metoclopramide given intravenously

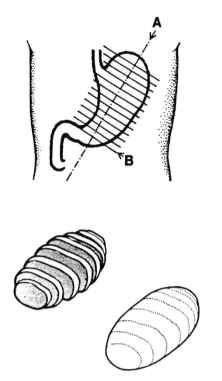

Fig. 17.1 Diagrams to illustrate the calculation of stomach volume by representing the stomach as a series of parallel cross-sectional slices (**B**) at regular intervals along its long axis (**A**). (Reproduced with permission from Bateman & Whittingham 1982.)

10 min before the drink (Bateman & Whittingham 1982).

Holt et al (1980, 1986) developed a rotating transducer-type ultrasonic scanner probe. They mounted four transducers of 2.5 MHz on a wheel rotating in an oil-filled plastic cylinder. The advantage of this technique was that the use of gantry to constrain the plane of the scan (which restricts the movement of the subject during the study) was avoided; instead the transducer was strapped to the patient's abdomen over the region of interest. Using this device, they showed regular antral contractions occurring approximately every 20 s after drinking 500 ml of orange juice. King et al (1984, 1985) also used this technique to study the relationship between human antroduodenal motility and transpyloric fluid movement. They studied the temporal relationships among contractions of the terminal antrum, pylorus and proximal duodenum. They observed that the gastroduodenal peristaltic cycles occured at a rate of about 3 cycles per minute (cpm) and noted contraction of the terminal antrum in 98% of

cycles. Two-thirds of the cycles were phase-locked with proximal duodenal contractions.

Bolondi et al (1985) from Italy were first to demonstrate a close correlation between gastric emptying time measured by gastric ultrasound vs. radioisotope γ-camera scintiscanning technique. They, however, restricted their measurements to assessing the volume of the antrum rather than the whole stomach, and based their calculations on the assumption that every section of the antrum was elliptical. The major difficulty, however, in clinical application with this technique was the cumbersome and time-consuming nature of the data recording and subsequent analysis. Holt et al (1986) noted that estimating gastric volume by serial transverse sections along the long axis of the organ was liable to introduce inaccuracies from inadvertently recording overlapping sections of the stomach and, therefore, measured gastric volume from 'serial near-longitudinal' sections of the whole stomach. Marzio et al (1989) more recently ultrasonically evaluated gastric emptying by calculating the percentage decrease in the diameter of the antrum in one plane and found a close correlation with that evaluated using scintigraphy. They calculated the diameter as an average of that measured anteroposteriorly and laterolaterally.

In recent years application of this technique has been further extended beyond measurement of gastric emptying to study antral peristaltic contraction characteristics (Thompson et al 1989, Hausken et al 1991). Duplex sonography has more recently been employed to observe to-and-fro movement of luminal contents in relation to the antroduodenal peristaltic cycle (Hausken et al 1992).

At present ultrasound is employed to:

1. Non-invasively assess gastric and antral emptying;
2. Study antral rhythmicity and contraction characteristics;
3. To assess antroduodenal coordination, gastroduodenal flow and luminal reflux.

APPARATUS REQUIRED

The ultrasound machine

To study antral motor characteristics a real-time high-resolution ultrasound machine, is required. A 5.0 MHz linear array probe is suitable for most studies.

Ultrasonics

The modern-day ultrasound machine has a dynamic

computer lens which results in a high definition that provides accurate quantitative measurement of the ultrasonic image of the antral circumference. It provides 128 independent channels and all the channels of the array are processed by the system to form the ultrasound image.

The facility of pulsed Doppler and colour Doppler modes in this machine allows for quantitative measurement of velocity in the former mode and the direction of flow can be visualized in different colours in the latter.

Plotting and measurement of the region of interest

Apart from providing a high-resolution image, the modern ultrasound machine also provides an in-built plotting and flow volume calculating facility. In earlier studies, before this plotting facility became available, the cross-section of the antrum was assumed to be circular or elliptical for calculating the area or volume of the antrum. The plotting facility permits the measurement of the circumference or area of the antrum exactly as it is visualized in the image and no assumptions of its being elliptical or circular are required for calculation, while the flow volume calculation facility allows accurate quantitative assessment of the direction, flow volume and velocity of luminal contents.

Recording and storage of images

In order to study antral motor characteristics the real-time images of the relaxed and contracted antrum need to be recorded on a videotape for retrospective quantitative analysis. Although most modern ultrasound machines have the facility to freeze any frame as the images are being recorded, an attempt to analyse these images at the time of recording is liable to introduce errors from selection of inappropriate frames for measurement. In order to study antral contraction characteristics and relate antral excursion to distension, it is important to measure the relaxed and contracted antral circumferences that belong to the same peristaltic cycle. Since the relaxed state lasts about 16 s and contracted for about 4 s in a single peristaltic cycle (King et al 1985), it is impractical to freeze the most appropriate relaxed frame, plot around it, record the antral circumference, unfreeze it and then be able to do the same for the antral image during the contracted state of the same peristaltic cycle. Furthermore, in order to average out the possible variation in the amplitudes of relaxed and contracted circumferences of suc-

cessive cycles (Jacobs et al 1982, Stacher et al 1984), it is important to take measurements of more than one consecutive cycle. All this is possible only if the images are recorded at the time of the study and replayed retrospectively to obtain the respective measurements. The real-time display on the monitor is also recorded, which during replay provides the time after the ingestion of the meal as well as in quantifying the interval in seconds between successive peristaltic contractions.

The test meal

Selection of the test meal depends upon the purpose of the study. Different meals have been used in different studies and countries. Ideally, a test meal should fulfil the following criteria:

1. It should be appropriately sonolucent with medium echogenicity. A sono-opaque meal is likely to obscure the images of the posterior antral wall while a highly sonolucent meal is likely to make it difficult to distinguish the antral image from its surroundings;
2. It should be palatable and culturally acceptable;
3. The nature and the composition of the meal should be such that it allows adequate time to carry out the study within the confinements of practicality and acceptability;
4. The volume and nature of the test meal ingested should be such that it does not induce undue sensation of nausea or bloating.

If the aim of the study is to relate the flow of the luminal contents to antro-pyloroduodenal peristalsis, a test meal with enough echogenic particles is required so that direction of flow can be observed. With the advent of coloured Doppler machines which recognize the direction of flow and display it in different colours, it is, however, not necesary to rely on visual images of the flow of particles for this purpose.

Different meals have been employed in different laboratories for studying gastric emptying. Orange cordial (Bateman & Whittingham 1982), water flavoured with orange juice containing fine bran particles as sonic markers (King et al 1984), a mixture of pasta, tomato sauce, vegetables and meat in 300 ml water (Bolondi et al 1985), isotonic saline or skimmed milk (Marzio et al 1989) have been used. The problem with using a solid meal to assess gastric emptying is that the study is likely to last unacceptably long. Using an Italian pasta meal, Bolondi et al (1985) found an empty-

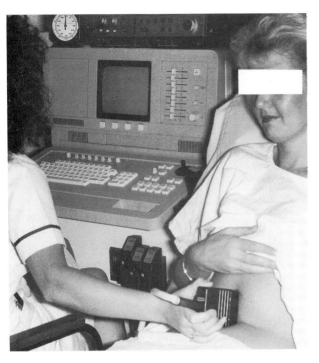

Fig. 17.2 A study in progress. Note the longitudinal position of the ultrasound probe to measure antral circumference in transverse section. A video is used to record all the images during the study.

ing time of 3–5 h in normal subjects and 4–8 h in patients with functional dyspepsia.

For the sake of convenience, easy commercial availability, and, not least, acceptability to most subjects, 'Cream of Chicken' soup (H J Heinz and Co Ltd; 200 Kcal; 11.5 g fat, 5.5 g protein) is a suitable test-meal to study antral contraction characteristics. This meal is sonolucent with medium echogenicity and has a $T\frac{1}{2}$ of 45 ± 10 min as measured by γ-camera technique after radiolabelling with ^{99m}Tc-pertechnetate. This test meal has a linear emptying profile with no lag phase. Hausken et al (1991) used meat soup and found it satisfactory for studying both antral contraction characteristics as well as luminal flow.

THE TECHNIQUE AND MEASUREMENTS

Technique

The subject lies comfortably at a 45° angle on the examination couch, exposed to the waist (Fig. 17.2). This, as opposed to the conventional lying down posi-

tion for other abdominal ultrasound examinations, has a distinct advantage of avoiding the intragastric gas from the path of the ultrasound beam. The gas being lighter than the meal shifts higher up in the fundus (Holm 1971).

The ultrasound probe is first placed gently in the longitudinal plane of the distal stomach. This allows simultaneous visualization of the antrum, pylorus and the proximal duodenum and orientation of the adjoining structures such as the aorta and the superior mesenteric vein (Fig. 17.3). This plane also allows direct observation of the passage of peristaltic contractions along the antral wall, traversing from the corpus to the antroduodenal area (King et al 1985, Hausken et al 1992). Prolonged studies in this plane are required to study antroduodenal coordination as well as assessment of direction of flow and its velocity and volume. The direction of flow is visualized in different colours and this can be temporally related to the antroduodenal contractions (Hausken et al 1992).

The probe is then rotated by about 90° to lie in a fixed vertical anatomical plane of the vascular structures, such as the aorta or the superior mesenteric vein (Fig. 17.4). In this plane, a cross-sectional image of the antrum is visualized (Fig. 17.5).

Measurements

After the completion of the study, the videotape is replayed and frame-by-frame images retrieved on the ultrasound machine monitor. For assessment of rhythmicity, a fixed recognizable point in the peristaltic cycle, such as the onset of the contraction is noted for successive cycles and the interval calculated from the time display for each successive point noted on the monitor. For assessment of antral contraction characteristics, the minimum circumference during the passage of peristaltic contraction and maximum during the relaxed state are plotted using the plotting facility (Fig. 17.5) and circumference or area obtained from the direct calculation and display made by the computer for the enclosed plotted antral image. Most ultrasonographers trace around the outermost layer of the antral image as the contrast of the serosal lining provides the sharpest image of the antrum as opposed to the slightly fuzzier image of the inner layer of the antral wall. The mean of the relaxed and contracted circumferences of several consecutive peristaltic cycles is obtained to average out the variation between the amplitude of successive contractions (see below). For the purpose of assessing antral contraction characteristics or antral emptying, it is immaterial whether the readings are obtained as circumference or area, as

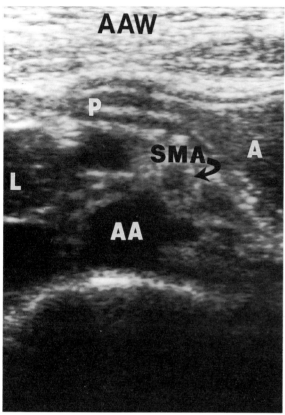

Fig. 17.3   Ultrasonic appearance of the longitudinal section of the gastric antrum. A = antrum, AAW = anterior abdominal wall, AA = abdominal aorta, L = liver, P = pylorus, SMA = superior mesenteric artery.

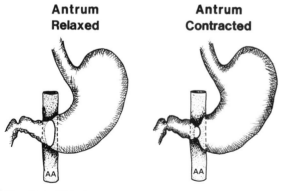

Fig. 17.4   This diagram illustrates the antral plane used for measurement of cross-sectional antral circumference both between peristalsis when the antrum is relaxed and during the passage of a peristaltic contraction. 'AA' identifies the abdominal aorta.

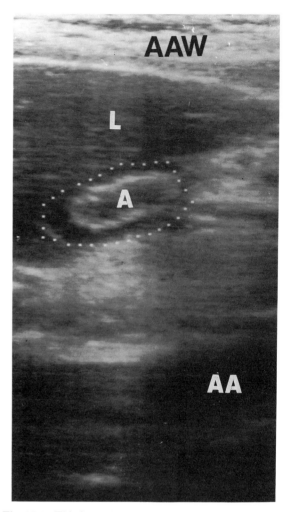

Fig. 17.5   This figure shows a typical ultrasound image. The dotted line shows the cursor marks placed around the outer wall of the antrum. AAW = anterior abdominal wall, A = antrum, L = left lobe of the liver. The hypo-echoic area just below 'AA' is the abdominal aorta in its longitudinal plane.

there is a direct mathematical relationship between the two and the results obtained will vary by the same mathematical correlate. In order to make the comparison of results between different centres easy, one or the other should be chosen uniformly by all investigators.

Using the above technique and measurements, the ultrasound has been used to study the following antral motor functions:

- Gastric and antral emptying
- Antral rhythmicity and contraction characteristics
  - Antral peristaltic rhythmicity

– Antral excursion/distension characteristics
- Antroduodenal coordination, luminal flow and gastroduodenal reflux.

STUDY OF GASTRIC AND ANTRAL EMPTYING

Gastric emptying

The role of gastric ultrasound as a test for measuring gastric emptying has already been partly alluded to above in the discussion of relaxed antral circumference. Earlier studies on gastric ultrasound first concentrated on exploiting its potential, as a noninvasive test for studying gastric emptying. However, the cumbersome nature of the measurement of the gastric or antral volume, prevented its widespread application as a tool for measuring gastric emptying (Bateman & Whittingham 1982, Holt et al 1986). Bolondi et al (1985) from Italy found that the slope of the measurements of gastric antrum in one plane, correlated closely with γ-camera studies. Although in normal subjects it has been shown that the slope of decrease in the gastric volume measured by ultrasound correlates closely with that of gastric emptying time measured by isotope technique, comparative studies in patients with delayed gastric emptying are lacking. It has recently been reported, using scintigraphic techniques, that in some patients the antral contents retropulse back into the fundus particularly at the beginning of the study (Troncon et al 1992). It is thus possible that in such patients the profile of antral emptying as measured by the ultrasound technique may not correlate with isotope gastric emptying techniques, and that intragastric redistribution of food in the stomach may make the slope of antral emptying different from that of gastric emptying measured by isotope technique. Such comparative studies are now indicated to understand more about the underlying pathophysiological mechanisms in such patients.

Antral filling and emptying

The factors modulating intragastric food distribution are not fully known. It is likely that the volume of food distributed to the distal stomach depends on several factors such as gastric tone, compliance, feedback regulation from the small bowel, composition of the meal itself in terms of viscosity and nutrients (Pröve & Ehrlein 1982, Azpiroz & Malagelada 1985). The magnitude of antral distension immediately after meal inges-

tion is, therefore, likely to depend upon all these factors, independent of the gastric emptying to follow. The decrease in relaxed antral circumference as emptying progresses may depend upon all these factors as well as the rate of disappearance of antral contents, be it to the small bowel as gastric emptying or to the proximal stomach as intragastric redistribution.

Slope of relaxed antral circumference, therefore, gives an index of antral emptying irrespective of whether antral contents get propelled out into the duodenum or retropulse back into the corpus and fundus. Unless further synchronous ultrasound and isotope studies are conducted in patients with delayed gastric emptying, any relationship between the rate of antral emptying measured by ultrasound and rate of isotope gastric emptying remains speculative.

STUDY OF ANTRAL RHYTHMICITY AND CONTRACTION CHARACTERISTICS

Antral peristaltic rhythmicity

During the interdigestive stage, it is difficult to appreciate any change in the antral circumference with peristalsis (Holt et al 1980). However after feeding a meal, whether liquid, solid or mixed, continuous antral contractions once every 20 s, are clearly visualized by the ultrasound technique (King et al 1985, Hausken et al 1991) (Fig. 17.6).

The interperistaltic contraction interval ranges between 16–29 s, representing 2.0–3.3 cpm and a mean of 3 ± 0.6 (mean $\pm$ SEM) cpm (King et al 1985). Similar rhythmicity is observed using other techniques such as 'antral wall motion detector', although manometry fails to pick up almost half of these contractions (White et al 1981, Fone et al 1990). Since gastric slow waves also occur at the same rate as antral peristaltic contractions, it appears that there is complete electromechanical coupling during the fed state.

This pattern of 3 cpm rhythmicity of antral contractions is observed throughout emptying, although it becomes technically increasingly difficult to accurately measure the regularity of this rhythm as the meal emptying progresses, and the antral circumferences both relaxed and contracted decrease making it difficult to recognize the precise point of onset of the contraction (Fig. 17.7). Electrical and manometric dysrrhythmias have been reported in patients with functional dyspepsia (You et al 1980, Malagelada & Stanghellini 1985, Geldof et al 1986). Studies on antral rhythmicity, using gastric ultrasound, are now

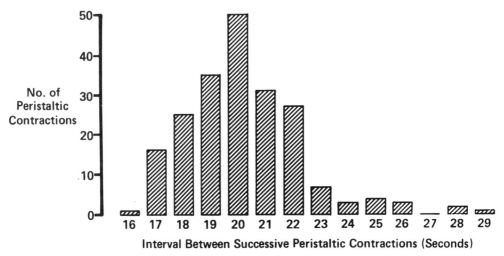

Fig. 17.6 This histogram shows the distribution of the interval between successive antral peristaltic contractions (excursions).

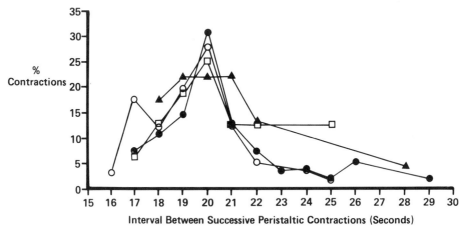

Fig. 17.7 Distribution of peristaltic frequency measured at different intervals. There is little difference in the pattern of rhythmicity at four different recording intervals after meal ingestion: ● = 0 min, ○ = 15 min, ▲ = 30 min, □ = 45 min.

indicated in such patients to see if there is accompanying mechanical dysrrhythmia.

Antral contraction characteristics

Prolonged studies have been conducted by several groups with the probe positioned longitudinally, which have shown that during the period between successive peristaltic contractions, the relaxed antral dimensions remain unchanged (Holt et al 1980, Bolondi et al 1985, King et al 1985, Hausken et al 1991). With the passage of each peristaltic wave the antral circumference decreases at the point where the wave is traversing. Thus at any given plane, the antrum stays

relaxed for about 15–16 s followed by a contraction lasting about 4 s. This cycle repeats approximately every 20 s throughout emptying (Bateman et al 1977, King et al 1985, Hausken et al 1992). This is the same as the frequency of the electrical pacesetter potentials in human distal stomach (Daniel & Chapman 1963), thus indicating that the antral excursion observed by gastric ultrasound is a true contraction of the antral smooth muscle initiated by the electrical potentials.

Relaxed antral circumference

After meal ingestion the antrum increases in size; the

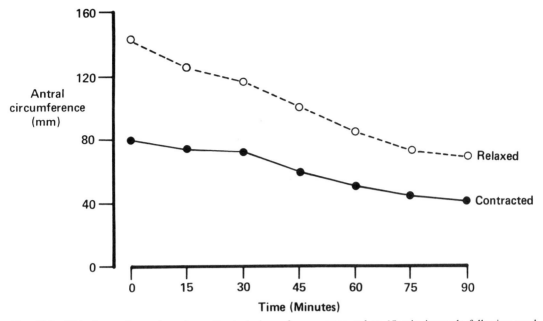

Fig. 17.8 This figure shows the values of antral circumference measured at 15 min intervals following meal ingestion in one subject. The open circles show relaxed, and the closed circles show contracted, antral circumference. The difference between the relaxed and contracted antral circumference is the antral excursion.

degree of antral distension evidently depending upon the volume of the antral contents. The amount of antral contents, in turn is likely to depend upon several interrelated factors such as the tone of the proximal and distal stomach, the nature and composition of the meal ingested and the neuroenteric feedback effect from the small intestine on gastric motor functions (Azpiroz & Malagelada 1985) and not least the volume of the meal ingested.

The relaxed antral circumference is maximal immediately after ingestion of the meal (Fig. 17.8) and declines progressively and linearly with time as emptying progresses.

Contracted antral circumference

The antral circumference diminishes approximately every 20 s, for 4–5 s with the passage of each peristaltic wave. The magnitude of the contracted antral circumference, like the relaxed, is also maximal immediately post-meal and thereafter decreases linearly as emptying progresses (Fig. 17.8).

Antral excursion and excursion vs. distension

The magnitude of change between relaxed and contracted antral circumference with each contraction rep-

resents antral excursion. As expected from a linear decrease in both relaxed and contracted antral circumferences with emptying, the magnitude of antral excursion also decreases linearly. For a given peristaltic contraction, there is a linear relationship between the degree of antral excursion and the degree of antral wall distension (Fig. 17.9).

Excursion/distension ratio

Excursion/distension ratio remains constant independent of the state of gastric emptying or the degree of distension of the antrum (Fig. 17.10). Using measurement of antral area, this ratio is about 0.4 (Hausken et al 1991).

It is not known whether these antral contraction characteristics are due to an inherent property of the smooth muscle itself or due to its intrinsic and extrinsic innervation. There is indirect evidence from manometric studies in animals, that this distension-dependent contraction characteristic of the antrum may be modulated by the intrinsic (Deloof & Rousseau 1985) as well as extrinsic innervation (Andrews et al 1980a, b, Grundy et al 1986). Distension-dependent increased antral manometric activity in antral pouches constructed in vagotomized and splanchniectomized rab-

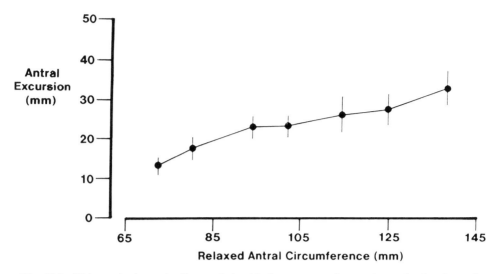

Fig. 17.9 This graph shows the linear relationship between antral excursion and relaxed antral circumference in 15 normal subjects. The ● represents mean and bars SEM.

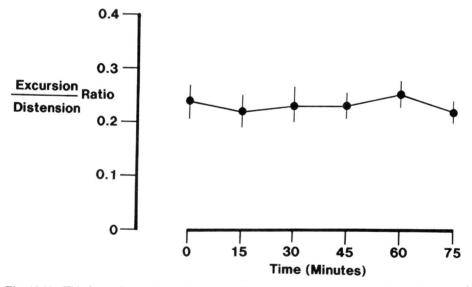

Fig. 17.10 This figure shows the antral excursion/distension ratio at each of the 15 min intervals, for 15 normal subjects. Note the ratio remains consistent throughout the study.

bits suggests either myogenic or myenteric mechanisms may control this response (Deloof & Rousseau 1985). The increased activity in vagal afferent and efferent fibres on antral and fundal distension, and the modulation of antral distension-dependent manometric response by fundal distension, suggests that this response is at least in part modulated by extrinsic vagal pathways (Andrews et al 1980a, Grundy et al 1989).

STUDY OF ANTRODUODENAL COORDINATION, LUMINAL FLOW AND GASTRODUODENAL REFLUX

Temporal relationships between the progression of the peristaltic wave across the antrum and onset of duodenal contraction have been studied, using real-time ultrasonography (King et al 1985). Approximately every 20 s, the terminal antrum contracts and remains so for about 4 s. The pylorus closure occurs at the midpoint of the terminal antrum contraction and remains so until the terminal antrum relaxes. Two-thirds of these antral contractions are temporally phase-locked with the onset of duodenal contractions, which occurs 1 s after the pyloric closure and lasts about 5 s. Using Doppler sonography, duodenogastric reflux is seen more often with these coordinated antroduodenal contractions than with those antral contractions which are not phase-locked with the following duodenal contractions.

With the advancements in technology, Hausken et al (1992) have employed coloured Doppler sonography to study both the temporal relationship between antropyloroduodenal contractions as well as luminal flow. They made quantitative assessment of propulsive and retropulsive flow in the antral region. Since retropulsive flow is visualized in a different colour from propulsive, the degree and timing of gastroduodenal reflux in relation to antroduodenal cycles can be measured. Using this technique, propulsive pendulating flow (pulsed to-and-fro movement of luminal contents across the pylorus synchronous with aortic pulsation) superimposed upon propulsive peristaltic-related flow (due to antral peristalsis) is clearly noted. Additionally, retropulsive flow (due to duodenogastric reflux) is observed during and just before the end of an antral peristaltic cycle. End-cycle reflux, seen at the end of the peristaltic cycle immediately before the closure of the terminal antrum and the pylorus, lasting about 2 s is seen in almost 50% of the cycles, more frequently (about 70%) with coordinated antropyloroduodenal contractions. The mid-cycle reflux occurs between and unrelated to the coordinated antroduodenal contractions in 45% of all cycles, and 32% of these are associated with a synchronous duodenal contraction unrelated to any antral peristaltic cycle. In this study, the peak velocity for both anterograde and retrograde luminal flow was 60 cm/s. From these observations it appears that the end-cycle reflux is physiological, constituting a hallmark of coordinated antroduodenal peristalsis. The exact nature of the mid-cycle reflux is uncertain and requires further investigations.

RELIABILITY OF MEASUREMENTS

Variability of the amplitude of successive antral excursions

The amplitude of relaxed and contracted antral circumference varies little between successive peristaltic contractions (Fig. 17.11). The median coefficient of variation of the relaxed and contracted antral circumference is about 3–5% which results in a variability of

about 15% in the amplitude of successive antral excursions. Albeit small, this variation in the magnitude of antral contractions, makes it important that the mean of several consecutive peristaltic contractions be taken to assess antral contractility using the ultrasound technique.

Inter- and intra-observer variability

A knowledge of the magnitude of inter- and intra-observer error is paramount for any technique that relies on the investigator to take measurements, and gastric ultrasound is no exception. In vitro ultrasound studies on water-filled balloons showed an error of about 4% in the measurement of the volume in a balloon from the actual volume, across a range of volumes assessed between 50–600 ml (Bateman & Whittingham 1982). The inter- and intra-observer error in measurement of the antral circumference using the ultrasound varies between 2–8% (Marzio et al 1989), which is very similar to that for measurement of gallbladder dimensions (Everson et al 1980).

Reproducibility between different laboratories

There are now several reports on measurement of gastric emptying, assessment of excursion/distension ratio and study of antroduodenal coordination from different centres, and the results on all the parameters measured have been very consistent (King et al 1985, Ahluwalia et al 1990, Hausken et al 1991).

Reproducibility and subject variability

There is a paucity of reports on reproducibility of the technique and day-to-day subject variability. In a repeat study on 10 healthy volunteers, the median coefficient of variation in assessing the excursion/distension ratio was about 10% suggesting both consistent performance of the antrum, given ingestion of the same meal and volume as well as good reproducibility of the technique. Similar information about the consistency of performance in patients with suspected gastric motor abnormalities is not available. It is common clinical experience that symptoms fluctuate from day to day in patients with functional dyspepsia (Nyrén 1992), it is equally possible that antral performance as assessed by ultrasound may vary too. Such studies are therefore, now indicated.

Lateral movement of the antrum after feeding

The gastric antrum is a somewhat conical structure with an ellipsoid base (Bolondi et al 1985) and if

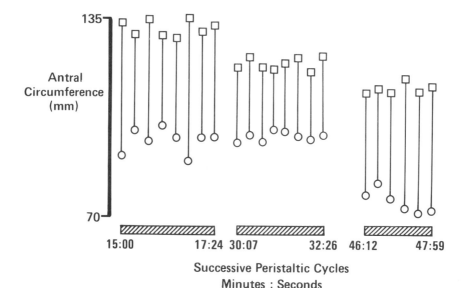

Fig. 17.11 This figure shows the relaxed and contracted antral circumferences of successive peristaltic contractions in a subject, at three separate recording intervals. Note the slight variation in the amplitude of successive excursions.

feeding the test meal were to significantly shift the antrum to the right and then it were to gradually return left to its fasting position with emptying, then the ultrasonic probe which is fixed to record antral circumference opposite the plane of the aorta is likely to record different planes of the antrum as it shifted back to the left. This would then result in recording of increasingly smaller planes of a cone as the tip approached the plane of recording. Little information in the literature exists on this topic. In a detailed study on six subjects although the distance between the pylorus and aorta varied from 2.3–3.2 cm between subjects, the median coefficient of variation during a study, including the fasting state, was less than 8%. This indicates that in an individual there is only a small shift in the transverse pre-aortic plane of the antrum after feeding and as emptying progresses. The ultrasound measurements during emptying therefore, represent a true decrease in the relaxed circumference and this small shift is unlikely to represent a spurious decrease.

HOW LONG SHOULD THE STUDY LAST?

This depends entirely upon the purpose of the study. If the aim of the study is to assess antral and gastric emptying, then it has to be performed until complete meal emptying.

Regarding studying luminal flow of antral contents,

there is at present not enough information about the pattern during the entire period of emptying and further work needs to be done to characterize the flow parameters during the entire period of emptying.

However, the study need not last as long if the purpose is to assess antral contraction characteristics. Since the excursion/distension ratio is constant throughout emptying and the pattern of antral rhythmicity does not change with emptying, theoretically there is no reason why only one set of measurements after meal ingestion should not suffice. However, a 10% variability in excursion/distension ratio over the period of emptying, albeit small, makes it important to make more than one set of measurements in a study. Hausken et al (1991) reported studies conducted over a 15-min period after meal ingestion. We currently perform five measurements at 15-min interval after meal ingestion over a period of 60 min. An index of variability of antral performance with emptying in patient group is not known. It is therefore difficult to decide the optimal period of duration for the study in patients.

FUTURE APPLICATIONS

Gastric ultrasound is a relatively new technique among the investigations available to study gastric motor functions. In the space of 20 years ultrasound has become an indispensable tool in the investigation of patients with structural problems in the abdomen. This has mainly been due to its safety, ready availability, and not least because it is noninvasive. For the same reasons, and the fact that other modalities for studying gastric motor functions involve inconvenience to the subject due to intubation of multi-lumen catheters or radiation hazard it is likely that gastric ultrasound may be increasingly used for assessing gut motor functions.

More work needs to be done however, before considering it as a clinically useful investigation. It is important to understand the physiology of antral motor functions in normal subjects before considering the pathophysiology in patients.

Physiological considerations

Studies in animals have shown that the amplitude of antral contractions is modulated by fundal distension (Andrews et al 1980a, Grundy et al 1989), feedback intestinal mechanisms (Azpiroz & Malagelada 1985), viscosity and the composition of the meal itself (Pröve & Ehrlein 1982, Houghton et al 1988a,b). Factors modulating the magnitude of antral contraction as a function of antral distension in humans, however, are not known. There is some preliminary evidence that volume of the meal or distension of the fundus do not, while increase in lipid composition does, modulate these characteristics. It is possible that decreased antral contractility is one of the factors responsible for dose-dependent delayed gastric emptying observed after lipids (Hunt & Knox 1968). Gastric ultrasound studies using different meal volume and composition or a distensible fundal balloon to alter the volume and tone of the fundus are now indicated to assess their influence on antral contraction characteristics.

To date, the studies conducted for assessing antral contraction characteristics have not employed a solid meal. Using the radio-labelled isotope scintiscanning technique, solid emptying characterizes an initial lag phase followed by a linear emptying phase (Azpiroz & Malagelada 1987, Smout et al 1987). The duration of the lag phase and the slope of emptying phase varies among individuals. It is possible that antral contraction characteristics may vary in these two phases. To answer this question prolonged studies of antral contraction characteristics after a solid meal until complete emptying are required.

Pharmacological considerations

The non-invasive nature of this technique lends itself as an ideal technique to study the effect of drugs on antral motor functions, which quite often require repeated studies with varying doses. In one study a therapeutic dose of 35 μg enprostil, a prostaglandin E_2 analogue, 60 min before the study resulted in decreased excursion/distension ratio and frequency of antral contractions (Hausken et al 1991). No doubt, reports on the effect of other prokinetic drugs on antral motor functions using gastric ultrasound will emerge in the future.

Clinical applications

Several reports suggest abnormalities of antral motor functions in patients with gastroparesis due to functional dyspepsia and idiopathic nausea and vomiting (You et al 1980). Manometric evaluation of such patients shows abnormalities such as decreased frequency and amplitude of antral manometric events (Malagelada & Stanghellini 1985, Camilleri et al 1986). Electrogastrographic studies show dysrrhythmias of antral myoelectrical activity (Geldof et al 1986). It is possible that these patients also have antral contractile abnormalities. Since gastric ultrasound non-invasively provides direct evaluation of both antral contraction characteristics as well as rhythmicity, similar studies are now indicated in such patients using gastric ultrasound. As these patients frequently complain of worsening of symptoms after certain foods, particularly those with high lipid content, gastric ultrasound evaluation using varying lipid composition of the meal are likely to be useful in understanding the pathophysiological mechanisms.

Since the gastric ultrasound technique is safe, and noninvasive, it can be repeated as often as clinically indicated. It can be used to assess the progress of such patients and monitor the effects of any treatment. This technique also provides a valuable tool to study the effect of prokinetic drugs, such as erythromycin, that are known to improve gastroparesis, on antral motor functions. Similarly, progress of the disease in patients with gastroparesis can be monitored.

The recent advent of colour Doppler ultrasonography opens up a new chapter for the understanding of the mechanisms underlying gastroduodenal reflux. Studies need to be conducted in a variety of patients presenting with biliary gastritis, oesophagitis as well as those with gastroparesis, including the effect of 'prokinetic drugs' on different types of gastroduodenal reflux observed using this technique.

Ultrasonography elsewhere in the gastrointestinal tract

Prompted by anecdotal reports of observations of antral contractions (Weighall et al 1979) and ultrasonic assessment of tumours in the gastric wall (Walls 1976) while using the stomach merely as an 'acoustic window' to study pancreas, researchers have concentrated on studying antral contraction characteristics and emptying. There is, however, no reason why other areas of the gut should not be ultrasonically accessible for studying their motor functions. The area under study, however, should be anatomically fixed and not be obscured by other sonopaque structures.

Caecum and colon appear to fulfil these criteria and studies to investigate the potential of assessing the contraction characteristics of the large bowel are indicated.

ADVANTAGES AND LIMITATIONS OF GASTRIC ULTRASOUND

Advantages

Certain features of this technique make it attractive to study the motor functions of the distal stomach.

It is safe, noninvasive, reliable, reproducible, easily repeatable and of relatively short duration. Antral motor functions studied over a 15–30 min postprandial period, provide adequate and reliable measure of antral contraction and luminal flow characteristics. The information provided is not influenced by factors such as anxiety and the possible effects of intubation, as in manometric evaluation (Read et al 1983). Most important, the information obtained relates to direct visual evaluation of a mechanical peristaltic contraction of the antrum and not an indirect effect of these contrac-

tions on the antral pressure activity which is likely to be influenced by factors such as incomplete apposition of the antral wall on the catheter and effect of pressure gradient between the fundus and duodenum (White et al 1981, Fone et al 1990).

Limitations

The accuracy of the results obtained by this technique relies heavily on the quality of the images obtained. This technique will be limited in those subjects where the quality of antral images obtained is compromised by anatomical factors such as obesity or a high location of the antrum under the thoracic cage. Patients after gastric surgery may be difficult to evaluate by this technique.

SUMMARY

Percutaneous high-resolution real-time ultrasound is a safe, readily available, noninvasive and reproducible technique to study gastric motor functions. It can be used to evaluate gastric emptying, antral peristaltic rhythmicity and contractility, to study the flow of luminal contents and to assess antroduodenal coordination. Its potential as a technique that directly evaluates mechanical contraction of the antrum, pylorus and duodenum needs to be tapped to study factors modulating gastric emptying, antral contractility and gastroduodenal reflux in clinical situations relating to gastroparesis, functional dyspepsia and reflux diseases.

REFERENCES

Ahluwalia N K, Thompson D G, Mamtora H, Clenton M 1990 Direct demonstration of 'Heterometric Autoregulation' of human antral peristalsis using real-time ultrasound 'Starling's law and the stomach'. Gastroenterology 98: A321

AIUM (American Institute of Ultrasound in Medicine) 1984 Safety considerations for diagnostic ultrasound. AIUM, Bethesda, Maryland

Andrews PLR, Grundy D, Scratcherd T 1980a Reflex excitation of antral motility induced by gastric distention in the ferret. J Physiol 298: 79–84

Andrews PLR, Grundy D, Scratcherd T 1980b Vagal afferent discharge from mechanoreceptors in different regions of the ferret stomach. J Physiol 298: 513–524

Azpiroz F, Malagelada J-R 1985 Intestinal control of gastric tone. Am J Physiol 249: G501–G509

Azpiroz F, Malagelada J-R 1987 Gastric tone measured by an electronic basostat in health and postsurgical gastroparesis. Gastroenterology 92: 934–943

Bateman D N, Whittingham T A 1982 Measurement of gastric emptying by real-time ultrasound. Gut 23: 524–527

Bateman D N, Leeman S, Metrewli C, Wilson K 1977 A non-invasive technique for gastric motility measurement. Br J Radiol 50: 526–527

Bolondi L, Bortolotti M, Santi V, Salletti T, Gaiani S, Labo G 1985 Measurement of gastric emptying time by real-time ultrasonography. Gastroenterology 89: 752–759

Camilleri M, Brown ML, Malagelada J-R 1986 Relationship between impaired gastric emptying and abnormal gastrointestinal motility. Gastroenterology 91: 94–99

Cartwright R A, McKinney P A, Hopton P A et al 1984 Ultrasound examinations in pregnancy and childhood cancer. Lancet ii: 999–1000

Daniel E E, Chapman K M 1963 Electrical activity of the gastrointestinal tract as an indication of mechanical activity. Am J Dig Dis 8: 54–102

Deloof S, Rousseau J P 1985 Neural control of electrical gastric activity in response to inflation of the antrum in rabbit. J Physiol 367: 13–25

Donald I, MacVicar J, Brown T G 1958 Investigation of abdominal masses by pulsed ultrasound. Lancet i: 1188–1195

Evans D H, McDicken W N, Skidmore R, Woodock J P

1989 Doppler ultrasound – physics, instrumentation and clinical applications, John Wiley, New York

Everson G T, Braverman D Z, Johnson M L et al 1980 A critical evaluation of real-time ultrasonography for the study of gallbladder volume and contraction. Gastroenterology 79: 40–46

Fleischer A, Muhletaler C, James A 1981 Sonographic assessment of the bowel wall. Am J Roentgenol 136: 887–891

Fone D R, Akkermans L M, Dent J, Horowitz M, Van der Schee E J 1990 Evaluation of patterns of human antral and pyloric motility with an antral wall motion detector. Am J Physiol 258: G616–G623

Geldof H, Van der Schee E J, Van Blankenstein M, Grashuis J L 1986 Electrogastrographic study of gastric myoelectrical activity in patients with unexplained nausea and vomiting. Gut 27: 799–808

Grundy D, Hutson D, Scratcherd T 1986 A permissive role of the vagus nerve in the genesis of antro-antral reflexes in the anaesthetised ferret. J Physiol 381: 377–384

Grundy D, Hutson D, Rudge L J, Scratcherd T 1989 Pre-pyloric mechanisms regulating gastric motor functions in the conscious dog. Q J Exp Physiol 74: 857–865

Hausken T, Odegaard S, Berstad A 1991 Antroduodenal motility studied by real-time ultrasonography. Gastroenterology 100: 59–63

Hausken T, Odegaard S, Matre K, Berstad A 1992 Antroduodenal motility and movements of luminal contents studied by duplex sonography. Gastroenterology 102: 1583–1590

Holm H H 1971 Ultrasonic scanning in the diagnosis of space-occupying lesions of the upper abdomen. Br J Radiol 44: 24–36

Holt S, McDicken W N, Anderson T, Stewart I C, Heading R C 1980 Dynamic imaging of the stomach by real-time ultrasound – a method for the study of gastric motility. Gut 21: 597–601

Holt S, Cervantes J, Wilkinson A A, Kirkwallace J H 1986 Measurement of gastric emptying rate in humans by real-time ultrasound. Gastroenterology 90: 918–923

Houghton L A, Read N W, Heddle R et al 1988a Motor activity of the gastric antrum, pylorus and duodenum under fasted conditions and after a liquid meal. Gastroenterology 94: 1276–1284

Houghton L A, Read N W, Heddle R et al 1988b Relationship of the motor activity of the gastric antrum, pylorus and duodenum to gastric emptying of a solid-liquid mixed meal. Gastroenterology 94: 1285–1291

Hunt J N, Knox M T 1968 A relation between the chain length of fatty acids and the slowing of gastric emptying. J Physiol 194: 327–336

Jacobs F, Akkermans L M A, You O H, Hoekstra A, Wittebol P 1982 A radioisotope method to quantify the functions of fundus, antrum and their contractile activity in gastric emptying of a semi-solid and solid meal in: Wienbeck M (ed.) Motility of the digestive tract, Raven Press, New York, pp 233–240

Kinnear Wilson L M, Waterhouse J A H 1984 Obstetric ultrasound and childhood malignancies. Lancet ii: 997–999

King P M, Adam R D, Pryde A, McDicken W N, Heading R C 1984 Relationships of human antroduodenal motility and transpyloric fluid movement: non-invasive

observations with real-time ultrasound. Gut 25: 1384–1391

King P M, Heading R C, Pryde A 1985 Co-ordinated motor activity of the human gastroduodenal region. Dig Dis Sci 30: 219–224

Langevin P, Chilowski M 1916 Procédés et appareils pour la production designaux sous-marins diriges et pour la localisation à distance d'obstacles sous-marins. Brevet français 502: 913

McMahon H, Bowie J, Beeshold C 1979 Erect scanning of the pancreas using a gastric window. Am J Gastroenterol 132: 587

Malagelada J-R, Stanghellini V 1985 Manometric evaluation of functional upper gut symptoms. Gastroenterology 88: 1223–1231

Marzio L, Giacobbe A, Conoscitore P, Facciorusso D, Frusciante V, Modoni S 1989 Evaluation of the use of ultrasonography in the study of liquid gastric emptying. Am J Gastroenterol 84: 496–500

Nyrén O 1992 Functional dyspepsia – a disease of the stomach in: Gustavsson S, Kumar D, Graham D Y (eds) The stomach. Churchill Livingstone, Edinburg, pp 385–415

Pröve J, Ehrlein H-J 1982 Motor function of gastric antrum and pylorus for evacuation of low and high viscosity meals in dogs. Gut 23: 150–156

Read N W, Al-Janabi M N, Bates T E, Barber D C 1983 Effect of gastrointestinal intubation on the passage of a solid meal through the stomach and small intestine of humans. Gastroenterology 84: 1468–1572

Smout A J P M, Akkermans L M A, Roelofs J M M, Pasma F G, Oei H Y, Wittebol P 1987 Gastric emptying and postprandial symptoms after Billroth II resection. Surgery 101: 27–34

Stacher G, Bergmann H, Haulik E, Schmiorer G, Schneider C 1984 Effect of oral cyclotroprium bromide, hyoscine N-butylbromide and placebo on gastric emptying and antral motor activity in healthy man. Gut 25: 485–490

Thompson D G, Mamtora H, Gait K 1989 Measurement of antral motor function by real-time ultrasound in health and in gastric diseases. Gastroenterology 96: A510

Troncon L E A, Bennett R J M, Ahluwalia N K, Thompson D G 1992 Abnormal intragastric distribution of food during gastric emptying in functional dyspepsia. Gastroenterology 102: A528

Walls W J 1976 The evaluation of malignant gastric neoplasms by ultrasonic B-scanning. Radiology 118: 159–163

Warren P S, Garrett W J, Kossoff G 1978 The liquid-filled stomach – an ultrasonic window to the upper abdomen. J Clin Ultrasound 6: 315–320

Weighall S L, Wolfman N T, Watson N 1979 The fluid-filled stomach: a new sonic window. J Clin Ultrasound 7: 353–356

White C M, Poxon V, Alexander-Williams J 1981 A study of motility of normal human gastroduodenal region. Dig Dis Sci 26: 609–617

You C H, Lee K Y, Chey W Y, Menguy R 1980 Electrogastrographic study of patients with unexplained nausea, bloating, and vomiting. Gastroenterology 79: 311–314

18. Electromyography

G. Coremans

One of the key observations in gastrointestinal motility research was the discovery of slow waves – electrical phenomena exhibited by smooth muscle cells. This rhythmic cycle of changes in membrane potential, with a repetition rate specific to different bowel segments, can occur either with or without associated action potential discharge activity and muscle contraction (Alvarez & Mahoney 1922, Bortoff & Ghalab 1972, Richter 1924, Bozler 1946, Armstrong et al 1956, McCoy & Bass 1963). Slow waves, also termed basal electrical rhythm, pacesetter potentials or electrical control activity are considered to be a myogenic mechanism controlling motility (Sarna 1975, Daniel & Sarna 1978). Slow waves occur continuously, without interruption, in stomach, small bowel and colon. Only when spikes, also called action potentials or electrical response activity are superimposed upon the plateau of the slow waves, do contractions occur (Sarna 1975, Bortoff & Ghalab 1972). Spike activity is normally initiated during maximal membrane depolarization. As contractions are triggered by spike bursts, which only occur during a limited part of the slow wave cycle, timing, maximal rate, direction and velocity of propagation are determined by the temporal and spatial organization of the slow waves (Bortoff & Ghalab 1972) (Fig. 18.1).

The factors that determine the occurrence of spikes and spike burst patterns, and thus of the accompanying contractions and organized motility patterns, are probably mainly neurohumoral responses to stimulation of chemo-, thermo- and mechanoreceptors in the gastrointestinal wall (Kosterlitz 1968).

RECORDING OF SMOOTH MUSCLE ELECTRICAL ACTIVITY

The electrical changes across the smooth muscle cell membranes generate intracellular and extracellular potentials which can be recorded both intracellularly and extracellularly using sophisticated technology (Bortoff 1975, Daniel & Chapman 1963). With the intracellular

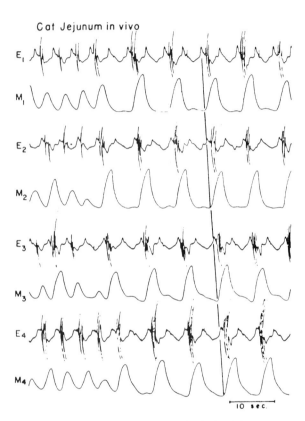

Fig. 18.1 Electrical (E_1–E_4) and mechanical activity (M_1–M_4) recorded along the cat jejunum in vivo at 2 cm intervals. Contractile wave propagates aborally at the same velocity as the corresponding slow waves and spike bursts. Solid line drawn to show propagation. (Reproduced with permission from Bortoff 1975.)

technique, a microelectrode is positioned in the cytoplasm of the cell making it possible to record the myoelectrical activity of a single cell (Bülbring & Hooton 1954). With the extracellular approach the electrodes are placed in the extracellular fluid surround-

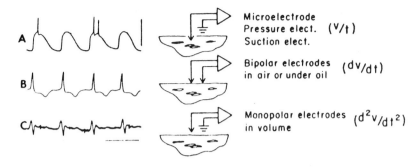

Fig. 18.2 Configuration of changes in membrane potential (slow waves) recorded from cat jejunum in vitro recorded by the methods indicated. (Reproduced with permission from Bortoff 1975.)

ing the smooth muscle cell mass which is organized as a syncytium. Extracellular electrodes record myoelectrical potentials reflecting the synchronized electrical activity generated by hundreds of cells which are in close contact with the surface electrodes. These electrodes can be used in both in vitro experiments and in vivo studies in experimental animals and humans. Intracellular electrodes can only be applied in vitro (Bortoff 1961).

While recording the electromyogram (EMG) both monopolar and bipolar techniques can be used (Bortoff 1975). In the monopolar technique the potentials are recorded by means of an active electrode and are referred to an indifferent electrode located in an area of weak electrical activity (Christensen et al 1964). In the bipolar technique the potential difference between the contact areas of a pair of electrodes is recorded. In in vivo studies, bipolar leads have the advantage of reducing cardiac, respiratory and movement artefacts, which can easily disturb monopolar recordings (Monges & Salducci 1970a).

The configuration of the recorded slow wave will be largely influenced by the method used to obtain it. Using glass tube suction microelectrodes in vitro, the rhythmic depolarizations of the smooth muscle cell membranes are recorded as monophasic slow waves. By recording with surface bipolar or monopolar electrodes in a volume conductor, such as intestinal fluid, the slow waves have a configuration approximating to the first and second time derivative respectively (Bortoff 1975, Bozler 1946) (Fig. 18.2).

The second electrical event, characterized by fast depolarizations and commonly named spike activity, can also be detected on the surface of the smooth muscle mass by means of external electrodes. Spike bursts are superimposed on the slow wave cycle and represent the summated action potentials of several individual smooth muscle cells (McCoy & Bass 1963,

Fleckenstein & Øigaard 1976, Sarna et al 1980, 1981).

RATIONALE FOR ELECTROMYOGRAPHY OF THE GASTROINTESTINAL TRACT

Electromyography with electrodes implanted in the smooth muscle through the serosa at operation has become an important and popular tool for measuring motility (Duthie et al 1972, Sarna et al 1981, Waterfall 1983). It is an accurate technique that can clearly identify slow waves and spike bursts, as well as their temporal and spatial organization, particularly in the stomach and small intestine and to a lesser extent in the colon (Sarna et al 1973, Sarna et al 1978). Although the rhythmic slow depolarizations of the smooth muscle cell membranes, recorded as slow waves, are not normally a contractile event, the registration of both electrical phenomena is meaningful in the study of motility, as the slow waves control the appearance of the spike bursts, and hence the contractions, in time and space along the gastrointestinal tract (Bortoff & Ghalab 1972). The occurrence of smooth muscle cell action potentials, that can be detected as the appearance of spike bursts on the slow wave cycle, is a sensitive indicator of muscular contractile activity and wall motion, as these spike potentials are a local phenomenon in the wall reflecting contraction of smooth muscle cells (Daniel & Chapman 1963, Bass & Wiley 1965, Kocylowski et al 1979) (Fig. 18.3). Short spike bursts may represent weak mechanical activity, not necessarily reflected in a rise of intraluminal pressure (Øigaard & Dorph 1974 a, b).

The simultaneous recordings of slow waves and spike bursts at closely spaced electrodes combined with intraluminal pressure measurements may contribute to a better understanding of the relation between segmental and propagated contractions and flow along

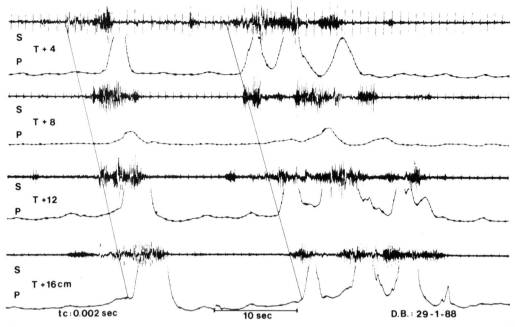

Fig. 18.3 Simultaneous recording, using closely spaced sensors, of spike activity (**S**) and pressure waves (**P**) in the human proximal jejunum during phase II of the MMC. A single propagated spike burst, accompanied by a single peak pressure wave is followed by propagated repetitive bursts of action potentials, accompanied by a cluster of repetitive pressure waves (**T + 4**: 4 cm past ligament of Treitz; **tc**: time constant).

the intestine (Bortoff & Sacco 1974, Summers & Dusdieker 1981, Sarna et al 1982, Fioramonti et al 1980b).

Electromyography allowed the characterization of the myogenic gradients along the intestine and of several motility patterns including the migrating myo-electrical complex (MMC), repetitive bursts of action potentials (RBAPs) and minute rhythm (Szurszewski 1969, Fleckenstein & Øigaard 1978, Diamant & Bortoff 1969, Vantrappen et al 1986, Coremans 1987, Coremans et al 1987). It also led to the discovery of abnormalities of myogenic control such as gastric dysrhythmias and inversion of the slow wave frequency gradient in patients with pseudo-obstruction and Roux-en-Y syndrome and to the detection of abnormal motor patterns, of which the migrating action potential complex (MAPC) and the stationary phase III (or pseudofront) are the best known (You et al 1981, Waterfall et al 1981, Coremans 1987, 1988, Coremans et al 1987, Vantrappen et al 1991) (Fig 18.4, 18.5). Recording of the electrical activity in pathological conditions also allows differentiation between myogenic and neural abnormalities of the gut. Absence of slow waves indicates smooth muscle cell damage (Lewis et al 1978, Sullivan et al 1977).

The simultaneous recording of slow waves and spikes was the first step in the long development of a less confusing terminology. Electromyography allowed a better characterization and classification of motility patterns based on the characteristics of the myoelectrical activity controlling them (Coremans 1987, Vantrappen et al 1986, Sarna 1975, Summers & Dusdieker 1981). By passing the electrical signals through filters and using adequate filter characteristics, a clear and stable baseline can be obtained allowing the determination of the exact beginning and end of the spike bursts and the accompanying contractile events (Code 1979, Marlett & Code 1979, Mathias et al 1976, Atchison et al 1978, Burns et al 1978) (Fig. 18.6).

INTRALUMINAL RECORDINGS OF MYOELECTRIC ACTIVITY IN MAN

The best and most reliable gastrointestinal EMGs in man have been obtained with implanted serosal electrodes in a 5–10-day period following an operation requiring laparotomy (Couturier et al 1972, Duthie et al 1972, Sarna et al 1978, 1981, Waterfall et al 1981, Waterfall 1983, Cucchiara et al 1986). Apart from ethical implications, the recording of electrical activity

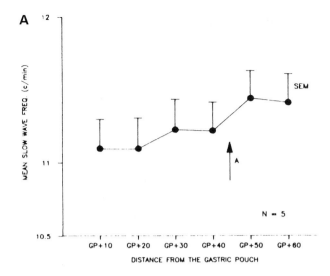

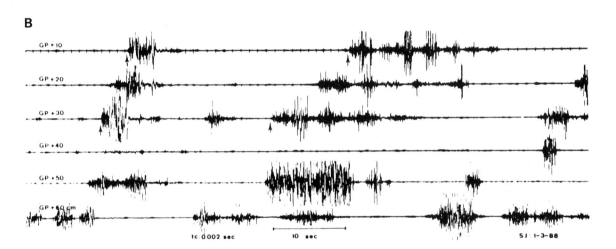

Fig. 18.4 **A** Inverse slow wave frequency gradient in the Roux limb of symptomatic patients with Roux-en Y reconstruction. **A**: level of end-to-side anastomosis; **GP + 10**: 10 cm below gastroenterostomy. **B** Single orally propagating contraction (arrows) followed by aborally propagating repetitive contractions (arrows) recorded during phase II of the MMC in the Roux limb of a patient with severe symptoms and delayed emptying. **GP + 10**: 10 cm below the gastric pouch; **tc**: time constant.

in a period in which motility may still be partially disrupted is a problem, as it may lead to erroneous conclusions about normal gastrointestinal motility. Therefore considerable efforts have been made to record the electrical events in a non-invasive way, i.e. from the mucosal surface by means of intraluminal electrodes (Fig. 18.7). The electrodes have been refined and perfected, and probes with reduced diameters are better tolerated for long periods of time by both healthy volunteers and sick patients (Coremans 1987, Coremans et al 1987).

Intraluminal electromyography of the gastrointestinal tract in man poses two types of problems: those inherent to motility studies in general and those related to the recording of the actual electrical events. Problems inherent to motility studies are related to the location and function of the gastrointestinal segment studied. The oesophagus and stomach can easily be reached. In contrast, the introduction of electrodes in regions where access is difficult, such as the jejunum, ileum and colon, is much more time-consuming. Positioning of a probe provided with electrodes in the colon using endoscopy is even potentially hazardous for the subject.

Problems due to gastrointestinal function are related to cyclic variations in gastrointestinal motor events. Ideally, due to the slow recycling of the MMC in the interdigestive phase, the duration of the postprandial pattern, and the slow movements and the circadian rhythm of the colon, the recording should last 24 h and include standard meals, but this exacerbates the discomfort for the subject (Vantrappen et al 1977, Frexinos et al 1985, Fleckenstein & Øigaard 1978). The

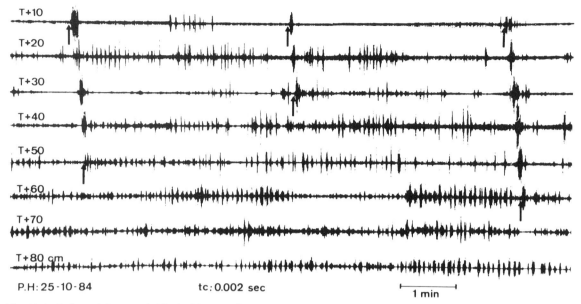

Fig. 18.5 Spike activity recorded in the jejunum of a patient with secretory diarrhoea. In addition to phase II activity of the MMC, three intensive spike bursts described as 'migrating action potential complexes' (➡) can be observed. These bursts progress distally over a distance of 40, 20 and 50 cm respectively. **T + 10**: 10 cm below ligament of Treitz; **tc**: time constant.

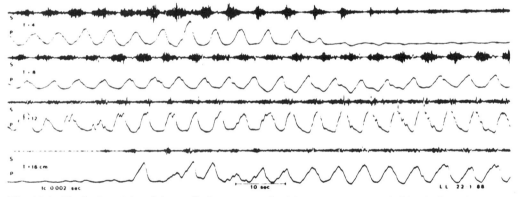

Fig. 18.6 Rhythmic activity of short spike bursts at maximal frequency, accompanied by single peak pressure waves recorded in the human jejunum during phase III of the MMC. **S**: spike activity; **P**: pressure waves; **T + 4**: 4 cm below ligament of Treitz; **tc**: time constant.

wide variation in motor patterns and periodicity even in healthy subjects also require prolonged recording in order to distinguish between health and disease (McRae et al 1982, Thompson et al 1980, Kumar et al 1986).

Different types of electrodes for recording the extracellular potentials from the mucosal face of the gastrointestinal tract have been reported. They all have their inherent advantages and limitations. Major problems are: intermittent signal loss precluding simultaneous recordings at different sites, artefacts caused by

movements or by strong contractions, excessively voluminous and complex construction, and inadequate slow wave detection. To aid analysis of the slow waves the electrical signals have to be passed through filters with a high time constant (lower frequency limit), necessitating uninterrupted, close contact between the electrodes and the gastrointestinal wall, that can only be obtained with suction or clip electrodes or with ring electrodes held against the mucosa by the use of magnetic force (Abell & Malagelada 1985). Various types of electrodes are suitable for incorporation in a single tube

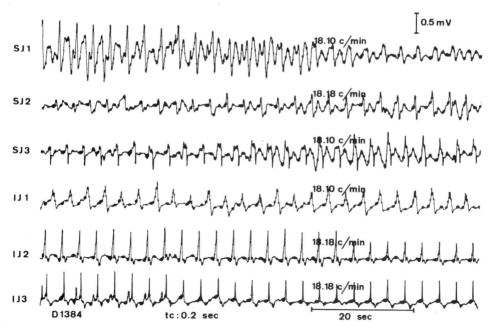

Fig. 18.7 Slow waves simultaneously recorded 10 cm apart with intraluminal suction electrodes (**SJ1–SJ3**) and implanted electrodes (**IJ1–IJ3**) in the dog in vivo. Notice the waxing and waning of the amplitude of the slow waves recorded with suction electrodes, probably as the consequence of the varying distance between the electrical source and electrode, due to changes in contact. The amplitude of the slow waves recorded with implanted electrodes is much more stable. **SJ1** and **IJ1**: 5 cm below ligament of Treitz. **SJ2** and **IJ2**: 15 cm below ligament of Treitz. **SJ3** and **IJ3**: 25 cm below ligament of Treitz.

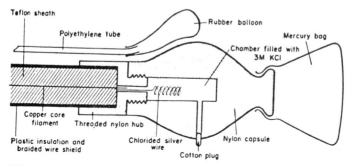

Fig. 18.8 Diagram of a complex monopolar silver–silver chloride KCl salt-bridge electrode. (Reprinted with permission from Christensen et al 1964.)

at a chosen spacing, allowing not only the recording of the electrical phenomena, but also the direction and propagation of the slow waves and spike bursts (Coremans 1987, Sarna et al 1982).

The various electrodes described include wick, needle, suction, ring and clip electrodes. In wick (salt bridge) electrodes the electrical contact between the wall and a chlorided silver wire electrode is effected by a cotton wick impregnated with saline or KCl. Unipolar wick electrodes with a cutaneous reference electrode are characterized by the absence of an injury potential, but do not usually allow simultaneous recordings and are prone to movement artefacts (Morton 1954). A bipolar silver–silver chloride KCl salt-bridge electrode has been employed for recording in the duodenum and jejunum, but is too complex to allow simultaneous recordings (Christensen et al 1964, 1966) (Fig. 18.8).

Needle or punctate electrodes usually provide reliable recordings (Kwong et al 1970, Monges & Salducci 1970a, b) (Fig. 18.9). Different materials that have been successfully used include platinum, stainless

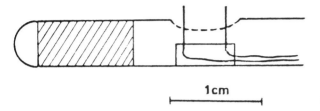

Fig. 18.9 Bipolar electrode composed of two stainless-steel electrodes, 4 mm apart, mounted in a side opening of a nasogastric tube and fixed to the mucosa by suction. (Reprinted with permission from Kwong et al 1970.)

steel and chlorided silver. Unipolar needle electrodes can be used with ECG skin electrodes as the reference (Couturier et al 1973). With bipolar electrodes containing needles up to 10 mm apart, the amplitude of the spike bursts increases with the distance between the needles. Needle electrodes are always mounted in a side hole of a tube or in a capsule made of rubber, PVC or plexiglas, in order to protect the needles and to apply negative pressure by suction to ensure contact of the electrode with the mucosal surface. Multiple needle electrodes can be incorporated in a single tube, but increasing the number of suction holes in the tube results in a more frequent loss of contact because of the presence of a more or less rigid segment between the suction orifices (Altaparmakov 1983, Hellemans et al 1968, Taylor et al 1978, Frieri et al 1983). Suction electrodes may also be simple contact bipolar electrodes comprising silver dots fixed at either side of lateral openings in a suction tube. They allow the recording of both types of electrical events (Coremans 1987, Coremans et al 1987) (Fig. 18.10).

Ring or circumferential wire electrodes are bipolar and consist of copper or nickel-chrome (80–20%) wires wound around the circumference of a tube, 5–6 mm in diameter, with a space of 4–5 mm between the wires. Series of ring electrodes can be easily mounted in a single tube allowing simultaneous recordings at adjacent sites (Fig. 18.11). But, as these electrodes move freely in the lumen of the intestine and as they are exposed to the liquid or semi-solid contents of the intestine, they are only adequate for recording spike bursts (Fleckenstein & Øigaard 1978, Fioramonti et al 1980a, b, Kolrep-Dechauffour et al 1989, Tokita et al 1970).

Clip electrodes containing stainless steel or silver–silver chloride parts have to be attached to the mucosa through an endoscope. They allow recording of both slow waves and spike activity. However, recordings at different levels simultaneously require repeated intubations of the subjects, as only one electrode can be passed at the time (Snape et al 1977a, b) (Fig. 18.12).

ELECTROMYOGRAPHY OF THE OESOPHAGUS

Although the oesophagus is an easily accessible segment of the intestinal tract, its electrical activity has not been extensively studied and electromyography is not yet an important method of assessment of oesophageal function. Nevertheless it has been shown that this technique allows the study of electrical events in the striated muscle of the upper oesophageal segment and in the smooth muscle of the distal oesophagus, the latter being of greater clinical interest since most motility disorders involve the distal oesophagus. At the present time only patterns of electrical activity that are closely related to the well-known mechanical responses to deglutition, such as the peristaltic pressure complex and the phenomenon of deglutitive inhibition, have been described. Electromyography, if combined with manometry, also allows the study of electromechanical coupling in the oesophagus in health and disease.

The best tracings in the human oesophagus have so far been obtained with suction electrodes (Monges et al 1968, Hellemans et al 1968, Bortolotti et al 1989). Bipolar electrodes consisting of a capsule of rubber or plexiglas containing silver or platinum-covered stainless steel needles, 0.1 mm in diameter, with an interelectrode distance of 2–6 mm were used by Hellemans et al (Fig. 18.13). In order to obtain simultaneous recordings at multiple levels, multiple electrodes have to be

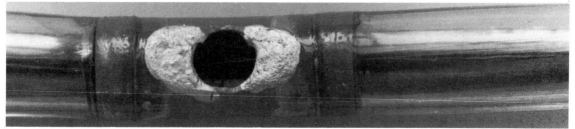

Fig. 18.10 Electrode with two silver conductive surfaces located on each side of a lateral suction opening incorporated in a polyvinyl tube. Insulated connecting wires shielded by polyvinyl tubing are lying in the lumen of the probe.

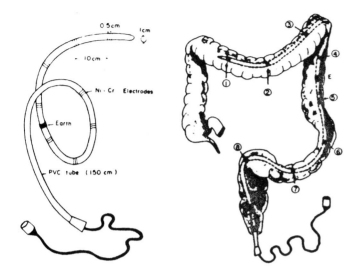

Fig. 18.11 EMG probe consisting of polyvinyl tube, 1 cm in diameter, carrying groups of bipolar ring electrodes of nichrome wire. The tube is introduced via the anus by colonoscope. (Reprinted with permission from Bueno et al 1980.)

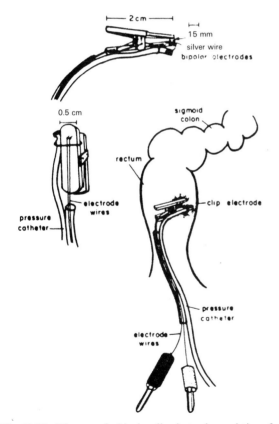

Fig. 18.12 Diagram of a bipolar clip electrode consisting of two silver wires 2 mm apart. The electrodes have to be introduced one by one in the distal colon through the proctoscope. (Reproduced with permission from Snape et al 1977b.)

introduced separately (Fig. 18.14). The incorporation of several suction capsules in a single probe will inevitably result in movement artefacts at the level of the distal electrode because of the upward and downward movements of the proximal segment during swallowing. This problem can be overcome to some extent by using multiple bipolar ring electrodes mounted on an intraluminal probe (Tokita et al 1970, Goodman et al 1966). However, after the probe has been swallowed, frequent manipulations of the probe are necessary to bring the electrodes in close contact with the oesophageal wall in order to record spike activity.

At rest, using implanted electrodes in animals with an oesophagus that resembles that of humans, and with intraluminal electrodes in humans, neither slow wave nor spike potentials can be recorded in the striated and smooth muscle part of the oesophageal body; electromyographic activity has to be studied on repetitive deglutitions (Hellemans et al 1968, 1970).

To study the electrical events accompanying peristalsis, three electrodes 5 cm apart in the oesophageal body and one electrode in the lower oesophageal sphincter are ideally used, so as to cover the entire smooth muscle segment. Adequate evaluation of oesophageal motility necessitates the performance of a series of wet swallows with intervals of more than 20 s, with recording of deglutition by an effective external automatic signal.

At the present time electromyography allows only a qualitative study of oesophageal motility. It is possible to record the spike potentials, organized in distally progressing bursts upon deglutition. Two types of

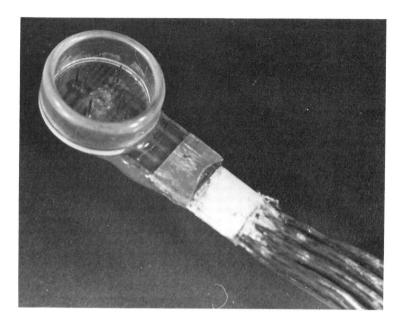

Fig. 18.13 Suction capsule for recording electrical activity in the human oesophagus. The plexiglas capsule contains eight platinum needles with a length of 4 mm and a diameter of 0.1 mm at the top. Via an external switching device it is possible to choose a number of bipolar combinations with distances between the recording electrodes varying from 2–6 mm. (Reprinted with permission from Hellemans Vantrappen 1974.)

A

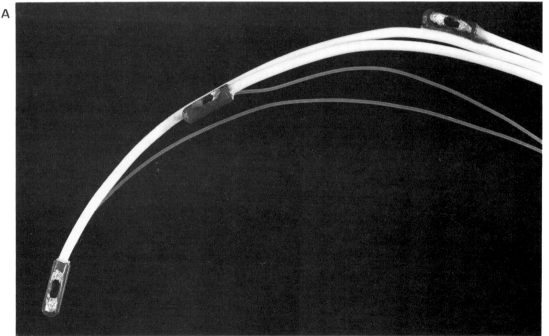

B

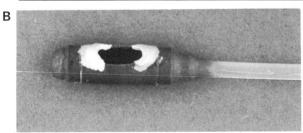

Fig. 18.14 **A** Three bipolar silver dot suction electrodes incorporated in three different poly-vinyl suction tubes for recording electrical activity in the human oesophagus. **B** Detail of suction capsule with two discrete conductive surfaces located at the two poles of the orifice.

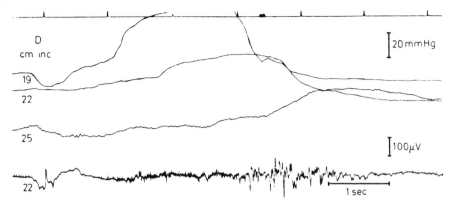

Fig. 18.15 EMG recorded in the human oesophagus with bipolar suction needle electrodes in the transitional zone between striated and smooth muscle portions at 22 cm from the incisors (cm inc). Simultaneous intraluminal pressure measurement at 19, 22 and 25 cm from the incisors. The electrical tracing shows initially the striated muscle type spike potentials followed by the smooth muscle type spike potentials. **D**: deglutition. (Reprinted with permission from Hellemans & Vantrappen 1974.)

action potentials upon deglutition may be observed, corresponding to smooth muscle and striated muscle (Monges et al 1968, Hellemans et al 1970). In the transitional zone both types of spike potentials occur (Fig. 18.15). The EMG of the LOS is difficult to obtain because of the technical problems of fastening the electrodes in the high pressure zone. Thus far, an electrical equivalent of sphincter relaxation has not been described in man (Monges et al 1968, Hellemans et al 1970). In contrast the electromyographic equivalent of the phenomenon of the deglutitive inhibition, in both the striated and smooth muscle part of the oesophagus, has been clearly characterized (Hellemans et al 1970).

ELECTROMYOGRAPHY OF THE STOMACH

Gastric myoelectrical activity can be recorded by means of implanted serosal electrodes, different types of intraluminal electrodes or by using cutaneous electrodes (Couturier et al 1972, 1973, Brown et al 1975, Hamilton et al 1986).

Recordings with serosal electrodes clearly show that the slow waves with a cycling frequency of 3 cpm originate on the greater curvature in the proximal corpus, propagating aborally in the distal corpus and antrum to the pylorus, either accompanied by spike activity or not (Hinder & Kelly 1977) (Fig. 18.16). As it is known from studies with serosal implanted electrodes that the gastric fundus does not exhibit typical slow waves, all the reported intraluminal recordings of

gastric electrical activity were obtained in the gastric body and antrum distal to the pacemaker region (Sarna et al 1972).

Surface electrodes are attractive, as they allow the recording of slow waves and their propagation in a non-invasive way. However, this method does not record spike activity (Smout et al 1980, Hamilton et al 1988).

Myoelectrical activity of the stomach has successfully been recorded simultaneously at adjacent areas using different types of intraluminal electrodes mounted on an intraluminal probe (Fig. 18.17). The probe with the electrodes can easily be positioned in the antrum along the greater curvature under fluoroscopic control. Wick, suction, circumferential wire and clip electrodes have been used with success (Morton 1954, Kwong et al 1970, Monges & Salducci 1970a, b, Couturier et al 1973, Fleckenstein & Øigaard 1978, Stoddard et al 1981).

Bipolar contact or needle electrodes which are fixed to the gastric mucosa by suction provided good tracings of both slow waves and spikes (Monges & Salducci 1970a). Bipolar stainless steel or silver chloride electrodes were incorporated in suction capsules or in the lateral holes of a tube, with a distance of 2–10 mm between the electrode parts. However, loss of contact due to strong antral contractions, particularly when multiple suction electrodes are incorporated in the same tube remains a difficult problem. Nickel–chrome or copper ring electrodes mounted on a polyvinyl tube, the wires being 5 mm apart to form bipolar

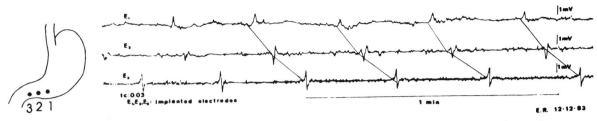

Fig. 18.16 Gastric slow waves recorded in a patient using three bipolar electrodes, surgically implanted on the antral serosa. Slow waves at a regular rhythm of 3 cpm propagate from the antrum to the pylorus. E_1, E_2, E_3: electrode sites at a distance of respectively 2.5, 1.5 and 0.5 cm from the pylorus. (Reproduced with permission from Cucchiara et al 1986.)

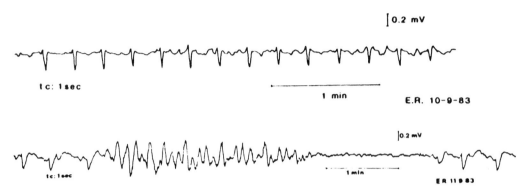

Fig. 18.17 Gastric electrical activity recorded by an intraluminal bipolar silver suction electrode in the gastric antrum of a girl with chronic intractable vomiting. Regular slow wave rhythm at 3 cpm (upper tracing) is followed by an episode of tachyarrhythmia characterized by irregular fast slow wave activity followed by a pause (**tc**: time constant). (Reproduced with permission from Cucchiara et al 1986.)

electrodes, allowed reliable spike burst detection. However, recordings of the slow waves were poor (Fleckenstein & Øigaard 1978). Small stainless steel clip electrodes of which the two parts are insulated from each other and soldered to conducting wires provided good contact with the gastric wall and reliable detection of slow waves. These electrodes have to be introduced by a flexible endoscope and fixed to the wall using a special device and seem to be less effective in recording spike bursts.

ELECTROMYOGRAPHY OF THE SMALL INTESTINE

There are a number of problems inherent in motility studies of the small bowel. They include the introduction of an array of electrodes in the jejunum or ileum, the long cycling period of the interdigestive motor activity and the duration of the fed pattern necessitating long recording periods and the occurrence of strong uncoordinated contractions during phase II of the MMC and the postprandial activity.

The intubation of the jejunum or ileal segments to be investigated is usually not difficult in healthy subjects. In contrast, in patients with disordered motility such as pseudo-obstruction, it may be a problem. In order to facilitate the passage of the electrodes through the stomach, a latex balloon, partially filled with mercury, may be attached to the distal end of the probe. Usually it suffices to turn the subject on his or her right side on the fluoroscopy table to see the bag slip into the duodenum. In most healthy subjects the electrodes then reach the angle of Treitz in a few minutes and it is not necessary to stimulate propulsive contractions by means of gastrokinetic drugs such as dopamine antagonists or cisapride. In difficult cases the probe can be passed over a guide wire, introduced into the distal duodenum via the biopsy channel of an endoscope. In order to hasten the passage of the probe down the small intestine, an inflatable balloon may be

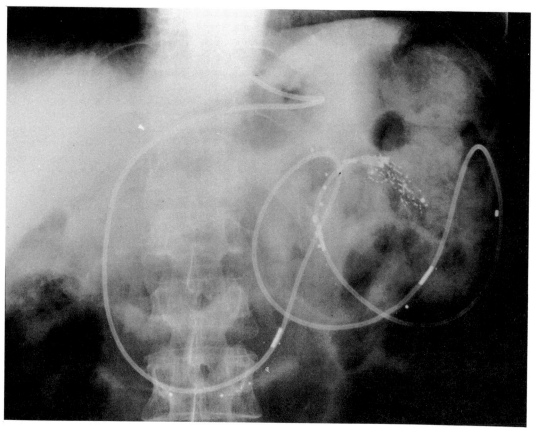

Fig. 18.18   EMG probe, 6 mm in diameter, carrying three suction electrodes, 40 cm apart, placed in the jejunum with the tip approximately 80 cm past the ligament of Treitz.

attached to the distal end of the probe. Once the probe has reached the desired level, the balloon should be deflated, so that it is not propelled aborally and no longer acts as an artificial stimulus of motility.

The same balloon can be used for both mercury and air filling. Reaspiration of mercury is facilitated if two catheters end inside the balloon, one for aspiration of mercury, the other for simultaneous inflation of air so that collapse of the latex balloon does not prevent aspiration. Frequently, the most difficult part of the intubation is to pass the probe over the angle of Treitz and down the first jejunal loop. In many subjects this loop turns from the angle of Treitz to the right before descending. We usually inflate the balloon with air only after it has passed one or two proximal jejunal loops (Fig. 18.18). Positioning of the probe with the distal end 80 cm below the angle of Treitz usually takes about 30 min (Coremans et al 1987).

Not only is the introduction of the probe in the small bowel demanding, but also the long recording time may contribute to the discomfort of the patient. Due to the slow recycling activity of the MMC, fasted motor activity in the small bowel should be recorded for at least 6 h before it is concluded that typical MMC activity is absent. As the first MMC after a meal starts ectopically in the jejunum and the first few MMCs are often more irregular than those developing after a longer fast, it is advisable to start the recording after a fast of at least 12 h (Fig. 18.19). The typical fed pattern after a standard meal of 450 kcal is seen from 5–210 min postprandially. Ideally the recording of the postprandial activity is continued until the MMCs reappear.

A complete study of the myoelectrical activity of the small bowel not only requires the continuous recording of the spike activity, but also of the slow waves from a large number of sites along the duodenum and the small bowel to identify both the motility patterns and

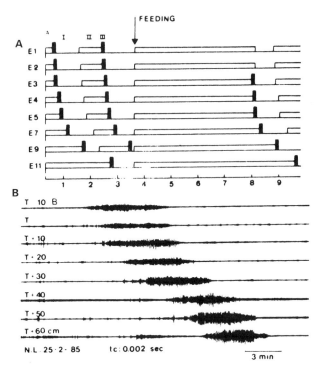

Fig. 18.19 A Histogram representing the number of spike bursts per minute during a complete MMC cycle with phase I, II and III in the duodenum and proximal jejunum (E1–E11). Feeding disrupted MMC activity for about 4 h. Note that the first MMC at the end of the 'fed' pattern started ectopically in the jejunum. **B** Interdigestive spike activity recorded in the human jejunum with intraluminal electrodes. Phase II, that is characterized by irregular spike activity, is followed by phase III, consisting of a migrating burst of rhythmic spike activity and phase I, during which no spike activity is detected. **T + 10**: cm below the ligament of Treitz.

the exact configuration of the slow wave frequency gradient, the latter determining the maximum frequency and polarity of the contractions (Coremans 1987, Coremans et al 1987, 1988, Vantrappen et al 1986) (Fig. 18.20).

Studies in man have been performed previously either with one single salt bridge electrode providing tracings that are not suitable for the study of slow wave coupling between different locations in the small bowel (Christensen et al 1966), or with an array of ring electrodes that allowed 24-h recording of spikes and analysis of phase III of the MMC; the latter technique is completely unsuitable for the detection of slow waves (Fleckenstein & Øigaard 1978). Since the pioneering work of Fleckenstein and Christensen on the small bowel the technique of intraluminal recording of myo-

electrical activity in the small intestine has been considerably improved. Coremans et al (1987) designed a probe that can contain up to eight bipolar electrodes mounted on either side of the lateral openings of a suction canal. The electrodes are held in close contact with the mucosa by the continuous application of slight negative pressure. The probe consists of a polyvinyl tube with an outer diameter of 6 mm and a length of 300 cm (Fig. 18.21), with a small latex balloon attached to the tip. The two discrete conductive surfaces of the electrodes are located at the two poles of the oval suction orifices, which measure 3 mm x 4 mm (Fig. 18.10). The conductive surfaces consist of silver powder dispersed in a mixture of tetrahydrofuran and polyvinyl chloride and are connected to the exterior with fine insulated copper wires in the lumen of the tube. The connecting wires of each pair of electrodes are doubled so that each bipolar electrode can be connected to two preamplifiers with different frequency characteristics. In this way the electrical activity picked up by each electrode is displayed in two different recordings, one well suited for slow wave activity, the other for spike activity. Slow waves and spikes can also be displayed simultaneously (Fig. 18.22). As might be expected, the amplitude of the electrical activity frequently varies in time and from electrode to electrode, probably as the consequence of the varying distance between the electrical source and recording electrode due to changes in contact between electrode surfaces and bowel wall, and to bowel contractions. To obtain uninterrupted detection of the electrical signals a negative pressure of only 25–50 cm water applied on the proximal end of the tube is sufficient (Fig. 18.23).

ELECTROMYOGRAPHY OF THE COLON

The electrophysiological basis of colonic motility is poorly understood. There are four main reasons for this: the relative inaccessibility of the colon, the occurrence of circadian rhythms requiring long recording periods, a longitudinal muscle that is not continuous but typically arranged in taeniae, and the irregularity of the slow waves making visual analysis impossible for most of the time. Intraluminal electrodes can be introduced perorally or via the anus. The passage of an array of electrodes through the small intestine into the colon is difficult and time-consuming. Colonoscopy makes it possible to introduce several electrodes mounted on a flexible tube allowing the simultaneous recording of myoelectrical activity at different levels in the colon (Bueno et al 1980) (Fig. 18.11). Drawbacks of the introduction of electrodes using the colonoscope

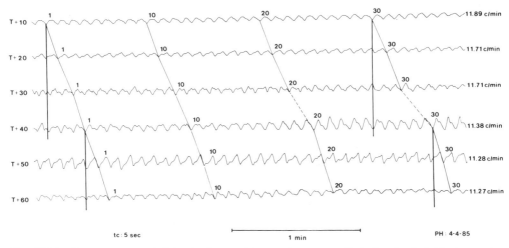

Fig. 18.20 Slow wave recorded in the human jejunum by means of six intraluminal bipolar suction electrodes during 30 consecutive slow wave cycles in phase I of the MMC. During the recording period the slow waves remained phase locked between **T + 10, T + 20** and **T + 30**. The slow waves at **T + 40** (11.38 c/min) became phase unlocked with the slow waves at **T + 10** (11.89 c/min) after about 20 cycles, as the increase in phase lag was more than one cycle. **T + 10**: 10 cm below ligament of Treitz; **tc**: time constant; solid oblique lines: phase locking; dotted oblique lines: phase unlocking; vertical lines drawn to show the phase lag.

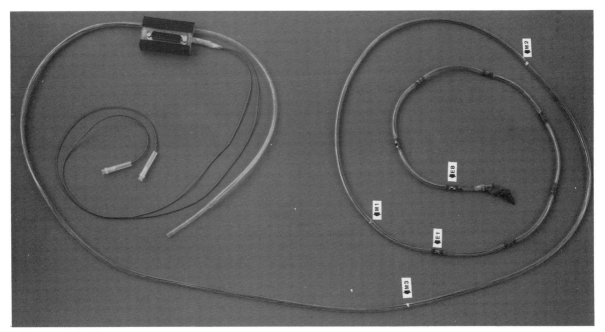

Fig. 18.21 Probe for small bowel electromyography with eight bipolar (**E1–E8**) suction electrodes, 10 cm apart. **M1–M3**: radiopaque markers 10, 60 and 110 cm proximal to **E1**.

are the need for bowel preparation to empty the colon, premedication and air insufflation, which are likely to interfere with normal electrical activity. Colonic spike

activity may undergo marked variation from one moment to another. It is influenced by physical activity and food intake, and shows a typical circadian rhythm

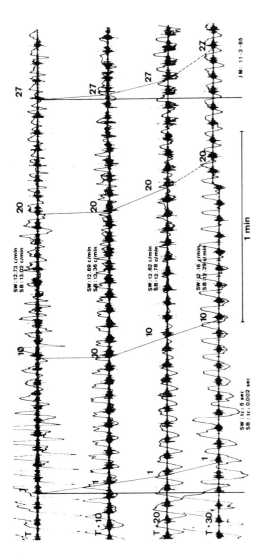

Fig. 18.22   Simultaneous recording of slow waves and spike burst activity in the human jejunum at the end of phase III of the MMC. The tracing is characterized by the occurrence of a spike burst in association with every slow wave cycle. Slow waves and spike bursts remain phase locked during 27 consecutive cycles between **T** and **T + 20** (solid lines); they became phase unlocked after 20 cycles between **T + 20** and **T + 30** (dotted lines). **T**: level of ligament of Treitz; **T + 10**: 30 cm below ligaments of Treitz; **tc**: time constant.

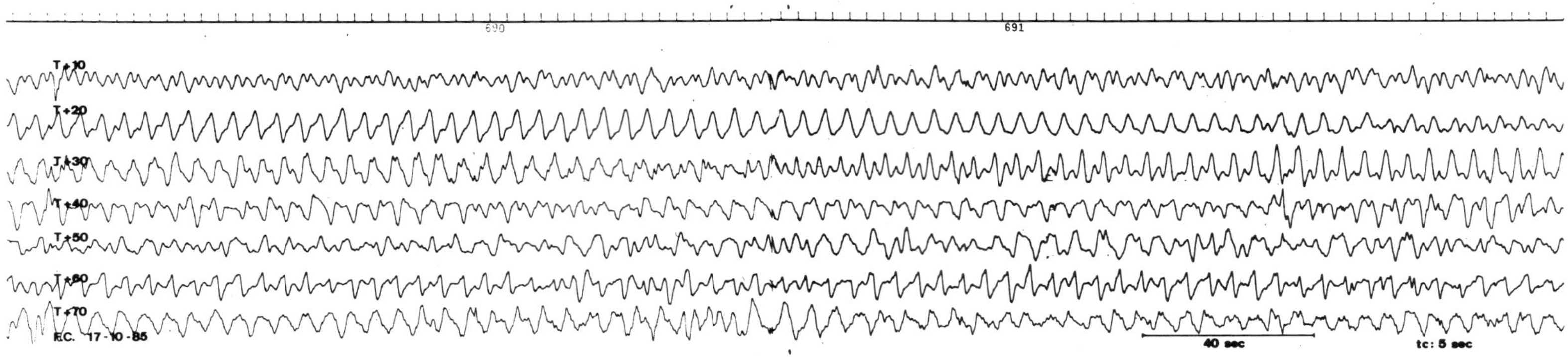

Fig. 18.23   Uninterrupted slow wave activity recorded simultaneously at seven locations in the jejunum of a healthy subject using suction electrodes 10 cm apart. Myoelectric activity was recorded during phase I and early phase II of the MMC.

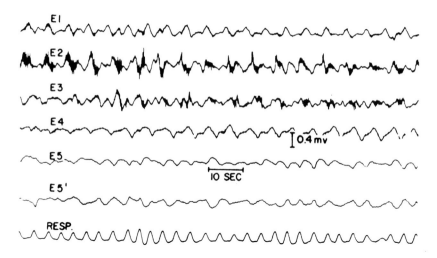

Fig. 18.24 Slow waves and intermittent irregular discrete spike bursts occurring within a slow wave cycle, recorded with surgically implanted serosal electrodes in the human transverse colon. Note that in this region approximate visual analysis of the dominant slow wave frequency is possible (Reprinted with permission from Sarna et al 1980.)

with mass movements occurring only a few times per day (Frexinos et al 1985, Sarna et al 1981). 24-h recordings seem to be inevitable, as short time recordings may lead to erroneous conclusions as a consequence of this marked variability.

The electrical communications between the continuous circular muscle layer and the longitudinal layer that is arranged in taeniae is up to now, poorly understood (El-Sharhawy 1978). The coupling of the slow waves in the different axes of the colon can only be studied with implanted electrodes, as the spatial relationship between the two muscle layers and intraluminal electrodes cannot be determined. In man, even with postoperatively implanted electrodes, the reported slow wave characteristics have been inconsistent, probably because of the variability in slow wave frequency, amplitude and coordination in time and space in the different colonic segments and in the two muscle layers (Sarna et al 1980). A wide spectrum of slow wave frequencies ranging from 2–13 cpm with different dominant frequencies have been obtained, and slow wave frequency gradients in the various parts of the colon have been demonstrated, without a consistent pattern of phase locking in either the circular or longitudinal direction (Bardakjian & Sarna 1980, Sarna et al 1980, Huizinga et al 1985) (Fig. 18.24). Depending on the method used to analyse the typically irregular slow waves, fundamental frequencies between 2 and 13 cpm have been detected (Taylor et al 1975, Provenciale & Pisano 1971, Sarna et al 1980). In addition to slow waves, surgically implanted electrodes in the human colon allowed the detection of different types of burst

patterns. Spike activity in the colon not only occurs as discrete bursts within one slow wave cycle, but also as continuous activity extending over several slow waves (Fig. 18.24). Furthermore the spike bursts may be both orally and aborally propagated (Sarna et al 1981).

Intraluminal recordings of colonic myoelectric activity have been obtained with needle electrodes attached by suction to the mucosa, clip and ring electrodes (Couturier et al 1967, 1979, Provenciale & Pisano 1971, Taylor et al 1978, Snape 1977a, b, Altaparmakov 1983, Frexinos et al 1985, Fioramonti et al 1980, a, b, Schang & Devroede 1983). As it was believed that abnormalities of the slow waves were directly related to colonic motor disorders, a lot of attention was focused on the development of electrodes allowing the recording of slow waves (Snape 1977a, b, Taylor et al 1978). Since recording of slow waves requires the use of a long time constant, suction electrodes or clip electrodes were developed to assure close contact to the colonic wall. Stainless steel or silver chloride pin electrodes mounted in side holes in a tube and attached by suction have been used (Taylor et al 1975, Sarna et al 1980), but are easily detached from the mucosa during wall movements.

The technique of using simple bipolar contact electrodes to record myoelectrical activity in the small bowel, may also be used to record both slow waves and spikes in the human colon (Coremans 1987a, b) (Fig. 18.25). Clip electrodes, giving good contact with the wall, have to be introduced one by one through a rigid proctoscope or a flexible endoscope, and have been successful in recording both slow waves and spike bursts (Snape 1977a). With needle and clip

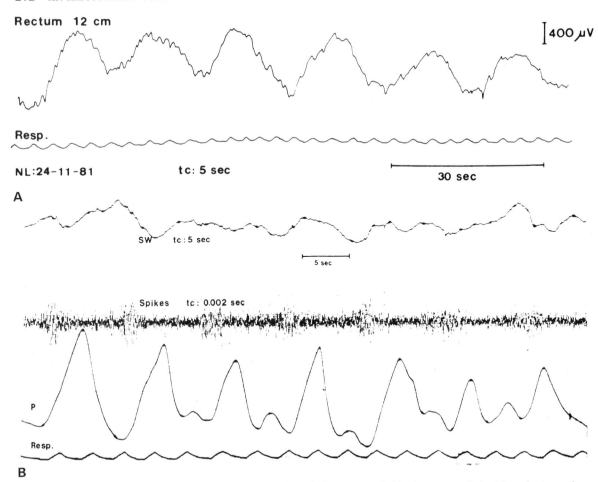

Fig. 18.25 **A** Regular slow waves, at a frequency of approximately 3 cpm, recorded in the rectum of a healthy volunteer using a bipolar silver dot suction electrode. **B** Simultaneous recordings of slow waves, spike activity and pressure waves (**P**) in the sigmoid colon of a healthy volunteer, 15 cm above the anus. Variability in slow wave characteristics makes visual analysis impossible. Slow waves and spikes were recorded with a biopolar silver dot electrode held against the wall by suction. Pressure was recorded with a perfused catheter at the level of the electrode. A contraction frequency of about 7 per min is clearly seen. **Resp.**: respiration; **tc**: time constant.

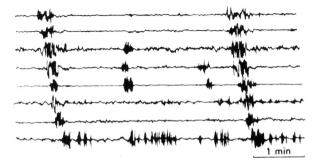

Fig. 18.26 Postprandial spike burst activity in the human descending colon with eight bipolar intraluminal ring electrodes at 10 cm distances, showing strong spike bursts propagating distally over at least 70 cm distance. (Reprinted with permission from Bueno et al 1980.)

electrodes slow wave activity was only recorded intermittently. The exact cause of the isoelectric periods, not found with implanted electrodes, is not known.

More recently attention has been focused on the recording of spike activity in different colonic segments with multiple closely-spaced electrodes, to study the variability and circadian rhythm of colonic motor activity. This method, although unsuitable for the recording of slow waves, can provide tracings of different motility patterns and even a complete 24-h motility profile of the colon (Bueno et al 1980, Fioramonti et al 1980a, b, Frexinos et al 1985) (Fig. 18.26) and is described in Chapter 28.

REFERENCES

Abell T L, Malagelada J R 1985 Glucagon-evoked gastric dysrhythmias in humans shown by an improved electrogastrographic technique. Gastroenterology 88: 1932–1940

Altaparmakov A 1983 Probe for multipositional intraluminal electromyography and colonomanometry. Comptes rendus de l'Académie Bulgare des Sciences 36: 987–990

Alvarez W C, Mahoney L J 1922 Action currents in the stomach and small intestine. Am J Physiol 58: 476–493

Armstrong H I O, Milton G W, Smith A W M 1956 Electropotential changes of the small intestine. J Physiol (London) 131: 147–153

Atchison W D, Stewart J J, Bass P 1978 A unique distribution of laxative-induced spike potentials from the small intestine of the dog. Dig Dis 23: 513–520

Bardakjian B L, Sarna S K 1980 A computer model of human colonic electrical control activity (ECA). IEEE Trans Biomed Eng 27: 193–202

Bass P, Wiley J 1965 Electrical and extraluminal contractile force activity of the duodenum of the dog. Am J Dig Dis 10: 183–200

Bortoff A 1961 Slow potential variation of small intestine. Am J Physiol 20: 203–208

Bortoff A 1975 Electrical activity of gastrointestinal muscle in: Friedman M H F (ed.) Functions of the stomach and intestine. University Park Press, Baltimore pp 17–30

Bortoff A, Ghalab E 1972 Temporal relationship between electrical and mechanical activity of longitudinal and circular muscle during intestinal peristalsis. Am J Dig Dis 17: 317–325

Bortoff A, Sacco J 1974 Myogenic control of intestinal peristalsis in: Daniel E E (ed.) Proc IV Int Symp Gastrointestinal Motility, Mitchell Press, Vancouver, pp 53–63

Bortolotti A, Pinotti R, Sarti P et al 1989 Esophageal electromyography in scleroderma patients with functional dysphagia. Am J Gastroenterol 84: 1497–1502

Bozler E 1946 The relation of action potentials to mechanical activity in intestinal muscle. Am J Physiol 146: 496–501

Brown B H, Smallwood R H, Duthie H L et al 1975 Intestinal smooth muscle electrical potentials recorded from surface electrodes. Med Biol Eng 13: 97–103

Bueno L, Fioramonti J, Ruckebusch J et al 1980 Evaluation of colonic myoelectrical activity in health and functional disorders. Gut 21: 480–485

Bülbring E, Hooton I N 1954 Membrane potentials in smooth muscle fibres in the rabbit's sphincter pupillae. J Physiol (London) 125: 292–301

Burns T W, Mathias J R, Carlson G M et al 1978 Effects of toxigenic Escherichia coli on myoelectric activity of small intestine. Am J Physiol 235 (3): E311–E315

Christensen J, Schedl H P, Clifton J A 1964 The basic electrical rhythm of the duodenum in normal human subjects and in patients with thyroid disease. J Clin Invest 43: 1659–1667

Christensen J, Schedl H P, Clifton J A 1966 The small intestinal basic electrical rhythm (slow wave) frequency gradient in normal man and in patients with a variety of diseases. Gastroenterology 50: 309–315

Code C F 1979 Diarrheogenic motor and electrical patterns of the bowel in: Janowitz H D, Sachar D B (eds) Frontiers of knowledge of diarrheal diseases. Projects in Health, Upper Montclair, New Jersey pp 227–241

Coremans G 1987 Myogenic control and motility patterns of the human small bowel. PhD Thesis, Acco Leuven, Belgium

Coremans G, Janssens J, Vantrappen G 1987 Migrating action potential complexes in a patient with secretory diarrhea. Dig Dis Sci 32: 1201–1206

Coremans G, Chaussade S, Janssens J et al 1988 Cisapride stimulates propulsive motility patterns in the human jejunum. Dig Dis Sci 33: 1512–1519

Couturier D, Rozé C, Couturier-Turpin M H et al 1967 Electromyographie par électrode unipolaire du côlon humain in situ. CR Acad Sci 264: 352–355

Couturier D, Rozé C, Paolaggi J et al 1972 Electrical activity of the normal human stomach. A comparative study of recordings obtained from the serosal and mucosal sides. Am J Dig Dis 17: 969–976

Couturier D, Rozé C, Vasconcellos D et al 1973 Effects of acid in stomach and duodenum upon the gastric myoelectrical activity in man. Digestion 9: 502–513

Couturier D, Rozé C, Courturier-Turpin M H et al 1979 Electromyography of the colon in situ. An experimental study in man and in the rabbit. Gastroenterology 56: 317–322

Cucchiara S, Janssens J, Vantrappen G et al 1986 Gastric electrical dysrhythmia in a girl with chronic intractable vomiting. J Pediatr 108: 264–267

Daniel E E, Chapman K M 1963 Electrical activity of the gastrointestinal tract as an indication of mechanical activity. Am J Dig Dis 8: 54–102

Daniel E E, Sarna S 1978 The generation and conduction of activity in smooth muscle. Ann Rev Pharmacol Toxicol 18: 145–166

Diamant N A, Bortoff A 1969 Nature of the intestinal slow wave frequency gradient. Am J Physiol 216: 301–307

Duthie H L, Brown B H, Robertson B 1972 Electrical activity in the gastroduodenal area. Slow waves in the proximal duodenum. A comparison of man and dog. Dig Dis 17: 344–351

El-Sharkarwy T Y 1978 Electrophysiological control of motility in canine colon in: Duthie H L (ed.) Gastrointestinal motility in health and disease, MTP, Lancaster pp. 387–396

Fioramonti J, Bueno L, Frexinos J 1980a Sonde endoluminale pour l'exploration électromyographique de la motricité colique chez l'homme. Gastroenterol Clin Biol 4: 546–550

Fioramonti J, Garcia-Villaz B S R, Bueno L et al 1980b Colonic myoelectric activity and propulsion in the dog. Dis Dig Sci 25: 641–646

Fleckenstein P, Øigaard A 1976 Electrical spike potentials of small bowel. A comparative study of the recordings obtained from muscular implanted and intraluminal suction electrodes. Dig Dis Sci 21: 996–999

Fleckenstein P, Øigaard A 1978 Electrical spike activity in the human small intestine. A multiple electrode study of fasting diurnal variations. Dig Dis Sci 23: 776–780

Frexinos J, Bueno L, Fioramonti J 1985 Diurnal changes in myoelectric spiking activity of the human colon. Gastroenterology 88: 1104–1110

Frieri G, Parisi F, Corazziari E et al 1983 Colonic electromyography in chronic constipation. Gastroenterology 84: 737–740

Goodman E N, Flood C A, Sandler B T et al 1966 A method of studying motility in the esophagus by recording electrical potentials. Am J Dig Dis 11: 958–962

Hamilton J W, Bellahsene B E, Reichelderger M et al 1986

Human electrogastrograms: Comparison of surface and mucosal recordings. Dig Dis Sci 31: 33–39

Hamilton J W, Bellahsene B E, Cascio D S et al 1988 Human electrogastrograms: comparison of techniques of recording. Am J Gastroenterol 83: 806–811

Hellemans J, Vantrappen G, Valembois G et al 1968 Electrical activity of striated and smooth muscle of the esophagus. Am J Dig Dis 13: 320–334

Hellemans J, Vantrappen G, Vandenbroucke J 1970 The electrical activity of the human esophagus. Gastroenterology 58: 959

Hellemans J, Vantrappen G, Janssens J 1974 Electromyography of the esophagus in: Vantrappen G, Hellemans J (eds) Handbuch der inneren Medizin. Springer-Verlag, Berlin–Heidelberg–New York, pp 270–285

Hinder R A, Kelly K A 1977 Human gastric pacesetter potentials site of origin, spread and response to gastric transection and proximal gastric vagotomy. Am J Surg 133: 29–33

Huizinga J D, Stern S, Chow E et al 1985 Electrophysiological control of motility in the human colon. Gastroenterology 88: 500–511

Kocylowski M, Bowes K L, Kingma Y J 1979 Electrical and mechanical activity in the ex vivo perfused total canine colon. Gastroenterology 77: 1021–1026

Kolrep-Dechauffour S, Cherbout C, Bruley Des Varannes S et al 1989 Les électrodes annulaires endoluminales sont-elles fiables pour le receuil de l'activité myoélectrique de l'intestin grêle? Gastroenterol Clin Biol 13: 602–606

Kosterlitz N W 1968 Intrinsic and extrinsic nervous control of motility of the stomach and the intestines in: Code C F (ed.) Handbook of physiology: a critical, comprehensive presentation of physiological knowledge and concepts. Section 6. Alimentary Canal, vol 4 Motility. Am Physiol Soc, Washington DC pp 2147–2171

Kumar D, Wingate D, Ruckebusch Y 1986 Circadian variation in the propagation velocity of migrating motor complex. Gastroenterology 91: 926–930

Kwong N K, Brown B H, Whittaker G E et al 1970 Electrical activity of the gastric antrum in man. Br J Surg 57: 913–916

Lewis T S, Daniel E E, Sarna S K et al 1978 Idiopathic intestinal pseudo obstruction. Report of a case, with intraluminal studies of mechanical and electrical activity, and response to drugs. Gastroenterology 74: 107–111

McCoy E J, Bass P 1963 Chronic electrical activity of the gastroduodenal area: effects of food and certain catecholamines. Am J Physiol 205: 439–445

McRae S, Younger K, Thompson D G et al 1982 Sustained mental stress alters human jejunal motor activity. Gut 23: 404–409

Marlett J A, Code J F 1979 Effects of celiac and superior mesenteric ganglionectomy on interdigestive myoelectric complex in dogs, Am J Physiol 237: 432–436

Mathias J R, Carlson G M, Marino D I et al 1976 Intestinal myoelectric activity in response to live Vibria cholerae and cholera enterotoxin. J Clin Invest 58: 91–96

Monges H, Salducci H 1970a A method of recording the gastric electrical activity in man. Dig Dis 15: 271–276

Monges H, Salducci J 1970b Etude électromyographique de la motricité duodénale chez l'homme normale. Arch Fr Mal App Dig 59: 19–28

Monges H, Salducci J, Roman C 1968 Etude électromyographique de la contraction oesophagienne chez l'homme normal. Arch Fr Mal App Dig 57: 545–560

Morton R S 1954 Potentialities of the electrogastrograph. Ann Roy Coll Surg 15: 351–373

Ǿigaard A, Dorph S 1974a The relative significance of electrical spike potentials and intraluminal pressure waves as quantitative indicators of motility. Am J Dig Dis 19: 797–803

Ǿigaard A, Dorph S 1974b Quantitative analysis of motility recordings in the human small intestine. Am J Dig Dis 19: 804–810

Provenciale L, Pisano M 1971 Methods for recording electrical activity of the human colon in vivo. Am J Dig Dis 16: 712–722

Richter C P 1924 Action currents from the stomach. Am J Physiol 67: 612–633

Sarna S K 1975 Gastrointestinal electrical activity: terminology. Gastroenterology 68: 1631–1635

Sarna S K, Bowes K L, Daniel E E 1973 Post-operative gastric electrical control activity (ECA) in man in: Daniel E E (ed.) Proc of the IV Int Symp on Gastrointestinal Motility, Mitchell Press Vancouver pp 73–83

Sarna S K, Daniel E E, Kingma Y J 1972 Simulation of the electrical control activity of the stomach by an array of relaxation oscillators. Am J Dig Dis 17: 299–310

Sarna S K, Daniel E E, Lewis T D et al 1978 Postoperative gastrointestinal electrical and mechanical activities in a patient with idiopathic intestinal pseudo obstruction. Gastroenterology 74: 112–120

Sarna S K, Latimer P, Cambell D et al 1982 Electrical and contractile activities of the human rectosigmoid. Gut 23: 698–705

Sarna S K, Waterfall W A, Bardakjian B L et al 1980 Human colonic electrical control activity (ECA). Gastroenterology 78: 1526–1536

Sarna S K, Waterfall W E, Bardakjian B L et al 1981 Types of human colonic electrical activity recorded postoperatively. Gastroenterology 81: 61–70

Schang J C, Devroede G 1983 Fasting and postprandial myoelectric spiking activity in the human sigmoid colon. Gastroenterology 85: 1048–1053

Smout A J P M, Van der Schee E J, Grashuis J L 1980 What is measured in electrogastrography? Dig Dis Sci 25: 179–187

Snape W J Jr, Carlson G M, Cohen S 1977a Human colonic myoelectric activity in response to prostigmin and the gastrointestinal hormones. Gastroenterology 22: 881–887

Snape W J Jr, Carlson G M, Matarazzo S A et al 1977b evidence that abnormal myoelectrical activity produces colonic motor dysfunction in the irritable bowel syndrome. Gastroenterology 72: 383–387

Stoddard C J, Smallwood R H, Duthie H L 1981 Electrical arrhythmias in the human stomach. Gut 22: 705–712

Sullivan M A, Snape W J Jr, Matarazzo S A et al 1977 Gastrointestinal electrical activity in idiopathic intestinal pseudo-obstruction. N Engl J Med 297: 233–238

Summers R W, Dusdieker N S 1981 Patterns of spike burst spread and flow in the canine small intestine. Gastroenterology 81: 742–750

Szurszewski J H 1969 A migrating electrical complex of the canine small intestine. Am J Physiol 217: 1757–1763

Taylor I, Duthie H L, Smallwood R et al 1975 Large bowel myoelectrical activity in man. Gut 16: 808–814

Taylor I, Darby C, Hammond P et al 1978 Is there a

myoelectrical abnormality in the irritable colon syndrome? Gut 19: 391–395

Thompson D G, Wingate D L, Archer L et al 1980 Normal patterns of human upper small bowel motor activity recorded by prolonged radiotelemetry. Gut 21: 500–506

Tokita T, Tashiro K, Kato K 1970 Electromyography of the esophagus and its clinical applications. Acta Otolaryng 70: 269–278

Vantrappen G, Coremans G, Janssens J et al 1991 Inversion of the slow-wave frequency gradient in symptomatic patients with Roux-en-Y anastomosis. Gastroenterology 101: 1282–1288

Vantrappen G, Janssens J, Coremans G et al 1986 Gastrointestinal motility disorders. Dig Dis Sci 31: 5S–25S

Vantrappen G, Janssens J, Hellemans J et al 1977 The interdigestive motor complex of normal subjects and patients with bacterial overgrowth of the small intestine. J Clin Invest 59: 1158–1166

Waterfall W A 1983 Electrical patterns in the human jejunum with and without vagotomy: migrating myoelectric complexes and the influence of morphine. Surgery 94: 186–190

Waterfall W A, Cameron G W, Sarna S K et al 1981 Disorganized electrical activity in a child with idiopathic intestinal pseudo obstruction. Gut 22: 77–93

You C H, Chey W Y, Lee K Y et al 1981 Gastric and small intestinal myoelectric dysrhythmia associated with intractable nausea and vomiting. Ann Int Med 95: 449–451

19. Electrical impedance measurements

N. M. Spyrou   F. D. Castillo

INTRODUCTION

Studies of gastric motility using electrical impedance methods are relatively recent (Sutton 1988). However, the application of non-ionizing electromagnetic radiation in medical diagnosis was first reported in 1926 (Lambert & Gremels) for a technique based on electrical impedance measurements that monitored the development of pulmonary oedema. There is an extensive body of literature related to biomedical impedance measurement techniques and applications (recommended articles: Schwan 1963, Plonsey 1969, Geddes & Baker 1975, and Brown 1983).

Two non-invasive methods of estimating gastric emptying that depend on such measurements have emerged –impedance epigastrography and applied potential tomography – and more recently the usefulness of the former has also been explored in the determination of gastric contractions. Since interest in employing these techniques is likely to grow in the field of gastric motility, it is perhaps useful to provide a guide to understanding some of the underlying mechanisms and models which attempt to explain the coupling of biological tissues to non-ionizing electromagnetic radiation; indicate what the measurements entail; and report work in which the techniques have been applied in different areas.

BACKGROUND

Electrical impedance measurements involve the monitoring of surface potentials created across a body when an external current source is applied. Thus a physiological event of interest, taking place between the measuring points and altering the current flow through the body, will manifest itself as a change of impedance. This event may be due, for example, to a change in breathing, in blood flow or the introduction of a meal into the stomach. In this respect, impedance epigastrography which makes use of two current injecting electrodes, one anterior and one posterior to the stomach, and two (or four) voltage sensing electrodes to measure the potential difference between them is not essentially different from applied potential tomography which employs 16 electrodes on a belt around the stomach to record these potential differences. The former provides a record of impedance changes with time, whereas the latter through reconstruction of the data will produce a series of tomographic images of a thick cross-section through the abdomen, representing changes in electrical resistivity from which a profile of gastric emptying can be extracted (Mangnall et al 1988). In this context electrogastrography (EGG), which picks up electrical activity through surface electrodes and detects, for example, changes in gastric myoelectric activity that can be related to the contractile activity of the stomach (Read 1989) is different and will not be discussed here.

Permittivity and Conductivity

The parameters which describe the macroscopic interaction of biological material with an applied current are the conductivity, σ, and the complex permittivity, $\varepsilon^\star$. The complex permeability, $\mu^\star$, describing the interaction with the magnetic field, can be neglected since for biological substances it is virtually identical to the permeability of free space. Although some biological materials have the ability to actively transport ions, for example, in the process of neural transmission, such processes occur within the low energy range up to a few Hz in frequency and therefore do not interfere with measurements at higher frequencies. All biological materials are considered to be 'polar' in nature and the magnitude of their associated dipole moment depends significantly on the size of the molecule and the charge distribution through it (Grant et al 1978). A molecule will, in general, respond to an applied field according to three types of polarization: (1) electrostatic: caused by the displacement of an electron orbital

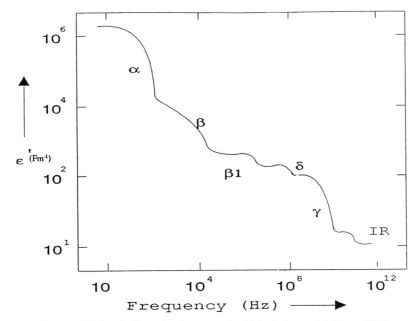

Fig. 19.1 Dielectric dispersion for a complex biological material (Grant 1984).

relative to the nucleus to generate an induced dipole moment, (2) atomic: caused by the mutual displacement of atoms of different electronegativities within a polar molecule to generate a second form of induced dipole moment and (3) orientational: caused by the tendency of dipolar molecules having permanent dipole moments to align with the field, a tendency opposed by thermal agitation and the interaction of neighbouring molecules.

The permittivity of a material reflects the extent to which local charge distribution can be distorted under the influence of an electric field and can be expressed in terms of its real, ε', and imaginary, ε'', components as follows:

$$\varepsilon^\star = \varepsilon' - j\varepsilon''$$

where j is the square root of -1, ε' is known as the relative permittivity, sometimes called the dielectric constant, and ε'' is the dielectric loss which is proportional to the energy absorbed by the material from the electric field applied. For polar substances the permittivity is a function of the frequency of the applied field and depends on, for example, temperature and pressure. Conductivity, σ, or its inverse, resistivity, ρ, is a measure of a material's ability to allow or resist the flow of electricity and reflects the ease with which delocalized charge can migrate through the material under the influence of the applied field.

It might be expected, from the complexity of biologi-cal tissues, in both composition and structure, that several different polarization mechanisms should exist to explain the interactions with the applied electromagnetic radiation in different regions of its spectrum. Each process can then be expected to be characterized by measurement and analysis of the variation of the magnitude of dielectric parameters within its particular frequency or time domain region of response, known as dispersion, to expose the underlying biophysics (Schwan 1957, 1977, Grant et al 1978, Pethig 1979, Stuchly 1979). The dielectric dispersions known to exist for typical biological tissues for audio frequencies through microwave to infra-red frequencies are shown in Figure 19.1.

As the frequency of the applied field is raised, the relative permittivity decreases in stages, at the same time the conductivity increases. This occurs because the molecular dipole motion becomes progressively unable to keep up with the alternating field direction (Grant et al 1978). The drop in ε' is accompanied by an absorption of energy from the field described by ε''. Larger molecules are generally responsible for the dispersion at the lower end of the frequency spectrum and the dominance of different polarization mechanisms in different frequency regions are due to induced, orientational and ionic polarizations. For clarity the dispersions in Figure 19.1 will be described separately, although there is overlap.

α-dispersion

The relaxation of counterions surrounding charged cell membrances are thought to cause α-dispersion. A membrane with a net charge will electrostatically attract an adjacent layer of electrolyte counterions. The applied field will tend to cause these counterions to move along the membrane since movement normal to the surface is inhibited by the electrostatic attraction. A large dipole moment is consequently induced due to the resulting space–charge polarization. Movement of the counterions is unable to keep up with an alternating field at fairly low frequencies and hence the α-dispersion is observed.

β-dispersion

The heterogeneity of biological material is responsible for this type of dispersion. Charge accumulates at the boundaries between regions of different permittivity and conductivity, taking a finite time to reach equilibrium. The apparent permittivity and conductivity of the whole medium therefore depends on the frequency of the applied field. Analysis of the subsequent dispersion can give information on the structure and width of the cell membranes which effectively act as boundaries between different materials. The first indication of the molecular thickness of cell membranes came from the study of the dielectric properties of red blood cells (Fricke 1925).

β_1-dispersion

This dispersion is not always clearly distinct from β-dispersion. It originates principally from the torque experienced in solution by biological macromolecules, such as proteins, possessing large dipole moments; this tends to align them in the direction of an applied field, a tendency opposed by the randomizing influence of thermal, or Brownian, motion (Grant et al 1978). As the frequency of oscillation of the applied field increases, the motion of polar dipoles becomes increasingly out of phase with the field until a stage is reached where orientational polarization is no longer possible.

δ-dispersion

There is evidence to suggest that δ-dispersion is due to the relaxation of water molecules in the immediate environment of the biological macromolecules; the water is known as bound water or water of hydration. Water which is intimately associated with solute protein molecules will have a restricted rotational freedom and will consequently relax at lower frequencies than that of bulk, or free, water at the same temperature. Although any pathological condition which perturbs the amount or properties of protein-bound water will modify the δ-dispersion of physiological fluids such as blood sera, with more heterogeneous material like biological tissues, the amount of unambiguous information which can be derived from dielectric data in the frequency range of the δ-dispersion is limited still further (Grant 1984).

γ-dispersion

There is lack of consensus about the relative quality and universality of the bound water in various tissues. Despite the uncertainty for many purposes the γ-dispersion can be considered to be overwhelmingly dictated simply by the total tissue water content and the dispersion to be caused by the relaxation of free water molecules, i.e. water which is effectively isolated from the influence of biological macromolecules. The high frequency limit permittivity is assumed comparable to that of pure water and the relaxation frequency of tissue bulk water is taken as identical to that of pure water, 25 GHz at 37°C.

Accurate extension of some theoretical models and equations, particularly those of α-dispersion, to tissues has not yet been achieved. This is not surprising since biological tissues are generally of elaborate architecture consisting of non-uniform cells in intimate contact and high cell volume fraction. However, much tissue data is in broad agreement to the idealistic theory (Schwan 1957) and the general form of any biodielectric perturbations can be at least conjectured by application of the known physical and biological characteristics of normal and pathological tissues to the model systems and their equations (Grant & Spyrou 1985).

Conduction and displacement currents

When biological material is subjected to an alternating current, its free and bound charges give rise to a conduction current I_c and a displacement current, I_d, respectively. The extent to which each of these occurs depends on the frequency, f, which for a potential applied between the opposite faces of a unit cube of material is (Brown 1983):

$$I_c = V(t)\sigma(f)$$

$$I_d = \left(\frac{dV(t)}{dt}\right)\varepsilon'(f)\varepsilon_o$$

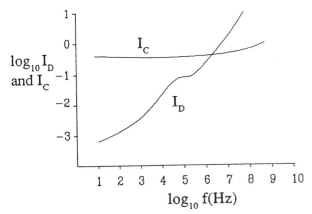

Fig. 19.2 Conduction and displacement current variations with frequency for a typical soft biological tissue (Brown 1983).

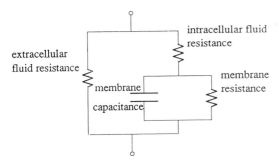

Fig. 19.3 Electrical equivalent circuit for biological tissue (Grant 1984).

and follows Ohm's law. Where V(t) is the applied voltage (V), t is the time (s), ε_o is the permittivity of freespace, ε' is the permittivity of the material (Fm^{-1}), $\sigma(f)$ is the conductivity of the material (S) and f is the frequency in Hz. The consequent variations of both the conduction and displacement currents with frequency in a typical soft tissue are shown in Figure 19.2.

The conduction current varies relatively little with frequency and is virtually constant below 100 kHz whereas the displacement current exhibits three main regions of change about the frequencies of 10 Hz, 1 MHz and 10^{10} Hz. These regions are caused by the dielectric dispersion associated with tissue interferences, the capacitive effects of the cell membrane and the dielectric dispersion associated with the polarization of tissue held water, respectively. Conductive effects dominate and I_d is very small with respect to I_c. This is equivalent to saying that capacitive effects are

insignificant in comparison to conductive effects at these low frequencies. The conductance, G, and the capacitance, C, for a material being held between parallel plate electrodes of surface area A, separated by a distance d, are given by:

$$G = \sigma(f)\frac{A}{d}$$

and

$$C = \varepsilon_o\varepsilon'(f)\frac{A}{d}$$

The electrical properties of body tissues are then dictated by the existence of free charge carriers, essentially ions. Body fluids, muscle and neural tissue thus show conductivities higher than those of fatty tissue and bone, where the organic nature of the former and the complex matrix of the latter restrict the freedom of any ions present.

Some physical insight into the behaviour of the tissues at these frequencies, incorporating α- and β-dispersions, can be acquired through consideration of a well-used equivalent circuit (Schwan 1957, Schwan & Foster 1980, Presman 1970, Grant 1984), as shown in Figure 19.3. At the low frequencies of the α-dispersion the cell membrane acts as a good insulator and the current is primarily supported by the extracellular fluid which can be thought of as a volume conductor. Likewise the dielectric properties of living tissue are associated mainly with the cell membrane. As frequency is increased the cell ionic atmospheres can no longer follow the applied field so the permittivity diminishes and there is a concomitant increase in conductivity. As frequency increases further, the characterization of the β-dispersion becomes dominated by the cell membrane capacitance.

THE IMPEDANCE OF THE ABDOMINAL REGION

It is possible to change the net electrical impedance (where impedance is a measure of the resistive and capacitive effects combined) across the torso at the stomach level by introducing into the latter a meal of different impedance to that of the body tissue in the region of interest. If the impedance is measured at frequencies lower than say 100 kHz, then capacitive effects are not significant and changes in impedance are essentially changes in resistivity. For a homogeneous tissue in the form of a cylinder of length l and cross-sectional area A, the impedance Z, of the tissue is given by:

Table 19.1   Resistivity of various body parts

Tissue	Resistivity (Ω cm)	Frequency (Hz)	Reference
Blood	165	1 k	Rosenthal & Tobias 1948
Heart muscle	456	120 k	Kinnen et al 1964
Lung	1 345–2 100	100 k	Kinnen et al 1964
Liver	817	< 100 k	Geddes & Baker 1967
Spleen	885	< 100 k	Geddes & Baker 1967
Fat	2 000	< 100 k	Price 1979
Bone (thorax)	16 000	< 100 k	Lepeschkin 1951
Skin	220	100 k	Rosell et al 1988

$$Z = \rho l / A$$

where ρ is the specific resistivity of the tissue, which is the reciprocal of the conductivity σ. The abdomen however is a region composed of different types of tissue and the overall impedance will be a function of the specific resistivities of each tissue and the amount of each tissue type situated in the region between the electrodes.

It is difficult to measure the resistivity of electrically heterogeneous materials and a number of other biological tissues. Consequently, a wide range of different tissue resistivities has been reported (Geddes & Baker 1967) but there is no obvious consistency of methods. There is a lack of in vivo information on tissue resistivities in the 20–100 kHz range. A selection of collected data is shown in Table 19.1 (Fenlon 1992) although the variations in applied frequency and the in vitro nature of the measurements should be noted.

The introduction of a new material into the abdominal region would then change the overall impedance as measured by the electrodes, provided the resistivity or conductivity of the material was sufficiently different to that of the surrounding tissue. This is the basis of gastric emptying studies.

APPLICATIONS

Overview

As we have shown, a rigorous theoretical basis already exists to model the interaction of electrical fields with biological tissues, and the associated electrical impedance measurements would seem to offer distinct advantages in clinical applications. Nonetheless, the use of these measurements in gastrointestinal motility has for many years been confined to the research laboratory.

Historically, one of the first clinical applications of electrical impedance measurements in gastrointestinal motility appears to be by Hunt and his coworkers (Challis et al 1976) who were able to measure the change in potential difference along the human oesophagus with an array of electrodes which had been equidistantly mounted on a thin flexible catheter. Using this arrangement it was possible to follow the transit of a liquid meal bolus along the oesophagus. At about the same time, the possibilities of using impedance measurements to monitor the movements of the smooth muscle which surrounds the gut in rats, was under investigation (Postaire et al 1975), and an indication of the contractile activity in the region was obtained. Application of the technique was explored once more (Darby et al 1982) during in vivo investigations in man by carrying out a combination of myoelectric and resistance measurements in the human colon and compared with pressure recordings. Therefore, until the mid-1980s there were parallel attempts to use the techniques for both transit measurement and contractile monitoring.

Gastric emptying measurements

Epigastrography

It was only a matter of time before the possibility of using electrodes on the surface of the body to record changes in impedance from more remote sites was attempted and Sutton et al (1985) began to make measurements to follow the filling and subsequent emptying of simple liquid meals. The 'epigastrograph', as it was to become known, applied an alternating current of about 1 mA peak-to-peak at a frequency of 100 kHz or less across the epigastric region of the body using a pair of standard ECG type Ag/AgCl adhesive electrodes, with a second pair of electrodes employed to monitor the fluctuations in the potential difference across the same region of the body (Fig. 19.4). The liquid meal, water flavoured with an orange cordial, presented a higher electrical impedance than that of the surrounding tissue. Therefore, on ingestion, a rise in the measured impedance could be clearly followed by a slow fall back to baseline, normally

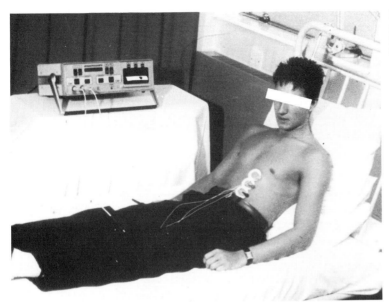

Fig. 19.4 Photograph illustrating the placement of electrodes on the surface of the subjects skin, posterior positions mirror those shown anteriorly.

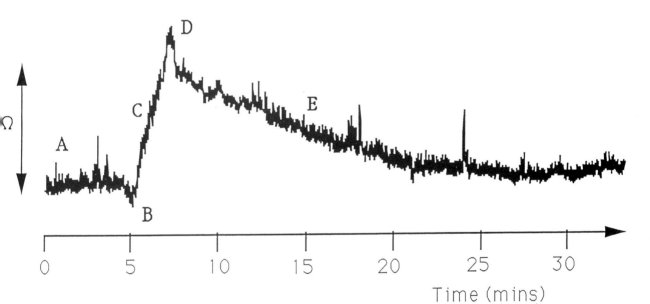

Fig. 19.5 Example gastric emptying trace from the epigastrograph. Positive excursion (**C**) from baseline impedance level (**A**) caused by ingestion of a liquid meal with a lower electrical conductivity than the body tissues surrounding the stomach. During the initial stage of consumption of the fluid it is common to see a slight dip in the measured impedance (**B**) and a similar effect once the peak has been reached (**D**) both contribute to uncertainty. Ideally, after consumption of the meal a gradual return to the initial baseline is observed (**E**).

within about 40 min (Fig. 19.5). This configuration has been used successfully in a range of areas both for pharmacological assessment and clinical measurements and a selection of normal values are illustrated in Table 19.2.

Applied Potential Tomography [APT]

APT is a technique (Brown et al 1983) which upgrades the simple tetrapolar mode of measurement, described above, to a multi-electrode array, circumferentially

Table 19.2   Measure gastric half-emptying times

Subjects	Age in years	Number	$t_{\frac{1}{2}}$	Reference
Children	8.9 (0.6–17)†	45	13.6 (4–29)†	Smith et al 1989
Children	7.7†	7	18.2 (7–34)†	Lamont et al 1988
Adults	30.5 ± 5.1*	9	8 (3–17)†	Gilbey & Watkins 1987
Adults	(20–26)	7	13 (10.7–17)†	Rainbird et al 1987
Women	28.6 ± 1.1*	15	8.3 ± 0.9*	O'Sullivan et al 1987

† median and range (if available); * mean and SEM (if available)

enclosing the region to be investigated. As with the epigastrograph, a constant alternating current passes into the body and the potential difference is detected by separate pairs of electrodes. However, in this case, not only are 14 other electrodes used, but these are multiplexed in such a way that the potential difference between all combinations of pairs of electrodes is measured. Once the full combination of measurements has been executed, the electrodes used to input the current are altered and a new set of measurements multiplex around the array. This process continues until all possible configurations have been used. The resulting arrays of data can then be transformed by a number of algorithms so that a representation of the distribution of the physical quantity (conductivity in this case) which gave rise to the measurements is obtained.

This reconstructed image on a grey scale plot represents the conductivity distribution of a slice through the abdomen in the epigastric region over the period of time when a cycle of measurements is taken. There is some uncertainty about the thickness and uniformity of this slice. Multiple images, reconstructed from data acquired at regular intervals, can then produce a dynamic representation of the changes taking place and form the basis for monitoring the filling and emptying of the stomach, provided there is sufficient contrast between the conductivity of the meal and that of the surrounding tissues.

In order to derive a gastric emptying curve from the data, a region of interest is defined by the user in the first few image frames and changes in the integrated pixel intensity over time, normalized with respect to initial baseline recording frames, provide the gastric emptying profile (Fig. 19.6).

Sources of errors

Impedance measurements of gastric emptying are not without problems. Not only do they rely on certain assumptions but the measurements themselves have an inherently low specificity to the measurement of volume changes within the stomach which must be overcome. To understand the nature of the problem it is important to consider the assumptions.

First, the technique assumes that a linear relationship exists between the volume of fluid consumed by the subject and the subsequent change in impedance. Given the complex and variable nature of the underlying tissue through which the current must pass this assumption does, at first, appear very simplistic. Nevertheless, a range of different studies aimed at validating this linearity seem to indicate that the system does indeed react in a linear fashion, although departures from this response do occur (Fig. 19.7).

The second assumption is that the electrodes are accurately positioned to reliably detect the changes which do take place. This is one of the main problems associated with the technique and arises from the wide anatomical variations which are known to exist between individuals with respect to the position and size of the stomach, if X-ray imaging for locating the stomach is to be avoided. Electrodes which are poorly positioned may not only miss the emptying process of the stomach, but may provide misleading information due to a fall off in the linearity when the stomach is further away from the recording electrodes. For this reason later versions of the epigastrograph were designed to incorporate an additional pair of recording electrodes so that whichever of the two independent electrode pairs has the greatest response to the filling of the stomach, is used for all subsequent calculations. Even so, epigastrography is greatly dependent on the subject's anatomy for its sensitivity and obese individuals are liable to provide poor results due to a fall off in the achievable sensitivity with body weight (Fig. 19.8). This reliance on the positioning of the electrodes with respect to the stomach is similarly important in APT. However, the spatial component of the visual information obtained does provide the potential to reduce this effect.

Further inaccuracies occur due to the assumption

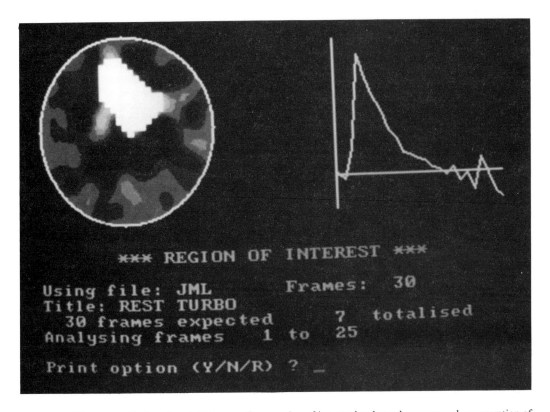

Fig. 19.6 The screen display of an APT image after a region of interest has been drawn around a summation of initial images. The curve on the right represents the calculated emptying profile for the resulting data after ingestion of a low conductivity liquid meal.

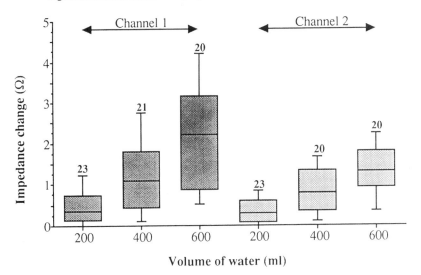

Fig. 19.7 Box and whisker plots indicate the median, interquartile, 10th and 90th centile values of maximum impedance deflection as a result of ingestion of three volumes (200 ml, 400 ml, 600 ml) of water. Data shown for two separate channels of the epigastrograph. The number above each box represents the number of subjects successfully measured.

that the contents of the stomach remain at a constant conductivity throughout the emptying of the meal, and that the impedance measured at the point when the stomach has fully emptied is always the same as the original baseline value. Clearly, the result of gastric secretion, blood perfusion, muscular tone and body posture all present possible factors to affect this final value.

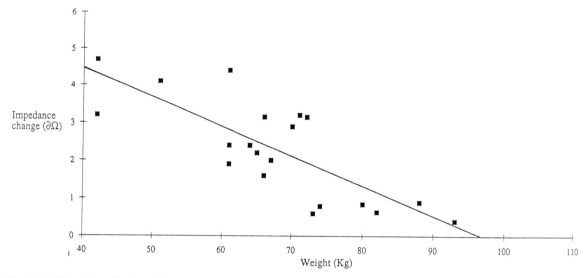

Fig. 19.8 The effect of body weight on the resulting maximum impedance change induced by 600 ml of water.

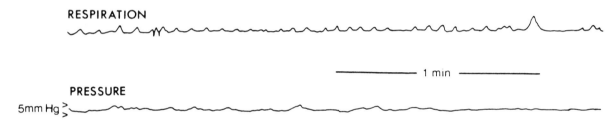

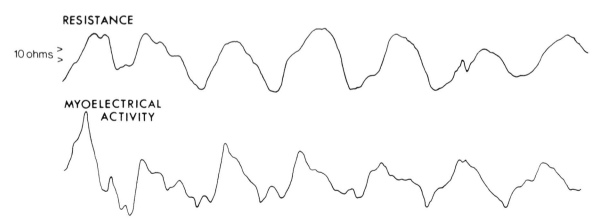

Fig. 19.9 Recording from a normal subject showing clear waves of resistance change at 2–3 cpm. There are simultaneous myoelectrical slow waves at the same frequency. (Morris et al 1983)

Monitoring contractile activity

Although emphasis has been placed on the measurement of transit through the stomach, impedance meas-

urements have also been used as a method of monitoring contractile activity within the gut. Despite the difficulty in relating the measured values obtained to absolute pressure changes within the gut, the potential

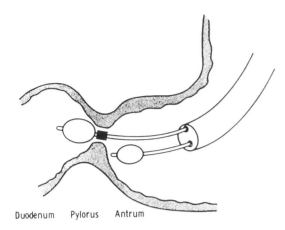

Fig. 19.10 Arrangement of antral and duodenal balloons at endoscopy. The impedance electrodes lie in the pyloric canal. (Johnson et al 1983)

advantages of impedance techniques have led to a number of different measuring modalities. In humans, the first example of these measurements being used successfully appears to be in the colon (Morris et al 1983). This is a difficult organ to investigate since the positioning of sensors is problematic and, once in position, pressure measurements may be inaccurate due to the non-occlusive nature of contractions. The measurement of electrical impedance changes, from a catheter placed within the colon, was compared with measurements derived from the same site simultaneously using both manometric and electromyographic measurements (Fig. 19.9). Although the method of analysis of the results was crude, the potential advantages of impedance in its plethysmographic qualities were highlighted. The impedance technique is able to detect changes in a volume of tissue and is not limited to a specific point measurement, thus enabling the detection of contractions which may not in themselves be directly in contact with the site of measurement.

Similar systems of measurement have been used for measurement in the upper gut. The relationship between pyloric sphincter closure and contractions in both the antrum and the proximal duodenum was assessed (Johnson et al 1983) using a circumferential arrangement of four silver electrodes positioned at the pyloric ring (Fig. 19.10). The impedance measured across opposing pairs of electrodes provided a measure of the degree of closure of the sphincter, producing a fall in impedance when all four electrodes came in contact with the pyloric ring (Fig. 19.11).

More recently, an electrical model for the oesophagus has been proposed (Silny 1991) that predicts the relationship between the measured potential differ-

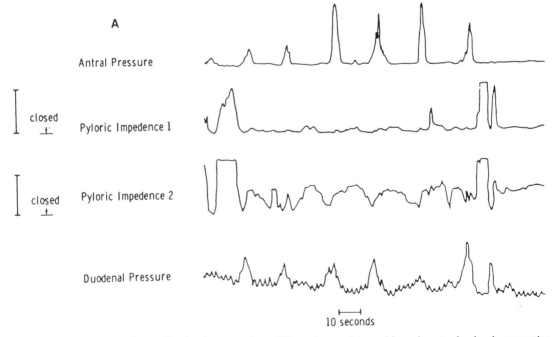

Fig. 19.11 Coordinated antroduodenal contractions. The pylorus closes with each antroduodenal contraction (Johnson et al 1983).

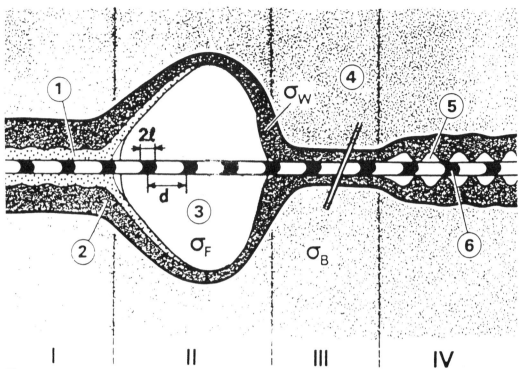

Fig. 19.12 Intraluminal electrical impedance catheter in the oesophageal tube during deglutition with characteristics of the catheter and the volume conductor, and electric conductivities of the body σ_B, the wall σ_W, and the bolus σ_F. 1 = saliva film, 2 = organ wall, 3 = bolus, 4 = body, 5 = air, 6 = impedance catheter electrode. The distance between adjacent cylindrical electrodes of length 2l is d. (Silny 1991.)

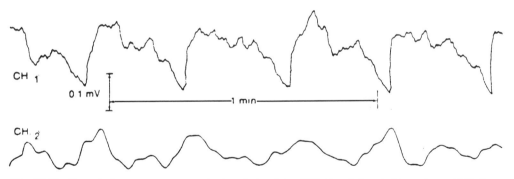

Fig. 19.13 Record of transcutaneous gastric electrical activity (CH. 1) and electrical impedance (CH. 2). (Familani et al 1987.)

ences and the mechanical action of the gut. Using an array of electrodes, similar to that employed by Hunt for oesophageal transit, the progress of intestinal contractions may be monitored because a difference in the electrical conductivity between the bolus within the lumen of the gut and the body surrounding the gut exists (Fig. 19.12). The impedance is measured in this case using a bipolar configuration, with one electrode in the lumen of the gut and the second reference electrode either longitudinally adjacent along the catheter or placed on the surface of the skin. The model assumes that the conductivity of the wall of the gut is similar to that of the bolus; in the oesophagus at least, this does not appear to be so, as the walls are particularly

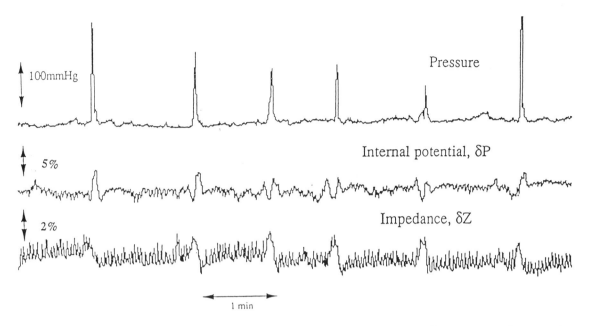

Fig. 19.14 Impedance measured transcutaneously, and intraluminal potential and manometris measurements from transducers positioned in the gastric antrum.

non-conductive. However, it does not change the general relationship between the bolus size and the impedance changes although it does affect the sensitivity. In practice, the configuration of electrodes in which both are located within the lumen appears to be the more sensitive.

The use of electrical impedance measurements for the recording of contractions from electrodes placed on the surface of the skin, with no need to use invasive catheters, would provide potentially the greatest benefits. A system for the simultaneous measurement of electrical and mechanical activity was developed (Familoni et al 1987) using an impedance plethysmograph similar to the epigastrograph, coupled with an additional low pass filter to enable the gastric electrical activity to be extracted from electrical impedance measurements (Fig. 19.13). The question of correlating the measured epigastric impedance changes with pressure changes in the gastric antrum was addressed by Castillo (1987) when simultaneous measurements of intraluminal pressure recorded by perfused tube manometry was compared with epigastric electrical impedance measurements. The presence of a clear correlation between the two signals in 3 cycles per minute (cpm) activity, further reinforced the suggestion that electrical impedance measurements could provide information with respect to the underlying contractility of the stomach. Skouras (1988) took this one stage further,

using one pair of measuring electrodes within the gastric antrum separated by 1 cm, a second pair of measuring electrodes on the skin surface and an input current injected again from a pair of electrodes on the skin surface. Pressure changes were recorded simultaneously using a perfused tube with its outlet positioned midway between the two intraluminal electrodes. Both forms of electrical measurement were able to detect events which corresponded to manometric pressure events. However, the amplitude of individual impedance fluctuations did not appear to relate to that of the manometric system (Fig. 19.14). The physiological variables inherent in the measurement of impedance make an accurate calibration of this form of measurement particularly difficult.

Compliance measurement

Since impedance measurements are sensitive to many physical changes within the tissues, it may seem that the best way to make use of such measurements is to closely control all interfering variables. Gregersen, (1988) placed a water filled balloon within the lumen of the gut and measured the impedance between two electrodes mounted on a catheter within this balloon. The contents of the balloon were easily controlled and the distribution of the electric field was considered to be totally contained within the insulating rubber boundary of the balloon. Therefore, the only significant changes in the electrical medium were geometric.

Measurement of the impedance, Z, between two electrodes separated along a 1 cm length of catheter, within this balloon, provides an estimation of the cross-sectional area, A, of the balloon between the electrode pair. Re-writing the equation on page 280 and substituting the conductivity of water, σ, for the specific resistivity, ρ, which are inversely related, the cross-sectional area can be expressed as:

$$A = \frac{l}{(Z\sigma)}$$

where l is the electrode separation. By using a water perfusion system in which both control of internal pressure and its measurement were possible, the values of the cross-sectional area, A, and pressure, P, could be obtained and hence the compliance of the surrounding wall calculated using the relationship:

$$\text{Compliance} = \frac{dA}{dP}$$

where dA is the change in cross-sectional area and dP is the change in pressure.

CONCLUSION

The prospect of being able to obtain relevant information about gastric emptying and contractile activity, simultaneously, is worthy of serious consideration. Despite the general problems that have been highlighted, with respect to electrical impedance measurements, and others that remain dormant only to arise when the technique is applied to a specific application, the advantages of using a non-invasive and easily repeated technique that provides a continuous record of changes in gastric motility are attractive. The emptying curve and the contraction pattern can be read and 'half-emptying' time and frequency extracted.

The relative ease with which impedance measurements are made is counterbalanced by the difficulty in interpretation of the magnitude of the signal and the attempts to relate this to pressure and volume changes, which may play a part but are not the only contributory sources. However, the body of work being carried out on the models and mechanisms that try to explain the underlying interactions of non-ionizing electromagnetic radiation with biological tissues is both significant and a basis for optimism. The 'inverse problem', where an observation or measurement is made outside a body in order to detect a structure or change in some property within it, is common in many branches of science and provides a continuing challenge.

REFERENCES

Brown B H 1983 Tissue impedance methods in: Jackson D F (ed.) Imaging with non-ionising radiations. Surrey University Press/Blackie, Glasgow pp 83–110

Castillo F D 1987 An investigation into the use of the gastric impedance monitor system for detecting gastric contractions. MSc Medical Physics, University of Surrey, Guildford.

Challis R E, Fisher M, Hunt J N 1976 The oesophagus as an electric cable. J Physiol 266: 1P–2P

Darby C F, Hammond P, Taylor I, Morris I R 1982 A method for the simultaneous detection of motility and myoelectric activity in smooth muscle. Clin Phys Physiol Meas 3: (4) 283–291

Eyre-Brook I A, Linhardt G E, Smallwood R H, Johnson A G 1983 The timing of pyloric closure in man: studies with impedance electrodes in: Roman C (ed.) Gastrointestinal motility. MTP Press, Lancaster pp 119–120

Familoni B O, Kingma Y J, Bowes K L 1987 Noninvasive assessment of human gastric motor function. IEEE Trans Biomed Eng BME-34: 30–36

Fenlon T J 1992 Medical applications of electrical impedance measurements. PhD thesis, University of Surrey, Guildford.

Fricke H 1925 A mathematical treatment of the electrical conductivity and capacity of disperse systems. Phys Rev 26: 678–681

Geddes L A, Baker L E 1967 The specific resistance of biological material – a compendium of data for the biomedical engineer and physiologist. Med Biol Eng 5: 271–293

Geddes L A, Baker L E 1975 Principles of applied biomedical instrumentation. Wiley-Interscience, New York

Gilbey S G, Watkins P J 1987 Measurement by epigastric impedance of gastric emptying in diabetic autonomic neuropathy. Diabetic Medicine 4: 122–126

Grant E H, Shephard R, South S 1978 Dielectric behaviour of biological molecules in solution. Oxford University Press, Oxford.

Grant J P, 1984 Measurements, medical significance and applications of dielectric properties of biological materials. PhD thesis, University of Surrey, Guildford.

Grant J P, Spyrou N M 1985 Complex permittivity differences between normal and pathological tissues: mechanisms and medical significance. J Bioelectricity 4: 419–458

Gregersen H, Jensen L S, Djurhuus J C 1988 Changes in oesophageal wall biomechanics after portal vein banding and variceal sclerotherapy measured by a new technique. An experimental study in rabbits. Gut 29: 1699–1704

Johnson A G, Eyre-Brook I A, Linhardt G E, Smallwood R H 1983 Does the human pylorus close in response to an isolated duodenal cap contraction? Studies with a new technique in: Labo G, Bortolotti M (eds) Gastrointestinal motility. Cortina International, Verona pp 251–254

Kinnen E, Kubecik W, Hill P, Turton G 1964 Thoracic cage impedance measurements: tissue resistivity in vivo and transthoracic impedance at 110 kc. USAF school of aerospace medicine technical documentary report, SAM-TDR-64–5, Brooks Airforce Base, Texas

Lambert R K, Gremels H 1926 The factors concerned in the production of pulmonary oedema. J Physiol 61: 98–112

Lamont G L, Wright J W, Evans D F, Kapila L 1988 An evaluation of applied potential tomography in the diagnosis of infantile hypertropic pyloric stenosis. Clin Phys Physiol Meas 9: A65–A70

Lepeschkin E 1951 Modern electrocardiography, vol 1, Williams & Wilkins, Baltimore.

Mangnall Y F, Barnish C, Brown B H, Barber D C, Johnson A G, Read N W 1988 Comparison of applied potential tomography and impedance epigastrography as methods of measuring gastric emptying. Clin Phys Physiol Meas 9 (3): 249–254

Morris I R, Hammond P, Darby C, Taylor I 1983 Simultaneous recording of myoelectrical activity and resistance from the human colon. Digestion 26: 33–42

O'Sullivan G M, Sutton A J, Thompson S A, Carrie L E, Bullingham R E 1987 Noninvasive measurement of gastric emptying in obstetric patients. Anesth Analg 66: 505–511

Pethig R 1979 Dielectric and electronic properties of biological materials, Wiley, Chichester

Plonsey R 1969 Bioelectric phenomena. McGraw Hill, New York

Postaire J -G, Devroede G, van Houtte N, Gerard J 1975 An improved instrument to record potential differences and impedance from the gastrointestinal tract. Med Biol Eng 13: 649–653

Presman A S 1970 Electromagnetic fields and life. Plenum Press, New York

Price L R 1979 Electrical impedance computed tomography (ICT): a new CT imaging technique. IEEE Trans Nucl Sci NS26: 2736–2739

Rainbird A L, Pickworth M J W, Lightowler C, Mitchell M, Wingate D L 1987 Effect of posture and cold stress on impedance measurements of gastric emptying. Pharmaceut Med 2: 35–42

Read N W (ed) 1989 Gastrointestinal motility. Which test? Wrightson Biomedical Publishing, Petersfield

Rosell J, Colomina J, Riu P, Pallasar R, Webster J G 1988 Skin impedance from 1 Hz to 1 MHz. IEEE Trans Biomed Eng 25: (8) 649–651

Rosenthal R L, Tobias C W 1948 Measurement of the electrical resistance of human blood use in coagulation studies and cell volume determination. J Lab Clin Med 80: 1110–1122

Schwan H P 1957 Electrical properties of tissue and cell suspensions, Adv Biol Med Phys, 5: 147–209

Schwan H P 1963 Determination of biological impedances in: Nastruk W L (ed.) Physical techniques in biological research vol. VI Academic Press, New York pp 323–407

Schwan H P 1977 Field interaction with biological matter. Ann N Y Acad Sci 303: 198–213

Schwan H P, Foster K R 1980 R F field interactions with biological systems – electrical properties and biophysical mechanisms. Proc IEEE 68 (1): 104–113

Silny J 1991 Intraluminal multiple electric impedance procedure for measurement of gastrointestinal motility. J Gastrointest Motility 3 (3): 151–162

Skouras T D 1988 An investigation into the potential of the gastric impedance monitor for detecting gastric contractions. MSc Medical Physics, University of Surrey, Guildford.

Smith H L, Newell S J, Puntis J W L, Hollins G W, Booth I W 1989 Use of epigastric impedance recording to measure gastric emptying in two infants with dumping syndrome. Euro J Gastroenterol Hepatol 1: 125–128

Stuchly M A 1979 Interaction of radiofrequency and microwave radiation with living systems: a review of mechanisms. Rad Environ Biophys 16: 1–14

Sutton J A 1988 Impedance in: Kumar D, Gustavsson S (eds) An illustrated guide to gastrointestinal motility, 1st edn Wiley, Chichester pp 113–117

Sutton J A, Thompson S, Sobnack R 1985 Measurement of gastric emptying rates by radioactive isotope scanning and epigastric impedance. Lancet 2: 898–900

20. Electrogastrography

K. L. Koch   R. M. Stern

INTRODUCTION

Electrogastrography refers to the recording of electrogastrograms (EGGs), which reflect gastric myoelectrical activity as it is recorded from the abdominal surface with electrodes placed on the skin. EGGs are more or less sinusoidal waves recurring at a rate of 3 per minute in man. This predominant frequency is usually discernible by visual inspection of the signal, but computer analysis is very helpful in the qualitative and quantitative study of EGG records.

The stomach is also the source of abnormally fast or slow myoelectrical signals, the tachygastrias and bradygastrias. Acute or chronic shifts from normal 3 cycles per minute (cpm) EGG signals to the gastric dysrhythmias are associated with a variety of clinical syndromes and symptoms, particularly nausea. In contrast to the abnormalities in frequency such as the gastric dysrhythmias, the amplitude, duration, wave form and wave propagation characteristics of the EGG have been infrequently studied or not investigated at all.

Physiological, pathophysiological and psychophysiological investigations of EGG characteristics in health and disease are increasing in number. In this chapter, the normal myoelectrical events of the stomach are reviewed, and methods of recording EGGs and EGG patterns in health and disease are discussed.

BASIC MYOELECTRICAL ACTIVITIES OF THE STOMACH

Slow waves

The stomach is a neuromuscular organ which has intrinsic electrical activities termed 'gastric slow waves'. Gastric slow waves are also described as 'pacesetter potentials' and as 'electrical control activity' (Sarna 1989) (Fig. 20.1A). The actual origin of the gastric slow waves remains controversial. The outer layer of the circular muscle of the stomach wall is considered a source of these electrical oscillations; the interstitial cells of Cajal may also be the primary generator of the gastric slow wave.

Gastric slow waves originate in a 'pacemaker region' located on the greater curvature of the stomach near the junction of the fundus and proximal gastric corpus (Hinder & Kelly 1977). The slow waves are propagated distally and towards the pylorus at a rate of one wave front every 20 s in man (Fig. 20.2) (Sarna 1989, Hinder & Kelly 1977, Nelson & Kohatsu 1968). Thus, the normal gastric slow wave frequency is approximately 3 cpm and ranges from 2.4–3.6 cpm (Hinder & Kelly 1977, Nelson & Kohatsu 1968, Smout et al 1980, Hamilton et al 1986, Geldof et al 1986a, Alvarez 1922). The gastric slow wave itself generates little or no circular muscle layer contraction. As the gastric slow wave approaches the distal antrum and pylorus, a new slow wave develops in the pacemaker region.

Thus, the slow wave controls the timing and propagation of gastric peristalses, which are produced by the contraction of the circular muscle layer (Fig. 20.1). Contractions of the circular muscle layer may range from very gentle, as seen in the postprandial state when the majority of gastric contractions may not occlude the lumen, to strong lumen-obliterating contractions which occur in the fasting state during phases II and III.

Spike and plateau potentials

Spike and plateau potentials, or electrical response activity, are the electrical events which occur during circular muscle contraction (Fig. 20.1B). Spike potentials occur only when slow wave depolarization has brought the circular muscle to its excitation threshold. If the excitation threshold is reached, then spike potential activity occurs and contraction of the circular muscle layer begins (Hinder & Kelly 1977). Thus, the linkage of the slow wave with spike potential activity

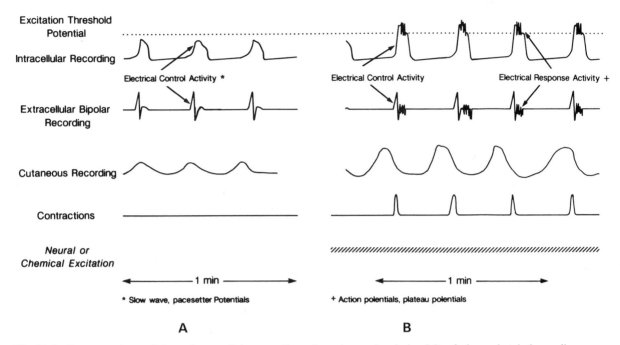

Fig. 20.1 Cutaneous, intracellular and extracellular recordings of gastric myoelectrical activity. **A** shows electrical recordings during motor quiescence. Electrical control activity is shown in intracellular and extracellular recordings. The cutaneous recording is an EGG which shows a 3 cpm pattern. **B** shows gastric electrical–contractile activity initiated by neural or chemical excitation. Electrical response activity is linked to electrical control activity. Thus, contractions occur at the normal 3 cpm rate. The additional electrical activity linked to electrical control activity is represented in the cutaneous recording as 3 cpm waves of increased amplitude. (Modified from Sarna 1989).

underlies gastric peristaltic contractions which migrate from proximal stomach to pylorus at a rate of 3 per minute (Fig. 20.2). EGG signals usually increase in amplitude during gastric contractions when spike activity is linked to slow waves (Smout et al 1980, Hamilton et al 1986, Geldof et al 1986b).

Slow wave, spike activity and gastric contractility are modulated by a host of factors including parasympathetic and sympathetic nervous system activity, ongoing hormonal changes in the fasting or postprandial state, a wide range of physical and nutrient factors which stimulate the stomach by intragastric or extragastric mechanisms, and a variety of emotional or stress-related stimuli. All of these factors influence gastric neuromuscular activity, and therefore, affect gastric myoelectrical and EGG patterns.

METHODS OF RECORDING EGGs

Myoelectrical activity of the stomach recorded from cutaneous electrodes was reported by Alvarez in 1922 (Alvarez 1922). Using a modified instrument for recording electrocardiograms which was obtained from

Einthoven's laboratory, Alvarez measured sinusoidal 3 cpm waves with electrodes placed on the upper abdomen. He called these recordings EGGs, and hypothesized that abnormalities of the myoelectrical rhythm may be related to upper gastrointestinal symptoms and gastric dysfunction. Since 1921, a variety of researchers have been interested in gastric myoelectrical events as recorded with electrodes placed on the skin, mucosa and serosa, or combinations of the above. The history of electrogastrography has been reviewed (Stern 1985).

EGG studies in man, utilizing suction-type electrodes applied to the gastric mucosa, have consistently shown 3 cpm gastric slow waves and 3 cpm EGG waves (Hamilton et al 1986, Abell & Malagelada 1985), as shown in Figure 20.3. Electrodes sewn to the serosa of the gastric body or antrum at the time of jejunostomy tube insertion or other abdominal operations have also recorded 3 cpm slow waves and EGG waves (Nelson & Kohatsu 1968, Familoni et al 1991). As shown in Figure 20.3, these studies have consistently shown that the frequency of the EGG is identical to the slow wave signal recorded with mucosal or serosal

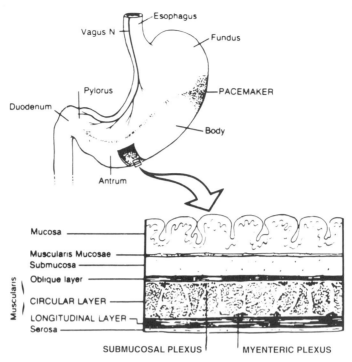

Fig. 20.2 Anatomical regions of the stomach, including the general area of pacemaker region, which generates electrical control activity. Pacesetter potentials migrate distally to the pylorus at a rate of 3 cpm and coordinate gastric peristalses.

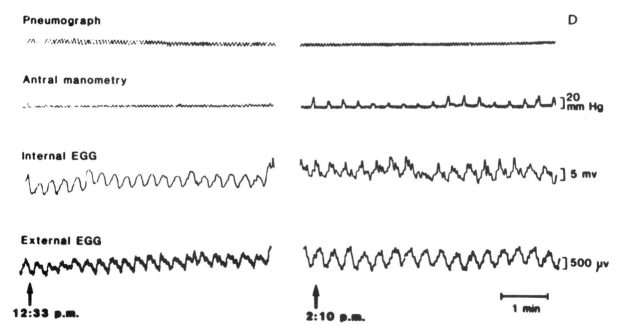

Fig. 20.3 Simultaneous recordings from mucosal (internal EGG) and cutaneous electrodes (external EGG) in man show similarity of 3 cpm gastric slow waves (Abell & Malagelada 1985). Pneumograph shows respiratory rate and antral manometry shows intraluminal contractions.

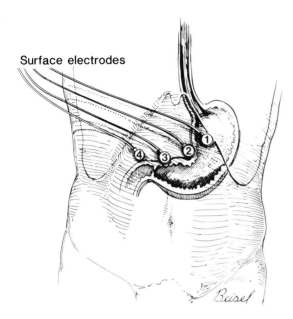

Surface electrodes

Fig. 20.4 Placement of cutaneous electrodes on the upper abdominal surface for recording ECGs (Koch et al 1989).

electrodes (Nelson & Kohatsu 1968, Hamilton et al 1986, Abell & Malagelada 1985, Familoni et al 1991).

The standard placement of EGG electrodes on the upper abdomen is shown in Figure 20.4. Descriptions of electrode placement, filter selection and equipment necessary for recording EGGs have been published (Stern & Koch 1985, Koch et al 1989, Stern et al 1987b). Briefly, four standard Ag–AgCl electrodes are positioned on the upper abdomen. The skin is abraded gently before placement of the electrodes. The first electrode is positioned below the left costal margin in the midclavicular line; the third electrode is placed between the xiphoid and umbilicus; the second electrode is placed between the first and third electrodes; the fourth electrode is the reference electrode and is placed below the right costal margin in line with the other three electrodes. This arrangement of electrodes, generally parallel with the long axis of the antrum, yields EGGs with the largest amplitudes when compared with other electrode positions (Mirizzi & Scafoglieri 1983). Ultrasound may be optionally used to locate the corpus and antrum.

The electrodes are connected through direct nystagmus couplers (Coupler 9859, SensorMedics, Anaheim, California) to a rectilinear recorder (Beckman R611, SensorMedics) for hard copy. Low pass filters to eliminate drift and frequencies less than 1 cpm (0.016 Hz) and high pass filters to eliminate signals greater than

18 cpm (0.3 Hz) provide the filters needed to admit frequencies from approximately 1–18 cpm, a range well within physiological and pathophysiological electrical activities of the stomach. The EGG signal may also be recorded on magnetic tape for later computer analysis or digitized online.

We have recently demonstrated (Stern et al 1991a) that EGGs can be recorded for up to 24 h from freely moving subjects. Ambulatory EGG recording presents the opportunity for clinicians to be able to obtain EGG data from patients during their normal activities and relate periodic reports of pain, nausea, or other symptoms to EGG patterns.

ANALYSIS OF EGGs

EGGs may be scored visually. However, with the aid of a desktop computer, spectral analysis programs provide quantification of the amount of power in EGG frequency bands that is not possible by manual analysis. The Fourier transform may be used to compute the power and frequencies contained in the EGG signal (van der Schee 1987). The power at a given EGG frequency is a unitless number that reflects the amplitude of electrical activity at that particular frequency relative to other frequencies contained in the raw EGG signal. The amplitude of EGG waves increases after sham feeding (Stern et al 1989), barium meals (Koch et al 1987), and bethanechol (Ignaszewski et al 1990), indicating that gastric distention alone does not account for the increase in EGG amplitude during gastric contractions. As shown in Figure 20.5, a single EGG wave corresponds with one gastric peristaltic wave. After the ingestion of nutrient or non-nutrient liquids, the amplitude of the EGG wave also increases as shown in Fig. 20.6 (Koch et al 1987). In the dog, postprandial increases in EGG amplitude are coincident with spike activity associated with gastric contractions (Smout et al 1980). Cutaneous electrodes positioned in standard fashion with typical amplification and filters do not detect spike potentials or direction of propagation (Familoni et al 1991). Changes in the EGG power in different frequency ranges over a time period may be displayed as a three-dimensional (Fig. 20.6) or a grey-scale plot (van der Schee 1987) (Fig. 20.7). The height of the peaks (Fig. 20.6) or darkness in the grey scale (Fig. 20.7) indicates the strength of the signal at a particular frequency. In Figure 20.6, each line in the plot represents the frequencies present in 4 min of raw EGG signal. The running spectral plot is obtained by adding 1 min of new EGG signal to the previous 3 min of EGG signal.

Changes in power may be described quantitatively in

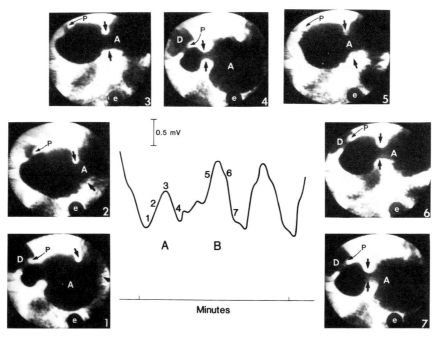

Fig. 20.5 EGG waves A and B recorded during fluoroscopy of the stomach after healthy subject ingested 5 ounces of a barium suspension. During the formation of 'wave A' a gastric peristaltic contraction began moving from the corpus (frame 1 and 2) through the antrum (A) (see frame 3 and 4) as shown by the arrows. As the peristaltic wave ends in the distal antrum the duodenal bulb (D) fills with barium (frame 4). During EGG 'wave B', the next peristaltic wave exhibits a similar sequence of events (frames 5, 6 and 7) (Koch et al 1987). The EGG electrode is labelled 'e', 'P' indicates pylorus.

terms of the percentage of total power in the various frequency bands designated in Figure 20.6. For example, in our laboratory 2.4–3.6 cpm is the normal gastric frequency range for quantitative analysis of the EGG (Stern et al 1987b, Koch et al 1987). The percentage of total EGG power which is within this normal range can be calculated using the spectral analysis data. Other frequency ranges of interest are 3.6–9.9 cpm, an abnormally rapid frequency range termed tachygastria. The EGG frequencies from 1–2.4 cpm are slower than normal, and may be abnormal if they dominate the EGG activity. These very slow EGG rhythms are termed bradygastrias. Finally, the 10–15 cpm range encompasses the known duodenal frequencies in man, which range from 10–13 cpm. In addition to frequency analysis and the percentage of power in the various frequency bands, the power in these bands can be compared before and after a stimulus (such as a meal or drug) to obtain a power ratio. Geldof et al (1986a) also determined the stability of the EGG signal around a selected frequency and described this as a stability or variance factor.

NORMAL ELECTROGASTROGRAPHIC ACTIVITY OF THE STOMACH

Fasting conditions

Very few EGG investigations have formally studied the fasting state. During fasting three stereotyped phases of gastric contractility have been identified (Szurszewski 1979). Phase I is a period of quiescence or no contractile activity. During phase I the stomach's electrical activity is in a normal 3 cpm EGG rhythm (Geldof et al 1986a). Duration of phase I is approximately 30 min. Phase II is a period of intermittent contractions of the gastric body and antrum. The contractions may be of moderate strength (20–80 mmHg) but there is no particular pattern to the contractile activity. During these irregular periods of strong antral contractions (> 25 mmHg) intermittent large amplitude electrical waves at a frequency of 1–2 per minute are recorded in the EGG (Geldof et al 1986a, van der Schee et al 1983). Phase III is characterized by 2–10-min periods of regular, strong, gastric contractions which occur at 3 per minute. During phase III contrac-

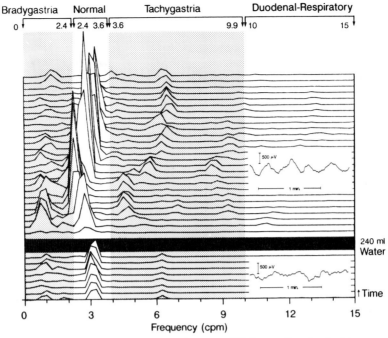

Fig. 20.6 Effect of ingesting 240 ml of water on EGG recordings in a healthy subject. X-axis indicates frequency in cpm, Y-axis indicates time in minutes (see text) and the Z-axis is EGG power. Descriptive and numerical frequency ranges of interest are listed above the spectral analysis. Baseline EGG tracing (inset) shows some 3 cpm waves, which are much clearer as 3 cpm peaks in the running spectral analysis. After water was ingested, there is a decrease in frequency to approximately 2 cpm, followed by clear 3 cpm peaks. 3 cpm waves of increased amplitude are also seen in the EGG tracing (inset) after ingestion of water.

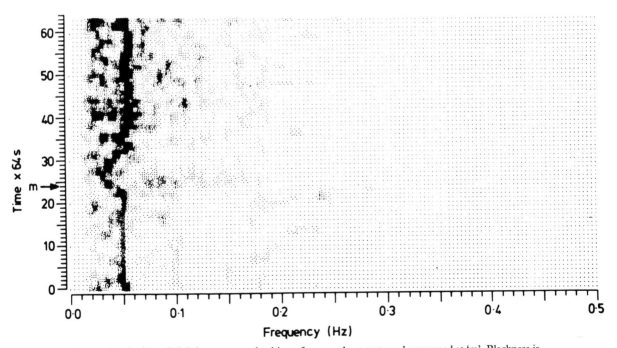

Fig. 20.7 Grey scale plot of an EGG from a control subject after a yoghurt test meal consumed at 'm'. Blackness is proportional to the power of the EGG signal. Immediately after the meal, note the temporary decrease in frequency (the 'frequency dip') and the increased blackness in the 0.05 Hz range (3 cpm) which follows the dip (Geldof et al 1986).

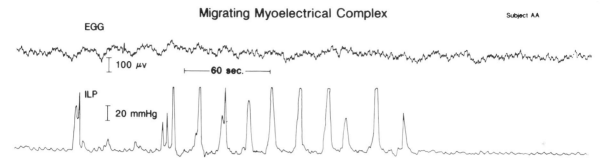

Fig. 20.8   EGG and intraluminal pressure recordings (ILP) from the antrum in a healthy subject during a phase III. Note the increased amplitude of the EGG signal during phase III antral contractions.

tions there is an increase in amplitude of the 3 cpm EGG waves approximately 50% of the time, as shown in Fig. 20.8 (Geldof et al 1986).

Postprandial patterns

A number of investigators have reported the effects of nutrient meals on EGG patterns. Yogurt or pancake meals increase the amplitude of the 3-cpm EGG wave (Geldof et al 1986a). Initially, the increase in amplitude occurs at a slower frequency, 2.2–2.5 cpm, a so-called frequency dip, as shown in Figures 20.6 and 20.7; after approximately 10–15 min, the EGG frequency gradually shifts back to the 3-cpm range as shown. Ingestion of whole milk increases the amplitude of 3 cpm EGG waves (Hamilton et al 1986) (Fig. 20.9), whereas 10% milk or cream diminishes the amplitude of the 3 cpm EGG wave (Chen & McCallum 1990). A technetium-labelled omelette meal evokes a complex series of events including increased 3 cpm waves in the first 15 min after ingestion, followed by an increase in the 1–2 cpm EGG activity during the linear phase of gastric emptying (Koch et al 1991b).

Non-nutrient meals such as barium sulphate or water loads stimulate 3 cpm waves of increased amplitude (Figs. 20.5 and 20.6). The EGG waves with increased amplitude correspond with gastric peristaltic waves which empty barium into the duodenum (Koch et al 1987). The increase in amplitude of EGG waves reflects increased myoelectrical events associated with contraction, i.e. plateau potentials linked to slow waves.

Few investigations of changes in EGG amplitude have been reported. Stern et al (1989) reported that sham feeding increased the amplitude of 3 cpm EGG signals in healthy subjects, but not in patients with previous vagotomies. Subjects who found sham feeding 'disgusting' did not have an increase in amplitude of 3

cpm EGG activity (Stern et al 1989). On the other hand, cold pressor tests which evoke increased sympathetic nervous system activity decrease 3 cpm wave amplitude significantly (Stern et al 1991b). Erythromycin increases the amplitude of EGG signals in the lower frequency ranges of 2.4–2.8 cpm (Chen et al 1992). Many other stimuli may affect the amplitude of the 3 cpm EGG waves. Physiologic and pathophysiologic changes in EGG amplitude in the 3 cpm or other frequency bands requires much further exploration.

ABNORMAL ELECTROGASTROGRAPHIC RHYTHMS OF THE STOMACH

The normal gastric slow wave rhythm in dog is 5 cpm, the rate at which canine gastric peristalses occur (Sarna 1989). However, Code and Marlett (1974) found that a variety of faster rhythms occurred spontaneously in the dog antrum, and they termed these abnormally fast rhythms tachygastrias. More recently, Kim showed that infusions of adrenaline in man (Kim et al 1989) and dogs (Kim et al 1987) induced arrhythmias or bradygastrias. Tachygastrias generally occur in the antrum, whereas the bradygastrias were recorded in the gastric corpus (Kim et al 1987).

As mentioned above, Alvarez predicted that electrical abnormalities of the stomach may be related to abnormal digestive symptoms and abnormal gastric function. In 1980, You et al described a series of patients with unexplained nausea and vomiting in whom conventional clinical investigation showed no abnormality (You et al 1980). However, these patients had antral dysrhythmias as recorded with mucosal electrodes; the rhythms ranged from regular 6–7 cpm tachygastrias to very chaotic, fast rhythms termed tachyarrhythmias. Periods of arrhythmia were also found

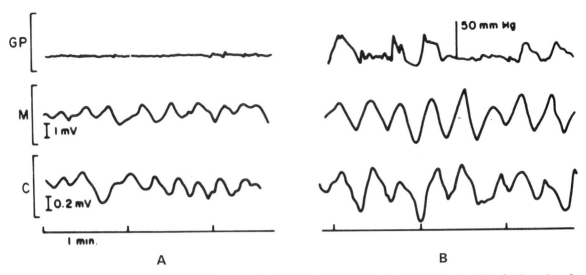

Fig. 20.9 Increased amplitude of the 3 cpm EGG signal recorded from mucosal and cutaneous electrodes after ingestion of milk (Hamilton et al 1986). **A** shows gastric pressure (GP), mucosal electrode (M) and cutaneous electrode (C). Note the similarity in frequency of electrical waves from M and C. After ingestion of milk (**B**), the increase in amplitude of electrical waves (M and C) and onset of gastric pressures are seen.

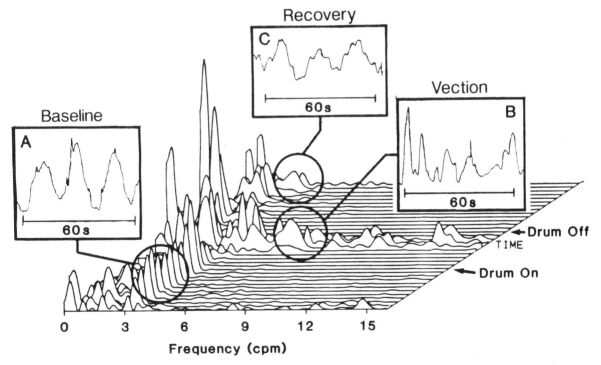

Fig. 20.10 EGG traces (A, B and C) and running spectral analysis of the EGG recording during motion sickness experiment. 3 cpm waves and peaks are seen at baseline (A) before the drum is rotated to create an illusion of motion (vection). During vection, gastric tachyarrhythmias develop in association with the onset of nausea (B). Peaks in the tachygastria range are seen in the running spectral analysis. After the drum is turned off, the tachyarrhythmias disappear; by the end of the recovery period, 3 cpm EGG rhythms are re-established (C).

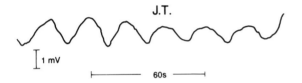

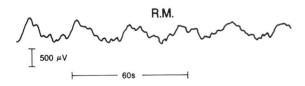

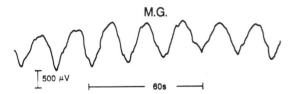

Fig. 20.11 EGGs recorded from patients JT, RM and MG with gastric outlet obstruction from pyloric or duodenal stenosis. The patients presented with nausea, vomiting and delayed solid phase gastric emptying. Note the obvious 3 cpm EGG recordings from each patient. The normal 3 cpm pattern raised the suspicion that the gastroparesis was *not* from a neuromuscular disorder.

in these patients. The authors associated the persistent symptoms of nausea and vomiting with the abnormal gastric electrical activity.

Stern and Koch (1985) induced nausea and motion sickness by creating vection (illusory self-motion) with a rotating optokinetic drum while simultaneously recording gastric electrical activity with cutaneous electrodes. These investigators showed that the shift from the normal 3 cpm EGG rhythm to tachyarrhythmias during vection (Fig. 20.10), was associated with onset of nausea. Abell et al (1985) showed that glucagon infusions evoked gastric dysrhythmias and nausea in healthy volunteers. Thus, acute or chronic gastric dysrhythmias such as tachygastrias or bradygastrias appear to be markers of gastric neuromuscular dysfunction from diverse causes. Tachygastrias recorded with EGG electrodes were identified 93% of the time, a percentage similar to that found with serosal electrodes (Familoni et al 1991). Tachygastrias recorded from patients with various clinical disorders are described below and summarized in Table 20.1.

Tachygastrias

Tachygastrias are abnormally fast gastric electrical activity ranging from 3.6–9.9 cpm. Tachygastrias have been recorded from patients with a wide range of diseases and disorders associated with nausea and gastric dysfunction. The clinical syndromes in which tachygastrias have been recorded are described below.

Table 20.1 Gastric dysrhymias associated with clinical conditions

Tachygastrias (3.6–9.9 cpm myoelectrical pattern)	Tachyarrhythmias (mix of tachygastrias and bradygastrias)	Bradygastrias (1–2.4 cpm myoelectrical pattern)	Arrhythmia (flatline EGG pattern)
Gastroparesis	Motion sickness	Gastroparesis	Nausea of pregnancy
Diabetic	Idiopathic gastroparesis	Diabetic	Hyperemesis
Idiopathic		Idiopathic	gravidarum
Ischaemic		Ischaemic	Drug-induced
Intestinal pseudo-obstruction		Post-operative (*see* tachygastrias)	adrenaline
Nausea of pregnancy		Intestinal pseudo-obstruction	Postoperative
Functional dyspepsia – dysmotility		Nausea of pregnancy	Billroth I, II and
type with normal gastric emptying		Functional dyspepsia – dysmotility	Roux-en-Y
Gastric ulcers (acute) with nausea		type with normal gastric emptying	Total gastrectomy
Postoperative		Bulimia nervosa	
Postoperative ileus		Drug-induced – adrenaline	
Post-cholecystectomy		– morphine sulphate	
Anorexia nervosa			
Premature infants			
Drug-induced			
Glucagon			
Adrenaline			
Morphine sulphate			

Month 0-Baseline

A

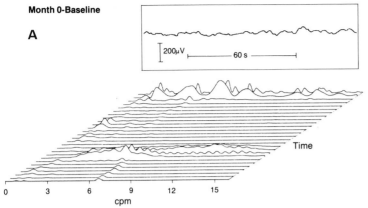

Month 6

B

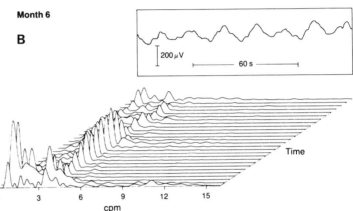

Fig. 20.12 EGGs and running spectral analyses from a patient with diabetic gastroparesis, nausea and vomiting. **A** (Month 0) shows a flatline pattern EGG signal (inset) and 6 cpm peaks in the spectral plot (baseline) when patient had significant nausea. **B** (Month 6) shows a 3 cpm EGG pattern in the same patient after 6 months of treatment with domperidone. Many regular peaks at 3 cpm are seen in the running spectral plot (from Koch et al 1989). The patient's symptoms resolved.

Gastroparesis

Obstructive gastroparesis Gastroparesis due to a fixed obstructive lesion, such as pyloric outlet obstruction or duodenal obstruction from peptic disease due to adhesions is associated with *normal 3 cpm EGG activity* (Koch et al 1991a) (Fig. 20.11). In these cases of obstructive lesions, the normal 3 cpm gastric myoelectrical activity suggested the possibility that the gastroparesis was *not* on the basis of neural or muscular dysfunction. Thus, a 3 cpm EGG pattern in a patient with documented gastroparesis suggests the possibility of a mechanical cause of the gastroparesis.

Diabetic gastroparesis Tachygastrias have been recorded in patients with symptomatic diabetic gastroparesis. Koch et al (1989) showed that treatment with domperidone converted gastric dysrhythmias to normal 3 cpm EGG rhythms (Koch et al 1989) (Fig. 20.12). This pharmacologic 'gastroversion' from tachygastria and bradygastria to normal 3 cpm gastric electrical activity was associated with significant improvement in symptoms. Hamilton et al (1986) recorded gastric dysrhythmias in some diabetics under

circumstances in which there were no upper gastrointestinal symptoms; but Abell et al (1991) found many tachygastrias which were associated with gastroparesis. Further studies are needed to determine the gastric electrical and contractile activities in diabetics with and without gastroparesis.

Idiopathic gastroparesis Tachygastrias have been recorded with mucosal electrodes in patients with idiopathic gastroparesis (Bortolotti et al 1990). These electrical recordings were obtained in the fasting state. Tachygastrias during fasting and after a water load were reported in patients with idiopathic gastroparesis (Koch et al 1991a). We have observed that metoclopramide converts tachygastria associated with idiopathic gastroparesis to a normal 3 cpm electrical activity (Fig. 20.13) and cisapride converts bradygastria to normal 3 cpm EGG patterns (Fig. 20.14).

Ischaemic gastroparesis Tachygastria and gastroparesis due to chronic mesenteric ischaemia were described in two patients (Liberski et al 1990). The gastric dysrhythmia and gastroparesis were completely reversed following mesenteric revascularization (Fig. 20.15). Five additional cases have been added to this

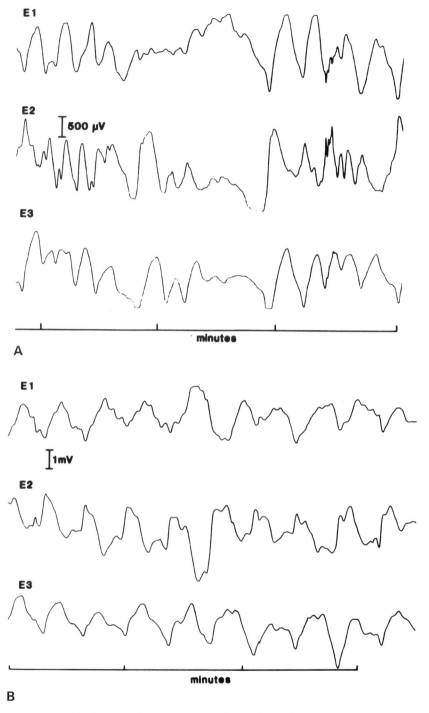

Fig. 20.13 EGG tracings showing 'gastroversion' in a patient with idiopathic gastroparesis.
A shows a 5–6 cpm tachygastria. **B** shows a 3 cpm EGG recorded from the same patient 20
min after metoclopramide (20 mg per os). Patient noticed decreased nausea after receiving
the metoclopramide and converting from tachygastria to normal 3 cpm pattern.

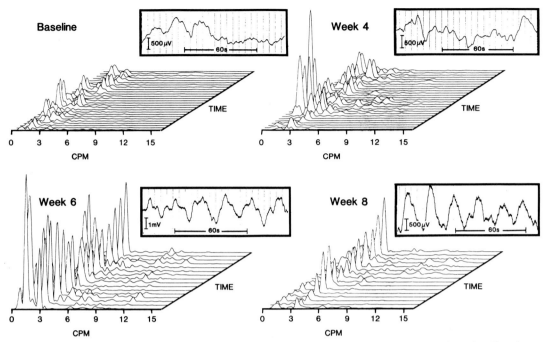

Fig. 20.14 EGGs (insets) and running spectral plots from a patient with idiopathic gastroparesis. At baseline, the EGG shows predominantly large amplitude slow waves consistent with bradygastria. The running spectral analysis also shows the most power in the 1–2 cpm range, but some 3 cpm peaks are apparent. The 3 cpm EGG pattern becomes increasingly clear during weeks 4, 6 and 8 of cisapride therapy. Similarly, the power of the peaks at 3 cpm becomes more obvious. By week 8 the patient had markedly decreased symptoms of nausea and epigastric distress and normal 3 cpm EGG pattern.

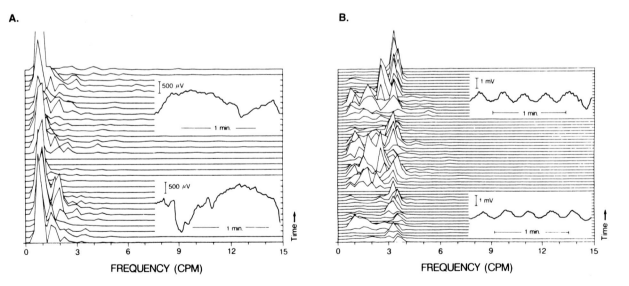

Fig. 20.15 **A** shows EGG traces and running spectral analysis of 30 minutes of EGG data in patient with chronic mesenteric ischaemia and gastroparesis. The EGG tracings show very large slow waves consistent with 1–2 cpm waves or bradygastrias. **B** shows EGGs and running spectral analyses approximately 6 months after mesenteric artery bypass surgery. The patient's symptoms had resolved and his gastric emptying study was normal. The EGG showed normal 3 cpm waves and many peaks in the 3 cpm range (Liberski et al 1990).

A.

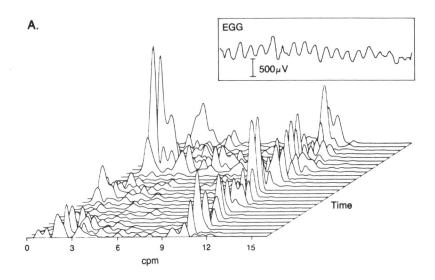

B.

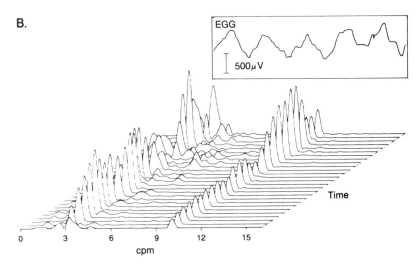

Fig. 20.16 EGGs and running spectral analyses from a patient with symptomatic chronic idiopathic intestinal pseudo-obstruction. Baseline EGG (**A**) shows a tachygastria with a steady 9–10 cpm rhythm and almost no normal 3 cpm signals. After treatment with metoclopramide for 4 months, the EGG shows a clear 3 cpm rhythm (**B**). The running spectral analysis also shows consistent peaks in the 3 cpm range. The 9–10 cpm rhythms remain, raising the possibility of a continuing ectopic antral pacemaker focus or a rhythm of duodenal origin. The patient's nausea, vomiting and gastroparesis resolved while on metoclopramide treatment.

patient group. In these additional patients the gastric dysrhythmias converted to a normal 3 cpm rhythm and gastric emptying became normal 3–6 months after revascularization (unpublished observations).

Intestinal Pseudo-obstruction

Intestinal pseudo-obstruction relates to a diverse variety of disorders involving damage to the muscular and/or neural elements of the gastrointestinal tract. Tachygastrias have been reported in the neuropathic form of intestinal pseudo-obstruction in children, while EGG recordings from the myopathic form revealed chaotic tachyarrhythmias (Bisset et al 1989). In an adolescent with intestinal pseudo-obstruction, regular 9 cpm tachygastrias were recorded when gastroparesis was present; treatment with metoclopramide resulted in improved symptoms, conversion of the

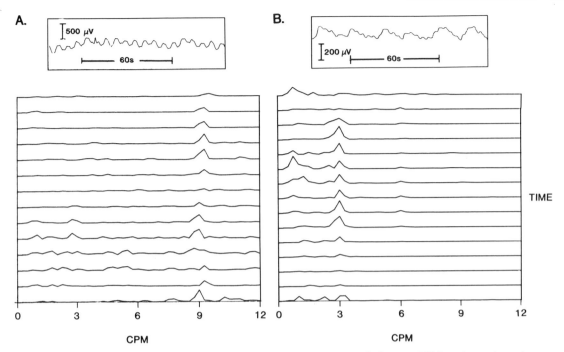

A.

500 µV

60s

B.

200 µV

60s

TIME

0   3   6   9   12   0   3   6   9   12

CPM

CPM

Fig. 20.17 EGGs and running spectral analyses before and after pregnancy. **A** shows an EGG tracing and running spectral plot from a patient with nausea in the first trimester of pregnancy. EGG and the running spectral plot show a tachygastria at approximately 9 cpm. 6 weeks after delivery, the patient had another EGG (**B**) which shows a normal 3 cpm EGG pattern in the raw EGG as well as in the running spectal plot (Koch et al 1990b).

tachygastria to a predominant 3 cpm gastric electrical pattern, and normalization of gastric emptying (Fig. 20.16).

Nausea of pregnancy and hyperemesis gravidarum

Tachygastrias were found in the majority of 32 women who had nausea during the first trimester of pregnancy (Koch et al 1990). The four pregnant women who did not have nausea on the study day had normal 3 cpm myoelectrical activity. Furthermore, six women returned for EGG recordings after their deliveries and their EGGs showed normal 3 cpm rhythm compared with gastric dysrhythmias and nausea during the first trimester (Fig. 20.17).

Functional dyspepsia–dysmotility type (*with normal gastric emptying*)

The symptoms of functional dyspepsia are vague and include early satiety, upper abdominal discomfort, nausea, and the absence of any obvious cause for these symptoms. 30–50% of these patients have gastric dysrhythmias and delayed gastric emptying. Recently, Koch et al (1992) reported that 9 of 13 subjects with

functional dyspepsia and *normal* gastric emptying studies had gastric dysrhythmias; two had tachygastrias and seven had bradygastrias. Gastric dysrhythmias have been reported in children with functional dyspepsia (Cucchiara et al 1992b) and cisapride treatment converted gastric dysrhythmias to normal 3 cpm signals (Cucchiara et al 1992a).

Gastric ulcers

Many patients with gastric ulceration have upper abdominal burning discomfort. Some patients also have considerable nausea associated with gastric ulcers. Smout et al (1980) showed that patients with acute gastric ulcers and nausea had tachygastrias as recorded by cutaneous electrodes, whereas those subjects with no nausea had normal 3-cpm rhythms (Geldof et al 1989).

Postoperative conditions

Postoperative ileus. Patients with postoperative ileus have few if any gastric dysrhythmias (Clevers et al 1992). The presence or absence of gastric dysrhythmias did not correlate with postoperative nausea symptoms.

Post-cholecystectomy. In the immediate postoperative days after cholecystectomy, a variety of tachygastrias were recorded with serosal electrodes. Others reported no gastric dysrhythmias after cholecystectomy (Pezzolla et al 1991). The presence of tachygastrias did not correlate with reports of gastrointestinal symptoms. These postoperative studies indicate that tachygastrias may be present, but they are apparently not related to symptoms. Specific characteristics of the postoperative tachygastrias and the complex neural, hormonal and psychological responses in the postoperative state may all contribute to the paucity of symptoms associated with postoperative tachygastrias.

The presence of a tachygastria or bradygastria may not always be clinically significant. The *duration* of the tachygastria, the *frequency* of tachygastria, and the threshold of an individual's perception of the dysrhythmia are all factors which may affect clinical significance. For example, premature ventricular contractions (PVCs) are clearly abnormal cardiac rhythms, but if PVCs occur sporadically each minute the dysrhythmia may never reach conscious perception and are clinically irrelevant. On the other hand, if 3–4 PVCs occur in a row, the event may reach consciousness as 'skipped beats' or 'palpitations', and are clinically relevant.

Billroth I and II and Roux-en-Y reconstructions. Patients with Roux-en-Y reconstructions often show a predominance of the duodenal frequencies from 10–13 cpm as recorded with cutaneous electrodes. These patients had significant nausea, vomiting and upper abdominal discomfort after their Roux-en-Y reconstructions. In patients with Billroth I and II reconstructions after partial gastrectomy, 1–2.4 cpm EGG waves predominate and duodenal rhythms may also be recorded (personal observation).

Total gastrectomy. In patients with total gastrectomy, no regular 3 cpm electrical signals are recorded in the EGG (Pezzolla et al 1989). Jejunal and colonic electrical activity may be recorded.

Anorexia nervosa

Patients with anorexia nervosa often have delayed gastric emptying. Abell et al (1987) showed that patients with anorexia nervosa also have a variety of tachygastrias. The gastric dysrhythmias did not improve with inpatient psychiatric treatment, although the patients' dietary intake was improved by behavioural modification.

Premature infants

In infants ranging from 22 weeks to term, no significant differences in the EGG frequencies were found according to gestational age. However, compared with adult controls, the infants had less 3 cpm activity and more tachygastria activity (Koch et al 1993). The infants also showed no consistent change in gastric myoelectrical activity in response to formula feedings.

Drug-induced tachygastrias

Glucagon, adrenaline and morphine sulfate have been shown to induce tachygastrias as well as bradygastrias in man, as described above.

Tachyarrhythmias

Tachyarrhythmias are a form of tachygastria that encompass a chaotic mixture of irregularly fast frequencies and bradygastrias. Conditions in which tachyarrhythmias have been recorded are described below.

Motion sickness

Tachyarrhythmias have been recorded during motion sickness induced by the illusion of self-motion (vection). During vection, 50–60% of healthy subjects experience the acute onset of nausea, which is preceded by an abrupt shift from the normal 3 cpm EGG signal to gastric tachyarrhythmias (Stern et al 1987a, 1985) (Fig. 20.10). The frequency of the tachyarrhythmias ranges irregularly from 4–9 cpm. Such tachyarrhythmias also have been reported during nausea induced by a rotating chair (Stewart et al 1989) and in subjects who develop nausea in the KC135 (Vomit Comet) during recurrent exposures to hypergravity and weightlessness (Harm et al 1987).

Idiopathic gastroparesis

Patients with idiopathic gastroparesis also may have tachyarrhythmias ranging from tachygastria to bradygastria to arrhythmia as described above.

Bradygastrias

Bradygastrias are abnormally slow 1–2 cpm myoelectrical waves. These EGG waves are usually of greater amplitude than the normal 3 cpm signals. The precise origin of bradygastria waves has not been determined. One per minute rhythms have been detected in the human antrum after fundic transection (Hinder & Kelly 1977). In a neonate with gastroparesis, 1 per minute waves were recorded simultaneously from electrodes on the antral serosa and from cutaneous electrodes (unpublished observations). Thus, it is not clear if the 1 per minute waves originate primarily in the corpus or antrum.

Bradygastrias have been recorded in patients with diabetic, idiopathic, ischaemic and postoperative gastroparesis, intestinal pseudo-obstruction, nausea of pregnancy, and functional dyspepsia – dysmotility type. Bulimia nervosa patients also have a predominance of bradygastrias before and after ingesting a water load (Koch et al 1990a). Adrenaline generally induces bradygastria. Figure 20.14 shows a bradygastria at baseline recorded from a 38-year-old woman with idiopathic gastroparesis. During the course of therapy with cisapride, the bradygastria was eradicated and a clear 3 cpm rhythm was recorded in the EGG. The gastroversion was associated with resolution of symptoms.

Arrhythmias

Arrhythmias are flat line patterns of gastric electrical activity as shown in Figure 20.12. Increasing sensitivity of the recording instrument does not reveal any rhythmic pattern of myoelectrical activity. Arrhythmias have been recorded in patients with entities described in Table 20.1.

SUMMARY

EGGs recorded from healthy subjects reflect gastric slow wave activity which appears as 3 cpm sinusoidal waves. Although the slow wave frequency is generally 3 cpm, tthe rhythm is not fixed but may fluctuate from moment to moment. Persistent gastric dysrhythmias, however, are recorded in a variety of clinical syndromes in which gastric motility disorders and symptoms of nausea are predominant. Furthermore, the eradication of the tachygastria, tachyarrhythmia or bradygastria and the restoration of normal 3 cpm gastric electrical activity have been associated with improvement in symptoms.

Gastric dysrhythmias also interfere with the circular muscular activity required for the normal mixing and emptying of a meal; thus, depending on the severity of the dysrhythmia, gastric emptying may be delayed. In special cases, such as ischaemic gastroparesis, both normal electrical activity (3 cpm patterns) and normal gastric emptying rates are restored after appropriate treatment. On the other hand, gastric dysrhythmias alone may elicit a sense of nausea and vague upper abdominal discomfort or dyspepsia.

The clinical importance of electrogastrography is emerging. Much additional work is necessary to understand the control of normal gastric myoelectrical activity. More study is needed to determine the mechanisms underlying gastric dysrhythmias and to investigate therapies designed to eradicate abnormal gastric myoelectrical events. The extent to which eradication of gastric dysrhythmias leads to the improvement in symptoms such as early satiety, vague epigastric distress, and nausea and vomiting will further indicate the clinical importance of gastric dysrhythmias and the noninvasive EGG methods to detect them.

REFERENCES

Abell T L, Malagelada J-R 1985 Glucagon-evoked gastric dysrhythmias in humans shown by an improved electrogastrographic technique. Gastroenterology 88: 1932–1940

Abell T L, Camilleri M, Hench V S, Malagelada J-R 1991 Gastric electromechanical function and gastric emptying in diabetic gastroparesis. Eur J Gastroenterol Hepatol 3: 163–167

Abell T L, Malagelada J-R, Lucas A R et al 1987 Gastric electromechanical and neurohormonal function in anorexia nervosa. Gastroenterology 93: 958–965

Alvarez W C 1922 The electrogastrogram and what it shows. JAMA 78: 1116–1119

Bisset W M, Devane S P, Milla P J 1989 Gastric antral dysrhythmias in children with idiopathic intestinal pseudo-obstruction. J Gastrointestinal Motility 1: 53 (abstract)

Bortolotti M, Sarti P, Barbara L, Brunelli F 1990 Gastric myoelectrical activity in patients with chronic idiopathic gastroparesis. J Gastrointestinal Motility 2: 104–108

Chen J, McCallum R W 1990 Milk suppresses the gastric slow wave. Gastroenterology 99: 1207 (abstr)

Chen J, Yeaton P, McCallum R W 1992 Effect of erythromycin on gastric myoelectrical activity in normal human subjects. Am J Physiol 263: G24–G28

Clevers G J, Smout A J P M, van der Schee E J, Akkermans L M A 1992 Changes in gastric electrical activity in patients with severe post-operative nausea and vomiting. J Gastrointestinal Motility 4: 61–69

Code C F, Marlett J A 1974 Canine tachygastria. Mayo Clin Proc 49: 325–332

Cucchiara S, Minella R, Riezzo G, Vallone P, Castellone F,

Auricchio S 1992a Reversal of gastric electrical dysrhythmias by cisapride in children with functional dyspepsia: report of three cases. Dig Dis Sci 37: 1136–1140

Cucchiara S, Riezzo G, Minella R, Pezzolla F, Auricchio S 1992b Electrogastrography in non-ulcer dyspepsia. Arch Dis Child 67: 613–617

Familoni B O, Bowes K L, Kingma Y J, Cote K R 1991 Can transcutaneous recordings detect gastric electrical abnormalities? Gut 32: 141–146

Geldof H, van der Schee E J, van Blankenstein M, Grashuis J L 1986a Electrogastrographic study of gastric myoelectrical activity in patients with unexplained nausea and vomiting. Gut 27: 799–808

Geldof H, van der Schee E J, Grashuis J L 1986b Electrogastrographic characteristics of the interdigestive migrating complex in humans. Am J Physiol 250: G165–G171

Geldof H, van der Schee E J, Smout A J P M, van de Merwe J P, van Blankenstein M, Grashuis J L 1989 Myoelectrical activity of the stomach in gastric ulcer patients: An electrogastrographic study. J Gastrointestinal Motility 1: 122–130

Hamilton J W, Bellhsene B E, Reicherlderfer M, Webster J H, Bass P 1986 Human electrogastrograms. Comparison of surface and mucosal recordings. Dg Dis Sci 31: 33–39

Harm D L, Stern R M, Koch K L, Vasey M W 187 Tachygastria during paraboli flight. Space ife Scince Sposium: Three decades of life science research in space. NASA Headquarters, Washington, D C

Hinder R A, Kelly K A 1977 Human gastric pacesetter potential: site of origin, spread and response to gastric transection and proximal gastric vagotomy. Am J Surg 133: 29–33

Ignaszewski L, Burrows C, Koch K L 1990 Effect of bethanechol on the canine electrogastrogram (EGG). Gastroenterology 99: 1206 (abstr)

Kim C H, Hanson R B, Abell T L, Malagelada J-R 1989 Effect of inhibition of prostaglandin synthesis on epinephrine-induced gastroduodenal electromechanical changes in humans. Mayo Clin Proc 64: 149–157

Kim C H, Zinmeister A R, Malagelada J R 1987 Mechanisms of canine gastric dysrhythmias. Gastroenterology 92: 993–999

Koch K L, Stewart W R, Stern R M 1987 Effect of barium meals on gastric electromechanical activity in man. A fluoroscopic-electrogastrographic study. Dig Dis Sci 32: 1217–1222

Koch K L, Stern R M, Stewart W R, Vasey M W, Sullivan M L 1989 Gastric emptying and gastric myoelectrical activity in patients with symptomatic diabetic gastroparesis: effect of long-term domperidone treatment. Am J Gastroenterol 84: 1069–1075

Koch K L, Bingaman S, Tan L et al 1990a Visceral perceptions and gastric myoelectrical activity in healthy women and in patients with bulimia. Gastroenterology 98: A367 (abstr)

Koch K L, Stern R M, Vasey M, Botti J J, Creasy G W, Dwyer A 1990b Gastric dysrhythmias and nausea of pregnancy. Dig Dis Sci 35: 961–968

Koch K L, Bingaman S, Sperry N, Stern R M, 1991a Electrogastrography differentiates mechanical vs idiopathic

gastroparesis in patients with nausea and vomiting. Gastroenterology 100: A99

Koch K L, Stern R M, Bingama S, Eggli D 1991b Satiety, stomach volume and gastric myoelectrical activity during solid-phase gastric emptying: A study of healthy individuals. J Gastrointestinal Motility 3: 187 (abstract)

Koch, K L, Medina M, Bingaman S, Stern R M 1992 Gastric dysrhythmias and visceral sensations in patients with functional dyspepsia. Gastroenterology 102: A469

Koch K C, Tran T N, Stern R M, Bingaman S, Sperry N 1993 Gastric myoelectrical activity in premature and term. J Gastrointest Motil 5: 41–47

Liberski S M, Koch K L, Atnip R G et al 1990 Ischemic gastroparesis: resolution of nausea, vomiting and gastroparesis after mesenteric artery revascularization. Gastroenterology 99: 252–257

Mirizzi N, Scafoglieri V 1983 Optional direction of the electrogastrographic signal in man. Med & Biol Eng & Comput 21: 385–389

Nelson T S, Kohatsu S 1968 Clinical electrogastrography and its relationship to gastric surgery. Am J Surg 116: 215–222

Pezzolla F, Riezzo G, Maselli M A, Giorgio I 1989 Electrical activity recorded from abdominal surface after gastrectomy or colectomy in humans. Gastroenterology 97: 313–320

Pezzolla F, Riezzo G, Maselli M A, Giorgio I 1991 Gastric electrical dysrhythmia following cholecystectomy in humans. Digestion 49: 134–139

Sarna S 1989 In vivo myoelectrical activity: methods, analysis, and interpretation in: Schultz S, Wood J D (eds) Handbook of physiology, the gastrointestinal system. Waverly Press, Baltimore pp 817–863

Smout A J P M, van der Schee E J, Grashuis J L 1980 What is measured in electrogastrography? Dig Dis Sci 25: 179–187

Stern R M 1985 A brief history of the electrogastrogram in: Electrogastrography: methodology, validation and applications in: Stern R M, Koch K L (eds) Praeger, New York pp 3–9

Stern R M, Koch K L 1985 Electrogastrography: Methodology, validation and applications. Praeger, New York

Stern R M, Koch K L, Leibowitz H W, Lindblad M S, Shupert C L, Stewart W R 1985 Tachygastria and motion sickness. Aviat Space Environ Med 56: 1074–1077

Stern R M, Koch K L, Stewart W R, Lindblad I M 1987a Spectral analysis of tachygastria recorded during motion sickness. Gastroenterology 93: 92–97

Stern R M, Koch K L, Stewart W R, Vasey M W 1987b Electrogastrography: current issues in validation and methodology. Psychophysiology 24: 55–64

Stern R M, Crawford H E, Stewart W R, Vasey M W, Koch K L 1989 Sham feeding. Cephalic-vagal influences on gastric myoelectrical activity. Dig Dis Sci 34: 521–527

Stern R M, Hu S, and Koch K L 1991a Effects of cold stress on gastric myoelectrical activity. J Gastrointestinal Motility 3: 225–228

Stern R M, Uijtdehaage S H J, Koch K L, Hanish H 1991b Ambulatory recording of the electrogastrogram. J Gastrointestinal Motility 3: 202 (abstract)

Stewart J J, Wood M J, Wood C D 1989 Electrogastrograms

during motion sickness in fasted and fed subjects. Aviat Space Environ Med 60: 214–217

Szurszewski J H 1979 A migrating electrical complex of the canine small intestine. Am J Physiol 217: 1757–1763

van der Schee E J, Grashuis J L 1983 Contraction-related, low-frequency components in canine electrogastrographic signals. Am J Physiol 245: G470–G475

van der Schee E J, Grashuis J L 1987 Running spectrum analysis as an aid in the representation and interpretation of electrogastrographic signals. Med & Biol Eng & Comput 25: 57–62

You C H, Lee K Y, Chey W Y et al 1980 Electrogastrographic study of patients with unexplained nausea, bloating and vomiting. Gastroenterology 79: 311–314

21. Chemical detection of transit

R. C. Spiller

INTRODUCTION

Indirect, inexpensive, non-invasive and hence readily repeatable tests have an obvious appeal for the investigation of transit in both clinical and research practice. The techniques described below have been developed with these requirements in mind but their advantages are often obtained at the cost of either low reproducibility or problems with interpretation.

Principle

Chemical methods rely on the ingestion of some substance which will travel with normal chyme and provide a signal when it reaches predetermined regions of the gastrointestinal tract. Such substances should ideally not alter transit and should be easily and accurately measurable. The rapid absorption of probe molecules from the duodenum but not the stomach means that a range of substances have been used to assess gastric emptying.

USE OF PARACETAMOL TO ASSESS GASTRIC EMPTYING

Paracetamol has a number of desirable properties as a probe molecule including a relatively easy chromatographic assay, lack of any effect on gastric emptying, and slow metabolism so that it accumulates in the blood allowing a sem-quantitative measure of emptying (Heading et al 1973).

Method

After an overnight fast subjects are given 1.5 g paracetamol with 200 ml of water. Blood samples are then collected at 30–min intervals and plasma paracetamol levels measured over 4–8 hours. A number of measures have been shown to correlate well with scintigraphic assessement of gastric emptying, including time to maximum plasma concentration ($r = +0.76$), maximum plasma concentration ($r = \pm 0.77$) and plasma paracetamol at 30 min ($r = \pm 0.72$) (Heading et al 1973). This has been used to show the delaying effect of narcotic analgesia on gastric emptying (Fig. 21.1). Paracetamol is better than glucose for this assessement because its clearance is slower, less variable and the basal values are zero.

The studies mentioned above have measured emptying from the fasting stomach but the method could also be used to measure emptying of a liquid test meal since paracetamol is water-soluble and provided it is mixed well with the test meal should empty at the same rate. Giving the drug in a solution should also improve reproducibility since it removes the variables of drug dissolution and dispersion which might influence drug absorption. This simple technique could be a useful way of monitoring the response to treatment of patients with gastric stasis without the expense of repeated scintigraphic studies.

MEASUREMENT OF OROCAECAL TRANSIT TIME

Measurement of transit through the small bowel relies on the enormous change in the intraluminal anaerobic bacterial count distal to the ileocaecal valve (Fig. 21.2). The caecal environment differs from the upper gut in being anaerobic, this permits a number of reactions including the fermentation of carbohydrate to H_2, CH_4, CO_2 and short-chain fatty acids, and the reduction of azo-bonds causing the liberation of sulphapyridine from salazopyrine. These reaction products can be readily measured and the production of H_2 and sulphapyridine are both used to assess mouth to caecum transit. Coated capsules which require bacterial enzymes to dissolve are now readily available and would allow the use of other probe drugs which are absorbed from the colon as indictors of mouth–caecum transit. The disadvantage of such a system would be that

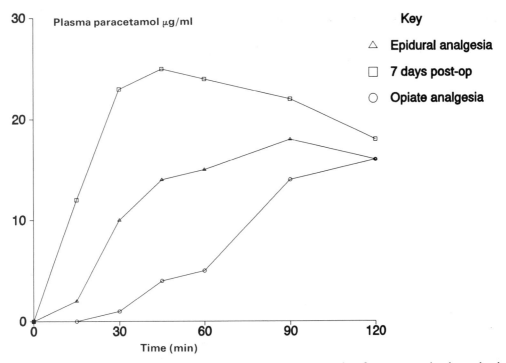

Fig. 21.1 Mean plasma paracetamol after oral dose of 1.5 g paracetamol on first postoperative day under the influence of either opiate analgesia or epidural analgesia compared with plasma curve on day 7 postoperatively (after Nimmo et al 1978).

transit of capsules may differ from normal chyme depending on their size, though microcapsules (< 2 mm) might well give a good assessment of normal chyme transit.

In practice the breath hydrogen technique is the most widely used and will be considered in the most detail.

BREATH HYDROGEN TEST FOR ASSESSING MONTH–CAECUM TRANSIT

Principle

This test relies on the fact that hydrogen is only produced by bacterial anaerobic fermentation which usually only occurs in the colon (Levitt 1969). Hydrogen, being highly diffusible, rapidly (< 1 mm) enters the blood stream and is exhaled in the breath within 1–2 min. Oral ingestion of a poorly absorbable carbohydrate therefore results in a rise in breath hydrogen which occurs within a few minutes of the substrate entering the anaerobic region, usually the caecum. This was demonstrated by Bond and Levitt (1975) by intubating normal volounteers and aspirating samples

from the terminal ileum. Subjects were given 10 or 20 g lactulose together with 2–3 g polyethylene glycol (PEG) and breath hydrogen was measured at 10-min intervals. The results (Fig. 21.3) demonstrate that within a few minutes of the non-absorbable marker, PEG, reaching the terminal ileum breath hydrogen rose. Furthermore in the same study direct instillation of 10 g lactulose into the caecum shows that the lag between entry into the colon and the resulting rise in breath hydrogen is only 4–5 min (Bond & Levitt 1975). Similar findings were reported by Read and colleagues (Read et al 1985) who also noted that as little as 0.5 g lactulose infused directly into the caecum could produce a rise in breath hydrogen of 5–10 ppm. These small doses produced short-lived rises (< 5 min), increasing the dose to 5 g prolonged the rises to 172 ± 32 min (Mean ± SEM).

Method of breath sampling

The earliest studies measured total breath hydrogen production by having subjects breathe into a closed rebreathing system. This was tedious and arduous for

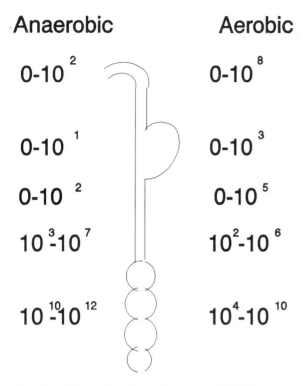

Fig. 21.2   Figures from Simon & Gorbach (1984) illustrating the rapid rise in anaerobic counts on passing the ileocaecal valve.

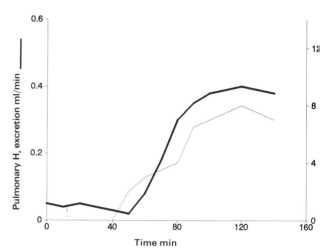

Fig. 21.3   Comparison of the arrival of the non-absorbable meal marker polyethylene glycol (PEG) in the terminal ileum with the rise in breath hydrogen after ingesting 10 g lactulose and 2 g PEG (after Bond & Levitt 1975).

the subject and it is fortunate that subsequent studies by Metz and colleagues (Metz et al 1976) showed that breath hydrogen production correlates very closely with end expiratory breath hydrogen concentration. This is best obtained by having the subjects breathe out through a washable plastic mouthpiece into a 1.7 m, wide bore (1.2 cm diameter) tube, sampling gas from the proximal part of the tube using a three-way tap (Fig. 21.4). It is important to emphasize to the subjects that they must not hyperventilate nor exercise vigorously during the test since this lowers breath hydrogen concentration (Thompson et al 1985). It is worth having a few practice samples to make sure all the instructions are understood before measuring basal values. After 4–5 steady breaths through the mouthpiece with their nasal passage gently occluded by pinching between finger and thumb, sujects should be asked to breath out and then hold their breath while 20 ml of gas is aspirated from the three-way tap. It often helps if subjects indicate by raising their thumb that they have breathed out and are ready for a sample to be taken. Obviously it is important that they do not

remove the tube from their mouth to avoid contamination of the gas sample by room air. End-expiratory gas can be more simply collected in subjects such as children who would have difficulty complying with such a complex schedule, by simply aspirating during expiration via a plastic tube placed in the oropharynx. These simpler techniques are more likely, however, to yield samples contaminated by room air, and hence to give less accurate measures. A recent modification of the original technique has been described which perhaps requires less patient cooperation (Cloarec et al 1990). This involves the use of two gas bags connected via a three-way tap. Subjects are asked to exhale into the first 500 ml bag and once this is full the three-way tap is switched so the remainder of the breath is collected in a larger 1000 ml bag which is then used to provide the gas for analysis.

Adaptation for animal studies

Studies can also be done on animals using this technique, modified by keeping the animals in an airtight container into which air is infused at a constant rate and passed out through a flow meter, gas samples being taken at intervals from the container (Brown et al 1987). This allows assessment of total hydrogen production and, providing the air flow is constant, this is directly proportional to the hydrogen concentration in parts per million.

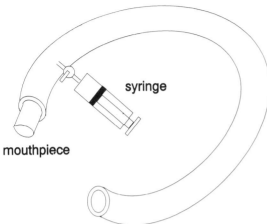

170cm rubber tube

syringe

mouthpiece

Fig. 21.4 Modified Haldane-Priestly tube used to collect end-expiratory breath sample for measuring breath hydrogen without contamination (after Metz et al 1976).

Measurement techniques for breath hydrogen

The earliest studies measured breath hydrogen concentrations using gas chromatography with a thermal conductivity detector (Bond & Levitt 1975). This has been largely superseded by the electrochemical method (Bartlett et al 1980). This consists of a hydrogen-sensitive polarographic cell. The gas sample (10–20 ml) is injected into the measurement chamber from which hydrogen diffuses through a metalized membrane at a rate proportional to its concentration. Hydrogen is oxidized at the membrane thus generating an electromotive force which can be detected and displayed on a digital readout scale as a concentration measured in parts per million. Some authors have continued to use gas chromatography where other gases such a methane are also being evaluated (Cloarec et al 1990), but where only hydrogen is of interest the polarographic cell is much more practical, being simple to use and very compact (Fig. 21.5) compared with gas chromatographic equipment.

Problems in perfoming test and how to avoid them

The early peak and how to reduce it

Many authors have noted that there is often a transient rise in breath hydrogen within 30 min of ingestion of

the test meal which occurs long before the carbohydrate substrate reaches the caecum. The hydrogen concentration then usually falls only to rise again as the meal residue reaches the caecum (Fig. 21.6). If this early rise is large it may obscure any subsequent rise and make interpretation of the breath hydrogen profile difficult, so most authors have endeavoured to minimize it. There are probably two main sources of the early peak, oral fermentation and increased delivery of the previous meal's residue from the terminal ileum into the colon.

Oral fermentation

The oral cavity has a large bacterial flora (10^6–10^9), largely facultative aerobes, but deep within the gingival crevases anaerobes are also common. Carbohydrates can therefore undergo fermentation with the production of hydrogen in the mouth. This will produce a transient, but misleading, initial rise in breath hydrogen within 10–20 min of ingestion of a meal containing either slowly fermented carbohydrate (Thompson et al 1986) or lactulose (Mastropaolo & Rees 1987). In both studies the initial rise could be abolished by careful oral hygiene, while sham feeding of carbohydrate simulated the rise seen after meal ingestion.

Ileal emptying as a cause of early rise in breath hydrogen

Other interpretations have been put on this early rise including the concept that this represents emptying of poorly digested carbohydrate remaining in the terminal ileum after the previous meal (Read et al 1985). These authors showed that the early peak was larger if the subjects ate a meal containing poorly digested carbohydrate (100 g baked beans) the night before the study, compared with that seen if they ate a meal low in unabsorbable carbohydrate. Furthermore, in studies with ileostomists who ate a test meal labelled with radioisotope, they showed that eating an unlabelled test meal some 9 h later, induced a significant rise in ileal output of radioactivity within 30 min (Read et al 1985).

It seems likely that depending upon the precise circumstances either or both of the effects could contribute to the early rise in breath hydrogen and in practice it is best to try to minimize both sources by restricting the intake of poorly absorbable carbohydrate the night before and attempting to minimize the bacterial population of the mouth by vigorous oral hygiene on the morning of the study.

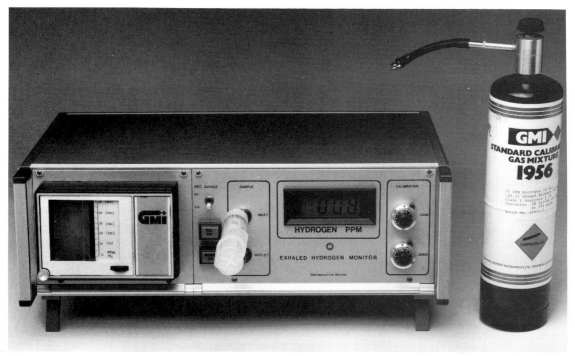

Fig. 21.5 Electrochemical polarographic hydrogen meter. Gas samples are injected into the port just to the left of the digital readout LCD. The meter is calibrated before use each day using the gas standard containing 100 ppm of hydrogen.

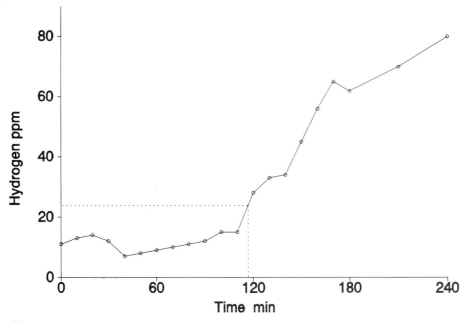

Fig. 21.6 Breath hydrogen profile after ingesting a 400 kcal liquid test meal labelled with 16 g lactulose. Note initial transient rise in breath hydrogen which then falls until a steep rise at about 120 min. Mouth–caecum transit is 119 min, the time to reach 21 ppm, 10 ppm above baseline (11 ppm).

High basal breath hydrogen

A substantial proportion of dietary starch in various legumes and grains resists digestion, and breath hydrogen the following day can be markedly raised. This makes interpretation of the breath hydrogen curve difficult since there is a declining baseline which may obscure any subsequent rise due to the test substrate reaching the caecum. Furthermore very high fluctuating basal breath hydrogen concentrations may dwarf the response that is sought and make it difficult to determine exactly when a rise occurs. This problem is best avoided by instructing subjects to take a diet low in poorly absorbable carbohydrate the night before (Kotler et al 1982, Cloarec et al 1990), avoiding legumes and green vegetables, and using rice as the main source of carbohydrate since this is very well absorbed. One difficulty here in using this test clinically is that patients with untreated coeliac disease and contaminated small bowel syndrome exhibit high basal breath hydrogen concentrations, in the range 6–60 ppm (normal controls 2–12 ppm) a feature which persists in spite of diets low in poorly absorbed carbohydrate the night before (Corazza et al 1987).

False high breath hydrogen due to smoking

Smoking leads to an acute rise in apparent breath hydrogen, mean rise being 70 ± 48 ppm (mean ± SD), lasting 5–10 min (Thompson et al 1985). The cause of this is uncertain but it is known that increased amounts of the reducing gas carbon monoxide are exhaled during smoking, the rise being 3–27 ppm. Electrochemical cells will detect carbon monoxide, 100 ppm giving a reading of 8 ppm hydrogen. When both carbon monoxide and hydrogen have been measured by gas chromatography the rise in carbon monoxide concentration accounts for only a small fraction of the increase in apparent breath hydrogen so there must be other reducing substances in cigarette smoke (Thompson et al 1985). Whatever the cause, subjects should be instructed not to smoke on the study day to avoid rapid and confusing changes in basal values.

Failure to produce hydrogen in response to unabsorbed carbohydrate

Non-hydrogen producers. A rise of less than 20 ppm above baseline in response to 10 g lactulose indicates non-hydrogen producer status, most such subjects producing large amounts of methane instead

(Cloarec et al 1990). Other causes of failure to produce hydrogen include recent bowel preparation for colonoscopy and broad-spectrum antibiotics (Gilat et al 1978) and profuse diarrhoea which disturbs the anaerobic flora of the colon (Solomons et al 1979). Under such circumstances the technique cannot be used; this is particulary restricting with sick patients since they are often exposed to broad spectrum antibiotics.

Contaminated small bowel syndrome

This leads to fermentation within the small bowel and production of hydrogen if the fermentation is anaerobic. This requirement is most often encountered in the 'blind loop' syndromes seen after Polya gastrectomy or the naturally occurring blind loops seen in jejunal diverticulae. Other situations characterized by hydrogen production within the small bowel in response to oral carbohydrate include pseudo-obstruction and ileal resection with loss of the ileocaecal valve (King & Toskes 1986, Kerlin & Wong 1988). These situations result in early rises in breath hydrogen as carbohydrate enters the contaminated small intestine preventing any meaningful assessment of transit.

Performing the test

Practical details

1. Subjects should be instructed to take a diet low in poorly absorbable carbohydrate the night before avoiding peas, beans, lentils, root vegetables and excessive fruit. A rice-based meal is ideal since this is virtually completely absorbed in normal individuals.

2. Subjects should ideally have already provided a breath sample to demonstrate that they do produce hydrogen; usually a random non-fasting sample is sufficient since most subjects will have values in the range 5–50 ppm. Methane producers and individuals who have recently taken broad spectrum antibiotics or had a bowel preparation may fail to ferment carbohydrate to hydrogen and hence have undetectable levels of hydrogen in a random sample. If there is any doubt then the response to 20 g lactulose after an overnight fast should make it clear whether the subject is suitable for study, since normal subjects will produce rises in breath hydrogen of 50–200 ppm within 1–2 hours of ingestion.

3. After an overnight fast subjects should arrive in the morning with their own toothbrush. They should then brush their teeth thoroughly and rinse their mouth

with chlorhexidine mouthwash to minimize the oral cavity bacterial flora.

4. Two basal end-expiratory breath samples should then be obtained at 5-min intervals and assayed for hydrogen, using either a gas chromatograph or more conveniently an electrochemical cell which gives a direct readout of hydrogen concentrations in parts per million.

5. The test meal is then ingested together with the marker substance which will be fermented to hydrogen when it reaches the caecum.

6. End-expiratory breath samples are then taken at predetermined intervals, generally every 5–10 min for the first 90 min and then less frequently until the test is finished. The more frequent the sampling the more accurate the measurement. A typical breath hydrogen versus time profile is shown in Figure 21.6.

7. Smoking is not allowed on the study day.

Calculation of mouth–caecum transit time

The arival of lactulose in the caecum is followed within 5 min by a sustained rise in breath hydrogen. The time for the breath hydrogen to achieve a sustained rise of > 10 ppm above baseline is the most common measure of transit (LaBrooy et al 1983, Cloarec et al 1990) though other authors have used a rise of 15 ppm (Staniforth & Rose 1989). Single, isolated high values are discounted, the rise must be sustained for 30 min to provide a valid measure of transit time.

Reproducibility

Using these criteria the coefficient of variation of repeated measures ranges from a mean of 18% for lactulose when given alone, to 4% when given with a meal (Staniforth & Rose 1989). At least part of the variability in mouth–caecum transit of lactulose test doses is due to the cyclical variability in fasting gastric and small bowel motility. Early studies at Central Middlesex Hospital showed that the variability could be substantially reduced by giving the lactulose as part of a nutrient meal (LaBroy et al 1983). More recently studies have been performed in which the lactulose was given during different phases of the fasting cycle (Di Lorenzo et al 1991). When lactulose was given the fasting cycle was not disrupted. Mouth–caecum transit was, as expected, slower when lactulose was given during the quiescent phase I (155 ± 26 min, n = 6, Mean ± SD) and fastest when given just before phase III (94 ± 14 min), in keeping with current concepts of the propulsive nature of late phase II and phase III. Thus most authors now agree that transit should be

assessed in the fed state for maximum reproducibility when, for example, looking at drug effects.

A recent paper (Staniforth & Rose 1989) which assessed reproducibility provides tables to assess the number of subjects needed to demonstrate drug effects on transit with acceptable beta errors. Substantial changes in transit (> 30%) can be demonstrated using this technique in as few as 14 subjects with a beta error of 20% and an alpha level of 5%. Greater power to avoid missing any effect requires larger numbers though in practice many papers have used much smaller numbers, perhaps reflecting a failure to appreciate the variability of the method.

Type of non-absorbable carbohydrate used

Although many of the early studies utilized lactulose because it provides a large easily detectable rise in breath hydrogen, there are inherent disadvantages in using such a low molecular weight, and hence osmotically active substance. On entry into the small intestine profuse water and salt secretion occurs into the hypertonic, low sodium fluid, increasing the ingested volume 3–4 fold. This secretion accelerates transit in proportion to the dose. Thus Read et al (1980) found transit of the residue of a solid/liquid test meal to be accelerated by adding increasing doses of lactulose (10–40 g), the highest dose halving the transit time (Fig. 21.7). The fact that the measurement technique actually alters the variable being measured is undesirable and a number of alternatives have been suggested. Baked beans (120 g) contains sufficient poorly absorbable carbohydrate to yield a rise in breath hydrogen of 20–40 ppm starting 3–4 h after ingestion. Other authors have documented similar rises after 70–100 g of barley groats that, like baked beans, deliver complex, polymerized carbohydrate to the colon without exerting any appreciable osmotic effect in the small bowel and hence not accelerating transit (De Vries et al 1988). This advantage is somewhat offset by the fact that transit times then become very prolonged, averaging 8.4 ± 0.4 h (Mean ± SEM) making the recording process very tedious if gas samples are taken at 15-min intervals. It also makes such a test impracticable for most ambulant patients.

Correlation of breath hydrogen technique with other methods for measuring mouth–caecum transit

A number of studies have compared the use of the breath hydrogen technique with scintigraphic methods (Caride et al 1984, Read et al 1985). These have shown a close correlation between the onset of the rise in

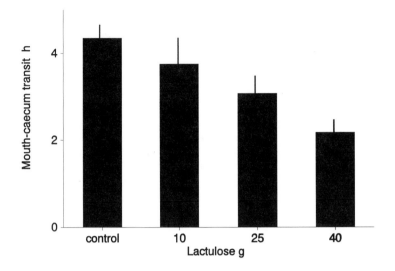

Fig. 21.7 Effect of increasing doses of lactulose on ileocaecal transit (mean ± SEM) assessed by the breath hydrogen technique demonstrating that lactulose accelerates mouth–caecum transit. The control meal contained 120 g baked beans which provided enough non-absorbable carbohydrate to give a rise in breath hydrogen without added lactulose.

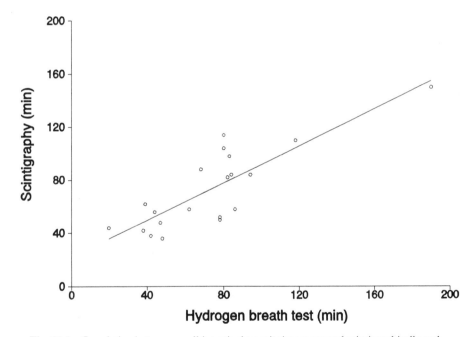

Fig. 21.8 Correlation between small intestinal transit time measured scintigraphically and mouth–caecum transit measured by the breath hydrogen method. Scintigraphy was used to define the time elapsed between isotope first entering the small intestine and reaching the caecum. In this study isotope always entered the duodenum within 5 min of ingestion and so small intestinal transit and mouth–caecum transit were virtually identical (Caride et al 1984).

breath hydrogen and the appearance of isotope in the caecum or ascending colon (Fig. 21.8). Unfortunately the time to peak of breath hydrogen does not reliably correlate with the arrival of meal residue in the caecum (Read et al 1985), depending as it does not only on the rate of delivery of lactulose to the colon but also the speed with which the caecum degrades lactulose. Thus if lactulose is infused directly into the caecum at a rate of 0.15 g/min then the peak breath hydrogen is observed shortly after all the lactulose enters the caecum.

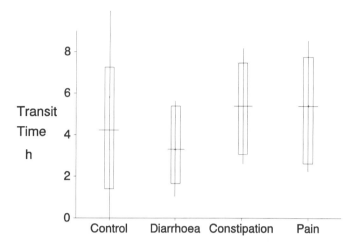

Fig. 21.9 Mouth–caecum transit measured using the breath hydrogen technique in 53 normal controls and 61 patients with irritable bowel syndrome (17 diarrhoea-predominant, 23 constipation-predominant, and 17 with pain and distension as their main symptom). The box includes all the patient data points, the whisker indicates Mean ± 2SD. As can be seen there is a very wide overlap between the different patient groups.

However this is an unrealistically high rate of entry, unlikely to be obtained when lactulose is given orally. At lower, more physiological rates of entry (0.075 g/ min), the peak usually occurs before the infusion ceases, levels declining as the caecal lactulose concentration falls with bacterial degradation (Read et al 1985).

On occasions, overlapping of loops of ileum over the caecum make precise determination of the caecal entry of isotope difficult. This can largely be overcome by also looking for the arrival of isotope in more distal regions of the right colon (Caride et al 1984) since isotope usually spreads rapidly throughout the ascending colon whose contents are fairly fluid. These authors found that usually < 4 min elapsed between isotope entering the caecum and reaching the hepatic flexure.

Isotopic measures have the obvious advantage of not relying on bacterial fermentation and hence can be used in situations where this is abnormal, such as after antibiotic therapy, and also in the contaminated small bowel syndrome. An important disadvantage is that unless the ileocaecal anatomy is well understood, difficulties can be experienced in interpreting the movement of isotope in this region; this can be problematic in up to one third of normal subjects. In the presence of significant disease such as terminal ileitis or small bowel resection one would anticipate even greater difficulties.

Clinical and research utility of breath hydrogen technique

Although the breath test has been widely used in a research setting to examine changes in small bowel motility both under experimental conditions (Read et

al 1984) and in disease (Cann et al 1983, Spiller et al 1987), it is not generally used in everday clinical practice. A glance at the scatter of small bowel transit in both normal subjects and patients with the irritable bowel syndrome (Fig. 21.9) should make it clear that a single measurement, unless extraordinarily extreme, is unlikely to be useful clinically in categorizing patients with symptoms suggestive of abnormal small bowel motility. Furthermore in most cases disordered transit is merely one manifestation of an underlying disease which can be better diagnosed by other means. Thus symptoms of delayed small bowel transit due to an ileal Crohn's stricture would be investigated by means of a barium follow through rather than assessing transit time. Where anatomy is normal but function is abnormal as in pseudo-obstruction, the breath test might be expected to be helpful but is in fact disappointing. This is because many such patients, once their symptoms are severe enough to require clinical investigation, suffer from small bowel bacterial contamination (Vantrappen et al 1977). Loss of the normal fasting cycle, the so-called 'interdigestive housekeeper', allows bacterial overgrowth which leads to rapid rises in breath hydrogen soon after the meal enters the small intestine, rendering assessment of small bowel transit impossible. Transit under such circumstances is much better assessed using scintigraphic techniques (see chapter 16). The breath hydrogen rise which occurs in the dumping syndrome after the ingestion of a glucose test meal is in most cases an indication of very rapid small bowel transit (O'Brien et al 1988) but even in these cases interpretation can be difficult as such patients with low acid output and often a blind afferent limb of a gastroenterostomy frequently suffer from small bowel contamination.

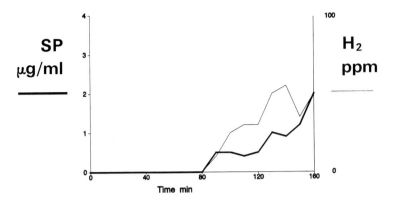

Fig. 21.10 Plasma sulphapyridine levels in μg/ml and breath hydrogen concentration plotted against time after ingestion of 50 ml water together with 2 g salazopyrine and 25 g lactulose in one individual showing good concordance between the rise in the two measures as the two substrates reach the caecum (Kellow et al 1986).

MEASUREMENT OF MOUTH–CAEUM TRANSIT USING SUPHASALAZINE

Sulphasalazine is degraded by a wide range of colonic bacteria under the reducing conditions usually found in the caecum (Soleim & Scheline 1972), undergoing azoreduction to yield the poorly absorbable 5-amino-salicylic acid and sulphapyridine which is rapidly absorbed and can then be detected in peripheral plasma. Initial studies (Kennedy et al 1979) used a spectrophotometric method (Bratton & Marshall 1939) but more recently a rapid automated HPLC assay has been described (Shaw et al 1983).

The time to the first detection of sulphapyridine can be used to assess mouth–caecum transit time, an idea first promoted by Kennedy and colleagues (Kennedy et al 1979).

Method

After an overnight fast, 2 g of salazopyrine are ingested as a suspension in 50 ml water. Plasma samples are then obtained at 10-min intervals for 1–2 h and at less frequent intervals thereafter depending on the expected transit time. Analysis by HPLC requires only 0.5 ml of plasma (Shaw et al 1983). Transit time is taken to be the time from ingestion to the first detection of sulphapyridine. Since the reaction depends on anaerobic conditions the test resembles the breath hydrogen method in being invalidated by small bowel contamination or broad spectrum antibiotics, bowel preparation or profuse infective diarrhoea.

Comparison with other methods

When this was directly compared with the lactulose breath hydrogen technique (Kellow et al 1986) there was good correlation ($r = 0.72$). When the sulphapyridine method was compared with scintigraphy it was apparent that there was a slight lag of about 5 min between the appearance of isotope in the caecum and the detection of sulphapyridine in plasma (Kellow et al 1986) (Fig. 21.10). This is in keeping with the observation by the same authors that after direct intracaecal infusion of both lactulose and salazopyrine, breath hydrogen rose within 1–6 min while plasma sulphapyridine lagged somewhat rising within 6–10 min

Though in theory a useful alternative to the breath hydrogen technique, the sulphasalazine method suffers from all its disadvantages and is very much more tedious to do since it involves obtaining and analysing many plasma samples for each test. This may explain why this test is in practice rarely used.

REFERENCES

Bartlett K, Dobson J V, Eastham E 1980 A new method for the detection of hydrogen in breath and its application to acquired and inborn sugar malabsorption. Clin Chim Acta 108: 189–194

Bond J H, Levitt M D 1975 Investigation of small bowel transit time in man utilizing pulmonary hydrogen (H₂) measurements. J Lab Clin Med 85: 546–555

Bratton A C, Marshall E K 1939 A new coupling component for sulfanilamide determination. J Biol Chem 128: 537–550

Brown N J, Rumsey R D E, Read N W 1987 Adaptation of hydrogen analysis to measure stomach to caecum transit time in the rat. Gut 28: 849–854

Cann P A, Read N W, Brown C, Hobson N, Holdsworth C D 1983 Irritable bowel syndrome: relationship of disorders in the transit of a single solid meal to symptom patterns. Gut 24: 405–411

Caride V J, Prokop K, Troncale F J, Buddoura W, Winchenbach K, McCallum R W 1984 Scintigraphic determination of small intestinal transit time: comparison with the hydrogen breath technique. Gastroenterology 86: 714–720

Cloarec D, Bornet F, Gouilloud S, Barry J L, Salim B, Galmiche J P 1990 Breath hydrogen response to lactulose in healthy subjects: relationship to methane producing status. Gut 31: 300–304

Corazza G R, Strocchi A, Gasbarrini G 1987 Fasting breath hydrogen in coeliac disease. Gastroenterology 93: 53–58

De Vries J J, Collin T, Bijleveld C M A, Kleibeuker J H 1988 The use of complex carbohydrates in barley groats for determination of mouth-to-caecum transit time. Scand J Gastroenterol 23: 905–912

Di Lorenzo C, Dooley C P, Valenzuela J E 1991 Role of fasting gastrointestinal motility in the variability of gastrointestinal transit time assessed by hydrogen breath test. Gut 32: 1127–1130

Gilat T, BenHur H, Gelman-Malachi E, Terdiman R, Pelad Y 1978 Alterations of the colonic flora and their effect on the hydrogen breath test. Gut 19: 602–605

Heading R C, Nimmo J, Prescott L F, Tothill P 1973 The dependence of paracetamol absorption on the rate of gastric emptying. Br J Pharmacol 47: 415–421

Kellow J E, Borody T J, Phillips S F, Haddad A C, Brown M L 1986 Sulfapyridine appearance in plasma after salicylazosulfapyridine. Another simple measure of intestinal transit. Gastroenterology 91: 396–400

Kennedy M, Chinwah P, Wade D N 1979 A pharmacological method of measuring mouth–caecum transit time in man. Br J Clin Pharmac 8: 372–373

Kerlin P, Wong L 1988 Breath hydrogen testing in bacterial overgrowth of the small intestine. Gastroenterology 95: 982–988

King C E, Toskes P P 1986 Comparison of the 1-gram[14C]xylose, 10-gram lactulose-H_2, and 80-gram glucose-H_2 breath tests in patients with small intestine bacterial overgrowth. Gastroenterology 91: 1447–1451

Kotler D P, Holt P R, Rosenweig N S 1982 Modification of the breath hydrogen test: increased sensitivity for the detection of carbohydrate malabsorption. J Lab Clin Med 100: 798–805

LaBrooy S J, Male P-J, Beavis A K, Misiewicz J J 1983 Assessment of the reproducibility of the lactulose H_2 breath test as a measure of mouth to caecum transit time. Gut 24: 893–896

Levitt M D 1969 Production and excretion of hydrogen gas in man. New Engl J Med 281: 122–127

Mastropolo G, Rees W D W 1987 Evaluation of the breath hydrogen test in man: definition and elimination of the early hydrogen peak. Gut 28: 721–725

Metz G, Gassul M A, Leeds A R, Blendis L M, Jenkins D J A 1976 A simple method of measuring breath hydrogen in

carbohydrate malabsorption by end-expiratory sampling. Clin Sci Mol Med 50: 237–240

Nimmo W S, Littlewood D G, Scott D B, Prescott L F 1978 Gastric emptying following hysterectomy with extradural analgesia. Br J Anaesth 50: 559–561

O'Brien J D, Thompson D G, McIntyre A, Burnham W R, Walker E 1988 The effect of codeine and loperamide on upper intestinal transit and absorption in normal subjects and patients with postvagotomy diarrhoea. Gut 29: 312–318

Read N W, Al-Janabi M N, Bates T E et al 1985 Interpretation of the breath hydrogen profile obtained after ingesting a solid meal containing unabsorbable carbohydrate. Gut 26: 834–842

Read N W, McFarlane A, Kinsman R I et al 1984 Effect of an infusion of nutrient solutions into the ileum on gastrointestinal transit and plasma levels of neurotensin and enteroglucagon. Gastroenterology 86: 274–280

Read N W, Miles C A, Fisher D et al 1980 Transit of a meal through the stomach, small intestine, and colon in normal subjects and its role in the pathogenesis of diarhhoea. Gastroenterology 79: 1276–1282

Shaw P N, Sivner A L, Aarons L, Houston J B 1983 A rapid method for the simultaneous determination of the major metabolites of sulphasalazine in plasma. J Chromatogr 274: 393–397

Simon G L, Gorbach S L 1984 Intestinal flora in health and disease. Gastroenterology 86: 174–193

Soleim H A, Scheline R R 1972 Metabolism of xenobiotics by strains of intestinal bacteria. Acta Pharmacol Toxicol 31: 471–480

Solomons N W, Garcia R, Schneider R, Viteri F E, VonKaemel V A 1979 H_2 breathtest during diarrhoea. Acta Paediatr Scand 68: 171–172

Spiller R C, Lee Y C, Edge C et al 1987 Delayed mouth–caecum transit of a lactulose-labelled liquid test meal in patients with steatorrhoea due to partially treated coeliac disease. Gut 28: 1275–1282

Staniforth D H, Rose D 1989 Statistical analysis of the lactulose/breath hydrogen test in the measurement of orocaecal transit: its variability and predictive value in assessing drug action. Gut 30: 171–175

Thompson D G, Binfield P, De Belder A, O'Brien J, Warren S, Wilson M 1985 Extraintestinal influences on exhaled breath hydrogen measurement during the investigation of gastrointestinal disease. Gut 26: 1349–1352

Thompson D G, O'Brien J D, Hardie J M 1986 Influence of the oropharyngeal microflora on the measurement of exhaled breath hydrogen. Gastroenteroloogy 91: 853–860

Vantrappen G, Janssens J, Hellemans J, Ghoos Y 1977 The interdigestive motor complex of normal subjects and patients with bacterial overgrowth of the small intestine. J Clin Invest 59: 1158–1166

22. Computerized data analysis

R. B. Hanson

INTRODUCTION

Motility recordings often last for many hours with multiple recording channels used creating large amounts of data to be analysed. Hand scoring the polygraph paper chart recording is subjective, time consuming and very boring. The initial role of the computer in motility analysis is to remove this drudgery and subjectivity by automatically finding and quantifying the motility patterns of interest.

Computers can do very exact repetitive measurements quickly. They can be programmed to do measurements and calculations that would take too much effort to do by hand. The calculation of individual contraction propagation with multiple recording sites requires accurate placement of the contraction in time, something that is easy for a computer but very difficult for a human. The computer can calculate thousands of events while a human is scoring one.

The use of computers for more than replacement of hand scoring analyses is limited only by the researcher's imagination. Computers can be used to model biological processes. Subtle patterns can be recognized by computer programs that would be missed by humans. New computer techniques for imaging and visualization may help create less invasive procedures for examining motility. The past decade has concentrated on the replacement and extension of manual motility analysis. This decade, with its inexpensive and powerful desktop workstations and the wide variety of new computer analysis and visualization software, promises rapid steps forward in computer assisted motility analysis.

This chapter will cover the basic parts of a computer system to collect, display, analyse and report on pressure, strain gauge and myoelectric waveforms. Over the past 5 years, several companies have marketed clinical motility computer systems that are of varying quality. The first available systems concentrated on the oesophagus: recording swallows and calculating pressures and peristalsis. Ambulatory oesophageal

pressure and pH monitoring followed. Now one can buy systems to record and analyse gastric, small bowel and anal/rectal motility. Some packages are tied to companies who sell recorders with computers added. Others have removed the expensive recorder and placed a 'black box' between the computer and the subject.

The market for clinical motility computer systems is small but growing and the number of companies producing computer solutions is increasing. We strongly recommend a trial period before purchasing any system, as the systems are in their infancy and the types of analyses needed to make use of motility recordings in diagnosis of disease are still under discussion.

DATA ACQUISITION

Signals coming from the body or instrumentation in the body consist of varying electrical voltage where the voltage changes represent some change in physiologic state. The changes commonly measured are: pressure within the gastrointestinal tract; wall movement as measured by strain gauges, balloons or bags; and electrical activity from gut wall muscles. The changes in the signal over time are usually what is important, so we need to record the value at regular intervals.

Computers record signals by measuring the voltage amplitude at selected time intervals and storing the voltage value in the computer (digitization). An electronic device, called an analogue-to-digital (A/D) converter, must be placed between the sensor and the computer to digitize the signal. Usually the A/D converter is a computer circuit board that plugs inside the computer with a connector outside the computer. A wire goes from the connector to each sensor to bring the signal into the A/D converter.

Digitization must be done often enough to reconstruct the original signal without loss of information critical to the analysis. To choose the digitization rate, find the time it takes for the fastest event of interest in the signal to occur. If a pressure change caused by a contraction in the small bowel of a human takes as little as 2 s to occur, and it takes eight points to properly show the shape of the contraction, then store four values per second. The term Hertz (Hz), is the unit of measurement used to describe the digitization rate, i.e. four values per second is described as 4 Hz.

The mathematics of signal analysis or waveform analysis as used in physics and electronics has precisely defined terminology. In motility, the terminology of waveforms is sometimes used less precisely and adds confusion to the already complicated and somewhat jumbled motility terminology. In giving a definition of a waveform, an electrical engineer or physicist differs in terminology with much that is published in motility research. For a pure sine wave, where the change in amplitude is above and below an equilibrium value, the period of the wave is defined as the time for one cycle to occur, the frequency as the number of cycles per second. The frequency is equal to the reciprocal of the period. The amplitude is the maximum displacement from the equilibrium position, and the wavelength is the shortest distance between two parts of the wave that are in phase.

Computer analysis techniques that use frequency finding or filtering calculations like the Fast Fourier Transform (FFT) and the associated spectral analysis give frequencies as defined above, not a count of contractions per time interval. For example, if an individual contraction lasts 4 s, its frequency can be found by calculating the reciprocal of the period, 0.25 Hz or 15 cycles per minute. If five of these occurred in 1 min, the frequency would not be five per minute (0.083 Hz), but would still be 0.25 Hz. One must be careful to be sure that what is being communicated between people is understood. With the marvellous variety of terminology seen in motility it is easy to get confused!

At Mayo, we digitize pressure and volume recordings from 2–10 Hz depending on the fidelity needed. Faster rates give more details about the shape of the contraction and are better to pinpoint the height and time maxima. We do ambulatory anal/rectal recordings at 2 Hz because we want to store seven channels of data for 24 h in a very small portable data logger that is limited in memory. Most of the time we record at 4 Hz. Calculation of contraction propagation with closely spaced ports in the canine small bowel would be recorded at 8 or 10 Hz to separate the events more precisely in time. Recording electrical activity from the gut requires a much faster rate so as to record high frequency electrical oscillations. We are currently re-

cording at 100 Hz although this may not be fast enough to see all of the electrical spikes.

A problem with digitizing data at regular intervals can occur when a high frequency masquerades as a lower one through a phenomena called aliasing (Fig. 22.1). This must be prevented by making sure that the signal is filtered electronically before it reaches the A/D board. The filter must cut out frequencies greater than $\frac{1}{2}$ the sampling rate (the Nyquist frequency). If the sampling rate is 100 Hz, the outside electronic filter needs to cut out frequencies of 50 Hz and greater. This is essential in high frequency myoelectric recordings due to the prevalence of electrical signals coming from the immediate surroundings (electrical noise) and the very small amplitude of the signal.

Pressure and strain gauge recordings have less aliasing and noise problems, with high signal to noise ratios. To learn more about aliasing problems and signal preprocessing consult free literature from companies that sell A/D converters.

Any computer that can be fitted with an A/D converter can be used as a recording computer. We use IBM personal computers (PCs) and clones, and Digital Equipment Corporation (DEC) Vax computers. The Vax machines are mostly used for specialized programs written for data analysis and for centralized data storage and review. The PCs are inexpensive and easy to set up for data collection and many commercial A/D converters and computer programs to collect data are available. Most programs plot the signals to the screen during recording and give flexibility in sampling rates and number of channels. Most A/D converters give the option of 16 channels and 12-bit recording. The user can select 1–16 channels and store the voltage values in the computer with 12 bits of accuracy. A 12-bit A/D divides the input signal amplitudes into a 4096 steps, more than sufficient where a pressure signal might range from 1 to 300 mmHg with accuracy of 0.5 mmHg adequate for analysis.

The voltages of signals coming from electrodes within the patient are often in the millivolt range and need to be amplified before they come into the A/D converter. The signal may have to be filtered to prevent aliasing. The patient must be electrically isolated from the computer/recorder equipment in conformity with safety criteria to make sure that no electrical current flows from the equipment to endanger the patient. A polygraph chart recorder is often used to take care of the preprocessing of the signal. Many recorders include electrical isolation and have filters and amplification adjustable from the front panel, and most also provide for a computer output signal ready for digitization. They are usually quite expensive, on the order of

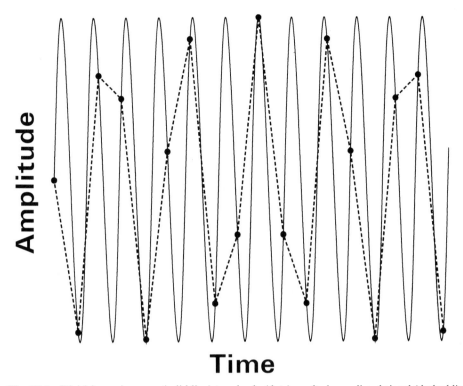

Fig. 22.1 Digitizing a sine wave (solid line) too slowly (dots) results in an aliased signal (dashed line) which masquerades as a lower frequency waveform.

$2000–4000 per channel. They are not really needed, as the electronics to amplify, filter, electrically isolate and provide electrical sensor activation can be built into a preprocessing electronics box for much less money. A/D card vendors sell preprocessing electronics that cost a few hundred dollars per channel and will often advise on the correct configuration appropriate for the signal.

The signal should be plotted on the computer screen as it is digitized (a real-time display) to make sure the computer is recording successfully. If there is no paper record being made this is especially important. A very useful feature is the ability to quickly review earlier waveforms during a study. This is easy to do on DEC Vax computers that serve multiple users and can do multiple functions simultaneously. The Vax computers have a real-time operating system that allows us to set the priority of data acquisition at a high level compared to other processes running in the computer. When it is time for the computer to read the voltages, the acquisition program gets full use of the computer, and the other users have to wait (the wait is a few milliseconds and is

not noticeable). IBM PCs, Macintoshes, and Unix computers do not have a real-time operating system, and thus cannot guarantee continuous lossless data acquisition while other computer functions are occuring. A few expensive data acquisition programs for PCs and Macintoshes do allow some simultaneous functions. The newer PC based operating systems that allow multiple programs to run such as OS/2 from IBM and Windows NT from Microsoft may improve the situation and allow data acquisition to coexist with other use of the computer.

A powerful computer can do real-time analysis, that is it can record and analyse the signal simultaneously. In a cardiovascular intensive care unit, computers process the ECG in real-time to make sure the patient has no life-threatening patterns. Most motility systems have been set up as 'record now, analyse later'. The long duration of most motility recordings and the lack of any need to make immediate clinical decisions on the data obtained allow this to work, but if future requirements change, real-time analysis could be done.

DATA VISUALIZATION

After the signal has been digitized and stored, the computer should be able to review the waveforms. The viewing process should allow scaling of the amplitudes and the time displayed on the screen. Paper chart recordings can be spread down a long hallway and a stroll along its length conveys an overall impression. Duplicating this on a computer screen requires condensing the time axis and compressing the waveforms. Computer screens vary in the amount of points (pixels) that can be displayed. The higher the resolution, the more the detail that can be seen in a compressed plot. Some computer workstation screens can plot 100 dots per inch (DPI) while a laser printer might plot 300 DPI making a printed plot much better than the visual display. A good system can display and print the waveform rapidly with flexibility in channel selection, position, filtering and compression (Fig. 22.2).

In addition to printing out portions of the waveforms for review or for permanent records, researchers need to create annotated plots for publication or slide making. All of the figures in this chapter were created directly from our computer system. Figure 22.3 contains 12 min of recording at 4 Hz on 7 channels (selected from 12 recorded channels) with over 20 000 points plotted. Most drawing and graphics programs are not able to handle this many points. We wrote our own program to handle several million points per plot on our Vax computers.

A printed record of part or the whole study can be made with any time scale desired. We print studies on a laser printer at user selected times per page so the study may be stored in a three-ring binder.

DATA FILTERING

Computer frequency filters can be set to remove frequencies above or below a given value. A low pass filter removes high frequencies and a high pass filter removes low frequencies. A bandpass filter removes both low and high frequencies. A smoothing filter acts like a low pass filter in that it smooths out the high frequencies. Often high frequency electrical noise from the circuitry in the recording room will be seen superimposed on the desired signal. A filter can improve a poor quality signal (Fig. 22.4).

A frequency filter can also be used to separate mixed signals such as electrical slow waves and electrical spikes from gut wall myoelectric recordings (Fig. 22.5). Computer filters are calculations made by taking into consideration surrounding points by averaging or fit-

ting curves to smooth the data, or decomposing the signal into component frequencies (spectral analysis). These calculations make each filtered point the result of a calculation with dozens of terms taking hours of calculation to process long multiple channel recordings. A powerful computer with efficiently written computer programs will speed this up to a few minutes.

Filter programs on a computer must be applied with care. Each filter has restrictions that determine when it should be used. Read the instructions on how and where to use the filter, then try it under varying conditions on a known signal before publishing!

ANALYSIS OF CONTRACTIONS

Measurements of electrical resistance in strain gauges sewn to the gastrointestinal tract serosal surface, or attached intraluminal tubes may be treated similarly, and can be recorded at rates of a few Hertz. Both can be analysed for individual contractile events. Intraluminal pressure consists of an underlying tone with phasic contraction pressure changes superimposed. Strain gauge recordings, while not showing tone, will show additional phasic wall movement that is not occlusive to the lumen and may not be detected by intraluminal pressure recording.

The digitized data stored on the computer is not in standard measurement units as it comes from the A/D converter. A calibration is done at the beginning of a pressure recording by applying a known pressure to the measuring device. This value and a zero pressure value are used to convert the digital units to actual pressure units. Myoelectric electrodes and strain gauges are also calibrated by applying known signals or forces.

Easy analyses of the converted data include finding mean, median, maximum and minimum pressures, area under curve values per time interval, and any other calculations that can be done with a table of numbers. One can also apply frequency techniques such as spectral analysis to try and determine the underlying frequencies present.

Pressure waveforms generally have two components that are noticeable on inspection; the fast, short pressure peaks due to contractions that occur at the measurement site (phasic changes) and the slower changes in the baseline (tonic changes). Measuring tone with a perfusion system is uncertain since changes in the height of the perfusion outlet point with respect to the transducer height will cause changes in the baseline pressure that may suggest a physiological change but are due to a shift in the posture of the patient. Solid

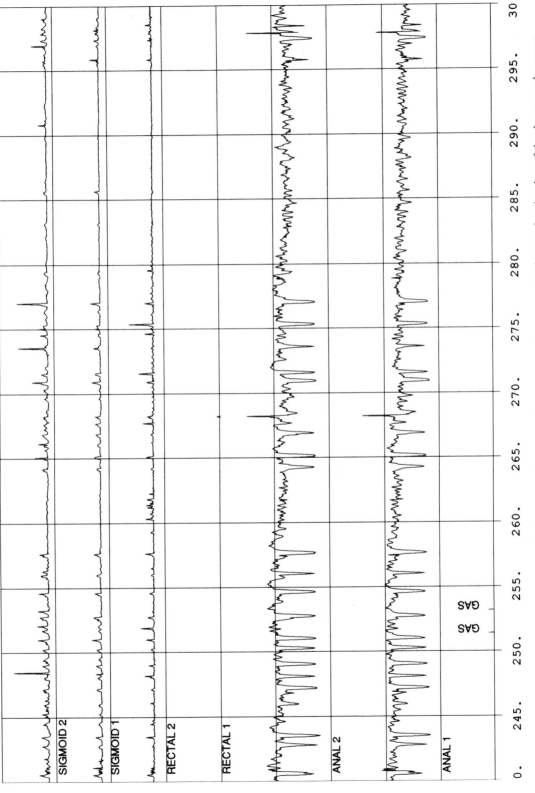

Fig. 22.2 One hour laser print of pressure recording from an ambulatory anal/rectal study. The computer printout takes the place of the chart recorder paper record. The patient records events of interest on the data logger. Rectal channel 1 was not working.

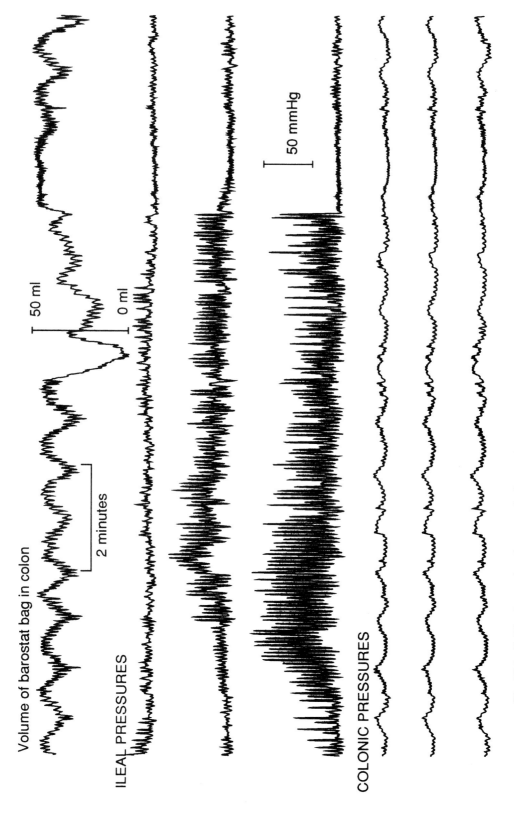

Volume of barostat bag in colon

50 ml

0 ml

2 minutes

ILEAL PRESSURES

50 mmHg

COLONIC PRESSURES

Fig. 22.3 Publication ready printout made directly from computer recording of barostat and manometry done simultaneously.

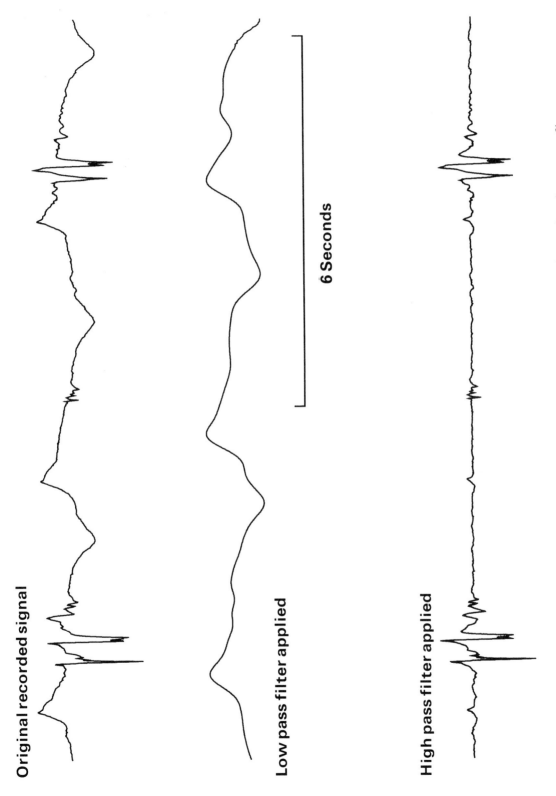

Fig. 22.5 Myoelectric signal filtered to remove high frequencies and then to remove low frequencies using computer filter.

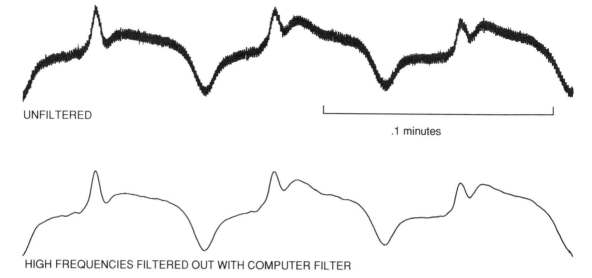

Fig. 22.4 The top trace shows an enlarged segment of channel 13 from a myoelectric recording (Fig. 22.8) with electrical noise present. The lower trace has had a low pass filter applied by computer.

Table 22.1   Stored peak values from Fig. 22.6

Peak #	Time [min]	Width [sec]	Base mmHg	Height mmHg	Area mmHg*sec	Separation [sec]
1	226.09	3.50	20.00	104.0	358.50	5.00
2	226.17	3.00	20.00	34.0	84.75	4.50
3	226.23	2.25	20.00	26.0	74.75	3.75
4	226.29	2.25	20.00	17.0	56.50	3.50
5	226.34	2.25	20.00	26.0	73.75	3.00
6	226.39	2.25	20.00	43.0	112.75	3.25
7	226.48	2.50	20.00	70.0	165.25	5.50
8	226.55	2.50	20.00	26.0	69.25	3.75
9	226.60	2.75	20.00	53.9	118.26	3.50
10	226.66	2.50	20.00	29.0	66.00	3.25
11	226.74	2.25	20.00	44.1	100.33	5.00
12	226.81	3.75	20.00	81.0	274.00	4.25

[Recorded at 4 Hertz]

state catheters are immune to this problem, but may present baseline problems when used in prolonged studies due to their fragility.

Since it is usually the contractile activity of the gut that is being studied, an early step in analysis is to find contractions that show up as peaks occurring above a variable baseline in a pressure recording. When a perfusion system is used, we define the amplitude of the contractile peak as a height above a floating baseline rather than an absolute height. A smoothing filter removes high frequency artifact before calculations. The peak finding algorithm looks at the change in amplitude between successive points and determines if the waveform is going up, down or is at baseline, and stores peak height, baseline height, area, width, and start and end heights and times. A smoothing filter has an amplitude shortening effect on the contractions, so the unsmoothed height is kept. A computer file is made to store the peak information of the peaks that exceed a minimum height and width (Fig. 22.6, Table 22.1).

Peak finding algorithms are the most difficult part of motility analysis due to the wide variation of peak shapes and baseline movement. Peaks in the stomach are different in shape and size from those in small bowel. Pressure changes in the colon and rectum are

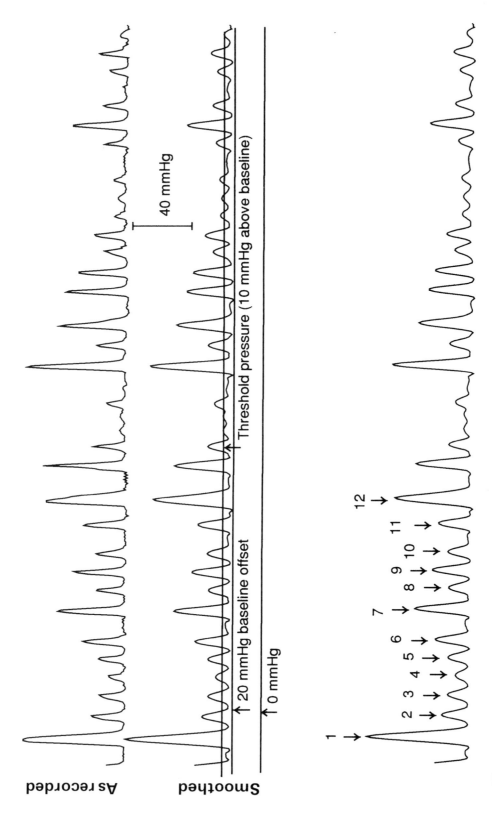

Fig. 22.6 Canine duodenal motility recorded by perfusion manometry. The waveform is smoothed, the baseline offset found and a minimum height above baseline threshold set. Peaks are found and stored for later analysis.

also different. The peak finding algorithm must be adjusted to the area of the gut where the recording is being made, and to the type of recording transducer used. Respiration, coughs, and movements may be present in the recording as peak-like shapes and must be excluded from the analysis.

Artifact peaks may be excluded by using threshold criteria such as minimum height, minimum and maximum duration, minimum separation and rise time. If recordings are made simultaneously over several sites, activity that is simultaneous over the sites may be excluded as artifact (Fig. 22.7). Peaks that are very close together can be combined into a single peak if the pressure drop between them is less than a predetermined minimum. The peak finding process is relatively slow and calculation-intensive, but since it is done once only for each study this is not really a problem.

After peaks are found and artifact removed, the peak file is available for calculations of peak statistics per time epoch such as motility index, peak count, peak area, mean amplitude, mean peak width, peak intervals, etc. The output files should be stored in text form so as to be easily imported into spreadsheet, statistics and graphing programs. Higher level analyses include peak propagation, cluster finding and propagation, migrating motor complex (MMC) location, other pattern finding and cross-channel correlations of activity. We wrote our own programs to do all of these functions since only very recently have they appeared as part of any commercial systems.

The peak file is less than one tenth the size of the original digitized waveform file. This reduction greatly speeds up the calculations that use it. Most of these calculations are cumulative summing or time comparisons and are rapidly calculated on the computer. Taking care with the peak finding process means that the subsequent analysis will be valid and relatively straightforward.

Classifying contractions into categories such as clusters, MMCs, propagated contractions and antropyloric-duodenal requires a great deal of attention to getting correct sensor spacing, to accuracy of the peak time location and to setting appropriate criteria for peak finding and time windows. It is easy to make errors in computer algorithms that can lead to wrong conclusions. The computer applies the rules the programmer puts into the program but does not make subjective judgements. It is also easy to include slight programming errors (bugs) that can subtly change the results of an analysis. Human judgement must verify that the computer calculations are appropriate and correct!

MYOELECTRIC ANALYSIS

Recording myoelectric activity from the gut muscle wall is done by placing electrodes directly into the muscle. The very low voltage signal is amplified and filtered by a recorder or direct interface device and digitized and stored in the computer. The high frequency of the electrical activity requires sampling at rates of 100 Hz or more. Since the amplitude is so low, noise is a problem and careful application of electronic filters is needed to preserve the signal.

The electrical recording is often divided into two portions, the omnipresent electrical slow wave and the spike bursts that correlate with contractions in the muscle wall (Fig. 22.8). The slow waves have a characteristic shape and may be recognized by using a program similar to peak finding (Fig. 22.9). The spikes may be located by finding areas of very rapid point to point slope changes.

If slow waves are identified accurately, the times may be used to examine slow wave propagation in the gut. The slow wave to slow wave interval varies slightly and this variation can be used to determine propagation between pairs of adjacent channels.

Spike bursts are seen in conjunction with contractions. Since the recording is a summation of potential changes from many cells, there are often multiple spikes seen. Finding the number of spikes, their amplitudes, the width of the burst, and the time that the burst occurred, and storing these in a spike file gives similar analysis capability as the peak file does for contractions.

Spectral analysis (with FFT) gives useful information with slow waves due to their regularity. The frequencies seen with this type of analysis include the slow wave rate, the spike frequency (but not a count) and the frequencies corresponding to different shaped portions of the slow wave. We use FFT analysis occasionally but prefer to find individual events such as peaks, slow waves and spikes and use their individual characteristics and temporal relationships in analysing the records.

ELECTROGASTROGRAPHY

Electrogastrography (EGG), the recording of the electrical activity of the stomach from the surface of the body is a technique that has been used for many years with varying success. Since most techniques for recording gastric activity are invasive or require radiation, investigators have used EGG in the hope that it will emulate the success of ECG recordings.

EGG signal strength is variable in amplitude

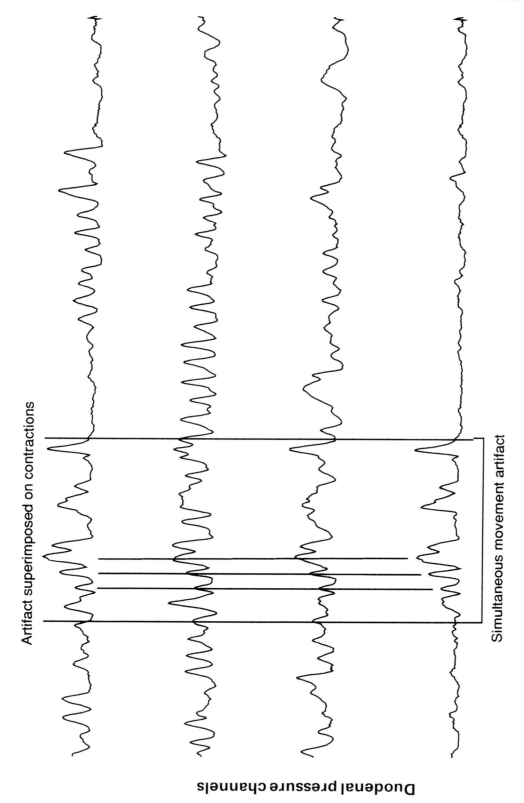

Fig. 22.7   Preterm human infant pressure recording showing an area of artifact caused by movement or crying. Simultaneous peaks are likely to be artifact and should be excluded from analysis.

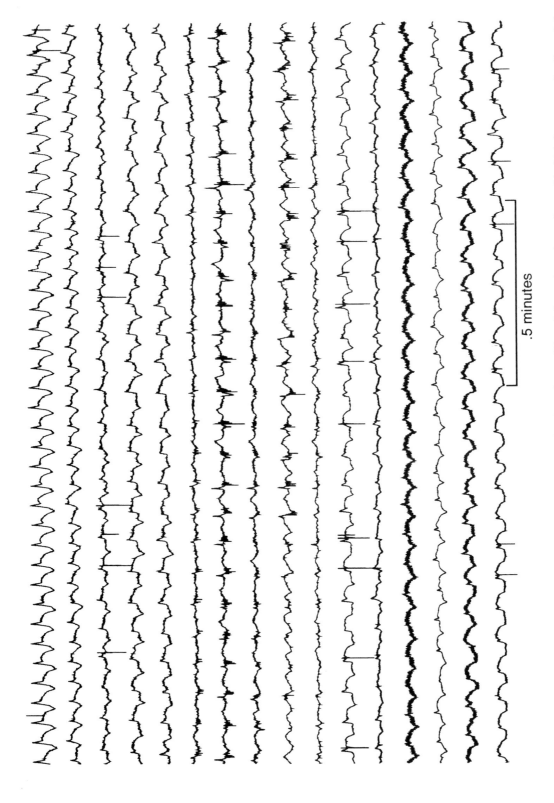

Fig. 22.8 Condensed computer printout of 16 channel myoelectric recording in canine small bowel. Some channels are obscured by high frequency noise. Recorded with interface box taking the place of a 16 channel polygraph recorder.

.5 minutes

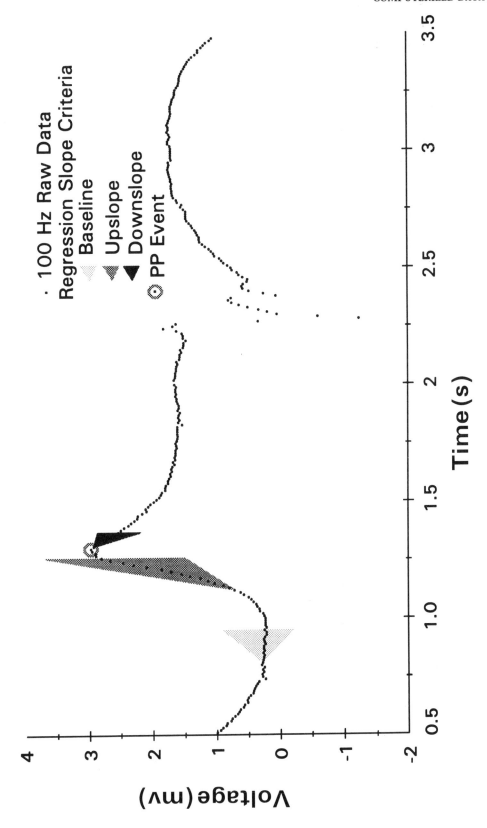

Fig. 22.9 Myoelectric recording showing one slow wave (pacesetter potential). The computer program recognizes the event by examining the slopes of selected portions of the baseline, up and downslope. If they fall within the shaded ranges, the time at the top is stored as the event time. Note that the speed of rapid changes in potential is too fast to give a continuous record at this sampling frequency.

between patients with different body builds. We have obtained excellent recordings from thin patients with the stomach located low in the abdomen. With heavier patients and those with the stomach behind the rib cage the signal quality varies from poor to almost unrecognizable, even with spectral analysis.

The problem of signal quality makes analysis difficult. Rather than look at discrete events, we have used spectral analysis techniques on longer segments of the recording to determine frequencies and strength (power). The results are reported as frequency and frequency changes with time, and power and power changes with time. Interpreting the meaning of changes in frequency and power is a matter for the physician or researcher!

The typical computer analyses techniques applied to the EGG include filtering to remove frequencies that are not in the known gastric range and 'running spectral analysis' to look at time dependent frequency changes. Remembering the caveat about the frequency of a waveform versus its shape the human EGG generally shows a power spectrum that will show frequency changes with time. The amplitude of the power spectrum may be influenced by distension of the stomach, or may reflect changes in contractile activity.

We have made some attempts at EGG analysis on the computer, but have been unenthusiastic about its values. With problems in signal to noise ratio, uncertainty about the significance of power and frequency shifts of the EGG, and the overall lack of detail produced in looking at discrete events, we are uncertain about the place of EGG. There are several research groups throughout the world, working on EGG hoping to succeed in making EGG a useful non-invasive diagnostic tool.

AMBULATORY RECORDING

The electronics for computers and A/D converters are basically a set of computer chips. These can be packed tightly together into a small package to make an ambulatory recording system. Our engineering department built a portable computer system to collect 27 h of data from seven channels for an ambulatory anal/rectal/sigmoid study. The system is 17 cm by 11 cm by 4 cm with a weight of about 1 kg. It is powered by six AA cells and collects data from three and six channel transducer solid state probes purchased from Galtec (Scotland) and Millar (Texas, USA).

One recording channel is used to mark events by the patient, with multiple pushes on a button indicating different events (Fig. 22.2). The box can be connected to a PC to watch the data during recording and to transfer the data to computer for further analysis at the end of recording. The weakness of this system is that the multiple channel solid state pressure probes are very easily damaged and quite expensive to replace or repair.

Portable data loggers are marketed by several companies. Solid state transducers are also available from several sources. When the transducers become less expensive or more robust, this method of data acquisition will probably be very widely used. Removing the perfusion portion of recording systems simplifies the system and makes calibration much easier.

VOLUME MEASUREMENTS

Placing a plastic bag in the stomach, colon or rectum has been used with a barostat, to measure wall motion and cavity volume. The barostat built by Mayo Section of Engineering in the early 1980s for Drs Azpiroz and Malagelada has been used to supplement intraluminal pressure recordings (Fig. 22.3). The barostat can measure volume changes that occur in the gastric fundus, colon and rectum that are not reflected by changes in pressure.

The Mayo barostat consists of a pumping bellows with sensitive feedback pressure control. A motor moves the bellows to inflate the plastic bag to maintain it at a set pressure. A barostat bag located in the colon might be set at 6 mmHg to inflate the bag to expand to fill the space available. A low pressure setting is used to prevent the bag from distending the viscus. As the colon volume decreases in size, a pressure sensor activates the motor on the bellows to remove air so as to maintain the set pressure. The movement of air in and out of the bag is sent out as a varying voltage signal that can be calibrated to measure volume changes in millilitres. As with all invasive monitoring devices, care must be taken in the interpretation of the results as measurement devices do influence the measurements being taken.

Computer analysis consists of descriptive statistics for bag volumes and pressures over selected time periods, and with varying interventions to the subject. Discrete volume changes can be found using a peak finding program with similar analyses made. Comparison of volume changes with intraluminal pressure changes recorded simultaneously elsewhere in the gastrointestinal tract have been used to look at gut function.

At least two companies make barostats for sale. An added feature is a computer control input so that barostat pressure and volume changes can be preprogrammed for automatically scheduled changes.

FUTURE DIRECTIONS

Over the past two decades many researchers have worked on computerizing motility analysis. Until the mid 1980s with the advent of inexpensive computers and A/D converters the data collection costs limited the development to a few research sites. During the past few years we have seen many gastrointestinal groups creating their own computerized motility systems and several companies beginning to market systems that automate the hand counting and measuring of motility contractions.

An ideal computerized motility system should not require a paper recorder, nor a perfusion system and should be able to measure contractions and tone accurately. An inexpensive one-use multiple site pressure transducer system should be attached to the computer with filtering, amplification, isolation and transducer excitation coming from an interface box. Waveforms should be displayed as they are recorded with the ability to review earlier parts of the recording without stopping data acquisition. Analysis should be done as the data is recorded with the computer screen divided up into windows that show graphical summaries of the analyses that are underway, as well as the incoming data.

Alternatively, the recording system might be an ambulatory system for a 'normal life' recording over a day or two. The patient would return at the end of the study, the data would be transferred to an analysis computer and a report written with summary motility values included.

The ideal motility computer system would not only present the basic calculated parameters of motility, but be able to compare how the incoming data matches that of normal patients as well as those with known motility problems. With a database of patients, the next step would be to suggest diagnoses, further tests, and evaluate and improve its ability to do these functions. In some areas in medicine, computers are beginning to be used to do preliminary diagnostic functions. Progress has been slow in gastrointestinal motility due to the limited effort being made which is in turn related to the limited demand for clinical motility tests. Much of the programming has been done by research groups using different incompatible computer systems resulting in much duplication of effort to get no more than the basic techniques available for each group.

Motility systems have become less costly as computers replace recorders. The elimination of perfusion systems will make the process much less complicated. Ambulatory systems will give real-life results that should be more useful in diagnosis. Computer analysis will help interpret the recordings by providing the pertinent values to the physician. All of these changes are underway and are giving motility a new perspective.

SELECT BIBIOGRAPHY

Benson M J, Castillo F D, Wingate D L, Demetrakopolos J, Spyrou N M The computer as referee in the analysis of human small bowel motility. Am J Physiol (in press)

Castell J A, Castell D O 1986 Computer analysis of human esophageal peristalsis and lower esophageal sphincter pressure. II An interactive system for on-line data collection and analysis. Dig Dis Sci 31: 1211–1216

Castrell D O, Dubois A, Davis C R, Cordova C M, Norman D O 1984 Computer-aided analysis of human esophgeal peristalsis. I. Technical description and comparison with manual analysis. Dig Dis Sci 29: 65–72

Christensen J, Glover, J R, Macagno E O, Singerman R B, Weisbrodt N W 1972 Statistics of contractions at a point in the human duodenum. Am J Physiol 221: 1818–1823

Crenner F, Lambert A, Angel F, Schang J C, Grenier J F 1982 Analogue automated analysis of small intestinal electromyogram. Med Biol Eng Comput 20: 151–158

Ehrlein H-J, Hiesinger E 1982 Computer analysis of mechanical activity of gastroduodenal junction in unanaesthetized dogs. QJ Exp Physiol 67: 17–29

Engstrom E, Webster, J, Bass P 1979 Analysis of duodenal contractility in the unanaesthetized dog. IEEE Trans, Biomed Eng BME 26: 517–523

Groh W J, Takahashi I, Sarna S, Dodds W J, Hogan W J 1984 Computerized analysis of spike-burst activity of the upper gastrointestinal tract. Dig Dis Sci 29: 442–446

Kingma Y J 1987 Spectral analysis of gastrointestinal electrical signals. Automedica 7: 237–248

Latour A 1973, Un dispositif simple d'analyse quantiatif de l'électro-myogramme intestinal chronique. Ann Rech Vet 4: 347–353

Misiewicz J J, Walker S L, Healy M J R, Piper E A 1968 Computer analysis of intraluminal pressure records. Gut 9: 232–236

Pousse A, Mendel C, Kashelhoffer J, Grenier J F 1979 Computer program for intestinal spike bursts recognition. Pflugers Archiv 381: 15–18

Reddy S N, Dumpala S R, Sarna S K, Northcott P G 1981 Pattern recognition of canine duodenal contractile activity. IEEE Trans. Biomed Eng BME 28: 696–701

Summers R W, Dusdieker N S 1981 Patterns of spike burst spread in the canine small intestine. Gastroenterology 81: 742–750

Wingate D L, Barnett T 1978 The logical analysis of the electroenterogram. Am J Dig Dis 23: 553–558

Wingate D L, Barnett T, Green R, Armstrong J M 1977 Automated high speed analysis of gastrointestinal myoelectric activity. Am J Dig Dis 22: 243–251

Normal gastrointestinal motility

23. The oesophagus

G. Vantrappen J. Janssens

The main function of the oesophagus is the transport of food and drink from the pharynx into the stomach. Swallowing induces a contraction wave which starts high up in the pharynx and progresses down the oesophagus until it reaches the cardia. This primary peristaltic contraction pushes a solid bolus down the oesophagus into the stomach. Fluids taken in the upright position reach the cardia prior to the arrival of the primary peristaltic contraction due to gravity forces, but in the head-down position fluids are also propelled by the deglutitive contractions. In the resting state, in between deglutitions, the oesophagus is closed at both ends by sphincter mechanisms. The upper oesophageal (pharyngo-oesophageal) sphincter (UOS) prevents air from entering the oesophagus during inspiration. The lower oesophageal (gastro-oesophageal) sphincter (LOS) is of primary importance in the prevention of gastro-oesophageal reflux. Both sphincters relax temporarily after deglutition to allow the passage of the swallowed bolus. If reflux occurs, it gives rise to a secondary peristaltic contraction which propels the refluxed material back into the stomach (Hellemans & Vantrappen 1974, Christensen 1987).

EXAMINATION TECHNIQUES

The motor function of the oesophagus can be studied in several ways.

Radiology with contrast material

Using contrast material that coats the mucosa and high speed cine or videorecording, radiographic methods will show, apart from morphologic abnormalities, flow of intraluminal material and motion of the wall. The technique is at present essential to study normal and disordered motor function of the pharynx and pharyngo-oesophageal region, and may yield important information on the motility of the oesphageal body

and LOS as well, especially when combined with manometry (mano-fluorography).

Manometry

Manometric techniques have been widely used to examine the motor function of the oesophagus and its sphincters. For clinical purposes a bundle of tubes having distal lateral openings at different levels is used in connection with externally placed strain-gauges and a continuous low compliance perfusion technique (Arndorfer et al 1977). Details of the manometric methods have been published in many recent publications and are discussed in section 4. Intraluminal pressure measurements yield information on tension developed in circular muscles, but not on changes in longitudinal muscle tension. Modern pressure transducers have a compliance of only 0.05 μl/mmHg; therefore, it is the pump-catheter assembly which is responsible for the compliance of the system. Commercially available capillary perfusion systems can provide a pressure rise rate of 300–400 mmHg/s, which is adequate for faithful recordings in the oesophageal body and LOS, but insufficient to cope with the very fast pressure rise rates in pharynx and pharyngo-oesophageal sphincter (Knauer et al 1990). Intraluminal solid state transducers have a much higher frequency response and prevent the need for perfusion, but they are more expensive and vulnerable. Solid state transducers are used in ambulatory recording systems that monitor oesophageal pressures (and pH) for prolonged periods of time in patients with angina-like chest pain of noncardiac origin (Fig. 23.1) (Vantrappen et al 1982, Janssens et al 1986).

Several software programs have been developed to automatically analyse the large amount of motility data obtained during prolonged recording (Castell & Castell 1986, Tijskens et al 1989).

As the LOS moves with respiration and swallowing, it is virtually impossible to accurately monitor maximal

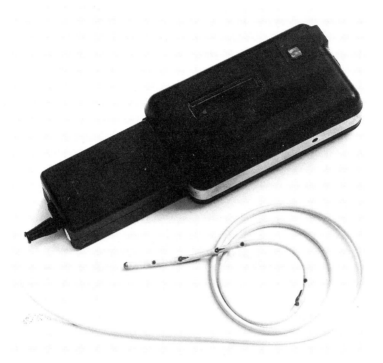

Fig. 23.1   Ambulatory 24-hour pH and pressure recording system.

sphincter pressure with a single pressure recording orifice. The Dent sleeve device (Dent 1976), which is approximately 4 cm long, accurately measures maximal pressure exerted anywhere over its length. Because of its pressure characteristics the sleeve is able to accurately measure the resting LOS pressure and LOS relaxations, but it is less well suited for sphincteric contractions.

Electromyography

Electromyographic techniques are the only way to distinguish contractile activity of striated muscles in the upper part of the oesophagus from that of smooth muscles in the lower gullet. The best recordings in man are currently obtained with small sized bipolar suction electrodes. This technique, however, is still in the experimental stage. (Fig. 23.2) (Hellemans et al 1974).

Scintiscanning

Scintiscanning over the oesophageal region with the gamma-camera during the passage of a radiolabelled bolus has been proved to be a reliable technique to quantitatively measure oesphageal transit.

Gastro-oesophageal reflux is best evaluated by intra-oesophageal pH-measurements or by scintiscanning. Several systems using small sized intraluminal glass electrodes with a combined intraluminal reference electrode and capable of recording intraoesophageal pH over a 24-h period in ambulatory patients are now commercially available. Scintiscanning over the oesophageal region after the administration of a radiolabelled meal is another way to detect reflux especially in children because it avoids the use of an intraoesophageal tube. The limited duration of the recording period, however, is a major disadvantage of the technique.

PHARYNGEAL AND OESOPHAGEAL MOTILITY 'AT REST'

Pharynx

Striated muscles of pharynx and parapharyngeal structures exhibit some activity during the respiratory cycle giving rise to intrapharyngeal pressure variations in between +1.4 mmHg (expiration) and −0.2 mmHg (inspiration) (Goyal et al 1970). This activity is best demonstrated by electromyography.

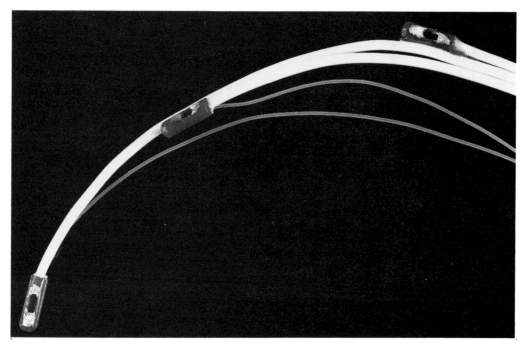

Fig. 23.2   Assembly of small-sized bipolar suction electrodes suitable for electromyographic recording in the human oesophagus.

Upper oesophageal sphincter

The upper oesophageal sphincter zone begins immediately below the hypopharyngeal air column and is 2–4 cm in length. It exhibits marked radial and axial asymmetry, pressures being higher anteriorly and posteriorly than laterally. (Figs 23.3, 23.4) (Welch et al 1979, Hellemans et al 1981).

Its normal maximal value during the resting state is fairly high, up to 100–130 mmHg above atmospheric pressure. The striated musculature of the sphincter generates continuous spiking activity which varies somewhat with respiration. The number of spike potentials is directly proportional with the resting pressure (Figs 23.5, 23.6).

Oesophageal body

The oesophageal body exhibits no rhythmic or tonic contractions at rest. Pressures are passively transmitted by respiratory variations (the intra-oesophageal pressure reflecting closely the intrapleural pressure), from −5 to −15 mmHg at inspiration to −2 to +5 mmHg at expiration, and by cardiovascular pulsations from aorta, left atrium and ventricle (Code & Schlegel 1968). Electromyographically the oesophageal body is quiescent at rest.

It is generally accepted that spontaneous contractions, not induced by deglutition or by the presence of an intraluminal bolus, are abnormal in the tubular oesophagus. Recent studies, however, have shown that non-deglutitive simultaneous repetitive contractions may be observed in most normal subjects during the gastric phase III of the migrating motor complex (MMC). In some individuals their number may be relatively high and their amplitude quite impressive (Fig. 23.7) (Janssens et al 1993).

Lower oesophageal sphincter

The high pressure zone of the LOS shows a bell-shaped configuration and is 2–4 cm in length. The sphincter has radial asymmetry with maximal pressures left laterally, primarily due to the crus sinistra of the diaphragm and the angled aspect of the lower oesophagus (Fig. 23.8) (Welch & Drake 1980).

Some asymmetry, however, persists even in hiatal hernia patients and may be related to the spiral nature of the circular muscle fibres of the LOS. Because of this asymmetry LOS resting pressures are to be evaluated manometrically with three to four tubes, the lateral openings of which face different directions 120° or 90° apart. In most instances the LOS is situated around

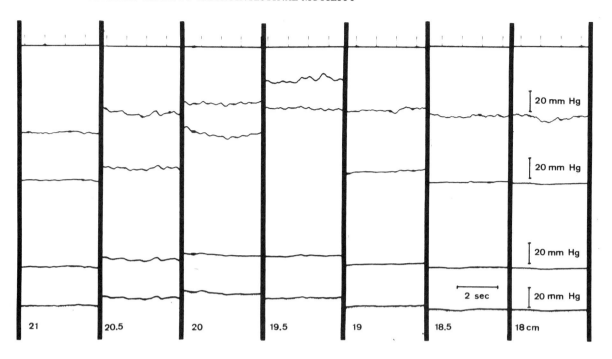

Fig. 23.3 Manometric profile of upper oesophageal sphincter in control subject, using four radially oriented continuously perfused catheters and a stepwise pull-through technique (steps indicated cm from incisors). Line 1: dorsally; 2: anteriorly; 3: left laterally; 4: right laterally.

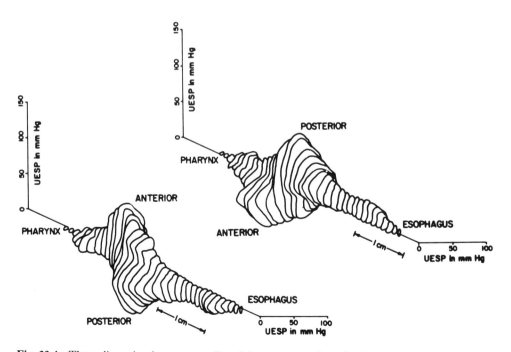

Fig. 23.4 Three-dimensional pressure profiles of the upper oesophageal sphincter. Pressures are higher in anterio-posterior position than laterally. (Welch et al 1979.)

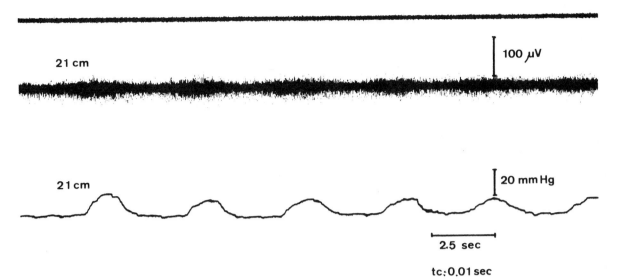

Fig. 23.5 Simultaneous recording of electromyographic and intraluminal pressure in the human upper oesophageal sphincter at rest (21 cm from the incisors). The continuous spiking activity fluctuates with respiration.

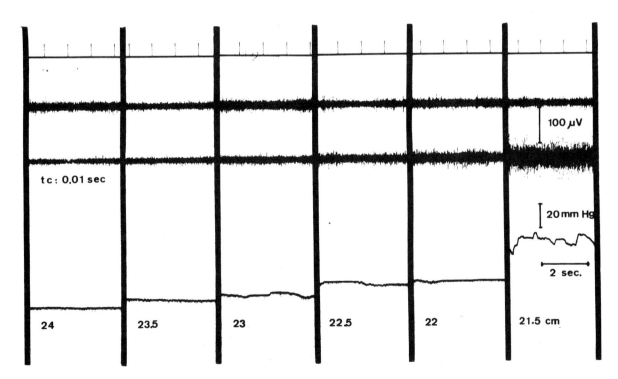

Fig. 23.6 Simultaneous recording of electromyographic and intraluminal pressure in the human upper oesophageal sphincter at rest; stepwise pull-through from 24 to 21.5 cm from incisors. Line 1: EMG of the suprahyoid muscle showing the absence of deglutition. Line 2: EMG of the upper oesophageal sphincter showing an increase in number and amplitude of spike potentials together with an increase in sphincter pressure (line 3).

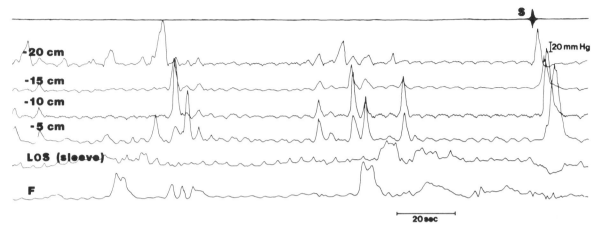

Fig. 23.7 Manometric recording in the gastric fundus (F), at 4 levels in the oesophageal body at 20, 15, 10 and 5 cm above the lower oesophageal sphincter (LOS) and in the sphincter, which was monitored with a sleeve device. Representative example of the non-deglutitive activity consisting of bursts of repetitive non-sequential pressure peaks in the oesophageal body. The bursts occur together with phasic contractions in the LOS and end with the occurrence of a secondary peristaltic contraction. The last pressure complex represents the primary peristaltic contraction induced by swallowing (S).

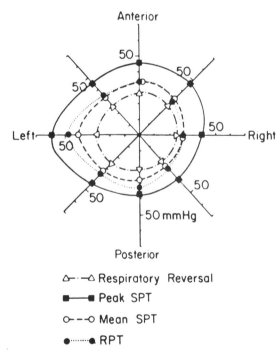

Fig. 23.8 Radial asymmetry of the lower oesophageal sphincter in 18 normal subjects. SPT: slow pull-through; RPT: rapid pull-through. With all methods pressures leftwards were significantly greater than rightwards (From Welch & Drake 1980.)

the pressure inversion point (PIP). This is the point at which the respiratory pressure swings with respiration changes from inspiratory positive (intra-abdominal) to inspiratory negative (intrathoracic), and which usually corresponds to the level of the diaphragm (Fig. 23.9). In case of a hiatus hernia a double PIP may exist (Fig. 23.10) (Harris & Pope 1966).

It is known that the LOS pressure increases during increased intra-abdominal pressure to protect the oesophagus against gastro-oesophageal reflux favoured by the increased abdomino-thoracic pressure gradient. Mittal and co-workers have shown that tonic activity of the crural diaphragm contributes to the increase in LOS pressure that accompanies a rise in intra-abdominal pressure provoked by leg raising and abdominal compression (Mittal et al 1988).

In addition to the respiratory-related pressure changes, the LOS pressure may also vary with the different phases of the MMC, pressures being highest during phase III and lowest during phase I (Fig. 23.11) (Dent et al 1983, Smout et al 1985).

The LOS pressure can also be evaluated by means of a rapid pull-through, which usually measures a slightly higher LOS pressure than the slow step-wise pull-through (Welch & Drake 1980) (Fig. 23.12). The best way to continuously monitor maximal LOS pressure over a prolonged period of time is performed with the Dent sleeve (Dent 1976).

Apart from intra-individual variations (i.e. due to the MMC cycle) the normal LOS pressure shows also marked variations between different subjects. Normal values are accepted to vary from + 10 to + 40 mmHg (as compared to the intrafundic zero level).

Electromyographic data obtained in man are scarce. It is still debated whether or not the human LOS

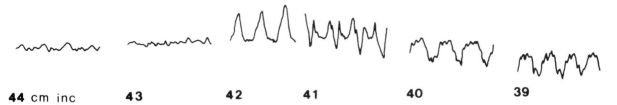

Fig. 23.9 Stepwise pull-through of the lower oesophageal sphincter showing the pressure inversion point (PIP) at the level of 41 cm from incisors.

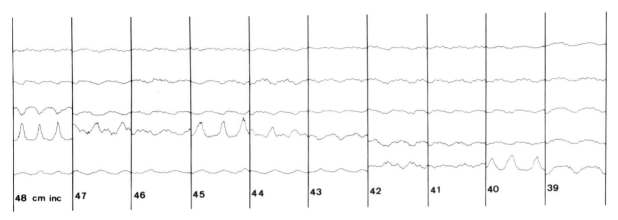

Fig. 23.10 Stepwise pull-through of the lower oesophageal sphincter in a patient with hiatal hernia. Catheter assembly with five perfused catheters with side openings 5 cm apart. Cm from incisors indicated for the most distally located side opening. A double pressure inversion point (double PIP) is observed at 42 and 39 cm from incisors at line 5 and at 41 and 38 cm (46–5 cm and 43–5 cm) at line 4.

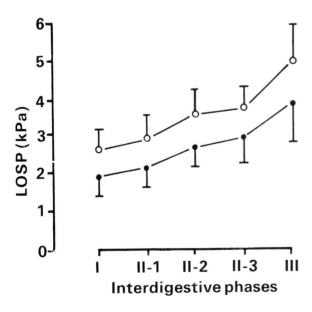

Fig. 23.11 Mean lower oesophageal sphincter pressure (± SEM) in six healthy patients during various phases of the migrating motor complex after placebo (●) and cisapride (○) (0.5 mg/h IV). (From Smout et al 1985.)

generates spontaneous electrical signals at rest (Hellemans et al 1974, Asoh & Goyal 1978).

The competence of the LOS in the prevention of gastro-oesophageal reflux is best evaluated by intra-oesophageal 24-h pH measurements. A few reflux episodes (less than 50 peaks/24 h, or pH < 4 less than 42% of time per 24 h) especially during the postprandial period reflects so-called physiologic reflux (Fig. 23.13) (De Meester et al 1974, Galmiche et al 1980, Johnson & De Meester 1986). The vast majority of these reflux episodes occur during so-called transient relaxations of the LOS (Dodds et al 1982). Transient LOS relaxations are complete relaxations whose onset does not directly follow a swallow. They may occur independently of the resting pressure of the LOS. Transient LOS relaxations usually last longer (from 5–30 s) than swallow-induced LOS relaxations. Their relatively long duration together with the fact that they occur while the oesophageal body is not sealed by a peristaltic wave clearly favours the occurrence of reflux (Fig. 23.14).

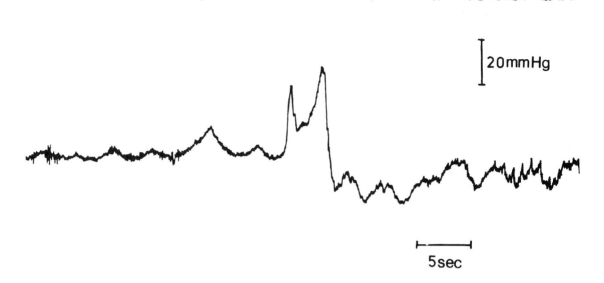

Fig. 23.12 Lower oesophageal sphincter pressure evaluated by rapid pull-through from stomach (left) to oesophageal body (right).

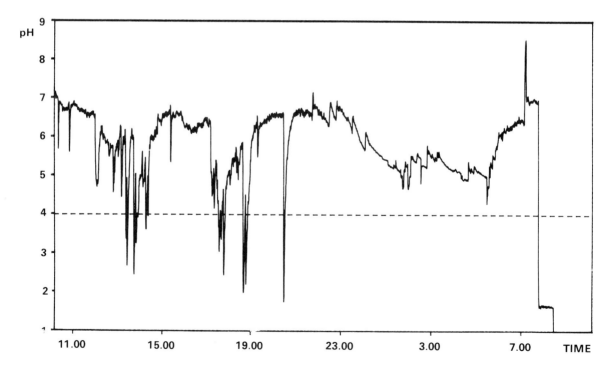

Fig. 23.13 24-h pH plot showing intra-oesophageal pH (measured at 5 cm above the lower oesophageal sphincter) versus time in a patient with minimal complaints of heartburn during the postprandial period.

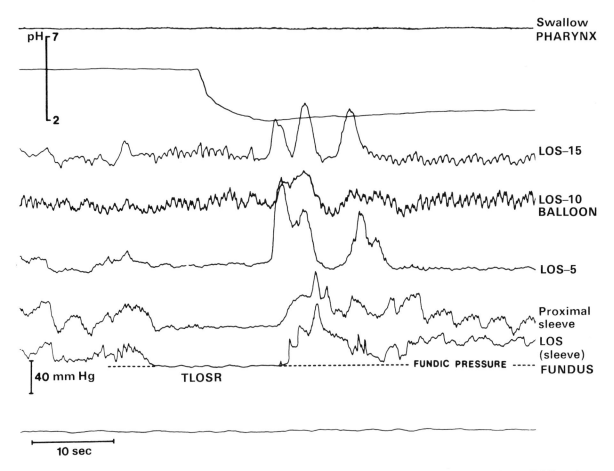

Fig. 23.14 Manometric recording in oesophageal body at 15, 10 and 5 cm above the lower oesophageal sphincter (LOS), and in the sphincter (monitored with a sleeve). A transient lower oesophageal sphincter relaxation occurs in the absence of swallowing and is accompanied by reflux as shown on the pH recording at 5 cm above the lower oesophageal sphincter.

PHARYNGEAL AND OESOPHAGEAL MOTILITY AFTER SWALLOWING

Pharynx

The swallowing movement starts with the onset of activity in the mylohioid muscle.

The sequence of pharyngeal and extrapharyngeal muscle contractions that occurs after swallowing, gives rise to a wave of pharyngeal peristalsis that travels down the oropharynx and hypopharynx at a speed of about 15 cm/s to reach the upper oesophageal sphincter after about 0.7 s. The hypopharyngeal peristaltic wave has a peak amplitude of about 200 ± 150 mmHg and a mean duration of 0.3–0.5 s (Fig. 23.15) (Dodds et al 1975).

Upper oesophageal sphincter

The upper oesophageal sphincter relaxes after deglutition to allow easy passage of the swallowed bolus. The relaxation may even reach subatmospheric pressures. It starts upon swallowing, lasts for about 0.5–1.0 s and is followed by a contraction which is the start of the primary peristaltic contraction in the oesophageal body.

Electromyographically the relaxation is accompanied by a cessation of all spiking activity; during the post-deglutitive contraction there is an increase in spiking activity which lasts as long as the contraction itself (Fig. 23.16) (Fyke & Code 1955, Pelemans 1983).

At the onset of deglutition the larynx and thus the

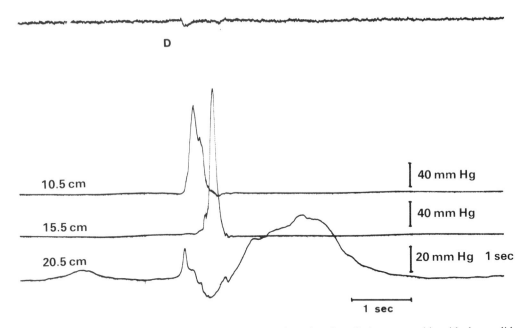

Fig. 23.15 Pressure measurement in the pharyngo-oesophageal region. Catheter assembly with three solid state intraluminal microtransducers at 10.5, 15.5 and 20.5 cm from incisors. The most distal catheter is located in the upper oesophageal sphincter.

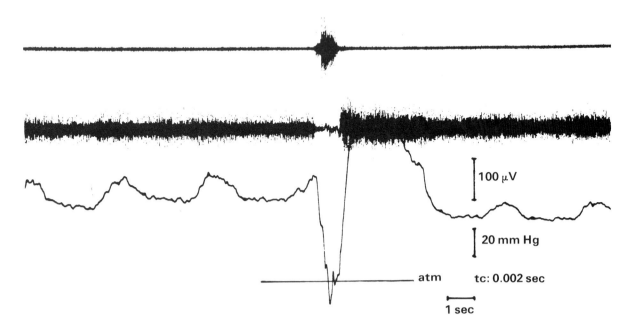

Fig. 23.16 Simultaneous electromyographic (line 2) and intraluminal pressure (line 3) recording in the human upper oesophageal sphincter. Line 1 is the deglutitive signal (EMG of the suprahyoideal muscle.)

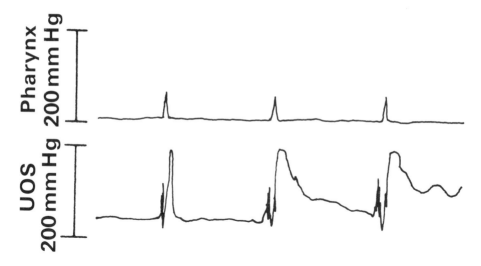

Fig. 23.17 Tracing of three swallows with transducers placed to allow accurate recording of pharyngeal UOS pressure dynamics. Sphincter transducer is positioned in the proximal extent of the UOS before a swallow. Note 'M' configuration seen at UOS as sphincter moves upward onto transducer before relaxation. (From Castell et al 1990.)

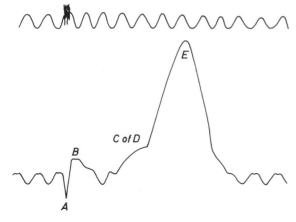

Fig. 23.18 Schematic representation of the various components of the deglutitive contractions in the oesophageal body.

upper oesophageal sphincter moves upwards to protect it from aspiration. It is, therefore, virtually impossible to keep a pressure measuring device other than a sleeve in the sphincter. The sleeve pressure dynamics, however, are highly inadequate to accurately measure the fast pressure transients during swallowing. The best recordings are obtained with the pressure sensor in the hypopharynx just above the level of the sphincter. The first positive deflection reflects the resting pressure of the sphincter which moves upwards, the downward reflection represents the sphincter relaxation and the second positive reflection is related to the post-deglutitive sphincter contraction (Fig. 23.17) (Castell et al 1990).

Oesophageal body

The manometrically recorded deglutitive contraction of the oesophageal body may comprise several components (Fig. 23.18) (Vantrappen & Hellemans 1967; Goyal & Cobb 1981).

The initial pressure change (A-wave) is a negative deflection which starts about 0.2 s after the onset of swallowing and lasts for about 0.3–0.5 s. It is probably due to a short inspiration just prior to the swallowing movement ('Schluckatmung') (Fig. 23.19).

In about 87% of the swallows this initial negative deflection is followed by a positive pressure change (B-wave), probably caused by the transmission of pharyngeal pressure through the swallowed bolus (Butin et al 1953). A second positive wave (C-wave) is recorded in the distal part of the oesophagus after about one-third of the swallows and is probably caused by the increase in pressure between the advancing bolus and the LOS (Fig. 23.20) (Vantrappen & Hellemans 1967, Hellemans 1970). A, B and C-waves are passively transmitted pressure phenomena, not related to the peristaltic contraction itself. If present they start simultaneously in the different segments of the oesophageal body.

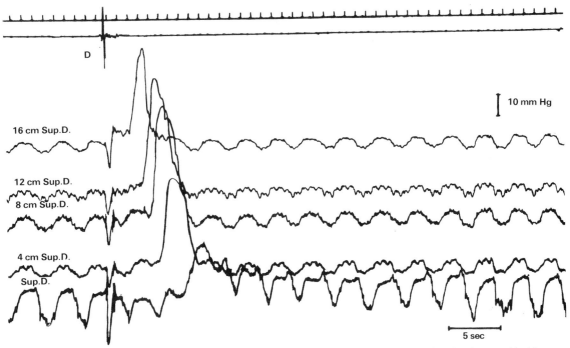

Fig. 23.19 Intraluminal pressure measurement with a catheter assembly consisting of five perfused catheters with side openings at different levels above the supradiaphragm (sup D). The post deglutitive (D) contraction shows an example of an A-wave ('Schluckatmung').

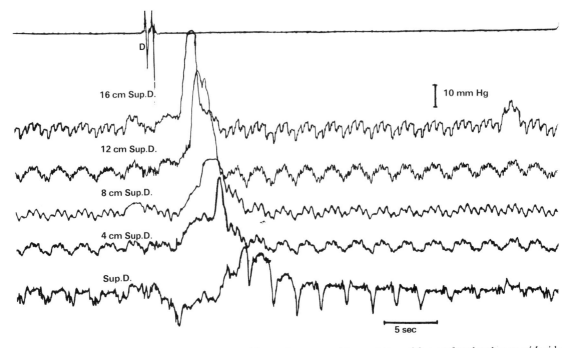

Fig. 23.20 Intraluminal pressure measurement with a catheter assembly consisting of five perfused catheters with side openings at different levels above the supradiaphragm (sup D). The post deglutitive (D) contraction shows an example of a C-wave at the level of 12, 8 and 4 cm sup D.

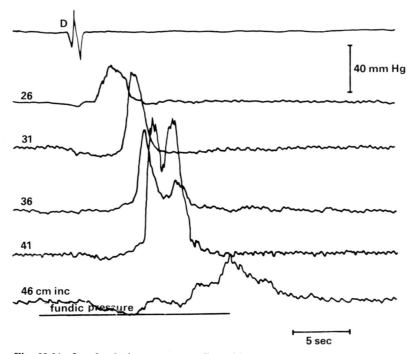

Fig. 23.21 Intraluminal pressure recording with a catheter assembly consisting of five perfused catheters with side openings 5 cm apart. The post deglutitive (D) peristaltic contraction shows an M-shaped pressure wave at the level of 41 cm from the incisors. (cm inc: cm from incisors)

The main pressure component of the normal deglutition complex is a large positive pressure wave which represents the peristaltic contraction. In most instances it is a single-peaked wave (E-wave) but double-peaked waves (M-waves) are seen in healthy volunteers after about 11% of wet swallows (Fig. 23.21) (Richter et al 1987).

The amplitude of the peristaltic contraction varies considerably from one individual to another and, in the same individual, from one segment of the oesophageal body to another. Measured with intraluminal solid state transducers the amplitude was found to be 69.5 ± 12.1 mmHg in the lower oesophagus, 53.4 ± 9.0 mmHg in the upper gullet and 35.0 ± 6.4 mmHg in the mid-oesophageal segment which corresponds to the transition zone between striated and smooth oesophageal muscle (Humphries & Castell 1977).

The speed of progression of the peristaltic wave increases from 3 cm/s in the upper segment to 5 cm/s in the lower oesophagus, but slows down again to 2.5 cm/s just above the LOS. The peristaltic contraction reaches the LOS 5–6 s after swallowing. The duration of a single peaked peristaltic wave varies from 2–4 s but never exceeds 6.5 s (Vantrappen & Hellemans 1967).

Richter et al (1987) have published the range of normal values of oesophageal contractions recorded in a large number of 95 healthy volunteers. Amplitude but not duration was greater after wet compared to dry swallows. Double peaked contractions frequently occurred after both wet (11.3%) and dry (18.1%) swallows, but triple peaked waves were rare. Non-peristaltic contractions were more common after dry (12.6%) than after wet (4.1%) swallows.

Some parameters of the normal deglutition complex may change with age. The most consistent finding is an increase in the number of non-peristaltic contractions (up to 30% of the deglutitive contractions being simultaneous) and in the number of repetitive (triple or more) waves, up to 7%. The manometric tracing may even appear as diffuse oesophageal spasm. The amplitude of the contractions may decrease somewhat with age but this is certainly not a consistent finding (Hellemans 1970, Richter et al 1987).

In the supine position the peristaltic contraction is responsible for the propulsion of the swallowed bolus. In this respect the peristaltic character of the contraction is more important than its amplitude provided a

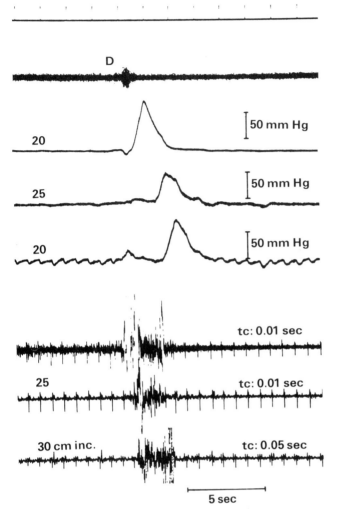

Fig. 23.22 Simultaneous electromyographic (lower part) and intraluminal pressure (upper part) measurements at three different levels in the human oesophagus. (cm inc: cm from incisors; D: deglutitive signal)

minimum amplitude of 12 mmHg in the upper and of 25 mmHg in the lower oesophagus is reached (Kahrilas et al 1988).

Electromyographic studies with intraluminal suction electrodes have shown that the contraction in the upper oesophagus is accompanied by a burst of striated muscle spikes, the intensity of which is directly proportional to the amplitude of the contraction; the spike burst lasts as long as the contraction.

In the lower oesophageal segment the spike burst that accompanies the contraction wave is of the smooth muscle type: smooth muscle spikes have a greater amplitude and a markedly longer duration and their rhythm is much slower than that of striated muscle spikes. In contrast with the response in the striated muscle oesophagus, smooth muscle action potentials never occur after the peak pressure of the deglutitive pressure wave has been reached (Fig. 23.22).

At the level of the transition zone between striated and smooth muscles both types of spikes occur intermingled, the tracing usually beginning with spikes of the striated muscle type (Fig. 23.23) (Hellemans et al 1974).

If swallows are taken in rapid succession, no peristaltic wave appears until after the last swallow because a new deglutition inhibits the activity of the previous swallow (Fig. 23.24).

In the zone where the spike burst consists entirely of striated muscle spikes, a second deglutition results in the immediate disappearance of all spiking activity of the previous swallow and is accompanied by a decrease in intraluminal pressure. Swallowing also inhibits the spiking activity in the transitional zone where striated and smooth muscles are intermingled. In the distal segment consisting of smooth muscles, the pattern is different. If the second deglutition occurs immediately before or during the initial phase of a spike burst, it does not interrupt the spiking activity in this oesophageal segment; yet the distal progression of the spike burst is halted and the deglutitive wave does not proceed further distally (Fig. 23.25) (Hellemans et al 1974, Janssens 1978).

The inhibitory phenomena which become apparent after paired swallows are caused by the wave of inhibition which has been shown to precede primary and secondary peristaltic contractions. In humans the characteristics of this inhibitory wave in the body of the oesophagus cannot be studied by simple manometry due to the absence of basal tone. Sifrim et al (1992) developed a method to study the inhibitory wave. An artificial high pressure zone is induced in the tubular oesophagus by inflation of an intraluminal balloon to a critical level. By measuring the pressure changes at the interface between the balloon and the oesophageal wall, they showed the presence of a deglutition-induced relaxation in this artificial high pressure zone beginning simultaneously at various levels of the oesophagus but lasting progressively longer in progressively more distal segments (Figs 23.26, 23.27).

Lower Oesophageal Sphincter (LOS)

The LOS relaxes upon deglutition to allow easy passage of the swallowed bolus. The relaxation may start with the onset of deglutition but in many

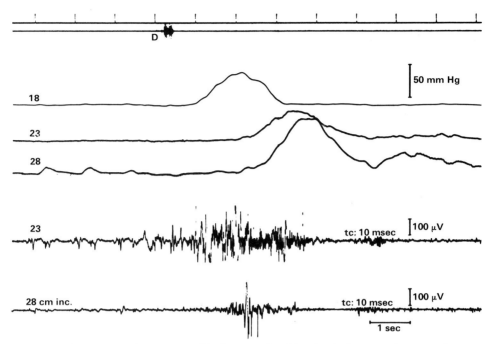

Fig. 23.23 Simultaneous electromyographic (lower part) and intraluminal pressure (upper part) recording in the human oesophagus. The electrical tracing at 23 cm from incisors was recorded in the transitional zone where striated and smooth muscle spikes occur intermingled. (cm inc: cm from incisors; D: deglutitive signal)

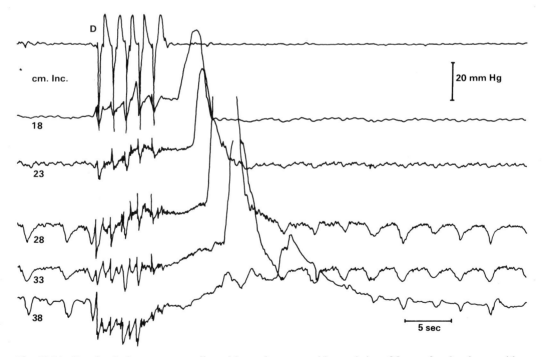

Fig. 23.24 Intraluminal pressure recording with a catheter assembly consisting of five perfused catheters with side openings 5 cm apart. When a series of deglutitions is taken in rapid succession, only one oesophageal contraction is elicited starting after the last swallow. (cm inc: cm from incisors; D: deglutitive signal)

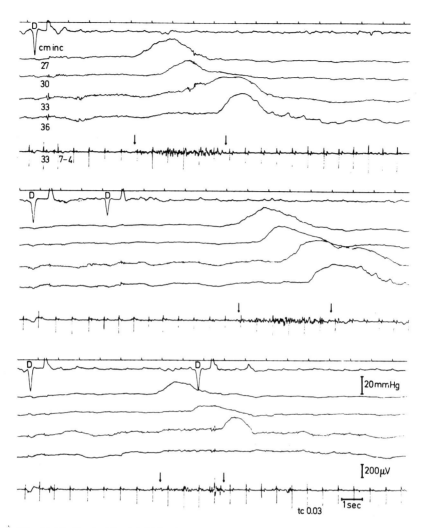

Fig. 23.25 Deglutitive inhibition in the human oesophagus. Simultaneous intraluminal pressure measurements at 27, 30, 33 and 36 cm from incisors and EMG at 33 cm. Upper part: normal deglutitive response. Middle part: a deglutition 3.5 cm after a previous swallow eliminates the deglutitive response to the first deglutition. Lower part: if the second deglutition occurs during the spike burst of a previous swallow, it does not inhibit the spiking activity in this oesophageal segment but the distal progression is halted. (D: deglutitive signal). (From Hellemans et al 1974.)

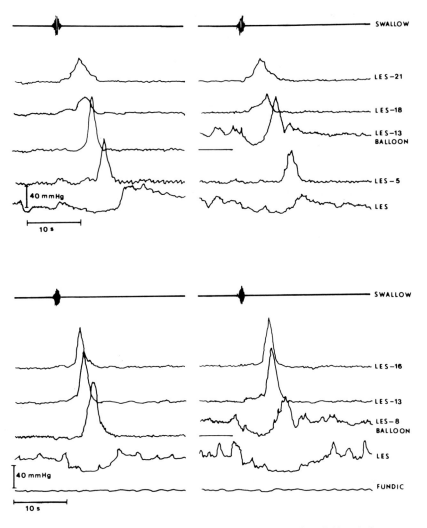

Fig. 23.26 Resting pressure and deglutitive pressure waves before (left) and after (right) balloon inflation with balloons 13 cm and 8 cm above the LOS, respectively. The deglutitive inhibition in the oesophageal body is shown by the fall in pressure at the level of the artificial high pressure zone created by balloon inflation. (From Sifrim et al 1992.)

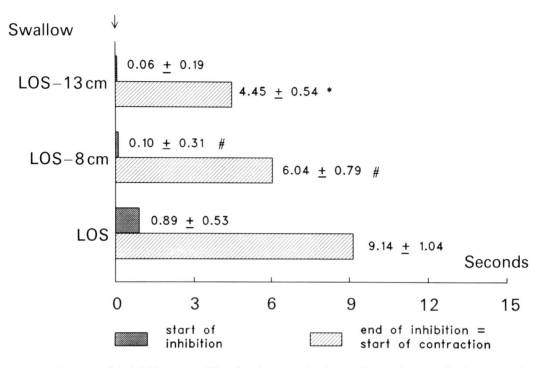

Fig. 23.27 Duration of the inhibitory wave. The relaxation starts simultaneously over the entire distal oesophageal body but lasts progressively longer in the progressively more distal segments. (▨, Start of inhibition; ▨, end of inhibition (start of contraction); * p < 0.001 vs. 8 cm above LOS, # p < 0.001 vs. LOS). (From Sifrim et al 1992.)

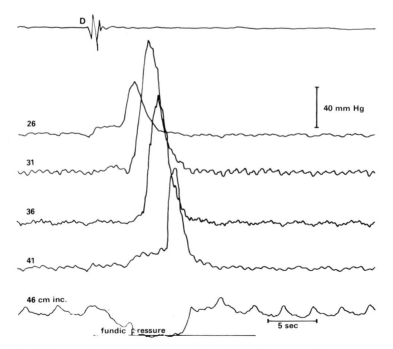

Fig. 23.28 Intraluminal pressure recording with a catheter assembly consisting of five perfused catheters with side openings 5 cm apart. The distal opening is located in the lower part of the lower oesophageal sphincter. The pressure returns to baseline level after the relaxation without the presence of an after-contraction.

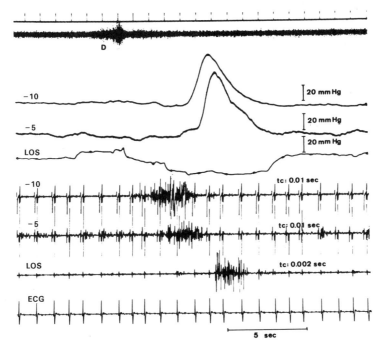

Fig. 23.29 Simultaneous electromyographic (lower part) and intraluminal pressure (upper part) recording at two different levels in the oesophagus (5 and 10 cm above the lower oesophageal sphincter) and in the lower oesophageal sphincter in a normal subject. There is no clear correlate for the sphincter relaxation. (ECG: electrocardiogram; D: deglutitive signal)

instances it is delayed for 2–3 s after the initiation of swallowing.

In normal individuals the relaxation is complete (or almost complete) with a mean reduction of 85% ± 5% of the resting LOS pressure. The relaxation lasts 5–10 s and is followed in the upper part of the sphincter by an aftercontraction which also lasts 7–10 s. In the lower part of the sphincter the pressure returns to baseline level after the relaxation without the presence of an after-contraction (Fig. 23.28)

(Goyal & Cobb 1981, Christensen 1987, Jian et al 1987).

Electromyographic studies in the human oesophagus were unable to demonstrate a clear electromyographic correlate for the sphincter relaxation, although in the opossum a cessation of the continuous spiking activity was described. The after-contraction is accompanied by a spike burst of the smooth muscle type, as in the oesophageal body (Fig. 23.29) (Hellemans et al 1968, Hellemans et al 1974, Asoh & Goyal 1978).

REFERENCES

Arndorfer R C, Stef J J, Dodds W J, Linehan J H, Hogan W J 1977 Improved infusion system for intraluminal esophageal manometry. Gastroenterology 73: 23–27

Asoh R, Goyal R K 1978 Electrical activity of the opossum lower esophageal sphincter in vivo. Gastroenterology 74: 835–840

Butin J W, Olsen A M, Moersh H J, Code C F 1953 A study of esophageal pressures in normal persons and patients with cardiospasm. Gastroenterology 23: 278–293

Castell J A, Castell D O 1986 Computer analysis of human peristalsis and lower esophageal sphincter pressure: 2. An

interactive system for on-line data collection and analysis. Dig Dis Sci 31: 1211–1216

Castell J A, Dalton C B, Castell D O 1990 Pharyngeal and upper esophageal sphincter manometry in humans. Am J Physiol 258: G173–G178

Christensen J 1987 Motor functions of the pharynx and esophagus in: Johnson L R (ed.) Physiology of the gastrointestinal tract. Raven Press, New York, pp 595–612

Code C F, Schlegel J F 1968 Motor actions of the esophagus and its sphincters in: Handbook of physiology, Section 6, Alimentary canal, Vol IV Motility. American Physiological Society, Washington DC, pp 1821–1839

De Meester T R, Johnson L F, Kent A H 1974 Evaluation

of current operations for the prevention of gastroesophageal reflux. Ann Surg 180: 511–525

Dent J 1976 A new technique for continuous sphincter pressure measurement. Gastroenterology 71: 263–267

Dent J, Dodds W J, Sekiguchi T, Hogan W J, Arndorfer R C 1983 Interdigestive phasic contractions of the human lower esophageal sphincter. Gastroenterology 84: 453–460

Dodds W J, Dent J, Hogan W et al 1982 Mechanism of gastroesophageal reflux in patients with reflux esophagitis. N Engl J Med 307: 1547–1552

Dodds W J, Hogan W J, Lyden S B, Stewart E T, Steff J J, Arndorfer R C 1975 Quantitation of pharyngeal motor function in normal human subjects. J Appl Physiol 39: 692–696

Fyke F E, Code C F 1955 Resting and deglutition pressures in the pharyngoesophageal region. Gastroenterology 29: 24–34

Galmiche J P, Guillard J F, Denis P, Boussakr K, Lefrançois R, Colon R 1980 Etude du pH oesophagien en période post-prandiale chez le sujet normal et au cours de syndrome de reflux gastro-oesophagien. Intérêt diagnostique d'un score de reflux acide. Gastroenterol Clin Biol 4: 531–539

Goyal R K, Cobb B W 1981 Motility of the pharynx, esophagus and esophageal sphincters in: Johnson L R (ed.) Physiology of the gastrointestinal tract. Raven Press, New York, pp 359–391

Goyal R K, Sangree M H, Hersh T 1970 Pressure inversion point at the upper high pressure zone and its genesis. Gastroenterology 59: 754–759

Harris L D, Pope C E II 1966 The pressure inversion point: its genesis and reliability. Gastroenterology 51: 641–648

Hellemans J 1970 Invloed van de leeftijd op de motorische functie van de slokdarm. Thesis, Lannoo pvba., Tielt.

Hellemans J, Pelemans W, Vantrappen G 1981 Pharyngoesophageal swallowing disorders and the pharyngoesophageal sphincter. Med Clin North Am 65: 1149–1171

Hellemans J, Vantrappen G 1974 Physiology in: Vantrappen G, Hellemans J (eds) Handbuch der Inneren Medizin, Diseases of the Esophagus. Springer-Verlag, Berlin, pp 40–102

Hellemans J, Vantrappen G, Janssens J 1974 Electromyography of the esophagus in: Vantrappen G, Hellemans J (eds) Handbuch der Inneren Medizin, Diseases of the Esophagus. Springer-Verlag, Berlin, pp 270–285

Hellemans J, Vantrappen G, Valembois P, Janssens J, Vandenbroucke J 1968 Electrical activity of striated and smooth muscle of the esophagus. Am J Dig Dis 13: 320–334

Humphries T J, Castell D O 1977 Pressure profile of esophageal peristalsis in normal humans as measured by direct intraesophageal transducers. Am J Dig Dis 22: 641–645

Janssens J 1978 The peristaltic mechanism of the esophagus. PhD thesis, University of Leuven, Belgium

Janssens J, Annese V, Vantrappen G 1993 Bursts of non-deglutitive simultaneous contractions may be a normal esophageal motility pattern. Gut 34: 1021–1024

Janssens J, Vantrappen G, Ghillebert G 1986 24-hour recording of esophageal pressure and pH in patients with noncardiac chest pain. Gastroenterology 90: 1978–1984

Jian R, Janssens J, Vantrappen G, Ceccatelli P 1987 Influence of metenkephalin analogue on motor activity of the gastrointestinal tract. Gastroenterology 93: 114–120

Johnson L F, De Meester T R 1986 Development of the 24-hour intraesophageal pH monitoring composite scoring system. J Clin Gastroenterol 8 (suppl. 1): 52–58

Kahrilas P J, Dodds W J, Hogan W J 1988 Effect of peristaltic dysfunction on esophageal volume clearance. Gastroenterology 94: 73–80

Knauer C M, Castell J A, Dalton C B, Nowak L, Castell D O 1990 Pharyngeal/upper esophageal sphincter pressure dynamics in humans: Effects of pharmacological agents and thermal stimulation. Dig Dis Sci 35: 774–780

Mittal R K, Rochester D F, McCallum R W 1988 Electrical and mechanical activity in the human esophageal sphincter during diaphragmatic contraction. J Clin Invest 81: 1182–1189

Pelemans W 1983 Functie van de faryngo-esofageale overgangszone en dysfunctie bij bejaarden. PhD thesis, University of Leuven, Belgium

Richter J E, Wu W C, Johns D N et al 1987 Esophageal manometry in 95 healthy adult volunteers: variability of pressures with age and frequency of 'abnormal' contractions. Dig Dis Sci 32: 583–592

Sifrim D, Janssens J, Vantrappen G 1992 A wave of inhibition precedes primary peristaltic contractions in the human esophagus. Gastroenterology 103: 876–882

Smout A J P M, Bogaard J W, Grade A C et al 1985 Effects of cisapride, a new gastrointestinal prokinetic substance, on interdigestive and postprandial motor activity of the distal oesophagus in man. Gut 26: 246–251

Tijskens G, Janssens J, Vantrappen G, De Bondt F 1989 Validation of a fully automated analysis of esophageal body contractility and lower esophageal sphincter function: A study on the effect of the PGE$_1$ analogue Rioprostil on human esophageal motility. J Gastrointest Motil 1: 21–28

Vantrappen G, Hellemans J 1967 Studies on the normal deglutition complex. Am J Dig Dis 12: 255–266

Vantrappen G, Servaes J, Janssens J, Peeters T 1982 Twenty-four hour esophageal pH- and pressure recording in outpatients in: Wienbeck M (ed.) Motility of the digestive tract. Raven, New York, pp 293–297

Welch R W, Drake S T 1980 Normal lower esophageal sphincter: a comparison of rapid vs slow pull through techniques. Gastroenterology 78: 1446–1451

Welch R W, Luckmann K, Ricks P M, Drake S T, Gates G A 1979 Manometry of the normal esophageal sphincter and its alteration in laryngectomy. J Clin Invest 63: 1036–1041

24. The proximal sphincters

J. A. Wilson   R. C. Heading

INTRODUCTION

The upper oesophageal sphincter (UOS) and lower oesophageal sphincter (LOS) usually operate as a functional unit – the deglutition reflex involves not only UOS relaxation but also, within 2–3 s of the initiation of swallowing, relaxation of the LOS. The two oesophageal sphincters also share a fundamental barrier function. Both are closed at rest – the UOS to prevent the ingress of air to the intrathoracic oesophagus with each respiration and the LOS to prevent reflux of gastric contents down a similar pressure gradient.

THE UPPER OESOPHAGEAL SPHINCTER

Anatomy

The principal component of the UOS is the horizontal portion of the inferior constrictor of the pharynx – the cricopharyngeus muscle. This arises bilaterally from the lateral arches of the cricoid cartilage, forming a sling behind the lamina of the cricoid which, therefore,

comprises the anterior of wall of the pharyngo-oesophageal junction. This muscle is only 1 cm broad, while the upper high-pressure zone is 2–4 cm. The other structures which may contribute muscular force to the area are the oblique portion of the inferior constrictor (thyropharyngeus muscle) and the upper circular fibres of the striated oesophageal muscle. (Fig. 24.1). The evidence for the contribution of these accessory muscles to the UOS is indirect and the existence of an oesophageal component remains controversial (Goyal & Cobb 1981). Nonetheless the upper oesophageal fibres have been observed intraoperatively to exert a circular 'squeeze' and division of at least the upper 1 cm of the cervical oesophageal musculative is advocated during 'cricopharyngeal' myotomy.

The persistence of a residual pressure in this area following myotomy emphasizes the important contribution of the laryngeal cartilage framework to the observed pressures. The presence of the bulky larynx anterior to the UOS, sandwiching it against the prevertebral fascia, accounts for the marked radial asymmetry of the sphincter (Fig. 24.2).

Anteroposterior UOS pressures are thus two to three times greater than those in the lateral planes; and this asymmetry is abolished following total laryngectomy, when the sphincter is found to be completely annular (Gates 1980). Down to the level of the cricopharyngeus, the pharyngeal constrictors possess a posterior midline raphe. This seems to stop at the lower border of the thyropharyngeus, which is separated from the cricopharygeus by only a thin layer of connective tissue – Killian's dehiscence. The existence of this dehiscence, the site of pharyngeal posterior midline pulsion (Zenker's) diverticula, has however been disputed by Lund (1965) who was unable to confirm its presence during human anatomical dissection. The dehiscence per se is unlikely to explain entirely the presence of such diverticula, which have a 2:1 male preponderance (Maran et al 1986). The well-known gender differences in laryngeal anatomy seem likely also to play a part.

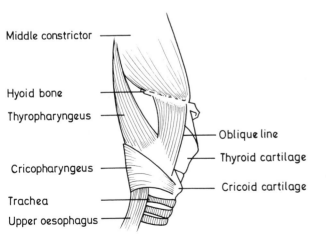

Middle constrictor

Hyoid bone

Thyropharyngeus

Oblique line

Thyroid cartilage

Cricopharyngeus

Cricoid cartilage

Trachea

Upper oesophagus

Fig. 24.1   Anatomy of the UOS.

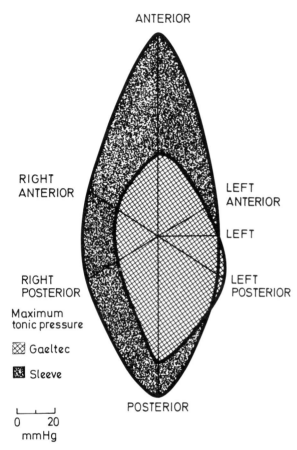

ANTERIOR

RIGHT
ANTERIOR

LEFT
ANTERIOR

LEFT

RIGHT
POSTERIOR

LEFT
POSTERIOR

Maximum
tonic pressure

⊠ Gaeltec

◼ Sleeve

POSTERIOR

0   20
mmHg

Fig. 24.2 Diagram of UOS pressure profiles in 50 healthy volunteers showing (1) marked radial asymmetry and (2) the differences in pressures recorded using a strain gauge assembly (2.8 mm diameter) (Gaeltec) and a sleeve catheter (7.2 mm diameter).

It is known that the pharyngeal musculature has a rich innervation comparable to that of the extraocular muscles, but the precise vagal branches through which these nerves are distributed to the UOS in man remain unknown. In this respect, animal experiments are unhelpful – the dog, for example has a separate pharyngo-oesophageal nerve arising from its common vagosympathetic trunk. A recent autopsy study suggests that both the pharyngeal plexus and the recurrent laryngeal nerve contribute to the innervation of the pharyngo-oesophageal junction (Mebis et al 1991). The area also has a rich arterial supply from the inferior thyroid artery which is necessary to supply the predominantly type 1, richly oxidative slow-twitch fibres of the cricopharyngeus.

Centrally, the motor innervation for the palatal, pharyngeal, oesophageal and laryngeal muscles originates within the nucleus ambiguus. The dendrites of motoneurones serving the pharyngo-oesophageal junction project widely into the adjacent reticular formation (Altschuler et al 1991) reflecting the complex requirements for functional synchronization of deglutition with associated phenomena, notably respiration.

Physiology

As there is only one, common upper aerodigestive tract as far down as the hypopharyngeus, respiration must be suspended transiently during each swallow. The pharyngeal phase of swallowing is, therefore, accomplished in about 0.5 s. It is important to understand the accompanying laryngeal events, not least because they influence greatly the observation of events in the pharyngo-oesophageal segment. A recent study of normal swallowing using concurrent transnasal videolaryngoscopy and pharyngeal manometry showed that the onset of vocal cord closure is the first recordable event in the normal swallow sequence, preceding even genioglossus electromyographic (EMG) activity (Shaker et al 1990). Similarly the supraglottic structures of the larynx – principally aryepiglottic folds and false cords – can be regarded as forming an accessory 'proximal sphincter' for it is this contraction which forms the principal barrier to the ingress of ingested material. The propulsion by the tongue of the food bolus into the oropharyngeal region (Fig. 24.3) marks the end of the voluntary phase of swallowing and the onset of the deglutition reflex. Laryngeal penetration is prevented not only by closure of the inlet but also by the marked laryngeal elevation (Isberg et al 1985).

This upward excursion of the larynx, which becomes tucked up in the concavity of the hyoid bone, beneath the base of the tongue is a sine qua non of the normal swallow (which the reader can test by trying to effect a dry swallow while anchoring the larynx).

What is in physiological terms an invaluable protective mechanism is to the investigator, however, a source of two confusing artifacts. Firstly, the elevation of the larynx is largely achieved by shortening of the thyrohyoid muscle. The cricoid cartilage and its attached cricopharyngeus muscle must, therefore, also elevate. This results in an average of 12 mm of sphincter-on-catheter movement during manometry (Isberg et al 1985). Secondly, the larynx moves forwards as it rises (which can be confirmed by self-palpation). This also subserves a useful physiological function, as it helps to lift the larynx framework off what may be an unyielding bolus. There is, therefore, a clear distinction between anatomical opening of the UOS and its muscular relaxation. Measurement of the completeness of UOS relaxation is also rendered difficult by its upward move-

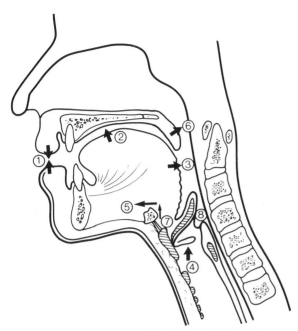

Fig. 24.3 Principal events of deglutition: (1) lips seal to achieve oral competence during mastication; (2) tongue pushes food bolus posteriorly; (3) base of tongue transmits 'driving force' to bolus – initiation of swallow reflex; (4) vocal cord apposition; (5) hyoid moves forward and upward; (6) soft palate closes off nasopharynx; (7) thyrohyoid membrane shortens; (8) epiglottis flips down over laryngeal inlet.

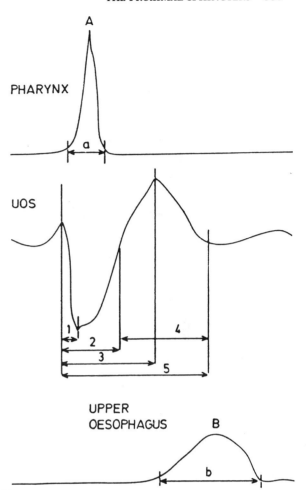

Fig. 24.4 Pressure events in the pharyngo-oesophageal segment during swallowing: **A** amplitude of pharyngeal contraction; **B** amplitude of upper oesophageal contraction; AB = pharyngo-oesophageal velocity; 1–5, a and b = various temporal parameters of UOS swallow dynamics which can be measured.

ment, as the recording catheter tends to slip into the cervical oesophagus during the swallow.

The pressure phenomena observed in the pharyngo-oesophageal segment are summarized in Figure 24.4. The peak of the hypopharyngeal contraction wave coincides with the period of UOS relaxation although not necessarily with its nadir. The pharyngeal wave is believed to be a clearing wave which mops up residual bolus, rather than a propulsive peristaltic wave. The bolus is propelled by the posterior pressure of the tongue – the so-called 'tongue driving force' (McConnel et al 1988).

The pharyngeal contraction wave proceeds across the UOS, where it is marked as an after-contraction, into the upper oesophagus. The amplitude and duration of these waves is altered by bolus and subject factors. Increasing bolus volume prolongs UOS relaxation (Jacob et al 1989) while solid boluses provoke pharyngo-oesophageal waves of increased amplitude and duration (Wilson et al 1989). Increasing age is associated with a slight reduction in UOS resting pressure, an increase in pharyngeal contraction amplitude

and an increase in pharyngo-oesophageal wave velocity (Wilson et al 1990). These two latter phenomena may be thought of as compensatory mechanisms for impaired laryngeal inlet protection.

Radiology

While expert radiology can contribute significantly to the investigation of dysphagia, e.g. demonstrating delayed swallow initiation, inadequate palatal elevation, the presence of a diverticulum, pharyngeal pooling or laryngeal penetration; the contribution of radiology to the understanding of UOS function itself is more limited because of the speed of swallowing and multiple

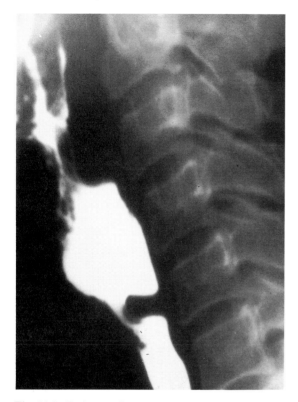

Fig. 24.5 Barium swallow examination showing marked cricopharyngeal impression

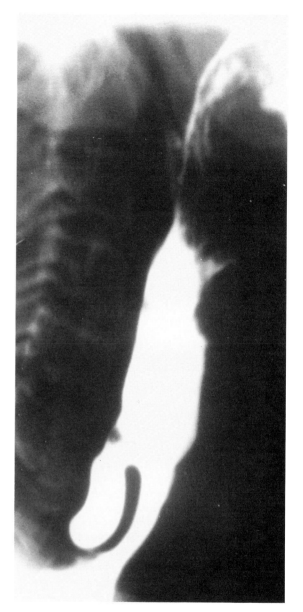

Fig. 24.6 Barium examination of a pharyngeal (Zenker's) diverticulum.

variables affecting UOS function (Curtis et al 1991). The most common reported UOS abnormality is variously described as 'cricopharyngeal impression', 'UOS achalasia' or 'UOS spasm' (Fig. 24.5). When a cricopharyngeal impression is observed, however, the video recording should firstly be rechecked, to ensure that the lesion is indeed a consistent functional or structural abnormality and not simply an impression caused by the occurrence of a double swallow. This is a frequent and normal manoeuvre, particularly during the ingestion of a solid or semi-solid bolus (Wilson et al 1989).

The second swallow shortens the duration of the original swallow complex and generates the appearance of an impression on the column of barium passing through the (hitherto) open UOS. If a video-recording is not available, the tell-tale sign on review of still films is the persistent elevation of the soft palate. Despite the limitations of contrast radiology in the UOS area, barium examination remains the principal method of following bolus progression, of demonstrating a pharyngeal web or diverticulum (Fig. 24.6), and

allowing detection of the wide variety of distal oesophageal structural and motor abnormalities which can give rise to cervical dysphagia (Ott et al 1986).

Manometry

The demands of reliable manometric measurement are considerable. Traditional perfused techniques are un-

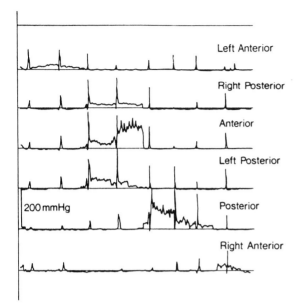

Fig. 24.7 Station pull-through of the UOS showing radial and axial asymmetry.

Left Anterior

Right Posterior

Anterior

Left Posterior

200 mmHg   Posterior

Right Anterior

suitable because of the sensitivity of the pharynx to infused water and the inadequate responsiveness of the external transducers to the rapid rise of pharyngeal pressure during dynamic motility studies. The UOS demonstrates not only the marked radial asymmetry resulting from its retrolaryngeal location but also shows axial asymmetry (Fig. 24.7) with peak posterior pressure 0.55 cm more distal than anterior pressure in normal subjects (Gerhardt et al 1980a). UOS axial asymmetry appears to be more marked in males than females, perhaps because of the sex difference in normal laryngeal anatomy (Wilson et al 1990). If adequate allowance is made for radial asymmetry, there is now considerable evidence that the recording of UOS pressure is similar whether continuous or station pull-through techniques are used (Gerhardt et al 1980a, Bretan et al 1990, Wilson et al 1992b).

Experimental UOS pressure measurement in dogs, however, indicates that greater UOS lengths are recorded during continuous rather than station pull-through (Bretan et al 1990). A radially orientated array of strain gauges mounted on a fine-bore catheter yields the most reproducible measure of tonic UOS pressure, with a mean value of around 40 mmHg in healthy volunteers (Wilson et al 1989). There is a problem of sphincter-on-catheter movement, however, during dynamic swallow studies which the sleeve catheter was designed to circumvent.

The sleeve has a 6 cm pressure-sensitive diaphragm which continues to register UOS pressure during its vertical excursions in swallowing and makes it a useful method for prolonged studies of UOS pressure during experiments such as Bernstein testing. The disadvantages of the sleeve are its broad diameter which produces a reflex increase in UOS pressure due to the length/tension relationship of striated muscle, such that UOS tonic pressures are twice as great when measured by a 7 mm sleeve sensor than by a 2.8 mm strain gauge assembly (Fig. 24.2). Also, recording fidelity is superior when the UOS is at its proximal end, nearest the point of perfusion as the inherent compliance of the sleeve membrane requires perfusion to give it necessary tension (Wilson et al 1989). Many studies also require the registration of pharyngeal pressure by a strain gauge which means either the passage of a second catheter (Kahrilas et al 1988) or the use of a multisensor strain gauge assembly for all of the measurements. Both the pharyngeal and UOS after contraction waves show an increase in amplitude (Fig. 24.8a) and duration (Fig. 24.8b) as the bolus swallowed is of increasingly thick consistency. This type of observation which can result from manometric study is of physiological interest, indicating in this instance the likely existence of peripheral feedback mechanisms which modify the deglutition reflex.

Of what value is manometry, used alone, as a clinical diagnostic tool? In practice, by no means the least important function of manometry is the identification of patients whose UOS tonic pressures are, in fact, normal. Some centres continue to advocate division of the cricopharyngeus on symptomatic grounds and myotomy is sometimes advocated for patients with cervical symptoms and a radiological cricopharyngeal impression (Fig. 24.5). Manometric study of 19 patients with such radiographic findings revealed UOS hypertonicity in only one-third, and failure of relaxation (UOS achalasia) was not identified manometrically (Wilson et al 1992a). Thus, manometry is a helpful prelude to myotomy in patients with cricopharyngeal 'impressions', whose abnormality may be a failure of UOS opening as opposed to failed relaxation (Dantas et al 1990). Occasionally, manometric findings show gross abnormality of the swallow mechanism (Fig. 24.9). In other situations, however, manometry in isolation is of relatively little value. This is in part because of the very wide range of normal values observed, coupled with a not inconsiderable measurement and biological variation. Over the past few years, therefore, many workers have attempted to combine radiology and manometry in a synchronous investigation.

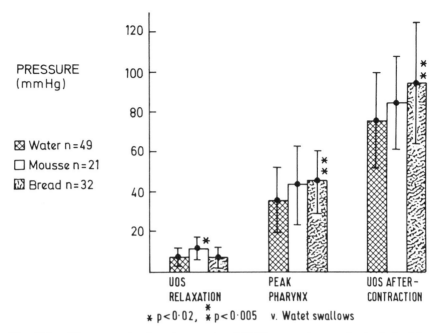

Fig. 24.8a Histograms showing pharyngeal and UOS contraction amplitudes in healthy volunteers swallowing boluses of different consistency.

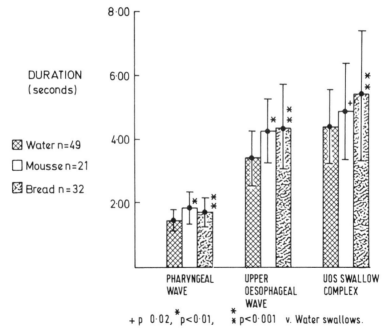

Fig. 24.8b Histograms in the same volunteers as Fig. 24.8 showing the interaction of bolus consistency with pharnygo-oesophageal wave duration.

Manofluorometry

The studies of Isberg et al (1985) to evaluate UOS movement during deglutition were among the first to combine manometry and radiology. The methods were developed extensively by McConnel et al (1988) in Atlanta, Georgia, whose techniques generate three

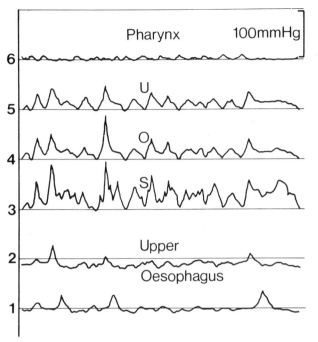

Fig. 24.9 Manometric tracing from a 79-year-old dysphagic male during attempted swallowing of a bread bolus. Despite multiple efforts, no adequate pharyngo-oesophageal segment reflex is achieved.

separate records of the investigation. The manofluorograph is a simultaneous presentation of manometry with the corresponding fluoroscopic image (Fig. 24.10).

This is used to derive both a manofluorogram, which tracks bolus passage in relation to the pressure tracing over an 8-s interval, and the pressure trace in isolation. The pressure sensors incorporate a radiopaque marker which allows visual determination of the point at which the pressure reading is made. A real-time resettable electronic counter marks 0.01 s on each frame. Analysis of normal swallows has shown that in some subjects the tongue driving force transmitted to the bolus develops with the pharyngeal clearing force at the level of the laryngeal inlet. Anterior elevation of the larynx is associated with a negative pressure in the UOS area which McConnel interprets as a 'hyopharyngeal suction pump'. The analysis of pharyngeal transit, bolus velocity and tongue during forces represents a major technological advance. Later studies by Isberg's group (Nilsson et al 1989) using cineradiography during manometry (with a skin marker on the cricoid arch) confirmed that UOS relaxation during deglutition was a genuine motor phenomenon, not an artefact and that the components of the upper high-pressure zone do

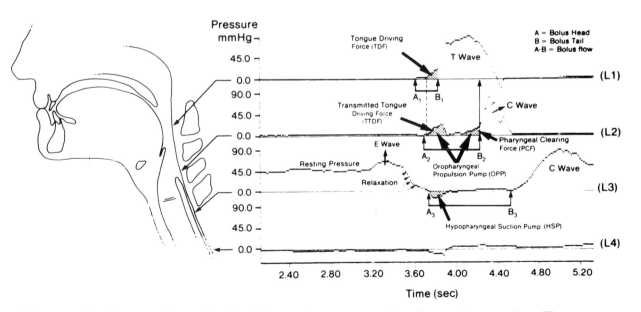

Fig. 24.10 Manofluorogram of a normal swallow. The normal pressure patterns from four transducers are shown. The pressures exercised on to the bolus over time (forces) are shaded. (From McConnel et al 1988, with permission.)

indeed include thyropharyngeus and upper oesophageal muscle fibres.

Manofluorometry has also shown that the UOS area moves 2–2.5 cm orally during swallowing, and that the extent of orad movement depends on the volume of barium swallowed (Kahrilas et al 1988). Larger boluses are accommodated by an increase in both the diameter and duration of UOS opening, and also by an increase in the interval between the onset of laryngeal elevation and hypopharyngeal contraction.

Tests of the ability of normal subjects to prolong volitionally the period of UOS opening by prolonging the anterior and superior displacement of the larynx at mid-swallow showed that the mechanics of swallowing could indeed be markedly altered in this way, indicating possibilities for biofeedback therapy for subjects with impaired UOS opening (Kahrilas et al 1990). UOS activity during swallowing can be divided into five phases: (1) relaxation; (2) opening; (3) distension; (4) collapse; and (5) closure (Jacob et al 1989). Relaxation precedes opening by an average of 0.1 s. Once open, UOS distension seems to be modified more by intrabolus pressure than by the degree of hyoid excursion, and the degree of opening is shown clearly by

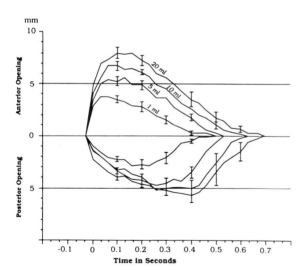

Fig. 24.11 UOS opening as a function of bolus volume. Time zero = first videoframe showing opening. Anterior opening occurred as the horizontal distance between the anterior UOS wall and a lead skin marked over the vertebral column increased and posterior opening as the distance between the posterior UOS wall and the skin marker decreased. Values are mean + SEM of two swallows for each of eight subjects. Anterior opening peaks with 0.13 s of opening onset, while posterior opening peaked later. (From Jacob et al 1989 with permission.)

manofluorometry to be a function of bolus volume (Fig. 24.11).

UOS responsiveness

In addition to its protective function against oesophageal distension by air, it has been suggested that a further function of the UOS is the prevention of oesophagopharyngeal reflux, which has been suggested to result from failure of UOS pressure augmentation in response to intraoesophageal fluid infusion (Gerhardt et al 1980b). While resting UOS tonic pressure seems likely to provide a barrier against pharyngeal reflux, several studies now confirm the absence of a UOS response to acid, either during experimental acid infusion (Fig. 24.12) or as a result of spontaneous gastro-oesophageal reflux (GOR) (Kahrilas et al 1987, Vakil et al 1989). The longstanding observation of a UOS response to upper oesophageal distension (Gerhardt et al 1978) has, on the other hand, stood the test of time. Animal experiments suggest the response to be at least in part vagally mediated (Freiman et al 1981). The sphincter appears, however, to respond to distension in two distinct ways.

While a fluid bolus causes a pressure augmentation, distension by air, as in belching, induces a prompt UOS relaxation (Kahrilas et al 1986) and these different responses are not impaired by topical anaesthesia of the oesophageal mucosa. Further balloon distension studies suggest it was the speed and spatial orientation of the stimulus which provoked the differential response. Proximal to the point of distension there is contractile activity of the oesophageal body, whose propogation is progressively inhibited as distension proceeds (Andreollo et al 1988).

Augmentation of UOS pressure can also be provoked by acute emotional stress (Cook et al 1987). During the first 2 min of a dichotic listening test, the mean increase in UOS pressure is over 20 mmHg. To date, there have been very few attempts to perform prolonged testing of UOS function. Kahrilas et al (1987) used a modified sleeve device to study UOS function during sleep and during a meal. Mean UOS pressure fell from 40 mmHg to 20 mmHg during stage 1 sleep, and to as low as 8 mmHg during deeper sleep. This implies a reduced barrier function to regurgitation and aspiration overnight. The significance of these early findings requires further evaluation by recently available techniques for ambulatory pharyngo-oesophageal manometry. These can be used with pharyngo-oesophageal dual probe pH-metry (Fig. 24.13) to assess oesophago-pharyngeal reflux.

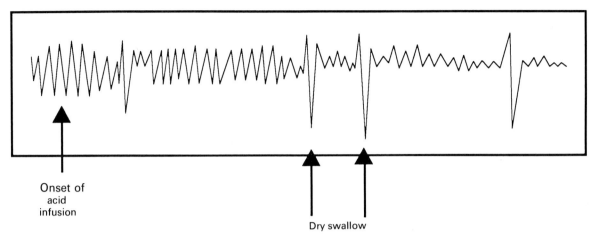

Fig. 24.12 Manometric tracing obtained from a sleeve sensor in the UOS showing (1) inspiratory UOS pressure augmentation (2) the absence of UOS pressure response during upper oesophageal infusion with 0.1M HCl, 8 cm below UOS.

The effects of cricopharyngeal myotomy

Surgical division of the UOS was introduced over 40 years ago for the treatment of dysphagia due to bulbar poliomyelitis and gradually gained in popularity for the treatment of elderly patients with radiological cricopharyngeus 'hypertrophy' (Helsper et al 1974, Calcaterra et al 1975). It remained widely used even once the rather negative correlates were made known – indeed Orringer (1980) in the report of his series of 40 myotomies suggested that the failure of manometry to show hypertonicity or achalasia was due to contemporary limitations in the technique. Careful pre-and postoperative manometric evaluation of 12 subjects with oculopharyngeal dystrophy (Fradet et al 1988) showed significant reductions not only in UOS resting pressure but also in the number of pharyngeal contractions required to generate an oesophageal pressure wave. In a heterogeneous group of patients undergoing the procedure in Malmö, only two of the four who had radiological cricopharyngeal achalasia improved symptomatically. Interestingly, there was no association between radiological and symptomatic improvement (Lindgren & Ekberg 1990).

LOWER OESOPHAGEAL SPHINCTER

Anatomy and physiology

The very existence of an anatomical LOS is debated. Most workers, however, consider that this dynamic, mobile high-pressure zone does have genuine muscular components, and that the thickening observed at autopsy is not, as has been suggested, merely a shrinkage artefact. The principal components of the LOS are the annular thickening of the distal oesophageal muscle, the oblique gastric fibres of the third gastric muscle layer and the musculofascial diaphragmatic sling. This sling contributes to the angle of His, between the distal oesophagus and gastric fundus, as described by Liebermann-Meffert et al (1979) (Fig. 24.14). Electron microscopic study of the LOS musculature reveals irregular evaginated muscle surfaces which may simply reflect the state of tonic sphincter contraction (Seelig & Goyal 1978). Myogenic features that may contribute to tonic contraction include a specialized calcium transport mechanism and continuous electrical spike activity. The myogenic tone of the sphincter is supported entirely by aerobic mechanisms in vitro (Christensen 1982). The LOS muscle mitochandria are large, centrally placed and have a low concentration of cytochrome oxidase. The distinctive biochemical characteristics support the concept of a sphincter independent of extrinsic innervation. The oesophagus is now believed to terminate as a single sac ('oesophageal vestibule'). Although the term 'phrenic ampulla' is used to designate the portion above the diaphragm and 'submerged vestibule', the subhiatal portion, the anatomical nature of these entities is constantly changed due to axial LOS movement. The squamocolumnar mucosal union (Z line) is not regarded as a reliable indicator of the gastro-oesophageal junction.

The upper margin of the manometric LOS corresponds to the tubulovestibular junction, while its lower margin approximates to the gastric sling fibres.

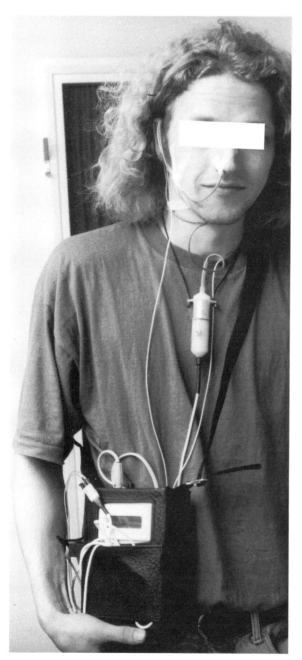

Fig. 24.13   Subject undergoing combined ambulatory UOS manometry and dual probe pharyngo-oesophageal pH-metry.

approaches the hiatus) and to the angulation of the terminal oesophagus as it joins the stomach. The cause of the residual asymmetry which persists when diaphragmatic factors have been excluded – as, for example, in hiatus hernia – remains unknown but may relate to the spiral LOS fibres and the pull of the gastric sling fibres.

LOS tonic pressure shows rhythmic inspiratory fluctuation. In the lower part of the human LOS, inspiration causes a pressure augmentation, while in the upper part, inspiration causes a pressure fall. The transition between the two segments of the LOS is the respiratory inversion point (Fig. 24.16), or more precisely respiratory inversion zone as it is often about 0.5 cm wide and has a somewhat variable location, usually the midpoint of the LOS (Harris & Pope 1966). The factors contributing to the phenomenon include inspiratory compression by the diaphragm, and the axial movement of the LOS (Welch & Gray 1982). The sphincter is 3–5 cm in length with a mean resting pressure of around 30 mmHg in normal volunteers (Richter et al 1987). As in the UOS, pressures recorded increase with the diameter of the recording catheter, a manifestation of the so-called Heisenberg uncertainty principle, that one cannot make a measurement without at the same time changing what one wishes to measure (Kaye & Showalter 1974).

In vitro analysis of the terminal oesophageal musculative of experimental animals has shown that resting LOS tone persists after total extrinsic denervation.

The closer to the diaphragm the vagotomy is performed the less the effect on LOS tone. Stimulation of the intramural oesophageal nerves causes contraction of the oesophagus and stomach, and LOS relaxation. The LOS response to balloon distension of the striated oesophagus was assessed by Price et al (1979) in dogs with and without vagosympathetic blockade. In the intact animals, distension produced relaxation, shortening and oral movement of the LOS. All of these responses were abolished by vagosympathetic blockade, implying that there is no intramural pathway for the reflex, at least in the dog. This finding is not applicable to species which have smooth muscle in the distal oesophagus and possess an intramural nervous mechanism which mediates descending inhibition, similar to that in the intestine. The vagus nerve is believed to mediate LOS relaxation after primary peristalsis is initiated in the swallowing centre, via noncholinergic non-adrenergic inhibitory neurones whose neurotransmitters may be vasoactive intestinal polypeptide, dopamine or dipeptide histidine–isoleucine The deglutition-induced LOS relaxation may occur almost simultaneously with that of the UOS at the onset of the reflex but is usually deferred for 2–3 s.

The LOS has a lesser degree of radial asymmetry than the UOS (Fig. 24.15). The greater pressures recorded on the left side probably relate to the indentation of the diaphragm (the oesophagus moves to the left as it

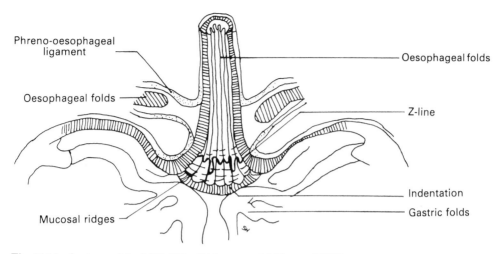

Fig. 24.14 Anatomy of the LOS. (After Liebermann-Meffert et al 1979)

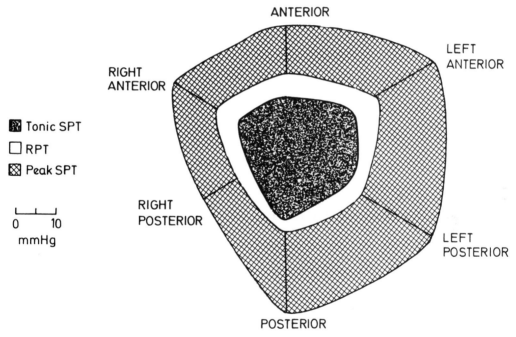

Fig. 24.15 Radial asymmetry of the LOS in 50 healthy volunteers, measured by rapid pull-through in full expiration at 1 cm/s and by station pull-through at 1 cm intervals.

Relaxation may be preceded by a brief pressure rise in the segment below the respiratory reversal zone. The relaxation lasts 5–10 s and is followed by an after-contraction which terminates the peristaltic wave of the oesophageal body. The occurrence of continuous spike activity which is inhibited by deglutition has been confirmed with EMG in the oppossum (Asoh & Goyal 1978).

Manometry

The variables influencing the accurate registration of LOS pressure include not only respiratory fluctuation but also catheter diameter, axial motion artefact, recording system fidelity and the type of pull-through used. Continuous or rapid pull-through has the advantage of generating a single readily measured pressure peak.

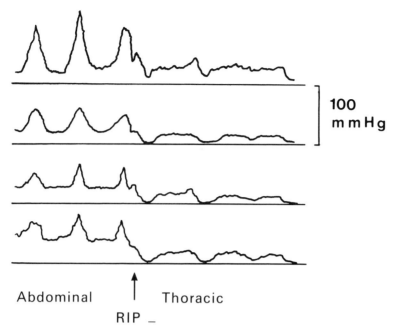

Fig. 24.16 Station pull-through of the LOS showing inspiratory pressure augmentation in the lower part of the sphincter, the respiratory inversion point (**RIP**) and the inspiratory pressure fall above this.

The analysis of tonic LOS pressure from a station pull-through is more open to observer error (if computerized wave form analysis is not available) because it requires the derivation of a mean pressure from a series of peaks, whose polarity and, therefore, configuration change during the test (Fig. 24.16). Richter et al (1987) report average normal values of LOS pressure of 29 mmHg for rapid pull-through, while station pull-through pressures were 39 mmHg at end inspiration, 24 mmHg at mid expiration and 15 mmHg at end expiration. Computerized manometric analysis readily allows not only the calculation of an accurate average pressure but also generates other parameters, e.g. area under the pressure curve or a three-dimensional vector volume analysis.

LOS achalasia

One cardinal feature of LOS achalasia is a poorly relaxing LOS. The defect involves the entire oesophageal body which shows failure of peristalsis. The disease has no extraoesophageal manifestations and its cause remains unknown. Both muscle and nerve abnormalities can be detected, but the neural lesions are thought to be of primary importance. There is a reduction in the number of ganglion cells in the intramural oesophageal nerve plexus.

Lewy bodies have been observed in the intramural plexuses of some patients with achalasia. Detailed electron microscopic examination has demonstrated degeneration of myelin sheaths and disruption of axon membranes. There is some thickening of the circular muscle of the lower oesophagus but this is thought secondary to the underlying neuropathy.

Functional impairment of the ganglion cells in the oesophageal body and LOS has been confirmed experimentally. For example, in achalasia patients, there is no response of isolated LOS muscle strips to ganglionic stimulation whereas exaggerated contractions can be measured in the oesophageal body and LOS in patients given acetylcholine analogues – an indication of denervation hypersensitivity. Also, cholecystokinin produces an unexpected increase in LOS pressure. The disease is of equal sex incidence affecting around one per 100,000 population. Onset is usually in the third to fifth decades and the predominant symptom is dysphagia, reflecting the failure of LOS relaxation and the gradual distension of the aperistaltic oesophagus. Peristalsis may return following successful reduction of LOS pressure. In the variant called vigorous achalasia, there are repetitive high-amplitude simultaneous contraction waves.

The length of the high-pressure zone is increased

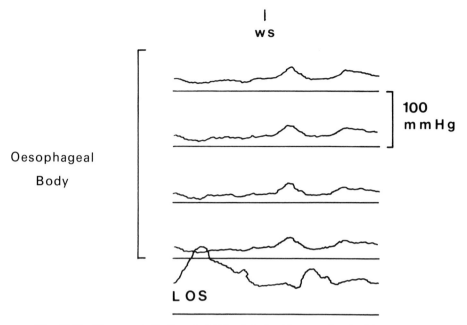

WS

Oesophageal

Body

100 mmHg

LOS

Fig. 24.17 Manometric findings in LOS achalasia. Absence of peristaltic response to water swallow (low-amplitude simultaneous contraction), hypertonic LOS with failure of swallow-induced relaxation.

compared with normal subjects, as is intraoesophageal resting pressure. The latter can be attributed to retained food and secretions within the oesophageal lumen. The classical manometric feature is the absence of swallow-induced LOS relaxation (Fig. 24.17). Manometry is the most useful diagnostic tool and barium examination serves essentially as screening function. Endoscopy is, however, valuable because it allows evaluation of the oesophageal mucosa before therapy. It also allows exclusion of so called 'pseudoachalasia' where there is an apparent failure of LOS relaxation due to a carcinoma of the gastric fundus.

Definitive treatment is by pneumatic dilatation or surgical myotomy. At present, the only role of medical therapy seems to be as a partial, temporary treatment in patients unfit for surgery and the hydrostatic bag technique, has become less popular (Stuart et al 1992). The most commonly used dilators are the Browne McHardy and Hurst-Tucker mercury pneumatic dilators which have a maximum external diameter of 3 cm. The inflation pressure required to obliterate the stricture which is visualized under fluoroscopic control may be as high as 600 mmHg. Some of the best results are, however, reported using progressive pneumatic dilatation, for example, with the Sippy dilating bag. Complications include pain, perforation, bleeding and aspiration.

The standard surgical procedure is oesophagomyotomy which remains the first-line treatment where there is severe oesophagitis or another associated pathology, e.g. epiphrenic diverticulum. It is also the method of choice in the rare young child or patient who cannot adequately be followed up. It is now almost 80 years since Heller described the original procedure which was an anterior and posterior myotomy. In patients with vigorous achalasia, the myotomy should extend to the level of the aortic arch. When the transabdominal approaches are used, an antireflux procedure is usually combined with the myotomy. Complications include mucosal perforation, failure to relieve symptoms, GOR and diaphragmatic herniation. The incidence of GOR following the transthoracic approach is about 8%. This is not much reduced by the addition of an anti-reflux procedure. An anti-reflux manoeuvre does, however, significantly reduce the incidence of GOR where the transabdominal approach is used.

Unfortunately, there has been only one prospective randomized trial comparing dilatation with myotomy and this was inconclusive. In a review of force dilatation therapy for achalasia, good or excellent results were achieved in about 80% of patients (Vantrappen & Janssens 1983). A not dissimilar figure was reported following Heller's procedure (Andreollo & Earlam 1987).

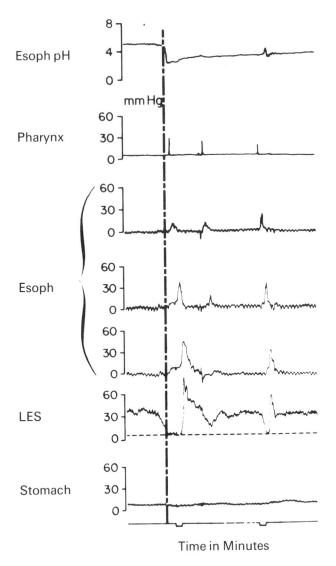

Esoph pH

Pharynx

Esoph

LES

Stomach

Time in Minutes

Fig. 24.18 GOR associated with a transient LOS relaxation in a patient with reflux oesophagitis. The relaxation *precedes* the pharyngeal swallow complex.

found less likely to generate a belch for any volume of air instilled into the mid-oesophagus. Indeed, such patients are more likely to have an augmentation rather than a fall of UOS pressure in response to air injection. This deficiency may contribute to some of the chest and upper airway symptoms reported by some patients during acute oesophageal distension.

LOS sphincter as an anti-reflux barrier

Use of a sleeve device for the measurement of LOS pressure circumvents the problem of relative axial motion between the side hole of the manometric catheter and the LOS during the respiration as the basis for the observed pressure oscillations.

There is an increase in LOS pressure with each inspiration associated with an increase in crural diaphragm EMG activity. The increase in LOS pressure is directly proportional to the depth of inspiration and the force of diaphragmatic contraction, and occurs very rapidly because of the fast rate of force generation by the striated muscle. While it is clearly important that the anti-reflux barrier increases when the intra-abdominal pressure rises, it is not clear whether the increase in LOS pressure is the result of a reflex LOS contraction or simply to the passive transmission of a rise in intra-abdominal pressure. There is some evidence, however, that the rate of increase in LOS pressure is faster than the corresponding rate of increase of intragastric pressure (Mittal 1990). The positive pressure caused by oesophageal contraction protects against GOR whereas the negative intrathoracic and intraoesophageal pressure will tend to promote GOR. It has been suggested that there are two functional sphincteric mechanisms at the lower end of the oesophagus such that the pressure gradients caused by the smooth muscle of the stomach and oesophagus are counteracted by the smooth muscle of the LOS while the skeletal muscle pressure gradients are counteracted by the diaphragmatic crura.

Transient LOS relaxations and GOR

In addition to the LOS relaxation induced by deglutition and oesophageal distension, the sphincter is also subject to frequent, abrupt, spontaneous relaxations. A study comparing the characteristics of such relaxations in healthy volunteers with those in patients suffering from GOR showed that the events comprised the only mechanism for reflux in healthy volunteers (Mittal & McCallum 1988). They also were found to account for 73% of reflux episodes in patients with GORD.

One interesting recent observation in patients with achalasia is that 95% report difficulty with belching (Massey et al 1992). In normal belching, there is transient relaxation of the LOS followed immediately by relaxation of the UOS to allow passage of gas to the hypopharynx. Many patients with achalasia report a difficulty with belching even after drinking carbonated beverages which it is thought release gas directly into the oesophagus, thus bypassing the need for GOR in order to generate a belch. Achalasia patients have been

The relaxations are characterized by an attenuation of the sub-mental EMG complex, a small pharyngeal contraction and an oesophageal contraction. The distinguishing feature between healthy individuals and those with GOR appears not to be the frequency of the relaxations as originally proposed (Dodds et al 1982) (Fig. 24.18) but the extent to which they are associated with reflux. Their frequency diminishes during sleep and possibly also during recumbency. The pattern of manometric events which accompanies repetitive episodes of spontaneous GOR and clearance has been termed cycling (Shay et al 1989).

Only a minority of reflux episodes occur because of a chronic absence of LOS pressure. In patients with erosive or ulcerative oesophagitis, only about two-thirds of reflux episodes occur during transient relaxation, in contrast to the almost exclusive relationship between transient relaxations and reflux in healthy volunteers. In other words, the more severe the GOR, the less effective the resting LOS barrier and the less the importance of transient LOS relaxations. Perhaps surprisingly, reflux is uncommon during swallow-induced LOS relaxation associated with a normal peristaltic sequence and this mechanism accounts for only 5–10% of reflux episodes (Holloway & Dent 1990). Not only does the peristaltic wave tend to clear the oesophagus of any refluxed material very rapidly but also the duration of LOS relaxation in response to a swallow is very brief, usually lasting for less than 5 s. Thus the majority of reflux episodes which are related to swallow-induced LOS relaxations are associated with defective oesophageal peristalsis (Dent et al 1980).

Transient LOS relaxations are usually of longer duration by up to 30 s and their recurrence appears to be unrelated to basal LOS pressure. In asymptomatic volunteers only about 35% of transient relaxations are reflux associated and the factors which determine the occurrence of reflux during relaxations are incompletely understood.

Occasionally reflux is prevented by a swallow manoeuvre which intervenes between the onset of relaxation and the onset of the consequent reflux. The abrupt onset, brief duration and abolition by vagosympathetic blockade in animal experiments confirm the neural mediation of the transient relaxations. They are probably triggered by gastric distension but their stimulation by a pharyngeal activity which is a variation of swallowing remains controversial. It is interesting to speculate that it is defective control of transient LOS relaxations which causes pathological GOR but little is known about the precise mechanisms of control of the relaxations.

The basis for defective basal LOS pressure is poorly understood. Impaired vagal cholinergic input, smooth muscle weakness and defects in the mechanical LOS properties have all been proposed. Extrasphincteric factors such as increased abdominal pressure, either steady state due to obesity or transient during straining, are also likely to play a part. The presence of hiatus hernia with displacement of the LOS into the chest causes a loss of the belching effect of the diaphragmatic crura. The sphincter area also moves away from the abdominal pressure transients which might help to maintain sphincter closure.

REFERENCES

Altschuler S M, Bao X M, Miselis R R 1991 Dendritic architecture of nucleus ambiguus motoneurons projecting to the upper alimentary tract in the rat. J Comp Neurol 309: 402–414

Andreollo N A, Earlam R J 1987 Heller's myotomy for achalasia: is an anti-reflux procedure necessary? Br J Surg 74: 765–769

Andreollo N A, Thompson D G, Kendall G P N 1988 Functional relationships between cricopharyngeal sphincter and oesophageal body in response to graded intraluminal distension. Gut 29: 161–166

Asoh R, Goyal R K 1978 Electrical activity of the opossum lower esophageal sphincter in vivo. Gastroenterology 74: 835–840

Bretan O, Henry M A C A, Cury P R 1990 Techniques in electromanometry of the upper esophageal sphincter. Arch Otolaryngol Head Neck Surg 116: 914–916

Calcaterra T C, Kadell B M, Ward P H 1975 Dysphagia secondary to cricopharyngeal muscle dysfunction. Arch Otolaryngol 101: 726–729

Christensen J 1982 Oxygen dependence of contraction in esophageal and gastric pyloric and ileocecal muscle of opossum. Proc Soc Exp Biol Med 170: 194–202

Cook I J, Dent J, Shannon S et al 1987 Measurement of upper esophageal sphincter pressure: effect of acute emotional stress. Gastroenterology 93: 526–532

Curtis D J, Ekberg O, Montesi A 1991 Swallowing: a radiological perspective. Gastroenterol Int 4: 47–54

Dantas R O, Cook I J, Dodds W J et al 1990 Biomechanics of cricopharyngeal bars. Gastroenterology 99: 1269–1274

Dent J, Dodds W J, Friedman R H, Sekiguchi T, Hogan W, Arndorfer R 1980 Mechanism of gastroesophageal reflux in recumbent asymptomatic human subjects. J Clin Invest 65: 256–267

Dodds W J, Dent J, Hogan W J et al 1982 Mechanisms of gastroesophageal reflux in patients with reflux esophagitis. New Engl J Med 307: 1547–1552

Fradet G, Pouliot D, Lavoie S et al 1988 Inferior constrictor myotomy in oculopharyngeal muscular dystrophy: clinical and manometric evaluation. J Otolaryngol 17: 68–73

Freiman, J M, El-Sharkawy T Y, Diamant N E 1981 Effect of bilateral vagosympathetic nerve blockade and response of the dog upper esophageal sphincter (UES) to intraesophageal distension and acid. Gastroenterology 81: 78–84

Gates G A 1980 Upper esophageal sphincter: pre and post-laryngectomy – a normative study. Laryngoscope 90: 454–464

Gerhardt D C, Schuck T J, Bordeaux R A et al 1978 Human upper esophageal sphincter. Response to volume, osmotic and acid stimuli. Gastroenterology 75: 268–274

Gerhardt D, Hewett J, Moeschberger M et al 1980a Human upper esophageal sphincter pressure profile. Am J Physiol 239: G49–G52

Gerhardt D C, Castell D O, Winship D H et al 1980b Esophageal dysfunction in esophagopharyngeal regurgitation. Gastroenterology 78: 893–897

Goyal R K, Cobb B W 1981 Motility of the pharynx, esophagus and oesophageal sphincters in: Johnson L R (ed.) Physiology of the gastrointestinal tract. New York, Raven Press, pp 359–391

Harris L D, Pope C E 1966 The pressure inversion point: its genesis and reliability. Gastroenterology 51: 641–648

Helsper J T, Lance J S, Baldridge E T et al 1974 Cricopharyngeal achalasia. Am J Surg 128: 521–526

Holloway R H, Dent J 1990 Pathophysiology of gastroesophageal reflux. Gastroenterol Clin North Am 19: 517–535

Isberg A, Nilsson M E, Schiratzki H 1985 Movement of the upper esophageal sphincter and a manometric device during deglutition. Acta Radiol Diag 26: 381–388

Jacob P, Kahrilas P J, Logemann J A et al 1989 Upper esophageal sphincter opening and modulation during swallowing. Gastroenterology 97: 1469–1478

Kahrilas P J, Dodds W J, Dent J et al 1986 Upper esophageal sphincter function during belching. Gastroenterology 91: 133–140

Kahrilas P J, Dodds W J, Dent J et al 1987 Effect of sleep, spontaneous gastroesophageal reflux and a meal on upper esophageal sphincter pressure in normal human volunteers. Gastroenterology 92: 466–471

Kahrilas P J, Dodds W J, Dent J et al 1988 Upper esophageal sphincter function during deglutition. Gastroenterology 95: 52–62

Kahrilas P J, Logemann J A, Krugler C et al 1990 Volitional prolongation of upper esophageal sphincter opening during swallowing. Gastroenterology 97: (abstract) A363

Kaye M D, Showalter J P 1974 Measurement of pressure in the lower esophageal sphincter. Am J Dig Dis 19: 860–863

Liebermann-Meffert D, Allgower M, Schmid P, Blum A L 1979 Muscular equivalent of the lower esophageal sphincter. Gastroenterology 76: 31–38

Lindgren S, Ekberg O 1990 Cricopharyngeal myotomy in the treatment of dysphagia. Clin Otolaryngol 15: 221–227

Lund W S 1965 A study of the cricopharyngeal sphincter in man and in the dog. Ann R Coll Surg Eng 37: 225–240

McConnel F M S, Cerenko D, Mendelsohn M S 1988 Manofluorographic analysis of swallowing. Otolaryngol Clin North Am 21: 625–635

Maran A G D, Wilson J A, Al Muhanna A H 1986 Pharyngeal diverticula. Clin Otolaryngol 11: 219–225

Massey B T, Hogan W J, Dodds W J et al 1992 Alteration of the upper esophageal sphincter belch reflex in patients with achalasia. Gastroenterology 103: 1574–1579

Mebis J, Ramaekers D, Geboes V et al 1991 The human pharyngo oesophageal sphincter has a characteristic neural and vascular supply. Gastroenterology 100: (abstract) A468

Mittal R K, McCallum R W 1988 Characteristics and frequency of transient relaxations of the lower esophageal sphincter in patients with reflux esophagitis. Gastroenterology 95: 593–599

Mittal R K 1990 Current concepts of the antireflux barrier. Gastroenterol Clin North Am 19: 501–516

Nilsson M E, Isberg A, Schiratzki H 1989 The location of the upper oesophageal sphincter and its behaviour during bolus propulsion – a simultaneous cineradiographic and manometric investigation. Clin Otolaryngol 14: 61–65

Orringer M B 1980 Extended cervical esophagomyotomy for cricopharyngeal dysfunction. J Thorac Cardiovasc Surg 80: 669–678

Ott D J, Gelfand D W, Wu W C et al 1986 Radiological evaluation of dysphagia. JAMA 256: 2718–2721

Price L M, El-Sharkawy T Y, Mui H Y et al 1979 Effect of bilateral cervical vagotomy on balloon-induced lower esophageal sphincter relaxation in the dog. Gastroenterology 77: 324–329

Richter J E, Wu W C, Johns D N et al 1987 Esophageal manometry in 95 healthy adult volunteers; variability of pressure with age and frequency of 'abnormal contractions'. Dig Dis Sci 32: 583–592

Robinson B A, Percy W H, Christensen J 1984 Differences in cytochrome C oxidase capacity in smooth muscle of opossum esophagus and lower esophageal sphincter. Gastroenterology 87: 1009–1013

Seelig L L, Goyal R K 1978 Morphological evaluation of opossum lower esophageal sphincter. Gastroenterology 75: 51–58

Shaker R, Dodds W J, Dantas R O et al 1990 Coordination of deglutitive glottis closure with oropharyngeal closure. Gastroenterology 98: 1478–1484

Shay S S, Eggli D, Oliver G et al 1989 Cycling, a manometric phenomenon due to repetitive episodes of gastroesophageal reflux and clearance. Dig Dis Sci 34: 1340–1348

Stuart R C, O'Sullivan G C, Hennessy T P J 1992 Oesophageal motility disorders in: Hennessy T P J, Cuschieri A (eds) Surgery of the oesophagus. Butterworths Heinemann, Oxford pp 109–169

Vakil N B, Kahrilas P J, Dodds W J et al 1989 Absence of an upper esophageal sphincter response to acid reflux. Am J Gastroenterol 84: 606–610

Vantrappen G, Janssen S J 1983 To dilate or to operate? That is the question. Gut 24: 1013–1019

Welch R W, Gray J E 1982 Influence of respiration on recordings of lower esophageal sphincter pressure in humans. Gastroenterology 83: 590–594

Wilson J A, Pryde A, Macintyre C C A et al 1989 Normal pharyngoesophageal motility: a study of 50 healthy subjects. Dig Dis Sci 34: 1590–1599

Wilson J A, Pryde A, Macintyre C C A et al 1990 The effects of age, sex and smoking on normal pharyngoesophageal motility. Am J Gastroenterol 85: 686–691

Wilson J A, Pryde A, Allan P L et al 1992a Cricopharyngeal dysfunction. Otolaryngol Head Neck Surg 106: 163–168

Wilson J A, Pryde A, Maher L et al 1992b The influence of biological and recording variables on pharyngeal pressure measurement. Gullet 2: 116–120

Wolf B S 1970 The inferior esophageal sphincter – anatomic, roentgenologic and manometric correlation, contradictions and terminology. A J R 110: 1260–277

25. The stomach, pylorus and duodenum

S. S. C. Rao   K. Schulze-Delrieu

The stomach: receives and stores food; grinds solid boluses into smaller particles; mixes its contents with saliva, pepsin and hydrochloric acid; discriminates between solid, liquid, fat and protein contents; and selectively delivers chyme into the duodenum at an optimal rate for digestion and absorption of food. The duodenum also participates in the regulation of gastric emptying by varying its resistance to outward flow. These complex events are carried out by the coordinated motor activity of the distinct muscular components of the stomach and duodenum. This activity is regulated by the electromechanical properties of the gastric and duodenal smooth muscle, the gastroduodenal nerve plexuses and reflexes, the intrinsic and extrinsic nerves and hormones. In this chapter we discuss the neuromuscular properties of the stomach and duodenum and their role in the storage, digestion and emptying of food.

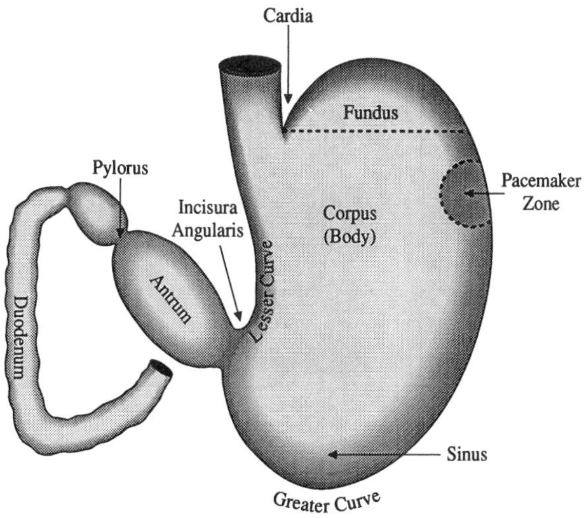

FUNCTIONAL MORPHOLOGY

Neuromuscular anatomy

Stomach

The stomach is anatomically divided into the fundus, body (corpus) and antrum. However, functionally there are only two distinct regions; the proximal and the distal stomach (Fig. 25.1). The proximal stomach includes the fundus and a segment of the body, and largely serves as a reservoir. It is electrically silent (Kelly 1981) and its musculature exhibits tonic mechanical activity (Schulze-Delrieu & Wall 1985). The proximal stomach muscle produces very little change in muscle tension even when stretched to about twice its length (Schulze-Delrieu & Shirazi 1987). This phenomenon of gastric accommodation is also known as adaptive relaxation. The distal stomach consists of the lower two-thirds of the body and antrum and is electrically active and can generate intense peristaltic contractions. It serves as a pump for grinding and emulsifying food and for delivering chyme to the small bowel.

Fig. 25.1 Schematic diagram of the stomach and duodenum. The segment orad to the cardia is the fundus. The fundus has a distensible muscle layer and serves as a reservoir. The segment between the incisura angularis and the pyloric orifice is the antrum. This has a thick muscle coat and serves as a pump. The segment between the fundus and the antrum is called the gastric body (corpus) and is a transition zone. The gastric sinus is the most dependent segment of the stomach in the upright position and is situated opposite the incisura. The gastric pacemaker zone is located in the body along the greater curvature.

Muscle layers of the stomach

The smooth muscle of the stomach (Fig. 25.2) is loosely organized into an outer longitudinal layer, a middle circular layer and an inner oblique layer (Torgersen 1942). The thickness of the gastric muscle coat increases from the cardia to the pylorus and from the greater to the lesser curve (Schulze-Delrieu 1983). The longitudinal muscle is arrayed in thick bundles

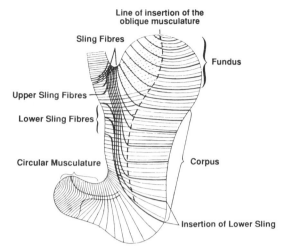

Fig. 25.2 An illustration of the arrangement of the smooth muscle layers of the stomach. The circular muscle layer is the most constant and is particularly thick and dense around the antrum. In the proximal stomach there is a third layer, the oblique muscle, which is the innermost muscle layer and forms an upper and lower sling. Not shown in this figure is the outer longitudinal muscle layer which covers the curvatures of the proximal stomach and the circumference of the antrum. (Modified from Torgerson 1942.)

over the curvatures, but only in thin strands across the anterior and posterior surfaces. In contrast, the circular muscle is more uniformly distributed throughout the stomach. The oblique muscle is the least complete and consists of muscle fibres which originate from the lower oesophageal sphincter area and fans across the proximal stomach forming two slings. An upper sling consists of fibres which spread across the fundus and a lower sling which radiates caudally to the incisura angularis (Fig. 25.2). At the incisura they split and radiate towards the greater curvature, penetrate the gastric wall and are inserted into the submucosal and serosal planes of the stomach.

Pyloric structure and closure

The pylorus is a butterfly shaped specialized muscular zone (Fig. 25.3A) which begins with the proximal loop of the pyloric sphincter (PPL) and terminates with the distal loop of the pyloric sphincter (DPL). The pyloric orifice, which is the narrowest segment of the gastroduodenal junction, is situated within the DPL and is anchored by the convergence of all the muscular layers of the stomach, and is reinforced by a septum of connective tissue. At this juncture, the submucosa

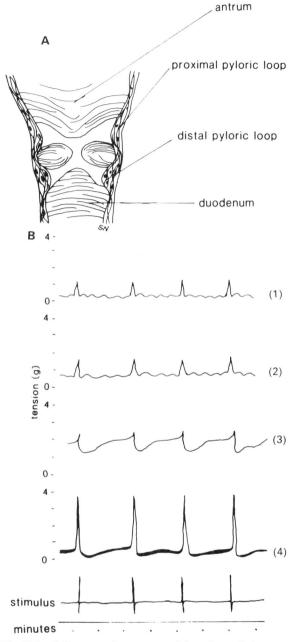

Fig. 25.3 **A** illustrates the structure of the pylorus. **B** shows differences in antroduodenal muscle responses to spontaneous and nerve-mediated stimulation. (See text for details.)

virtually disappears and the muscularis mucosae fuses with the circular muscle.

The individual muscular structures of the gastroduodenal junction differ in their spontaneous and nerve-

RELAXED

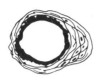
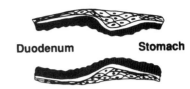

Duodenum   Stomach

CONTRACTED

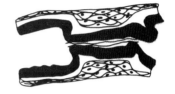

Transverse Section   **Longitudinal Section**

Fig. 25.4 Transverse and longitudinal sections through the relaxed and the contracted gastroduodenal junction. At rest, the distal pyloric loop produces a waist like indentation of the junction. When both loops contract, the pyloric orifice is obliterated and its mucosa is thrown up into multiple folds forming a star like slit. (Modified from Williams 1962.)

mediated mechanical activity (Fig. 25.3B). Spontaneous activity of the circular muscle from the antrum (1) and the proximal pyloric loop (2) consists of phasic contractions with little baseline tension. Nerve stimulation causes powerful phasic contractions. In contrast, nerve stimulation of the distal pyloric loop (3) markedly increases baseline tension, and minute contraction response, followed by prominent relaxation (4). Stimulation of the duodenal muscle however generates a marked contraction followed by a minute relaxation without any change in basal tension (Schulze-Delrieu & Shirazi 1987).

The pyloric closure is accomplished by contractions of both the pyloric sphincters and the muscularis mucosae (Williams 1962). Closure begins when the gastric ring contraction reaches the PPL. Immediately, both the PPL and the DPL contract, which causes a sharp reduction in the luminal diameter. The aperture is further reduced by the prolapse of the antral mucosal folds (Fig. 25.4), which project through the pyloric orifice into the base of the duodenal bulb, forming a mucosal plug and a watertight seal for the gastric outlet (Williams 1962, Biancani et al 1980).

The duodenum

The duodenum is a hollow 25-cm long muscular tube, and anatomically has four parts. The first part (bulb) is intraperitoneal and lacks circular folds. It exhibits contractile activity largely in coordination with the antral pump (Houghton et al 1988a). The remaining three portions are retroperitoneal with prominent plicae circulares. The duodenal contractile activity may serve as a mechanical brake for gastric emptying and for the downstream movement of the gastric chyme (Schulze-Delrieu 1992). In addition, they may produce retrograde flow which could further slow gastric emptying (Schulze-Delrieu 1992; Houghton et al 1988a).

Electrophysiological properties of the gastric smooth muscle and the gastric pacesetter potential

The contractile activity of the gastric smooth muscle is a mechanical manifestation of its electrophysiological and excitable properties. Fundal smooth muscle potentials are stable with a resting membrane potential of

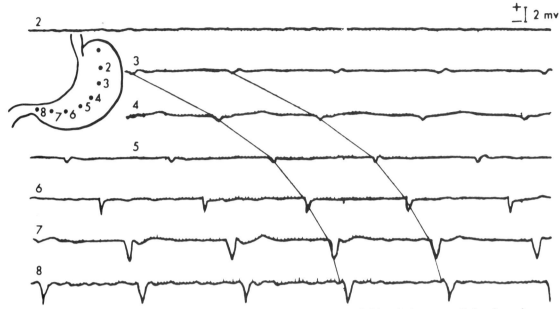

Fig. 25.5   Electrical activity of the smooth muscle of the stomach as recorded by placing extracellular electrodes on the serosal surface. The proximal stomach exhibits very little change in the membrane potential whereas the distal two thirds of the stomach generates continuous oscillations at 10–20 s intervals, which propagate towards the duodenum. (Reproduced with permission from Kelly 1981.)

− 50 mV, whereas those from the antropyloric region exhibit bursts of spontaneous oscillations with a resting potential of ± 70 mV (Papasova et al 1968; Morgan et al 1978a, 1978b). The highest frequency of electrical slow wave activity is generated from an area in the midcorpus along the greater curvature (Fig. 25.1), and this zone is considered to be the gastric pacemaker (Kelly & Code 1971; Hinder & Kelly 1977b). The slow waves are generated by cells which are situated in close proximity to the myenteric plexus (Bauer et al 1985a), and it is suspected that they are interstitial cells of Cajal (Christensen 1992). Slow waves propagate aborally and circumferentially along the longitudinal axis of the circular muscle, towards the duodenum. The conduction velocity is seven times greater along the longitudinal axis than the transverse axis (Publicover & Sanders 1985), possibly due to the arrangement of the smooth muscle cells; electrical propagation is more rapid along the length of the cell wall than across the cell, as fewer cell junctions are involved. These cells exhibit a gradient for the frequency and amplitude of contraction, and the threshold for excitability and initiation of a propagation potential, which increases from the proximal to the distal stomach (Fig. 25.5). This facilitates entrainment of the antral cells by the pacesetter potentials which originate from the proximal stomach.

In the stomach, the rate of contraction is approximately 3 cycles per minute (cpm) in man and 5 cpm in dogs (Kelly & Code 1971; Hinder & Kelly 1977b). The characteristics of gastric electrical activity depend on the method of recording (Fig. 25.6).

Intracellular recording shows a biphasic response comprising an upstroke (spike) potential and a plateau potential (Fig. 25.6). Extracellular recording reveals that a slow wave consists of a triphasic potential complex (positive–negative–positive deflection) and an isopotential segment (Szurszewski 1981, McCallum 1989). These slow waves are not associated with a gastric contraction. Contraction of a gastric smooth muscle fibre is triggered by the generation of an action potential which increases the size of the plateau potential of the slow wave. These electrical potentials are called pacesetter potentials (Fig. 25.6). This consists of a rapid initial upstroke (depolarization) followed by a plateau phase and a slower repolarization potential (Morgan & Szurszewski 1980). Thus, gastric contraction is a motor manifestation of the pacesetter potential generated by the gastric smooth muscle cells. Although muscle contraction is initiated by a pacesetter potential, not all of these potentials result in a contraction. Whether the smooth muscle cell is sensitive or insensitive to a pacesetter potential depends on the fasting or

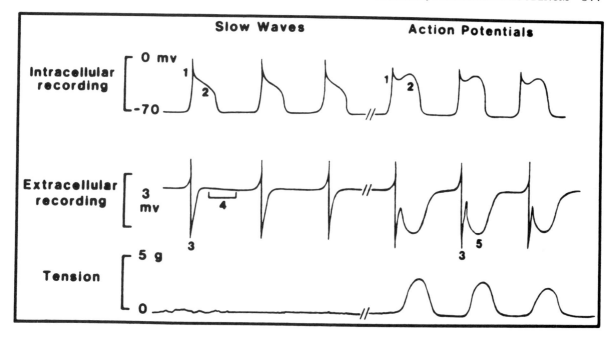

Fig. 25.6   Diagramatic illustration of the electromechanical activity of the stomach. During intracellular recording each slow wave consists of an upstroke potential (1) and a plateau potential (2) followed by a return to baseline. Their counterparts during extracellular recording are the initial potential (3) and the isopotential segment (4). The shape of an action potential differs from that of slow waves in that during intracellular recording the amplitude of the plateau potential is greater and during extracellular recording, the isopotential segment is replaced by a negative potential deflection called the second potential (5). The peaks of gastric contractile activity coincide with the peaks of plateau and second potentials. (Reproduced with permission from McCallum 1989 and W. B. Saunders, Philadelphia.)

postprandial state of the stomach as well as neurohumoral input. For example, stretch, at least in vitro, increases the propagation velocity of the electrical slow waves (Bauer & Sanders 1985b) more than can be predicted from the change in length. Gastrin, cholecystokinin (CCK) and acetylcholine (ACH) enhance the amplitude and the duration of the plateau potential and the force and duration of rhythmic contractions (Kelly 1981), whereas, noradrenaline (NA) neurotensin, prostaglandin E_2 and (PGE_2) vasoactive intestinal polypephde (VIP) produce opposite effects (Morgan et al 1978a,b, Morgan & Szurszewski 1980, Sanders & Vogalis 1989). Vagal stimulation (cholinergic input) increases the amplitude and duration of the antral plateau potentials. Bombesin also produces contraction of smooth muscles (Mayer et al 1982). Thus, the force of gastric contraction is determined by the duration and amplitude of the plateau potentials.

Innervation of the stomach

Intrinsic

The stomach is richly innervated by intrinsic and extrinsic nerves. The intrinsic innervation is provided by neurones located in the ganglia of the myenteric plexus, and this is an important component of the enteric nervous system (ENS). The ganglia are more densely distributed in the antrum. The neurones synapse with other intrinsic neurones in the plexus as well as with the extrinsic nerves. The axons from these neurones synapse with the muscle and the glandular structures of the stomach. Several pleomorphic branching cells, the interstitial cells of Cajal, are distributed within the intrinsic nerve network. These are believed to possess pacemaking activity and also mediate nerve to muscle communication (Christensen 1992). In addition several paracrine and neurotransmitter substances are found within the cell bodies of the enteric plexus. Histochemical techniques have identified Ach, NA, serotonin, substance P (SP), VIP, ATP and enkephalins (Edin et al 1980, Crowe & Burnstock 1981, Gabella 1981, Hoyes et al 1982). These chemicals are important

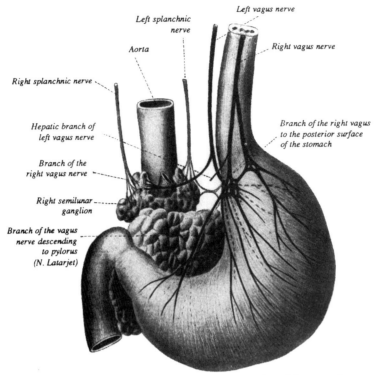

Left vagus nerve

Left splanchnic nerve

Aorta

Right vagus nerve

Right splanchnic nerve

Hepatic branch of left vagus nerve

Branch of the right vagus to the posterior surface of the stomach

Branch of the right vagus nerve

Right semilunar ganglion

Branch of the vagus nerve descending to pylorus (N. Latarjet)

Fig. 25.7   Diagram showing the extrinsic innervation of the stomach.

for neuro-muscular transmission and the regulation of motility.

Extrinsic

The extrinsic innervation is provided by the parasympathetic (vagus) and the sympathetic systems (Fig. 25.7). The cell bodies for the vagal nerve trunks are located in the brain stem, dorsal motor nuclei (Ewart & Wingate 1983), the nucleus ambiguus and the tractus solitarius. They enter the stomach wall along the lesser curve and form extensive ramifications across the stomach wall. There are two types of vagal efferents, the low-threshold excitatory fibres and the high-threshold inhibitory fibres (Roman & Gonella 1987). The low-threshold fibres are cholinergic and, when stimulated, increase gastric tone and contractility. They are blocked by atropine and hexamethonium. The high-threshold fibres are inhibitory and are not blocked by atropine or adrenergic blockers, and are therefore designated non-cholinergic non-adrenergic nerves. The preganglionic vagal fibres synapse with both the excitatory (cholinergic)andinhibitory(sympathetic)motorneurones

of the myenteric plexus. Thus vagal stimulation may have a biphasic response with both excitatory and inhibitory components. The net effect depends on the basal activity of the stomach as well as the type of vagal input. Of particular importance to normal gastric function is a tonic excitatory vagal input (Grundy et al 1986), which regulates the basal tone of the gastric muscle. This is achieved by providing a steady concentration of ACh. If this vagal input is removed, for example by severing the vagal nerves, the gastric tone is abolished and the mechanical responses are blunted. The postganglionic fibres serve as neuroeffectors for the control of gastric smooth muscle function.

The sympathetic input is provided by the preganglionic fibres arising from segments T6-T9 of the spinal cord. The fibres pass alongside the splanchnic nerves to reach the coeliac ganglion. Postganglionic adrenergic fibres form plexuses around the gastroduodenal branches of the coeliac artery and after entering the stomach synapse with the intramural ganglia. NA released from the sympathetic nerves inhibits the release of ACh from the cholinergic nerves (Daniel 1982), thereby inhibiting gastric smooth muscle activity.

A

PHASE-II   PHASE-III   PHASE-I

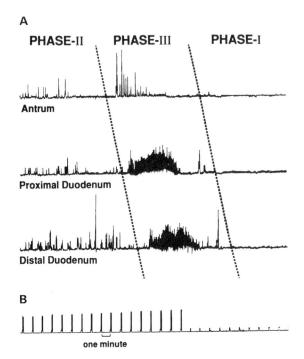

Antrum

Proximal Duodenum

Distal Duodenum

B

one minute

Fig. 25.8 Intraluminal pressure activity of the stomach and duodenum in humans during fasting (**A**) and during the post-prandial period (**B**). In the fasted state phasic non-propagating activity is seen in the antrum (phase II) and this is followed by a rapid burst of propagating activity (phase III) which migrates aborally. This is followed by a period of motor quiescence, phase I. (Courtesy of Dr E Soffer, University of Iowa Hospitals & Clinics.)

The pyloric segment appears to have specialized innervation. The vagus nerve gives off a special branch to the pylorus known as the Nerve of Latarjet. This encircles the pylorus. The pyloric musculature has numerous cholinergic ganglia and adrenergic nerve terminals (Behar et al 1979, Edin et al 1979). During nerve stimulation, the mechanical response of the pylorus consists of a contraction, a relaxation or both. Usually, nerve stimulation leads to an en bloc contraction of the pyloric segment and an increase in pyloric resistance. In this regard, the pylorus differs from other sphincters which predominantly show an inhibitory response to nerve stimulation.

Nevertheless, a high resting tension is characteristic of at least some of the pyloric musculature, and nerve inhibition can be prominent under specific circumstances (Schulze-Delrieu & Shirazi 1983). The nerve inhibition of the pylorus is of a long duration, and is not mediated by adrenergic mechanisms (Anuras et al 1974). Indeed, alpha-adrenergic mechanisms excite the

pylorus and contribute to the maintenance of resting tone by the pyloric muscle. There is also evidence for an enkephalinergic component to the vagal innervation of this segment (Edin et al 1980).

Sensory

The splanchnic and the vagus nerves primarily contain afferent nerve fibres which relay signals to the autonomic nervous system and the central nervous system (CNS) (Kosterlitz 1968; Mei et al 1989). After ingestion of a meal, the splanchnic nerves prevent a rise in intraperitoneal pressure, by bringing about a relaxation of the abdominal muscles. The mechanoreceptors are best classified according to their response and location. In the antral region, the stomach is densely supplied with tension receptors (Andrews et al 1980). These are stimulated both by distension (passive generation of wall tension) and by rhythmic contractions (active generation of wall tension) of the stomach. The tension receptors are slowly adapting whereas the mechanoreceptors located in the mucosal and submucosal layers of the stomach are rapidly adapting. The latter are activated by stroking the mucosa as well as by chemical stimuli (Grundy & Scratcherd 1984).

Extrinsic versus intrinsic control of gastric motility

It is widely assumed that vagal input controls gastric motor activity, with only a small contribution from the enteric neurones. However, the isolated stomach is capable of generating organized mechanical activity in vitro, which includes peristalsis (Schulze-Delrieu et al 1989), emptying of fluids (Schulze-Delrieu & Brown 1985) and volume adaptation to intraluminal distension (Sick & Tedesco 1908, Paton & Vane 1963, Haffner & Staadas 1972, Schulze-Delrieu & Wright 1985, Schulze-Delrieu & Shirazi 1987). Furthermore, stimulation of the intrinsic gastric neurons produces a more powerful mechanical response than is observed with stimulation of the vagus (Paton & Vane 1963). These findings imply that ENS is more important than hitherto acknowledged.

Normal motility of the stomach

Under fasting conditions, the antrum, pylorus and duodenum exhibit a distinct cyclical motor pattern, the migrating motor complex (MMC), or the interdigestive myoelectric complex (Fig. 25.8) (Code & Marlett 1975, Szurszewski 1981). The MMC migrates from the stomach sweeping down the entire small intestine every 90–120 min (Code & Marlett 1975). A full cycle

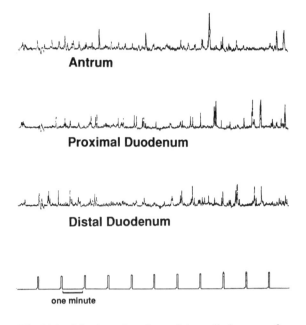

Antrum

Proximal Duodenum

Distal Duodenum

one minute

Fig. 25.9 After ingestion of a meal the cyclical pattern of fasting motor activity is replaced by irregular bursts of persistent phasic pressure activity. (Courtesy of Dr E Soffer, University of Iowa Hospitals & Clinics.)

consists of four phases. Phase I is the longest, lasting 45–60 min, and is a period of motor quiescence with little or no contractions. During phase I pacesetter potentials are generated and traverse the antrum, but are not associated with a contraction. Phase II consists of intermittent muscular contractions (approximately one per minute, which increase in frequency and amplitude over a period of 30 min progressively leading to a crescendo of activity and are coordinated with bursts of duodenal contractions (Houghton et al 1988a). Phase III is the most dynamic phase and consists of a burst of activity which lasts for 5–15 min. During this phase almost every pacesetter potential is followed by a forceful contraction which sweeps down the antrum and the small bowel. The antrum and the pylorus contract regularly at a frequency of 2.5–3.5 per minute; and the duodenum contracts at a frequency of 10–12 per minute (Houghton et al 1988a, Larsen & Osnes 1987). Phase IV is a brief transition period between the hyperactivity of phase III and the quiescence of phase I. This cyclical activity repeats itself until it is disrupted by the ingestion of a meal. There is a strong correlation between the MMC and the movement of gastric contents. During phase I there is no movement. During phase II there is some mixing of the gastric contents, but very little propulsion takes place. During phase III most of the aboral propulsion is observed (Ehrlein & Akkermans 1984), and during this period large undigestible residue may leave the stomach (Kelly 1981). Thus a MMC is associated with a 'cleansing' effect on the stomach and the small bowel and has been, therefore, called the 'housekeeper' of the gut (Code & Schlegel 1974). The control of this periodic activity is incompletely understood, but may be modulated by motilin, gastrin, prostaglandins and signals from the CNS (Weisbrodt 1984).

Feeding disrupts the MMC through as yet unknown mechanisms. The 'fed' or 'postprandial' pattern is non-cyclical, and consists of intermittent contractile activity resembling the fasting phase II pattern (Fig.25.9). Approximately 50% of pacesetter potentials are associated with submaximal contractions of the antral muscle. This pattern persists as long as the bulk of food remains in the stomach. Conversion from the fasting to the postprandial pattern is partly mediated by the vagus nerves, since experimental cooling of the vagus alters the 'fed' pattern to a phase III like activity (Hall et al 1986). However, other factors such as luminal distension, tone, chemical composition of nutrients, fat content, pH, and bulking agents such as cellulose may all affect this pattern (Meyer 1987).

GASTRIC DIGESTION AND EMPTYING

After ingestion of a meal, the stomach stores, grinds, digests and empties its contents. The sequence of events is determined by various factors: the reservoir capacity of the stomach; the trituration of food; the viscosity, nutrient and caloric content and the volume load of the meal; the phase of the interdigestive complex when food was ingested; and small intestinal feedback inhibition. If the meal is a non-caloric, isotonic solution, it may leave the stomach rapidly, bypassing storage and digestion, whereas a meal with large pieces of solid food may be retained until it is fragmented into fine particles.

Reservoir function

The stomach is an expansile reservoir. Its ability to store food allows the individual to pursue activities other than continuous ingestion of food. Swallowing and distension of the oesophagus induces a reflex relaxation of the fundus called receptive relaxation (Cannon & Lieb 1912, Azpiroz & Malagelada 1985a) which is abolished after vagotomy (Jansson 1969). This response is shortlived (Fig. 25.10) and is unlikely to be solely responsible for the reservoir function of the

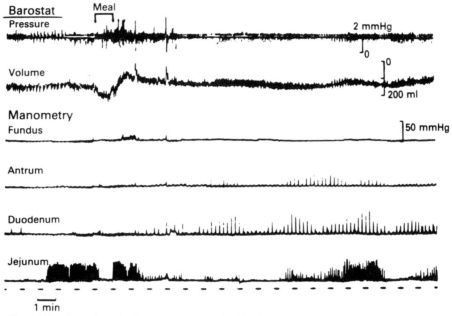

Fig. 25.10 Gastrointestinal motor response to feeding in dog as recorded by gastric barostat and manometry. The barostat's volume inversely measures changes in gastric tone. It can be seen that immediately after ingestion of a meal, there is a reflex relaxation of the proximal stomach (receptive and adaptive relaxation) due to a reduction in the gastric tone. After some time the tone recovers and transiently increases to aid emptying. The meal also stimulates phasic contractile activity in the antrum and duodenum. (With permission from Azpiroz & Malagelada 1985a and editor of Am J Physiology.)

stomach. The gastric fundus relaxes for extended periods of time in response to intragastric distension. This reflex relaxation is known as adaptive relaxation, which is most likely responsible for the accommodation of the stomach after ingestion of food and liquids (Kelly 1981).

Accommodation (in response to gastric filling), alters the configuration of the stomach from a collapsed tube to an inflated balloon (Groedel 1924). Most of this expansion is seen along the greater curvature of the proximal stomach with little change in the antrum and the lesser curvature (Groedel 1924, Haffner & Staadas 1972, Kelly 1981, Schulze-Delrieu 1983) (Fig. 25.11). This adaptation in the size of the stomach maintains the intraluminal pressure within a narrow range, even though the intragastric volume may fluctuate. If the stomach is filled rapidly, there is an initial increase in pressure, which quickly levels off and when contents are removed, the muscle shortens and contracts around the residual volume thereby maintaining enough intraluminal pressure to empty its contents. The mechanisms responsible for this adaptation are controversial. One important factor is the viscoelastic property of the

smooth muscle (Schulze-Delrieu & Shirazi 1987). Additional factors include stretch-induced modulation of the muscle tone through intramural and vagovagal reflexes.

Digestion and dispersion of food (trituration)

The breakdown of food in the stomach involves mechanical and chemical processes. The mechanical digestion occurs through repeated to and fro movements of the gastric contents in the distal stomach (Meyer et al 1979). The contents are propelled towards the gastric outlet by the propagating ring contraction of the corpus and antrum and retropelled by the closure of the pylorus (Cannon 1911, Carlson et al 1966, Ehrlein & Krais 1981, Prove & Ehrlein 1982, Ehrlein & Akkermans 1984). It is believed that the fragmentation of particles occurs as a result of the crushing of food against the narrow and rigid distal antrum (Dozois et al 1971, Ehrlein & Akkermans 1984) (Fig. 25.12). Additional disintegration occurs during retropulsion as a result of shearing forces. This force develops when the food particles are forcefully ejected back into

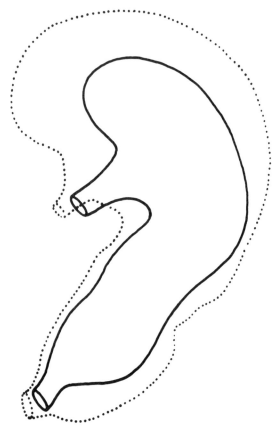

Fig. 25.11   Contour of the rabbit's stomach when empty (solid line) and during experimental filling (broken line). After filling it can be seen that there is very little change in the lesser curvature, but the fundus and the greater curvature expand to accommodate the contents. This bulging of the greater curvature to the left, increases the distance between the most dependent part of the stomach (the sinus) and the gastric outlet.

the stomach (by pyloric closure) through an advancing ring contraction (Carlson et al 1966). Large particles of food usually settle in the dependent portion of the stomach (the sinus, Fig. 25.1) and are likely to move at the periphery of the centrally moving jet stream of smaller particles. Hence, when the large particles are pushed against the narrow funnel shaped antrum, they tumble against the wall and are sheared by the sudden reversal of flow.

The digestion of food in the stomach requires a strong mechanical effort. A failure of this process can cause retention of solid material in the stomach (gastric stasis), which may lead to the formation of bezoars and an inability to maintain adequate nutrition (Malagelada et al 1980).

The chemical process consists of the splitting of starch and carbohydrate by parotid amylase, the emulsification of fat by lingual lipase and the breakdown of protein by gastric pepsin. Simple exposure of food to these chemicals is insufficient for digestion (Meyer 1987), clearly suggesting that chemical digestion is dependent on motor activity. Thus, it appears that mechanical factors enhance the chemical effects and vice versa. During this phase, the digestive juices penetrate food particles. This mechanochemical dispersion decreases the density of chyme and provides a larger surface area for further chemical digestion by pancreatic and intestinal enzymes. The suspension and emulsification of food in the chyme also enables the intraluminal contents to become isotonic with plasma (Meyer et al 1986a). The semi-digested particles are retained in the stomach until they are reduced to about 1 mm in diameter and only then are delivered to the small intestine. The undigested food is retained in the stomach until the resumption of the next fasting MMC, and during phase III of this cycle even large food particles are swept out.

Another physical property of the meal which affects emptying, is its viscosity. While aqueous solutions are rapidly evacuated from the stomach, viscous meals leave the stomach slowly (Houghton et al 1988b). This is nicely demonstrated during measurements of gastric emptying; solids produce a sigmoid-shaped curve whereas liquids empty rapidly and exponentially (Fig. 25.13).

Gastric emptying of liquids and particulate solids (sieving and decanting)

The stomach discriminates between solid and liquid contents and allows fluid to empty before smaller particles and the latter before larger particles. Thus, emptying is combined with sieving, wherein liquids and suspended particles leave the stomach early, while larger particles are retained until they are broken down and partially digested (Meyer 1980, Meyer et al 1985). Traditionally, entrapment of particles at the pylorus has been held as the primary mechanism for sieving, but it is likely that other mechanisms such as decanting may operate. According to the entrapment theory, all of the gastric contents are propelled into the antrum at the same time and at the same rate, but only liquids and smaller particles escape through the narrow pyloric orifice (Hinder & Kelly 1977a). Against this notion is the observation that sieving persists even after removal of the antrum and pylorus (Hinder & Sang-Garde 1983) and outflow into the duodenum occurs before the ring contraction reaches the pylorus and before

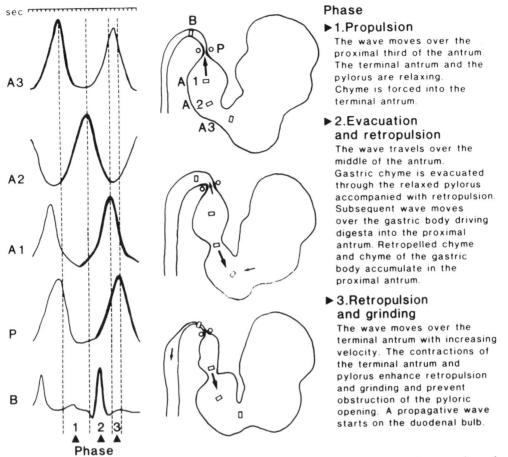

Phase

▶1.Propulsion

The wave moves over the proximal third of the antrum. The terminal antrum and the pylorus are relaxing. Chyme is forced into the terminal antrum.

▶2.Evacuation and retropulsion

The wave travels over the middle of the antrum. Gastric chyme is evacuated through the relaxed pylorus accompanied with retropulsion. Subsequent wave moves over the gastric body driving digesta into the proximal antrum. Retropelled chyme and chyme of the gastric body accumulate in the proximal antrum.

▶3.Retropulsion and grinding

The wave moves over the terminal antrum with increasing velocity. The contractions of the terminal antrum and pylorus enhance retropulsion and grinding and prevent obstruction of the pyloric opening. A propagative wave starts on the duodenal bulb.

Fig. 25.12 Diagrammatic illustration of the digestion and dispersion of food, as well as the propulsion, emptying and retropulsion and the development of shearing forces. (With permission from Ehrlein & Akkermans 1984.)

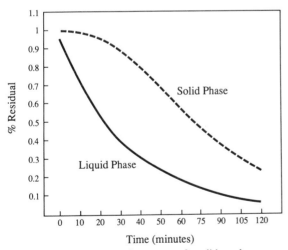

Fig. 25.13 Gastric emptying curves of a solid meal (Technetium sulphur colloid labelled scrambled egg) and a liquid meal (Technetium sulphur colloid labelled water). Liquids empty rapidly and in an exponential fashion. Solids, empty slowly after a lag phase and characteristically exhibit a sigmoid curve.

pyloric closure (Ehrlein & Akkermans 1984, Schulze-Delrieu & Brown 1985). One possible explanation for this discrepancy is that the process of sieving may more closely resemble decanting (Fig. 25.14).

Animal experiments have shown that after ingestion of a meal, the contour of the stomach changes (Fig. 25.11), such that the pyloric orifice is situated at a higher level than any other segment of the gastroduodenal junction (Schulze-Delrieu 1992). When a gastric contraction propels a bolus of food, fluids which are normally suspended above solids, flow over the pyloric border into the duodenum, whereas the solid particles fall back into the dependent portion of the stomach (Fig. 25.14). These observations have been recently confirmed in humans using ultrasonography to monitor accommodation, flow and emptying of food (Brown et al 1992). This study shows that both sieving and

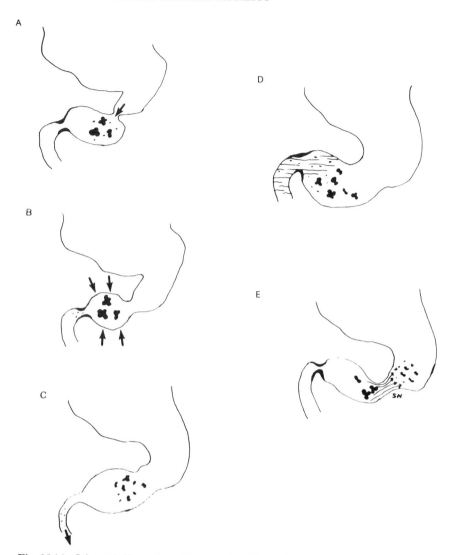

Fig. 25.14   Schematic illustration of the two views of gastric emptying; gastric sieving and decanting. **A**, **B** and **C** show how food is swept into the distal stomach and only small particles escape through the pylorus, whereas the larger particles are retained and crushed by the contraction of the distal antrum and pylorus. **D** and **E** depict how the pylorus owing to its anatomical location, forms a ridge over which fluids and smaller suspended particles are swept, whereas the larger particles sediment and lie in the dependent portion of the stomach. As large particles are retropelled into the proximal stomach by the antral contractions that occur against a closed pylorus, the resulting jet effects grinds them.

decanting may operate (Figs 25.15, 25.16). When garbanzo beans (chick peas) and broth are ingested together, at first, the greater curvature bulges and the antrum assumes a funnel shape. The beans are held in the mid portion of the stomach and do not enter the antrum, although fluids are intermittently propelled through the antrum and the patent pylorus. As the stomach empties and the antrum becomes more tubular, the beans are brought closer to the gastric outlet, and are then propelled towards the pyloric orifice by peristaltic contractions. The beans are initially entrapped at the pyloric orifice and are returned to the corpus by a retrograde jet stream. During this phase the larger beans disintegrate into a pasty material,

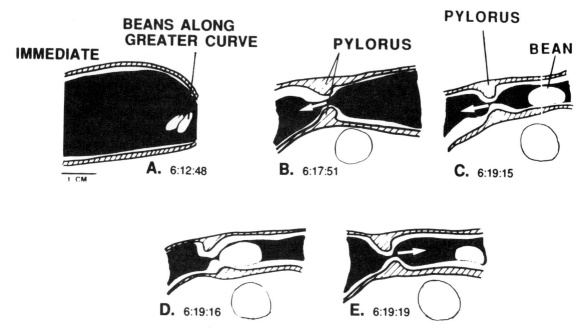

Fig. 25.15 Images were obtained from real-time ultrasonography approximately 60 min after ingestion of a meal. The meal consisted of chicken soup and beans. The beans were swallowed without mastication. The figures show a sequence of a longitudinal scan through the body, distal antrum, pylorus and duodenal bulb. In **A**, the beans are lying in the dependent portion of the proximal stomach. In **B**, pyloric closure begins as a contraction wave has reached the distal antrum. In **C**, the distal antrum is contracting and a bean has moved towards the pylorus. In **D**, the bean has been retained at the pyloric orifice (whose opening has now been reduced to a slit). In **E**, the bean is returned from the pyloric orifice towards the gastric reservoir by a retrograde jet stream. (Courtesy of Dr B Brown, Dept. of Radiology, University of Iowa Hospitals.)

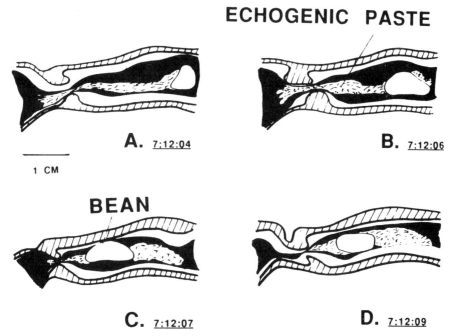

Fig. 25.16 Real-time ultrasonography images showing that 2 h after meal ingestion, the beans are largely fragmented into an 'echogenic paste' (**A**). Peristaltic contractions propel some of this paste together with gastric secretions across the pylorus (**B**). The remainder, including the unfragmented portion of the bean is retained (**C**) and retropulsed (**D**). (courtesy of Dr B. Brown, Dept. of Radiology, University of Iowa Hospitals.)

which is thereafter propelled through the pylorus by further peristaltic contractions of the distal half of the stomach.

Forces promoting gastric emptying

The process of gastric emptying is a balance between propulsive and non-propulsive motor activity. Gravity by itself cannot produce emptying, but the erect posture accelerates emptying when compared with the recumbent position, by increasing delivery to the antrum from where they are propelled distally (Kelly 1981, Ehrlein & Akkermans 1984). It has been suggested that the fundus controls liquid emptying by generating contractile activity which produces a gastroduodenal pressure gradient (Kelly 1980). However, this pressure gradient has not been demonstrated. Liquids empty from the stomach in gushes associated with coordinated contractions of the antrum, pylorus and duodenum (Houghton et al 1988b, Prove & Ehrlein 1982). The role of the fundus in liquid emptying is more likely to prime the antral pump and enhance its efficiency (Read & Houghton 1989).

Solid emptying from the stomach also occurs in surges. These surges are caused by ring contractions which develop in the distal stomach and move towards the gastric outlet separating a bolus from the intragastric contents and propelling it towards the duodenum (Ehrlein & Akkermans 1984, Schulze-Delrieu & Brown 1985). The bolus flow accelerates as the contents advance through the increasingly narrow and thick walled antrum and pylorus. As long as the pylorus is relaxed and the ring contraction is located in the antrum, maximal flow occurs. Once the ring contraction advances into the pre-pyloric area, the pylorus closes and a large fraction of the bolus is retropelled into the stomach (Carlson et al 1966, Code & Marlett 1975, Ehrlein & Akkermans 1984) while a small fraction is squeezed into the duodenum.

Gastric outflow resistance

The pylorus (Cannon 1911, Carlson et al 1966, Biancani et al 1980, Schulze-Delrieu & Brown 1985) and the duodenum (Schulze-Delrieu 1992, Miller et al 1981) serve as mechanical barriers for the efflux from the stomach. The pylorus acts as a restrictive resistor (Schulze-Delrieu & Wall 1983) and the duodenum as a capacitative resistor (Shirazi et al 1988). The pylorus is the narrowest segment of the upper gastrointestinal tract and, unlike the lower oesophageal sphincter

(LOS) and the internal anal sphincter, does not tonically occlude the lumen, at least in man. Furthermore, while the LOS relaxes ahead of the oesophageal peristaltic wave, the pyloric sphincter contracts either with or even ahead of the gastric peristaltic wave. Thus, pyloric closure traps part of the bolus propelled by antral contraction.

The pyloric segment provides an adaptable physiologic resistance to gastric outflow. Hence, at any given time, the pylorus offers equal resistance to both the gastric outflow as well as the gastric inflow from duodenogastric reflux, thus maintaining gastric continence and a barrier for biliary reflux. This resistance is maintained by both the tonic and the phasic contractile activity of the pyloric muscle (Biancani et al 1980, Schulze-Delrieu & Wall 1983, Ehrlein 1988). Recent studies have also shown that the pyloric segment exhibits isolated pyloric pressure waves (Fig. 25.17) which are more frequent after ingestion of a nutrient-dense drink, and this may be an important barrier for transpyloric flow (Houghton et al 1988b).

An interesting phenomenon relates to the relative diameters of the pyloric orifice and of the antral ring contraction (Prove & Ehrlein 1982). With meals of high viscosity, the pylorus remains narrow and antral contractions are shallow. With meals of low viscosity, the pylorus is widely patent, and contractions are deep and occlude the lumen. During digestion of a meal, there is a steady progression from a narrow to a wide pylorus, and from shallow to deep antral contractions. To what extent reflexes of other regulatory mechanisms lead to these changes in the baseline tone of the pyloric musculature and the force of the antral contractions is not clear.

Earlier studies often failed to show an effect of the pylorus on the rate of gastric emptying or on duodenogastric reflux. Recent studies have consistently shown that pyloroplasty or other procedures eliminating the pylorus increase both the rate of gastric outflow as well as the reflux of duodenal contents into the stomach (Muller-Lissner et al 1981, Hinder 1983).

The duodenum has a relatively small luminal capacity when compared to the volume of chyme which can be delivered from the gastric outlet. Hence the duodenum must empty its lumen before it can receive gastric contents. Duodenal clearance occurs during propagated duodenal contractions (Fig. 25.18). However, these contractions temporarily occlude the duodenal lumen offering further resistance to gastric outflow.

When there is a rapid filling of the duodenum, duodenal contractions are strong (Weisbrodt et al 1969, Buhner & Ehrlein 1989, Houghton et al 1988b) and involve long segments, thereby providing an effective

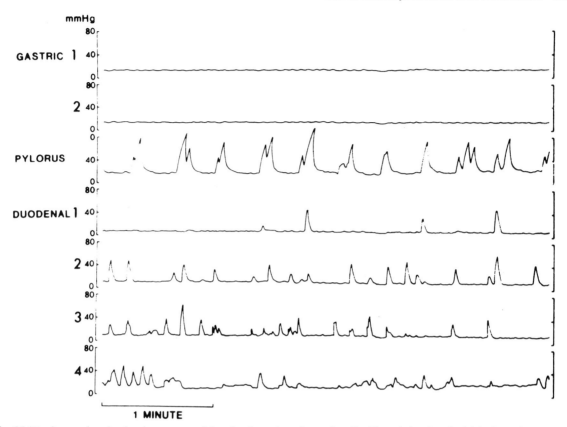

Fig. 25.17 Antropyloroduodenal pressure activity after ingestion of a nutrient liquid meal showing diminished antral contractions, stimulation of isolated pyloric pressure waves and random duodenal contractions. These isolated pyloric pressure waves may serve as an important barrier for transpyloric flow of liquids. (With permission from Houghton & Kerrigan 1989 and Wrightson Publications.)

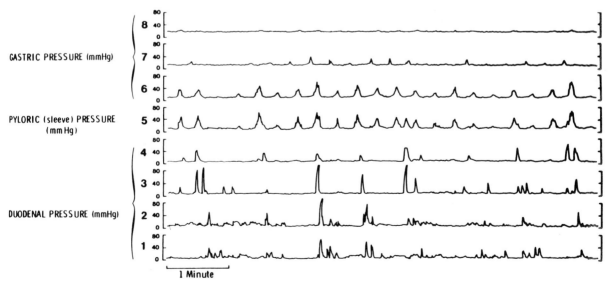

Fig. 25.18 Intraluminal pressure activity recorded at multiple sites in the body and antrum of the stomach, the pyloric canal and the duodenum in a healthy volunteer, during emptying of a solid meal. Frequent antropyloric and antropyloroduodenal contractile activity can be seen which appear to be coordinated and propagated caudally. (With permission from Houghton et al 1988a, and editor of Gastroenterology.)

impediment to gastric outflow and a safeguard against dumping. It has been recently shown that duodenal contractions are also capable of producing retrograde flow which could further retard gastric emptying (Schulze-Delrieu 1992, Houghton et al 1988b).

Effect of nutrients

Non-nutrient meals are steadily propelled out of the stomach whereas nutrient-rich meals are associated with a delay in gastric emptying (Hunt & Stubbs 1975, Brener et al 1983, Houghton et al 1988b). This slowing of gastric emptying is believed to be proportional to the energy density of the meal (Hunt & Stubbs 1975, Brener et al 1983), and is thought to be produced by the interaction of specific nutrients with small intestinal receptors. However, the effect of a powerful nutrient inhibitor such as fat may be mediated by its action on receptors at different sites in the stomach and small intestine and through several mechanisms. When a fatty solution or hyperosmotic glucose is infused into the duodenum the fundus relaxes (Azpiroz & Malagelada 1985b, Dooley et al 1984), facilitating redistribution of food from the distal to the proximal stomach (Collins et al 1986), and antral motility is suppressed (Heddle et al 1988, Keinke & Ehrlein 1983, White et al 1983), whereas pyloric tone and phasic pyloric contractions increase, interrupting the flow from the stomach to the duodenum (Heddle et al 1988, Houghton et al 1988b, Tongas et al 1987, White et al 1983). Furthermore, the pattern of duodenal motor activity also changes from propulsive contractions to those of mixing or stationary contractions. All of these mechanisms are important in regulating gastric emptying, but none of them are solely responsible. For example, disruption of any one mechanism, as produced experimentally by fundectomy or by pyloric stenting (Schulze-Delrieu & Brown 1985) has only a partial effect on gastric outflow.

Small intestinal feedback inhibition

It has been proposed that there are at least five types of chemoreceptors which play a role in the feedback control of gastric emptying, namely: lipid receptors (Cooke 1975), osmoreceptors (Meeroff et al 1975, Thompson & Wingate 1988), receptors for amino acids such as tryptophan (Cooke 1975) and phenylalanine (Grundy & Scratcherd 1989), glucoreceptors (Lin et al 1989, MacGregor et al 1976, Treacy et al 1988) and pH receptors (Hunt & Knox 1969, Gershon-Cohen & Shay 1937).

Infusion of lipid solutions into the small intestine causes a profound reduction in gastric contractile activity (Fig. 25.19) and a delay in gastric emptying (Keinke and Ehrlein 1983, Read et al 1984, Spiller et al 1984). One possible mechanism for this is the release of CCK from subepithelial endocrine cells in the proximal small intestine. CCK infusions delay gastric emptying (Debas et al 1975) and CCK antagonist L-364718 promotes gastric flow (Gould et al 1987). Fat in the ileum also delays gastric emptying (Fig. 25.20), but this is probably not mediated by CCK, but by peptide YY. Ileal infusion of lipids raises plasma PYY in dogs (Pappas et al 1985) and in man (Spiller et al 1988) and PYY administration also delays gastric emptying (Allen et al 1984).

How does fat reach the ileum? It is suggested that following ingestion of a meal, and before the stomach and small bowel switch over to a postprandial pattern of motor activity, a peculiar pattern of cluster contractions sweep food samples throughout the length of the small intestine (McHugh 1982, Keinke & Ehrlein 1983). The nutrients present in these food samples may stimulate specialized receptors such as lipid receptors in the distal small bowel. Similarly, pH of the ingested food and that of the chyme may influence gastric efflux. Recent studies have shown that infusion of acid into the duodenum suppresses antral contractility, induces phasic pyloric activity and reduces duodenal propulsive activity (Houghton et al 1987). How this effect is mediated is not known. In addition, experimental psychologic stress (Fone et al 1990a), distension and intubation of the small bowel (Fone et al 1988), and triglyceride infusion into the terminal ileum (Fone et al 1990b) have all been shown to retard gastric emptying and inhibit gastroduodenal motility. Finally, the length of the small intestinal segment exposed to a nutrient also determines the degree to which gastric outflow is inhibited (Lin et al 1989).

The mechanisms by which the physical properties of a meal affect gastric emptying are less clear. There is not only discrimination between solids and liquids, but also between particles of different density and and viscosity. For example, solid particles, which are of a lower and a higher density than that of water, empty

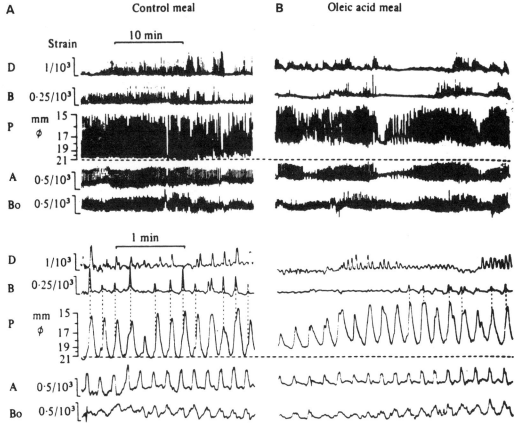

Fig. 25.19 Gastroduodenal contractile pressure activity after administration of a potato meal (**A**) and a mashed potato-oleic acid meal (**B**). The lower tracings are recorded with higher paper speed to show the sequence of the antral, pyloric and duodenal contractions. The oleic acid meal significantly reduced the frequency and amplitude of contractile activity, showing that fat is a potent inhibitor of gastric emptying. D = duodenum, B = bulb, P = pylorus, A = antrum, Bo = gastric body. (With permission from Keinke & Ehrlein 1983 & Editor of Q J Exp Physiol.)

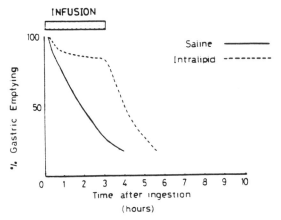

Fig. 25.20 Effect of ileal infusion of lipid on gastric emptying of a meal. During saline infusion the half time for gastric emptying ($t\frac{1}{2}$) was less than 2 h, whereas during lipid infusion the $t\frac{1}{2}$ was greater than 4 h demonstrating the ileal brake. (Modified from Read et al 1984, with permission of the author and Praeger Publishers, New York.)

more slowly than particles which are of the same density as water (Meyer 1987). An increase in the viscosity of the meal decreases the rate at which fluids empty from the stomach, but it also increases the size of the particles which leave the stomach (Meyer et al 1986b; Sirois 1990).

The normal stomach, pylorus and duodenum accomplish several diverse but interrelated motor functions in a smooth and coordinated fashion. This activity is closely monitored and regulated by the ENS with inputs from other nerves, the CNS, local gut hormones and other peptides, prostaglandins, as well as by the ingestion of a meal and the characteristics of a meal. The stomach and duodenum have several mechanisms which overlap, so that even if one system fails, the organ is capable of functioning adequately, at near optimal levels. An abnormal function results only when there is a serious disruption of several mechanisms, as occurs in diabetic gastroparesis, following vagotomy or with pyloric stenosis.

REFERENCES

Allen J M, Fitzpatrick M L, Yeats J C et al 1984 Effect of peptides YY and neuropeptide on gastric emptying in man. Digestion 30: 255–262

Andrews P L R, Grundy D, Scratcherd T 1980 Vagal afferent discharge from mechanoreceptors in different regions of the ferret stomach. J Physiol 298: 513–524

Anuras S, Cooke A, Christensen J (1974) An inhibitory innervation at the gastroduodenal junction. J. Clin Invest 54: 529–535

Azpiroz F, Malagelada J R 1985a Physiological variations in canine gastric tone measured by an electronic barostat. Am J Physiol 247: 229–237

Azpiroz F, Malagelada J R 1985b Intestinal control of gastric tone. Am J Physiol 249: G501–G509

Bauer A J, Publicover N G, Sanders K M 1985 Origin and spread of slow waves in canine gastric antral circular muscle. Am J Physiol 12: G800–G806

Bauer A J, Sanders K M 1985 Gradient in excitation-contraction coupling in canine gastric antral circular muscle. J Physiol 369: 283–294

Behar J, Biancani P. Zabinski M P (1979) Characterisation of feline gastroduodenal junction by neural and hormonal stimulation. Am J Physiol 236: E45–E51

Biancani P, Kerstein M D, Zabinski M P et al 1980 Mechanical characteristics of the cat pylorus. Gastroenterology 78: 301–309

Brener W, Hendrix T R, McHugh P R 1983 Regulation of gastric emptying of glucose. Gastroenterology 85: 76–82

Brown B P, Schulze-Delrieu K, Schrier J E, Abu-Yousef M M 1993 The configuration of the human gastroduodenal junction in the separate emptying of liquids and solids. Gastroenterology 105: 433–440

Buhner S, Ehrlein H J 1989 Characteristics of postprandial duodenal motor patterns in dogs. Dig Dis Sci 34(12): 1873–1881

Cannon W B 1911 The nature of gastric peristalsis. Am J Physiol 29: 250–266

Cannon W B, Lieb C 1912 The receptive relaxation of the stomach. Am J Psysiol 29: 267–273

Carlson H C, Code C F, Nelson R A 1966 Motor action of the canine gastroduodenal junction; a cineradiographic, pressure, and electric study. Am J Dig Dis 2: 155–172

Christensen J 1992 A commentary on the morphological identification of interstitial cells of Cajal in the gut. J Auton Nerv Syst 37: 75–88

Code C F, Marlett J A 1975 The interdigestive myoelectric complex of the stomach and small bowel of dogs. J Physiol 246: 289–309

Code C F, Schlegel T F 1974 The gastrointestinal housekeeper in: Daniel E E (ed.) Gastrointestinal motility. Mitchell Press, Vancouver pp 631–633

Collins P J, Heddle R, Horowitz M et al 1986 The effect of intraduodenal lipid on gastric emptying and intragastric distribution of a solid meal. Gastroenterology 90: 1377

Cooke A R 1975 Control of gastric emptying and motility. Gastroenterology 68: 804–816

Crowe R, Burnstock G 1981 Comparative studies of quinarcine positive neurons in myenteric plexus of stomach and intestine of guinea pig, rabbit and rat. Cell Tissue Res 221: 93–107

Daniel E E 1982 Pharmacology of adrenergic, cholinergic, and drugs acting on other receptors in gastrointestinal muscle in: Bertaccini G (ed.) Handbook of experimental

pharmacology. Springer Verlag, 59/II Berlin, 249–322

Debas H T, Farooq O, Grossman M I 1975 Inhibition of gastric emptying as a physiological action of cholecystokinin. Gastroenterology 68: 1211–1217

Dooley C P, Reznick J B, Valenzuela J E 1984 Variations in gastric and duodenal motility during gastric emptying of liquid meals in humans. Gastroenterology 87: 1114–1119

Dozois R R, Code D F, Kelly K A 1971 Effect of distal antrectomy on gastric emptying of liquids and solids. Gastroenterology 61: 675–681

Edin R, Ahlman H, Kewenter J 1979 The vagal control of the feline pyloric sphincter. Acta Physiol Scand. 107: 169–174

Edin R, Lundberg J, Terenius L et al 1980 Evidence for vagal enkephalinergic neural control of the feline pylorus and stomach. Gastroenterology 78: 492–497

Ehrlein H J 1988 Motility of the pyloric sphincter studied by the inductograph method in conscious dogs. Am J Physiol 254: G650–G657

Ehrlein H J and Akkermans L M A 1984 Gastric emptying in gastric and gastroduodenal motility in: Akkermans L M A et al (ed.) Gastric and gastroduodenal motility Praeger Scientific, New York pp 74–84

Ehrlein H J, Krais J 1981 Untersuchungen uber die Magenmotorik des Kaninchens. D T W 88: 415–419

Ewart WR, Wingate D L 1983 Central representation and opioid modulation of gastric mechanoreceptor activity in the rat. Am J Physiol 244: G27–G32

Fone D R, Horowitz M, Maddox A et al 1990a Gastroduodenal motility during the delayed gastric emptying induced by cold stress. Gastroenterology 98: 1155–1161

Fone D R, Horowitz M, Read N W et al 1990b The effect of terminal ileal triglyceride infusion on gastroduodenal motility and the intragastric distribution of a solid meal. Gastroenterology 98: 568–575

Fone, D R, Meddle R, Horowitz M et al 1988 Comparative effects of duodenal and ileal intubation on gastric emptying and antropyloric motility. Gastroenterology 94: A133

Gabella G 1981 Musculature of the gastrointestinal tract of the guinea pig. Anat Embryol 163: 135–156

Gershon-Cohen J, Shay H 1937 Experimental studies on gastric physiology in man. III. A study on pyloric control. The role of milk and cream in the normal and in subjects with quiescent duodenal ulcer. Am J Roentgenol 38: 427–446

Gould R J, Cook P G, Fiorvanti C et al 1987 L364 718 A cholecystokinin antagonist, promotes gastric emptying in cats. Clin Res 35: 590

Groedel F 1924 Die Rontgenuntersuchung des Magens in: Groedel F M (ed.) Rontgendiagnostik in der Inneren Medizin Medizinische Atlanten, vol 7. München, Lehmann Verlag, 500–732.

Grundy D, Hutson D, Scratcherd T 1986 A permissive role of the vagus nerve in the genesis of antro-antral reflexes in the anaesthetized ferret. J Physiol (Lond) 381: 377–384

Grundy D, Scratcherd T 1984 The role of the vagus and sympathetic nerves in the control of gastric motility in Akkermans L M A et al (ed.) Gastric and gastroduodenal motility. Praeger Scientific, New York, 21–34

Grundy D, Scratcherd T 1989 Sensory afferents from the gastrointestinal tract in: Wood J D (ed.) American Handbook of Physiology, Gastrointestinal System, 16, vol 1. American Physiological Society, Bethesda 593–620

Haffner J F W, Staadas J 1972 Pressure response to

cholinergic and adrenergic agents in the fundus, corpus and antrum of isolated rabbit stomachs. Acta Chir Scand 138: 713–719

Hall K E, Diamant N E, El-Sharkay T 1986 Vagal control of postprandial upper gastrointestinal motility. Am J Physiol 250(4): G501–G510

Heddle R, Dent J, Read N W et al 1988 Antropyloroduodenal motor responses to intraduodenal lipid infusion in healthy volunteers. Am J Physiol 259: G671–G679

Hinder R A, Kelly K A 1977a Canine gastric emptying of solids and liquids. Am J Physiol 233: E335–E340

Hinder R A, Kelly K A 1977b Human gastric pacesetter potential. Site of origin spread, and response to gastric transection and proximal gastric vagotomy. Am J Surg 133: 29–33

Hinder R A, San-Garde B A 1983 Individual and combined roles of the pylorus and antrum in the canine gastric emptying of a liquid and a digestible solid. Gastroenterology 84: 281–386

Houghton L A, Heddle R, Read N W et al 1988a Motor activity of the gastric antrum, pylorus and duodenum under fasted conditions and after a liquid meal. Gastroenterology 94: 1276–1284

Houghton L A, Heddle R, Read N W et al 1988b The relationship of the motor activity of the antrum, pylorus and duodenum to gastric emptying of a solid-liquid mixed meal. Gastroenterology 94: 1285–1291

Houghton L A, Kerrigan D D, Read N W et al 1987 Antropyloroduodenal motor responses to intraduodenal acid infusions in healthy volunteers. Dig Dis Sci 32: A16, 915

Houghton L A, Kerrigan D D 1989 Gastropyloroduodenal manometry in: Read N W (ed.) Gastrointestinal motility, which test? Wrightson Biomedical, Petersfield pp 105–112

Hoyes A D, Barber P, Sikri K L 1982 Localization of Substance-P like immunoactivity in the intraluminal nerve plexuses of the guinea-pig stomach using immunofluorescence and immunoperoxidase techniques. J Anat 135: 319–332

Hunt J N, Knox M T 1969 The slowing of gastric emptying by nine acids. J Physiol 201: 161–179

Hunt J N, Stubbs D F 1975 The volume and energy content of meals as determinants of gastric emptying. J Physiol 245: 209–225

Jansson G 1969 Extrinsic nervous control of gastric motility. An experimental study in the cat. Acta Physiol Scand (suppl) 326: 1–42

Keinke O, Ehrlein H J 1983 Effect of oleic acid on canine gastroduodenal motility, pyloric diameter and gastric emptying. Q J Exp Physiol 68: 675–686

Kelly K A 1980 Gastric emptying of liquids and solids. Role of proximal and distal stomach. Am J Physiol 217: 461–470

Kelly K A 1981 Motility of the stomach and gastroduodenal junction in: Johnson L R (ed.) Physiology of the gastrointestinal tract. Raven Press, New York, 393–410

Kelly K A, Code C F 1971 Canine gastric pacemaker. Am J Physiol 220: 112–118

Kosterlitz H W 1968 Intrinsic and extrinsic nervous control of motility of the stomach and the intestines in: Code C F (ed.) Handbook of physiology, section 6, Alimentary Canal, volume IV, Motility. Washington, D C, American Physiological Society pp 2147–2172

Lin H C, Doty J E, Ready T J et al 1989 Inhibition of gastric emptying by glucose depends on length of intestine exposed to nutrients. Am J Physiol 256: G404–G411

Larsen S, Osnes M 1987 The unstimulated duodenal pressure activity in healthy humans. Scand J Gastroenterol 22: 1–36

McCallum R W 1989 Motor function of the stomach in health and disease in: Sleisenger M H, Fordtran J S (eds) Gastrointestinal disease, pathophysiology, diagnosis, management. Saunders, Philadelphia pp 675–713

MacGregor I L, Gueller R, Watts H D et al 1976 The effects of acute hyperglycemia on gastric emptying in man. Gastroenterology 70: 190–196

McHugh P R, Moran T H, Wirth J B 1982 Post-pyloric regulation of gastric emptying in rhesus monkeys. Am J Physiol R408–R415

Malagelada J R, Longstreth G F, Summerskill W I H et al 1976 Measurement of gastric function during digestion of ordinary solid meals in man. Gastroenterology 70: 203–210

Malagelada J R, Mazzotta L G, Rees W D W et al 1980 Gastric motor abnormalities in diabetic and postvagotomy gastroparesis: Effect of metoclopramide and bethanechol. Gastroenterology 78: 286–293

Mayer E A, Jehn D, Thomson J B et al 1982 Gastric emptying of solid food and pancreatic and biliary secretions in patients with truncal vagotomy and antrectomy. Gastroenterology 83: 184–192

Meeroff J C, Go V L W, Phillips S D 1975 Control of gastric emptying by osmolality of duodenal contents in man. Gastroenterology 68: 1144–1151

Mei N, Boyer A, Condamin M 1989 The composition of the vagus nerve of the cat. Cell Tissue Res 209: 423–431

Meyer J H 1987 Motility of the stomach and the gastroduodenal junction in: Johnson L R Christensen J, Jackson M J, Jacobson E D, Walsh J H (eds) Physiology of the gastrointestinal tract. Raven Press, New York, 613–630

Meyer J H 1980 Gastric emptying of ordinary food: Effect of antrum on particle size. Am J Physiol 239: G133–G135

Meyer J H, Cohen M B, Thomson J B et al 1979 Sieving of food by the canine stomach and sieving after gastric surgery. Gastroenterology 76: 804–813

Meyer J H, Dressman J, Fink A S et al 1985 Effect of size and density on gastric emptying of indigestible solids. Gastroenterology 89: 805–813

Meyer J H, Dressman J, Gu Y G et al 1986a Effect of viscosity and flow rate on gastric emptying of solids. Am J Physiol 250: G161–G164

Meyer J H, Jehn D, Mayer E A et al 1986b Gastric emptying and processing of fat. Gastroenterology 90: 1176–1187

Miller J, Elashoff J, Kauffman G et al 1981 Search for resistances controlling gastric emptying of liquid meals. Am J Physiol 241: G403–G425

Morgan K G, Szurszewski J H 1980 Mechanism of phasic and tonic actions of pentagastrin on canine gastric smooth muscle. J Physiol 301: 229–242

Morgan K G, Schmalz P E, Szurszewski J H 1978a The inhibitory effects of vasoactive intestinal peptide on the mechanical and electrical activity of the canine antral smooth muscle. J Physiol 282: 437–450

Morgan K G, Schmalz P E, Szurszewski J H 1978b Electrical and mechanical effects of molecular variants of CCK on antral smooth muscle. Am J Physiol 235: E324–E329

Muller-Lissner S A, Schattermann G, Schenker G et al. 1981 Duodenogastric reflux in the fasting dog: role of pylorus and duodenal motility. Am J Physiol 241: G159–G162

Papasova M P, Nagai T, Prosser C L 1968 Two-component

slow waves in smooth muscle of cat stomach. Am J Physiol 214 (4): 695–702

Pappas T N, Debas H T, Goto Y et al (1985) Peptide YY inhibits meal stimulated pancreatic and gastric secretion. Am J Physiol 248: G118–G123

Paton W D M, Vane J R 1963 An analysis of the response of the isolated stomach to electrical stimulation and to drugs. J Physiol 165: 10–46

Prove J, Ehrlein H J 1982 Motor function of gastric antrum and pylorus for evacuation of low and high viscosity meals in dogs. Gut 23: 150–156

Publicover N G, Sanders K M 1985 Myogenic regulation of propagation in gastric smooth muscle. Am J Physiol 248: G512–G520

Read N W, Houghton L A 1989 Physiology of gastric emptying and pathophysiology of gastroparesis in: Motility disorders. Ouyang A (ed.) Gastroenterol Clin N Am 18 (2): 359–373

Read N W, Al-Jamali M N, Edwards C A 1984 The relationship between post prandial motor activity in the human small intestine and the gastrointestinal transit of food. Gastroenterology 86: 721–727

Roman C, Gonella J 1987 Extrinsic control of digestive tract motility in: Johnson L R Christensen J, Jackson M J, Jacobson E D, Walsh J H (eds) (ed.) Physiology of the gastrointestinal tract. Raven Press, New York pp 507–554

Sanders K M, Vogalis F 1989 Organization of electrical activity in the canine pyloric canal. J Physiol 416: 49–66

Schulze-Delrieu K 1983 Volume accommodation by distension of gastric fundus (rabbit) and gastric corpus (cat). Dig Dis Sci 28: 625–632

Schulze-Delrieu K 1992 Clearance patterns of the isolated guinea pig duodenum. Gastroenterology 102: 849–856

Schulze-Delrieu K, Brown K 1985 Gastric emptying as a function of pyloric resistance. Am J Physiol 248: G727–G732

Schulze-Delrieu K, Percy W H, Ren J et al 1989 Evidence for inhibition of opossum LES through intrinsic gastric nerves. Am J Physiol 256: G198–G205

Schulze-Delrieu K, Shirazi S S (1983) Neuromuscular differentiation of the human pylorus. Gastroenterology 84: 287–292

Schulze-Delrieu K, Shirazi S S 1987 Pressure and length adaptations in the isolated cat stomach. Am J Physiol 15: G92–G99

Schulze-Delrieu K, Wall J P 1983 Determinants of flow across the isolated gastroduodenal junction of cats and rabbits. Am J Physiol 245: G257–G264

Schulze-Delrieu K, Wall J P 1985 Mechanical activity of muscular patch pouches from cat and rabbit stomachs. Gastroenterology 88: 1012–1019

Schulze-Delrieu K, Wright B 1985 The ultrastructure of the gastric smooth muscle in relation to volume accommodation. Gastroenterology 88: A1577

Shirazi S S, Brown C K, Schulze-Delrieu K 1988 Duodenal resistance to the emptying of various solutions from the isolated cat stomach. J Lab Clin Med 111: 654–660

Sick K, Tedesko F 1908 Studien über Magenbewegung mit besonderer Berucksichtigung der Ausdehnungsfahigkeit des Hauptmagens (Fundus). Dtsch Arch Klin Med 92; 416–451

Sirois P J, Amidon G L, Meyer J H 1990 Gastric emptying of nondigestible solids in dogs: a hydrodynamic correlation. Am J Physiol 258: G65–G72

Spiller R C, Trotman I F, Higgins B E et al 1984 The ileal brake – inhibition of jejunal motility after ileal fat perfusion in man. Gut 25: 365–374

Spiller R C, Adrian T E, Trotman I F et al 1988 Further characterization of the 'ileal brake' reflex in man – effect of ileal infusion of partial digests of fat, protein and starch on jejunal motility and release of neurotensin, enteroglucagon and peptide YY. Gut 29: 1042–1051

Szurszewski J H 1981 Electrical basis for gastrointestinal motility in: Physiology of the gastrointestinal tract. Johnson L R, Christensen J, Jackson M J, Jacobson E D, Walsh J H (eds) Raven Press, New York pp 1435–1466

Thompson D G, Wingate D L 1988 Effects of osmoreceptor stimulation on human duodenal motor activity. Gut 29: 173–180

Tongas G, Anvari M, Richards D et al 1987 Relationship of pyloric motility to transpyloric flow in healthy subjects. Gastroenterology 92: A1673

Torgersen J 1942 The muscular build and movements of the stomach and duodenal bulb. Acta Radiol (Suppl) 45: 1–101

Treacy P J, Dent J, Jamieson G C et al 1988 Antropyloric pressure and isolated pyloric waves are major regulators of gastric emptying of liquids. Gastroenterology 94: A464

Weisbrodt N W 1984 Basic control mechanisms. In: Akkermans L M A (ed.) Gastric and gastroduodenal motility. Praeger, New York pp 3–20

Weisbrodt N W, Overholt B F, Wiley J N et al 1969 A relation between gastroduodenal muscle contractions and gastric emptying. Gut 10: 543–548

White C M, Alexander-Williams J, Poxon V 1983 Effect of nutrient liquids on human gastroduodenal motor activity. Gut 26: 1109–1116

Williams I 1962 Closure of the pylorus. Br J Radiol 35: 653–670

26. Biliary tract

J. Toouli

INTRODUCTION

The regulation of bile flow from the liver to the duodenum involves the interaction of motility of the gallbladder, bile duct and sphincter of Oddi that together determine the movement of fluid through the biliary tract. Furthermore, hepatic bile is modified by secretion and absorption via the lining mucosa. These functions are controlled by extrinsic and intrinsic neurones containing a number of regulatory peptides. In addition, a large number of hormones are released during the various stages of the interdigestive period and after the ingestion of food, and these influence the mechanisms which control bile flow.

The liver and the biliary tract are mentioned in the earliest recorded observations of man, having been described by the Babylonians as early as 2000 BC, (Glenn & Grafe 1966). However, it was not until the mid-1500s that the liver and its secretions were associated with digestion. Soon afterwards the role of the biliary tract in controlling the flow of bile from the liver to the duodenum was recognized, and Rugero Oddi (Oddi 1887) described the anatomy of the sphincteric mechanism which bears his name and subsequently demonstrated its function in controlling bile flow (Oddi 1888).

STUDY TECHNIQUES

Anatomy

Extrahepatic biliary tract anatomy has been determined from human cadaver dissections which have demonstrated the complex and variable relationships of its various components (Smadja & Blumgart 1988). Histological studies have further enhanced the appreciation of the relationships between the gallbladder biliary ducts, sphincter of Oddi (SO), nerves and blood vessels.

Standard histological techniques have been used to define the relationships between the smooth muscle layers, the mucosal lining, the serosa, the nerve plexuses and the vessels. The wholemount preparation (Costa & Furness 1983) has been used in order to examine nerves in the different layers of the viscus and nerve lesioning experiments (Furness & Costa 1987) as well as silver staining techniques which have provided data on neural pathway connections between different parts of the biliary tract and surrounding gastrointestinal tract.

Fluorescence immunohistochemistry techniques have been used on the biliary tracts of experimental animals and in some human specimens in order to define the presence and distribution of a variety of peptide-containing neurones (Padbury et al 1989). Detailed studies have been conducted in the Australian brush-tailed possum (*Trichosurus vulpecula*) systematically examining the gallbladder bile duct and SO. Tissue obtained from the possum or human cadavers is fixed in Zamboni's solution (2% formaldehyde in 0.1 M phosphate buffer + 15% picric acid) and sectioned (Costa et al 1987). Antisera to a variety of available neuropeptides are applied and labelled with fluorescein coupled to specific antibodies allowing observation of peptide localization with a fluorescence microscope. Further advances in these techniques have allowed double labelling of nerves and co-localization of neuropeptides in the nerve supply of the biliary tract has been determined (Costa et al 1986).

Resin casting techniques have been used to define the distribution and relationships of the blood supply to the biliary tract (Northover et al 1980). Arteries and veins are infused separately with coloured resin which hardens and is resistant to corrosion. The surrounding tissue can then be removed by tissue corrosives leaving the architecture of the vessels intact. Examination of the casts defines the distribution of the layers of small vessels in the biliary tract. Other methods used to define the vasculature of the biliary tract have included injection of indian ink (Shapiro & Robillard 1948) and the use of radio-opaque solutions which allow

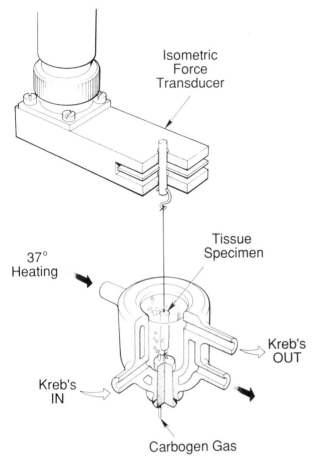

Fig. 26.1 A full-thickness strip of SO suspended in a muscle bath of Kreb's solution. The isometric force transducer records changes in length.

examination by radiographic methods (Munkacsi & Siklos 1962).

Motility studies

In vitro techniques

Studies conducted on biliary tract specimens in vitro have provided important understanding of the contractile activity of the gallbladder, bile ducts and SO. Representative tissue specimens from experimental animals or human speciments obtained at surgery have been studied by immersion in a bath solution of oxygenated Tyrode's or Kreb's solution (Toouli & Watts 1971). Under these conditions the tissue remains viable for up to 12 h and exhibits spontaneous contractile activity. The tissue is suspended at a fixed length

determined by a predetermined weight and the motility is recorded by force transducers (Fig. 26.1).

The specimens may be further stimulated via an electrical field applied by the immersion of electrodes in the bath. Electrical stimulation may selectively activate either the nerves or the smooth muscle. Using a variety of pharmacological agonists or antagonists, the function of various nerves associated with the specimen can be determined. Pharmacological experiments have been conducted using such in vitro techniques to determine the dose-response relationships for a number of potential agonists in the biliary tract (Helm et al 1985). The simultaneous recording of changes in tone and electrical activity from the smooth muscle has revealed the relationship between contraction and electrical events. Intracellular recordings from smooth muscle cells have also been made and illustrate that the muscle of the biliary tract behaves very much like that in other areas of the gastrointestinal tract (Bauer et al 1987).

Manometry of the gallbladder and SO

The recording of pressure changes from the lumen of the extrahepatic biliary tract has been a major technique in the understanding of biliary motility. Manometric techniques have been used for recording the motility of the gallbladder, bile duct and SO both in humans and a number of animal species.

Human manometry. Intraluminal pressure recordings from the human biliary tract were first made at the time of surgery on the biliary tract (Hess 1979). Pressure measurements from the bile ducts have been obtained by inserting a tube into the bile duct by way of the cystic duct. The pressure changes were read either directly from fluid-filled manometers or recorded by a transducer linked to a polygraph. Using these techniques, the opening, passage and closing pressures of the SO were determined by either increasing or decreasing the height of a fluid reservoir connected in series with the tube inside the bile duct (Cushieri et al 1972). Intraluminal pressure changes of the gallbladder were also recorded at operation by inserting a fluid-filled catheter in series with a transducer into the gallbladder (Csendes & Sepulveda 1980).

Accurate direct pressure measurements from the SO became possible with the miniaturization of manometry catheters and the development of fluid perfusion systems of low compliance (Arndorfer et al 1977). The polyethylene catheters have three lumens of 0.5 mm internal diameter making up a catheter of 1.7 mm outer diameter or a tapering catheter of 1.5 mm outer

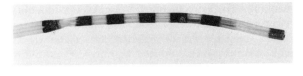

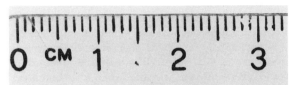

Fig. 26.2 SO manometry catheter. The triple lumen catheter is tapered to an outer diameter of 1.5 mm. Three recording ports are placed at 2 mm intervals. The black concentric rings are placed at 2 mm intervals.

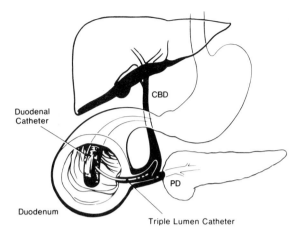

Fig. 26.4 Endoscopic SO manometry. The triple lumen catheter is introduced into either the bile duct or pancreatic duct. It is withdrawn so that the three recording ports are positioned in the sphincter. A separate catheter records duodenal pressure. (With permission from Toouli J, Roberts-Thomson I C, J Gastroenterol Hepatol 1987 2 431–442, Blackwell Scientific Publications.)

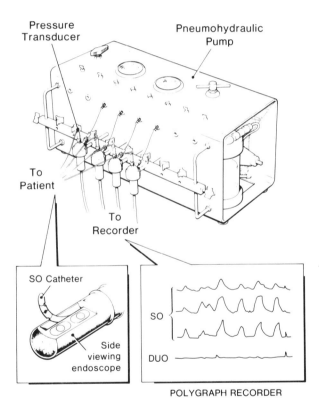

POLYGRAPH RECORDER

Fig. 26.3 Equipment used for biliary manometry. A triple lumen catheter is constantly perfused via a pneumohydraulic pump set at a pressure of 750 mmHg. For endoscopic manometry the tip of the catheter is introduced into the bile duct via the biopsy channel of a side viewing endoscope.

diameter (Fig. 26.2). Three side-holes are placed at 2 mm intervals starting at 10 mm from its distal tip. Therefore, the three lumens record across a length of

5 mm from within the SO. The catheter is 200 cm long and is perfused with deionized bubble-free water by way of a pneumohydraulic capillary system at a pressure of 750 mmHg. Water is perfused through the catheter at 0.125 ml/min and the whole system is capable of accurately recording pressure changes up to 300 mmHg/s (Fig. 26.3). The recording from three lumens allows the evaluation of the progressive nature of sphincter contractions as well as the determination of basal pressure, amplitude and frequency of contractions (Toouli et al 1982a).

Intraluminal recording of SO motility may be carried out under three different circumstances. The catheter may be introduced by way of an endoscope (Fig. 26.4) as in endoscopic retrograde cholangiopancreatography (Geenen et al 1980). The patient is mildly sedated and the oropharynx anaesthetized in order to assist the passage of the endoscope. The manometry catheter is introduced through the biopsy channel of the duodenoscope, through the papilla and into either the bile duct or the pancreatic duct. The catheter is then withdrawn so that all three recording ports are situated within the SO segment. In order to assist in the positioning of the catheter across the sphincter, circular markings are placed on the catheter at 2 mm intervals from the most proximal hole for a total length of 12 mm. Recordings are made for approximately 3–10 min. It is difficult to record for much longer by the endoscopic technique because patients often become intolerant of prolonged intubation.

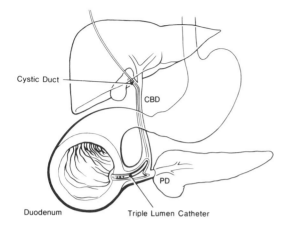

Fig. 26.5 Intraoperative SO manometry is performed by introducing the triple lumen manometry catheter via the cystic duct. The three recording lumens of the catheter are positioned across the sphincter of Oddi.

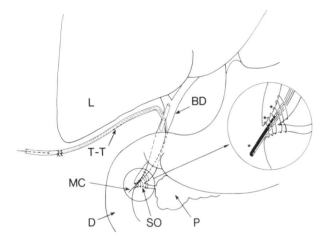

Fig. 26.6 Post-operative human T-tube (T–T) manometry. The manometry catheter (MC) is introduced via a modified T–T previously positioned in the bile duct (BD). The insert illustrates two of the ports positioned to record from the sphincter and the third records from the duodenum. L = liver; D = duodenum; SO = sphincter of Oddi; P = pancreas. (Worthley et al 1989.)

During elective operation for gallstones, recordings from the SO may be made by introducing the triple-lumen catheter through the cystic duct, into the bile duct and through the sphincter into the duodenum (Saccone et al 1988). The catheter is then withdrawn so that the three lumens are recording from the sphincter (Fig. 26.5). The duration of recording may be greater than that obtained at endoscopy but a major disadvantage is the fact that the patient is anaesthe-

tized. The effect of anaesthetic agents on biliary motility is unknown. However, in studies where manometry of the sphincter was obtained in both anaesthetized and awake patients, sphincter motility did not differ significantly when non-opiate anaesthetics were used (Toouli et al 1986a).

In order to conduct prolonged studies of SO motility, the catheter may be introduced through the T-tube in patients who have undergone exploration of the bile duct for stones (Worthley et al 1989). The manometry catheter is passed into the bile duct, through the sphincter and into the duodenum. It is then withdrawn so that it is positioned across the sphincter (Fig. 26.6). The position is confirmed fluoroscopically and by characteristic changes seen on the pressure tracings as the catheter is withdrawn from the duodenum into the sphincter. Recordings of up to 6–8 h may be made with this technique. The disadvantage is that, by necessity, only those patients who have had stones in the bile duct can be studied.

Animal manometry. Pressure changes from within the biliary tract have been studied in a variety of animal species including dogs, cats, possums, opossums, rabbits, pigs, prairie dogs and guinea pigs. The methods used are similar to those described above for man. An ingenious technique has been used to record the resistance to flow across the SO of the cat in acute experiments performed under anaesthesia. The catheter is inserted by way of the bile duct so that it is jammed above the sphincter. The catheter is ligated in this position and water is perfused. The resistance to flow is measured by a pressure transducer connected to the catheter (Behar & Biancani 1980).

Measurement of flow across the SO has been made via a complex model which records changes in reservoir volume of fluid perfused proximal to the sphincter and in addition fluid collected by a funnel positioned to catch the effluent (Fig. 26.7). This technique allows the study of mechanisms which control flow across the SO (Liu et al 1992). In addition the flow changes can be correlated with pressure changes recorded by a small catheter placed within the lumen of the sphincter.

Prolonged recordings of pressure have been made from conscious pigs following prior insertion of a non-perfused manometry catheter in the gallbladder and a T-tube in the bile duct which allows insertion of a triple lumen manometry catheter for measuring SO motility (McIntosh et al 1988). The technique is similar to that used in humans for prolonged studies.

An ingenious method for studying gallbladder tone has been developed by adapting the gastric barostat technique to the gallbladder (Fig. 26.8). The

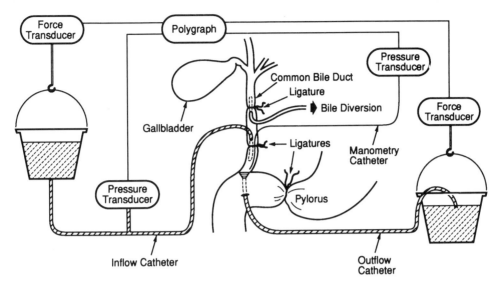

Fig. 26.7 Possum model for recording flow across the SO. Inflow is recorded by change in volume from the inflow reservoir. Outflow is also recorded by collecting the fluid via a funnel sutured to the opening of the bile duct in the duodenum. Simultaneous sphincter pressure changes are recorded via a single lumen manometry catheter. (Reproduced with permission from Liu et al 1992.)

gallbladder barostat is made up of a polyurethane bag that is connected by a double lumen polyvinyl tube to a strain gauge and a syringe air injection system. The bag is inserted into the gallbladder via a cannula, which has been previously implanted in the animal gallbladder and exteriorized. The balloon is inflated so that it takes up the gallbladder volume. The bag is maintained at a constant low pressure (2 mmHg) and at this pressure is able to register gallbladder wall contraction and relaxation by recording the changes in the volume of the bag. The studies are done by occluding the cystic duct via a previously implanted inflatable hydraulic occluding device, thus allowing study of gallbladder motility changes without influence by changes in SO motility (Tanaka et al 1990).

Electromyography

The electrical activity of the biliary tract has been recorded using extracellular bipolar or monopolar electrodes sutured to the outside surface of the gallbladder and the SO in animals (Sarles et al 1975). Extensive studies have been done in the American opossum SO as this animal has a long extraduodenal segment which allows for the attachment of electrodes. Bipolar electrodes sutured to the SO and gallbladder of the American opossum have shown that as in other parts of the gastrointestinal tract, the SO exhibits two forms of myoelectric activity; slow regular changes in mem-

brane potential, known as electrical slow waves and rapid depolarization spikes, called spike bursts. Spike bursts are virtually always associated with phasic smooth muscle contractions and therefore produce transient intraluminal pressure changes (Honda et al 1982).

Recordings of electrical signals from the human SO have been made by introducing electrodes into the lumen of the sphincter through the biopsy channel of a duodenoscope. Recordings so produced resemble those seen from recordings in experimental animals and are thought to reflect contractions of the human SO (Bortolotti et al 1985).

Ultrasonography

Techniques that make use of ultrasonography have been developed for measuring the volume of the gallbladder and the diameters of the biliary and pancreatic ducts. Following stimulation either by eating or by hormone infusion, changes in these measurements can be followed, thus providing a non-invasive means of evaluating the motility of the biliary and pancreatic ductal systems in clinical situations.

Human gallbladder volume is determined by measuring the maximal length and the maximal transverse diameter of the gallbladder. The volume is then calculated from the ultrasound images as the sum of a series of cylinders (Everson et al 1980). Serial measurements

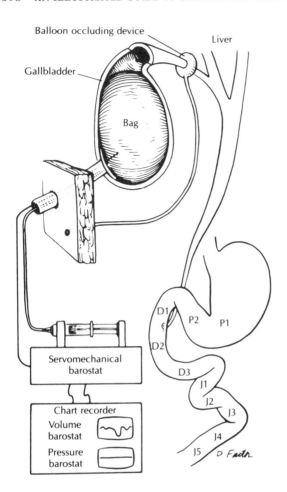

Fig. 26.8 A gallbladder barostat device. The bag has been positioned in the gallbladder and inflated so that changes in the gallbladder tone are recorded. D = duodenum, J = jejenum. (Toouli J 1991 Curr Opin Gastroenterol 7: 758–764.)

in normal persons is less than 1 mm. Following the infusion of secretin, there is an increase in ductal diameter followed by a rapid return to normal size within 30 min. If the ductal diameter remains in excess of 1.5 mm after 30 min, this suggests an increase in resistance to the outflow of pancreatic juice which may represent dysfunction of the SO (Bolondi et al 1984).

Isotope studies

^{99m}Tc IDA (iminodiacetic acid) compounds are cleared through the liver into bile after intravenous administration. ^{99m}Tc gives off 140 Kev gamma photons that are ideally suited for imaging and counting by a gamma camera. These properties of the ^{99m}Tc IDA compounds have been used to image the gallbladder (Shaffer et al 1980) and the biliary tract; by producing temporal profiles, monitoring of gallbladder emptying and flow across the bile duct in post-cholecystectomy subjects can be accomplished.

The motor function of the gallbladder can be evaluated by determining the gallbladder ejection fraction (GBEF). Following the concentration of ^{99m}Tc DIDA in the gallbladder, cholecystokinin (CCK) octapeptide is infused intravenously over 45 min. Gallbladder emptying of the ^{99m}Tc DIDA is monitored during the infusion period and for 15 min after cessation of infusion (Krishnamurthy et al 1981). The GBEF is determined by use of the formula:

$$\frac{\text{counts at specified time}}{\text{maximal counts prior to infusion}} \times 100$$

The mean GBEF at 15 min after infusion is normally 70%. Values <40% represent abnormalities in GBEF which reflect disorders in gallbladder motility (Yap et al 1991).

A similar evaluation of flow through the bile duct has been done in patients after cholecystectomy in order to determine the characteristics of flow across the SO (Roberts-Thomson et al 1986). Following the injection of ^{99m}Tc DIDA, the subject is positioned under a gamma camera and continuous recordings are made from the liver, biliary tract and duodenum. In order to analyse flow, areas of interest are outlined and the counts per second within those areas are determined and graphically displayed. The shape and slope of the curve of counts from the bile duct reflect flow through the biliary tree. Delay in outflow may represent a raised resistance to flow across the SO which is due to SO dysfunction.

of volume changes can reveal the effects of various stimuli on gallbladder volume.

The maximal diameter of the bile duct can also be measured using ultrasonography. A fixed point adjacent to the point where the right hepatic artery crosses the common hepatic duct has been taken as the point of maximal diameter. Following the ingestion of a fatty meal, it is expected that normal changes in SO motility will enhance bile flow into the duodenum and so the diameter of the common hepatic duct should decrease. An increase in ductal diameter is taken to reflect a resistance to outflow which may represent dysfunction of the SO (Darweesh et al 1988).

The diameter of the pancreatic duct as determined

ANATOMY OF THE BILIARY SYSTEM

Gross anatomy

Embryology

The gallbladder and bile ducts arise from the caudal portion of a diverticular anlage that originates from the ventral floor of the foregut. The pancreas develops from two foregut buds in the region of the future duodenum. In 1957 Boyden confirmed that the distal muscularis propria of the bile duct and pancreatic duct are independent from the duodenal musculature. In studies of the human foetus he showed that the SO musculature arises de novo from mesenchyme, appearing approximately 5 weeks after the intestinal musculature appears (Boyden 1957).

Morphology

Bile from the hepatocytes is secreted into canaliculi which communicate with numerous interlobular ducts; these, in turn, drain into two main hepatic ducts. The main right and left hepatic ducts fuse at the porta hepatis into the common hepatic duct and the cystic duct joins the common hepatic duct at a variable distance caudal to the porta hepatis to form the common bile duct (CBD) (Dowdy et al 1962).

The human gallbladder is a pear-shaped sac nestled along a fossa on the right inferior surface of the liver. The gallbladder is divided anatomically into the blunt fundus, the body, and the neck which leads to the cystic duct. A sacculation at the neck of the gallbladder is known as Hartmann's pouch. The cystic duct is of variable length, usually joining the common hepatic duct at an acute angle to form the CBD.

The CBD passes dorsal to the first part of the duodenum lying in a groove either within or posterior to the head of the pancreas (Lytle 1959) and enters the second part of the duodenum through the major duodenal papilla in association with the pancreatic duct of Wirsung. The junction of the terminal CBD, pancreatic duct and duodenum at the papilla assumes one of three configurations that may be likened to a Y, V or U. In approximately 70% of subjects the ducts open into a common channel and thus have a Y configuration. This common channel drains into the duodenum through a single orifice on the duodenal papilla of Vater. In approximately 20% of subjects the common channel is almost non-existent and the two ducts have a common V-shaped configuration as they approach the opening on the papilla. In 10% of subjects the CBD and pancreatic duct have separate openings on the tip of the papilla and these openings lie adjacent to

give the U-shaped configuration. The terminal parts of the CBD and pancreatic duct, the common channel and major duodenal papilla of Vater are invested by smooth muscle of varying thickness and together form the SO segment.

The major part of the human SO lies within the duodenal wall, and has been shown to be distinctly separated from it. Boyden (1937), in a series of publications on the anatomy of the SO, described distinct sphincters at the terminal end of the CBD (sphincter choledochus), the terminal end of the pancreatic duct (sphincter pancreaticus) and the common channel (sphincter ampullae). More recently, however, Hand (1963), using a combination of radiographic methods, duct casting techniques and histological sectioning methods, could not distinguish separate sphincters. Hand concluded from his human autopsy studies that the CBD and the pancreatic duct become fused in a common connective tissue sheath outside the duodenal wall and pass together through a slit in a duodenal muscle called the 'choledochal window'. The lumina, however, do not join at this level but are separated by a thick muscular septum. In most subjects fusion of the two lumina occurs in the submucosal layer of the duodenum to form a common channel varying in length between 2–17 mm. Before entering the duodenum, each duct becomes completely surrounded by circular muscle, some of which forms a figure-of-eight pattern around the two ducts. The point at which the smooth muscle starts on each duct is readily identified radiologically as a notch. Distal to the notch, each lumen becomes narrow as it traverses the duodenal wall; this narrowing is associated with a thickening of the duct wall consisting of smooth muscle, connective tissue and mucous glands. As the ducts pass through the duodenal wall, longitudinal muscle fibres interdigitate between the circular muscle fibres of the ducts and the duodenal muscle. The ducts emerge from the duodenal muscle layers to follow a course of variable length through the duodenal submucosa before opening on the papilla of Vater; throughout this submucosal course, the ducts are ensheathed by circularly-oriented smooth muscle bundles. Recent manometric studies in man support Hand's description of the SO in that separate sphincteric zones were not identified (Toouli et al 1982a).

The mucosal layer of the gallbladder consists of a lamina propria with connective tissue, blood vessels, nerves and lymphatics (Jansson 1979). There is neither a muscularis mucosae nor a submucosa (Sutherland 1966). The mucosa is usually folded and is lined by a single layer of columnar epithelium.

The cystic duct is similar in structure to the gall-

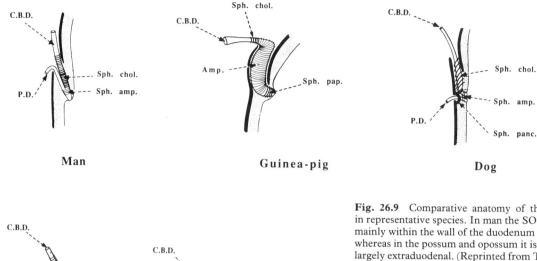

Fig. 26.9 Comparative anatomy of the SO in representative species. In man the SO is mainly within the wall of the duodenum whereas in the possum and opossum it is largely extraduodenal. (Reprinted from Toouli J & Baker R A, Pharmacol Therap 49: 269–281, with permission from Pergamon Press Ltd, Oxford, UK.)

bladder except that there are mucosal folds or valves which are oriented transverse to the long axis. These valves contain extensions of muscle from the fibromuscular layer (Scott & Otto 1979).

The bile duct is similar in structure to the gallbladder. The mucosa demonstrates numerous infoldings that create the appearance of intramural glands (Mahour et al 1967). The bile duct wall is fibromuscular with no distinct layers of muscle but smooth muscle cells are generally found scattered throughout the wall. Most of these muscle fibres are orientated in the longitudinal axis of the duct.

The mucosa of the SO segment in man is lined by a columnar epithelium and contains numerous mucus-secreting glands. The mucosa is thrown into longitudinal folds that have been called mucosal valvules (Tansy et al 1975). These folds are least marked proximally

and increase in prominence distally becoming maximal in the common channel. The mucosal folds may occasionally be seen projecting through the orifice of the duodenal papilla.

In order to study the motility of the biliary tract and its controlling mechanisms, investigators have used a variety of experimental animals. It should be noted, however, that the anatomical arrangements of the biliary tract differ between species and these differences probably reflect differences in function (Fig. 26.9).

Some species, such as the horse, rat, pigeon and pocket gopher, do not have gallbladders. These species also have a rudimentary SO (Hallenbeck 1967). In dogs, pigs and rabbits, the bile duct and pancreatic duct enter the duodenum separately. In these species the SO is present and, as in man, is mainly contained within the wall of the duodenum (Boyden 1937). The guinea pig bile duct and pancreatic duct enter a common ampulla which is situated within the duodenal wall. This animal has the most prominent ampulla of any species and a distinct sphincter is present at its junction with the duodenal papilla. The American opossum and the Australian possum are characterized by an extraduodenal SO. In both of these marsupials, the bile duct and pancreatic duct join to form a common channel of entry into the duodenum. In the American opossum, however, circular muscle encircles both ducts while in the Australian species the arrangement is that of a figure-of-eight, thus creating a muscular septum between the bile duct and the pancreatic duct.

The SO in cats, chimpanzees and monkeys appears most closely to approximate the human anatomy. In these species the bile duct and the pancreatic duct join together in a short common channel which is surrounded by a sphincter that lies largely in the wall of the duodenum.

Innervation

The extrahepatic bile ducts, gallbladder and SO are richly supplied by both extrinsic and intrinsic nerves. Recent studies have shown an extensive distribution of ganglia and nerve fibres in the biliary tract suggesting an important role for nerves in the control of biliary tract motility.

Extrinsic nerves

The extrinsic nerve supply of the biliary tract is similar in distribution to that of the small intestine and is made up of parasympathetic and sympathetic components. The parasympathetic innervation reaches the upper abdomen by way of the vagus nerves. Animal studies have demonstrated that 90% of fibres in the vagi are afferent and 10% efferent. 10% of these fibres supply the biliary tract (Harkins et al 1963). The cell bodies of the vagal efferent fibres are situated in the medulla oblongata while the afferent cell bodies are found in the jugular and nodose ganglia (Davison 1983). In addition to the well-described cholinergic effects of the actions of the vagi, studies have demonstrated the presence of a variety of peptide-containing nerves in the vagi. These peptides include substance P (SP), somatostatin (SOM), vasoactive intestinal polypeptide (VIP), galanin (GAL) and enkephalins (ENK) (Lundberg et al 1978).

The sympathetic fibres to the biliary tract project from the thoracic and lumbar spinal cord to the prevertebral sympathetic ganglia. The cell bodies of the major-ity of noradrenergic fibres which supply the gut are located here. In general the distribution of noradrenergic fibres to the biliary tract follows the pattern of the blood supply (Bingham et al 1950).

Parasympathetic and sympathetic extrinsic nerves which innervate the biliary tract form an anterior and posterior hepatic plexus which is situated in the porta hepatis, anterior and posterior to the bile duct, hepatic artery and portal vein. Contributions to the plexuses are made from the anterior and posterior vagi and from the coeliac ganglion. The relative proportions in the mix of fibres from each of these sources is uncertain. A further sympathetic contribution to the biliary tract arises from the superior mesenteric ganglion and supplies the SO by way of the inferior pancreaticoduodenal artery.

Intrinsic nerves

The architecture and distribution of intrinsic nerves of the biliary tract have not been fully characterized. However, studies from a number of different species have demonstrated variations between species and between individuals of one species.

The gallbladder is thought to be innervated from three ganglionated plexuses, an outer subserosal, an intramuscular and an innermost plexus in the lamina propria. This latter plexus has not been found in some studies and it may be a variable between species (Keast et al 1985). Nerve fibres in the gallbladder wall are densely distributed along a subepithelial plexus and a lesser concentration of fibres is found in the muscle coat with fibres oriented in the direction of the muscle bundles. Fluorescence histochemistry has demonstrated nonadrenergic fibres and nerves with cholinesterase reactivity among these fibres (Cai & Gabella 1983a). Furthermore, a relatively rich distribution of VIP and SP containing nerves has been described (Cai et al 1983). Lesser concentrations of other neuropeptide nerves have also been described and these include neuropeptide Y (NPY), SOM, gastrin releasing peptide (GRP), GAL and ENK (Allen et al 1984, Cai & Gabella 1983b).

The distribution of nerves to the common bile duct appears not to be so orderly as that seen for the gallbladder (Alexander 1940, Burnett et al 1964). A prominent feature, however, is the presence of two or more large nerve trunks which run along the length of the bile duct in the submucosal region. These nerve trunks may be important in the coordination of motor activities of the gallbladder and the SO. Histochemical studies of nerves to the bile duct have demonstrated noradrenergic fibres and some small cholinesterase-containing ganglia (Kyosola 1978). Sparsely situated VIP, ENK, SOM, NPY and GRP fibres have been identified in some species (Dancygier et al 1984).

The density of ganglia and fibres increases at the lower end of the bile duct in the region of the SO. The sphincter contains two ganglionated plexuses; an outer plexus between the muscle layers and a submucous plexus (Cai & Gabella 1983a, Van Buskirk & Boyden 1944). Most studies have described connections between these plexuses and those of the duodenum and the gallbladder. However, further studies are required to precisely define the connecting fibre circuitry. A dense distribution of nerve fibres supplies the sphincter muscle and is observed around blood vessels. Noradrenergic and cholinesterase-containing fibres have been described (Mori et al 1979). In addition, a dense innervation of the muscle by nerves containing VIP, SP, GRP and ENK has been demonstrated (Alumets et al 1979, Cai et al 1983). Nerves containing NPY and SOM have also been observed in separate studies (Allen et al 1984).

Blood supply

The biliary tract obtains oxygenated blood through two major routes, the hepatic artery and the gastroduodenal artery. There is marked variation in the origin and the distribution of these arteries in relation to the biliary tract. A common finding is that of an extensively-anastomosing arterial plexus which ensheaths the biliary tract and from which the intramural blood supply is derived.

For purposes of description the blood supply of the extrahepatic biliary tract is divided into anterior and posterior components relative to the bile duct (Northover & Terblanche 1979). However, it should be noted that this is an artificial division and a free anastomosis exists between the two plexuses. Anterior to the bile duct there are two to five ascending vessels which arise from the retroduodenal branch of the gastroduodenal artery. In addition, there are three or four vessels originating from the right hepatic artery and the cystic artery which anastomose with the ascending arteries. In particular, the ascending and descending vessels form two prominent arterial channels at the 3 o'clock and 9 o'clock aspects of the bile duct, and these arteries provide the major source of the axial blood supply to the biliary tract. In one study, (Northover & Terblanche 1979) it was concluded that the major axial blood supply of the biliary tract was derived from the gastroduodenal artery where 60% of the blood originated. 38% was supplied from the right hepatic artery and 2% from other sources.

A retroportal artery has been described posterior to the bile duct. This artery arises from either the coeliac axis or the superior mesenteric artery and runs upward on the back of the portal vein. It has a variable course, most commonly ending by joining the retroduodenal artery close to the lower end of the extraduodenal bile duct. Less frequently it joins the right hepatic artery.

An important factor regarding the position of these major arteries to the bile duct is the possibility of injury during operations on the biliary tract to produce relative ischaemia to a part of the bile duct. Furthermore, in view of the fact that most of the blood supply is derived from the right hepatic artery, it is recommended that anastomoses to the bile duct should be as close to the upper bile duct as possible.

The intrinsic blood supply of the bile duct is made up of arterioles which penetrate the wall and form two rich plexuses of capillaries (Parke & Michels 1963). The most superficial plexus is between the outer fibrous sheath and the lamina propria. The other plexus lies directly under the mucosa. Both of these plexuses form an extensive capillary network of fine vessels (Cho & Lunderquist 1983). The site of this vascular bed and its configuration suggests that it is probably involved in physiological absorption of substances from the lumen of the bile duct.

MOTILITY OF THE BILIARY TRACT

Gallbladder

The human gallbladder has been shown by ultrasound techniques to have a normal volume of approximately 17 ml. This volume however does not remain static during the fasting state. Studies in dogs and opossums have demonstrated that the gallbladder contracts up to 40% of maximal contractile capacity during the interdigestive period, and that these gallbladder contractions occur during phase II of the interdigestive cycle, just prior to phase III of the migrating motor complex (MMC). The periodic gallbladder contractions during fasting empty concentrated viscous bile and enable the gallbladder to refill with the more dilute hepatic bile (Takahashi et al 1982a).

Ultrasound studies in human volunteers have shown that a similar cyclical pattern of gallbladder volume changes also occurs in man (Toouli et al 1986b). Just as in the experimental animal studies, the gallbladder reduces its volume up to 40% of maximal volume just prior to phase III of the MMC in the duodenum (Fig. 26.10).

The mechanisms which control the gallbladder volume changes during the interdigestive cycle are

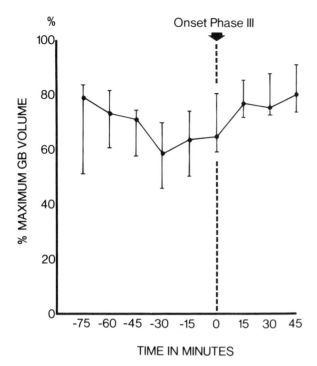

Fig. 26.10 Gallbladder volume changes during the interdigestive cycle. The human gallbladder partially empties just prior to the onset of duodenal phase III activity. (Reproduced with permission from Toouli et al 1986.)

unknown. However, it is postulated that both neuronal and hormonal factors may have a role. Serum motilin levels peak just before phase III of the MMC and animal studies have shown that motilin at physiological concentrations produces gallbladder contraction (Takahashi et al 1982b).

Following a meal the gallbladder empties by a steady contraction which delivers bile into the duodenum. This steady contraction generates a low intramural pressure which is only just above that registered in the bile ducts. This tonic contraction resembles that generated by the fundus of the stomach during gastric emptying. Gallbladder emptying following a meal is thought to be due to release of endogenous CCK from the mucosa of proximal small intestine. CCK is released by fat and protein entering the duodenum while carbohydrates have little to no effect (Weiner et al 1981).

The role of the enteric nervous system in regulating gallbladder volume is unclear. Vagotomy has been shown to produce increased fasting gallbladder volume (Johnson & Boyden 1952), thus suggesting a mechanism for the vagus in maintaining gallbladder tone.

However, direct stimulation of the vagus does not appear to produce consistently reproducible effects on gallbladder contraction, (Benevantano & Rosen 1969) and, similarly, stimulation of the sympathetic nerves does not appear to produce consistent results (Persson 1972).

Cystic duct

The role of the cystic duct in influencing flow in and out of the gallbladder has been debated. Currently the prevailing view suggests that a sphincter type mechanism does not have a major role. However the mucosal valves of Heister which produce prominent folds in the lumen of the cystic duct exert a variable resistor to flow. Studies in dogs have demonstrated resistance to flow across the cystic duct both into and out of the gallbladder (Scott & Otto 1979). Reductions in flow occur following either systemic or local intra-arterial injection of morphine or adrenaline, indicating that smooth muscle in the cystic duct may modulate flow through its lumen. In the prairie dog gallstone model, cystic duct resistance to flow increases before gallstone formation suggesting that disorders of cystic duct function may be associated with the formation of gallstones (Pitt et al 1981b). A role for the enteric nervous system (ENS) in controlling cystic duct resistance has not yet been identified.

Common bile duct

The human bile duct does not exhibit primary propulsile activity and its main role is thought to be that of providing a constant-tonic pressure. This is consistent with the histology of the bile duct which shows that it is mainly made up of elastic fibres and longitudinally orientated smooth muscle cells which are suited to fulfilling this function (Toouli & Watts 1971).

The diameter of the bile duct may change as a result of a change in resistance provided to outflow of bile by the SO. Following cholecystectomy, bile duct size does not alter significantly (Le Quesne et al 1959, Hunt & Scott 1989) and so the finding of an abnormally dilated duct in the absence of a clear pathological cause reflects increased resistance across the SO due to a motor disturbance of the sphincter.

Sphincter of Oddi

Manometric recordings from the SO of experimental animal species and man have shown that the SO is characterized by prominent pressure peaks representing phasic contractions (Fig. 26.11) which are

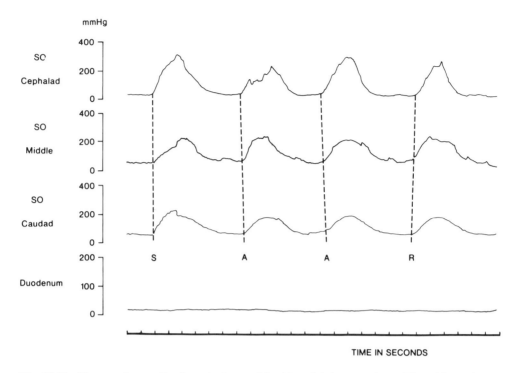

Fig. 26.11 Manometric recording from the human SO with a triple lumen catheter. The sphincter is characterized manometrically by prominent phasic contractions superimposed on a modest basal pressure (With permission from Toouli J, Roberts-Thomson I C, J Gastroenterol Hepatol 1987 2: 431–442, Blackwell Scientific Publications.)

superimposed on a low and stable basal pressure (tone). The function of these phasic contractions and their role in promoting flow from the bile duct and pancreas into the duodenum varies between the different species.

Studies have been done in the opossum SO in order to define the relationships between flow and contractions (Toouli et al 1983). Recordings using cineradiography and EMG to register contractions at the same time as flow have demonstrated that flow occurs both by active peristaltic propulsion and passively, between the phasic contractions (Fig. 26.12). In the opossum, the sphincter relaxes and bile flows from the bile duct into the sphincter segment. Some of this bile flows ahead passively from the SO segment on into the duodenum, but the major flow is accomplished by an active propulsive contraction which sweeps across the length of the SO segment, emptying its contents into the duodenum. This cycle then repeats and most of the net flow occurs through active propulsion, with a significant amount of flow still occurring passively.

In man, manometric and flow studies have demonstrated that, unlike the opossum, most of the flow

from the bile duct into the duodenum occurs between the contractions, hence passively (Worthley et al 1989). In addition, the phasic contractions expel a relatively small volume of bile across the SO segment (Hess 1979). However, when the sphincter contracts, the phasic pressure changes produce a transient resistance to flow between the bile duct and the duodenum, for each time the sphincter contracts the outflow from the bile duct is occluded. This action of the sphincter is no more obstructive in function than the action of the ventricle of the heart in obstructing blood flow out of the atria every time it contracts. Hence, the overall effect of the phasic contractions of the human SO is that of promoting flow from the ducts into the duodenum.

During the interdigestive period, the frequency of SO contractions demonstrates a periodicity that relates to the small intestine interdigestive cycle. However, unlike the small intestine, SO contractions do not pass through a phase I of absolute quiescence; they are omnipresent. In the opossum the frequency of contractions gradually increases during phase II and culmi-

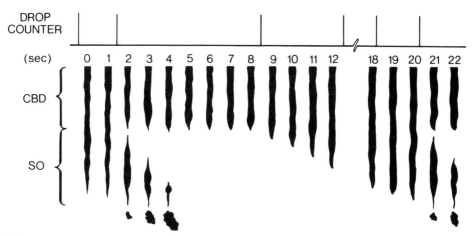

Fig. 26.12 Schematic representation of a cineradiographic sequence illustrating flow of contrast medium from the common bile duct (CBD) through the SO into the duodenum. The drop counter records drops of contrast medium from the reservoir into the CBD (Toouli et al 1989).

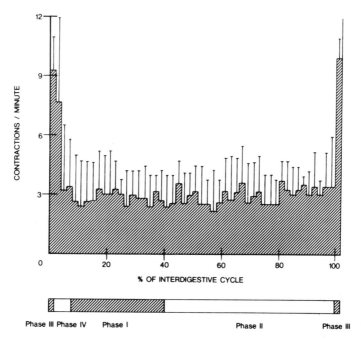

Fig. 26.13 Histogram demonstrating the frequency of human SO contractions in relation to the duodenum interdigestive activity (phase I to IV). SO contractions are omnipresent throughout the interdigestive period. The SO contraction frequency increases just prior to duodenal phase III (Worthley et al 1989.)

nates in a short burst of high-frequency contractions just before duodenal phase III activity (Honda et al 1982). In man the SO contractions are similarly constantly present during all phases of the interdigestive cycle (Worthley et al 1989). The SO frequency remains constant until just before phase III of the duodenal

MMC, when it increases to approximate the frequency of duodenal contractions. This burst of maximal activity lasts throughout the length of phase III of the duodenal MMC and the SO then returns to its normal contractile frequency after the passage of phase III of the duodenal MMC (Fig. 26.13).

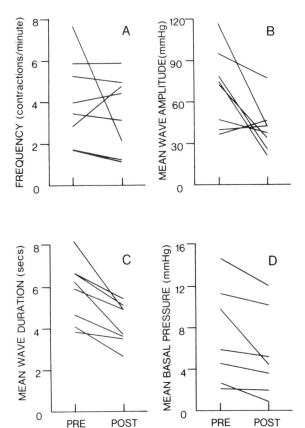

Fig. 26.14 Comparison of SO wave (A) frequency, (B) amplitude, (C) duration and (D) basal pressure, 10 min *before* versus 20 min *after* food ingestion in eight patients. There is a significant fall in SO amplitude, duration and basal pressure. There was no change in frequency. (Worthley et al 1989).

has recently become evident. The functional significance of the extrinsic nerves has not been clearly defined as yet. Vagotomy has been shown in some studies (Pitt et al 1981a) to increase resistance to flow across the SO while in other studies (Tansy et al 1974) little effect was seen. Stimulation of the vagus or sympathetic nerves have not demonstrated reproducibly consistent results. This may suggest that the extrinsic nerves only set a background tone for the superimposed contractile events, which are modulated at a peripheral site by the actions of intrinsic nerves and hormones.

Neural connections have been demonstrated between the gallbladder, cystic duct and SO, as well as between the gastric antrum and SO. Distension of the gallbladder has been shown to promote relaxation of the sphincter by way of a reflex mediated by these connections (Thune et al 1986, Thune et al 1991).

A role of gastrointestinal hormones in the control of motility in the SO is well established and the mechanism of action of CCK has been demonstrated in the cat (Behar & Biancani 1980). This hormone which is important for the control of biliary motility, has been shown to inhibit SO phasic contractions by an effect on non-adrenergic non-cholinergic inhibitory neurones (Fig. 26.15). Its action in man is thought to occur through a similar mechanism to produce inhibition of phasic contractions and a fall in SO basal pressure (Toouli et al 1982b). The action of other gastrointestinal hormones on the SO has not been so well established as has that of CCK. However, secretin, glucagon, histamine, gastrin, VIP and SP have all been shown to alter SO contractions in doses that may apply in the physiological state (Carr-Locke et al 1983, Dahlstrand et al 1988, Dahlstrand et al 1989).

Normal biliary motility

Gallbladder and SO motility is orchestrated during both fasting and after a meal by a combination of neural and hormonal actions. During fasting, bile is stored in the gallbladder and concentrated by the absorption of water. However, the gallbladder empties part of its contents every 100–120 min just prior to phase III of the interdigestive cycle, thus reducing the chance of supersaturated bile in the gallbladder producing stones. SO contractions also vary in frequency during the interdigestive period. During phase III, the frequency of SO contractions is similar to that of duodenal contractions, hence providing a powerful resistor to reflux of duodenal contents either into the bile duct or pancreatic duct.

After a meal the gallbladder contracts slowly, largely in response to release of CCK from the duodenum. SO

After a meal the responses of the opossum SO and the human SO differ in a way that may reflect the different functions of the contractions in the two species. In the opossum there is an increase in contractile frequency which enhances flow across the SO. In man, there is no alteration in the frequency but the amplitude of the contractions decreases so that the interval between contractions is increased (Fig. 26.14). In addition, the SO basal pressure is decreased and the overall effect is the promotion of passive flow of fluid from the ducts to the duodenum. It is, however, significant that the SO contractions are not abolished so that even in a weakened form they tend to maintain the SO segment free of debris and to promote flow towards the duodenum.

The role of the ENS in the control of SO activity

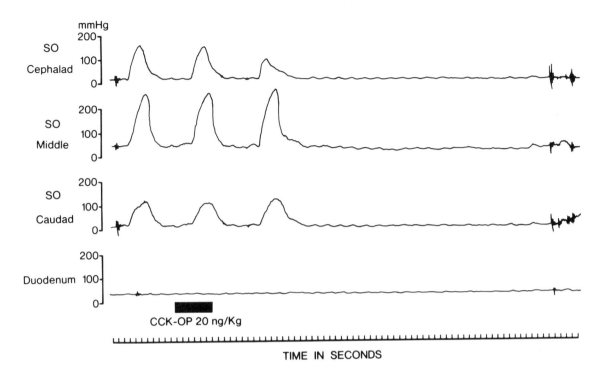

Fig. 26.15 Manometric recording demonstrating the effect of cholecystokinin octapeptide (CCK – OP) 20 ng/kg on SO activity. The phasic contractions are normally inhibited by CCK – OP. (Reproduced from Toouli J, Roberts-Thompson I C, J Gastroenterol Hepatol 1987 2: 431–442 with permission from Blackwell Scientific Publications.)

contractions are reduced in amplitude and basal pressure falls. These effects enhance the flow of bile from the gallbladder into the duodenum and promote flow of pancreatic juice. Disorders in the activity of either the gallbladder or SO may vary and result in clinical syndromes which will be discussed in chapter 33.

REFERENCES

Alexander W F 1940 The innervation of the biliary system. J Complete Neurol 72: 357–370

Allen J M, Gu J, Adrian T E, Polak J M, Bloom S R 1984 Neuropeptide Y in the guinea-pig biliary tract. Experentia 40: 765–767

Alumets J, Fahrenkrug J, Hakanson R, Schaffalitzky D E, Muckadell O, Sundler J, Uddman R 1979 A rich VIP nerve supply is characteristic of sphincters. Nature 280: 155–156

Arndorfer R C, Steff J J, Dodds W J, Linehan J H, Hogan W J 1977 Improved infusion system for intraluminal esophageal manometry. Gastroenterology 73: 23–27

Bauer A J, Go V L W, Koch T R, Szurszewski J 1987 Non-adrenergic, non-cholinergic (NANC) inhibitory innervation of the canine and opossum sphincter of Oddi. Gasteroenterology 92 (Part 2): 1311

Behar J, Biancani P 1980 Effect of cholecystokinin and the octapeptide of cholecystokinin on the feline sphincter of Oddi and gallbladder. Mechanisms of action. J Clin Invest 66: 1231–1239

Benevantano T C, Tosen R G 1969 The physiological effect of acute vagal section on canine biliary dynamics. J Surg Res 9: 331–334

Bingham J R, Ingelfinger F J, Smithwick R H 1950 The effects of sympathectomy on the motility of the human gastrointestinal and biliary tracts. Gastroenterology 15: 6–17

Bolondi L, Gaiani S, Gullo L, Labo G 1984 Secretin administration induces a dilatation of the main pancreatic duct. Dig Dis Sci 29: 802–808

Bortolotti M, Caletti G C, Brocchi E, Bersani G, Guizzardi G, Labo G 1985 Endoscopic electromyography and manometry of the human sphincter of Oddi. Hepatol Gastroenterol 32: 250–252

Boyden E A 1937 The sphincter of Oddi in man and certain representative mammals. Surgery 1: 25–37

Boyden E A 1957 The anatomy of the choledochoduodenal junction in man. Surg Gynecol Obstet 104: 641–652

Burnett W, Cairns F W, Bacsich P 1964 Some observations on the innervation of the extrahepatic biliary system in man. Ann Surg 159: 8–26

Cai W Q, Gabella G 1983a The musculature of the gallbladder and biliary pathways in the guinea pig. J Anat 136: 237–250

Cai W Q, Gabella G 1983b Innervation of the gallbladder and biliary pathways in the guinea-pig. J Anat 136: 97–109

Cai W Q, Gu J, Huang W et al 1983 Peptide immunoreactive nerves and cells of the guinea-pig gallbladder and biliary pathways. Gut 24: 1186–1193

Carr-Locke D L, Gregg J A, Auki T 1983 Effects of exogenous glucagon on pancreatic and biliary ductal and sphincteric pressures in man demonstrated by endoscopic manometry and correlation with plasma glucagon. Dig Dis Sci 28: 312–320

Cho K J, Lunderquist A 1983 The peribiliary vascular plexus: the microvascular architecture of the bile duct in the rabbit and in clinical cases. Radiology 147: 357–364

Costa M, Furness J B 1983 Immunohistochemistry on wholemount preparations in: Cuello A C (ed.) Methods of Neuroscience, Wiley, New York, (vol. 3 Immunohistochemistry), 373–398

Costa M, Furness J B, Gibbins I L 1986 Chemical coding of enteric neurones in: Hokfeldt T, Fuxe K, Pernow B (eds) Progress in brain research. Elsevier, Netherlands, 68.

Costa M, Furness J B, Llewellyn-Smith I J 1987 Histochemistry of the enteric nervous system in: Johnson L R (ed.) Physiology of the gastrointestinal tract, 2nd edn. Raven Press, New York 1–40

Csendes A, Sepulveda A 1980 Intraluminal gallbladder pressure measurements in patients with chronic or acute cholecystisis. Am J Surg 139: 383–384

Cuschieri A, Hughes J H, Cohen M 1972 Biliary pressure studies during cholecystectomy. Br J Surg 59: 267–273

Dahlstrand C, Bjorck S, Edin R, Dahlstrom A, Ahlman H 1988 Substance P in the control of extrahepatic biliary motility in the cat. Regul Pept 20: 11–24

Dahlstrand C, Dahlstrom A, Ahlman H 1989 Adrenergic and VIPergic relaxatory mechanisms of the feline extrahepatic biliary tree. J Auton Nerv Sys 26: 97–106

Dancygier H, Klein U, Leaschner U, Hubner K, Classen M 1984 Somatostatin containing cells in the extrahepatic biliary tract of humans. Gastroenterology 86: 892–896

Darweesh R M A, Dodds W J, Hogan W J et al 1988 Efficacy of quantiative hepatobiliary scintigraphy and fatty meal sonography for evaluating patients with suspected partial common bile duct obstruction. Gastroenterology 94: 779–786

Davison J S 1983 Innervation of the gastrointestinal tract in: Christensen L, Wingate D L (eds) A guide to gastrointestinal motility. Wright, New York, pp 1–47

Dowdy G S, Waldron G W, Brown W G 1962 Surgical anatomy of the pancreaticobiliary system: observations. Arch Surg 84: 229

Everson G T, Braverman D Z, Johnson M L, Kern F Jr 1980 A critical evaluation of real-time ultrasonography for the study of gallbladder volume and contraction. Gastroenterology 79: 40–46

Geenen J E, Hogan W J, Dodds W J, Steward E T, Arndorfer R C 1980 Intraluminal pressure recording from the human sphincter of Oddi. Gastroenterology 78: 317–324

Glenn F, Graffe Jr W R 1966 Historical events in biliary tract surgery. Arch Surg 93: 848–852

Hallenbeck G A 1967 Biliary and pancreatic intraductal pressures in: Code, C F (ed.) The handbook of physiology, Section 6, The alimentary canal, Volume 2, Secretion. Washington D C, American Physiological Society, pp 1007–1025

Hand B H 1963 The anatomical study of the choledochoduodenal area. Br J Sur 50: 486–494

Harkins H N, Stavney L S, Griffith C A, Savage L E, Kato T, Nyhus L M 1963 Selective gastric vagotomy. Ann Surg 158: 448–460

Helm J F, Dodds W J, Christensen J, Sarna S K 1985 Control mechanisms of spontaneous in-vitro contractions of the opossum sphincter of Oddi. Am J Physiol 249: G572–G579

Hess W 1979 Physiology of the sphincter of Oddi in: Classen M, Geenen J, Kawai K (eds) The papilla Vateri and its diseases. Proceedings of the International Workshop of the World Congress of Gastroenterology held in Madrid 1978. Verlag Gerhard Witzshock, Kohn pp 14–21

Honda R, Toouli J, Dodds W J, Sarna S, Hogan W J Itoh Z 1982 Relationship of sphincter of Oddi spike bursts to gastro-intestinal myoelectric activity in conscious opossums. J Clin Invest 69: 770–778

Hunt D R, Scott A J 1989 Changes in bile duct diameter after cholecystectomy: 15-year operative study. Gastroenterology 97: 1485–1486

Jansson R 1979 Effects of gastrointestinal hormones on concentrating function and motility in the gallbladder. Acta Physio Scand (suppl.): 456, 1–38

Johnson F E, Boyden E A, 1952 The effect of double vagotomy on the motor activity of the human gallbladder. Surgery 32: 591–601

Keast J R, Furness J B, Costa M 1985 Distribution of certain peptides containing nerve fibres and endocrine cells in the gastrointestinal mucosa in five mammalian species. J Complete Neurol 236: 413–422

Krishnamurthy G T, Bobba V R, Kingston E 1981 Radionuclide ejection fraction: a technique for the quantitative analysis of motor function of the human gallbladder. Gastroenterology 80: 482–490

Kyosola K 1978 Adrenergic and cholinergic innervation of the supraduodenal common bile duct. Am J Gastroenterol 70: 179–183

LeQuesne L P, Whiteside C G, Hand B T 1959 The common bile duct after cholecystectomy. Br Med J 1: 329–332

Liu Y F, Saccone G T P, Thune A, Baker R A, Harvey J, Toouli J 1992 The sphincter of Oddi regulates flow by acting as a passive resistor and not a pump. Am J Physiol 263: G683–G689

Lundberg J M, Hokfelt T, Nilsson G, et al 1978 Peptide neurones in the vagus, splanchnic and coeliac nerves. Acta Physiol Scand 104: 499–501

Lytle W J 1959 The common bile duct groove in the pancreas. Br J Surg 47: 209

McIntosh G H, Baker R A, Worthley C S, Iannos J, Saccone

G T P, Toouli J 1988 Motility of the biliary tract in a chronic pig model. Surg Res Commun 4: 93–102

Mahour G H, Wakin K G, Ferris D O, Soule E H 1967 The common bile duct after cholecystectomy. Ann Surg 166: 964–967

Mori J, Azuma H, Fujiwara M, 1979 Adrenergic innervation and receptors in the sphincter of Oddi. Eur J Pharmacol 14: 365–373

Munkacsi I, Siklos I 1962 Blood supply of the common bile duct. Acta Morphol 11: 179–188

Northover J, Terblanche J 1979 A new look at the arterial supply of the bile duct in man and its surgical implications. Br J Surg 66: 379–384

Northover J M A, Williams E D F, Terblanche J 1980 The investigation of small vessel anatomy by scanning electron microscopy of resin casts. J Anat 130(1): 43–54

Oddi R 1985 Ruggero Oddi and the sphincter (editorial). Ital J Gastroenterol 17: 109–111

Oddi R 1888 Sulla tonicita dello sfintere del coledoco. Arch Sci Med 12: 333–339

Padbury R T A, Furness J B, Toouli J 1989 Intrinsic catecholamine containing neurones in the sphincter of Oddi and duodenum of the Australian possum. Gastroenterology 96 (part 2): 381

Parke W W, Michels N A 1963 Blood supply of the common bile duct. Surg Gynecol Obstet 177: 47–55

Persson C G A 1972 Adrenoreceptors in the gallbladder. Acta Pharmacol 32: 177–185

Pitt H A, Doty J E, Roslyn J J, DenBesten L 1981a The role of altered extrahepatic biliary function in the pathogenesis of gallstones after vagotomy. Surgery 90: 418–425

Pitt H A, Roslyn J J, Kuchenbecker S L, Doty J E, DenBesten L 1981b The role of cystic duct resistance in the pathogenesis of cholesterol gallstones. J Surg Res 30: 508–514

Roberts-Thomson I C, Toouli J, Blanchett W, Lichtenstein M, Andrews J T 1986 Assessment of bile flow by radioscintigraphy in patients with biliary type pain after cholecystectomy. Aust N Z J Med 16: 788–793

Saccone G T P, Toouli J, Iannos J et al 1988 The effect of catheter diameter on sphincter of Oddi motility. Surg Res Commun 2: 315–321

Sarles J C, Midejean A, Devaux M A 1975 Electromyography of the sphincter of Oddi. Am J Gastroenterol 63: 221–231

Scott G W, Otto W J, 1979 Resistance and sphincter-like properties of the cystic duct. Surg Gynecol Obstet 149: 177–182

Shaffer E A, McOrmond P, Duggan H 1980 Quantitative cholescintigraphy: assessment of gallbladder filling and emptying and duodenogastric reflux. Gastroenterology 79: 899–906

Shapiro A L, Robillard G L 1948 The arterial blood supply of the common and hepatic bile ducts with reference to the problems of common duct injury and repair. Surgery 23: 1–11

Smadja C, Blumgart L H (eds) 1988 The biliary tract and the anatomy of biliary exposure in: Blumgart L M (ed.) Surgery of the liver and biliary tract. Churchill Livingstone, London, pp 11–22

Sutherland S D 1966 The intrinsic innervation of the gallbladder in Macaca rhesus and Cavia porcellus. J Anat 100: 261, 68.

Takahashi I, Nakaya M, Suzuki T, Itoh Z 1982a Postprandial changes in contractile activity and bile concentration in gallbladder of the dog. Am J Physiol 6: G365–G371

Takahaski I, Suzuki T, Aizawa I, Itoh Z 1982b Comparison of gallbladder contractions induced by motilin and cholecystokinin in dogs. Gastroenterology 82: 419–424

Tanaka M, Sarr M G, Miller L J, Malagelada J R 1990 Changes in tone of canine gallbladder measured by an electronic pneumatic barostat. Am J Physiol 259: G312–G320

Tansy M F, Innes D L, Martin J S, Kendall F M 1974 An evaluation of neural influences on the SO in the dog. Dig Dis Sci 19: 423–437

Tansy M F, Salkin L, Innes D L, Martin J S, Kendall F M, Litwack D 1975 The mucosal lining of the intramural common bile duct as a determinant of ductal opening pressure. Am J Dig Dis 20: 613–625

Thune A, Saccone G T P, Toouli J 1991 Distension of the gallbladder inhibits sphincter of Oddi motility in man. Gut 32: 690–693

Thune B A, Thornell E, Svanvik J 1986 Reflex regulation of flow resistance in the feline sphincter of Oddi by hydrostatic pressure in the biliary tree. Gastroenterology 91: 1364–1369

Toouli J, Bushell M, Iannos J, Collinson T, Wearne J, Kitchen D 1986a Peroperative sphincter of Oddi manometry: motility disorders in patients with cholelithiasis. Aust NZ J Surg 56: 625–629

Toouli J, Bushell M, Stevenson G, Dent J, Wycherley A, Iannos J 1986b Gallbladder emptying in man related to fasting duodenal migrating motor contractions. Aust NZ J Surg 56: 147–151

Toouli J, Dodds W J, Honda R et al 1983 Motor function of the opossum sphincter of Oddi. J Clin Invest 71: 208–220

Toouli J, Geenen J E, Hogan W J, Dodds W J, Arndorfer R C 1982a Sphincter of Oddi motor activity: a comparison between patients with common bile duct stones and controls. Gastroenterology 82: 111–117

Toouli J, Hogan W J, Geenen J E, Dodds W J, Arndorfer R C 1982b Action of cholecystokinin octapeptide on sphincter of Oddi basal pressure and phasic wave activity in humans. Surgery 92: 497–503

Toouli J, Watts J McK 1971 In-vitro motility studies on the canine and human extrahepatic biliary tracts. Aust N Z J Surg 40: 380–387

Van Buskirk C, Boyden E A 1944 The distribution of nerve cells and fibres to the choledochal-duodenal junction of the cat. Anat Recept 88: 423

Watts J McK, Dunphy J E 1966 The role of the common bile duct in biliary dynamics. Surg, Gynecol Obstet 122: 1207–1281

Weiner I, Kazutomo I, Fagan C J, Lilja P, Watson L C, Thompson J C 1981 Release of cholecystokinin in man, correlation of blood levels with gallbladder contraction. Ann Surg 194: 321–327

Worthley C S, Baker R A, Iannos J, Saccone G T P, Toouli J 1989 Human fasting and post-prandial sphincter of Oddi motility. Br J Surg 76: 709–714

Yap L, McGee M A, McKenzie J, Wycherley A, Toouli J 1991 Acalculous biliary pain: diagnostic use of choleycstokinin cholescintigraphy in the selection of patients for cholecystectomy. Gastroenterology 101: 786–793

27. The small bowel and the ileocaecal region

G. Basilisco   S. F. Phillips

INTRODUCTION

Motility is a rubric applied to the physiological consequences of the functions of gastrointestinal smooth muscle. It covers a full spectrum of phenomena: cellular properties, contractile activity, neurohumoral control, and net effects of muscular activity on transit of contents. Very important are the mechanisms whereby muscular contractions are coordinated. This sequence is of particular importance in the small intestine, for finely coordinated contractions are the means whereby the muscular layers achieve their key teleological effects – the transit of chyme in a way which optimizes digestion and absorption.

The thrust of this chapter is towards the applied aspects of motility, those which pertain to function of the *small intestine and the ileocaecal region as an organ.* Thus, no attention will be directed towards the intrinsic cellular properties of intestinal smooth muscle, to its intramural innervation by the enteric nervous system (ENS), and rather little to extrinsic innervation through the autonomic nervous system (ANS). Instead, the focus will be on the myoelectrical signals whereby the mechanical events, contractions of the tunica muscularis, are regulated. Attention will also be accorded to transit, this being the important end-result of contractions of individual cells as expressed by their groupings into tissues (e.g. segments of the longitudinal or circular muscle coats). Less can be said about the consequences of motility in the small intestine, the relationships that are presumed to exist between muscle contractions, transit and absorption. Unfortunately, data on these vital associations are sparse and incomplete.

Appreciation of the motor properties of the small bowel and the ileocaecal region requires an understanding of several basic physiological phenomena. These include: (1) the electrical 'slow wave', and the action potentials that are 'paced' by slow waves; these are the electrical equivalents of contractions; (2) coordination

or propagation of contractile activity; (3) interdigestive motility; (4) postprandial motility. The story is not yet complete in man, extrapolations are needed from one species to another, and it is known that differences among species are not trivial. However, a credible overview can be fashioned, with primary attention to man. Clues to the pathophysiology of some common gastroenterological diseases will be also provided. For those wishing more detailed analyses of certain aspects, the following reviews are recommended: Wingate (1981), Szurszewski (1987), Weisbrodt (1987), Camilleri & Phillips (1989), Sarna & Otterson (1989)

SLOW WAVES AND ACTION POTENTIALS

Designated variously (basal electrical rhythm, pacesetter potential, electrical control activity – ECA), 'slow waves' are rhythmic oscillations of the membrane potential of smooth muscle cells. The signals can be recorded by several techniques, including intracellular microelectrodes within individual cells in vitro; or from a group of cells, by extracellular electrodes in vitro or in vivo. Recordings in vivo are usually from needle electrodes placed within the tunica muscularis; for most experimental studies, electrodes are sewn onto the serosal surface of the bowel. Such approaches have had limited application in man, though they have been placed on the human bowel, when a laparotomy has been done for other reasons.

In man, most attention has been given to recording from mucosal electrodes incorporated in orointestinal tubes (Christensen et al 1966). Anatomical considerations however dictate that the mucosa is not the closest or most direct approach to the tunica muscularis, and few adequate electrical recordings from intact man are available. On the other hand, serosal electrodes have been used extensively in laboratory animals (Fig. 27.1).

Studies in the several species have established the principle of the 'gradient of the small intestine'. First

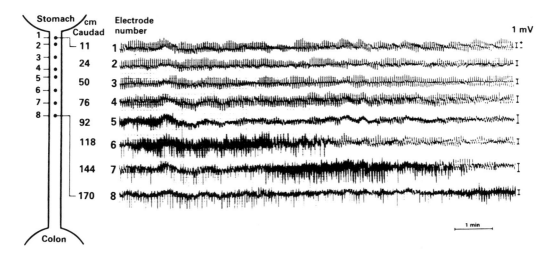

Fig. 27.1 Electrical recording from the canine small bowel, from serosal electrodes at the loci indicated to the left. Slow waves are omnipresent in all recordings. A band of action potentials begins at site 5, passes to sites 6 and 7 and is beginning at site 8. This is phase III of the interdigestive myoelectrical complex (Szurszewski 1969).

documented carefully by Alvarez (1928), this describes an intrinsic frequency of the slow wave which decreases distally, i.e. it is faster in the proximal than in the distal bowel. In the dog, this ranges from 14–18/min in the duodenum to 10–12/min in the ileum (Fig. 27.1). Comparable values in man are, duodenum 11–13/min and ileum 6–8/min. The human gradient was first described by electrical techniques (Christensen et al 1966) and has been confirmed (Kerlin & Phillips 1982) many times by mechanical tracings (Fig. 27.2). The universality of this phenomenon among species has led most authors to conclude that the intrinsic capacity of the proximal gut to contract faster than the distal gut is important in the normal orad to distal transit of contents. A 'pacemaker' has been localized in the duodenum of several species and, drawing an analogy from the conducting system in the heart, the faster proximal pacemaker is considered to be dominant. Pacemaker potentials could be generated by muscle cells under the influence of the nervous system or by some specialized tissue of origin. The interstitial cells of Cajal have been proposed as the origin of this property (Rumessen & Thuneberg 1991).

Given that the slow wave acts as a 'pace-setter', the maximal rate at which contractions can occur is established for each level of the bowel by the frequency of the slow waves. This is born out experimentally. When membrane depolarization occurs in association with a slow wave, an action potential (spike potential, electrical response activity – ERA) is recorded (Fig. 27.1).

When depolarization occurs in association with all slow waves, the small bowel contracts at its maximum rate and this shows the same gradient of frequency along the bowel as does the slow wave (Fig. 27.2). Alternatively, the bowel may contract in association with some or none of the slow waves. This capacity of the membrane potential to react or not to react (by firing or not firing an action potential) provides the basis whereby muscular contraction varies widely in intensity, and subtle patterns of motility are established. The basic concept that the small bowel can contract at the maximal frequency of the slow wave has, however, its exceptions. When chyme reaches the ileum, this segment of the small intestine contracted in dog at a rate (20–24/min), much greater than the rate of the slow wave at that site (13–15/min) (Fig. 27.3); (Fich et al 1989). This response shows that under special circumstances, e.g. the local contact of nutrients with the mucosa, the normally tight coupling between electrical and mechanical events can be altered.

COORDINATION OR PROPAGATION OF CONTRACTIONS

In addition to the gradient of frequency for slow waves (and the maximal contractile frequency) along the bowel, a 'phase-lag' exists so that slow waves appear to move in an aboral direction. By progressing along the length of the bowel, slow waves not only set the pace for contractile events at any one site, but offer the potential whereby mechanical activity may also be

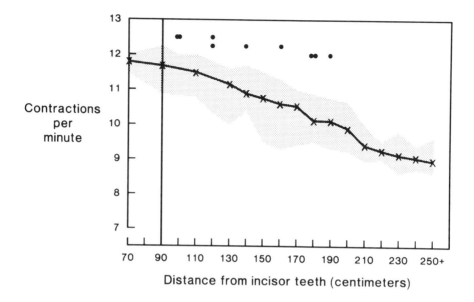

Fig. 27.2 Maximum frequency of phasic contractions in the human small intestine, as recorded from perfused catheter pressure sensors. The maximum contractile frequency is equivalent to the frequency of slow waves at that locus; note the gradient of decreasing frequency along the small bowel. The mean and SEM (shaded) are shown for a group of healthy subjects, the single symbols are from one subject who was outside the normal range. (Reproduced from Kerlin & Phillips (1982) with permission.)

propagated. Further, it is logical to assume that mechanical activity which is propagated will be more likely to propel contents, whereas stationary contractile rings might be expected to move contents in both directions simultaneously. Moreover, the greater the length over which contractions are propagated, the greater should be the potential to propel. These questions have been approached by several investigators, the work of Schemann and Ehrlein (1986a,b) being a good example (Fig. 27.4). Sophisticated computerized analysis of mechanical signals from strain gauges allowed transit of contents (as assessed by simultaneous monitoring of radio-opaque chyme) to be correlated with the numbers of motor events and the distances over which they propagated.

Though the cellular and biochemical mechanisms whereby these degrees of coordination can be regulated are not known, the ENS provides an integrated neural circuitry that can set in operation various patterns of motility. For normal function of the small intestine, the circuit that operates peristalsis is one of the most important. This programme coordinates the reciprocal behaviours of the circular and longitudinal muscle layer and establishes an overall contracted state above and relaxed state below any point at which a distention is applied (Grider 1989). Even if these circuits can

operate independently from the extrinsic nerve regulations, they are within the continuous influence of local factors (luminal contents), extrinsic nerves, and hormones (Fig. 27.5).

INTERDIGESTIVE MOTILITY

Prior to Szurszewski's (1969) description of a regular cycle of motility in the fasting small bowel, many confusing and at times contradictory observations had been recorded. In particular, some authors reported minimal motor activity when the small bowel was empty between meals, while others noted bursts of intense motility. When based only on short periods of recording, as most were, the fact that these were errors of sampling became obvious only when the cyclic nature of fasting motility was appreciated.

Though clearly conceived of by others, including Boldereff's observations in Pavlov's laboratory (for discussion, see Wingate 1981), Szurszewski's description of a migrating burst of intense spiking which passed from duodenum to ileum in the dog each 90–120 min during fasting first clearly identified this phenomenon (Fig. 27.1). This is now recognized as a general property of the mammalian small intestine. In

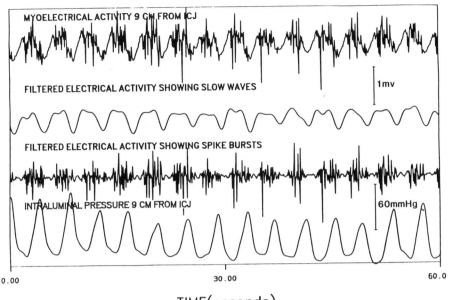

Fig. 27.3 Myoelectrical and intraluminal pressure recordings from the postprandial canine ileum. The top tracing is the unfiltered myoelectrical signal; the second was filtered to illustrate the slow wave; the third was filtered to illustrate spikes. At the bottom is intraluminal pressure activity. Note the equivalent frequency of spikes and pressures waves, both at 22/min. The slow wave rate is 14–15/min. (Reproduced from Fich et al (1989) with permission.)

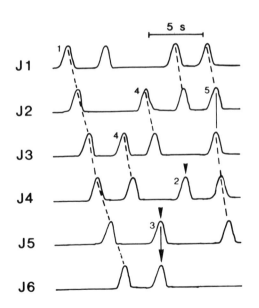

Fig. 27.4 Mechanical contractions recorded from six strain gauges sewn to the circular muscle of the canine jejunum, four centimetres between successive gauges. Some mechanical events propagate aborally (dotted lines), others appear simultaneously at two sites (full lines) or are solitary (arrows). (Reproduced from Schemann & Ehrlein 1986a with permission.)

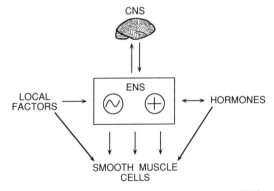

Fig. 27.5 Anatomically based neural circuits of the ENS programme and regulate the function of smooth muscle cells. However, these programmes are also under the influence of local factors from the intestinal lumen or mucosa, the extrinsic nerves, the CNS, and gastrointestinal (neuro-) peptides.

electrical terms, the interdigestive myoelectrical complex (IDMEC) is a short (several minutes) burst of spiking during which every slow wave shows an action potential. The complex migrates along the length of the small bowel, with a velocity and periodicity such that when one burst reaches the ileum, another

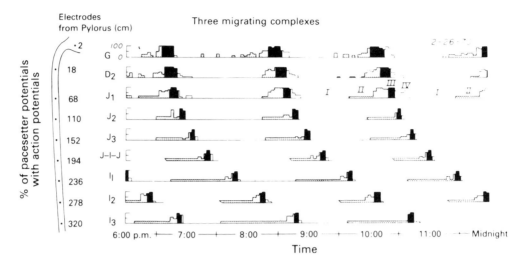

Fig. 27.6 Migration of the interdigestive cycle along the length of the canine small bowel, from gastric antrum to distal ileum over a 6-h period of recording. Phases of the cycle (I–IV) are indicated and migration of phase III (black blocks) is evident. Note that passage of the front slows in the distal bowel. (Reproduced from Code & Marlett (1975) with permission.)

Table 27.1 General characteristics of the MMC (phase III) in the human upper gastrointestinal tract

Site	Velocity of propagation (cm/min)	Maximum frequency of contractions (per min)	Duration (min)
D	–	11.7 ± 0.1	8.7 ± 1.0
J_1	4.3 ± 0.6	11.3 ± 0.1	9.1 ± 0.6
J_2	2.8 ± 0.4	10.7 ± 0.1	11.7 ± 0.6
J_3	2.0 ± 0.5	10.4 ± 0.2	14.7 ± 1.2
I_1	1.3 ± 0.2	9.8 ± 0.2	15.6 ± 1.6
I_2	0.9 ± 0.1	9.3 ± 0.2	15.3 ± 1.0
I_3	0.7 ± 0.2	8.9 ± 0.2	13.9 ± 1.1
I_4	0.6 ± 0.2	8.5 ± 0.2	13.8 ± 1.5
C	–	6.1 ± 0.2	–

Notes: D gives the characteristics in the duodenum, J_1–J_3 those in the jejunum
I_1–I_4 are values for the ileum and C is the caecum.

commences in the duodenum. Code and Marlett (1975) subsequently divided the cycle of 90–120 min into four parts: phase I, a period of quiescence when spikes were absent; phase II, during which sporadic spiking was recorded; phase III, the 'front' or migrating motor complex (MMC), when the bowel contracted at its maximal frequency; and phase IV, a transition period back to quiescence. This sequence can be displayed neatly to show the migration of the front (Fig. 27.6). Note that the MMC migrates more slowly in the distal bowel, and that feeding interrupts the sequence.

The IDMEC has its mechanical equivalent. During phase I very few contractions occur, sporadic mechanical activity is recorded during phase II (by either extraluminal strain gauges or sensors of intraluminal pressure), and phase III shows an intense burst of rhythmic mechanical events at the frequency of slow waves for that site (Fig. 27.7). Designation of a phase IV, which is often poorly developed, has largely been discontinued.

Variations on the interdigestive cycle

Though the general phenomenon of the interdigestive cycle has been recorded from most mammals, differences have been noted. In non-ruminants, the MMC is present only during fasting, but MMCs persist postprandially in ruminants. The pig has also been studied extensively, and it shows another variation; the MMC is present during fasting and after meals, but only when food is taken ad libitum. If the pig is fed only once a day, the pattern becomes that of non-ruminants, and meals disrupt the MMC cycle. The periodicity of the cycle varies widely; it can be correlated roughly with the size of the animal, and ranges from 15–120 min. In general, phase III is relatively brief, occupying 10% or less of the cycle. Phases I and II each comprise 30–80% of the cycle (Sarna 1985). Rather than attempt a catalogue of multiple species, focus will be given to the human interdigestive complex, with note being made

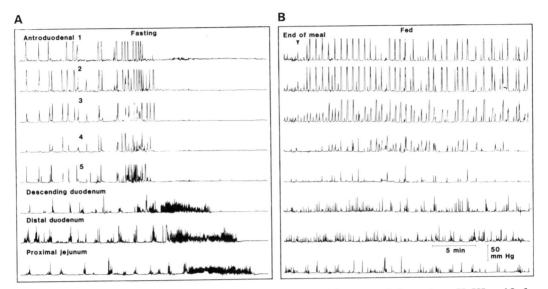

Fig. 27.7 Intraluminal pressures from the antroduodenum of a healthy person. **A** shows phases II, III, and I of a fasting cycle. Phase III consists of rhythmic contractions (3/min) in the antrum and duodenum (12–14/min). **B** shows a typical postprandial pattern; sporadic contractions are seen in the stomach and small bowel. (Reproduced from Malagelada et al (1986) with permission.)

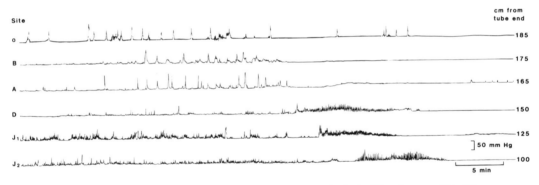

Fig. 27.8 Human MMC beginning in the oesophagus (**O**), involving the body (**B**) and antrum (**A**) of the stomach, the duodenum (**D**) and jejunum (**J**). The distances given are from the distal end of the tube which was in the proximal colon (Phillips 1988)

where the findings in man differ from those of the common experimental animals.

Our approach has been to use orocaecal tubes which are perfused by a low compliance system, and we utilize the overnight period for prolonged fasting recordings (Quigley et al 1984b, Kellow et al 1986). Table 27.1 give the general characteristics of the MMC in healthy man; it highlights: (1) the distal slowing of propagation velocity; (2) the lengthening of duration of the MMC with distal spread; (3) the rhythmic rate of contractions, equivalent to the frequency of the slow wave at each recording point.

The distal oesophagus and stomach participate in the human interdigestive cycle (Fig. 27.8), though not invariably; about 50% of cycles have an oesophageal and antral component, which often appear together. Conversely, in most species including man, a proportion of interdigestive cycles begins distally (e.g. in the proximal jejunum or even beyond). Thus, we found the maximal incidence of phase III in man to be in the proximal jejunum (Fig. 27.9). An important and consistent human variant is that MMCs 'die out' in the ileum; less than 20% were recorded from the mid-ileum and even fewer from the ileocaecal junction (Fig. 27.9).

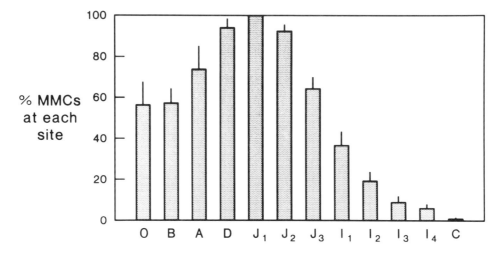

Fig. 27.9 Incidence of MMCs at various sites in the human bowel. The maximum number was recorded from the proximal jejunum (J_1), designated as 100%. **O** is oesophagus, **B** and **A** the body and antrum, of stomach; **D** is duodenum; **J**, **I** and **C** are jejunal, ileal and colonic sites. (Reproduced from Kellow et al 1986 with permission.)

Occasionally, the MMC appears to progress into the caecum and be represented there by a burst of phasic pressure waves.

Periodicity of the cycle fluctuates widely within and between individuals; thus, care must be used when interpreting recordings in which interdigestive cycling cannot be clearly demonstrated. Cycling as frequently as every 30 min is not uncommon in health, but intervals of 3 h or more are also common (Kerlin & Phillips 1982, Kellow et al 1986).

Periodicity of the cycle is shorter at night and the nocturnal phase III moves down the small bowel more slowly; phase II also virtually disappears during sleep and a greater proportion of the cycle is taken up by quiescence (Kellow et al 1986, 1987, 1990, Kumar et al 1986). Truncal vagotomy is also often associated with a short interval between phase III bursts and with a reduction in phase II activity; after coeliac and superior mesenteric ganglionectomy in dog, the interval between phase III is prolonged and an increase in action potential activity (phase II) is observed between the complexes (Marik & Code 1975, Marlett & Code 1979). Thus, the interdigestive cycle appears to be controlled primarily by the ENS but sleep, vagotomy or sympathectomy modify the exact way in which the cycle is expressed by the bowel.

Studies in low-birthweight infants showed the small intestine to continuously exhibit short bursts of contractions; periods of quiescence were absent. During later infancy the patterns matured towards those seen in adults, implying that an inhibitory innervation perhaps developed as a part of the maturation process (Berseth 1989, 1990).

Phase II has received less attention than have the more dramatic features of phase III. However, all apparently random activity of phase II *is not the same*. Within the sporadic contractions of phase II must be one of the keys to the major functions of the small intestine. Subtle differences within the patterns of phase II presumably determine that mixing, localized transit, absorption, and slow distal movement of contents will occur. Moreover, these variations on the underlying theme provide mechanisms whereby transit is not inadvertently hastened. The same can be said about the postprandial patterns. The techniques used in dogs to dissect phase II or the 'fed pattern' (Schemann & Ehrlein 1986a) are not easily applicable to intact man. However, even conventional recording techniques in man illustrate variations on the usual patterns of phase II. Discrete burst of contractions (Fig. 27.10) are often seen, and they appear to migrate. These have been described (Fleckenstein 1978, Fleckenstein & Øigaard 1978) to occur regularly ('minute rhythm'), and should probably be considered to be normal for approximately 25% of the total duration of phase II.

Special features of ileal motility

The human ileum does not usually participate in phase

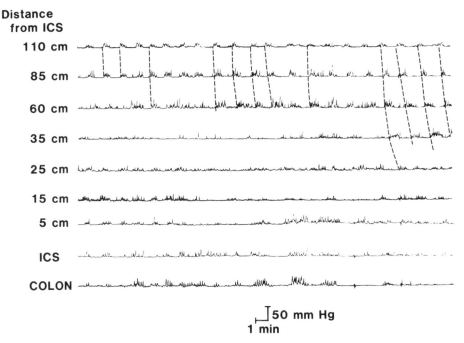

Fig. 27.10 Intraluminal pressures from the jejunum and ileum of a healthy person from sites proximal to the ileocaecal sphincter. In this recording phase II consists mainly of short bursts of phasic waves which appear to migrate. These are presumed to be the mechanical equivalent of 'minute rhythm' recorded electrically by Fleckenstein (1978) and Fleckenstein & Øigaard (1978).

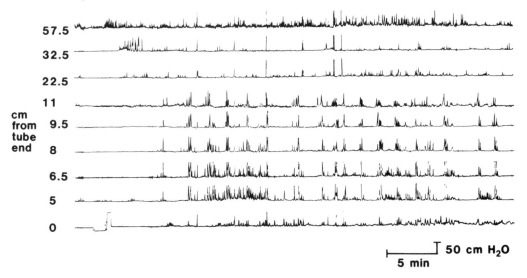

Fig. 27.11 Motor patterns in the fasting healthy human ileum, the recording assembly terminated in the proximal colon and the top eight tracings are from the ileum. No MMCs are recorded and the tracing show prominent clusters of phasic waves (Phillips 1988).

III of the MMC (Fig. 27.9) and phase II in the ileum also showed features different from those of the duodenum and jejunum (Borody et al 1985, Kellow et al 1986, Quigley et al 1984b). Motor activity was more often grouped into bursts of phasic waves lasting 1–2 min, some of which migrated but others of which appeared to be stationary or simultaneous (Fig. 27.11). A second motor phenomenon occurred infrequently,

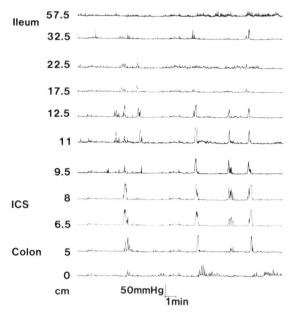

Ileum 57.5

32.5

22.5

17.5

12.5

11

9.5

ICS 8

6.5

Colon 5

0

cm

50mmHg
1min

Fig. 27.12 Motor patterns in the healthy human ileum and proximal colon. The striking feature is a series of broad-based ('prolonged', lasting 15–30 s) pressure waves which propagate rapidly through the ileum and into the proximal colon (PPCs) (Phillips 1988).

but predictably; we termed these 'prolonged propagated contractions' (PPCs) (Fig. 27.12). They were pressure waves of high amplitude (usually in excess of 50 mmHg, sometimes above 100 mmHg) and they lasted longer than the equivalent duration of the slow wave. Thus, they are probably *not* an event which is controlled by the slow wave. PPCs migrate very rapidly, so that at slow paper speed they may appear to be simultaneous; we even confused them initially with mechanical artefacts. These are peristaltic phenomena.

We studied PPCs in the dog and found that they can be stimulated reproducibly by instilling into the ileum small boluses of a short-chain (or volatile) fatty acid (SCFA) solution (Kamath et al 1987; Fig. 27.13); we used concentrations of SCFA similar to those recovered from canine stools. Thus, we proposed that PPCs may occur when SCFA reach the ileum as a result of coloileal reflux, since SCFA are universal constituents of colonic contents. SCFA reaching the ileum would then act as a chemical signal for a powerful motor response. The proximal small bowel can also develop PPCs when exposed to an appropriate intraluminal stimulus but in normal dogs and man PPCs are rarely recorded from the duodenum and jejunum.

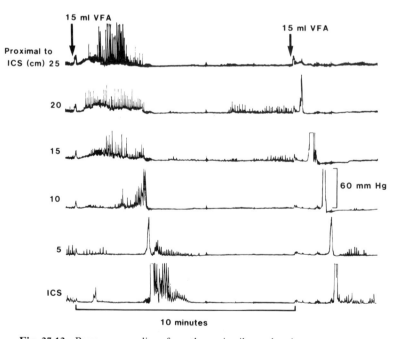

Fig. 27.13 Pressure recordings from the canine ileum showing responses to boluses of volatile (short-chain) fatty acids (VFA). The first bolus elicited a phasic burst which also showed features of a single, large contraction at the ileocolonic sphincter (ICS). The second bolus elicited a prolonged propagated contraction (Phillips 1988).

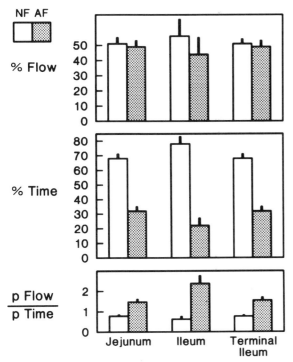

Fig. 27.14 Flow of fluid at three levels of the human small intestine during fasting. Total flow was approximately equal in non-front (NF) and activity front (AF) periods (**A**). However, AF periods comprised a third or less of total recording time (**B**) and the ratios of percentage flow to percentage time (**C**) were significantly greater for AF periods in the jejunum and terminal ileum. (Reproduced from Kerlin et al (1982) with permission.)

Flow and transit of contents in the interdigestive period

Code and Schlegel (1973) ascribed to the phase III of the interdigestive complex the role of sweeping the fasting gut clear of accumulated interdigestive debris, in preparation for the next meal; the so-called 'housekeeper' function. The concept has been modified somewhat by subsequent observations which suggest that transit rates are maximal just before phase III, in late phase II. However, flow of fasting intestinal contents is largely intermittent, in small boluses; 50% immediately before or during the activity front (phase III) and 50% during the phase I and II of the interdigestive complex (Fig. 27.14). Discrete bursts of phasic contractions (Fig. 27.15) and PPCs (Fig. 27.16) are also propulsive; they empty liquid contents rapidly from the ileum (Kruis et al 1985). The variety of motor patterns that can be recorded in the interdigestive period can therefore explain the marked variability in flow rate and transit during this period.

POSTPRANDIAL MOTILITY

Eating interrupts the interdigestive cycle, which is replaced by an apparently random occurrence of mechanical events. Figure 27.7 is a good example of the effect of food on the upper gut; the ileum behaves similarly except that, since MMCs are usually absent from the human ileum, the change is a less dramatic one. The lag time between the ingestion of the meal

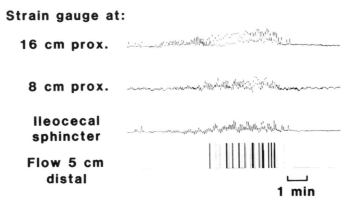

Fig. 27.15 Simultaneous recording of a propagated burst of rhythmic phasic activity (not related to interdigestive myoelectric complex) in canine ileum and flow from an end colostomy. This motor pattern was associated with prominent flow from colostomy. (Reproduced from Kruis et al 1985 with permission.)

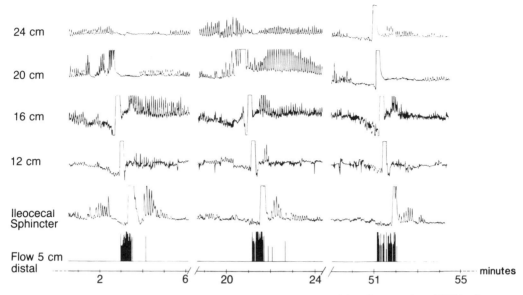

Fig. 27.16 Strain gauge recordings from the canine ileum. Three broad-based contractions (PPCs) migrate rapidly through the ileum as far as the ileocaecal sphincter. Each is associated with a bolus outflow of fluid from the ileum into the colon (Phillips 1988).

and the beginning of the fed pattern is short in the jejunum and longer in the ileum. The fed pattern starts when intraluminal nutrients are first in contact with the mucosa. In the dog distal ileum, high-frequency pressure waves (Fig. 27.3) develop 2–4 h after food but, if jejunal contents are diverted from the ileum, high-frequency waves do not develop. Local instillation of nutrients reproduce the fed pattern of contractions (Fich et al 1990). Thus, local afferent pathways appear to be important.

Postprandial motor patterns have received relatively little detailed analysis. Schemann and Ehrlein (1986b) examined the fed pattern in dogs given cellulose meals, to which were added a variety of nutrients. They analysed the mechanical response by methods described earlier in this chapter (Fig. 27.4) and reached several conclusions. Firstly, the non-nutrient, control (cellulose) meal was associated with contractions which migrated for the longest distances and which produced the most rapid transit. Secondly, various nutrients induced different contractile patterns; some migrated for short, and others for intermediate or long distances. Rates of transit were variable and were best correlated with the mean distance of migration. Thirdly, since nutrients induced shorter patterns of migration and slower rates of transit, the findings offer an explanation as to how the small bowel slows the transit of chyme, and presumably optimizes digestion and absorption concomitantly (Fig. 27.17).

The duration of the fed pattern also depends on the physicochemical characteristics of the meal. Fed patterns last longer after a caloric than a non-caloric meal (Schemann & Ehrlein 1986b) and are longest after fat than after other nutrients (DeWever et al 1978). However, in man we found that the duration of the fed pattern did not differ between isocaloric meals containing or not containing fat (Kellow et al 1986). After a meal, the human interdigestive cycle usually returns first in the mid-jejunum.

Ingestion of the meal and the concomitant changes in motility strikingly modify flow and transit along the small intestine. Ileal flow increases after a meal (4–6 ml/min in comparison to fasting, 1–2 ml/min) and, as in the fasting state, is discontinuous, occurring in discrete boluses (Fig. 27.18). Ileal infusion of fat after ingestion of a meal delays gastrointestinal transit and decreases motor activity of the proximal intestine (the 'ileal brake') (Read et al 1984); eating also stimulates an increase in motility in the distal ileum (the 'gastroileal reflex') (Kerlin et al 1983).

THE ILEOCOLONIC JUNCTION (ICJ)

The small intestine terminates in a specialized segment of bowel, the ileocolonic junction (or sphincter). Early anatomists recognized the possibility that this region had the anatomical basis whereby it might function as a 'valve'. Surgeons have even based surgical procedures

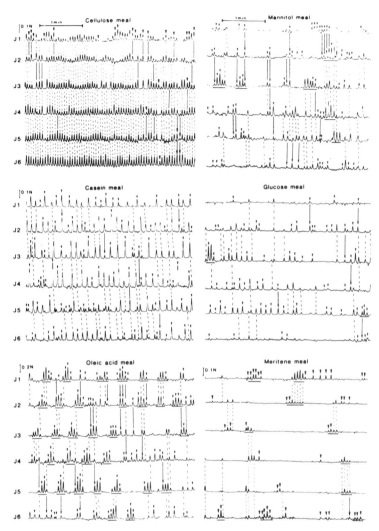

Fig. 27.17 Motor patterns from the canine jejunum after six different meals, recorded from serosal strain gauges. Propagated contractions are shown by dashed lines, simultaneous events by solid lines and single events by arrows. Different nutrients induced different motor patterns and different rates of transit. (Reproduced from Schemann & Ehrlein (1986b) with permission.)

on its functional importance, devising restorative procedures to be used for 'incompetent junctions' (Gazet & Kopp 1964). Later, properties of a physiological sphincter were identified, and attention swung more towards the importance of an ileocolonic sphincter (ICS).

Our studies confirmed that the dog possesses a specialized band of muscle which has a resting tone (Fig. 27.19); it relaxes in response to proximal distension and contracts when the proximal colon is stretched. However, the significant reduction in tonic pressure of the sphincter induced by extramucosal sphincterotomy in dog did not alter flow rates or

transit time of chyme across the ileocaecal junction (Neri et al 1991). Moreover, studies in healthy man have not always confirmed a comparable tonic sphincteric zone. Even under the influence of morphine, a pharmacological stimulus thought to elevate pressure at the ICS, no tonic zone could be clearly identified in man (Borody et al 1985); others have also failed to demonstrate anything other than a low tonic pressure at the human ICS (Nasmyth & Williams 1985). On the other hand, coloileal reflux occurred when the ligamentous bands that maintain acute angulation between ileum and colon were severed (Kumar et al 1987a,b).

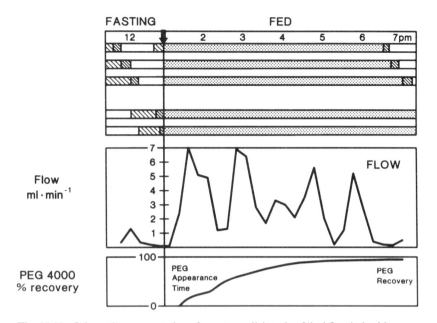

Fig. 27.18 Schematic representation of a postprandial study of ileal flow in healthy man. The fasting motor pattern is interrupted by the meal and the fed motor pattern (strippling) ensues for 6 h before phase III (heavy hatching) of an MMC signals a return to a fasting motor pattern. Ileal flow increases shortly after the liquid meal and fluctuates for 6 h. Polyethylene glycol in the meal appears rapidly and cumulative recovery is close to 100% by the return of fasting motility. (Reproduced from Kerlin et al (1982) with permission.)

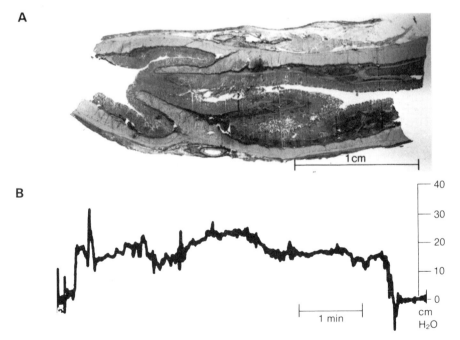

Fig. 27.19 A Histological section of the canine ileocolonic junction showing a thickened band of circular muscle. **B** shows a pull-through pressure tracing illustrating the zone of sphincteric tone (Phillips 1988).

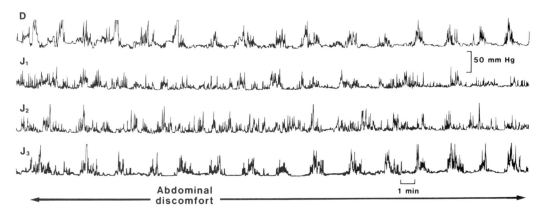

Fig. 27.20   Intraluminal pressures from duodenum and jejunum of a patient with IBS. Phase II shows prominent clusters of phasic bursts at all levels; these patterns occupy a greater proportion of phase II in IBS than in controls. (Reproduced from Kellow & Phillips 1987b with permission.)

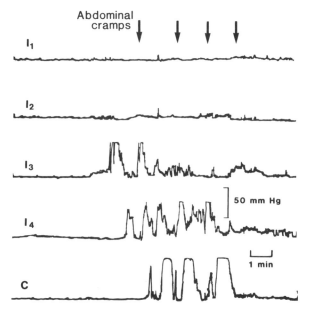

Fig. 27.21   Pressure waves from the ileum (I_{1-4} and caecum (C) from a patient with IBS. High pressure, broadly-based contractions (prolonged propagated contractions, PPCs) pass through the region and are accompanied by abdominal pain. (Reproduced from Kellow & Phillips 1987 with permission.)

Reconstruction of the angle by sutures restored competence. Perhaps, like other gastrointestinal 'gates' (e.g. pylorus, lower oesophageal sphincter), the ileocolonic junction should be considered as an integrated functional unit. We have proposed that the junctional region should be considered as including the terminal ileum, ICS and proximal colon, all of which act in concert to control input to the colon and reflux from

colon to ileum (Quigley et al 1983, 1984a,b, 1985, Phillips et al 1988).

MOTILITY OF THE SMALL INTESTINE IN DISEASE

The scope of this chapter permits only brief attention to pathophysiology. In irritable bowel syndrome (IBS), one consistent finding has been the presence of bursts of rhythmic activity in the jejunum and of prolonged propagated contractions in the distal ileum (Kellow & Phillips 1987). These motor patterns occur in health (Figs 27.10–27.12) but they were more common in patients with IBS and they were frequently concomitant with spontaneous complaints of abdominal pain (Figs 27.20, 27.21). Moreover, IBS patients with diarrhoea had shorter lengths of the interdigestive cycle than did control subjects and those with predominant constipation (Kellow & Phillips 1987). These findings were confirmed using ambulatory recording techniques that permitted the study of patients at home (Kellow et al 1990).

Unusual motility patterns in the small intestine might be anticipated in diarrhoeal disease, and various dysmotilities have been reported in clinical and experimental conditions (VanTrappen et al 1986). At this time, a coherent picture has not emerged and it is still unclear whether the unusual motilities observed in diarrhoeal states are causative, or merely reflect the increased volume of intraluminal fluid in diarrhoea. The review of VanTrappen et al should be consulted for an overview of this area.

Patients with idiopathic constipation due to colonic inertia may have delayed transit in the small intestine (Stivland et al 1991); moreover, partial colectomy for

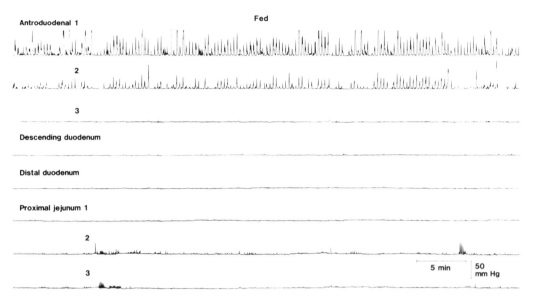

Fig. 27.22 Myogenic form of chronic intestinal pseudo-obstruction, from a person with a family history of hereditary hollow visceral myopathy. In this postprandial recording antropyloric activity is within normal limits but there are very few, weak contractions in the small bowel. (Reproduced from Malagelada et al (1986) with permission.)

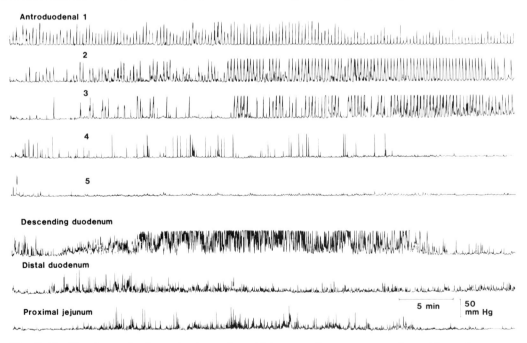

Fig. 27.23 Chronic pseudo-obstruction in a patient with long-standing symptoms and no evidence of mechanical obstruction. This postprandial record shows normal postprandial antroduodenal motility. The small intestine shows a prolonged burst of intense phasic pressures with tonic change. The distal channels show abnormal waxing and waning of the fed pattern. (Reproduced from Malagelada et al 1986 with permission.)

constipation is often complicated by small bowel obstruction (Whitehead et al 1991). Thus, some patients with colonic inertia may also suffer from a more general-ized motility disorder, including the small bowel. Indeed, these patients overlap those with intestinal pseudo-obstruction; this syndrome can be categorized

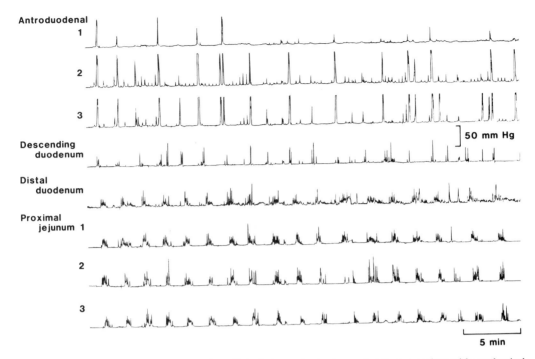

Antroduodenal
1

2

3

Descending
duodenum

Distal
duodenum

Proximal
jejunum 1

2

3

50 mm Hg

5 min

Fig. 27.24 Regular clusters, an exaggeration of the 'minute rhythm' recorded from a patient with mechanical obstruction of the small bowel. (Reproduced from Malagelada et al 1986 with permission.)

into those with myopathic (Fig. 27.22) and neuropathic (Fig. 27.23) disorders. Thus, the disorder can affect the muscle per se, or the integrating neural circuitry that regulates muscle action. Patients with pseudo-obstruction must be distinguished from those with mechanical obstruction (Fig. 27.24). However, Summers et al (1983) have drawn attention to the overlap of motor features between mechanical and pseudo-obstruction.

In summary, the most dramatic and reproducible facet of the small bowel's motor function is the MMC. Though a relatively constant finding among species, there are prominent variations on this major theme. Further, among individuals, wide differences are also seen. These must be kept in mind when small bowel motility is being recorded and analysed diagnostically. It is possible that abnormalities will be over-diagnosed

if the wide range of normality is not fully appreciated. The more subtle patterns of phase II of the fasting cycle and postprandial motility have received less attention, but are surely very important. It is also clear that abnormalities of motility can be recognized in some diseases, but closer pathophysiological correlations need to be established.

ACKNOWLEDGEMENTS

The work from the Mayo Gastroenterology Unit has been performed in conjunction with numerous research associates, whose contributions are acknowledged gratefully by extensive reference to their publications. This work was supported in part by grants from the National Institutes of Health, Bethesda, Maryland (AM32121, RR585).

REFERENCES

Alvarez W C 1928 The mechanics of the digestive tract. Hoeber, New York
Berseth C L 1989 Gestational evolution of small intestine motility in preterm and term infants. J Pediatr 115: 646–651
Berseth C L 1990 Neonatal small intestinal motility: motor responses to feeding in term and preterm infants. J Pediatr 117: 777–782

Borody J T, Quigley E M M, Phillips S F et al 1985 Effects of morphine and atropine on motility and transit in the human ileum. Gastroenterology 89: 562–570
Camilleri M, Phillips S F 1989 Disorders of small intestinal motility. Gastroenterol Clin North Am 18: 405–424
Christensen J, Schedl H P, Clifton J A 1966 The small intestinal basic electrical rhythm (slow wave) frequency gradient in normal men and in patients with a variety of diseases. Gastroenterology 50: 309–315
Code C F, Marlett J A 1975 The interdigestive myo-electric

complex of the stomach and small bowel of dogs. J Physiol 246: 289–309

Code C F, Schlegel J F 1973 The gastrointestinal interdigestive housekeeper: motor correlates of the interdigestive myoelectric complex of the dog in: Daniel E E (ed.) Proceedings of the Fourth International Symposium on GI Motility. Mitchell Press, Vancouver pp 631–634

DeWever I, Eeckhout C, VanTrappen G et al 1978 Disruptive effect of test meals on interdigestive motor complex in dogs. Am J Physiol 235: E661–E665

Fich A, Phillips S F, Hanson R B et al 1989 Rapid frequency rhythmic postprandial motility in the canine ileum. Am J Physiol 257: G766–G772

Fich A, Phillips S F, Neri M et al 1990 Regulation of postprandial motility in the canine ileum. Am J Physiol 259: G767–G774

Fleckenstein P 1978 Migrating electrical spike activity in the fasting human small intestine. Dig Dis Sci 23: 769–775

Fleckenstein P, Øigaard A 1978 Electrical spike activity in the human small intestine. A multiple electrode study of fasting diurnal variations. Dig Dis Sci 23: 776–780

Gazet J-C, Kopp J 1964 The surgical significance of the ileocecal junction. Surgery 56: 565–573

Grider J R 1989 Identification of neurotransmitters regulating intestinal peristaltic reflex in humans. Gastroenterology 97: 1414–1419

Kamath P S, Hoepfner M T, Phillips S F 1987 Short chain fatty acids stimulate motility of the canine ileum. Am J Physiol 253: G427-G433

Kellow J E, Borody T J, Phillips S F et al 1986 Human interdigestive motility: variations in patterns from esophagus to colon. Gastroenterology 91: 386–395

Kellow J E, Phillips S F 1987 Altered small bowel motility in irritable bowel syndrome is correlated with symptoms. Gastroenterology 92: 1885–1893

Kellow J E, Gill R C, Wingate D L 1990 Prolonged ambulant recordings of small bowel motility demonstrate abnormalities in the irritable bowel syndrome. Gastroenterology 98: 1208–1218

Kerlin P, Phillips S F 1982 Variability of motility of the ileum and jejunum in healthy man. Gastroenterology 82: 694–700

Kerlin P, Zinsmeister A, Phillips S F 1982 Relationship of motility to flow of contents in the human small intestine. Gastroenterology 82: 701–706

Kerlin P, Zinsmeister A, Phillips S F 1983 Motor responses to food of the ileum, proximal colon, and distal colon of healthy humans. Gastroenterology 84: 762–770

Kruis W, Azpiroz F, Phillips S F 1985 Contractile patterns and transit of fluid in canine terminal ileum. Am J Physiol 249: G264-G270

Kumar D, Phillips S F 1987a The contribution of external ligamentous attachments to function of the ileocecal junction. Dis Colon Rectum 30: 410–416

Kumar D, Phillips S F, Brown M L 1987b Reflux from ileum to colon in the dog. Role of external ligamentous attachments. Dig Dis Sci 33: 345–352

Kumar D, Wingate D L, Ruckebusch Y 1986 Circadian variation in the propagation velocity of the migrating motor complex. Gastroenterology 91: 926–930

Malagelada J-R, Camilleri M, Stanghellini V 1986 Manometric diagnoses of gastrointestinal motor disorders. Thieme, New York

Marik F, Code C F 1975 Control of the interdigestive myoelectric activity in dogs by the vagus nerves and pentagastrin. Gastroenterology 69: 387–395

Marlett J A, Code C F 1979 Effects of celiac and superior mesenteric ganglionectomy on interdigestive myoelectric complex in dogs. Am J Physiol 237: E432–E436

Nasmyth D G, Williams N S 1985 Pressure characteristics of the human ileocecal region – a key to its function. Gastroenterology 89: 345–351

Neri M, Phillips S F, Fich A et al 1991 Canine ileocolonic sphincter: flow, transit, and motility before and after sphincterotomy. Am J Physiol 260: G284–G289

Phillips S F 1988 Small Bowel. In: Kumar D, Gustavsson S (eds) An illustrated guide to gastrointestinal motility (edition 1). John Wiley & Sons, Chichester, pp 187–206

Phillips S F, Quigley E M M, Kumar D et al 1988 Motility of the ileocolonic junction. Gut 29: 390–406

Quigley E M M, Phillips S F, Dent J et al 1983 Myoelectric activity and intraluminal pressure of the canine ileocolonic sphincter. Gastroenterology 85: 1054–1062

Quigley E M M, Phillips S F, Dent J 1984a Distinctive patterns of interdigestive motility at the canine ileocolonic junction. Gastroenterology 87: 836–844

Quigley E M M, Borody T J, Phillips S F et al 1984b Motility of the terminal ileum and ileocecal sphincter in healthy humans. Gastroenterology 87: 857–866

Quigley E M M, Phillips S F, Cranley B et al 1985 Tone of canine ileocolonic junction: topography and response to phasic contractions. Am J Physiol 249: G350–G357

Read N W, McFarlane A, Kinsman R I et al 1984 Effect of infusion of nutrient solutions into the ileum on gastrointestinal transit and plasma levels of neurotensin and enteroglucagon. Gastroenterology 86: 274–280

Rumessen J J, Thuneberg L 1991 Interstitial cells of Cajal in human small intestine. Gastroenterology 100: 1417–1431

Sarna S K 1985 Cyclic motor activity: Migrating motor complex. Gastroenterology 89: 894–913

Sarna S K, Otterson M F 1989 Small intestinal physiology and pathophysiology. In: Motility Disorders. Gastroenterol Clin North Am 18: 375–404

Schemann M, Ehrlein H-J 1986a Mechanical characteristics of phase II and phase III of the interdigestive migrating motor complex in dogs. Gastroenterology 91: 117–123

Schemann M, Ehrlein H-J 1986b Postprandial patterns of canine jejunal motility and transit of luminal content. Gastroenterology 90: 991–1000

Stivland T, Camilleri M, Vassallo M et al 1991 Scintigraphic measurement of regional gut transit in idiopathic constipation. Gastroenterology 101: 107–115

Summers R W, Anuras S, Green J 1983 Jejunal manometry patterns in health, partial intestinal obstruction, and pseudo-obstruction. Gastroenterology 85: 1290–1300

Szurszewski J H 1969 A migrating electric complex of the canine small intestine. Am J Physiol 217: 1757–1763

Szurszewski J H 1987 Electrophysiological basis of gastrointestinal motility in: Physiology of the gastrointestinal tract. Raven Press, New York

VanTrappen G, Janssens J, Coremans G et al 1986 Gastrointestinal motility disorders. Dig Dis Sci 31: 5S–25S

Weisbrodt N T 1987 Motility of the small intestine. In: Johnson L R Physiology of the gastrointestinal tract. Raven Press, New York, pp 411–444

Whitehead W E, Chaussade S, Corazziari E et al 1991 Report of an international workshop on management of constipation. Gastroenterol Int 4: 99–113

Wingate D L 1981 Backwards and forwards with the migrating complex. Dig Dis Sci 26: 641–666

28. Colonic motility

J. Frexinos   M. Delvaux

INTRODUCTION

Up to now, despite numerous studies of colonic motor disorders and increasing knowledge of its physiology and control pathways, human colonic motility has not been completely understood. These difficulties may be explained in several ways:

1. the absence of a satisfactory and accessible animal model;
2. the extremely irregular activity of the organ, knowledge of which needs long time recordings – 90% of normal subjects have bowel movements at a frequency between three per day and three per week;
3. the technical problems of investigating the whole colon; most studies have been performed on the

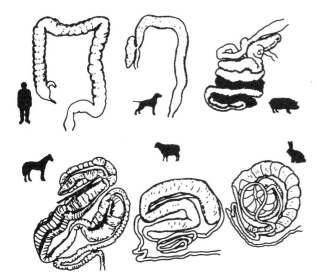

Fig. 28.1 Anatomical differences of the colon in various species (man, dog, pig, horse, sheep and rabbit). The anatomy of the colon is similar in dog and man. Helicoidal colon of the pig may also be considered as a functional 'single' colon.

rectosigmoid area because it is more accessible, but some investigators have concluded that their findings were characteristic of the motility in the rest of the colon.

Colonic motility is recognized as one of the three main functions of the colon, together with water and electrolytes absorption, and carbohydrate transformation by colonic flora. It must be kept in mind that colonic motility is related to the two latter functions, retaining intraluminal contents over long periods of time, in order to favour optimal bacterial growth and water absorption.

At the beginning of this century, radiological observations demonstrated that faeces were propelled by a series of infrequent large movements, known as mass movements or mass peristalsis, and that different patterns of movements could be described in various parts of the colon:

1. segmental localized contractions dividing the lumen and its content into haustra to promote mixing of the digesta;
2. propulsive contractions preceded by the disappearance of the haustral pattern, migrating distally along the colon and called 'mass movement';
3. 'antiperistalsis', which is the main motor activity of the proximal colon.

ANATOMICAL ASPECTS

The colon exhibits a wide anatomic variability among the different species (Fig. 28.1), and these structural variations reflect the major differences in colonic physiology observed from one species to another. Up to now, no single animal model has been identified that would enable studies directly consistent with the physiology of the human colon. The morphological gross structure closest to that of the human colon is found in the pig. In man, different regions can be described.

427

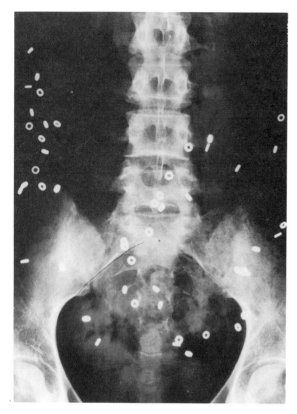

Fig. 28.2   Plain film of the abdomen showing the progression of radio-opaque markers of various shapes along the colon, in order to measure colonic transit time.

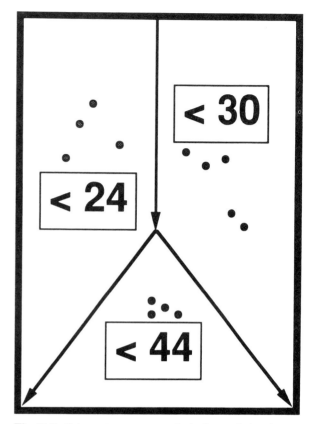

Fig. 28.3   Schematic assessment of colonic transit time by counting radio-opaque markers on plain films of the abdomen. 60 markers (20 × 3 successive days) are ingested and plain film are obtained at 4, 7 and 10 days after the first ingestion of the markers. The transit time (TT) in one segment is equal to the sum of the markers counted on the films: $TT = (n_{D4} + n_{D7} + n_{D10}) \times 1.2$. Numbers on the picture indicate the upper normal value of the transit time in each segment (adapted from Chaussade et al 1986).

The right colon is composed of the caecum which is about 6 cm in length – quite small in comparison to that of many animals – and the ascending colon which is about 12–20 cm long; the circumference of the latter is greater than that of the remainder of the colon. The transverse colon is about 50 cm long; the descending colon about 25 cm; the sigmoid about 40 cm; and the rectum 12 cm long. The whole human colon presents a sacculated appearance and exhibits an outer longitudinal muscle punched into three, 6–10 mm wide bundles, the taeniae. One of them is located along the mesenteric insertion. In the sigmoid colon the taeniae become less apparent, broaden and fuse in the distal part, the rectum, to form a longitudinal layer of uniform thickness (Hamilton 1984).

METHODS FOR STUDYING COLONIC MOTILITY

Colonic transit time

Colonic transit time accounts for about 90% of whole-gut transit time. It is extremely variable even in normal subjects. Ingestion of unabsorbable material (seeds or small stones) and stool collection has been used for centuries to evaluate digestive transit time. Later, carmine, charcoal, barium sulphate, ^{51}Cr-labelled sodium chromate etc. were also used in this way. At the present time the most commonly used method of investigating colonic transit time is measurement of the progression of radio-opaque markers, which can be detected, located and counted within the bowel on plain films of the abdomen (Fig. 28.2) or counted in successive stool samples. The first method allows determination of the transit time in different segments of the colon (Fig. 28.3), while the second only allows evaluation of the total transit time. Many techniques have been pro-

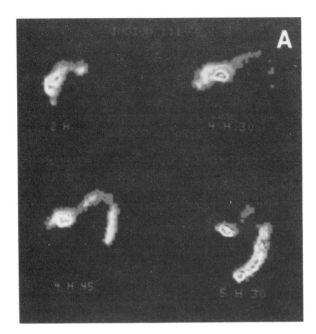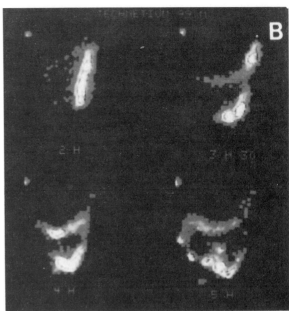

Fig. 28.4 Scintigraphic measurement of colonic transit time. The tracer is infused at the hepatic flexure and moves aborally in fasted state (**A**). In the fed state (**B**), the tracer injected at the splenic flexure moves in both aboral (antegrade) and aboral (retrograde) directions (from Picon et al 1992 with permission).

posed, the best being the simplest (Hinton et al 1969, Chaussade et al 1986). The evidence that the colon is able to mix the digesta has been demonstrated by giving single doses of differently shaped pellets on 3 consecutive days and then measuring their appearance in the stools (Wiggins & Cummings 1976). Obviously, colonic segmental transit time is especially useful in assessing the pathophysiology of transit disturbances in conditions like chronic constipation. Such studies have suggested that residues from different meals are mixed in the caecum and the right colon and then gradually transferred to the left and sigmoid colons where they are stored. However this widely accepted theory has been challenged by studies of colonic transit using scintigraphy. Scintigraphy is a safe physiological and quantitative method for evaluating colonic transit (Jian et al 1984) (Fig. 28.4). Mass movements can be observed and the distance from the caecum to the sigmoid may be traversed in less than 1 min. Some results (Krevsky et al 1986), suggest that the caecum and the ascending colon do not function as a storage area but that the transverse colon could be the primary site for storage, mixing and dehydratation of residues within the large intestine. 3 hours after a caecal instillation of 8 ml of ^{111}indium-diethylene-triamine-penta-acetic acid, the radioisotopic activity was fairly evenly distributed throughout all colonic segments, and the transverse colon showed a relatively rapid increase in activity which remained constant for 20–24 hours. Further studies (Moreno-Osset et al 1989) have confirmed the role of the transverse colon in mixing and storage. Recently, it has also been shown by this method (Fig. 28.4) that both antegrade and retrograde isotopic movements increase in the colon after eating, the antegrade movements being more frequent than the retrograde (Picon et al 1992).

Colonic manometry

Measurement of intraluminal pressure has been the major source of information on colonic motility, but most recordings have been limited to the distal colon and lasted only a few hours. Physiological interpretation of pressure waves has been difficult because of wide variability in morphology. Moreover, manometrically recorded activity does not correlate with colonic diameter as measured radiographically (Ritchie et al 1962). Until recently, manometric methods have not been generally accepted as useful either experimentally or clinically. However, the development of fine-bore, open-tip catheters perfused with water at a low rate by a low-compliance pump have allowed some progress.

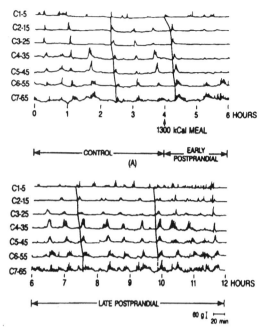

Fig. 28.5 Manometric recording of colonic motility showing the basal activity before the meal and the early and late response to a meal. Solid lines demonstrate the propagation of the pressure waves (from Sarna 1991 with permission).

Analysis of intraluminal pressures, recorded over a 24-h period from the ascending colon of healthy volunteers (Kerlin et al 1983), mainly showed irregular, isolated peaks of pressure during fasting and, sometimes, bursts of continuous activity occurring at a predominant frequency of 6 per min. In the distal colon, regular contractile activity occurred at a frequency of 2.5–3.5 per min, except in three subjects in whom a rate of 7 per min was recorded. No temporal relationship was observed between motor activity in ascending and distal colons. The motor activity of the transverse, descending and sigmoid colon was recorded during 24 h in 14 volunteers by Narducci et al (1987). The colonic motility index was low before lunch and dinner. In the fasting state, the motor activity was chiefly represented by low amplitude, non-propulsive segmental contractions, while peristaltic movements seldom occurred. After eating and in the morning upon wakening, a significant increase in colonic motility occurred, characterized by an irregular alternation of quiescences, sporadic non-propagating contractions, non-propagating bursts of contractions and high-amplitude propagated contractions (HAPCs) (Fig. 28.5).

These HAPCs were investigated more recently by

Bassoti and Gaburri (1988) in healthy volunteers with a colonoscopically positioned manometric probe and a low compliance infusion system. Diurnal changes in HAPCs were noted with a maximum frequency observed after meals and after wakening in the morning: the mean frequency was 6.1 ± 0.9 HAPC per subject per 24 h, the mean amplitude being 110.37 ± 6.3 mmHg, and mean duration about 14.15 ± 0.8 s. The velocity of propagation of these HAPCs was 1.11 ± 0.1 cm/s. No significant differences could be demonstrated between colonic segments.

Colonic myoelectrical activity

Slow wave activity

Slow waves are present in the colonic smooth muscle and correspond to rhythmic fluctuations in electrical potential (Fig. 28.6). An effective contraction is only initiated when a strong depolarization (a spike) occurs. It has been demonstrated in vitro, that the electrical oscillatory activity of the human colon determines the spacing of the spikes and the pattern of contractile activity (Huizinga et al 1985). However, few characteristics of the human colonic slow waves are identical to those observed in the small intestine or in the colon of the dog and the cat. Colonic slow waves are much more variable than those recorded from the stomach and the small intestine. Taylor et al (1975) and Snape et al (1976) observed along the large bowel, gradients in frequency and percentage of electrical activity using various types of electrodes: mucosal suction-electrodes, serosal and cutaneous electrodes. They reported that regular slow wave activity was not constantly present and that two rhythms could occur: a dominant rate of 6–12 cpm and, less frequently observed, a lower rate between and 2–4 cpm. These results have been disputed by other workers. The discrepancies in the frequency of colonic slow waves might be explained by differences in recording techniques and the complex methods (Fast Fourier Transform) of data analysis. Stoddard et al (1979) when analysing monopolar and bipolar recordings of human colonic myoelectrical activity found that the concordance between the two techniques was less than 50%. They noted that the incidence of both the 3 and 12 cpm rhythms in the transverse colon was approximately twice that in the ascending colon. In most cases, bipolar recording detected a lower incidence of slow waves than monopolar recording, but the difference in frequency incidence between monopolar and bipolar recordings was not sufficient to account for discrepancies between the various studies of colonic slow waves. They concluded

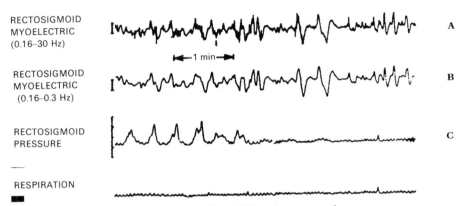

RECTOSIGMOID
MYOELECTRIC
(0.16–30 Hz)

◄——1 min——►

RECTOSIGMOID
MYOELECTRIC
(0.16–0.3 Hz)

RECTOSIGMOID
PRESSURE

RESPIRATION

A

B

C

Fig. 28.6 Electromyographic recording, filtered (**B**) to demonstrate slow waves. The fast electrical activity (**A**) is correlated with pressure (**C**) (from Sunshine et al 1989 with permission).

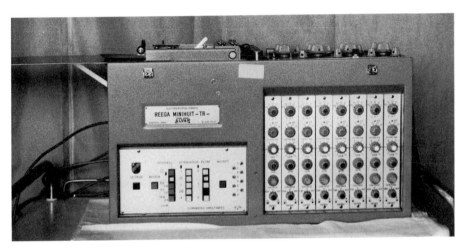

Fig. 28.7 Electroencephalograph (Minihuit Alvar®) for recording spiking activity of the colon. Low frequency filters are used to discriminate between slow waves and spikes.

that the main factor, accounting for differences in published results on electrical activity, could be the method of mathematical analysis used. Another explanation for the complexity of the electrical colonic activity is that the circular and longitudinal muscles have distinctly different electrical activities, and that in vivo recordings are composites of both activities. In vitro studies of human colonic muscle activity revealed that the circular layer of the human colon exhibits spontaneous electrical oscillatory activity with a wide range of frequencies (4–28 cpm) with or without superimposed spiking activity, while longitudinal muscle also shows only one type of activity at a frequency of 20–36 cpm (Huizinga et al 1985).

In current clinical practice and research, colonic slow waves are no longer studied and spike activity gives a better representation of colonic activity from a clinical point of view.

Spiking activity

Myoelectrical spiking activity appears to be the electrical counterpart of colonic contractile activity, contractions being marked by bursts of action potentials. In the human distal colon, Couturier et al (1969), using unipolar suction-type electrodes, recorded spike bursts and slow waves with a similar contraction frequency (10 per min).

In 1980, Bueno et al (1980a) reported a new technique for recording human colonic myoelectrical

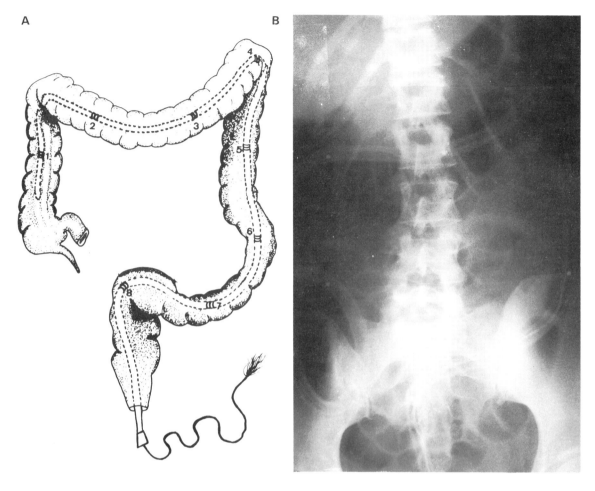

Fig. 28.8   A Schematic representation of an electromyographic (EMG) probe inserted into the colon, up to the caecum and bearing eight groups of three electrodes. **B** Plain film of the abdomen with EMG probe inserted up to the caecum.

Table 28.1   Comparative table of various nomenclatures used to describe colonic spiking activity

Bueno et al 1980	Sarna et al 1981	Schang & Devroede 1983
Short spike bursts (SSBs)	Discrete electrical response activity (DERA)	Rhythmic spike potentials
1.5–3.5 s 10–12/min	2.2 ± 1.3 s 11.4/min	3.0 ± 0.2 s 10.0 ± 0.1/min
Long spike bursts (LSBs)	Continuous electrical response activity (CERA)	Sporadic spike potentials
19.6 ± 2.5 s Non-propagated or short propagation	21.5 ± 5.1 s Non-propagated	12.1 ± 4.0 s Non-propagating
Migrating long spike bursts (MLSBs)	Contractile electrical complex 36.1 ± 34.2 sec May propagate	Sporadic spike potentials Propagating

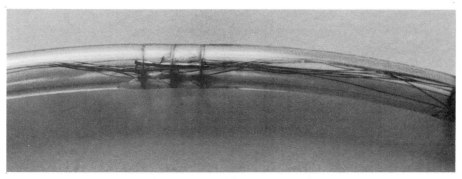

Fig. 28.9 Detailed view of an EMG probe: one group of three nickel-chrome electrodes for bipolar recording of myoelectrical activity.

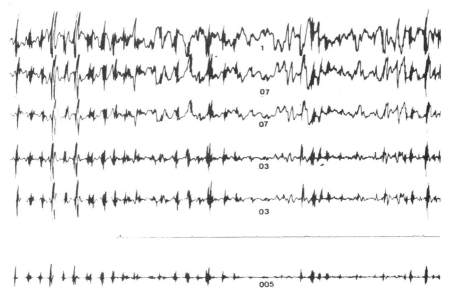

Fig. 28.10 Photograph of an EMG recording. Activity is recorded from the same group of electrodes but (from top to bottom) with filters of increasing sensitivity for low frequencies (1–0.05 Hz), resulting in progressive suppression of slow waves and enhancement of spiking activity.

activity, using an intraluminal probe with contact electrodes and an electroencephalograph (Fig. 28.7) allowing recording of left colonic activity for more than 8 h (Bueno et al 1980b). A few years later, an improvement in the method, which positioned the probe in the caecum (Fig. 28.8), permitted 24-h – and later 48-h – recordings of the whole colon (Frexinos et al 1985).

The probe (INRA no. 79 09 689) is made of a polyvinyl tube, 150 cm in length, supporting eight groups of three annular nickel-chrome electrodes (Fig. 28.9).

The probe is pulled up to the caecum under visual control – a thread is attached to the tip of the tube which passes through the biopsy channel of the colonoscope. As during the withdrawal of the endoscope, the probe may be displaced backwards by 10–20 cm, the position of the probe is checked at the end of the recording by a plain abdominal X-ray. Bipolar recordings are obtained with an eight-channel-electroencephalograph (Minihuit Alvar®) using a short time constant (0.03 s) to selectively detect spike bursts (Fig. 28.10).

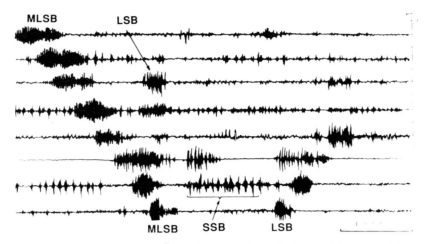

Fig. 28.11   Schematic representation of the three kinds of spiking activity recorded in the colon: short spike bursts (SSBS), long spike bursts (LSBs) and migrating long spike bursts (MLSBs).

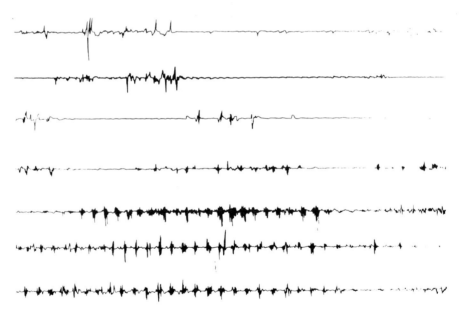

Fig. 28.12   EMG recording showing intense SSB activity, especially in the four lower traces which recorded activity from the left and sigmoid colons.

Two types of spike bursts, defined by their duration, appearance and propagation (Table 28.1) (Fig. 28.11), have been found in the colon of all mammalian species so far investigated (Fioramonti et al 1985).

Short spike bursts (SSBs) are characterized by a short duration of 1.5–4 s, are recorded at only one electrode site, and appear rhythmically at approxima-

tively 10 cpm, corresponding to weak non-propagated variations of pressure and probably to tonic activity (Fig. 28.12). SSBs were also described as 'discrete electrical response' by Sarna et al (1981) or 'rhythmic spike potentials' by Schang and Devroede (1983) (Table 28.1). In normal subjects, SSBs can be observed intermittently at any site in the colon, but predomi-

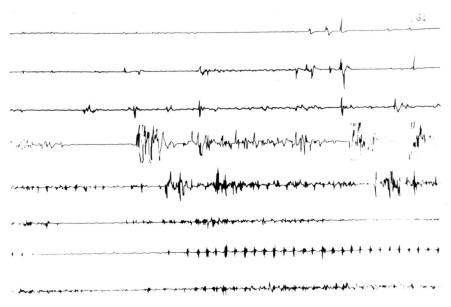

Fig. 28.13 Intense SSB activity predominant on the three lower traces and occurring regularly over periods of about 5 min. This SSB activity corresponds to the 'rectosigmoid brake'.

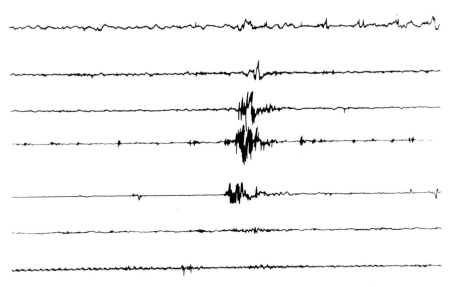

Fig. 28.14 LSB activity propagating orally over 50 cm. Groups of electrodes are 12 cm apart.

nantly in the rectosigmoid area with a characteristic frequency (Fig. 28.13). The rectosigmoid junction is characterized by SSBs appearing at a rate of 6–7 per min for long periods of 5–10 min, followed by periods of quiescence of 10–20 min (Bueno et al 1980b). The marked SSB activity at this level is consistent with the concept of a hyperactive segment acting as a 'brake', as are manometric recordings from the human colon that

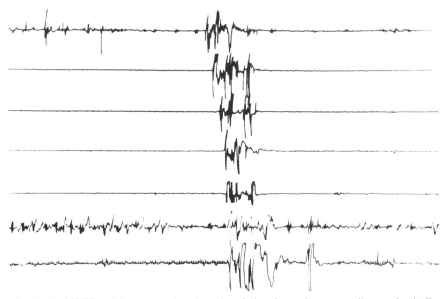

Fig. 28.15 MLSB activity propagating along the whole colon and corresponding mechanically to propulsive waves.

have shown the presence of a hyperactive pressure zone at the rectosigmoid junction in constipated subjects and more rarely in normal subjects (Connell 1962) in agreement with myoelectrical records (Bueno et al 1980b). Thus rectosigmoid activity is important in the maintenance of normal bowel habits by preventing premature passage of stools in the rectum (Chowdhury et al 1976).

Long spike bursts (LSBs) lasting 10.3 ± 0.4 s appear in one of three different patterns (Fig. 28.11): (1) bursts localized at one electrode site and sometimes occurring rhythmically at a rate of about 3 per min; (2) bursts propagated over a short distance (10–70 cm) at a speed of 4 cm/s, in aboral or oral direction (Fig. 28.14); (3) bursts migrating rapidly in aboral direction at a speed of 10 cm/s, over the whole length of the colon, and called migrating long spike bursts (MLSBs) (Fig. 28.15). MLSBs are most evident during colonic reponse to eating. LSB activity corresponds to phasic variations in intraluminal pressure, which are probably responsible for the mixing and propulsion of the stool, especially when propagated (Fig. 28.16). The amplitude of pressure changes associated with SSBs was approximately ten times lower than for the pressure peaks corresponding to LSBs (Bueno et al 1980b). LSB activity has been described as 'continuous electrical response activity' (CERA) or 'contractile electrical complex' (CEC) by Sarna et al (1981) and as 'sporadic spike potentials' by Schang and Devroede (1983)

(Table 28.1). The MLSBs correspond to the migrating spikes bursts described by Christensen (1984) in the cat colon 'in vitro'.

It has to be considered whether all recorded electrical activity is due to contraction of colonic muscle. Changes due to displacement of the probe or to the electrocardiogram can easily be detected on the records. The electromyogram does not appear to be affected either by respiratory movements or by colonic faecal loading.

In man loss of contact of the electrodes with the mucosa is a potential problem, but controlled experimental studies in dogs (Fioramonti et al 1985) did not reveal significant differences between mucosal contact or implanted serosal electrodes.

The effects of bowel preparation were studied by Dinoso et al (1983). The motility index (MI) of the cleansed and unwashed colon showed segmental differences. However significant differences were found in the mean MI per 3 h of recording but not in the basal activity. The MI was lower in the unwashed colon suggesting that cleansing enemas may indeed stimulate the basal myoelectrical activity (BMA) of the distal colon. The technique of Bueno et al (1980a) is not wholly physiological since emptying of the colon, air insufflation and analgesic drug injections are required to set up the probe, so an 8-h interval is needed as adaptation time before recording starts. Nevertheless, since normal meals are taken during

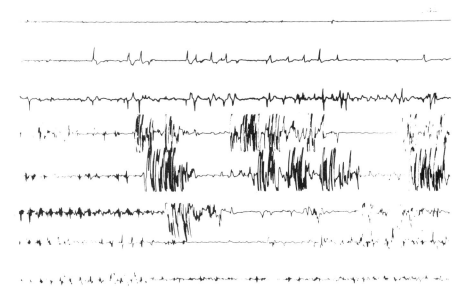

Fig. 28.16   LSB-type activity occurring on the transverse and left colon and propagating aborally over 10–30 cm.

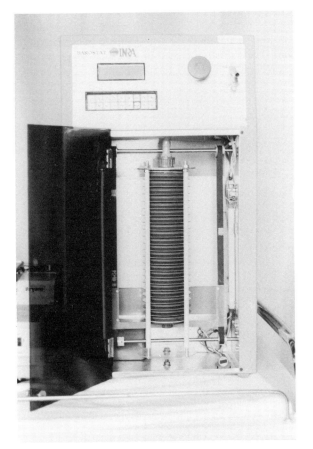

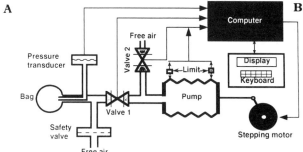

Fig. 28.17   **A** The electromechanical barostat. **B** Schematic diagram of the barostat. The pressure in the bag is continuously monitored by the computer and variations in volume needed to maintain the steady state-pressure are recorded. These variations reflect changes in tone of the studied organ.

the 48-h record period, the colon progressively fills during this time.

Measurement of colonic tone by the barostat technique

Muscle tone adapts to the arrival of large amounts of content by 'receptive relaxation' or increases to ensure emptying of the segment. Until recently little was known about visceral tone because manometric recording of intraluminal pressure reflects phasic contractions but not tonic relaxation of the gut. This is particularly true in large cavities like stomach, caecum and rectum. The electromechanical barostat (Fig. 28.17) was developed to study changes in visceral tone and validated in studies of the gastric fundus in dog and humans (Aspiroz & Malagelada 1985).

Colonic muscle maintains a continuous tone, which may vary in physiological conditions. When a barostat bag is placed in the left colon in man, allowing the bag to follow closely the contour of the colonic wall, the volume ranges between 50–150 ml (Steadman et al 1991, Staumont et al 1992). During fasting, balloon volumes are generally constant; small fluctuations in volume are not accompanied by phasic contractile activity (Steadman et al 1991).

PHYSIOLOGICAL REGULATION OF COLONIC MOTILITY

Diurnal changes in colonic motility

The human colon exhibits variation in the frequency of contractions. According to numerous studies, performed mainly in the rectosigmoid area (Snape 1977, Taylor et al 1978, Sarna et al 1982), basal colonic motility is characterized by long periods of quiescence interrupted by bursts of apparently spontaneous activity (Wyman et al 1978).

Electromyographic recordings involving proximal, transverse and distal colon over 24 h or more were obtained for the first time in 1985 (Frexinos et al 1985) and similar observations of pressure activity were made by Narducci et al (1987). However, these were carried out on resting patients or volunteers, and the effects of physical activity could not be studied. In these circumscribed conditions, two major events, eating and sleeping, dominate the 24-h cycle of colonic activity (Fig. 28.18). The colonic response to eating will be discussed below. Motor activity during sleep is dramatically decreased and can entirely disappear for

long periods (Fig. 28.19). Our experience of more than 300 electromyographic recordings over 24–48 h, performed in different clinical profiles of irritable bowel syndrome (IBS) is in accordance with the first results on healthy volunteers, published in 1985. The lowest values of spiking activity were observed from 22:00 to 06:00 and at any site of recording these values were significantly lower than those observed between 17:00 and 19:00, i.e. during the daytime and preceding the dinner served at 19:00. Propagated spiking activity is almost absent during sleep with the exception of some rare LSBs migrating aborally or orally. A moderate and intermittent SSB activity is often observed in the area of the rectosigmoid junction. However, it is accepted that nocturnal colonic activity is very low in healthy volunteers and patients with IBS, with the exception of patients with painless diarrhoea (Frexinos et al 1987) who have a significant increase in the number of MLSBs. The same pattern was observed in man several hours after the administration of sennosides (Frexinos et al 1989).

Colonic motor activity increases soon after wakening, reaching the basal level of spiking activity in the afternoon. A low-calorie continental breakfast (300 kcal) does not induce a true colonic response to eating. This small increase is not due to physical activity because it occurs in supine subjects; the first

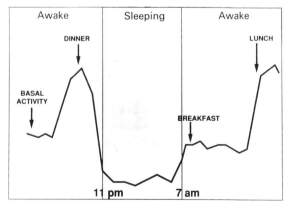

Fig. 28.18 Diurnal variations of colonic activity in man as observed during long-term recordings of EMG. Intense activity is observed after the two main meals (lunch and dinner). Basal activity is markedly higher during the day compared with the night. The lowest level of activity is recorded during the sleeping time.

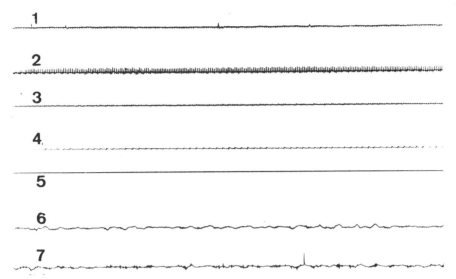

Fig. 28.19 Typical nocturnal EMG pattern characterized by the absence of activity. A few SSBs appear on the sigmoid colon. Note the presence of an artefact on trace 2, caused by interference from cardiac electrical activity.

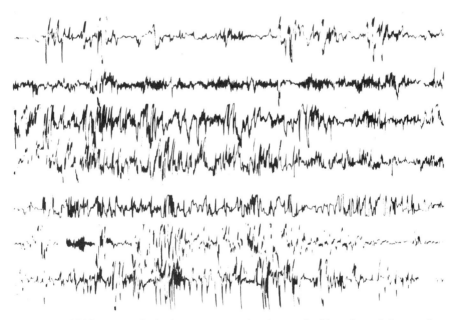

Fig. 28.20 EMG pattern of colonic response to eating characterized by a dramatic increase in spiking activity, predominantly involving the LSB type of activity. Colonic response to eating stimulates spiking activity in the entire colon.

major increase in colonic motility appears after lunch.

More recently, Soffer et al (1988) positioned three pressure sensors in the colon of nine healthy volunteers, allowing ambulant monitoring over sessions lasting each between 13 and 48 h. The results showed that contractile activity throughout the large bowel was dramatically reduced during sleep and was enhanced on waking whereas meals were non-constant stimuli of motor activity. Motor activity in the various colonic regions was characterized by scant and irregular contractions with infrequent bursts. Motor coordination was not obviously detected between the different regions studied. These results were supported by Wegman et al (1990) who demonstrated that regions of smooth muscle in the unstimulated human rectosigmoid area in vivo act independently and that there is no apparent common neuromuscular drive under these conditions.

Colonic response to eating (CRE)

Description

The gastrocolonic response consists of an increase in colonic motor activity after eating (Fig. 28.20). This stimulating effect is one of the most consistent findings in the diurnal changes of colonic motility and has been described in many species, mainly man, in the rectosigmoid area (Misiewicz 1984). In this segment the CRE is generally thought to occur in two phases: an early phase within 30 min of ingestion of a meal, previously called 'gastrocolonic reflex' and now described as the gastrocolonic response; and a late phase, occurring at least 1h later, which corresponds to the intestinal phase of digestion (Snape et al 1979). The literature concerning the mechanisms involved in the CRE is inconclusive probably due to the failure to define 'gastrocolonic reflex' and 'CRE', and also due to the problems, of recording sigmoid motor activity. A striking feature of rectosigmoid motor activity is the enormous variation at different recording sites in this region, which underlines the need to use multiple recording sites (Dinoso et al 1983). This may explain the differences between the various observations that have been reported.

The increase in rectosigmoid motor activity that occurs in response to a meal has been known for many years. Early studies were conducted by measuring pelvic colonic pressure before and after a meal in patients with non-specific diarrhoea or constipation. During the meal, colonic activity was strikingly increased in patients with diarrhoea, beginning immediately or within 3 min after the start of the meal but returning to basal level immediately after it; such a response was not observed in patients with constipation (Waller et al 1972).

Electromyographic studies (Frexinos et al 1985) show an increase in the number of LSBs and MLSBs starting less than 10 min after feeding and lasting 1–2 h. Food intake provokes a significant increase in both propagating and non-propagating spike bursts (Fig. 28.21). Localized LSB activity increases, the first peak appearing within 10–20 min after the beginning of the meal and the second appearing within 60–70 min after it. Propagated spiking activity (MLSB) increased only 70–80 min after the meal (Schang & Devroede 1983). In patients with IBS, the right colon exhibits a lower LSB activity than the rectosigmoid during the postprandial period (Dapoigny et al 1988). LSB activity propagating in the aboral direction is increased in the right colon while it is inhibited in the rectosigmoid colon. In contrast, LSB activity propagating orally is increased in both the right colon and the rectosigmoid. Furthermore, at the level of the rectosigmoid junction, a specific myoelectrical activity with a predominant frequency of 2.7–3.3 cpm (Fast Fourier Transform analysis) is observed (Dapoigny et al 1988).

Manometry (Moreno-Osset et al 1989), shows that the increase in motility during CRE consists predominantly of segmental and migrating contractions. The correlation between movements of the luminal content and changes in intraluminal pressure has been studied in healthy volunteers. This study showed that the movements of the tracer occurred during both types of pressure waves: the non-propagating contractions are associated with a gradual movement of the luminal content, the direction of the movement being determined by the differences in pressure in the various segments of the colon, whereas the propagating contractions are associated with rapid movements of intraluminal contents. Colonic scintigraphic studies have demonstrated that in fasting subjects the tracer remains in the splenic flexure, while after food (1000 kcal) it moves into the descending and the sigmoid colon as well as into the transverse, reaching the hepatic flexure and the ascending colon. These data show that, although the gastrocolonic response may promote colonic propulsion, retrograde transport of the luminal content can also occur and this is consistent with the increase of retrograde LSB activity observed during electromyographic recording (Frexinos et al 1985).

Modulation of CRE

The response of the colon to a meal depends on the

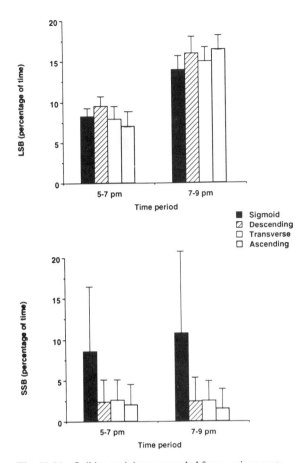

Fig. 28.21 Spiking activity as recorded from various parts of the colon during the basal period before the meal (17:00–19:00) and the 2-h period following the meal (19:00–21:00). The increase in spiking activity only concerns the LSB while the SSB type of activity is not altered after the meal.

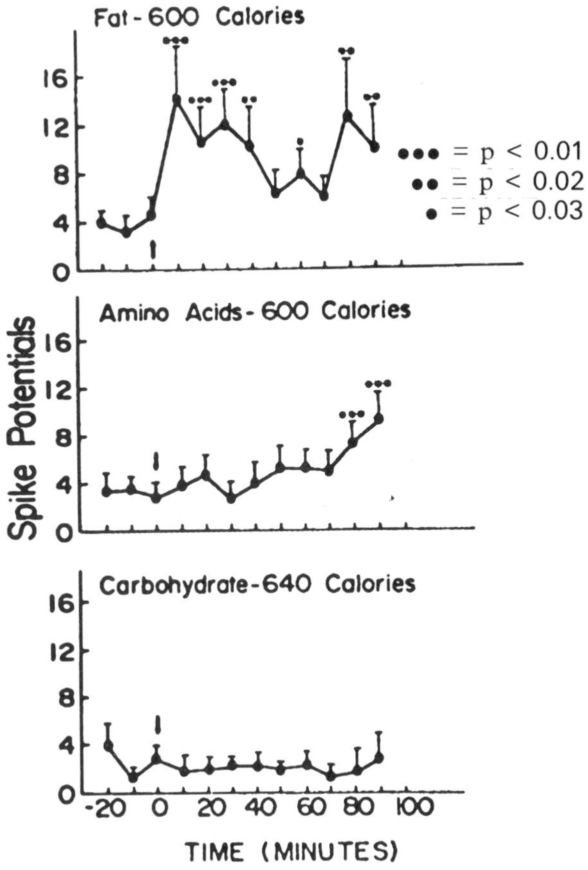

Fig. 28.22 Physiological control of the colonic response to eating. Role of ingestion of equicaloric amounts of individual dietary components: fat, amino acids and carbohydrate (from Battle et al 1980 with permission).

number of calories consumed and on the chemical composition of the meal.

The gastrocolonic response can be evoked by a standard 1000 kcal meal which significantly increases spiking and contractile activity while a 350 kcal meal is only a minimal stimulus (Snape et al 1978). Wright et al (1988) have suggested that the fatty component of the meal is the major stimulus of the CRE; other dietary components – proteins or carbohydrates – have little effect on colonic motility when they are ingested alone. However, the distal colonic spiking activity recorded after a 600 kcal fatty meal is quite different from the response to a 1000 kcal standard meal. After a fatty meal, two peaks of spiking activity are recorded as compared to the single peak induced by a standard and complete meal (Fig. 28.22). The first peak induced

by a fatty meal occurs within the first 10 min and the second peak within 70–90 min. Addition of proteins to a fatty meal converts the CRE to a pattern similar to that observed after a standardized meal: the early peak occurs but the late response is abolished. Moreover, the post prandial response to a fatty meal can be inhibited, both in normal subjects and in patients with IBS, by the administration of an amino acid mixture before the meal (Battle et al 1980) as well as by anticholinergic drugs (Sullivan et al 1978) or vagotomy (Connell & McKelvey 1970). Others (Levinson et al 1985) demonstrated that fat stimulates colonic motility only through direct mucosal contact, since intravenous administration of fat emulsion has no effect, while mixed amino acids, both enteral and parenteral, inhibit CRE.

The mechanism of CRE

The CRE may be mediated either by neural reflexes that originate in the upper part of the gastrointestinal tract or by gastrointestinal hormones. In the absence of a cephalic phase in man, the rapid appearance of the early component of the CRE suggests mediation by the stomach, although CRE still occurs in subjects with total gastrectomy (Holdstock & Misiewicz 1970). Vagotomy (Connell & McKelvey 1970) or anticholinergic drugs inhibit the CRE while complete transsection of the spinal cord does not disrupt the increase of colonic motility (Glick et al 1984).

A study performed by Sun et al (1982) with bipolar clip electrodes recording spiking activity of the distal colon in healthy volunteers showed that the afferent neural receptors that initiate the gastrocolonic response originate in the stomach or in the proximal duodenal mucosa. After sham feeding of a modified 1000 kcal meal, there is no increase in colonic motility which excludes the contribution of a cephalic phase in CRE. Naloxone inhibits the postprandial gastrocolonic response, but does not inhibit stimulation of colonic motility by neostigmine. Thus, the CRE may be mediated by both efferent cholinergic and opiate pathways.

Some recent observations (Wiley et al 1988) established the existence of a gastric phase in the human gastrocolonic response that can be generated by gastric mechanoreceptors. Distension of the stomach with increasing volumes of water (100, 200, 300 ml) produces a volume-dependent increase in rectosigmoid motility that is abolished by atropine. The possibility of a nutrient-specific intestinal phase in the control of the CRE was investigated by infusing various solutions – normal saline, lipid, glucose or essential amino acids – into the duodenum. Only the infusion of lipid caused an increase in rectosigmoid motility partially antagonized ($\pm 60\%$) by atropine. This response was independent of CCK release since intravenous infusion of high doses of CCK (20 ng/g/h), reaching plasma levels threefold higher than those measured during lipid infusion was needed to increase rectosigmoid motility. In contrast, Liberge et al (1991) suggested that, in rats, CCK is involved in the generation of the CRE to a meal, possibly through CCK receptors located in the ventromedial hypothalamic nuclei.

Tomling et al (1991) proposed that the close association between the time concordance of the rise in hydrogen in exhaled air (corresponding to the entry of ingesta in the caecum) and in rectosigmoid motor activity would support the assumption that the motor activity could be generated by chemical or mechanical stimulation of the proximal colon. After a 620 kcal meal they noted, within minutes of ingestion, a significant increase in motility index and a temporary rise in exhaled hydrogen. A late increase in motor activity occurring 123 ± 19 min after the meal, was temporarily related to the beginning of a second and larger rise in exhaled hydrogen. These results contradict ealier studies by Kerlin et al (1983) who could not demonstrate a clear relationship between maximal postprandial colonic activity and the initial rise or peak of H_2 expiration.

Colonic motility and physical exercise

Physical exercise may affect gastrointestinal function and it is well known that constipation is a major complaint in immobile patients or in elderly inactive subjects. In contrast, vigorous jogging and running may cause diarrhoea, abdominal cramps, etc. However, due to technical difficulties, there are very few studies on the effects of exercise on colonic motility. Early observations, by DeYoung et al in 1932, using water-filled balloons introduced through a caecostomy, showed that an exercise lasting a few minutes increased colonic motor activity in fasting subjects. Using radio-opaque markers, radiotelemetric capsules and scintigraphy, Holdstock et al (1970) observed in physically active patients that propulsion of colonic contents and intraluminal pressure significantly increased after meals, while in resting patients the increase of intraluminal pressure was rarely associated with propulsive activity.

Connell et al (1964) using manometric methods, showed only transient and variable effects of physical exercise on colonic motility in post-dysenteric patients studied lying down and sitting up. However in this study, the physical exercise was mild.

More recently, Bingham and Cummings (1989) reported in a controlled trial, that regular daily exercise without associated changes in diet, performed over a period of 9 weeks, had no effect on transit time and stool weight and frequency. They concluded that exercise has marked effects on physical fitness but no consistent effect on large bowel function. In contrast, Cordain et al (1986) showed that aerobic running by a group of healthy volunteers maintaining the same dietary habits, decreased bowel transit time and increased the predicted maximum oxygen consumption.

Dapoigny and Sarna (1991) investigating the effects of running in conscious dogs in both fasting and fed states, observed on the contrary that exercise had profound effects on colonic motility and that these effects depended on the timing of the exercise. Postprandial exercise disrupted colonic MMCs and replaced them by non-MMCs; exercise also increased the total duration of the contractile activity throughout the colon. Exercise initiated giant migrating contractions, mass movements and defaecation in both the fasted and fed states in the majority of dogs.

Physiological regulation of colonic tone

After a meal, the volume of a barostat bag placed in the colon consistently decreases. The decrease in bag volume, which corresponds to an enhanced colonic tone, occurs over 5–20 min after the meal and lasts up to 3 h. In the study by Steadman et al (1992), test meals increased colonic tone by 75% while filling the stomach with water increased it by no more than 20%. In contrast during nocturnal sleep, the colonic tone seems to be decreased since the bag volume may increase up to 60% above the basal volume. In this study, basal values in colonic tone were reached again after awakening of the subjects. These studies clearly show physiological changes in colonic tone that are independent of phasic contractile activity.

The variations of colonic tone observed in barostat studies closely correlate with those of contractile activity as recorded by intraluminal manometry or electromyography. After a meal, there is simultaneous increase in colonic tone and in contractile activity. Colonic tone has been considered to be due to SSB activity, but until recently no experimental evidence has been produced to support this assumption. We studied the effect of atropine on colonic motor activity in man, using both electromyographic recording and a barostat (Staumont et al 1992). Atropine provoked a decrease in colonic tone corresponding to a relative increase in the volume of the balloon in the order of 256% (Fig. 28.23). The effect of atropine was maximal after about 3 min and remained stable for at least 120 min. EMG recording showed a marked decrease in SSB activity (-61%) during the first 30 min following injection. In contrast, LSB activity, which corresponds to phasic contractions, was not affected after atropine injection (Fig. 28.24). Steadman et al (1992) reported that atropine not only inhibited colonic tone in fasted subjects but also impaired the postprandial increase.

Rectal tone also increases after a meal and may be modulated by pharmacological agents (Bell et al 1991); neostigmine increases rectal tone and induces phasic contractions whereas glucagon abolishes these contractions and decreases tone (Fig. 28.25).

THE PHYSIOLOGICAL CONTROL OF COLONIC MOTILITY

Cholinergic innervation of the colon is provided by both the vagus (ascending colon and transverse to left parts) and the sacral cholinergic supply (rectum to left colon and maybe some digitations to the transverse part). Afferent pathways include parasympathetic nerves but they mainly run with pelvic nerves and pass via the dorsal roots of the spinal cord (Gonella et al 1987). Both parasympathetic and sympathetic nerves terminate in the myenteric plexus, which is responsible for the intrinsic control of colonic motility (Fig. 28.26), through muscarinic cholinergic transmission and non-adrenergic non-cholinergic (NANC) transmission utilizing vasoactive intestinal peptick (VIP) or ATP or both as neurotransmitters (Daniel 1985).

Numerous biologically active peptides are present in the colon (Table 28.2). VIP is known to cause prolonged relaxation of gut musculature (Grider & Makhlouf 1988) and immunohistological studies have shown that VIP is present in nerve terminals close to muscle cells, indicating a direct myogenic effect of VIP (Ekblad et al 1988). VIP is also involved in the defaecation reflex (Fahrenkrug et al 1978). Substance P may be a neurotransmitter in the colon (Ekblad et al 1988) and stimulates colonic motility in many species (Hou et al 1989). There are no immunohistochemical data on the distribution of intrinsic nerves containing CCK in the colon. To regulate colonic motility, CCK and gastrin may act either at a local level by interacting directly with smooth muscle cells (Botella et al 1992), or at the level of the CNS (Liberge et al 1991). As circulating hormones, CCK and gastrin may be involved in the colonic response to eating. In man, some correlation has been obtained between gastrinaemia and increase in colonic motor activity after a meal (Snape et al 1978). Neurotensin may also stimulate colonic motility after a meal. Neurotensin promotes defaecation (Calam et al 1983) and stimulates colonic motility in healthy subjects (Thor & Rosell 1986). However, plasma levels of neurotensin in these studies were much higher than the physiological levels observed after a meal. Many other regulatory peptides, including enkephalins and motilin, have been thought to influence postprandial colonic motor activity. The early phase of the colonic response to food is under the control of cholinergic pathways and corresponds to the gastrocolonic reflex (Sullivan et al 1978); a delayed response may be under hormonal control (Snape et al 1979).

Recently, there has been increased interest in the effects of motilin on the motor activity of the gut.

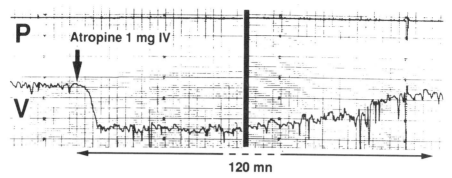

Fig. 28.23 Recording of the intra-bag pressure (**P**) and volume (**V**) as recorded in man before and after intravenous infusion of atropine. Constant pressure is maintained by the barostat. Variations in bag volume reflect variations in colonic tone, the larger the volume, the lower the tone. Volume scale increases from the top to the bottom of the picture. Atropine induces a relaxation of the colon marked by an increase in bag volume.

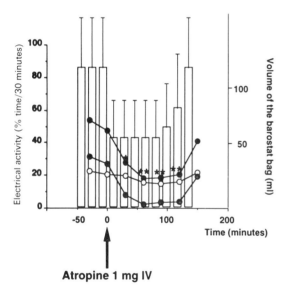

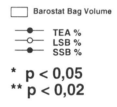

Fig. 28.24 Correlation between decrease in colonic tone measured by the barostat (open bars) and SSB activity. Electrical activity is expressed as percentage duration during 20-min epochs: TEA = total electrical activity; LSB = long spike burst; and SSB = short spike burst.

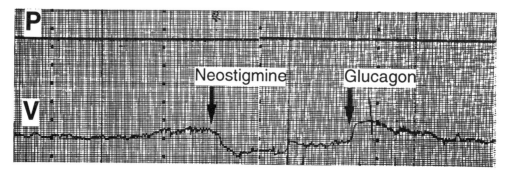

Fig. 28.25 Effect of neostigmine and glucagon on the tone of the left colon measured by barostat volume (**V**). Neostigmine increases tone, while glucagon reverses the effects of neostigmine and induces relaxation.

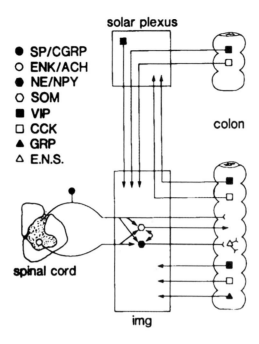

● SP/CGRP
○ ENK/ACH
● NE/NPY
○ SOM
■ VIP
□ CCK
▲ GRP
△ E.N.S.

solar plexus

colon

spinal cord

img

Fig. 28.26 Origin and distribution of neuropeptides involved in control of colonic motility. Peptides may be contained in the nerves arising from the solar (coeliac) plexus, the inferior mesenteric ganglion (img) or the spinal cord as well as in the nerve terminals of the myenteric plexus.
SP = substance P; CGRP = calcitonin gene related peptide; ENK = enkephalins; ACH = acetylcholine; NE = neurotensin; NPY = neuropeptide Y; SOM = somatostatin; VIP = vasoactive intestinal peptide; CCK = cholecystokinin; GRP = gastrin releasing peptide; E.N.S. = enteric nervous system. (Adapted from Gonella et al 1987.)

Table 28.2 Peptides involved in the regulation of colonic motility

	General effect	Regulation of CRE
CGRP	Excitatory	Not involved
CCK and related peptides	Excitatory	Probably
Enkephalins and opioids	Increase non-propulsive contractions	Possibly
Galanin	Excitatory in vitro	?
Motilin	Excitatory (controversial)	Possibly
Neuropeptide Y	Mainly inhibitory	?
Neurotensin	Excitatory	Probably involved especially after fat ingestion
Somatostatin	Excitatory and inhibitory in vitro	Not involved
Substance P	Excitatory	Possibly
VIP	Inhibitory	Not involved

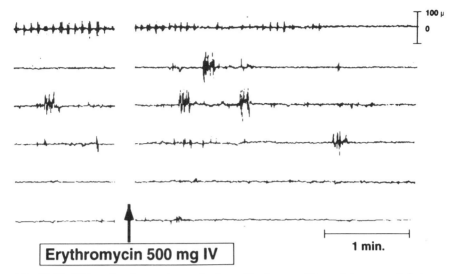

Fig. 28.27   Effect of erythromycin on colonic motility in man. After an intravenous infusion of erythromycin, LSB and SSB activity is not altered in the right colon (traces 1–3) nor in the left colon (traces 4–6).

Whereas its effects on gastric and intestinal motility are clear those on colonic motility remain controversial. Some authors report mild stimulation of left colon activity by motilin and erythromycin (Bradette et al 1991) while others did not observe any change in colonic motor activity after a perfusion of erythromycin (Delvaux et al 1991) (Fig. 28.27). No role for motilin in the colonic response to eating has been demonstrated.

Although the hormonal control of colonic motility is an exciting field of investigation, the bulk of experimental evidence emphasizes the dominant role of cholinergic and NANC neural pathways, and these are possible targets for new drugs designed to alter colonic motility.

REFERENCES

Aspiroz F, Malagelada J R 1985 Physiological variations in canine gastric tone measured by an electronic barostat. Am J Physiol 248: G229–G237

Bassoti G, Gaburri M 1988 Manometric investigation of high amplitude propagated contractile activity of the human colon. Am J Physiol 255: G660–G664

Battle W A, Cohen S, Snape W J 1980 Inhibition of postprandial colonic motility after ingestion of an amino acid mixture. Dig Dis Sci 25: 647–652

Bell A M, Pemberton J H, Hanson R B, Zinsmeister A R 1991 Variations in muscle tone of the human rectum: recordings with an electromechanical barostat. Am J Physiol 260: G17–G25

Bingham S A, Cummings J H 1989 Effect of exercise and physical fitness on large intestinal function. Gastroenterology 97: 1389–1399

Botella A, Delvaux M, Frexinos J et al 1992 CCK and gastrin induce contraction of pig ileum by interacting with different receptor subtypes. Gastroenterology 102: 779–786

Bradette M, Riberdy M, Raymond M C et al 1991 Effect of motilin on the contractile activity of the human colon. J Gastrointest Motility 3: 174 (abstract)

Bueno L, Fioramonti J, Frexinos J, Ruckebusch Y 1980a Colonic myoelectrical activity in diarrhoea and constipation. Hepatogastroenterology 27: 381–389

Bueno L, Fioramonti J, Ruckebusch Y et al 1980b Evaluation of colonic myoelectrical activity in health and functional disorders. Gut 27: 381–389

Burns T W 1980 Colonic motility in the irritable bowel syndrome. Arch Intern Med 140: 247–251

Calam J, Unwin R, Stanley-Pert W 1983 Neurotensin stimulates defecation. Lancet 1: 737–738

Chaussade S, Roche H, Khyari A et al 1986 Mesure du temps de transit colique: description et validation d'une nouvelle technique. Gastroenterol Clin Biol 10: 385–389

Chowdhury A B, Dinoso V P, Lorber S H 1976 Characterization of an hyperactive segment at the rectosigmoid junction. Gastroenterology 71: 584–588

Christensen J 1984 Colonic motor activity. Ital J Gastroenterol 16: 126–133

Connell A M 1962 Motility of the pelvic colon. Part II: Paradoxical motility in diarrhoea and constipation. Gut 3: 342–348

Connell A M, McKelvey S T D 1970 Influence of vagotomy on the colon. Proc Roy Soc Med 63: 7–9

Connell A M, Gaafer M, Hassanein M A, Khayal M A, 1964

Motility of the pelvic colon. Part III. Motility response in patients with symptoms following amoebic dysentery. Gut 5: 443–447

Cordain L, Latin R W, Behnke J J 1986 The effects of an aerobic running program on bowel transit time. J Sports Med 26: 101–104

Couturier D, Couturier-Turpin M H, Debray C 1969 Electromyography of the colon in situ. An experimental study in man and in the rabbit. Gastroenterology 56: 317–322

Daniel E E 1985 Non-adrenergic non-cholinergic neuronal inhibitory interactions with smooth muscle in: Grover A K, Daniel E E (eds) Calcium and contractility, Humana Press pp 385–426

Dapoigny M, Sarna S K 1991 Effects of exercise on colonic motor activity. Am J Physiol 260: G646–G652

Dapoigny M, Trolese J F, Bommelaer G, Tournut R 1988 Réponse colique au repas du colon droit, du colon gauche, du rectosigmoïde et de la charnière recto-sigmoïdienne au cours des troubles fonctionnels intestinaux. Gastroentérol Clin Biol 12: 361–367

Delvaux M, Fioramonti J, Staumont G et al 1991 Lack of effect of erythromycin on colonic muscle in man. J Gastrointest Motil 3: 179 (abstract)

DeYoung V R, Rice H A, Steinhaus A H 1932 Studies in the physiology of exercise. VII The modification of the colonic motility induced by exercise and some indications for a nervous mechanism. Am J Physiol 99: 52–63

Dinoso V P, Murthy S N S, Goldstein J, Rosner B 1983 Basal motor activty of the distal colon: a reappraisal. Gastroenterology 85: 637–642

Ekblad E, Ekman R, Hakanson R, Sundler F 1988 Projections of peptide-containing neurons in rat colon. Neuroscience 27: 655–674

Fahrenkrug J, Galbo H, Holst J J et al 1978 Influence of the autonomic nervous system on the release of vasoactive intestinal peptide porcine gastrointestinal tract. J Physiol 280: 405

Fioramonti J, Garcia-Villar R, Bueno L, Ruckebusch Y 1985 Colonic myoelectrical activity and propulsion in the dog. Dig Dis Sci 25: 641–646

Frexinos J, Bueno L, Fioramonti J 1985 Diurnal changes in myoelectrical spiking activity of human colon. Gastroenterology 88: 1104–1110

Frexinos J, Fioramonti J, Bueno L 1987 Colonic myoelectrical activity in IBS painless diarrhoea. Gut 28: 1613–1618

Frexinos J, Staumont G, Fioramonti J, Bueno L 1989 Effects of sennosides on colonic myoelectrical activity in man. Dig Dis Sci 34: 214–219

Glick M E, Meshkinpour H, Haldeman S et al 1984 Colonic dysfunction in patients with thoracic spinal cord injury. Gastroenterology 86: 287–294

Gonella J, Bouvier M, Blanquet F 1987 Extrinsic nervous control of motility of small and large intestines and related sphincters. Physiol Rev 67: 902–1053

Grider J, Makhlouf G 1988 Vasoactive intestinal polypeptide transmitter of inhibitory motor neurons of the gut. Am NY Acad Sci 527: 369–377

Hamilton S R 1984 Structure of the colon. Scand J Gastroenterol 19 (suppl 93): 13–23

Hinton J M, Lennard-Jones J E, Young A C 1969 A new method for studying gut transit times using radiopaque markers. Gut 10: 842–847

Holdstock D J, Misiewicz J J 1970 Factors controlling colonic motility, colonic pressures and transit after meals in patients with total gastrectomy, pernicious anemia or duodenal ulcer. Gut 11: 100–110

Holdstock D J, Misiewicz J J, Smith T, Rowlands E N 1970 Propulsions (mass movements) in the human colon and its relationship to meal and somatic activity. Gut 11: 91–99

Hou J, Otterson M F, Sarna S K 1989 Local effect of substance P on colonic motor activity in different experimental states. Am J Physiol 256: G997–G1004

Huizinga J D, Stern H S, Chow E, Diamant N E, El-Sharkawy T Y 1985 Electrophysiologic control of motility in the human colon. Gastroenterology 88: 500–511

Jian R, Najean Y, Bernier J J 1984 Measurement of intestinal progression of a meal and its residues in normal subjects and patients with functional diarrhoea by a dual isotope technique. Gut 25: 728–731

Kerlin P, Zinsmeister A, Phillips S 1983 Motor response to food of the ileum, proximal colon, and distal colon of healthy humans. Gastroenterology 84: 762–770

Krevsky B, Malmud L S, D'Ercole F et al 1986 Colonic transit scintigraphy. A physiologic approach to the quantitative measurements of colonic tranist in humans. Gastroenterology 91: 1102–1112

Levinson S, Bhasker M, Gibson T R et al 1985 Comparison of intraluminal and intravenous mediators of colonic response to eating. Dig Dis Sci 30: 33–39

Liberge M, Arruebo M P, Bueno L 1991 Role of hypothalamic cholecystokinin 8 in the colonic response to a meal in rats. Gastroenterology 100: 1001–1009

Misiewicz J J 1984 Human colonic motility. Scand J Gastroenterol 19 (suppl 93): 43–57

Moreno-Osset E, Bazzocchi G, Lo S et al 1989 Association between postprandial changes in colonic intraluminal pressure and transit. Gastroenterology 96: 1265–1273

Narducci F, Bassoti G, Gaburri M, Morelli A 1987 Twenty four hours manometric recording of colonic motor activity in healthy man. Gut 28: 17–25

Picon L, Lemann M, Flourié B et al 1992 Right and left colonic transit after eating assessed by a dual isotopic technique in healthy humans. Gastroenterology 103: 80–85

Ritchie J A, Ardran G M, Truelove S C 1962 Motor activity of the sigmoid colon of human. A combined study by intraluminal pressure recording and cineradiography. Gastroenterology 43: 642–668

Sarna S K 1991 Physiology and pathophysiology of colonic motility. Dig Dis Sci 36: 998–1018

Sarna S K, Latimer P, Campbell D, Waterfall W E 1982 Effect of stress, meal and neostigmine on restosigmoid electrical control activity (ECA) in normal and in irritable bowel syndrome patients. Dig Dis Sci 27: 582–591

Sarna S K, Waterfall W R, Bardakjian B L, Lind J F 1981 Types of human colonic electrical activities recorded post-operatively. Gastroenterology 81: 61–70

Schang J C, Devroede G 1983 Fasting and postprandial myoelectric spiking activity in the human sigmoid. Gastroenterology 85: 1048–1053

Snape W J 1977 Evidence that abnormal myoelectric activity produces colonic motor dysfunction in the irritable bowel syndrome. Gastroenterology 72: 382

Snape W J, Carlson G M, Cohen S 1976 Colonic myoelectric activity in the irritable bowel syndrome. Gastroenterology 70: 326–330

Snape W J, Stephen A, Matarazzo N, Cohen S 1978 Effect

of eating and gastrointestinal hormones on human myoelectrical and motor activity. Gastroenterology 75: 373–378

Snape W J, Wright S H, Battle W M, Cohen S 1979 The gastrocolonic reponse: evidence for a neural mechanism. Gastroenterology 77: 1235–1240

Soffer E E, Scalabrini P, Wingate D L 1988 Prolonged ambulant monitoring of human colonic motility. Am J Physiol 257: G601–G606

Staumont G, Delvaux M, Louvel D et al 1992 Effet de l'atropine sur le tonus et l'activité myoélectrique du côlon chez les patients atteints de troubles fonctionnels intestinaux. Gastroentérol Clin Biol 16: A134 (abstract)

Steadman C J, Phillips S F, Camilleri M et al 1991 Variations of muscle tone in the human colon. Gastroenterology 101: 373–381

Steadman C J, Phillips S F, Camilleri M et al 1992 Control of muscle tone in the human colon. Gut 33: 541–546

Stoddard C J, Duthie H L, Smallwood R H et al 1979 Colonic myoelectric activity in man: comparison of recording techniques and method of analysis. Gut 29: 476–483

Sullivan M A, Cohen S, Snape W J 1978 Colonic myoelectrical activity in irritable bowel syndrome. Effect of eating and anticholinergics. N Engl J Med 298: 878–883

Sun E A, Snape W J, Cohen S, Renny A 1982 The role of opiate receptors and cholinergic neurons in the gastrocolonic response. Gastroenterology 82: 689–693

Sunshine A G, Perry R, Reynolds J C, Cohen S, Ouyang A 1989 Colonic slow waves analysis. Limitations of usefulness of Fast Fourier Transform. Dig Dis Sci 34: 1173–1179

Taylor I, Duthie H L, Smallwood R, Linkens D 1975 Large bowel myoelectrical activity in man. Gut 16: 808–814

Taylor I, Darby C, Hammond P et al 1978 Is there a myoelectrical abnormality in the irritable colon syndrome. Gut 19: 391–395

Thor K, Rosell S 1986 Neurotensine increases colonic motility. Gastroenterology 90: 27–31

Tomling J, Brown S R, Cann P A, Read N W 1991 Is rectosigmoid response to food modulated by proximal colon stimulation? Dig Dis Sci 36: 1481–1485

Waller S L, Misiewicz J J, Kiley N 1972 Effect of eating on motility of the pelvic colon in constipation and diarrhoea. Gut 13: 805–811

Wegman E A, Gandevia S C, Anis A M 1990 Concordance between colonic myoelectrical signals recorded with intramuscular electrodes in the human rectosigmoid in vivo. Gut 31: 1289–1293

Wiggins H S, Cummings J H 1976 Evidence for the mixing of residue in the human gut. Gut 17: 1007–1011

Wiley J, Tatum D, Keinath R et al 1988 Participation of gastric mechanoreceptors and intestinal chemoreceptors in the gastrocolonic response. Gastroenterology 94: 1144–1149

Wright S H, Snape W J, Battle W et al 1988 Effect of dietary components on gastrocolonic response. Am J Physiol 238: G228–G232

Wyman J B, Heaton K W, Manning A P et al 1978 Variability of colonic function in healthy subjects. Gut 19: 146–150

29. The anorectum

R. Farouk   D. C. C. Bartolo

ANATOMICAL CONSIDERATIONS

The rectum

The rectum usually makes three curves in its course, two lesser curves to the right superiorly and inferiorly, and a prominent loop to the left, extending as far as the tip of the coccyx. Inferiorly it widens and forms the rectal ampulla. On distension the rectum normally presents the three valves of Houston, two on the left and one on the right side. The middle valve, to the right, is the most constant and is situated at the level of the anterior peritoneal fold.

The anal canal

The 3–4 cm long anal canal is the terminal part of the alimentary tract (Fig. 29.1). It descends as the continuation of the rectum but turns posteriorly through the pelvic floor and opens externally at the anus. It commences at the ampullary part of the rectum at the level of the anorectal angle, and corresponds physiologically with the zone of intraluminal high pressure described by Bennett and Duthie in 1964.

Anteriorly the perineal body separates it: in the

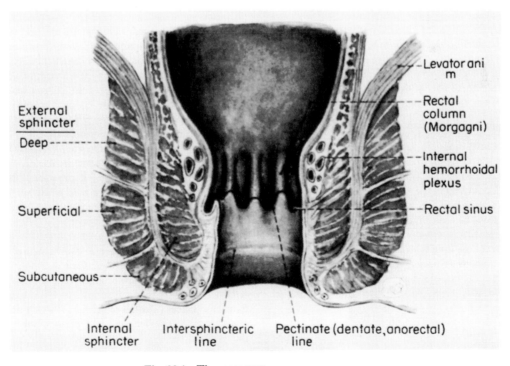

Fig. 29.1 The anorectum.

female, from the lower end of the vagina; and in the male, from the bulb of the penis and the prostate gland. The anal canal is surrounded by the internal and external anal sphincter muscles.

A transitional area of epithelium separates the columnar epithelium of the upper anal canal (UAC), from the squamous epithelium of the lower anal canal (LAC). This, the transitional zone, extends 1–9 mm in length with a mixed picture of stratified squamous and stratified columnar epithelium. There are in addition patches of rectal-type epithelium and other areas with urogenital type transitional epithelium (Walls 1959).

The internal anal sphincter (IAS)

The IAS, an involuntary muscle, is the continuation of the circular muscle coat of the rectum. It surrounds the upper two-thirds of the anal canal. The thickness of the IAS varies between 0.1–0.5 cm and is 3–4 cm long, extending distally to a well-defined rounded edge 8–12 mm below the pectinate line. There has been macroscopic and histological evidence of the IAS continuing to the anal verge (Eisenhammer 1953).

The external anal sphincter (EAS)

The EAS is striated and has traditionally been divided into a subcutaneous, superficial and deep layer (Milligan & Morgan 1934). The superficial components are attached anteriorly to the perineal body and posteriorly to the coccyx. The deep and subcutaneous parts are annular. Descriptions by Kerremans (1969), Duthie (1971) and Shafik (1987) have confirmed the attachments of the caudal part of the muscle.

The conjoined longitudinal muscle

At the anorectal junction this longitudinal muscle layer joins with fibres from the pubococcygeus and then splits to pass on either side of the EAS. The band between the IAS and the EAS presents as an intersphincteric plane and forms an intermuscular septum. Interpretation of the fate of this intersphincteric muscle band differs, but some workers claim that it is responsible for the intersphincteric groove which is palpable in conscious subjects (Milligan & Morgan 1934).

Caudally, the muscle fans out as the 'corrugator cutis ani' passing through the EAS and inserting in the perianal skin.

The pelvic floor

The levator ani is a thin broad muscle which is attached laterally to the back of the body of the pubis, the pelvic surface of the ischial spine and the fascia covering the muscle obturator internus. Medially, its fibres descend to the midline and meet the fibres of the opposite side in a midline raphe. The anterior fibres pass backwards around the prostate or vagina to the fibrous perineal body. The middle fibres pass backwards and downwards around the rectum to the fibrous anococcygeal body. The posterior fibres pass to the coccyx and a midline raphe between it and the anococcygeal body. This muscle is thought to act as a muscular support for the pelvic viscera, particularly when intra-abdominal pressure is raised as in defaecation, micturition and parturition. The sling created by the puborectalis component of this muscle creates the anorectal angle which is acute at rest and becomes more obtuse on defaecation in normal subjects secondary to puborectalis relaxation.

Innervation of the anorectum

Rectum and anal canal

The innervation of the rectum and anal canal has been considered along the traditional lines of sensory and motor components. Much of the understanding concerning sensory innervation was the product of investigations by Duthie and Gairns (1960). In the rectum, only one intra-epithelial receptor has been identified with abundant beaded, non-myelinated nerve fibres in the mucosa. This distribution is found until about 10–15 mm above the anal valves; the epithelium is then found to have a rich sensory nerve supply consisting of Meissner's corpuscles, genital corpuscles, Golgi–Mazzoni bodies, Krause end-bulbs, Pacinian corpuscles and endings which are not readily categorized. The distribution of these nerve endings appear to be most numerous in the region of the anal valves (Duthie & Gairns 1960, Gould 1960). Rectal distension stimulates sensory afferents which travel via the pelvic splanchnic nerves to S2 and S3. Nocioceptive pathways travel in both parasympathetic and sympathetic systems via the inferior and superior hypogastric plexus to L1 and L2.

The anal canal is sensitive to touch, pain, temperature and movement (Duthie & Gairns 1960). This has been suggested as an important mechanism which aids continence by allowing discrimination between fluid, flatus and faeces (Duthie & Bennett 1963). The cutaneous sensation experienced in the perianal region and in the wall of the anal canal below the dentate line is conveyed by afferent fibres via the inferior rectal nerve. The sensory endings in the hairy perianal skin are similar to those in hairy skin elsewhere, comprising both free and organized nerve endings.

Patients who have undergone rectal resection and coloanal anastamosis retain a degree of sensation indicating that sensory receptors may also lie in the pelvic floor fascia or musculature (Lane & Parks 1977).

The motor innervation of the rectum and anal canal is classified according to its intrinsic and extrinsic motor supplies. The intrinsic nerve supply is via the myenteric and submucosal plexus. The ganglia of these two plexuses are interconnected by numerous nerve fibres and form a part of the enteric nervous system (ENS) which extends uninterrupted throughout the gastrointestinal tract (Furness & Costa 1987). Towards the distal end of the rectum the ENS becomes less pronounced and investigations in man have revealed very few, if any, ganglia cells in the IAS (Aldridge & Campbell 1968, Baumgarten et al 1971). The effects of cholinergic or adrenergic agents on the electrical activity of the IAS differ from those observed in non-sphincteric gastrointestinal smooth muscle cells. The cell bodies of the sympathetic preganglionic neurons are in the lumbar spinal cord (L2–L4). Their axons leave the cord by the lumbar ventral roots, run in the lumbar splanchnic nerves and synapse in the inferior mesenteric plexus with postganglionic noradrenergic neurons whose axons reach the rectum and IAS via the hypogastric nerves (Carlstedt et al 1988). The studies by Denny-Brown and Robertson (1935) concluded that the IAS was under both inhibitory and excitatory control although stimulation of the sympathetic nerves at various places along this pathway has been shown to have an excitatory action in both animals and humans (Langley & Anderson 1895, Schuster et al 1963).

The parasympathetic nerve supply of the anorectum has its origin in the sacral segments of the spinal cord (S2–S4). The axons leave the spinal cord by sacral ventral roots, run in the pelvic nerves and synapse with postganglionic intramural receptors.

The IAS is pharmacologically characterized by the presence of alpha-excitatory and beta-inhibitory adrenergic receptors. The effect of acetylcholine (ACh) via muscarinic receptors is unclear although there is evidence that stimulation of the parasympathetic nerves in the pelvic nerves relaxes the IAS in humans (Shepherd & Wright 1968). The presence of a non-adrenergic non-cholinergic (NANC) nervous system with an inhibitory effect on the IAS has been demonstrated by use of electrical field stimulation (Burleigh et al 1979). The putative neurotransmitter has previously been suggested to be ATP, neuropeptide (NPY) and/or nitric oxide (NO).

EAS and pelvic floor

The autonomic (visceral) and somatic nervous systems are often described separately but have to function in an integrated manner. Evidence exists of some interplay between the two systems (Gonella et al 1987). The cell bodies of the EAS somatic nerves and the striated muscles of the pelvic floor lie in the ventral horn of the sacral spinal cord (S1–S3), the so-called Onuf's nucleus (Onuf 1901, Parks et al 1961). The EAS is supplied by the pudendal nerve (Milligan & Morgan 1934, Lawson 1974b, Ayoub 1979, Sato 1980, Gagnard et al 1986). Sato (1980) found that the posterior sphincter received, in addition, a direct branch from the perineal branch of S4.

The levator ani group of muscles are innervated by the third and fourth sacral nerves (S3, S4) and the pudendal nerve (S2) (Percy et al 1981). Occasionally there is a contribution from S5 (Lawson 1974a, Sato 1980). These fibres pass anteriorly over the cranial surface of the muscle to terminate in the posterior urethra.

PHYSIOLOGICAL CONSIDERATIONS

Anal canal pressure

Resting anal pressure undergoes regular fluctuations with an amplitude of 5–25 cm H_2O and a frequency of 10–20 fluctuations per minute (Wankling et al 1968, Kerremans 1969) (Fig 29.2). These fluctuations are termed 'slow waves' and are thought to be generated by the IAS (Kerremans 1969). The frequency of the slow wave is higher in the LAC providing for a mechanism which propels small amounts of anal canal contents cephalad into the rectum (Kerremans 1969). A gender difference does exist, males generally having higher pressures.

A zone of high pressure does exist approximately 2 cm from the anal verge (Bennett & Duthie 1964) which is caudal to the puborectalis sling. Zones of low pressure have also been identified within the anal canal (Taylor et al 1984). The anterior aspect of the upper one-third of the anal canal, which corresponds to the area not closely applied to the puborectalis sling, and the posterior aspect of the lower one-third of the anal canal are areas of relatively low pressures.

The relative contribution of the various sphincters has been identified by pudendal nerve block (Frenckner & von Euler 1975). There is a direct relationship between the electromyographic frequency of the IAS and the resting anal canal pressures (Duthie et al 1990). The IAS contributes up to 85% of resting anal pressure (Frenckner & von Euler 1975). The

cm Water

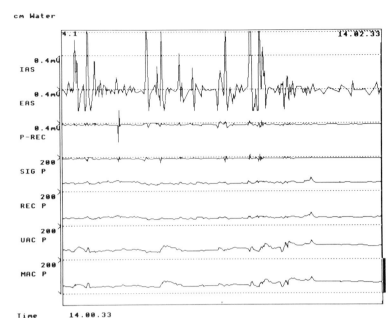

Fig. 29.2 A 2-min recording from a 74-year-old normal control. Note the fluctuation in rectal and anal pressures. IAS = internal anal sphincter EMG; EAS = external anal sphincter EMG; P-REC = puborectalis EMG; Sig P = recto-sigmoid pressure; REC = mid-rectal pressure; UACP = upper anal canal pressure; MACP = mid-anal canal pressure.

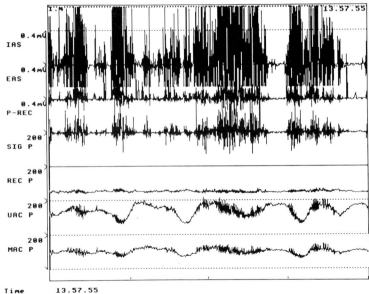

Fig. 29.3 A 4-min recording from a patient with chronic anal fissure. Note the ultra-slow waves in the anal canal. IAS = internal anal sphincter EMG; EAS = external anal sphincter EMG; P-REC = puborectalis EMG; Sig P = recto-sigmoid pressure; REC = mid-rectal pressure; UACP = upper anal canal pressure; MACP = mid-anal canal pressure.

haemorrhoidal plexuses have a minor contribution to resting pressures (Lestar et al 1984). However this increases in patients with haemorrhoids who generally have high resting anal pressures and exhibit ultra-slow anal pressure waves (Hancock & Smith 1975). Patients

with anal fissures (Hancock & Smith 1975) and those with idiopathic chronic constipation (Arhan et al 1983) have also been shown to have such ultra-slow wave activity (Fig. 29.3).

When a subject is asked to voluntarily contract their

anal sphincters, the anal canal pressures rise by between 175–270%. The distribution of the contraction is generally symmetrical, except at about 3 cm anteriorly where it is significantly lower compared to the pressures posteriorly at a similar level (Taylor et al 1984).

The length of the anal canal can be assessed by manometric measurements (Nivatongs et al 1981). The pressure probe is inserted and allowed to rest for 30 s to allow the pressure to fall to a steady level. The probe is then slowly withdrawn and the pressure will rise sharply when the anal canal is entered. This is termed the 'pull-through' technique. The anal canal using this technique is 2.5–4 cm long in normal controls.

Rectal pressure

Basal pressures within the rectum range between 5–25 cm H_2O. The inflation of an intrarectal balloon is associated with an initial rise in pressure, often followed by an increase in pressure secondary to rectal contraction. A degree of accommodation then occurs and the rectal pressure gradually falls to a baseline value. Increasing the distending volume eventually results in failure to further accommodate, and a large increase in rectal pressure results which may be associated with pain (Arhan et al 1976). The contractile response of the rectum to distension is decreased or absent in patients with a spinal cord lesion suggesting a spinal input to this reflex (Denny-Brown & Robertson 1935). Efferent stimulation of the pelvic nerves by the ventral roots of S2, S3 and S4 produces isolated rectal contractions, peristaltic waves and an increased rectal tone (Varma et al 1986). Such motor effects may constitute the final extrinsic pathway of the autonomic 'defaecation reflex'.

Normal values

The range of normal values for anal canal pressures is dependent on the manometric method. In our laboratory the normal range is between 70–110 cm H_2O.

The rectoanal inhibitory reflex

Distension of the rectum with a small volume of air causes transient IAS relaxation. This is accompanied by a transient but significant fall in resting anal pressures (Gowers 1877, Denny-Brown & Robertson 1935). The reduction in anal canal pressure is due to IAS relaxation since it is associated with attenuation of electrical activity in the IAS but not in the EAS (Kerremans 1968, 1969). Increasing the amount of air/water instilled will result in prolonged inhibition of the IAS accompanied by a similar fall in anal pressures (Kerremans 1969, Ihre 1974). This reflex is termed the rectoanal inhibitory reflex (Fig. 29.4).

The rectal receptors responsible for this reflex are located near the mucosa because topical anaesthesia of the rectal mucosa blocks the reflex (Gaston 1948). Rectal distension results in descending inhibition of the muscle fibres mediated possibly by vasoactive intestinal peptide (Burleigh 1983).

Anal motility and basal pressure recover after intermittent as well as during continuous submaximal rectal distension. In contrast, the IAS remains relaxed during continuous supramaximal stimulation. Anal relaxation may be absent however during progressive rectal distension with low infusion rates. This suggests that the IAS can maintain continence when the rectum is slowly filling (Sun et al 1990).

This reflex is absent after circumferential rectal myotomy and in patients with Hirschsprung's disease (Lubowski et al 1987) suggesting that intrinsic myenteric nerve plexuses play a major role in this reflex. In patients with faecal incontinence and rectal prolapse there is heightened sensitivity of the reflex (Orrom et al 1991).

The 'sampling reflex'

Distension of the rectum and the subsequent relaxation of the IAS results in the anal canal becoming funnel shaped to allow rectal contents access to the specialized sensory epithelium (Duthie & Gairns 1960). This allows for 'sampling', a process (Miller et al 1988) which is usually covered by EAS recruitment (Fig. 29.5). Further rectal distension with increasing volumes results in non-recovery of the anal sphincter. The EAS, if intact, will maintain continence for a short period of time before defaecation ensues. If defaecation is not appropriate and the external sphincters have avoided incontinence, the lower rectal contents are returned cephalad by contraction of the pelvic floor muscles. This allows IAS recovery from the rectoanal inhibitory reflex. IAS relaxation will also occur following propulsive activity in the lower sigmoid colon in the presence of an empty rectum (Miller et al 1989). Some of the fall in anal pressures recorded during ambulatory recordings may be related to contractile episodes in the sigmoid colon.

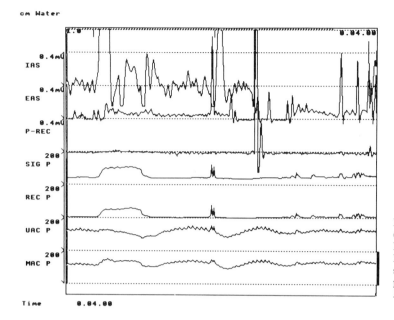

Fig. 29.4 The rectoanal inhibitory reflex (arrow). IAS = internal anal sphincter EMG; EAS = external anal sphincter EMG; P-REC = puborectalis EMG; Sig P = recto-sigmoid pressure; REC = mid-rectal pressure; UACP = upper anal canal pressure; MACP = mid-anal canal pressure.

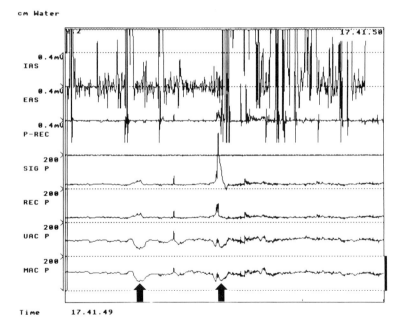

Fig. 29.5 Two episodes of the sampling reflex in a patient with haemorrhoids (↑). IAS = internal anal sphincter EMG; EAS = external anal sphincter EMG; P-REC = puborectalis EMG; Sig P = recto-sigmoid pressure; REC = mid-rectal pressure; UACP = upper anal canal pressure; MACP = mid-anal canal pressure.

The internal anal sphincter

Examination of the IAS reveals electrical slow wave activity which is sinusoidal in nature at a frequency of 15–25 cpm in normal controls (Kerremans 1969, Wankling et al 1968, Monges et al 1980) (Fig. 29.6). Several groups of pacemaker cells are present within the lower sphincteric portion, each group generating a slightly different frequency (Penninckx 1981). This slow-wave activity is not disrupted by general anaesthesia or by pudendal nerve blockade (Frenckner & von Euler 1974). The frequency of the IAS slow wave has a linear relationship with resting anal canal pressures and is reduced in patients with neurogenic faecal incon-

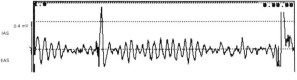

Normal internal sphincter EMG

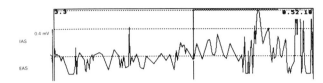

Post-rectopexy internal sphincter EMG

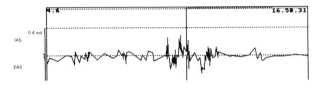

Pre-rectopexy internal sphincter EMG

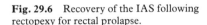

Fig. 29.6 Recovery of the IAS following rectopexy for rectal prolapse.

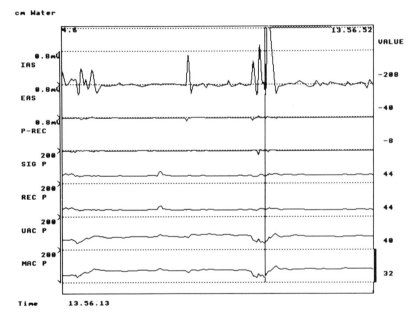

Fig. 29.7 A 1-min recording from a patient with faecal incontinence. Note the low frequency of the IAS EMG and low anal pressures. An abnormal sampling reflex is marked by the cursor. IAS = internal anal sphincter EMG; EAS = external anal sphincter EMG; P-REC = puborectalis EMG; Sig P = recto-sigmoid pressure; REC = mid-rectal pressure; UACP = upper anal canal pressure; MACP = mid-anal canal pressure.

tinence (Duthie et al 1990) and full thickness rectal prolapse (Figs 29.6 and 29.7).

The IAS is continuously active (Kerremans 1969). In vitro examination of isolated strips of sphincter muscle reveal it to be in a continuously tonic state (Burleigh et al 1979). Activity of the IAS slow wave is not constant and recruitment occurs following events that challenge the continence mechanism, e.g. coughing. There is diminished activity during sleep which is accompanied by a fall in resting anal canal pressure. Abolition of IAS electrical activity occurs during rectal distension (Denny-Brown & Robertson 1935). Should the rectal distension be sufficient, this abolition in activity becomes prolonged. The basal tension or tone of isolated strips of IAS preparations is related to the spontaneous rhythmic activity observed.

The external anal sphincter

The EAS is continuously active, even in subjects who are asleep, but the amount of activity is dependent on posture and activity (Floyd & Walls 1953). It is a fatigable muscle however and voluntary contraction to maintain maximal squeeze and therefore continence lasts for less than a minute.

Rectal distension with 50 ml of air results in the recruitment of EAS electromyographic (EMG) activity which precedes IAS inhibition (Gaston 1948). Continued distension of the rectum results in sustained EMG activity of the EAS until 150–200 ml of air has been used to inflate the rectal balloon. This results in complete inhibition of EAS activity. Such activity of the EAS can be inhibited by a pudendal nerve block (Frenckner & von Euler 1974). Patients with spinal transection above the third lumbar segment have normal resting EAS EMG activity with good recruitment while the patient is coughing (Parks et al 1962; Porter 1962).

The puborectalis muscle forms a part of the pelvic floor musculature and exhibits almost identical electrophysiological characteristics with the EAS during coughing and straining. Pudendal nerve blockade does not abolish pelvic floor contraction (Frenckner & von Euler 1974).

Ihre (1974) studied pressure and EMG changes during evacuation of a rectal balloon in 11 patients. EAS and puborectalis activity was inhibited in eight subjects while the remainder exhibited continued sphincter activity during straining. Duthie and Bartolo (1992) have studied 12 patients who displayed inappropriate pelvic muscle contraction exceeding 50% of basal activity of these muscles while straining in the laboratory. Ambulatory monitoring did not exhibit such inappropriate contraction on defaecation in nine of these patients during defaecation (Bartolo & Duthie 1992).

Rectal compliance

Rectal capacity determines the frequency and degree of urgency for defaecation. Appreciation of rectal filling occurs with volumes as small as 10 ml but its capacity often approaches 300 ml before there is an urgent desire to defaecate. Specific for rectal musculature is the property of receptive relaxation. Given a slow filling rate the intraluminal pressure does not increase until the maximum tolerated volume is approached. On rapid distension of the rectum however, a rectal contraction can be demonstrated in the majority of normal subjects before the maximal tolerated volume is achieved. Poor rectal compliance is usually observed in patients with a rectal prolapse, radiation proctitis, colitis and rectal neoplasms.

The continence mechanism

Normal continence is dependent on a complex interaction between local and reflex mechanisms and voluntary intervention. Important factors are sensation of rectal filling and urge to defaecate, and the ability to discriminate between gas, fluid and solid faeces. The ability to retain faeces while passing flatus requires an awareness of rectal contents. Goligher and Hughes (1951) suggested flatus caused less increase in intrarectal pressure and that this was important for discrimination. Rectal filling is thought to depend on the stretch receptors in the pelvic floor muscles (Lane & Parks 1977, Winckler 1958), although Oresland et al (1990) suggest a rectal component. Filling of the rectum results in fullness felt in the pelvis and that sensation persists after coloanal anastomosis (Lane & Parks 1977) or restorative proctocolectomy (Keighley et al 1988). It is however blunted and less reliable pointing to the rectum as an important source of sensory input. It seems likely that both the rectum and pelvic floor are involved in the sensory process.

Defaecation can occur as part of colonic and rectal peristalsis. This process usually includes anal relaxation. Rectal evacuation is assisted by adopting the squatting position ʰhich is associated with an increase in the anorectal angle. Increasing the volume of a simulated faecal bolus, to the point where the sensation of urge is attained, facilitates this evacuation process.

Theories of cotinence

There are eveal different theories of anorectal continence.

The flutter valve. This theory when first proposed was basedon ʰe ʳinciples of the gastro-oesophaeal continence mechanis fo th prevention of ʲcid reflux (Philips & Edwads ⁹965). A inre in intraabdominal pressure would occlude the lower rectum which itself is at high pressure, thereby preventing any contact of rectal contents with the anal canal. Anal sphincteric activity was largely limited to fine control of continence and against urgent, short-lived increases of rectal pressure. The only high-pressure zone that has been consistently observed in the anorectum however is in the mid-portion of the anal canal (Duthie 1971). Furthermore, there is evidence that the intrarectal pressure during straining is close to 0 cm H_2O (McDonald et al 1992).

The flap-valve theory. Sir A. Parks in 1975 popularized the concept of a flap-valve mechanism of continence which is maintained by an acute resting anorectal angle. According to this, intra-abdominal forces are applied to the anterior rectal wall. Any rise in intra-abdominal pressure, the proximal anus would be plugged by anterior rectal mucosa thereby preventing rectal contents from entering the anal canal. Incontinence resulted from an obtuse anorectal angle and was associated with perineal descent (Parks 1975). The concept of a post-anal repair for faecal incontinence was based on this theory. Some doubt on the validity of this theory has been cast by the findings from videoproctography combined with EMG of the anal sphincter (Bartolo et al 1986). By this method, it has been shown that there is no contact between the anterior rectal wall and the anal canal during the valsalva manoeuvre. In addition, Miller et al (1988, 1989) reported that improvement in continence status following anal sphincter repair for incontinence was not associated with the acuity of the anorectal angle.

Sphincteric mechanism. Bartolo et al (1986) found that continence was maintained in subjects when the rectum was filled with liquid during the valsalva manoeuvre by recruitment of the EAS and puborectalis muscle. Bannister et al (1987) confirmed the sphincteric nature of continence.

The high-pressure zone of the anal canal at rest presents a barrier to rectal contents. This high-pressure zone is largely generated by the IAS (Bennett & Duthie 1964, Frenckner & Ihre 1976, Lestar et al 1989). The anal canal at rest is an antero-posterior slit. It does appear that the IAS alone is not able to maintain complete occlusion of the anal canal. There is some evidence that the anal endocushions assist in the occlusion of the anal canal at rest (Lestar et al 1992). These anal cushions are estimated to generate up to 15% of resting anal pressures (Lestar et al 1989).

CLINICAL MEASUREMENT OF ANORECTAL FUNCTION

The use of various methods of measurement to assess anorectal function has increasingly been used in an attempt to provide objective appraisal of activity together with a method of measuring outcome following treatment. Furthermore, these methods would allow comparison between various conditions and also comparison of outcome between different treatment options. Such methods have contributed to a better understanding of the physiology of continence and the treatment of its disorders, e.g. the anorectal angle and the development of post-anal repair for the treatment of faecal incontinence. It also forms the scientific basis for comparison of results between different units in the evaluation of treatments.

Manometric assessment

Perfused catheters

These are usually multiport systems. Each port is perfused with water at a constant rate which is sufficient to keep the port open, but low enough to prevent errors arising because of anorectal filling. The pressure recorded in each catheter is an index of the resistance to flow of fluid out of the catheter. Leakage may result in sphincter contractions. Large-bore catheters also record falsely-high pressures (Lestar et al 1989). Perfusion systems are dependent on the compliance of the system and the rate of perfusion. These systems are simple and relatively cheap to use. Computerized multiport analysis allows for three-dimensional imaging of the anal canal (Coller 1987). Lack of uniformity concerning materials and methods has reduced the value of interunit comparisons of results.

Microballoon catheters

Similar alterations in anorectal contractility as seen with perfused systems may arise when using balloon systems. Large balloons are to be avoided because of a false increase in pressure. Balloon catheters avoid the potential of artefacts caused by leakage seen in perfused catheters however, and are multidirectional, rather than unidirectional. Air or water may be used with microballoon systems. Miller et al (1989) have shown a good correlation between air- and water-filled systems, and Sun & Read (1989) have shown the systems to be very similar in action.

Sleeve catheters

Fluid is perfused through a sleeve formed by silastic material glued over a silastic base (Dent 1976). In the anal canal, the sleeve spans the sphincter so that a contraction anywhere along its length will cause an increased resistance to the flow of fluid and is measured as an increase in pressure in the catheter. The sleeve catheters are unable to distinguish between the activities of the IAS and EAS.

Microtransducers

These avoid many of the problems due to sleeve catheters by minimizing distension of the anus. They do however suffer from being unidirectional, fragile and expensive. They may be converted to an omnidirectional system by sealing the microtransducers in an air-filled microballoon. This increases the diameter of the probe but causes distension of the anus.

Rectal function

This can be assessed by instilling air or water at a

steady rate (40 ml/min) into a rectal balloon and comparing with the rate of change of rectal pressure. Initially the proctometrogram shows small increases in rectal pressure per unit volume instilled but the rise in pressure becomes progressively steeper as the maximum tolerated volume is approached. Thus, values can be recorded of volumes causing the initial sensation of distension, a desire to defaecate, urgency and the maximum tolerated volume. This provides for the estimation of rectal compliance which is calculated by plotting volume versus pressure and calculating the gradient.

Variability of rectal compliance because of age, sex, and/or the presence of faeces in the rectum has been demonstrated (Sorensen et al 1990).

A more accurate method of measuring rectal tone involves the insertion of a large capacitance plastic bag into the rectum, filling the bag with water and connecting it to an external fluid reservoir. Rectal pressures are kept constant in this system while rectal volume is varied (Akervall et al 1988).

The continence mechanism can also be assessed by infusing saline at 37°C intrarectally in the presence of an anorectal manometer and recording the volume at which a subject becomes incontinent. Normal subjects could be expected to retain volumes of up to 1500 ml of saline (Haynes & Read 1982).

The rectoanal inhibitory reflex

As the rectum is filled the IAS relaxes. This 'rectoanal inhibitory reflex' (Gowers 1887), or 'rectosphincteric reflex' is altered in disease. It can be detected using any of the previously mentioned manometry systems.

Electromyography

Methodology

Individual muscle fibres, derived from a motor unit, summate to form the motor unit action potential which can be recorded at a distance greater than that required to record individual muscle fiber activity (small action potentials of brief duration). A motor unit consists of the anterior horn cell, its axon and terminal branches, and the muscle fibres it supplies. The number of muscle fibres innervated by each anterior horn cell varies between 10–200, dependent on whether the muscle is used for fine or coarse control of function. Each motor unit potential will have the characteristics of amplitude, duration and shape of electrical response. Analysis of duration and shape are of physiological value (Bartolo 1984).

Concentric needle EMG. Concentric needle electrodes are commonly used and consist of bare-tipped steel wire of 0.1 mm diameter with an insulating resin. The area of uptake of the electrode is small and any electrical activity recorded is that into which the electrode is inserted. Individual muscle fixer action potentials cannot however be identified reliably using concentric needle electrodes.

Single firer EMG. The single fixer EMG electrode which has an uptake radius of 270 μ can record the activity of individual muscle fibres within a motor unit. The electrode consists of a needle slightly narrower than 0.1 mm filled with resin. A central wire opens at the mid-shaft of the electrode through a 25 μm leading-off surface. The cannula of the electrode represents the reference electrode and a separate ground electrode is also required. An amplifier with a 500 Hz low-frequency filter setting and a trigger delay line are required with the amplifier set at 2–5 ms per division. The mean duration of motor unit potentials consisting of more than one component recorded by this method is less than 8 ms. The following method is used: right and left lateral stabs are made without anaesthetic and 20 different recordings are taken from each muscle. The fixer density is assessed by counting the number of peaks recorded per stab. The 20 recordings are totalled and then averaged. The potentials are recorded on a Medelec Mystro.

Following injury to the motor unit, re-innervation will result in an increase in fixer density as there will be more fibres innervated by a single axon within the uptake area. In normal subjects the fixer density of most muscles is less than two though this increases slightly with age (Neill & Swash 1984).

Pudendal nerve assessment

Technique. Pudendal nerve stimulation transanally provides for a method of assessing pelvic floor neuropathy. A glove-mounted electrode (St Mark's Pudendal Electrode 13L40, Dantec Electronics, Bristol, UK) is connected to a pulsed stimulus generator (Medelec Mystro) and the pudendal nerve is stimulated transanally as it passes over the ischial spines. The latent period between pudendal nerve stimulation and electromechanical response of the muscle is measured using an oscilloscope (Medelec Mystro).

Interpretation. Prolonged pudendal nerve terminal motor latency is seen in the majority of patients with idiopathic faecal incontinence (Swash & Snooks 1992), patients with a rectal prolapse (Parks et al 1977, Swash & Snooks 1992), double anorectal and urinary incontinence (Snooks et al 1984), and in certain neurological disorders (Snooks et al 1984). Damage to the pudendal nerves is thought to occur in 60% of women who have sustained injury to the EAS. Furthermore, 20% of women undergoing vaginal delivery with no apparent injury to the EAS have prolonged pudendal nerve terminal motor latencies with recovery occurring in 15% (Snooks et al 1985). Normal subjects record latencies of 1.9–2.3 ms (Swash & Snooks 1992).

Anal sensitivity

A Gauge 14 Nelaton catheter is used for this purpose by attaching two copper electrodes spaced 1 cm apart at the tip. Copper wires are connected to the electrodes and a constant current generator (Department of Medical Physics, Bristol Royal Infirmary, Bristol, UK) is used to apply a stimulus at 5 pulses per second in increasing strength between 1–25 mA. The threshold sensation, which is usually a throbbing or burning type feeling, is measured at the lower, mid-, and upper anal canal (Roe et al 1987).

Radiological methods

The use of radiological methods in the investigation of defaecatory disorders can largely be divided into two categories, namely techniques to exclude pathologies which may present with altered bowel habit such as a carcinoma, and secondly, methods which are primarily used to determine the presence of benign pathologies are primarily a motility disorder. Examples of the former investigation would be a barium enema whereas examples of the latter include colonic transit studies, videoproctography, and endoanal ultrasound.

Cinedefaecography

An attempt to investigate defaecation and its disorders in a physiological manner was described by Burhenne in 1964. Proctography was then modified by Mahieu (1984) in order to obtain a more dynamic recording of defaecation.

A 50 ml semi-solid barium sulphate and potato starch mixture may be instilled directly into the rectum. Use of a semi-solid mixture allows for simulation of stool. Furthermore, a liquid mixture would be evacuated in 2 s whereas a semi-solid mixture is evacuated by the rectum over 10–15 s allowing better radiological visualization. Fluoroscopic techniques are generally used with cineradiographic or video recording to reduce radiation dosage in defaecography. The technique is coupled with synchronous anorectal manometry and striated muscle electromyography to allow

integrated assessment. A dilute solution of barium sulphate is infused into the rectum until the subject reports a desire to defaecate. The anorectum is visualized using a 100 mm camera (Sircam 106, Siemens), and 0.6 mm focus from an X-ray source generating 125 kV at 1000 mA. The image in addition to being displayed on the image intensifier is stored for further study on a Sony Umatic videotape recorder.

Interpretation

The anorectal angle is often assessed by proponents of the 'flap valve theory' (Parks 1975) and for the assessment of patients' other defaecation-related problems such as the perineal descent syndrome, suspected rectal prolapse, rectoceles and the solitary ulcer syndrome. The interpretation of results is notoriously plagued by a large overlap of results with apparently normal symptomless subjects (Shorvon et al 1989). It is therefore a possibility that these findings may represent an epiphenomenon in patients with defaecation problems.

There is also a lack of uniformity on defining the anorectal angle. Some authors have used the angle at the posterior rectal border. Others measure the anorectal angle between the axis of the anal canal and the central axis of the rectum. The variation in technique requires normal values to be generated individually.

Normal values. Using the central anorectal angle, the average angle at rest is around 80° with hip flexion increasing this angle to over 90°. During defaecation this angle opens to about 115°. Squeezing the anus and the Valsalva manoeuvre decrease the anorectal angle to between 85–100°, with the angle being more acute in the former action. Changing position from lateral decubitus to sitting straightens the resting angle, with no change from sitting to standing.

The position of the anorectal junction is another parameter which may be assessed by defaecography or scintigraphy in the measurement of perineal descent. Similar problems as for the anorectal angle exist for the assessment of the perineal plane because of varying interpretations of which anatomical landmarks should be used. The anorectal angle at rest lies closest to a line joining the tip of the coccyx to the most anterior part of the symphysis pubis and this is the line of the perineal plane used in this unit. Radiological assessment of descent is superior to use of a perineometer (Oettle et al 1986). Perineal descent of between 1–3 cm occurs on straining in all cases. Descent in excess of this range is defined as a clinical entity, i.e. 'the descending perineal syndrome'.

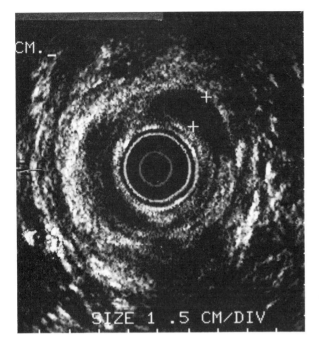

Fig. 29.8 Division of the IAS following fistula surgery demonstrated by endosonography.

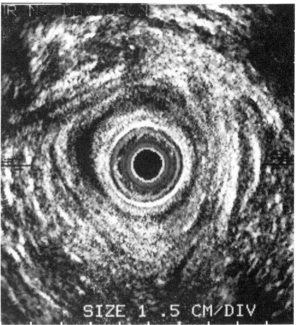

Fig. 29.9 Injury to the IAS following anal stretch. Note that the IAS has wasted away.

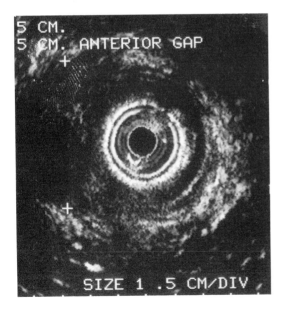

Fig. 29.10 An anterior sphincter defect resulting from obstetric injury.

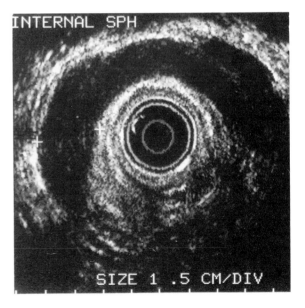

Fig. 29.11 Complete division of the IAS resulting in incontinence following sphincterotomy for fissure.

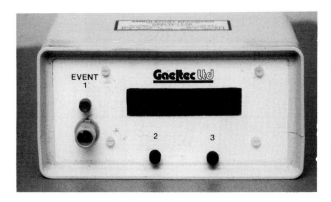

Fig. 29.12 The 7-MPR recorder.

Endoanal ultrasound

Bruel & Kjaer (Naerum, Denmark) have developed a rotating 7 MHz transducer which is covered by a screw-on plastic cone and acoustically coupled by instilling degassed water. The external diameter of the cone is 1.7 cm. To perform this examination, the patient is asked to lie in the left lateral position, and the lubricated cone is inserted into the anal canal, protected by a condom. No bowel preparation is necessary. Using this technique, the integrity of the IAS, EAS, perineal body and to a lesser extent puborectalis may be assessed (Bartram & Mahieu 1992) (Figs 28.8, 28.9, 28.10, 28.11). As the probe is withdrawn from the anal canal, serial images may be recorded (Law & Bartram 1989).

In addition, endoanal ultrasonography has been used

to assess fistula-in-ano. Good correlation between the preoperative and endosonography findings and those at surgery has been reported in a previous study of 22 patients (Law et al 1989).

Ambulatory monitoring

In order to assess the patient in the more physiological environment of their own homes, digital and analogue systems have been developed which are capable of EMG and manometric recordings over 24 hours of anorectal motility. The following method described is that which is used in our own laboratory.

Method of ambulatory assessment

Equipment. The ambulatory recorder used was the 7MPR recorder (Fig. 29.12) manufactured by Gaeltec Ltd, Isle of Skye Scotland. This recorder has a memory capacity of 512 kbytes and has the potential of displaying seven separate channels at any one time (Fig. 29.6). Three channels were used for the recording of EMG activity and the remaining channels were used for manometry (Fig. 29.13). The recorder samples the information from each channel at a minimum rate of 8 times per second.

In essence, the recording program has the facility to scan the 7-channel recording on a second-to-second basis. If the recording value per channel remained constant in 1 s only the first and last points of the recording were stored and a presumption is made of a straight-line recording between these points. Should

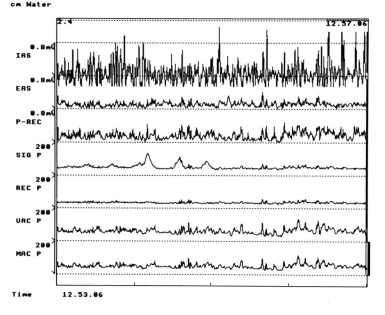

Fig. 29.13 A 4-min recording from a 34-year old male control at rest in the laboratory. IAS = internal anal sphincter EMG; EAS = external anal sphincter EMG; Sig P = recto-sigmoid pressure; REC = mid-rectal pressure; UAC = upper anal canal pressure; MAC = mid-anal canal pressure.

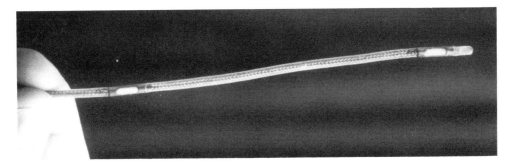

Fig. 29.14   Pressure microtransducers mounted on a probe 3 mm in diameter.

there have been a change of values in that 1 s, the recorder logs the intervening points to reconstruct the record. Pressure channels were accurate to within 2 cmH$_2$O and the EMG channels accurate to within 2 μV.

A single non-integrated channel recorded IAS EMG activity at a frequency response of between 0.1–10 Hz while the two remaining EMG channels (EAS and puborectalis) recorded activity between 10–1.5 kHz. The latter two channels were integrated for this function. In addition, the channels were gated to exclude 50 Hz, the national mains frequency.

In the laboratory, the recorder is connected in serial to a personal computer (BBC or IBM compatible) which uses software programmed by the manufacturers of the ambulatory system. Our own system utilized a desktop Acorn Archimedes computer, version 420, with an addition of 1 Mbyte of RAM; the software used the Forth language modified by Gaeltec. A separate facility allowing the entry of the current time according to a 24-h clock enables the display of the time on the ambulatory recorder. An event button facility enables the subject being studied to mark events on the recording. This allows for accurate records of the time to be made during events such as passage of flatus or defaecation on the recording as well as for entries made in a diary provided.

The manometer (Fig. 29.14) used consists of four solid-state pressure microtransducers mounted on a silicon probe 3 mm in diameter. The microtransducers are at 2 cm, 8 cm, 12 cm and 14 cm from the probe tip which once inserted will respectively record upper rectal, mid-rectal, upper anal and mid-anal canal pressures (Type CTG-4). The probe is connected to the ambulatory recorder which in turn is attached to the personal computer allowing real-time display of the recordings.

To obtain the EMGs, three pairs of sterilized fine Teflon-coated steel wires (0.15 mm diameter) which have been bared, barbed at the tip, and off-set by 1 mm are mounted on a gauge 21 hypodermic needle.

Method. The subject is asked to attempt defaecation prior to assessment. Topical lignocaine is applied to the anal verge and a gauze pad secured over the area. The patient returns 60 min later to commence the study. The subject is asked to lie in the left-lateral position. An intradermal injection of 1% lignocaine is delivered to the anal verge. The gloved index finger of the assessor's left hand is placed in the anal canal to identify the anal sphincters, by identifying the intersphincteric ring and the anorectal angle. Each pair of EMG wires is inserted into the IAS, EAS and puborectalis respectively. These wires are then connected to a preamplifier board which is firmly secured to the patient's skin with tape. A paediatric ECG electrode is used as an earth electrode – this is also attached to the preamplifier board and applied to the patient's skin.

The manometer is lubricated and then inserted into the anorectum without the aid of a proctoscope. The manometer is inserted 8 cm from the anal verge and withdrawn at 30-s intervals. The position at which there is a maximum increase in pressure (by at least 10 cm H$_2$O) is considered to be the zone of high pressure and the length of the anal canal is measured from this point to the anal verge. A similar process is used for the measurement of maximum voluntary contraction and the position of the probe is then readjusted so that the channel which displays the highest resting anal pressure coincides with the pressure microtransducer mounted 12 cm from the catheter tip. Once in position, the position of the catheter at the anal verge is marked to determine any subsequent dislocation, and the catheter itself is taped to the perineum.

The whole process of insertion of the electrodes takes approximately 20 min to perform and, once completed, simple manoeuvres such as the responses to cough and squeeze are assessed. The subject is then asked to attempt defaecation on a commode. This allows additional detection of any tendency for catheter displacement prior to commencement of ambulatory recording.

The subject is then instructed to complete a diary of such events as a desire to open bowels, passage of flatus, micturition and defaecation. Each event is also marked on the recorder's memory by pressing an event marker facility and noting the time on the recorder's clock.

On completion of the recording, the subject returns to the laboratory and the equipment is removed. The recording is down-loaded to the personal computer and can be stored on floppy or hard disk for analysis. An analysis program for the assessment of EMG frequencies and pressure channels is available based on Fouriers analysis to ease reporting. The first hour of recordings are ignored to allow for any potential effect of the lignocaine on sphincter function.

REFERENCES

Akervall S, Fasth S, Nordgren S, Oresland T, Hulten L 1988 Manovolumetry: a new method for investigation of anorectal function. Gut 29: 614–623

Aldridge R T, Campbell P E 1968 Ganglion cell distribution in the normal rectum and anal canal. A basis for the diagnosis of Hirschsprung's disease by anorectal biopsy. Journal of Paediatric Surgery 3: 475–490

Arhan P, Faverdin C, Devroede G 1976a Manometric assessment of continence after surgery for imperforate anus. Journal of Paediatric Surgery 11: 157–166

Arhan P, Faverdin C, Persoz B 1976b Relationship between viscoelastic properties of the rectum and anal pressure in man. Journal of Applied Physiology 41: 677–682

Arhan P, Devroede G, Jehannin B 1983 Idiopathic disorders of fecal incontinence in children. Pediatrics 71: 774–779

Attwood S E A 1990 Manometric diagnosis of anal sphincter injuries. American Journal of Surgery 159: 112–117

Bannister J J, Abozekri, Read N W 1987a Effect of aging on anorectal function. Gut 28: 353–357

Bannister J J, Davison P, Timms J M, Gibbons C, Read N W 1987b Effect of stool size and consistency on defaecation. Gut 28: 1246–1250

Bannister J J, Gibbons C, Read N W 1987c Preservation of faecal continence during rises in intra-abdominal pressure: is there a role for the flap-valve? Gut 28: 1242–1245

Bartolo D C C 1984 A comparative study of the pelvic floor musculature in disorders of defaecation and idiopathic faecal incontinence. MS thesis, Universty of London

Bartolo D C C, Roe A M, Locke-Edmunds J C, Virjee J, Mortensen N J M 1986 Flap-valve theory of anorectal continence. British Journal of Surgery 73: 1012–1014

Bartram C I, Mahieu P H G 1992 Evacuation proctography and endosonography in: Henry M M, Swash M (eds) Coloproctology and the pelvic floor. Butterworth, London pp. 146–172

Baumgarten H G, Holsten A F, Stelzner F 1983 Nervous elements in the human colon of Hirschsprung's disease. Virchows Archiv. A Pathological Anatomy and Histology 358: 113–136

Bennett R C, Duthie H L 1964 The functional importance of the internal anal sphincter. British Journal of Surgery 51: 355–357

Burhenne H J 1964 Intestinal evacuation study: a new roentgenologic technique. Radiology Clinics 33: 79–84

Burleigh D E, D'Mello A 1983 Neural and pharmacologic factors affecting motility of the internal anal sphincter muscle. Gastroenterology 84: 409–417

Burleigh D E, D'Mello A, Parks A G 1979 Responses of isolated human internal anal sphincter to drugs and electrical field stimulation. Gastroenterology 77: 484–490

Carlstedt A, Nordgren S, Fasth S, Appelgren L, Hulten L 1988 Sympathetic nervous influence on the internal anal sphincter and rectum in man. International Journal of Colorectal Disease 3: 90–95

Coller J A 1987 Clinical application of anorectal manometry. Surgical Clinics of North America 16: 17–33

Denny-Brown D, Robertson E G 1935 An investigation of the nervous control of defaecation. Brain 58: 256–310

Dent J A 1976 A new technique for continuous sphincter pressure measurement. Gastroenterology 71: 263–267

Duthie H L 1971 Anal continence. Gut 12: 844–852

Duthie H L, Bennett R C 1963 The relation of sensation in the anal canal to the functional anal sphincter: a possible factor in anal continence. Gut 4: 179–182

Duthie H L, Gairns F W 1960 Sensory nerve endings and sensation in the anal region of man. British Journal of Surgery 47: 585–595

Eisenhammer S 1953 The internal anal sphincter: its surgical importance. South African Medical Journal. 27: 266–270

Floyd W, Walls E 1953 Electromyography of the sphincter ani externus in man. Journal of Physiology 16: 638–644

Frenckner B, Ihre T 1976 Influence of autonomic nerves on the internal anal sphincter in man. Gut 17: 306–312

Frenckner B, von Euler C 1975 Influence of pudendal nerve block on the function of the anal sphincters. Gut 16: 482–489

Gagnard C, Godlewski G, Prat D, Lan O, Cousineau J, Maklouf Y 1986 The nerve supply to the external anal sphincter: the macroscopic supply and microscopic structure. Surgery Radiology & Anatomy 8: 115–119

Gaston E A 1948 The physiology of faecal continence. Surgery, Gynaecology and Obstetrics 87: 280–290

Gaston E 1951. Physiological basis for preservation of faecal continence after resection of the rectum. Journal of the American Medical Association 146: 1486–1489

Goligher J C, Leacock A G, Brossy J J 1955 The surgical anatomy of the anal canal. British Journal of Surgery 43: 51–61

Gould R P 1960 Sensory innervation of the anal canal. Nature 187: 337–338

Gowers W R 1877 The autonomic action of the sphincter ani. Proceedings of the Royal Society of Medicine London 26: 77–84

Hancock B D, Smith K 1975 The internal anal sphincter and Lord's procedure for haemorrhoids. British Journal of Surgery 64: 92–95

Haynes W G, Read N W 1982 Anorectal activity in man during rectal infusion of saline: a dynamic assessment of the anal continence mechanism. Journal of Physiology (London) 330: 45–56

Ihre T 1974 Studies on anal function in continent and incontinent patients. Scandinavian Journal of Gastroenterology 9 (supplement 25): 1–64

Keighley M R B, Yoshoka K, Kmiot W A, Heyen F 1988 Physiological parameters influencing the function in restorative proctocolectomy and ileo-pouch-anal anastomosis. British Journal of Surgery 75: 997–1002

Kerremans R 1969 Morphological and physiological aspects of anal continence and defaecation, Arscia, Brussels

Lane R H S, Parks A G 1977 Function of the anal sphincters following colo-anal anastomosis. British Journal of Surgery 64: 596–599

Law P J, Bartram C I 1989 Anal endosonography: technique and normal anatomy. Gastrointestinal Radiology 14: 349–353

Lestar B, Penninckx F, Kerremans R 1989 The composition of anal basal pressure. An in-vivo and in-vitro study in man. International Journal of Colorectal Disease 4: 118–122

Lestar B, Penninckx F, Kerremans R 1989 Defaecometry, a new method for determining the parameters of rectal evacuation. Diseases of the Colon & Rectum 32: 197–201

Lestar B, Penninckx F, Rigauts H, Kerremans R 1992 The internal anal sphincter cannot close the anal canal completely. International Journal of Colorectal Disease 7: 159–161

Lubowski D Z, Nicholls R J, Swash M, Jordan M J 1987 Neural control of internal sphincter function. British Journal of Surgery 74: 668–670

Mahieu P, Pringot J, Bodart P 1984 Defaecography: 1. Description of a new procedure and results in normal patients. Gastroenterological Radiology 9: 247–251

Mahieu P, Pringot J, Bodart P 1984 Defaecography: 2. Contribution to the diagnosis of defaecation disorders. Gastroenterological Radiology 9: 253–261

Miller R, Bartolo D C C, Roe A M, Mortensen N J 1988 Assessment of microtransducers in anorectal manometry. British Journal of Surgery 75: 40–43

Miller R, Bartolo D C C, Cervero F, Mortensen N J 1988 Anorectal sampling: a comparison of normal and incontinent patients. British Journal of Surgery 75: 44–47

Miller R, Bartolo D C C, James D, Mortensen N J M 1988 Air-filled microballoon manometry for use in anorectal physiology. British Journal of Surgery 76: 72–75

Miller R, Bartolo D C C, Locke-Edmunds J C, Mortensen N J 1988 Prospective study of conservative and operative treatment for faecal incontinence. British Journal of Surgery 75: 101–105

Miller R, Lewis G T, Bartolo D C C, Cervero F, Mortensen N J 1988 Sensory discrimination and dynamic activity in the anorectum: evidence using a new ambulatory technique. British Journal of Surgery 75: 1003–1007

Miller R, Orrom W J, Cornes H, Duthie G S, Bartolo D C C 1989 Anterior sphincter plication and levatorplasty in the treatment of faecal incontinence. British Journal of Surgery 76: 1058–1060

Milligan E T C, Morgan C N 1934 Surgical anatomy of the anal canal. Lancet 2: 1150–1156, 1213–1217

Monges H, Salducci J, Naudi B et al 1980 Electrical activity of internal anal sphincter. A comparative study in man and

cat in: Christensen J M (ed) Gastrointestinal motility, Raven Press, New York pp. 495–502

Nivatongs S, Stern H S, Fryd D S 1981 The length of the anal canal. Diseases of the Colon & Rectum 24: 600–601

Oettle G J, Roe A M, Bartolo D C C, Mortensen N J M 1985 What is the best way of measuring perineal descent? A comparison of radiographic and clinical methods. British Journal of Surgery 72: 999–1001

Onuf B 1901 On the arrangement and function of the cell groups of the sacral region of the spinal cord in man. Archives of Neurology and Psychopathology 3: 387–412

Oresland T, Fasth S, Akervall S, Nordgren S, Hulten L 1990 Manovolumetric and sensory characteristics of the ileoanal pouch compared with the healthy rectum. British Journal of Surgery 77: 803–806

Orrom W J, Miller R, Cornes H, Duthie G S, Mortensen N J M, Bartolo D C C 1991 Comparison of anterior sphincteroplasty and postanal repair in the treatment of idiopathic faecal incontinence. Diseases of the Colon & Rectum 34: 305–310

Parks A G, Porter N H, Melzack J 1962 Experimental study of the reflex mechanism controlling the muscle of the pelvic floor. Diseases of the Colon & Rectum 5: 407–414

Parks A G 1975 Anorectal incontinence. Proceedings of the Royal Society of Medicine 68: 681–690

Parks A G, Swash M, Urich A B 1977 Sphincter denervation in anorectal incontinence and rectal prolapse. Gut 18: 656–665

Penninckx F 1981 Morphological and physiological aspects of anal function. PhD thesis, Katholieke Univeritiet, Leuven

Percy J P, Neill M E, Swash M, Parks A G 1981 Electrophysiological study of the motor supply of the pelvic floor. Lancet i: 16–17

Porter N H 1962 Physiological studies of the pelvic floor in rectal prolapse. Annals of the Royal Society of Medicine 286: 379–404

Sato K 1980 A morphological analysis of the nerve supply of the sphincter ani externus, levator ani and coccygeus. Acta Anatomica Nipponica 55: 187–223

Schuster M M, Hendrix T R, Mendeloff A I 1963 The internal anal sphincter response: manometric studies on its normal physiology, neural pathways and alteration in bowel disorders. Journal of Clinical Investigation 42: 196–207

Shafik A 1987 A concept of the anatomy of the anal sphincter. Mechanism and the physiology of defaecation. Diseases of the Colon and Rectum 30: 970–982

Shorvon P J, McHugh F, Somers S, Stevenson G W 1989 Defaecography in normal volunteers: results and implications. Gut 30: 1737–1749

Snooks S J, Barnes R P H, Swash M 1984 Damage to the voluntary anal and urinary sphincter musculature in childbirth. Journal of Neurology, Neurosurgery and Psychiatry 47: 1269–1273

Snooks S J, Setchell M, Swash M, Henry M M 1985 Injury to the innervation of the pelvic floor musculature in childbirth. Lancet 2: 546–550

Snooks S J, Henry M M, Swash M 1985 Faecal incontinence due to external anal sphincter division in childbirth is associated with damage to the innervation of the pelvic floor musculature: a double pathology. British Journal of Obstetrics and Gynaecology 92: 824–828

Sun W M, Read N W 1989 Anorectal function in normal subjects: effect of age and gender. International Journal of Colorectal Disease 4: 188–196

Sun W M, Read N W, Miner P B, Kerrigan D D, Donnelly T C 1990 The role of transient internal sphincter relaxation in faecal incontinence. International Journal of Colorectal Disease 5: 31–36

Sun W M, Read N W, Prior A et al 1990 Sensory and motor resonses to rectal distension vary according to the rate and pattern of balloon inflation. Gastroenterology 99: 1008–1015

Swash M, Snooks S J 1992 Motor nerve conduction studies of the pelvic floor innervation in: Henry M M, Swash M (eds) Coloproctology and the pelvic floor. Butterworth-Heinnemann, Oxford pp 196–206

Varma J S, Smith A N 1986 Reproducibility of the proctometrogram. Gut 27: 288–292

Walls E W 1959 Recent observations on the anatomy of the anal canal. Proceedings of the Royal Society of Medicine 52 (supplement): 85–87

Wankling W J, Brown B H, Collins C D, Duthie H L 1968 Basal electrical activity in the anal canal in man. Gut 9: 457–460

Winckler G 1958 Remarques sur la morphologie et l'innervation du muscle releveur de l'anus. Archives d'Anatomie, d'Histologie et d'Embryologie 41: 77–95

FURTHER READING

Akervall S, Fasth S, Nordgren S, Oresland T, Hulten L 1989 Rectal reservoir and sensory function studied by graded isobaric distension in normal man. Gut 30: 496–502

Allan A, Ambrose N S, Silverman S, Keighley M R B 1987 Physiological study of pruritis ani. British Journal of Surgery 74: 576–579

Arabi Y, Alexander-Williams J, Keighley M R B 1977 Anal pressures in haemorrhoids and anal fissure. American Journal of Surgery 134: 608–610

Arhan P, Devroede G, Persoz B, Faverdin C, Dornic C, Pellerin D 1979 Response of the anal canal to repeated distension of the rectum. Clinical Investigation in Medicine 2: 83–88

Bannister J J, Timms J M, Banfield C J, Read N W 1986 Physiological studies in young women with chronic constipation. International Journal of Colorectal Disease 1: 175–182

Bannister J J, Read N W, Donnelly T C, Sun W M 1989 External and internal anal sphincter responses to rectal distension in normal subjects and in patients with idiopathic faecal incontinence. British Journal of Surgery 76: 617–621

Bartolo D C C, Read N W, Jarrat J A et al 1983 Difference in anal sphincter function and clinical presentation in patients with pelvic floor descent. Gastroenterology 85: 68–75

Bartolo D C C, Jarrett J A, Read M G, Donnelly T C, Read N W 1983 The role of partial denervation of the puborectalis in idiopathic faecal incontinence. British Journal of Surgery 70: 664–667

Bartolo D C C, Roe A M, Virjee J, Mortensen N J M, Locke-Edmunds J C 1988 An analysis of rectal morphology in obstructed defaecation. International Journal of Colorectal Disease 3: 17–22

Batignani G, Monaci I, Ficari F, Tonelli F 1991 What affects continence after anterior resection of the rectum? Diseases of the Colon & Rectum 34: 329–335

Becker J M 1984 Anal sphincter function after colectomy, mucosal proctectomy, and endorectal ileoanal pull-through. Archives of Surgery 119: 526–531

Bell A M, Pemberton J H, Hanson R B, Zinsmeister A R 1991 Variations in muscle tone of the human rectum: recordings with an electro-mechanical barostat. American Journal of Physiology 260: G17–G25

Biancani P, Walsh J, Behar J 1985 Vasoactive intestinal peptide: a neurotransmitter for relaxation of the rabbit internal anal sphincter. Gastroenterology 89: 867–874

Bielefeldt K, Enck P, Erkenbrecht J F 1990 Sensory and motor function in the maintenance of anal continence. Diseases of the Colon & Rectum 33: 674–678

Blatchford G J, Perry R E, Christiansen M A, Thorson A G 1990 The effect of sphincteroplasty on manometric vector symmetry. Diseases of the Colon & Rectum 33: 22

Bleijenberg G, Kuijpers H C 1987 Treatment of the spastic-pelvic floor syndrome with biofeedback. Diseases of the Colon & Rectum 30: 108–111

Bouvier M, Kirschner G, Gonella J 1986 Action of morphine and enkephalins on the internal anal sphincter of the cat: relevance for the physiological role of opiates. Journal of the Autonomic Nervous System 16: 219–232

Bouvier M, Gonella J 1981 Nervous control of the internal anal sphincter of the cat. Journal of Physiology (London) 310: 457–469

Bouvier M, Grimaud J C, Naudy B, Salducci J 1987 Effects of morphine on electrical activity of the rectum in man. Journal of Physiology (London) 388: 153–161

Bowyer A, McColl I 1970 A study of 200 patients with pruritis ani. Proceedings of the Royal Society of Medicine 63: 96–98

Braun J, Truetner K H, Harder M et al 1991 Anal sphincter function after intersphincteric resection and stapled ileal-pouch anastomosis. Diseases of the Colon & Rectum 34: 8–16

Broden B, Snellman B 1968 Procidentia of the rectum studied with cine radiography: a contribution to the discussion of causative mechanism. Diseases of the Colon & Rectum 11: 330–347

Broden G, Dolk A, Holmstrom B 1988 Recovery of the internal anal sphincter following rectopexy: a possible explanation for continence improvement. International Journal of Colorectal Disease 3: 23–28

Brown A C, Sumfest J M, Rozwadowski J V 1989 Histopathology of the internal anal sphincter in chronic anal fissure. Diseases of the Colon & Rectum 32: 680–683

Browning G G P, Parks A G 1982 Effect of colonic motor activity on the internal anal sphincter. Gut 23: A914

Burleigh D E 1983 Non-cholinergic, non-adrenergic inhibitory neurons in human internal anal sphincter muscle. Journal of Pharmacy and Pharmacology 35: 258–260

Buser W D, Miner P B 1986 Delayed rectal sensation with faecal incontinence. Successful treatment using anorectal manometry. Gastroenterology 91: 1186–1191

Caplan R M 1966 The irritant role of faeces in the genesis of perianal itch. Gastroenterology 50: 19–23

Carlstedt A, Nordgren S, Fasth S, Hulten L 1989 The influence of the pelvic nerves on anorectal motility in the cat. Acta Physiologica Scandinavia 135: 57–64

Caruana B J, Wald A, Hinds J P, Eidelman B H 1991 Anorectal sensory and motor function in neurogenic faecal incontinence. Comparison between multiple sclerosis and diabetes mellitus. Gastroenterology 100: 465–470

Chiou A W H, Lin J K, Wang F M 1989 Anorectal abnormalities in progressive systemic sclerosis. Diseases of the Colon & Rectum 32: 417–421

Chowcat N L, Araujo J G, Boulos P B 1986 Internal sphincterotomy for chronic anal fissure: long-term effects on anal pressure. British Journal of Surgery 73: 915–916

Corazziari E, Cucchiara S, Staiano A et al 1985 Gastrointestinal transit time, frequency of defaecation, and anorectal manometry in healthy and constipated children. Journal of Paediatrics 106: 379–382

Cornes H, Bartolo D C C, Stirrat G M 1991 Changes in anal canal sensation after childbirth. British Journal of Surgery 78: 74–77

Cortesini C, Pucciani F, Carassale G, Paparozzi C 1983 Anorectal physiology after anterior resection and pull-through operation. European Surgical Research 15: 176–183

Courtney H 1950 Anatomy of the pelvis diaphgram and anorectal musculature as related to sphincter preservation in anorectal surgery. American Journal of Surgery 79: 155–173

Deutsch A A, Moshkowitz M, Nudelman I, Dinari G, Reiss R 1987 Anal pressure measurements in the study of haemorrhoid aetiology and their relation to treatment. Diseases of the Colon & Rectum 30: 855–857

Devroede G, Lamarche J 1974 Functional importance of extrinsic parasympathetic innervation to the distal colon and rectum in man. Gastroenterology 66: 273–280

Duthie H L, Watts J 1965 Contribution of the external anal sphincter to the pressure zone in the anal canal. Gut 6: 64–68

Duthie H L 1975 Dynamics of the rectum and anus. Clinical Gastroenterology. 4: 467–477

Duthie G S, Bartolo D C C, Miller R 1991 Laboratory tests grossly overestimate the incidence of anismus. British Journal of Surgery 78 (abstract): 747

Eckhardt V F, Nix W 1991 The anal sphincter in patients with myotonic sphincter dystrophy. Gastroenterology 100: 424–430

Enck P, Kuhlbusch R, Lubke H, Frieling T, Erckenbrecht J F 1989 Age and sex and anorectal manometry in incontinence. Diseases of the Colon & Rectum 32: 1026–1030

Eyres A A, Thompson J P S 1979 Pruritis ani: Is anal sphincter dysfunction important in aetiology? British Medical Journal 2: 1549–1551

Farthing M J G, Lennard-Jones J E 1978 Sensibility of the rectum to distension and the anorectal distension reflex in ulcerative colitis. Gut 19: 64–69

Fasth S, Hulten L, Nordgren S 1980 Evidence for a dual pelvic nerve influence on large bowel motility in the cat. Journal of Physiology 298: 156–169

Felt-Bersma R J F, Klinkenberg-Knol E C, Meuwissen S G M 1990 Anorectal function investigations in incontinent and continent patients. Diseases of the Colon & Rectum 33: 479–486

Ferrara A, Pemberton J H, Levin K E, Hanson R B 1991 A new ambulatory recording system of sigmoid, rectal and anal canal motor activity. Gastroenterology 100: 442–446

Ferrara A, Pemberton J H, Hanson R B 1992 Preservation of continence after ileoanal anastomosis by coordination of ileal pouch and anal canal motor activity. American Journal of Surgery 162: 83–89

Finlay I G, Carter K, McLeod I 1986 A comparison of intra-rectal infusion of gas and mass on anorectal angle and anal canal pressure. British Journal of Surgery 73: 1025 A

Frenckner B 1975 Function of the anal sphincters in spinal man. Gut 16: 638–644

Frenckner B, Molander M L 1979 Influence of general anaesthesia on anorectal manometry in healthy children. Acta Paediatrica Scandinavica 68: 97–101

Friedmann C A 1968 The action of nicotine and catecholamines on the human internal anal sphincter. American Journal of Digestive Diseases 13: 428–431

Frykman H M, Goldberg 1969 The surgical treatment of rectal procidentia. Surgery, Obstetrics & Gynaecology 129: 1225–1230

Garrett J R, Howard E R, Jones W 1974 The internal anal sphincter of the cat: a study of nervous mechanisms affecting tone and reflex activity. Journal of Physiology London 243: 153–166

Gibbons C P, Trowbridge E A, Bannister J J, Read N W 1986 Role of the anal cushions in maintaining anal continence. Lancet i: 886–887

Gibbons C P, Read N W 1986. Anal hypertonia in fissures: cause or effect? British Journal of Surgery 73: 443–445

Gibbons C P, Bannister J J, Trowbridge E, Read N W 1988 An analysis of anal sphincter pressure and anal compliance in normal subjects. International Journal of Colorectal Disease 1: 231–237

Gibbons C P, Trowbridge E, Bannister J J, Read N W 1988 The mechanics of the anal sphincter complex. Journal of Biomechanics 21: 601–604

Gill R C, Kellow J E, Browning C, Wingate D L 1990 The use of intraluminal strain gauges for recording ambulant small bowel motility. American Journal of Physiology 258: G610–615

Goligher J C, Hughes E S R 1951 Sensibility of the colon and rectum. Its role in the mechanism of anal continence. Lancet i: 543–547

Gunterberg B, Kewenter J, Petersen I, Stener B 1976 Anorectal function after major resections of the sacrum with bilateral or unilateral sacrifice of the sacral nerves. British Journal of Surgery 63: 546–554

Hancock B D 1976 Measurement of anal pressure and motility. Gut 17: 645–651

Hancock B D 1977 The internal anal sphincter and anal fissure. British Journal of Surgery 64: 92–95

Harrison M J, Tomlinson P A, Ubhi C S, Wright J, Hardcastle J D 1988 Changes in anal sphincter tone at induction of anaesthesia. Annals of the Royal College of Surgeons of England 70: 61–63

Henry M M, Parks A G, Swash M 1982. The pelvic floor musculature in the descending perineum syndrome. British Journal of Surgery 69: 470–472

Hiltunen K M 1985 Anal manometric findings in patients with anal incontinence. Diseases of the Colon & Rectum 28: 925–928

Holmes A M 1961 Observations of the intrinsic innervation of the rectum and anal canal. Journal of Anatomy 85: 416–422

Holmstrom B, Broden G, Dolk A 1986 Increased anal resting pressure following the Ripstein operation: a contribution to continence? Diseases of the Colon & Rectum 29: 45–47

Horgan P G, O'Connell P R, Shinkwin C A, Kirwan W O 1989 Effect of anterior resection on anal sphincter function. British Journal of Surgery 76: 783–786

Johnson G P, Pemberton J H, Ness J, Samson M, Zinsmeister A R 1990 Transducer manometry and the effect of body position on anal canal pressures. Diseases of the Colon and Rectum 33: 469–475

Johnston D, Holdsworth P J, Naysmyth D G et al 1987 Preservation of the entire anal canal in conservative proctocolectomy for ulcerative colitis: a pilot study comparing end to end ileo-anal anastomosis without mucosal resection with mucosal proctectomy and endoanal anastomosis. British Journal of Surgery 74: 940–944

Kamm M A, Hawley P R, Lennard-Jones J E 1988 Lateral division of the puborectalis muscle in the management of severe constipation. British Journal of Surgery 75: 661–663

Kamm M A, Hawley P R, Lennard-Jones J E 1988 Outcome of colectomy for severe idiopathic constipation. British Journal of Surgery 75: 969–973

Kamm M A, Lennard-Jones, R J Nicholls 1989 Evaluation of the intrinsic innervation of the internal anal sphincter using electrical stimulation. Gut 30: 935–938

Kamm M A, Lennard-Jones J E 1990 Rectal mucosal electrosensory testing: evidence of a rectal sensory neuropathy in idiopathic constipation. Diseases of the Colon and Rectum 33: 419–423

Keighley M R B, Fieldings W L, Alexander-Williams J A 1983 Results of Marlex mesh abdominal rectopexy for rectal prolapse in 100 consecutive patients. British Journal of Surgery 70: 229–232

Keighley M R B, Fielding J W L 1983 Management of faecal incontinence and results of surgical treatment. British Journal of Surgery 70: 463–468

Keighley M R B, Shoulder P J 1984 Abnormalities of colonic function in patients with rectal prolapse and rectal incontinence. British Journal of Surgery 71: 892–895

Keighley M R B, Winslet M C, Yoshioka K, Lightwood R 1987 Discrimination is not impaired by excision of the anal transition zone after restorative proctocolectomy. British Journal of Surgery 74: 1118–1121

Keighley M R B, Henry M M, Bartolo D C C, Mortensen N J M 1988 Anorectal physiology assessment: report of a working party. British Journal of Surgery 76: 356–357

Kerremans R 1968 Electrical activity and motility of the internal anal sphincter. Acta Gastroenterologica Belgica 31: 465–482

Kiff E S, Barnes P R H, Swash M 1984 Evidence of pudendal neuropathy in patients with perineal descent and chronic straining at stool. Gut 1279–1282

Kiff E S, Swash M, Urich A B 1984 Slowed conduction in the pudendal nerves in idiopathic (neurogenic) faecal incontinence. British Journal of Surgery 71: 614–616

Krogh, Pedersen I, Christiansen J 1989. A study of the physiological variation in anal manometry. British Journal of Surgery 76: 69–71

Kuijpers H C, Bleijenberg G 1985 The spastic pelvic floor syndrome. A cause of constipation. Diseases of the Colon and Rectum 669–672

Kuijpers H C, Scheuer M 1990 Disorders of impaired faecal control. A clinical and manometric study. Diseases of the Colon & Rectum 33: 207–211

Kumar D, Waldron D L, Williams N S 1989 Home assessment of anorectal motility and external sphincter EMG in idiopathic faecal incontinence. British Journal of Surgery 76: 635–636

Kumar D, Waldron D, Williams N S et al 1990 Prolonged anorectal manometry and external sphincter electromyography in ambulant human subjects. Digestive Diseases and Sciences 35: 641–648

Kumar D, Thompson P D, Wingate D L 1990 Absence of synchrony between human small intestinal migrating motor complex and rectal motor complex. American Journal of Physiology 258: G171–G172

Lavery I C, Tuckson W B, Easley K A 1989 Internal anal sphincter function after total abdominal colectomy and stapled ileal pouch-anal anastomosis without mucosal proctectomy. Diseases of the Colon & Rectum 32: 950–953

Law P J, Kamm M A, Bartram C I 1991 Anal endosonography in the investigation of faecal incontinence. British Journal of Surgery 78: 312–314

Legino L J, Woods M P, Rayburn W F, McGoogan L S 1988 Third and fourth degree tears: experience at a university hospital. Journal of Reproductive Medicine 33: 423–426

Loening-Baucke V, Anuras S 1985 Effects of age and sex on anorectal manometry. American Journal of Gastroenterology 80: 50–53

Lorentzen M, Thagaard C, Christiansen J 1989 Influence of gastrointestinal neuropeptides on the anal canal. Diseases of the Colon & Rectum 32: 293–295

Lubowski D Z, Nicholls R J, Burleigh D E, Swash M 1988 The internal anal sphincter in neurogenic faecal incontinence. Gastroenterology 95: 997–1002

Lubowski D Z, Nicholls R J 1988 Faecal incontinence associated with reduced pelvic sensation. British Journal of Surgery 75: 1086–1088

Madoff R D, Williams J G, Wong W D et al 1992 Long-term functional results of colon resection and rectopexy for overt rectal prolapse. American Journal of Gastroenterology 87: 101–104

Mann C V, Hoffman C 1988 Complete rectal prolapse: the anatomical and functional results of treatment by extended abdominal rectopexy. British Journal of Surgery 75: 34–37

Marks M M 1968 The influence of intestinal pH on anal pruritis. Southern Medical Journal 61: 1005–1006

Matheson D M, Keighley M R B 1981 Manometric evaluation of rectal prolapse and faecal incontinence. Gut 22: 126–129

McHugh S M, Diamant N E 1987 Effect of age, gender, and parity on anal canal pressures: Contribution of impaired anal sphincter function to faecal incontinence. Digestive Diseases and Sciences 32: 726–736

McNamara M J, Percy J P, Fielding I R 1990 A manometric study of anal fissure treated by subcutaneous lateral internal sphincterotomy. Annals of Surgery 211: 235–238

Mellerup-Sorensen S, Bondesen H, Istre O, Villeman P 1988 Perineal rupture following vaginal delivery. Long-term consequences. Acta Obstetrica Gynecologica Scandinavia 67: 315–318

Mellerup-Sorensen S, Gregersen H, Sorensen S, Djurhuus J C 1989 Spontaneous anorectal pressure activity.

Evidence of internal anal sphincter contractions in response to rectal pressure waves. Scandinavian Journal of Gastroenterology 24: 115–200

Melzack J, Porter N H 1964 Studies on the reflex activity of the external sphincter ani in spinal man. Paraplegia 1: 277–296.

Miller R, Bartolo D C C, Cervero F, Mortensen N J 1987 Anorectal temperature sensation: a comparison of normal and incontinent patients. British Journal of Surgery 74: 511–515

Miller R, Bartolo D C C, Cervero F, Mortensen N J M 1987 Anorectal temperature sensation: a comparison of normal and incontinent patients. British Journal of Surgery 74: 511–515

Morgan C N 1936 The surgical anatomy of the anal canal and rectum. Postgraduate Medical Journal 12: 287–301.

Moschowitz A V 1912 The pathogenesis, anatomy and cure of prolapse of the rectum. Surgery Gynaecology and Obstetrics 15: 7–21

Murrie J A, Sim A G W, MacKenzie I 1981 The importance of pain, pruritis ani and soiling as symptoms of haemorrhoids and their response to haemorrhoidectomy or rubber band ligation. British Journal of Surgery 68: 279–289

Nakahara S, Itoh H, Mibu R, Ikeda S, Oohata Y, Kitana K, Nakamura Y 1988 Clinical and manometric evaluation of anorectal function following low anterior resection with low anastomotic line using an EEA stapler for rectal cancer. Diseases of the Colon & Rectum 31: 762–766

Naysmyth D G, Johnston D, Godwin P G R, Dixon M F, Smith A, Williams N S 1986 Factors influencing bowel function after ileal pouch-anal anastomosis. British Journal of Surgery 73: 469–473

Neill M H, Swash M 1980 Increased motor unit fiber density in the external anal sphincter muscle in anorectal incontinence: a single fiber EMG study. Journal of Neurology, Neurosurgery and Psychiatry 43: 343–347

Neill M E, Parks A G, Swash M 1981 Physiological studies of the pelvic floor in idiopathic faecal incontinence and rectal prolapse. British Journal of Surgery 68: 531–536

Nurko S, Dunn B M, Rattan S 1989 Peptide histidine isoleucine and vasoactive intestinal polypeptide cause relaxation of opposum internal anal sphincter via two distinct receptors. Gastroenterology 96: 403–413

O'Connell P R, Stryker S J, Metcalf A M, Pemberton J H, Kelly K A 1988 Anal canal pressure and motility after ileo-anal anastomosis. Surgery, Gynaecology and Obstetrics 166: 47–54

Oh C, Kark A E 1972 Anatomy of the external anal sphincter. British Journal of Surgery 59: 717–723

Orkin A B, Hanson R B, Kelly K A 1989 The rectal motor complex. Journal of Gastrointestinal Motility 1: 5–8

Orkin B A, Hanson R B, Kelly K A, Phillips S F, Dent J 1991 Human anal motility while fasting, after feeding and during sleep. Gastroenterology 100: 1016–1023

Pappalardo G, Toccaceli S, Dionisio P, Castrini G, Ravo B 1988 Preoperative and postoperative evaluation by manometric study of the anal sphincter after coloanal anastomosis for carcinoma. Diseases of the Colon and Rectum 31: 119–122

Parks A G, Porter N H, Hardcastle J D 1966 The syndrome of the descending perineum. Proceedings of the Royal Society of Medicine 59: 477–482

Parks A G, Fishlock D J, Cameron J D H, May H 1969

Preliminary investigation of the pharmacology of the internal anal sphincter. Gut 10: 674–677

Pedersen I K, Christiansen J 1985 The effect of glucagon and glucagon 1–21 on anal sphincter function. Diseases of the Colon & Rectum 28: 235–237

Pedersen B K, Huit K, Olsen J et al 1986 Anorectal function after low anterior resection for carcinoma. Annals of Surgery 204: 133–135

Penninckx F, Mebis J, Kerremans R 1982 The recto-anal reflex in cats analysed in-vitro. Scandinavian Journal of Gastroenterology 17 (supplement 71): 147–149

Penninckx F, Lestar B, Kerremans R 1989 A new balloon-retaining test for evaluation of anorectal function in incontinent patients. Diseases of the Colon & Rectum 32: 202–205

Percy J P, Neill M E, Kandiah T K, Swash M 1982 A neurogenic factor in faecal incontinence in the elderly. Age and Ageing 11: 175–179

Pescatori M, Parks A G 1984 The sphincteric and sensory components of preserved continence after colectomy, mucosal proctectomy, and ileo-anal anastomosis. Surgery, Gynaecology and Obstetrics 158: 517–521

Pinho M, Yoshioka K, Keighley M R B 1900 Long-term results of anorectal myectomy for chronic constipation. Diseases of the Colon & Rectum 33: 795–797

Pinho M, Yoshioka K, Ortiz J, Oya M, Keighley M R B 1990 The effect of age on pelvic floor dynamics. International Journal of Colorectal Diseases 5: 207–208

Poos R J, Frank J, Bittner R, Berger H G 1986 Influence of age and sex on anal sphincters: manometric evaluation of anorectal continence. European Surgical Research 18: 3443–3448

Prior A, Fearn U J, Read N W 1991 Intermittent rectal motor activity: a rectal motor complex? Gut 32: 1360–1363

Read N W, Harford W V, Schmulen A C, Read M G, Santa Ana C, Fordtran J S 1979 A clinical study of patients with faecal incontinence and diarrhoea. Gastroenterology 76: 747–756

Read M G, Read N W 1982 Role of anorectal sensation in preserving continence. Gut 23: 345–347

Read M G, Read N W, Barber D C, Duthie H L 1982 Effects of loperamide on anal sphincter function in patients complaining of chronic diarrhoea with faecal incontinence and urgency. Digestive Diseases and Sciences 27: 807–814

Read M G, Read N W, Haynes W G, Donnelly T C, Johnson A G 1982 A prospective study of the effect of haemorrhoidectomy on sphincter function and continence British Journal of Surgery 69: 396–398

Read N W, Haynes W G, Bartolo D C C, Hall J, Read M G, Donnelly T C, Johnson A G 1983 Use of anorectal manometry during rectal infusion of saline to investigate sphincter function in incontinent patients. Gastroenterology 85: 105–113

Read N W, Bartolo D C C, Read M G, Hall J, Haynes W G, Johnson A G 1983 Differences in anorectal manometry between patients with haemorrhoids and patients with descending perineum syndrome: implications for management. British Journal of Surgery 70: 656–659

Read N W, Bartolo D C C, Read M G 1984 Differences in anal function in patients with incontinence to solids and in patients with incontinence to liquids. British Journal of Surgery 71: 39–42

Read N W, Abouzekry L 1986 Why do patients with faecal impaction have faecal incontinence? Gut 27: 283–287

Ripstein C B, Lanter B 1963 Aetiology and surgical therapy of massive prolapse of the rectum. Annals of Surgery 157: 259–264

Roe A M, Bartolo D C C, Mortensen N J M 1986 New method for the assessment of anal sensation in various anorectal disorders. British Journal of Surgery 73: 854–861

Roe A M, Bartolo D C C, Mortensen N J M 1986 Diagnosis and management of intractable constipation. British Journal of Surgery 73: 854–861

Rogers J, Henry M M, Misiewicz J J 1988 Combined sensory and motor deficit in primary neuropathic faecal incontinence Gut 29: 5–9

Rogers J, Hayward M P, Henry M M, Misiewicz J J 1988 Temperature gradient between the rectum and anal canal: evidence against the role of temperature sensation as a sensory modality in the anal canal of normal subjects. British Journal of Surgery 75: 1083–1085

Sagar P M, Holdsworth P J, Johnston D 1991 Correlation between laboratory findings and clinical outcome after restorative proctocolectomy: serial studies in 20 patients with end-to-end pouch anastomosis. British Journal of Surgery 78: 67–70

Sainio A P, Voutilainen P E, Husa Ai 1991 Recovery of anal sphincter function following transabdominal repair of rectal prolapse: cause of improved continence? Diseases of the Colon & Rectum 34: 816–821

Schang J C, Devroede G 1988 Myoelectric propagating spike bursts in the sigmoid colon elicits the recto-anal inhibitory reflex. Gastroenterology 94: A403

Schiller L R, Santa Ana C A, Schmulen A C et al 1982 Pathogenesis of faecal incontinence in diabetes mellitus: evidence for internal anal sphincter dysfunction. New England Journal of Medicine 307: 1666–1671

Schouten W R, Blankensteijn J D 1991 Ultra-slow wave pressure variations in the anal canal before and after lateral internal sphincterotomy. Diseases of the Colon and Rectum 34: P17

Schuster M M 1975 The riddle of the sphincters. Gastroenterology 69: 249–262

Schwiger M 1979 Method for determining individual contributions of voluntary and involuntary anal sphincters to resting tone. Diseases of the Colon & Rectum 22: 415–416

Seow-Choen, Tsunoda A, Nicholls R J 1991 Prospective randomised trial comparing anal function after hand sewn ileoanal anastomosis with mucosectomy versus stapled ileoanal anastomosis without mucosectomy in restorative proctocolectomy. British Journal of Surgery 78: 430–434

Shouler P, Keighley M R B 1986 Changes in colorectal function in severe idiopathic chronic constipation. Gastroenterology 90: 414–420

Smith L E, Henrichs D, McCullah R D 1982 Prospective studies in the aetiology and treatment of pruritis ani. Diseases of the Colon & Rectum 25: 358–363

Snooks S J, Henry M M, Swash M 1981 Anorectal incontinence and rectal prolapse: differential assessment of the innervation of the puborectalis and external anal sphincter muscles. Gut 26: 470–476

Snooks S J, Swash M, Mathers S, Henry M M 1990 Effect of vaginal delivery on the pelvic floor: a 5 year follow-up. British Journal of Surgery 77: 1358–1360

Sorensen M, Tetzschner T, Rasmussen O O, Christiansen J 1991 Relation between electromyography and anal manometry of the external anal sphincter. Gut 32: 1031–1034

Sorensen M, Rasmussen O O, Tetzschner T, Christiansen J 1992 Physiological variation in rectal compliance. British Journal of Surgery 79: 1106–1108

Speakman C T M, Hoyle C H V, Kamm M A et al 1990 Adrenergic control in the internal anal sphincter is abnormal in patients with idiopathic faecal incontinence. British Journal of Surgery 77: 1342–1344

Spencer R J 1984 Manometric studies in rectal prolapse. Diseases of the Colon & Rectum 27: 523–525

Stryker S J, Phillips S F, Dozois R R, Beart R W, Kelly K A 1986 Anal and neorectal function after ileal pouch anastomosis. Annals of Surgery 203: 55–61

Sun W M, Read N W, Donnelly T C, Bannister J J, Shorthouse A J 1989 A common pathophysiology for full-thickness rectal prolapse, anterior mucosal prolapse and solitary rectal ulcer. British Journal of Surgery 76: 290–295

Suzuki H, Matsumoto K, Fujioka M, Honzumi M 1980 Anorectal pressure and rectal compliance after low anterior resection. British Journal of Surgery 67: 655–657

Swash M, Gray A, Lubowski D Z, Nicholls R J 1988 Ultrastructural changes in internal anal sphincter in neurogenic faecal incontinence. Gut 29: 1692–1698

Symington J 1889 The rectum and the anus. Journal of Anatomy, London 23: 106–115

Taylor B M, Beart R W, Phillips S F 1984 Longitudinal and radial variations of pressure in the human anal canal. Gastroenterology 86: 693–697

Teramoto T, Parks A G, Swash M 1981 Hypertrophy of the external anal sphincter. Gut 22: 45–48

Tuckson W B, Fazio V W, Lavery I C et al 1991 Do anal sphincter pressures improve with time following total proctocolectomy and ileal pouch-anal anastomosis? Diseases of the Colon & Rectum 34: P26

Ustasch T J, Tobon F, Hambrecht T, Bass D D, Schuster M M 1970 Electrophysiological aspects of human sphincter function. Journal of Clinical Investigation 49: 41–48

Vantrappen G, Janssens J, Hellemans J, Ghoos Y 1977 The interdigestive motor complex of normal subjects and patients with bacterial overgrowth of the small intestine. Journal of Clinical Investigation 22: 117–124

Waldron D J, Kumar D, Hallan R I, Williams N S 1989 Prolonged ambulant assessment of anorectal function in patients with prolapsing haemorrhoids. Diseases of the Colon & Rectum 32: 968–974

Watts J D, Rothenberger D A, Buls J G, Goldberg S M, Nivatongs S 1985 The management of procidentia. 30 years experience. Diseases of the Colon & Rectum 28: 96–102

Wells C 1959 New operation for rectal prolapse. Proceedings of the Royal Society of Medicine 52: 602–603

Weinbeck M, Altaparmacov I 1980 Is the internal anal sphincter controlled by a myoelectrical mechanism? in: Christiansen J (ed.) Gastrointestinal Motility, Raven Press, New York, pp 487–493

Wexner S D, Marchetti F, Jagelman D G 1991 The role of sphincteroplasty for faecal incontinence reevaluated: a prospective physiologic and functional review. Diseases of the Colon and Rectum 34: 22–30

Williams N S, Price R, Johnston D 1980 The long term effect of sphincter preserving operations for rectal carcinoma on function of the anal sphincter in man. British Journal of Surgery 67: 203–208

Williams N S, Marzou D E M M, Hallan R I, Waldron D J 1989 Function after ileal-pouch and stapled anastomosis for ulcerative colitis. British Journal of Surgery 76: 1168–1171

Williams J G, Wong W D, Jensen L, Rothenberger D A, Goldberg S M 1991 Incontinence and rectal prolapse: a prospective manometric study. Diseases of the Colon & Rectum 34: 209–216

Womack N R, Williams N S, Holmsfield J H M, Morrison J F B, Simpkins K C. New method for the dynamic assessment of anorectal function in constipation. British Journal of Surgery 72: 994–998

Yoshioka K, Hyland G, Keighley M R B 1989 Anorectal function after abdominal rectopexy: parameters of predictive value in identifying return of continence. British Journal of Surgery 76: 64–68

Yoshioka K, Helen F, Keighley M R B 1989 Functional results after posterior abdominal rectopexy for rectal prolapse. Diseases of the Colon & Rectum 32: 835–838

Disorders of gastrointestinal motility

30. Motor disorders of the oesophagus

C. E. Pope II

As was discussed in Chapter 23, the motor functions of the oesophagus are a coordinated series of events involving the pharynx, larynx, upper oesophageal sphincter (UOS) the striated and smooth musculature of the body of the oesophagus, the smooth muscle of the lower oesophageal sphincter (LOS) and the crural fibres of the diaphragm. Motor disorder occurs as a result of primary muscle disease (myotonia, scleroderma), metabolic disorder which affects muscle function (hypothyroidism), defects in the central nervous system (CNS) (stroke), enteric nervous system (ENS) (achalasia) or failure in coordination (non-specific motor disorder, NSMD).

When the orderly progression of an oesophageal swallow is affected by any of the problems mentioned above, clinical symptoms may occur. Dysphagia manifested either as difficulty in initiating deglutition or an awareness that bolus arrest has occurred is a common presentation of an oesophageal motor disorder. Chest pain of several types may signify that an oesophageal motor disorder is present. Tracheal aspiration can occur when there is failure in coordination of the pharynx or UOS during swallowing, from retrograde transport of a fluid oesophageal bolus during a simultaneous contraction of the entire oesophageal body, or from reflux of retained food and fluid from a dilated achalasic oesophagus.

Oesophageal motor function can be evaluated by studying luminal transport of solids or liquids (X-ray, scintigraphy), by recording intraluminal pressures which can measure force of closure and muscular coordination (manometry), or with research tools such as intraluminal force transducers, electromyography (EMG) or impedance changes. Some motor disorders such as achalasia have fairly well-established pathophysiology, symptoms and diagnostic test results. In other disorders, such as chest pain, associated with abnormal contractions of the oesophagus, there is a lack of pathophysiological information, clinical cause and even stability of diagnostic features. This chapter will discuss two main groups of motor disorders. The first group involves the pharynx, the UOS, and the upper striated muscle of the oesophagus. The second group presents with involvement of the smooth muscle portion of the oesophagus.

PHARYNGEAL – UPPER OESOPHAGEAL BODY DISORDERS

The initial phases of swallowing depend on precise coordination of pharyngeal, laryngeal and striated oesophageal muscles. This coordination is managed by pre-programmed neural pathways controlled by the CNS. Defects in the striated muscle or in the CNS can produce difficulties. Modern combinations of combined cinefluorography and strain gauge manometry have not yet been reported in many of the clinical syndromes to be discussed, so current knowledge depends on technology which is sometimes inadequate. Many of these studies were reported in two excellent review articles in 1976 (Kilman & Goyal 1976, Palmer 1976), unfortunately, not a great deal of progress has been made since then.

Striated muscle disorders

The following list shows the clinical syndromes in which muscular involvement of the pharyngeal and striated oesophageal body musculature may lead to oesophageal symptoms.

- Myotonic muscular dystrophy
- Oculopharyngeal muscular dystrophy
- Polymyositis
- Dermatomyositis
- Systemic lupus erythematosus
- Myasthenia gravis
- Hypothyroidism
- Hyperthyroidism

Both dysphagia for solids and liquids and symptoms of

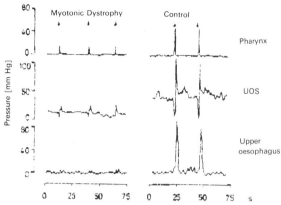

Fig. 30.1 Manometric tracings from the pharynx and proximal oesophagus in a patient with myotonic dystrophy and a control subject. The patient's tracing shows a decrease in UOS pressure and a decrease in peristaltic amplitude. (Reproduced with permission from Eckardt et al 1986.)

aspiration are common. Careful cinefluorographic studies may show laryngeal penetration or pharyngeal stasis. Often, the transfer of liquid contrast agent into the larynx and trachea does not provoke coughing. Reflux of barium into the nasopharynx occurs because of the inability of the soft palate to separate the nasopharynx from the oropharynx.

Manometric tracings obtained from patients with striated muscle diseases reveal low amplitude pressure waves in the pharyngeal and upper oesophageal body musculature. Resting UOS pressures tend to be low. Such changes are shown in Figure 30.1 from a patient with myotonic dystrophy (Eckardt et al 1986). Although the amplitudes are low, coordination between pharynx, UOS and upper body is maintained. The decrease in contraction amplitude of the striated muscle in myotonic dystrophy is also found in the smooth muscle portion of the oesophageal body. Patients with muscular dystrophy of other types than myotonic dystrophy show no decrease in oesophageal muscle amplitude of contraction. Clearance time of a radioisotopically labelled liquid from the oesophagus is also markedly prolonged in myotonic dystrophy (Horowitz et al 1987).

Treatment of diseases affecting striated muscle is usually ineffective. Swallowing difficulties secondary to myasthenia gravis may improve with anticholinesterase treatment, although manometric or cinefluorographic confirmation of clinical improvement is rare. If there are thyroid abnormalities, thyroid treatment will improve muscle function (Wright & Penner 1981). Cricopharyngeal myotomy will be discussed below.

Defects in neural control of swallowing

As has already been discussed, normal deglutition involves exact regulation of pharyngeal, laryngeal and upper striated muscle. Destruction of the swallowing centre in the pons and medulla or the motor nerve nuclei of the cranial nerves results in total inability to initiate swallowing. I have had the opportunity of studying one such patient with the Wallenberg syndrome (infarction of the nuclei of cranial nerves IX–XII). This unfortunate individual could neither initiate swallowing voluntarily or swallow involuntarily. He was forced to expectorate saliva constantly. Interestingly, he apparently did not aspirate while asleep – it is possible that other mechanisms of deglutition might have become active during sleep.

Since the pharynx receives bilateral innervation from the brain stem, it has always been tacitly assumed that a unilateral cerebrovascular accident should not produce swallowing difficulties. However, if patients are studied soon after a cerebrovascular accident, almost half of them are found to have dysphagia, even when computed tomography (CT) or necropsy shows that infarction is confined to only one hemisphere (Gordon et al 1987). Of clinical importance is the fact that those with dysphagia have a poor clinical outcome, with frequent pulmonary infection, presumably from aspiration. In another study, 44 out of 46 individuals who had recently sustained a cortical or subcortical infarct (confirmed by CT scan), were demonstrated by cinefluorography to have disorders of pharyngeal function (Chen et al 1990). 35 of these patients had unilateral infarcts. Pharyngeal stasis of liquid or paste barium, usually bilaterally, and laryngeal aspiration were the most common radiological findings.

The following are some of the neurological syndromes in which swallowing function is disordered. Sometimes, the first manifestation of amyotrophic lateral sclerosis or multiple sclerosis is dysphagia, and careful neurological examination is necessary to detect manifestations in other parts of the body.

- Cerebrovascular accidents, unilateral or bilateral
- Brain stem strokes
- Guillain-Barré
- Multiple sclerosis
- Parkinson's disease
- Amyotrophic lateral sclerosis
- Poliomyelitis

Most of these diseases will present with pharyngeal stasis, laryngeal aspiration, unilateral pharyngeal transport and abnormalities of tongue movements. There has been little manometric study of pharyngeal and cricopharyngeal function using modern strain gauge transducer technology.

Treatment of neuromuscular pharyngeal disease

Simple alterations in the consistency or viscosity of food and fluids can be shown to be of benefit. If a cine study shows unilateral pharyngeal paralysis as is seen with certain brain stem infarcts, then rotation of the head towards the weak side increases pharyngeal clearing, possibly by decreasing cricopharyngeal sphincter tension (Logemann et al 1989).

Pharmacological treatment can be of use in several specific diseases. As mentioned earlier, myasthenia gravis can be improved with anticholinesterase agents, and thyroid myopathies can also be successfully treated. Another disease in which drugs may be helpful is Parkinson's disease. In a study utilizing carefully graded cinefluorograms, five patients improved their performance when given levodopa; ten patients showed no improvement (Bushmann et al 1989). Whether this radiologic improvement would be of lasting benefit is uncertain, as cine findings and patient symptoms often did not correlate very well in this group of Parkinsonian patients.

Cricopharyngeal myotomy has been recommended for persistent dysphagia in neuromuscular diseases. A review published in 1978 reported that less than half of the patients having a myotomy for neurological diseases will have a 'good' result (marked improvement or disappearance of dysphagia) (Hurwitz & Duranceau 1978). More recent studies are a little more optimistic (Bonavina et al 1985, van Overbeek 1991) but not uniformly so (Lindgren & Ekberg 1990).

Patient selection may determine whether myotomy produces good results in this type of patient. Performing a cricopharyngeal myotomy in a patient with marked reflux may lead to terrible consequences because of aspiration. Using cine studies to predict which patients should have a cricopharyngeal myotomy has been advocated (Wilson & Bruce-Lockhart 1990). This group achieved excellent to good results in five of six patients who had poor function of the cricopharyngeal region but good tongue function. Since the patients with poor tongue function and poor cricopharyngeal function, were not subjected to operation, this method of selection has not been proven, but seems worthy of exploration.

Other conditions

Patients presenting with transfer dysphagia will often be found to have a prominent cricopharyngeal bar on barium swallow. Although this has been called cricopharyngeal achalasia, thus suggesting a motor disorder, manometric studies usually show no evidence of failure of relaxation of the upper sphincter (Dantas et al 1990). Some cases represent increased fibrosis of the cricopharyngeus muscle (Cruse et al 1979).

A sensation of a lump in the throat (globus hystericus) has also been attributed to spasm in the pharynx and/or cricopharyngeus muscle. Again, manometric studies fail to show elevated resting pressures in the UOS (Wilson et al 1989).

Whether or not patients with a Zenker's diverticulum (pharyngo-oesophageal pouch) have a motor disorder which might have produced the abnormality remains a controversial question. Earlier reports suggested an incoordination between the pharyngeal pressure spike and the period of UOS relaxation (Ellis et al 1969, Lichter 1978). However, low compliance recording systems have failed to document premature closure of the UOS (Frieling et al 1988).

SMOOTH MUSCLE OESOPHAGEAL BODY DISORDERS

Once the pharynx and upper striated muscle has transported a bolus into the smooth muscle portion of the oesophagus, a lumen-obliterating contraction sweeps the bolus down the length of the oesophagus, through the relaxed LOS, and into the stomach. Failure of the smooth muscle, or of its coordinating extrinsic and intrinsic nervous control, can lead to dysphagia, regurgitation, chest pain or oesophageal retention of contents. Some of the syndromes leading to these clinical manifestations are fairly well characterized (achalasia, scleroderma). Other syndromes (chest pain of unknown origin, dysphagia secondary to non-specific motor abnormalities) are of great clinical importance, but are not well understood in terms of pathophysiology, diagnosis or therapy. This section will begin with the syndromes best understood, then progress into the unknown.

Achalasia (cardiospasm)

First recognized in 1674, achalasia was the second oesophageal motor disorder described, the first motor disorder being rumination (1618). The striking clinical manifestations of dysphagia, regurgitation and pulmonary aspiration, weight loss and chest discomfort usually bring patients to medical attention relatively soon in their clinical course.

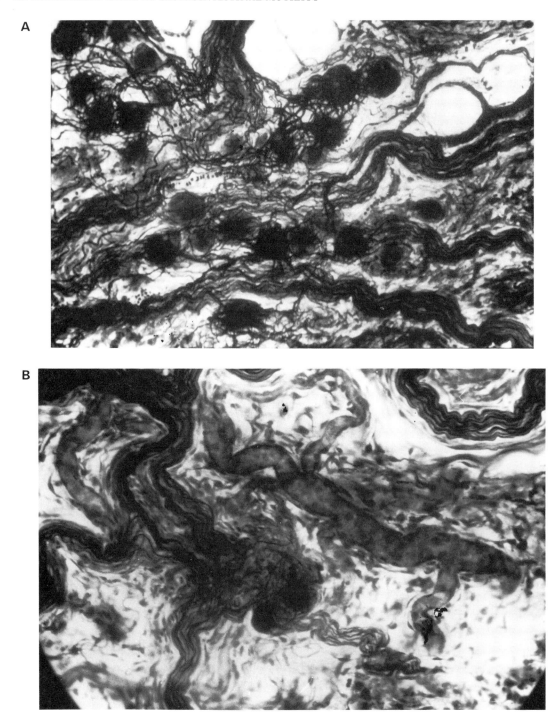

Fig. 30.2 **A** Photomicrograph of a section from a normal oesophagus. Numerous ganglion cells are seen, some taking up the silver stain (argyrophilic) and some staining only slightly (argyrophobic). **B** Photomicrograph of a section from the oesophagus of a patient with achalasia. Only two slightly shrunken ganglion cells are seen. (Courtesy of Dr Michael D. Schuffler)

Pathophysiology

There is a double defect present in achalasia. The LOS shows no or only partial relaxation on swallowing, and there are no peristaltic waves in the body of the oesophagus. The structural and physiological abnormalities producing failure of peristalsis and lack of relaxation of the LOS have been fairly well established. Least controversial is a disappearance of enteric neurons from the myenteric plexus of the oesophagus (Fig. 30.2). Remaining nerve bodies are often surrounded by an increased number of mononuclear inflammatory cells. Lewy bodies (intranuclear inclusions) are found both in the remaining neurons and in the brain stem nuclei responsible for swallowing (Qualman et al 1984). An older study reports dropout of nerve bodies in the dorsal motor nucleus of the vagus and evidence of degeneration in the vagal fibres (Cassella et al 1964). There are suggestions that these lesions in the vagal nuclei and trunks may have expressions elsewhere than in the oesophagus. Some patients with achalasia have blunted responses to sham feeding (decreased acid output and decreased polypeptide secretion) (Dooley et al 1983). The decrease in acid output in response to sham feeding was not confirmed by another study, but there was a slower rate of gastric emptying, suggesting vagal impairment (Eckardt et al 1989).

Other changes in structure have also been reported. There are fewer small nerve fibres (as seen by electron microscopy) in oesophageal muscle biopsies from patients with achalasia (Friesen et al 1983). There is also a paucity of interstitial cells of Cajal, whose oesophageal function is unknown (Faussone-Pellegrini & Cortesini 1985). Selective loss of fibres containing vasoactive intestinal polypeptide in the sphincter area suggests that this neuropeptide may be involved in LOS relaxation (Aggestrup et al 1983). Intact excitatory vagal input to the LOS is suggested by an increase in LOS pressure after edrophonium, a decrease in pressure after atropine, and presence of migrating motor complex (MMC) contractions in the LOS which require intact vagal innervation (Holloway et al 1986).

Investigations of motility changes in achalasia

Radiology has always been and remains the primary method of motor function evaluation in achalasia. It is easily available and well-tolerated. Radiographs of the LOS zone shows the classical 'bird-beak' appearance (Fig. 30.3). Also easily appreciated is the marked dilatation of the oesophageal body. Isolated non-propulsive contractions of the oesophageal body that do not obliter-

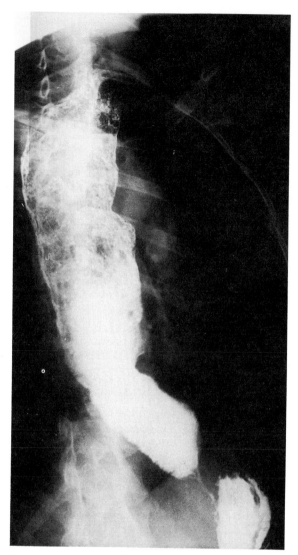

Fig. 30.3 Achalasia. A dilated oesophagus with filling defects representing retained food and secretions is seen. The oesophagus terminates in a smooth point or 'bird-beak'.

ate the lumen are commonly seen. Pharyngeal pouches may also be present, and have been observed in 11 of 21 patients with achalasia (Jones et al 1987).

Manometry shows absent or impaired relaxation of the LOS in response to a swallow (Fig. 30.4). This finding is an absolute requirement for the diagnosis of achalasia. The resting LOS pressure tends to be elevated (30–40 mmHg versus a normal value of 10–20 mmHg), but one in three patients with achalasia by all other criteria will have resting LOS pressures within the normal range. In addition to failure of relaxation

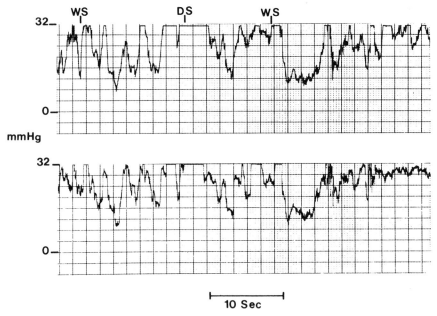

Fig. 30.4 Failure of LOS relaxation in achalasia. This record is obtained from two pressure tips at the same level. Neither a dry swallow (DS) nor two wet swallows (WS) cause more than a small drop in LOS pressure. This drop in pressure does not even approach the gastric base line of zero.

in response to swallowing, there are also no transient relaxations of the LOS in response to gastric distension with air as are observed in control subjects (Holloway et al 1989).

Motor activity in the body of the oesophagus usually consists of a low-amplitude long-duration simultaneous wave (Fig. 30.5). Occasionally, the simultaneous waves have normal amplitudes and durations. Rhythmic spontaneous simultaneous contractions are occasionally recorded. This finding has been dubbed 'active achalasia', but current opinion is that these patients follow the same clinical course as do those with classic achalasia (Todorczuk et al 1991). The baseline pressure recorded from the oesophageal body is often elevated and can exceed intragastric resting pressures. This is merely a reflection of retained fluid in the dilated oesophagus, and a return to negative baseline pressures can be accomplished by emptying the oesophageal fluid with a wide-bore tube.

Little attention has been paid to the striated portion of the oesophagus in achalasia but there are differences among patients who appear to have classic achalasia. In a study reported in abstract, 38 of 52 achalasic patients had a normal striated muscle response to swallowing (Fig. 30.6) (Russak & Pope 1990). The simultaneous contractions seen in the body of the oesophagus

followed the striated contraction; occasionally both types of wave were recorded from the same site. The remaining 14 patients with achalasia had no identifiable striated muscle contraction. Smooth muscle-type contractions were seen as the catheter was withdrawn until it reached the normally functioning UOS (Fig. 30.7). Perhaps these latter patients had some disturbance in the efferent nerve pathways from the brain to the striated muscle of the body of the oesophagus.

Radioisotopes can be used to measure the transport of fluid in achalasia. By administering radioisotope-labelled fluid collecting an oesophageal scintigram with a gamma camera and then dividing the oesophageal area of interest into segments, time-activity curves can be generated (Fig. 30.7). (Russell et al 1981). Such studies show that the majority of an ingested liquid bolus tends to linger in the mid-body, and only a small amount of radioactivity is seen in the gastric 'area of interest'.

Retention of oesophageal contents can also be easily documented by giving the patient a mixed radioactively labelled meal (Fig. 30.8) (Holloway et al 1983). This test helps in the evaluation of pharmacological or surgical therapy. A decreased oesophageal retention time of the meal correlates nicely with a decreased LOS pressure after balloon dilatation or myotomy.

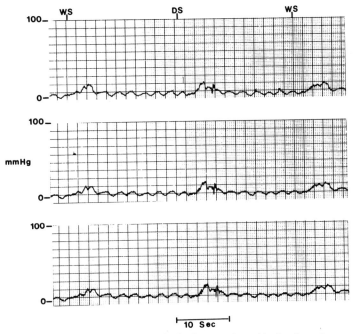

Fig. 30.5 Swallow-induced activity in the oesophageal body of a patient with achalasia. Three pressure sensors 5 cm apart record the effect of two wet swallows (**WS**) and one dry swallow (**DS**). Only a low-amplitude long-duration simultaneous contraction is seen.

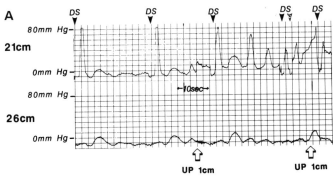

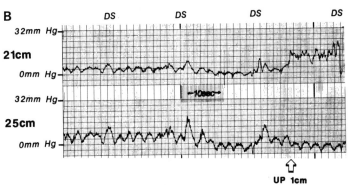

Fig. 30.6 Striated muscle activity in achalasia. **A** Dry swallowing (**DS**) causes a short high-amplitude wave to be recorded by the tip labelled 21 cm. Immediately following this, the low amplitude long duration contraction is seen in both leads. The catheter is pulled up by 1 cm increments until the pressure characteristics of the UOS are seen. **B** From a different patient with achalasia, swallowing causes only a smooth muscle type contraction in both leads. The catheter is then pulled up 1 cm and the elevated pressure and fall in response to a swallow is seen. No striated muscle-type contractions were seen in this patient.

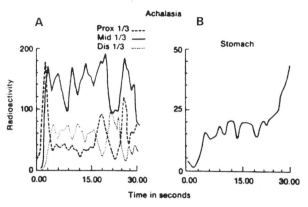

Fig. 30.7 Scintiscan of a patient with achalasia. **A** is from three separate areas of interest over the oesophagus. The radioisotope is cleared rapidly from the proximal site and remains in the mid-oesophagus. **B** Relatively little radioactivity enters the stomach by 30 s. (Reproduced with permission from Russell et al 1981)

Very limited EMG studies have been performed in achalasia (Bortolotti et al 1982, Tibbling et al 1986). Figure 30.9 shows a tracing obtained from an individual with achalasia who had a decompensated dilated oesophagus. Spike activity is detected in the upper striated portion of the oesophagus, whereas no spike activity is seen in the smooth muscle portion, even though a rise in pressure is recorded. This suggests that the rise in pressure is not due to local muscle contraction, but is transmitted from a common cavity.

Another interesting technique that can be used to evaluate the LOS in achalasia is measurement of the intragastric air pressure required to force open the sphincter (yield pressure) (McGouran et al 1988). With an endoscope in the retroflexed position, air is pumped into the stomach with simultaneous pressure monitoring until the cardia is observed to open and an audible belch is heard. Controls have a yield pressure of 7.5–9 mmHg, whereas patients with achalasia have a mean value of 21.3 mmHg. A fall to a yield pressure mean value of 1.8 mmHg after balloon dilatation has been documented.

Pseudoachalasia and other syndromes resembling achalasia

The term pseudoachalasia has been applied to patients presenting with dysphagia and a dilated oesophagus who are subsequently found to have a tumour infiltrating the LOS area. It may be very difficult to differentiate these patients from those with true achalasia. X-ray studies can be very similar, and manometric and

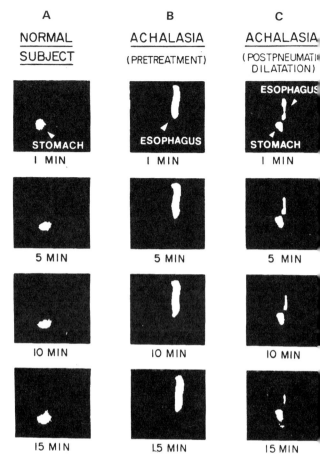

Fig. 30.8 Clearing of radioisotope from the oesophagus of patients with achalasia. A solid meal is rapidly cleared from the oesophagus of a control subject (**A**). **B** shows retention of the meal in the oesophagus. After dilation (**C**), there is marked improvement of oesophageal emptying. (Reproduced with permission from Holloway et al 1983.)

scintigraphic studies do not separate these two groups (Kahrilas et al 1987, Rozman & Achkar 1990). Endoscopy may show nodularity in the distal oesophagus, or it may be impossible to pass the endoscope into the stomach. A retroflexed view of the cardia may show an extraluminal mass compressing the gastro-oesophageal junction. Endoscopic ultrasonography can sometimes demonstrate an intramural tumour (Fig. 30.10) (Ziegler et al 1990). Inhalation of amyl nitrite may cause the sphincter of true achalasia to open (judged radiologically), whereas the oesophagogastric junction of pseudoachalasia will remain tightly closed (Dodds et al 1986).

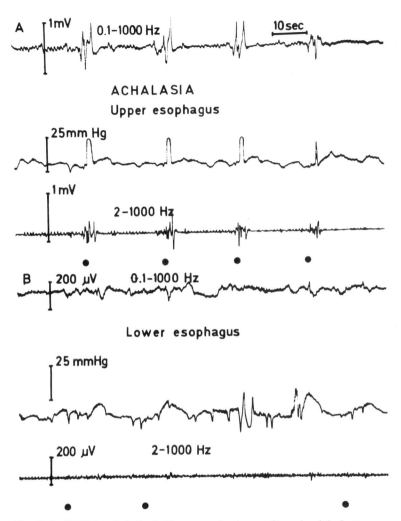

Fig. 30.9 EMG in achalasia. **A** The top tracing is an unfiltered and the bottom tracing a filtered EMG from the proximal striated muscle of a patient with achalasia. The middle tracing is a pressure tracing taken at the same level. Spike activity coincident with the pressure activity is seen. **B** In contrast, no spike activity is seen in response to a swallow (●) even though a low-amplitude long-duration pressure wave is recorded. (Tibbling et al 1986.)

Involvement of the ENS with the protozoan *Trypanosoma cruzi* produces Chagas' disease (Dantas 1988). The oesophageal manifestations are identical to those of idiopathic achalasia, although not all patients with Chagas' disease have elevated LOS pressures. The colon, small bowel and bladder can also be involved as well. Treatment is the same as in classic achalasia (see below).

Involvement of the oesophagus with amyloid, either primary or secondary, can also produce a clinical and radiological syndrome indistinguishable from classic achalasia (Costigan & Clouse 1983, Estrada et al 1990). The diagnosis can be made by oesophageal or gastric biopsy with subsequent demonstration of amyloid protein in the blood vessels by special stains.

In the paediatric literature, there are reports of achalasia of the oesophagus being associated with defects in tear production and problems with endocrine secretion (Feldman 1988). These defects seem to have an autosomal recessive inheritance, and involvement of the autonomic and peripheral nerves is also noted.

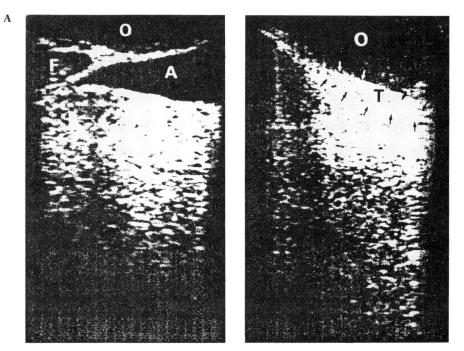

Fig. 30.10 Ultrasonography detects a tumour in pseudoachalasia. (**A**) Ultrasonogram of a normal gastro-oesophageal junction. **A** = aorta; **O** = oesophageal lumen; **F** = fundus. (**B**) Intramural tumour (**T**) is shown in oesophagogastric junction area. **O** = oesophageal lumen. (Reproduced with permission from Ziegler et al 1990.)

Treatment of achalasia

Three main approaches have been tried for treatment in achalasia: drug therapy, dilatation and surgical disruption of the LOS. Drug therapy has the advantage of being non-invasive, but requires excellent patient compliance. Dilatation offers the promise of a very short hospital experience, but may lead to an uncontrolled perforation. Surgery allows a definitive disruption of the muscle of the lower oesophagus, but at the price of increased morbidity and expense. Each of these options will be discussed.

Two main classes of drugs have been used in the

long-term therapy of achalasia (Table 30.1). Nitrites in the form of isosorbide 5 mg given before meals have been shown to decrease LOS pressures from high values to a normal level and to increase emptying of a test meal (Gelfond et al 1982). However, efficacy fades with time in a substantial number of patients. Nifedipine taken in 20 mg oral doses before meals also caused a fall in LOS pressure, but did not increase oesophageal emptying as measured by radioisotopes. Another group also showed no improvement in oesophageal emptying, and only modest clinical improvement (Robertson et al 1989). Yet a prospective trial of sublingual nifedipine versus pneumatic dilatation showed equivalent falls in LOS pressure and equivalent clinical improvement (Coccia et al 1991). My own experience with these two drugs has been rather disappointing, but there may still be a place for them in treating patients in whom more invasive procedures may pose an unacceptably high risk.

Brusque dilatation with a balloon has been employed for almost a century. A balloon constrained to expand to a fixed diameter is now used. When localized fluoroscopi-

Table 30.1 Pharmacologic agents for treatment of achalasia

Agent	Dose
Dicyclomine	10 mg tid
Nitroglycerine	0/4 mg with meals
Isosorbide	5 mg tid
Nifedipine	20 mg tid

cally, a waist can be seen as the balloon is slowly inflated. Disappearance of the waist-signals adequate dilatation of the LOS. Results of several series in which dilatation has been retrospectively compared to myotomy reveals good results in from 40–65% of patients (Csendes et al 1991).

Surgery of the gastro-oesophageal junction area in achalasia has a very high rate of success in relieving obstruction. In a large multicentre trial, 988 patients underwent surgery, with good results in 82%, fair results in 11%, and failure of obstruction relief in 7% (Gonzalez et al 1988).

There is only one truly randomized series in which balloon dilatation and myotomy were compared (Csendes et al 1989). The patients were well randomized and followed clinically with objective measurements for at least 2 years post-treatment. There was a 5% incidence of balloon perforation, but no deaths. 40 of 42 patients having surgery were relieved of dysphagia, whereas only 20 of 37 patients undergoing balloon dilatation were able to swallow normally. LOS pressure and oesophageal diameters decreased more in the surgical group than in the medical group. This was achieved at the cost of increased reflux (28% versus 8% in the balloon-treated patients). The authors feel that these results favour the choice of surgery as a method of relieving obstruction at the gastro-oesophageal junction in achalasia. Although I am impressed with these results, it still seems worthwhile to try pneumatic dilatation, but not to persist with this form of treatment if relief of dysphagia is not obtained on the first or second dilatation.

One of the most unexpected results of either type of therapy is the return of peristalsis after relief of lower-oesophageal obstruction by balloon dilatation or myotomy. Such return has been reported after both balloon dilatation (Vantrappen et al 1979) and Heller's myotomy (Bianco et al 1986, Ponce et al 1986) (Fig. 30.11). If the absence of peristalsis is due to lesions in the myenteric plexus, then return of peristalsis should not occur. In fact, it is very uncommon – less than 15% of the reported cases of achalasia have this documented. However, it should be noted that postoperative manometric studies are not done routinely.

Scleroderma and other connective tissue diseases

Progressive systemic sclerosis (scleroderma) is a disease in which problems with oesophageal motor function can lead to severe morbidity. Patients with scleroderma will complain of dysphagia for both solids and liquids, and these symptoms may predate the cutaneous manifestations of the disease. In addition to dysphagia, failure of the LOS may lead to severe reflux disease.

Motility studies in scleroderma

Plain films of the chest may show an air-filled oesophagus in those individuals with scleroderma who have had total LOS failure. On cine studies, the peristaltic wave will die out in mid-oesophagus, and retention of barium in the oesophagus in the supine position is common. If the patient is in an upright position, the oesophagus will empty by gravity.

Less attention has been paid to the pharyngeal area in scleroderma, but cine studies showed abnormal function in 13 of 51 patients studied (Montesi et al 1991). Pharyngeal retention and laryngeal penetration and aspiration were the most common abnormalities. These abnormalities were found in patients who also had motor abnormalities of the smooth muscle portion of the oesophagus.

Manometry shows either absence of contractions in the distal oesophagus (Fig. 30.12) or marked decrease in the amplitude of the peristaltic wave in 75–90% of patient studies (Carette et al 1985, Weihrauch et al 1978). A longitudinal study suggested that there is degeneration of the peristaltic wave amplitude with time (Hendel et al 1989). The reason for the decreased amplitude is not clear. Studies from the Mayo Clinic showed no sclerosis or fibrosis in oesophageal muscle of patients who earlier had been shown to have aperistalsis on manometry (Treacy et al 1963).

Scintigraphy has also been a popular method for quantifying muscle function in scleroderma. Studies show retention of isotope in the middle and distal thirds of the oesophagus (Fig. 30.13) (Carette et al 1985, Davidson et al 1985). Entry time of the isotope into the stomach is prolonged. Serial studies over time using scintigraphy reveal deterioration of oesophageal transit in over half of the patients followed for 3–5 years (Baron & Arzoumanian 1991).

Therapy for the oesophageal motor disorders in scleroderma remains disappointing. D-penicillamine did not prevent oesophageal function deterioration (Hendel et al 1989). Metoclopramide did include a transient improvement in LOS pressure as well as increases in oesophageal peristaltic amplitude values (Johnson et al 1987), but long-term studies of efficacy have not been reported.

Other collagen diseases have a lesser prevalence of oesophageal motor abnormalities. Mixed connective tissue disease (MCTD) is a syndrome with elements of progressive systemic sclerosis, lupus erythematosus and polymyositis, marked by circulating antibodies directed against a ribonucleoprotein. Two studies suggest that peristaltic abnormalities are quite common in mixed connective tissue disorders (Gutierrez et al 1982, Marshall et al 1990). The first study demonstrated

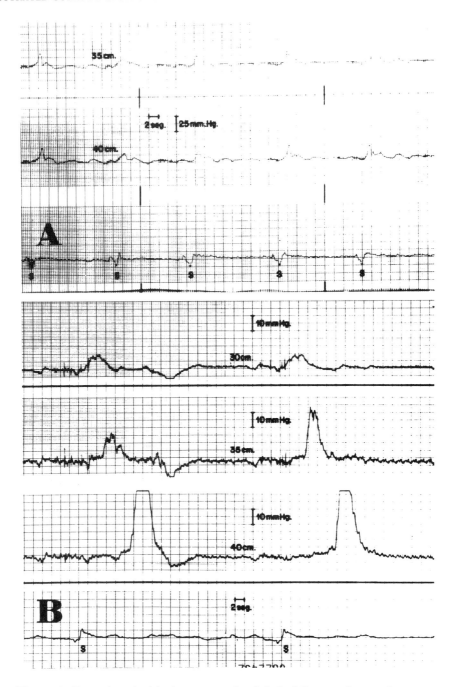

Fig. 30.11   Return in peristalsis after myotomy in achalasia. **A** Preoperative record showing only simultaneous low amplitude contraction. **S** marks swallowing activity. **B** After surgical myotomy of the LOS, peristaltic waves in response to swallowing are recorded. (Reproduced with permission from Ponce et al 1986.)

that patients with pure systemic lupus erythematosus had a rather low prevalence of manometric abnormali-

ties (3 of 14), whereas in the patients with MCTD, 14 of 17 had manometric abnormalities consisting of

Respiration

Swallow

Proximal

Middle

Distal

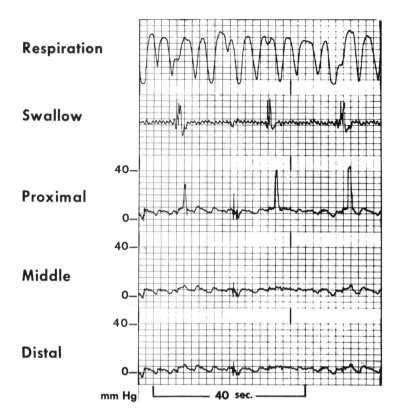

mm Hg | └── **40 sec.** ──┘

Fig. 30.12 Manometric pattern in scleroderma. The record from three recording tips 5 cm apart is shown. The proximal tip shows a normal striated muscle contraction. No contractions are recorded from the middle and distal tips which are located in the smooth muscle zone.

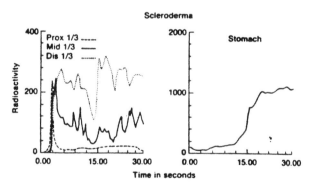

Fig. 30.13 Scintigraphy in scleroderma. The radioactive bolus is cleared promptly from the proximal oesophagus and mostly from the middle of the oesophagus. It remains in the distal oesophagus. More activity has entered the stomach than was seen in achalasia, but the entry was delayed. (Reproduced with permission from Russell et al 1981.)

either distal aperistalsis or total oesophageal body hypoperistalsis/aperistalsis. The second study suggested that steroid therapy improved both LOS pressure and peristaltic amplitude. It is not clear whether this caused clinical improvement as well.

CONTRACTION ABNORMALITIES ASSOCIATED WITH PAIN AND/OR DYSPHAGIA

It has long been recognized that pain resembling angina pectoris can be produced by the oesophagus. Chest pain and dysphagia of oesophageal origin have been given many descriptive names. Cardalgia, diffuse spasm, super-squeeze, nutcracker oesophagus, rosary-bead oesophagus, hypertensive LOS, hypercontracting LOS and non-specific motor disorder are a few of these terms that have been employed. In this lexicon of oesophageal diseases, I believe that one term deserves to be discarded – 'diffuse oesophageal spasm'. I say this because this term means so many things to different people. Many physicians assume any chest discomfort not attributable to coronary artery disease (CAD) must be 'oesophageal spasm'. The radiologist can often demonstrate multiple contraction waves occurring simultaneously in the oesophageal body (Fig. 30.14), and so this also is called oesophageal spasm whether or not the patient is actually having any chest symptoms during this radiologically demonstrated activity. Then the manometrist enters the scene, adding

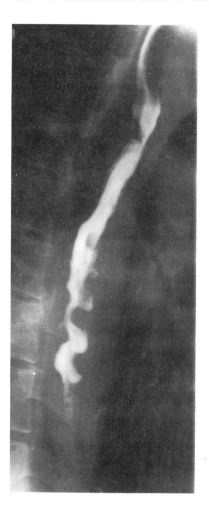
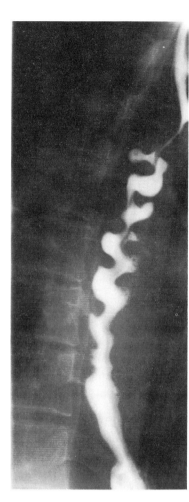

Fig. 30.14 Tertiary contractions in the oesophageal body. Two views of the same oesophagus taken several minutes apart. The oesophagus segments itself. Sometimes these segmentations are associated with chest pain. More often, they are asymptomatic. (Courtesy of C. Rohrmann MD.)

yet another circle to the Venn diagram. More unfortunately, the manometric fraternity cannot even agree within itself about the diagnostic criteria for diffuse spasm, the most important of which are:

1. Simultaneous contractions in response to a swallow intermixed with peristaltic waves after deglutition
2. Repetitive contractions
3. Spontaneous (not swallow-related) contractions
4. Prolonged baseline elevation after a swallow with superimposed multiple simultaneous contractions
5. High-amplitude long-duration peristaltic waves
6. Hypertensive sphincter
7. Incomplete LOS relaxation

Articles are now appearing which define and redefine diffuse oesophageal spasm (Richter & Castell 1984, Dalton et al 1991). Even when diffuse oesophageal spasm was redefined, it was found in only 56 of 1480 patients studied (Dalton et al 1991).

Another approach to classification which is much more appealing to me is to avoid these descriptive terms and describe the disorder by listing the type of motility pattern encountered. A scheme has been proposed by Clouse and Staiano which allows precise classification of oesophageal motor patterns (Clouse & Staiano 1992). Figure 30.15 shows the categories to which a tracing can be assigned. For instance, a normal tracing would be assigned to IA1a. According to the redefinition on diffuse spasm put forth by Richter and

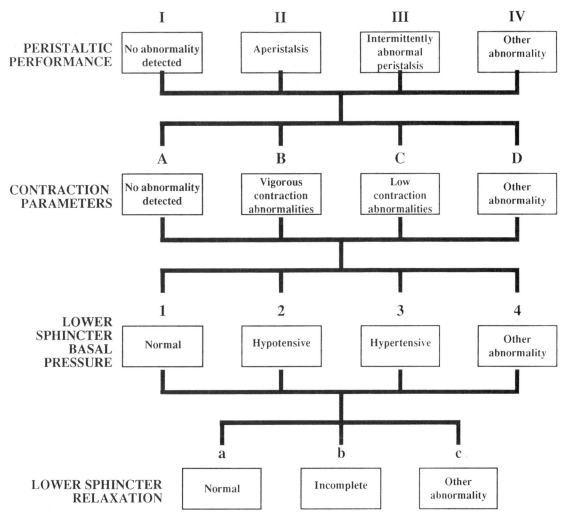

Fig. 30.15 Classification of oesophageal motor abnormalities. Each tracing is assigned a classification from each of four categories (peristaltic performance, contraction, LOS pressure and LOS relaxation). The classifications are mutually exclusive. (Clouse & Staiano 1992.)

Castell, a tracing would be coded IIIA or IIIB. There are 11 possibilities of coding depending on whether waves are of normal or high amplitude, and whether sphincter function is normal or abnormal. It is easily seen why the literature of diffuse spasm is so confused. Many studies have lumped several of these categories under one rubric; others have not even bothered to define or show manometric tracings of what is being described. To add to the confusion, many of the early papers used non-perfused manometric systems which underestimate peristaltic amplitudes, sphincter pressures and sphincteric relaxation. Better definitions as well as better instrumentation

will be of benefit in understanding this group of diseases.

Clinical manifestations of oesophageal body contraction abnormalities

Pain is certainly the most arresting symptom of oesophageal contraction abnormalities. Pain from contraction abnormalities can be easily confused with pain from myocardial ischaemia. Both types of pain can be brought on by exercise, radiate to the neck, jaw and left arm, and respond to sublingual nitroglycerin. Pain radiating straight through to the back seems to be much more common in patients with contraction abnormalities than in patients with CAD (Schofield et al 1988). Although both types of patients can have pain occur during exercise, patients with CAD often develop pain after the same amount of exercise, whereas oesophageal patients tend to vary widely in the exertion required to bring on chest pain. The delay in response to sublingual nitroglycerin also can differentiate between oesophageal and cardiac patients. Cardiac patients tend to note relief 3–5 min after sublingual nitroglycerin; the relief experienced by patients with oesophageal contraction abnormalities may require as long as 10–15 min for appearance. When all is said, differentiation of cardiac from oesophageal pain by clinical means alone can be difficult, if not impossible in an individual patient.

Dysphagia is the other primary manifestation of contraction abnormalities of the oesophageal body. Dysphagia is more characteristic of non-obstructive oesophageal disease. Liquid as well as solid boluses will arrest. Temperature of the bolus is also important; cold boluses give more symptoms and hot fluid will occasionally relieve dysphagia. If a solid bolus arrests, it is usually dislodged by re-swallowing or by a water chaser, rather than by being regurgitated. One very characteristic symptom of a contraction abnormality is the regurgitation of fluid back into the nasopharynx after a swallow of fluid has passed into the oesophagus. This presumably occurs when a lumen-obliterating contraction occurs over the entire fluid-filled oesophagus, forcing liquid both forwards and backwards. Unlike the situation in achalasia, patients with contraction abnormalities rarely lose weight.

Pathophysiology

How do the contraction abnormalities cause pain and dysphagia? At first, the answers to both questions seem obvious. However, more thought and experience shows this to be a difficult question to answer. Most studies investigating the relationship between chest pain and manometric abnormalities find high amplitude waves ('nutcracker oesophagus') to be the most common abnormality (Langevin & Castell 1991). Could tension receptors in the muscle wall explain the pain? Perhaps for those patients who complain of short 1–2 min episodes of chest pressure. However, more often the patient complains of a more prolonged episode of pain with waxing and waning of pain intensity and, in a few subjects I have observed during attacks, the increases in pain have correlated nicely with the increased pressure and duration of the high-amplitude waves. However, there is no manometric explanation

for the sustained background pain. An intriguing but untested possibility is prolonged contraction of the longitudinal muscle of the oesophagus.

Alternatively, do prolonged contractions of the oesophageal muscle lead to ischaemia? Since there is no single source of arterial input or outflow to the oesophagus, blood flow measurements are difficult to make by non-destructive methods. An intriguing paper by Mackenzie and colleagues measured the re-warming time of the distal oesophagus after cooling it with ice water (Mackenzie et al 1988). They found prolonged re-warming time in eight of nine patients thought to have oesophageal contraction abnormalities, and postulated that this prolongation was due to decreased blood flow to the oesophageal muscle. Some patients with microvascular angina (patients with no gross CAD who develop angina and increased myocardial vascular resistance during heart pacing and ergonovine stimulation) also have contraction abnormalities of the oesophagus (Cannon et al 1990). They also have increased vascular resistance of the small vessels in the forearm. Therefore, presumably these patients could have ischaemia during prolonged oesophageal contractions, and the effects of this ischaemia could produce prolonged discomfort.

Could the contraction abnormalities of the oesophagus merely be a clue to a more generalized problem with gut smooth muscle? Constipation has been reported in 10 of 54 patients with high-amplitude contractions (Clouse & Eckert 1986). Oesophageal contraction abnormalities have also been associated with irritable bowel syndrome (Whorwell et al 1981). In a patient with biliary dyskinesia, increased manometric resting and phasic pressure recordings from the sphincter of Oddi, as well as high amplitude oesophageal contractions have been reported (Johnson et al 1986). Since visceral pain is very poorly localized, it is possible that other smooth muscle groups (gallbladder, small bowel) are producing the chest pain instead of the oesophagus, thus explaining the poor correlation between oesophageal and pain records.

Dysphagia would seem to be easier to understand. Clearly, aperistalsis or amplitude of peristaltic waves under 30 mmHg are expected to be related to dysphagia. Why high amplitude waves are associated with dysphagia is less clear. Transport of barium and radioisotope can be either normal or abnormal (Chobanian et al 1986b, Drane et al 1987). Once the lumen of the oesophagus is occluded by a pressure of at least 30 mmHg, amplitude and duration values of the waves are not important (Massey et al 1991). It can only be surmised that high-amplitude waves may mark an oesophagus which can develop other motor abnormali-

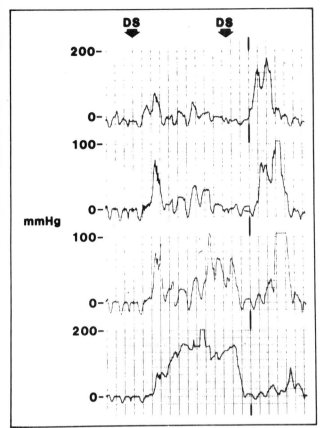

Fig. 30.16 Isolated contraction producing pain. In the distal tip, the first dry swallow produces a prolonged contraction (20 s) which was associated with chest pain. This was not seen elsewhere in the oesophageal body.

ties. Support for this idea is provided when long-term ambulatory monitoring demonstrates shifts in manometric patterns from progressive high-amplitude waves to simultaneous oesophageal contractions in the same individual (Stein et al 1991). Presumably, this same transition could occur during a meal, converting a wave from a high-amplitude peristaltic wave to a simultaneous wave, which might produce dysphagia. Another possibility is the occurrence of an isolated, prolonged contraction (Fig. 30.16) which might produce temporary bolus arrest.

Diagnosis

By definition, contraction abnormalities require recognition by a detection system. Historically, radiology was the method first used to detect contraction abnormalities associated with chest pain (Evans 1952), but

the short observation time possible with X-ray and the very intermittent nature of chest pain makes documentation by this method quite unusual. Occasionally, a patient will develop pain during a barium oesophagram, and demonstration of a lumen-obliterating contraction with retrograde transport of barium, or prolonged segmental spasm with bolus arrest will document a symptomatic contraction abnormality.

Oesophagoscopy is a relatively poor method for the evaluation of motor abnormalities of the oesophagus. It is an uncomfortable procedure, which is usually done under sedation and which produces only qualitative results. There are anecdotal reports of an oesophagoscope (or bougie) being gripped by a spastic oesophagus to the extent that withdrawal is difficult. This certainly must be taken as evidence for a contraction abnormality!

Manometry remains the mainstay of recognition of patients with oesophageal contraction abnormalities. Each laboratory should develop its own standard values for peristaltic amplitude, duration and velocity, but, in practice, values published in the literature are usually used (Clouse & Staiano 1983, Richter et al 1987b). Room-temperature water boluses are usually the stimuli for swallows but, occasionally, ice water or a solid bread bolus are used.

The most common abnormality associated with chest pain and/or dysphagia demonstrated in the manometric laboratory is high amplitude waves, sometimes of long duration and/or slow velocity (Fig. 30.17). Originally described in 1976 (Pope 1976), high-amplitude waves are the most common abnormality found in patient populations being evaluated for chest pain (Traube et al 1983, Brand et al 1977, Chobanian et al 1986a, Katz et al 1987).

The fact that a manometric abnormality is present in a patient with chest pain does not necessarily mean that a causal relationship exists. It is necessary to show that the manometric abnormality immediately precedes or coincides with the period of pain. Ideally, by examining a record taken during asymptomatic periods and periods of pain, the manometrist should be able to predict the onset, length and intensity of the period of pain. This ideal is very rarely attained. In one study, only 17 of 58 patients studied had pain during manometry; of these, only eight had abnormal waves (usually high-amplitude waves) coinciding with their pain (Brand et al 1977).

When the capability of performing ambulatory manometry became available, it was hoped that the yield would be increased by the longer period of observation. This prediction has only partially come true. In a combined study of 24-hour monitoring of pH and

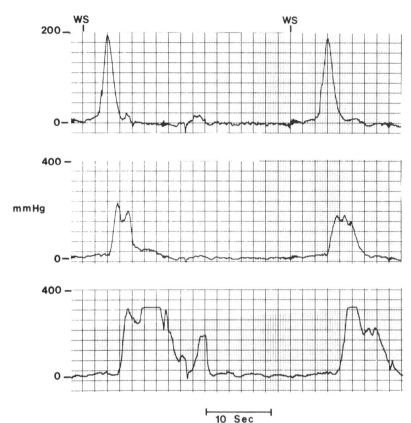

Fig. 30.17 High-amplitude long-duration waves associated with dysphagia and/or chest pain. This record was obtained from a patient with chest pain with a catheter with three tips 5 cm apart. Note that the scale is different. The distal tip has prolonged duration and a wave amplitude close to 400 mmHg.

pressure, abnormal results were detected during an episode of pain in 21 of 60 patients (35%) (Janssens et al 1986). Of these, nine patients had only motor abnormalities, four had only acid reflux, and eight had episodes of both abnormal reflux activity and acid reflux. In another study which required a pain-associated contraction abnormality to be significantly different than the asymptomatic motor activity recorded from the same patient, pain-associated contraction abnormalities were found in eight of 24 subjects tested (33%) (Peters et al 1988). If the total number of episodes of pain were used as the denominator instead of the number of patients, then only 12% of the episodes of pain were associated with contraction abnormalities. Both of these studies were performed on selected groups of individuals who had at least three episodes of pain a week and usually had daily discomfort.

One of the major problems is deciding whether an event (a high-amplitude wave, a drop in pH) is the cause of a symptom (chest pain). Long-term monitoring has shown that events are common, but events associated with symptoms are less common. Attempts have been made to surmount this problem by calculating a symptom index (the number of chest pain episodes associated with abnormal contractions divided by the number of chest pain episodes) (Wiener et al 1988). Another index, the symptom sensitivity index, calculates the number of abnormal contractions associated with pain divided by the number of episodes of abnormal contractions seen during monitoring (see Table 30.2) (Breumelhof & Smout 1991). One measures specificity, the other sensitivity. The correct index to confirm a causal relationship remains a matter of opinion. Indices below 25% have been interpreted as showing no relationship; above 75% suggest a causal relationship. These opinions will need to be validated by observing the effect of treatment. If treatment reverses abnormal contractions (currently a difficult feat) or acid reflux (somewhat easier), then a more precise value can be assigned to these two ratios.

If the yield of monitoring patients for spontaneous pain is low, then why not try to provoke pain by pharmacological or mechanical methods? Several pharmacological agents have been used:

Table 30.2 Calculation of symptoms sensitivity and specificity indices

Index	Calculation	Reference
Symptom sensitivity	$\dfrac{\text{Number of symptoms associated with event}}{\text{Number of events}}$	Breumelhof & Smout 1991
Symptom specificity	$\dfrac{\text{Number of symptoms associated with event}}{\text{Number of symptoms}}$	Wiener et al 1988

- Edrophonium
- Pentagastrin
- Vasopressin
- Hydrochloric acid
- Bethanechol
- Ergonovine

Edrophonium, a cholinesterase inhibitor (Langevin & Castell 1991), is the drug currently most in favour. It is safe, has a short period of action, and does not provoke pain in control subjects. In both control and chest pain patients, edrophonium increases contraction amplitudes. Therefore, a positive test requires both the reproduction of the patient's spontaneous pain and a change in oesophageal motility pattern.

Mechanical means have also been employed. Inflation of a balloon in the oesophagus has been used to provoke chest pain (Barish et al 1986, Richter et al 1986). Graded inflation of a balloon produced chest pain in 18 of 30 patients with chest pain and in six of 30 controls. Pain was produced at a lower balloon volume in the patients than in the controls; there was no overlap. In another study employing balloon distension in patients with chest pain, balloon distension not only produced chest pain, but also produced contractile activity distal to the balloon in 61% of the chest pain patients but in none of the control patients (Deschner et al 1990). This study did not note the clear separation of balloon volume threshold for pain reported earlier, but the authors did feel that balloon stimulation was more productive than pharmacological stimulation. This was not the experience of another group who found only a 5% yield with balloon stimulation and a 52% yield with pharmacologic stimulation (Ghillebert et al 1990).

There are several problems with the use of provocative tests. Pharmacologic stimulation is not specific for oesophageal muscle and may be stimulating other smooth muscle or vascular beds. Balloon distension is not 'physiological' in the sense that most patients with

chest pain of oesophageal origin are not eating at the time of pain, and so do not have localized distension from a bolus. Balloon size and wall characteristics may also vary from laboratory to laboratory. Most important, events such as abnormal contractions or acid reflux, detected during spontaneous pain, are not well predicted by the results of provocative tests. Patients responding to an acid drip may well show abnormal contractions but not reflux during spontaneous pain. Patients developing pain after edrophonium, a muscle stimulant, often do not show contraction abnormalities during spontaneous pain, but rather reflux. Provocative testing may be useful to determine threshold sensitivity or reactivity, but it cannot be used in an individual patient to predict the cause of chest pain.

Most of the foregoing discussion has focused on high amplitude waves as the contraction abnormality responsible for symptoms, but clearly there are other patterns which merit consideration. Prolonged elevations of the baseline on which are superimposed simultaneous contractions can also be associated with chest pain. This pattern is what I used to call diffuse oesophageal spasm (when I used to use the term!). Pain is experienced during the period of baseline elevation. Sometimes the baseline elevation is only 4–5 mmHg; it is difficult to imagine why such a small increase in pressure should provoke so much pain. Isolated contractions such as the one shown in Fig. 30.16 can also be associated with pain, usually short-lived.

Other patterns of abnormal motor activity can be found in patients with dysphagia. Some patients will have a peristaltic wave in response to a 'dry' rather than a 'wet' (water bolus) swallow, the exact opposite of the usual situation. Contraction of the upper half of the oesophagus as a unit, followed by contraction of the lower half of the oesophagus has been seen in a patient with dysphagia. Dropped peristalsis, when a wave begins normally but disappears before reaching the distal oesophagus, may also be observed in patients with mild dysphagia. Combined manometry with a bolus can be useful in sorting out some of these situations (Mellow 1983).

Other test modalities can be used in an attempt to understand dysphagia. An intraluminal force transducer can be used to measure the isometric contraction force of the oesophagus (Pope & Horton 1972). Both increased force and decreased force has been detected in patients whose simultaneous pressure motility tracing is normal. The intraluminal force transducer is undoubtedly responding to a combination of circular and longitudinal muscle contractions. Frictional forces also affect output of the transducer.

Scintigraphy is also a sensitive way to measure

oesophageal motor function. Abnormalities in radioactive bolus transport have been found in patients whose manometric tracings were within normal limits (Blackwell et al 1983, Kjellén et al 1984, Russell et al 1981). This is true whether a liquid or solid bolus is used as a test; solid boluses seem to have a higher sensitivity. Even in a paper which concluded that scintigraphy had little value, 11 of 33 patients with oesophageal symptoms and normal manometry had abnormal scintigraphic results (Mughal et al 1986). My own experience is that many patients with dysphagia as a prime symptom who are shown to have normal manometry will have abnormal scintigraphic results.

Treatment of contraction abnormalities

When the subject of painful oesophageal contractions is examined, it becomes apparent that a great deal more effort has been expended on diagnosis than on therapy. This may reflect the clinical observation that patients with painful contraction abnormalities are extremely difficult to manage. Many medications have been tried; few have proved useful. Most of the reported trials are open trials performed on patients whose manometric characteristics have not been carefully defined. The following are that some of the agents have been employed in treating painful contraction abnormalities of the oesophagus:

- Nitroglycerin
- Isosorbide
- Hydralazine
- Hyoscyamine
- Nifedipine
- Diltiazem
- Trazodone

When the relief of pain is the desired endpoint, then it is essential to employ a double-blind experimental design, as there is a strong placebo response in these conditions, at least initially. Most of the adequate trials have employed calcium-channel blockers such as nifedipine and diltiazem. Although these drugs can reduce peristaltic amplitude values in both control subjects and those with contraction abnormalities, their clinical results in relieving pain are somewhat disappointing. In a placebo-controlled trial, Nasrallah et al noted a clinical improvement in both chest pain and dysphagia in patients treated with nifedipine 10 mg three times a day (Nasrallah et al 1985). Most of those patients were described as having 'hypertensive LOSs'. In a trial of patients with high-amplitude contractions, no benefit over placebo was noted (Richter et al 1987a). A review paper also reports varying results in trials

with nifedipine (Baunack & Weirauch 1991). Diltiazem is another agent in which preliminary studies look promising. In a double-blind study completed by 14 patients, 60 mg or 90 mg of diltiazem given four times a day caused a significant decrease in the pain index (Cattau et al 1991). Dysphagia also improved, although the improvement did not reach statistical significance. There was also a slight decrease in peristaltic amplitude in the treated group. Another study with very small numbers was reported as showing no effect of diltiazem in the treatment of diffuse oesophageal spasm; however five of eight patients seemed to have an improvement in pain scores (Drenth et al 1990).

In an attempt to treat the possible psychological factors which seem to be linked to contraction abnormalities of the oesophagus, the antidepressant trazodone in doses of 100–150 mg/day was reported to improve chest patients' sense of well-being (Clouse et al 1987). However, the chest pain index showed no improvement over placebo; both groups improved significantly over the 6-week trial period.

Mechanical means have been used to treat patients with contraction disorders. In a trial of pneumatic dilatation, eight of nine patients with high LOS pressures and diffuse oesophageal spasm reported improvement in dysphagia and regurgitation after dilatation (Ebert et al 1983). Mean LOS pressure was reduced from 34 to 19 mmHg, and improvement persisted for at least 3 years. A trial of dilatation with either a large (54 French) or a small (24 French) bougie, led to equivalent clinical improvement in symptoms, leading the authors to believe that they were demonstrating a placebo effect (Winters et al 1984). An alternate explanation exists – perhaps dilatation really does help, no matter what sized dilator is used!

Surgical therapy has also been used, although there are very few modern series reporting good preoperative manometric data and good postoperative follow-up on a significant number of patients. One series with a heterogeneous population of contraction abnormalities reports 'good-quality' results in 32 of 34 patients subjected to long myotomy (Henderson et al 1987). Five patients with high amplitude contractions have been treated by extended myotomy; all benefited by the procedure (Horton & Goff 1986, Traube et al 1987). Yet Richter and Castell (1987) state they have never felt the need to refer anyone for a long myotomy for symptomatic relief.

With this rather discouraging and contradictory group of results of medical and surgical therapy, is there any point in pursuing the diagnosis of a contraction abnormality? One major benefit in reassuring the patient who is demonstrated to have an oesophageal cause for chest pain and understands this relationship, is much less apprehension. The reassured patient is less likely to seek repeated diagnostic tests than is the patient who has only been told that coronary disease is not present (Ward et al 1987).

SUMMARY

The study of oesophageal motor disorders has ad-vanced a great deal in the last 30 years. Advances in technology (low-compliance manometry, ambulatory manometry, scintigraphy, video-fluoroscopy) have led to better descriptions of oesophageal motility in health and disease. There is still a crying need for standardization of terminology and for controlled trials of therapy. I look forward to the next 30 years with anticipation!

REFERENCES

Aggestrup S, Uddman R, Sundler F et al 1983 Lack of vasoactive intestinal peptide nerves in esophageal achalasia. Gastroenterology 84: 924–927

Barish C F, Castell D O, Richter J E 1986 Graded esophageal balloon distension: a new provocative test for non-cardiac chest pain. Dig Dis Sci 31: 1292–1298

Baron M, Arzoumanian A 1991 Radionuclide esophageal transit studies in progressive systemic sclerosis: an analysis of longitudinal data. J Rheumatol 18: 1837–1840

Baunack A R, Weirauch T R 1991 Clinical efficacy of nifedipine and other calcium channel antagonists in patients with primary esophageal motor dysfunction. Arzneim-Forsch/Drug Res 41: 595–602

Bianco A, Cagossi M, Scrimieri D et al 1986 Appearance of esophageal peristalsis in treated idiopathic achalasia. Dig Dis Sci 31: 40–48

Blackwell J N, Hannan W J, Adam R D et al 1983 Radionuclide transit studies in the detection of oesophageal dysmotility. Gut 24: 421–426

Bonavina L, Khan N A, DeMeester T R 1985 Pharyngoesophageal dysfunction. Arch Surg 120: 541–549

Bortolotti M, Labo G, Bragaglia R B et al 1982 Electromyographic study in diffuse esophageal spasm and achalasia in: Wienbeck M (ed) Motility of the digestive tract. Raven Press, New York, pp 319–331

Brand D L, Martin D, Pope II C E 1977 Esophageal manometrics in patients with angina-like chest pain. Am J Dig Dis 22: 300–304

Breumelhof R, Smout A J P M 1991 The symptom sensitivity index: a valuable additional parameter in 24-hour esophageal pH recording. Am J Gastroenterol 86: 160–164

Bushmann M, Dobmeyer S M, Lecker L et al 1989 Swallowing abnormalities and their response to treatment in Parkinson's disease. Neurology 39: 1309–1314

Cannon R O, Cattau E L, Yakshe P N et al 1990 Coronary flow reserve, esophageal motility and chest pain with angiographically normal coronary arteries. Am J Med 88: 217–222

Carette S, Lacourciere Y, Lavoie S et al 1985 Radionuclide esophageal transit in progressive systemic sclerosis. J Rheumatol 12: 478–481

Cassella R R, Brown A L Jr, Sayre G P et al 1964 Achalasia of the esophagus: pathologic and etiologic conditions. Ann Surg 160: 474–487

Cattau E L, Castell D O, Johnson D A et al 1991 Diltiazem therapy for symptoms associated with nutcracker esophagus. Am J Gastroenterol 86: 272–276

Chen M Y M, Ott D J, Peele V N et al 1990 Oropharynx in patients with cerebrovascular disease: evaluation with video fluoroscopy. Radiology 176: 641–643

Chobanian S J, Benjamin S B, Curtis D J et al 1986a Systematic esophageal evaluation of patients with noncardiac chest pain. Arch Int Med 146: 1505–1508

Chobanian S J, Curtis D J, Benjamin S B et al 1986b Radiology of the nutcracker esophagus. J Clin Gastroenterol 8: 230–232

Clouse R E, Eckert T C 1986 Gastrointestinal symptoms of patients with esophageal contraction abnormalities. Dig Dis Sci 31: 236–240

Clouse R E, Staiano A 1983 Contraction abnormalities of the esophageal body in patients referred for manometry: a new approach to manometric classification. Dig Dis Sci 28: 784–791

Clouse R E, Staiano A 1992 Manometric patterns using esophageal body and lower sphincter characteristics. Dig Dis Sci 37: 289–296

Clouse R E, Lustman P J, Eckert T C et al 1987 Low-dose trazodone for symptomatic patients with esophageal contraction abnormalities: a double-blind, placebo-controlled trial. Gastroenterology 92: 1027–1036

Coccia G, Bortolotti M, Michetti P et al 1991 Prospective clinical and manometric study comparing pneumatic dilatation and sublingual nifedipine in the treatment of esophageal achalasia. Gut 32: 604–606

Costigan D J, Clouse R E 1983 Achalasia-like esophagus from amyloidosis: successful treatment with pneumatic bag dilatation. Dig Dis Sci 28: 763–765

Cruse J P, Edwards D A W, Smith J F et al 1979 The pathology of cricopharyngeal dysphagia. Histopathology 3: 223–232

Csendes A, Braghetto I, Henriquez A et al 1989 Late results of a prospective randomized study comparing forceful dilatation and oesophagomyotomy in patients with achalasia. Gut 30: 299–304

Csendes A, Braghetto I, Burdiles P et al 1991 Comparison of forceful dilatation and esophagomyotomy in patients with achalasia of the esophagus. Hepato Gastroenterol 38: 502–505

Dalton C B, Castell D O, Hewson E G et al 1991 Diffuse esophageal spasm. A rare motility disorder not characterized by high-amplitude contractions. Dig Dis Sci 36: 1025–1028

Dantas R O 1988 Idiopathic achalasia and chagasic megaesophagus. J Clin Gastroenterol 10: 13–15

Dantas R O, Cook I J, Dodds W J et al 1990 Biomechanics of cricopharyngeal bars. Gastroenterology 99: 1269–1274

Davidson A, Russell C, Littlejohn G O 1985 Assessment of esophageal abnormalities in progressive systemic sclerosis using radionuclide transit. J Rheumatol 12: 472–477

Deschner W K, Maher K A, Cattau E L et al 1990

Intraesophageal balloon distension versus drug provocation in the evaluation of noncardiac chest pain. Am J Gastroenterol 85: 938–943

Dodds W J, Stewart E T, Kishk S M et al 1986 Radiologic amyl nitrite test for distinguishing pseudoachalasia from idiopathic achalasia. A J R 146: 21–23

Dooley C P, Taylor I L, Valenzuela J E 1983 Impaired acid secretion and pancreatic polypeptide release in some patients with achalasia. Gastroenterology 84: 809–813

Drane W E, Johnson D A, Hagan D P et al 1987 'Nutcracker' esophagus: diagnosis with radionuclide esophageal scintigraphy versus manometry. Radiology 163: 33–37

Drenth J P H, Bos L P, Engels G J B 1990 Efficacy of diltiazem in the treatment of diffuse oesophageal spasm. Aliment Pharmacol Therapy 4: 411–416

Ebert E C, Ouyang A, Wright S H et al 1983 Pneumatic dilatation in patients with symptomatic diffuse esophageal spasm and lower esophageal sphincter dysfunction. Dig Dis Sci 28: 481–485

Eckardt V F, Nix W, Kraus W et al 1986 Esophageal motor function in patients with muscular dystrophy. Gastroenterology 90: 628–635

Eckardt V F, Krause J, Bolle D 1989 Gastrointestinal transit and gastric acid secretion in patients with achalasia. Dig Dis Sci 34: 665–671

Ellis F H, Schlegel J F, Lynch V P et al 1969 Cricopharyngeal myotomy for pharyngoesophageal diverticulum. Ann Surg 170: 340–349

Estrada C A, Lewandowski C, Schubert T T et al 1990 Esophageal involvement in secondary amyloidosis mimicking achalasia. J Clin Gastroenterol 12: 447–450

Evans W 1952 Oesophageal contraction and cardiac pain. Lancet 2: 1091–1097

Faussone-Pellegrini M S, Cortesini C 1985 The muscle coat of the lower esophageal sphincter in patients with achalasia and hypertensive sphincter. An electron microscopic study. J Submicrosc Cytol 17: 673–685

Feldman M 1988 Southwestern internal medicine conference: esophageal achalasia syndromes. Am J Med Sci 295: 60–81

Frieling T, Berges W, Lubke H J et al 1988 Upper esophageal sphincter function in patients with Zenker's diverticulum. Dysphagia 3: 90–92

Friesen D L, Henderson R D, Hanna W 1983 Ultrastructure of the oesophageal muscle in achalasia and diffuse spasm. AJCP 79: 119–125

Gelfond M, Rozen P, Gilat T 1982 Isosorbide dinitrate and nifedipine treatment of achalasia: a clinical, manometric and radionuclide evaluation. Gastroenterology 83: 963–969

Ghillebert G, Janssens J, Vantrappen G et al 1990 Ambulatory 24-hour intraoesophageal pH and pressure recordings and provocation tests in the diagnosis of chest pain of oesophageal origin. Gut 31: 738–744

Gonzalez E M, Alvarez A G, Garcia I L et al 1988 Results of surgical treatment of esophageal achalasia. Multicenter retrospective study of 1,856 cases. Int Surg 73: 69–77

Gordon C, Hewer R L, Wade D T 1987 Dysphagia in acute stroke. Brit Med J 295: 411–414

Gutierrez F, Valenzuela J E, Ehresmann G R et al 1982 Esophageal dysfunction in patients with mixed connective tissue diseases and systemic lupus erythematosus. Dig Dis Sci 27: 592–597

Hendel L, Stentoft P, Aggestrup S 1989 The progress of oesophageal involvement in progressive systemic sclerosis during D-penicillamine treatment. Scand J Rheumatology 18: 149–155

Henderson R D, Ryder D, Maryatt G 1987 Extended esophageal myotomy and short total fundoplication hernia repair in diffuse esophageal spasm: five year review in 34 patients. Ann Thorac Surg 43: 25–31

Holloway R H, Krosin G, Lange R C et al 1983 Radionuclide esophageal emptying of a solid meal to quantitate results of therapy in achalasia. Gastroenterology 84: 771–776

Holloway R H, Dodds W J, Helm J F et al 1986 Integrity of cholinergic innervation to the lower esophageal sphincter in achalasia. Gastroenterology 90: 924–929

Holloway R H, Wyman J B, Dent J 1989 Failure of transient lower oesophageal sphincter relaxation in response to gastric distension in patients with achalasia: evidence for neural mediation of transient lower oesophageal sphincter relaxation. Gut 30: 762–767

Horowitz M, Maddox A, Maddern G J et al 1987 Gastric and esophageal emptying in dystrophica myotonia. Gastroenterology 92: 570–577

Horton M, Goff J S 1986 Surgical treatment of nutcracker esophagus. Dig Dis Sci 31: 878–883

Hurwitz A L, Duranceau A 1978 Upper-esophageal sphincter dysfunction. Dig Dis Sci 23: 275–281

Janssens J, Vantrappen G, Ghillebert G 1986 24-hour recording of esophageal pressure and pH in patients with non-cardiac chest pain. Gastroenterology 90: 1978–1984

Johnson D A, Cattau E L, Winters C 1986 Biliary dyskinesia with associated high amplitude peristaltic contractions. Am J Gastroenterol 81: 254–256

Johnson D A, Drane W E, Curran J et al 1987 Metoclopramide response in patients with progressive systemic sclerosis. Arch Int Med 147: 1597–1601

Jones B, Donner M W, Rubesin S E et al 1987 Pharyngeal findings in 21 patients with achalasia of the esophagus. Dysphagia 2: 87–92

Kahrilas P J, Kishk S M, Helm J F et al 1987 Comparison of achalasia and pseudoachalasia. Am J Med 82: 439–446

Katz P O, Dalton C B, Richter J E et al 1987 Esophageal testing of patients with noncardiac chest pain or dysphagia. Ann Int Med 106: 593–597

Kilman W J, Goyal R K 1976 Disorders of pharyngeal and upper esophageal sphincter motor function. Arch Int Med 136: 592–601

Kjellén G, Svedberg J B, Tibbling L 1984 Solid bolus transit by esophageal scintigraphy in patients with dysphagia and normal manometry and radiography. Dig Dis Sci 29: 1–5

Langevin S, Castell D O 1991 Esophageal motility disorders and chest pain. Med Clin N Amer 75: 1045–1063

Lichter I 1978 Motor disorder in pharyngoesophageal pouch. J Thorac Cardiovasc Surg 76: 272–275

Lindgren S, Ekberg O 1990 Cricopharyngeal myotomy in the treatment of dysphagia. Clin Otolaryngol 15: 221–227

Logemann J A, Kahrilas P J, Kobara M et al 1989 The benefit of head rotation on pharyngoesophageal dysphagia. Arch Phys Med Rehabil 70: 767–771

McGouran R C M, Galloway J M, Spence D S et al 1988 Does measurement of yield pressure at the cardia during endoscopy provide information on the function of the lower oesophageal sphincter mechanism? Gut 29: 275–278

MacKenzie J, Belch J, Land D et al 1988 Oesophageal ischaemia in motility disorders associated with chest pain. Lancet ii: 592–595

Marshall J B, Kretschmar J M, Gerhardt D C et al 1990 Gastrointestinal manifestations of mixed connective tissue disease. Gastroenterology 98: 1232–1238

Massey B T, Dodds W J, Hogan W J et al 1991 Abnormal esophageal motility: an analysis of concurrent radiographic and manometric findings. Gastroenterology 101: 344–354

Mellow M H 1983 Esophageal motility during food ingestion: a physiologic test of esophageal motor function. Gastroenterology 85: 370–377

Montesi A, Pesaresi A, Cavalli M L et al 1991 Oropharyngeal and esophageal function in scleroderma. Dysphagia 6: 219–223

Mughal M M, Marples M, Bancewitz J 1986 Scintigraphic assessment of oesophageal motility: what does it show and how reliable is it? Gut 27: 946–953

Nasrallah S M, Tommaso C L, Singleton R T et al 1985 Primary esophageal motor disorders: clinical response to nifedipine. Southern Med J 78: 312–315

Palmer E D 1976 Disorders of the cricopharyngeal muscle: a review. Gastroenterology 71: 510–519

Peters L, Maas L, Petty D et al 1988 Spontaneous noncardiac chest pain: evaluation by 24-hour ambulatory esophageal motility and pH monitoring. Gastroenterology 94: 878–886

Ponce J, Miralbes M, Garrigues V et al 1986 Return of esophageal peristalsis after Heller's myotomy for idiopathic achalasia. Dig Dis Sci 31: 545–547

Pope II C E 1976 Abnormalities of esophageal amplitude and force – a clue to the etiology of chest pain? in: Vantrappen G (ed.) Proceedings of the Fifth International Symposium on Gastrointestinal Motility. Herentals Typoff Press, Herentals, Belgium pp 380–386

Pope II C E, Horton P F 1972 Intraluminal force transducer measurement of human oesophageal peristalsis. Gut 13: 464–470

Qualman S J, Haupt H M, Yang P et al 1984 Esophageal Lewy bodies associated with ganglion cell loss in achalasia. Gastroenterology 87: 848–856

Richter J E, Castell D O 1984 Diffuse esophageal spasm: a reappraisal. Ann Int Med 100: 242–245

Richter J E, Castell D O 1987 Surgical myotomy for nutcracker esophagus. Dig Dis Sci 32: 95–96

Richter J E, Barish C F, Castell D O 1986 Abnormal sensory perception in patients with esophageal chest pain. Gastroenterology 91: 845–852

Richter J E, Dalton C B, Bradley L A et al 1987a Oral nifedipine in the treatment of noncardiac chest pain in patients with the nutcracker esophagus. Gastroenterology 93: 21–28

Richter J E, Wu W C, Johns D N et al 1987b Esophageal manometry in 95 healthy adult volunteers: variability of pressures with age and frequency of 'abnormal' contractions. Dig Dis Sci 32: 583–592

Robertson C S, Hardy J G, Atkinson M 1989 Quantitative assessment of the response to therapy in achalasia of the cardia. Gut 30: 768–773

Rozman R W, Achkar E 1990 Features distinguishing secondary achalasia from primary achalasia. Am J Gastroenterol 85: 1327–1330

Russak E, Pope II C E 1990 Proximal esophageal

contractions suggest vagal integrity in achalasia. Gastroenterology 98: A386

Russell C O H, Hill L D, Holmes III E R et al 1981 Radionuclide transit: a sensitive screening test for esophageal dysfunction. Gastroenterology 80: 887–892

Schofield P M, Whorwell P J, Jones P E et al 1988 Differentiation of 'esophageal' and 'cardiac' chest pain. Am J Cardiol 62: 315–316

Stein H J, DeMeester P–R, Eypasch E P et al 1991 Ambulatory 24-hour esophageal manometry in the evaluation of esophageal motor disorders and noncardiac chest pain. Surgery 110: 753–763

Tibbling L, Ask P, Pope II C E 1986 Electromyography of human oesophageal smooth muscle. Scand J Gastroenterol 21: 559–567

Todorczuk J R, Aliperti G, Staiano A et al 1991 Reevaluation of manometric criteria for vigorous achalasia. Dig Dis Sci 36: 274–278

Traube M, Albibi R, McCallum R W 1983 High-amplitude peristaltic esophageal contractions associated with chest pain. J A M A 250: 2655–2659

Traube M, Tummala V, Baue E et al 1987 Surgical myotomy in patients with high-amplitude peristaltic esophageal contractions. Dig Dis Sci 32: 16–21

Treacy W L, Baggenstoss A H, Slocumb C H et al 1963 Scleroderma of the esophagus: a correlation of histologic and physiologic findings. Ann Intern Med 59: 351–356

van Overbeek J J M 1991 Upper esophageal sphincterotomy in dysphagic patients with and without a diverticulum. Dysphagia 6: 228–234

Vantrappen G, Janssens J, Hellemans J et al 1979 Achalasia, diffuse esophageal spasm, and related motility disorders. Gastroenterology 76: 450–457

Ward B W, Wu W C, Richter J E et al 1987 Long-term follow-up of symptomatic status of patients with non-cardiac chest pain: is diagnosis of esophageal etiology helpful? Am J Gastroenterol 82: 215–218

Weihrauch T R, Korting G W, Ewe K et al 1978 Esophageal dysfunction and its pathogenesis in progressive systemic sclerosis. Klin Wochenschr 56: 963–968

Whorwell P J, Clouter C, Smith C L 1981 Oesophageal motility in the irritable bowel syndrome. Brit Med J 282: 1101–1102

Wiener G J, Richter J E, Cooper J B et al 1988 The symptom index: a clinically important parameter of ambulatory 24-h esophageal pH monitoring. Am J Gastroenterology 83: 358–361

Wilson P S, Bruce-Lockhart F J 1990 Video fluoroscopy in motor neurone disease prior to cricopharyngeal myotomy. Ann Roy Coll Surg Engl 72: 375–377

Wilson J A, Pryde A, Piris J et al 1989 Pharyngoesophageal dysmotility in globus sensation. Arch Otolaryngol Head Neck Surg 115: 1086–1090

Winters C, Artnak E J, Benjamin S B et al 1984 Esophageal bouginage in symptomatic patients with the nutcracker esophagus. J A M A 252: 363–366

Wright R A, Penner D B 1981 Myxedema and upper esophageal dysmotility. Dig Dis Sci 26: 376–377

Ziegler K, Sanft C, Friedrich M et al 1990 Endosonographic appearance of the esophagus in achalasia. Endoscopy 22: 1–4

31. Gastro-oesophageal reflux disease

J. E. Richter

Gastro-oesophageal reflux (GOR) is a multifactorial process whose importance lies in its ubiquity, diverse clinical presentation, and potential morbidity. It is the most common malady afflicting the oesophagus and is probably the most prevalent clinical condition involving the alimentary tract.

Gastro-oesophageal reflux disease (GORD) is defined as the sequelae, both clinical and histopathologic, of the movement of gastroduodenal contents into the oesophagus. GORD, however, is a spectrum of disease. GOR occurs without adverse consequences, for example, in many healthy individuals. Episodes of 'physiological' reflux are typically postprandial, short-lived, asymptomatic, and almost never occur at night. 'Pathologic' reflux leads to histopathologic and clinical abnormalities. The term 'reflux oesophagitis' refers to mucosal injury, such as epithelial erosions, ulcerations, or hyperplasia, accompanied by inflammation. Generally, reflux oesophagitis is accompanied by clinical symptoms, but these histologic alterations may be asymptomatic.

EPIDEMIOLOGY

Heartburn is the classic symptom of GORD and, as such, may serve as a useful marker for epidemiologic studies. Nebel et al (1976) were the first to assess the prevalence of GORD in the general population. They found that 7% of 335 hospital employees noted heartburn at least daily and 15% experienced heartburn monthly. In a Gallup survey, even higher prevalence rates for heartburn were found; 25% of 800 randomly questioned adults noticed heartburn at least once in the previous month (Gallup 1988). Over 40% of the patients took antacids for their heartburn, but only a quarter sought medical attention from their physicians. The highest prevalence rates for heartburn are found in pregnant women with over 50% reportedly affected particularly in the last two trimesters (Castro 1967).

Although heartburn and 'oesophagitis' are often considered together, this may not be the case. Depending upon the 'gold standard' used for defining GORD, 30–79% of reflux patients have evidence of oesophagitis (DeMeester et al 1980, Johnsson et al 1987). These data suggest a 3–4% prevalence of oesophagitis in the general population with oesophagitis increasing dramatically after the age of 50 years (Brunnen et al 1969). Minimal information exists on the incidence of different stages of oesophagitis. Recent series suggest that the vast majority of patients suffer mild or moderate forms of oesophagitis (Weinbeck et al 1989). Analyses of the sex ratio of GORD show roughly equal portions of affected males and females but a male preponderance of oesophagitis (2:1–3:1) and Barrett's oesophagus (10:1) (Weinbeck & Barnert 1989). Although GORD does not affect longevity, it can impair quality of life prior to appropriate diagnosis and treatment. Moreover, the complications of GORD (oesophageal stricture, Barrett's oesophagus, oesophageal adenocarcinoma, gastrointestinal haemorrhage, pulmonary, or ear, nose and throat complications) may lead to considerable morbidity.

PATHOPHYSIOLOGY

In 1935, Winkelstein was the first to suggest that the common form of oesophagitis was related to the digestive action of gastric juices on the oesophageal mucosa (Winkelstein 1935). Before this time, oesophagitis was attributed to causes such as infection, chemical irritants, or a secondary effect of cardiospasm or neoplasia. The term 'reflux oesophagitis' was later introduced in 1946 by Allison, emphasizing that irritant gastric juices were refluxed from the stomach into the oesophagus (Allison 1946). The modern concept of reflux disease has since undergone a process of evolution. In the 1940s and 1950s, many investigators believed that reflux oesophagitis was caused by abnormal mechanical factors, primarily related to a sliding hiatal hernia. In the 1960s, attention shifted to the lower oesophageal

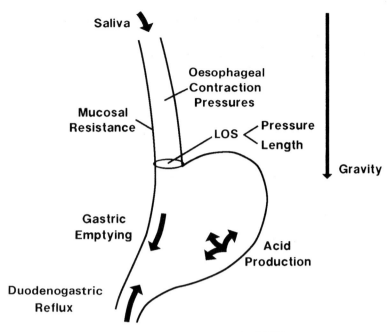

Fig. 31.1 The major factors involved in GORD.

sphincter (LOS) and the belief that a feeble or atonic sphincter was the major culprit in the production of oesophagitis. During the last few decades, consensus has developed that GORD is a multifactorial process whose pathogenesis may vary in a given patient. The multiple factors that may contribute to GORD include the barrier to reflux provided by the LOS, the ability of the oesophagus to clear refluxed material, the potential of refluxed material to damage the oesophagus, the role of the stomach in terms of gastric secretion, volume, distention and emptying, the intrinsic resistance of the oesophageal mucosa to damage, and hiatus hernia (Fig. 31.1). Symptomatic GORD results when the balance between aggressive factors (acid reflux, potency of refluxate) and defensive factors (oesophageal acid clearance, mucosal resistance), tilts in favour of the aggressive forces.

Lower oesophageal sphincter

The LOS is a high pressure zone at the gastro-oesophageal junction interposed between the positive intra-abdominal pressure and the negative intrathoracic pressure. Although this region can be identified readily by manometric studies, it is not a distinct anatomic sphincter. The high pressure zone results from the combined tonic activity of the distal oesophageal smooth muscle, smooth muscle fibres from the fundus of the stomach (gastric sling), and the pinchcock-like

activity of the crural portion of the diaphragm. In the resting state, the end expiratory pressure represents the contribution from the smooth muscle of the LOS while the end inspiratory pressure fluctuations are due to crural diaphragm activity (Fig. 31.2) (Mittal et al 1989). The LOS functions as the primary barrier to the reflux of gastroduodenal contents and accordingly is vital in preventing reflux.

The LOS is a dynamic sphincter. Tone of the LOS varies throughout the day, particularly in relation to ingested food such as fat, alcohol, or chocolate and after some medications (e.g. anticholinergics, theophylline, sedatives) and cigarette smoking (Castell 1975). Therefore, a single isolated determination of basal LOS pressure may not be an accurate representation of daily events. Historically, this has been a confusing issue because basal values of LOS pressures have correlated poorly with clinical evidence of reflux disease (Fig. 31.3). It was only with simultaneous prolonged monitoring of intraoesophageal pH and pressure that this controversy was resolved. Dent et al (1980) observed that reflux occurred primarily when LOS pressure was low but this could occur by one of three mechanisms: (1) spontaneous reflux associated with transient relaxation of the LOS; (2) transient increase in intra-abdominal pressure resulting in 'stress reflux'; and (3) free reflux (Fig. 31.4). Regardless of the mechanism generating a low LOS pressure, the common denominator permitting acid reflux is the creation of a

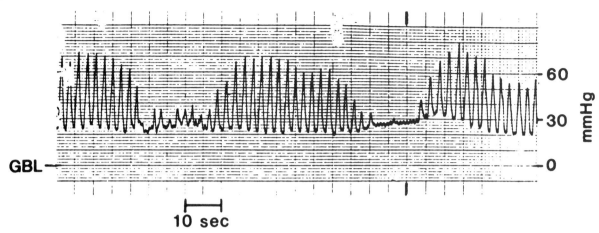

Fig. 31.2   Demonstration of the two major contributory factors to LOS pressure. In the resting state, the end expiratory pressure (30 mmHg) represents the contribution from the smooth muscle of the LOS. The respiratory pressure fluctuations are due to crural diaphragm activity with maximum pressures at end inspiration approaching 60 mmHg. Thus, the end expiration pressure may be the best indicator of true intrinsic sphincter tone.

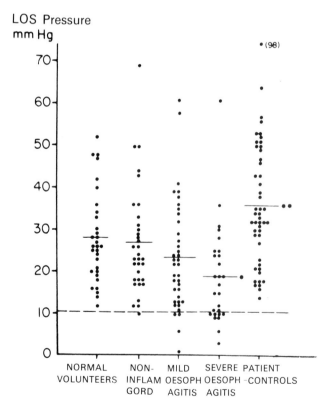

Fig. 31.3   Pull-through values of LOS pressures in 177 subjects. Overall, LOS pressures did not distinguish the five groups. Only the patient group with severe oesophagitis had a mean LOS pressure significantly lower than that of normal volunteers (p < 0.01). In this group, 8 patients had LOS pressures < 10 mmHg and two had LOS pressures < 6 mmHg. (Reprinted with permission from Kahrilas et al 1986.)

'common cavity phenomenon' equalization of intragastric and intraoesophageal pressures.

Transient LOS relaxation accounts for nearly all episodes of reflux in normal subjects and 65% of episodes in patients with GORD (Dent et al 1980, Dodds et al 1982). The descriptor 'transient' is used to distinguish this phenomena from swallow-induced LOS relaxation. As shown in Figure 31.5, transient LOS relaxations occur without an antecedent pharyngeal contraction, persist for longer periods (5–30 s) than do swallow-induced LOS relaxations and are generally unaccompanied by oesophageal peristalsis. The likelihood of reflux during a transient LOS relaxation is influenced by both the circumstance of the recording and the proximity to a meal with different investigators reporting reflux during as many as 95% (Dent et al 1980) or as few as 10–15% (Mittal & McCallum 1987) of transient LOS relaxations.

The aetiology of transient LOS relaxations is unclear. Some authors suggest that this is a variant of the belch reflex, or secondary to provocative sensory stimuli such as gastric distention or mechanical stimulation of the pharynx (Holloway et al 1985, Mittal et al 1990). The frequency of LOS relaxation is greatly increased by distention of the stomach by gas or after a meal (Fig. 31.6) in the upright but not the supine position (Holloway et al 1991). These relaxations are totally suppressed during deep sleep but may be present during the lighter stages of REM sleep (Freidin et al 1991). The absence of transient LOS relaxations in achalasia supports the hypothesis that they are mediated by peripheral nerves possibly located in the fundus of the stomach (Holloway et al 1989).

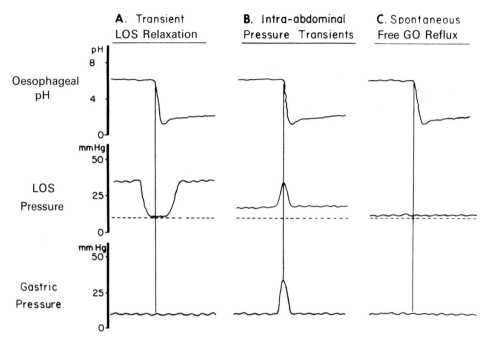

Fig. 31.4   Mechanisms of LOS dysfunction in GORD. **A** Transient LOS relaxation not preceded by a swallow. **B** An increase in intra-abdominal pressure that overcomes low resting LOS pressure, i.e. stress reflux. **C** Spontaneous free reflux across an atonic LOS. (Reprinted with permission from Dodds et al 1982.)

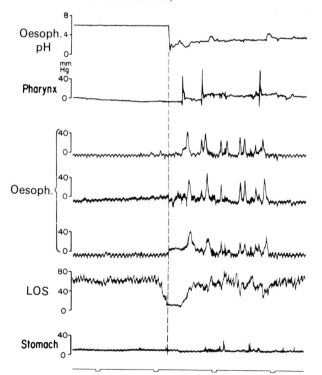

Time in Minutes

Fig. 31.5   GOR associated with a transient LOS relaxation. Before acid reflux, resting LOS pressure was stable at 50–60 mmHg. Reflux of acid into the oesophagus occurred during a transient LOS relaxation that was not related to swallowing (i.e. no pharyngeal activity before relaxation). LOS relaxation lasted approximately 20 s during which time there was no peristaltic activity in the body of the oesophagus. Acid reflux occurred during the transient LOS relaxation when oesophageal pressure equalled intragastric pressure. After the reflux episode, several swallow-induced peristaltic contractions were recorded in the body of the oesophagus which helped to clear the acid. (Reprinted by permission from Dodds et al 1982.)

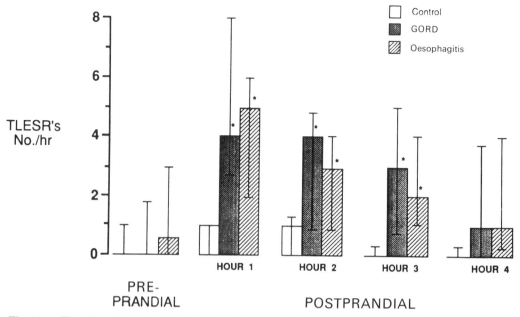

Fig. 31.6   The effect of a meal on the rate of transient LOS relaxation in control subjects and two groups of reflux patients – those without oesophagitis (GORD) and with oesophagitis. Preprandially all groups exhibited a low rate of transient LOS relaxation. Postprandially the rate of transient LOS relaxation did not change in controls, while the reflux patients experienced a fourfold increase in transient LOS relaxation during the first three postprandial hours. Data are expressed as median values and interquartile range p < 0.05. (Reprinted by permission from Holloway et al 1991.)

Diminished LOS pressure can be associated with GOR by two mechanisms: stress reflux and free reflux. Stress reflux results when a relatively hypotensive LOS is overcome and 'blown open' by an abrupt transient increase in intra-abdominal pressure. Substantial data has accumulated suggesting that stress reflux is unlikely when the LOS pressure is greater than 10 mmHg (Dodds et al 1982). The other mechanism by which diminished LOS pressure is associated with GOR is free reflux. Free reflux is characterized by a fall in intraoesophageal pH without an identifiable change in either intragastric or LOS pressure. Free reflux is seen when the resting LOS pressure is within 0–4 mmHg of intragastric pressure (Dodds et al 1982). The cause of LOS hypotonia allowing stress or free reflux in some patients with GORD is unknown. Clearly, LOS hypotonia may be secondary to reflux oesophagitis; but in the vast majority of cases, the LOS hypotension predates the development of reflux symptoms and generally persists after therapeutic resolution of histologic oesophagitis.

Oesophageal clearance

Reflux events determine the frequency and extent that gastric contents enter the oesophagus, but oesophageal clearance determines mucosal acid exposure time and probably severity of mucosal injury. Oesophageal clearance involves two related but separate processes. The first is volume clearance, which is the actual removal of refluxed material from the oesophagus. The second process, acid clearance, describes the restoration of normal pH in the oesophagus following acid exposure which is accompanied by titration with base (i.e. saliva) rather than true removal of the refluxed material. Three mechanisms are important in determining the efficacy of oesophageal clearance: peristalsis, saliva and gravity.

First, peristaltic oesophageal motor activity rapidly clears fluid volume from the oesophagus. Helm et al (1984) showed that one or two primary peristaltic sequences will completely clear a 15 ml fluid bolus from the oesophagus (Fig. 31.7). Primary peristalsis is elicited by swallowing, which occurs with a frequency of once per minute in awake subjects regardless of whether or not reflux occurs. Secondary peristalsis, initiated by oesophageal distention from acid reflux, is much less effective in promoting clearance of refluxate thus offering only an ancillary protective role.

Peristaltic dysfunction (failed primary peristalsis or hypotensive 'feeble' peristalsis) increases in frequency in direct relation to the degree of oesophagitis. As

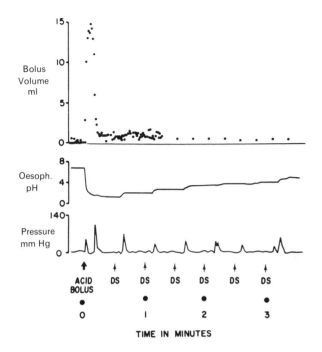

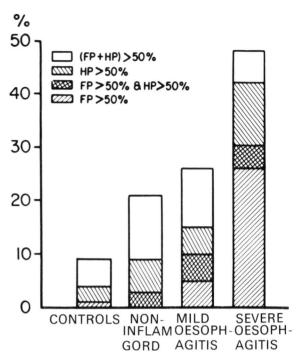

Fig. 31.7 Relationship among oesophageal peristalsis, distal oesophageal pH, oesophageal volume clearance, and oesophageal acid clearance during an acid clearance test done with radiolabelled 0.1N HCl. The calculation of bolus volume within the oesophagus is derived from scintiscanning over the chest. DS = dry swallow. Note that although all but about 1 ml of the infused fluid is cleared from the oesophagus by the first peristaltic contraction, the distal oesophageal pH remains unchanged. Stepwise increases in distal oesophageal pH occur with subsequent swallows. (Reprinted by permission from Helm et al 1984.)

Fig. 31.8 Bar graph indicating the prevalence of peristaltic dysfunction in controls and patients with increasing severity of GORD. The criteria for motility abnormalities was the occurrence of either failed primary peristalsis (FP) or regional hypotensive peristalsis (< 27 mmHg) in the distal oesophagus (HP) with more than half of the swallows. Note the increased prevalence of peristaltic dysfunction with increasing severity of GORD. (Reprinted with permission from Kahrilas et al 1986.)

shown in Figure 31.8, Kahrilas et al (1986) found that the prevalence of peristaltic dysfunction rose from 25% in individuals with mild oesophagitis to over 50% in patients with severe oesophagitis. Failed peristalsis results in very poor volume clearance while foci of feeble contractions clear most, but not all, refluxate from the oesophagus. Whether oesophagitis leads to peristaltic dysfunction, or an underlying motility disorder predisposes to development of reflux disease, is unclear. Both viewpoints have experimental support such that in any one patient, either factor may be operational. Current opinion, however, suggests that impaired motor function does not revert to normal following either effective medical or surgical therapies (Eckardt 1988).

Saliva is the second essential factor required for normal oesophageal clearance of acid. Saliva has a pH of 6.4–7.8 and, therefore, is a relative base compared to acidic gastric contents. The high rate of spontaneous swallowing results in saliva production of approximately 0.5 ml per min. Although saliva is ineffective in neutralizing large volumes of acid (5–10 ml), it can

neutralize small residual amounts of acid remaining in the oesophagus after the volume of reflux material has been cleared by several peristaltic contractions (Helm et al 1983). The importance of swallowed saliva is supported by findings that increased salivation induced by oral lozenges or bethanechol is associated with a significant decrease in acid clearance time. In contrast, suction aspiration of saliva (Helm et al 1982) is accompanied by a marked prolongation in oesophageal clearance, despite the presence of normal peristaltic contractions (Fig. 31.9).

Physiologic or pathologic compromise of salivation may contribute to the severity of GORD. Diminished salivation during sleep explains why reflux events during or immediately prior to going to sleep are associated with markedly prolonged acid clearance times (Orr et al 1981). Similarly, chronic xerostomia is associated with prolonged oesophageal acid clearance and oesophagitis (Korsten et al 1991). Cigarette smoking may promote GOR. This was originally attributed to the effects of nicotine on lowering LOS pressure but more recent studies suggest that cigarette smokers

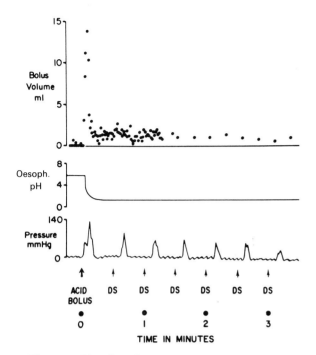

Fig. 31.9 The effect of aspirating oral saliva on oesophageal acid clearance and volume clearance. The experimental setup is the same as Fig. 31.7. Despite effective volume clearance by the initial peristaltic sequence, saliva aspiration markedly prolonged the process of acid clearance. (Reprinted by permission from Helm et al 1984.)

have hyposalivation which may also prolong oesophageal acid clearance (Kahrilas & Gupta 1989). Finally, the oesophagosalivary reflex may be impaired in people with reflux oesophagitis. This is a vaso-vagal reflex which can be demonstrated by perfusing acid into the oesophagus thereby stimulating increased salivation. This reflex may be the explanation for the symptom of water brash observed in some patients with reflux disease. The oesophagosalivary reflex is very active in healthy individuals with a doubling or tripling of the salivary rate on exposure to acid. However, this reflex is diminished in oesophagitis patients and in individuals with strictures (Sonnenberg et al 1982).

Utilization of gravity via elevation of the head of the bed is a time honoured treatment of GORD. This manoeuvre markedly improves acid clearance time and is most beneficial in those patients with aperistalsis (e.g. scleroderma) (Johnson & DeMeester 1981, Harvey et al 1987). Gravity is particularly important at night when the other oesophageal clearance mechanisms are inactive. Some data suggest, however, that gravity contributes little to oesophageal clearance in subjects with normal peristaltic stripping waves (Helm et al 1983).

Gastric factors

Gastric factors (particularly gastric volume and certain aggressive factors found in the refluxate) are potentially important in the production of reflux oesophagitis. Gastric volume is chiefly determined by the rate of gastric emptying, basal acid secretory rate, duodenogastric reflux, and the degree of gastric distention. Decreased gastric volume not only provides more gastric contents available for reflux but also increases the rate of transient LOS relaxations.

Controversy surrounds the importance of delayed gastric emptying in the pathogenesis of GORD. Early studies found gastric emptying of liquids to be normal, but solid emptying delayed in up to 41% of GORD patients (McCallum et al 1981). However, methodological concerns have arisen about these studies. These investigations usually took place with the patient supine, scanning was often done only in the anterior position, and the radiolabelled marker may have been unstable. More recent studies using solid-phase gastric emptying, performed in the upright position with both anterior and posterior imaging, have not consistently documented a higher prevalence of delayed gastric emptying in patients with GORD. Studies from the USA (Johnson et al 1986, Shay et al 1987) recently found only a 6–12% rate of delayed gastric emptying regardless of the severity of the reflux disease (Fig. 31.10). Somewhat higher results are reported in European studies. Thus, delayed gastric emptying contributes to GORD but probably only in a small subset of patients.

Recent studies raised the possibility that reflux patients not responding to conventional anti-secretory therapy may have higher rates of acid secretion than control subjects. In particular, this may apply to patients with Barrett's oesophagus. Mulholland et al (1989) found basal output of acid and secretion of acid in response to synthetic gastrin to be significantly greater in patients with Barrett's oesophagus when compared with healthy volunteers. Responses in patients with uncomplicated oesophagitis were intermittent between these two groups. Similarly, Collen et al (1990) found significantly higher basal output of acid in 13 patients with Barrett's oesophagus (11.9 ± 4.6 mEq/h) compared to 59 patients with GORD (5.8 ± 5.4 mEq/h) and 40 healthy volunteers (3.2 ± 2.7 mEq/h). Basal output of acid was greater than 10 mEq/h in 9 out of 13 (69%) patients with Barrett's oesophagus compared with 14 out of 59 (24%) of GORD patients. The above studies may have been flawed methodologically, however, by failure to consider other factors influencing acid secretion especially

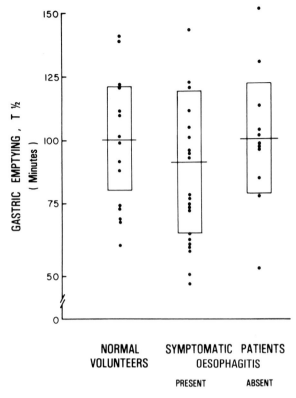

Fig. 31.10 Gastric emptying rates in normal volunteers and symptomatic patients with and without oesophagitis. Overall, there is no difference in gastric emptying rates between the groups. Data presented as individual values and mean ± 1 SD. (Reprinted by permission from Shay et al 1987.)

male gender and the presence of duodenal ulcer disease. Hirschowitz (1991) has analysed a very large series of patients with oesophagitis and Barrett's oesophagus finding that both groups have no greater outputs of gastric acid or pepsin than control patients without oesophagitis when all subjects were properly classified and matched for background (gender and the presence of duodenal ulcers) (Fig. 31.11).

Acid, pepsin, bile and possibly pancreatic enzymes have all been implicated in the development of reflux oesophagitis. The primary importance of acid is indisputable, but its mechanism may involve activation of pepsin more than direct damage from acid alone. In the cat, for example, acid causes minimal injury by protein denaturation at a pH less than 3.0; major damage does not occur unless pepsin is present (Goldbert et al 1969). Studies in animals demonstrate that conjugated bile salts produce their greatest injury in the presence of acid and pepsin, whereas trypsin, deconjugated bile salts and the conjugated bile salt taurode-

oxycholate are more damaging in the absence of acid (Lillemoe et al 1983). Despite the great interest in 'alkaline' reflux, there is meagre evidence that this is an important cause of GORD except in patients with postsurgical or resected stomachs.

Oesophageal epithelial resistance

The intrinsic defence mechanisms of the oesophageal epithelium are important factors in resisting injury from acid reflux. It is useful to separate oesophageal epithelial resistance into three categories: pre-epithelial, epithelial and postepithelial. Pre-epithelial defences include mucus, bicarbonate ions and the unstirred water layer that coats the mucosa. Mucus in the unstirred water layer confers gel-like properties that serve as a barrier to large molecules such as pepsin. Although hydrogen ions can readily enter the mucus fluid layer, they can be neutralized by bicarbonate ions within the unstirred fluid layer. Bicarbonate ions arise from two sources; saliva and submucosal oesophageal glands recently shown in animal (Hamilton & Orlando 1989) and human studies (Singh et al 1992) to produce bicarbonate ions in response to acid perfusion.

Epithelial defences consist of the stratified squamous epithelial cells and their tight intercellular junctions, which are initially impermeable to hydrogen ions. Postepithelial factors, including an active ionic transport mechanism, are able to maintain a normal intracellular pH even when hydrogen ions have penetrated the intracellar junctions and reach deeper epithelial cells. Quigley and Turberg (1987) demonstrated the effectiveness of this mechanism by finding that human oesophageal mucosa can maintain juxtamucosal pH at 4, while luminal pH is constant at 2. Other postepithelial factors that effect tissue resistance include mucosal blood flow and acid base status. Further protective mechanisms may involve increased esophageal cell replication in the face of acid exposure (Orlando 1986).

Hiatus hernia

The relationship between the sliding hiatus hernia and GORD remains controversial. While the majority of individuals with a sliding hernia do not have reflux disease, most patients with moderate to severe oesophagitis or Barrett's oesophagus have a sliding hiatus hernia. The mechanism whereby a hernia induces reflux is unclear. Most likely, the hiatus hernia acts as a fluid trap permitting the 're-reflux' of gastric contents from the hernia sac during swallowing (Fig. 31.12) (Mittal et al 1987). This is particularly marked in patients with non-reducible hernias, thereby limit-

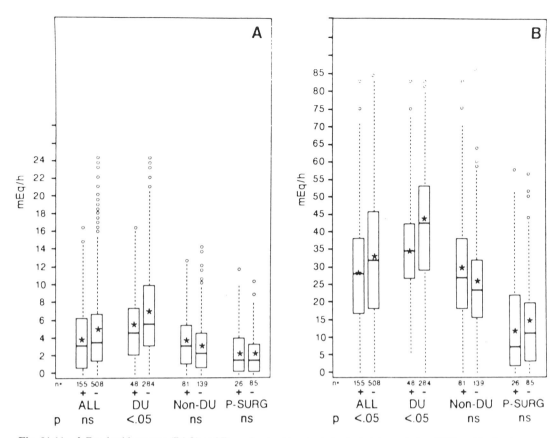

Fig. 31.11 **A** Basal acid outputs (BAO) and **B** maximal acid outputs in the total population (**All**) and in the three major diagnostic groups (**DU**: duodenal ulcers; **Non-DU**: no ulcer; **p-surg**: postgastric surgery) – comparing patients with (+) and without (−) oesophagitis (men and women combined). Significant differences primarily found in DU patients; i.e. those with DU and oesophagitis had lower BAO and MAO than DU patients without oesophagitis. Box-whisker plots give the median (bar), mean (star), and interquartile values, as well as the range of observed values. (Reprinted by permission from Hirschowitz 1991.)

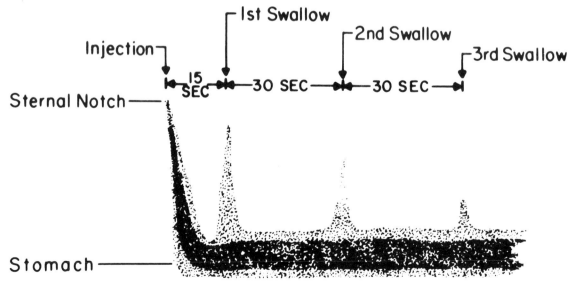

Fig. 31.12 Effect of a hiatal hernia on radionuclide acid clearance in a hernia patient. The subject swallowed at 30-s intervals after the injection of a 15 ml bolus of 0.1N HCl labelled with Tcn sulphur colloid. The vertical axis represents the region from the sternal notch to the stomach. The horizontal axis is the time scale. Black area represents radioactivity. Soon after injection, the radioactivity is cleared into the stomach. However, note the re-reflux event occurring with each of the first three swallows as the labelled acid transiently flows back into the oesophagus. (Reprinted by permission from Mittal et al 1987.)

ing the effectiveness of the lower oesophageal clearance mechanism. Other studies suggest that the hiatus hernia promotes transient LOS relaxations or that the hernia causes a reduction in the length of the high-pressure zone.

CLINICAL PRESENTATION

Classic presentations

Heartburn is a classic symptom of GORD (Table 31.1). The patient generally reports a retrosternal burning sensation, often describing the symptom with a vertical sweep of the hand. The burning also may be noted in the epigastrium, the neck, the throat and occasionally the back. Frequently, it occurs postprandially, particularly after consumption of spicy food, citrus fruits, fats, chocolates and alcohol. Recumbency and bending over may exacerbate heartburn. Recent weight gain, as little as 4.5–6.8 kg, is often a predisposing factor.

Other associated symptoms include dysphagia, odynophagia, regurgitation, water brash and belching. The most common cause of dysphagia in a patient with acid reflux is a peptic stricture. This usually occurs in the setting of long standing heartburn with slowly progressive dysphagia for solids followed by liquids. Oesophageal inflammation alone, peristaltic

dysfunction seen with the more severe forms of oesophagitis, and finally oesophageal cancer rising from Barrett's oesophagus may be other causes of dysphagia in GORD patients. Odynophagia is most commonly secondary to infectious oesophagitis, though some patients with reflux report this symptom if questioned specifically. In this setting, odynophagia is representative of more severe ulcerative oesophagitis. The effortless regurgitation of acid fluid, especially post-prandially and exacerbated by stooping or recumbency is highly suggestive of GORD. Water brash is the sudden appearance in the mouth of slightly sour or salty fluid. It is not regurgitated fluid, but rather secretions from the salivary gland in response to intraoesophageal acid exposure. Excessive belching, probably initiated by the increased swallowing of saliva as well as air brought about by acid reflux, may be an important symptom in some patients.

Atypical presentations

GORD may present with symptoms not immediately referable to the gastrointestinal tract, including chest pain, respiratory symptoms and ear, nose and throat problems (Table 31.1). Recent studies suggest that acid reflux is a major cause of non-cardiac chest pain, accounting for 20–50% of these cases (Fig. 31.3) (De-Meester et al 1982, Hewson et al 1991). Of particular importance is the demonstration of a temporal relationship between acid reflux and chest pain events, regardless of the total 24-h acid exposure time. Chronic persistent cough, recurrent aspiration, pneumonitis and asthma may be caused by GORD. Acid reflux may induce asthma either by microaspiration of acid

Table 31.1 Clinical presentations of GORD

Classic Symptoms	Frequency
Heartburn	Most common
Regurgitation	
Waterbrash	Less common
Dysphagia	
Atypical Symptoms*	
Oesophageal	
Non-cardiac chest pain	Uncommon
Odynophagia	
Epigastric pain	
Extraoesophageal	
Wheezing	
Chronic or nocturnal cough	
Sore throat	
Hoarseness	
Hiccups	
Belching	
Earache	

* These symptoms are not usually asked about in patients with GORD and thus may be more common than generally recognized.

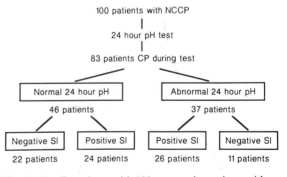

Fig. 31.13 Experience with 100 consecutive patients with noncardiac chest pain (NCCP) referred by cardiologists to the oesophageal laboratory. An equal portion of patients had abnormal reflux parameters by ambulatory oesophageal pH monitoring. More importantly, 50% had evidence of a positive symptom index (SI), confirming that acid reflux was a cause of some of their angina-like chest pain.

or via vagally mediated bronchospasm triggered by intraoesophageal acid exposure. Reflux disease should be considered in all refractory cases of asthma, particularly those with a nocturnal or exercise-related component (Fig. 31.14) (Sontag et al 1990). Hoarseness improving as the day progresses, sore throat, hiccups, dental injury and otitis media are all recognized head and neck manifestations of GORD. Animal studies suggest that direct injury to the larynx by a combination of acid and pepsin may be the mechanism of GORD-induced hoarseness ('peptic laryngitis'). Recent studies using 24-h pH monitoring confirmed these observations by finding an increased amount of supine reflux particularly high in the oesophagus of patients with laryngeal abnormalities (Fig. 31.15) (Jacobs et al 1991). Acid reflux and voice therapy may heal the oesophagitis and improve speech quality.

In contrast to the above symptomatic presentations, some patients with GORD are asymptomatic. Their oesophageal disease is discovered as an incidental finding, e.g. erosive oesophagitis found during endoscopy for a bleeding duodenal ulcer. Others present with complications of GORD without antecedent symptoms. Up to one-third of patients with Barrett's oesophagus are acid insensitive. This group in particular may present with oesophageal adenocarcinoma as their first and only manifestation of reflux disease.

DIAGNOSIS

In many patients, the history of heartburn and regurgitation is sufficiently typical to permit a trial of therapy without need for diagnostic tests. The following cases should be considered for early investigation: oesophageal symptoms not responding to medical therapy; dysphagia and atypical presentations of suspected GORD; those involving possible complications of reflux disease; and patients being considered for anti-reflux surgery. The specific tests employed in the diagnosis of GORD evaluate different variables in the disease spectrum such as potential for reflux, damage to the oesophagus and actual presence of reflux:

1. *Tests that demonstrate reflux potential*
   - Oesophageal manometry
   - Hiatal hernia
2. *Tests that indicate mucosal damage*
   - Endoscopy ± biopsy
   - Barium oesophagram
   - Bernstein test
3. *Tests that demonstrate reflux events*
   - Prolonged pH monitoring
   - Barium oesophagram with fluoroscopy

Radiology

Older studies suggested that the demonstration of GOR by fluoroscopy or cineradiography was an insensitive but fairly specific test for reflux. In a review of three series (Richter & Castell 1982), GOR demonstrated at the time of fluoroscopy had an average sensitivity of 40% and a specificity of 85%. Recent studies from our laboratory suggest that the sensitivity can be improved by the addition of the water siphon test without compromising specificity. In nearly 100 consecutive patients, we have compared fluoroscopic evidence of reflux with 24-h pH monitoring. Reflux induced spontaneously, by coughing, Valsalva manoeuvre or rolling side-to-side had a sensitivity of 44%, specificity of 89% and positive predictive value of 84% when compared to 24-h pH testing as the reference standard. The addition of the water siphon test improved the sensitivity to 65% without compromising specificity or positive predictive value (80% and 82%, respectively). Therefore, when reflux is seen by fluoroscopy, patients usually have other positive tests for reflux disease.

The barium oesophagram is an unreliable method for detecting reflux oesophagitis because most cases have mild morphologic changes that are not perceptible on radiographs. In a large prospective study correlating double contrast radiography with endoscopic evidence of oesophagitis, radiography was found to be quite insensitive (22%) for the diagnosis of mild degrees of inflammation (Ott et al 1981). Therefore, a normal oesophagram never rules out reflux disease. In cases of moderate to severe oesophagitis (erosions, ulcerations, strictures), sensitivity for oesophagography, however, approached 90%. Radiographic signs such as marginal irregularity in the fully distended oesophagus, ulcerations, incomplete oesophageal distensibility, and stricture formation were found to have the best correlation with severe endoscopic oesophagitis (Fig. 31.16).

When coupled with radiographic examinations of the stomach and duodenum, barium studies are quite useful in excluding other diagnoses (ulcers, cancer) and identifying possible complications of chronic reflux such as stricture or oesophageal ulcers, which are often associated with Barrett's oesophagus. As a general rule, the barium oesophagram with administration of a solid bolus challenge should be the initial diagnostic procedure in patients with dysphagia. Fluoroscopy or cineradiography also provides excellent information about oesophageal motor dysfunction that compares favourably with information obtained by oesophageal manometry; in fact, the tests are complimentary

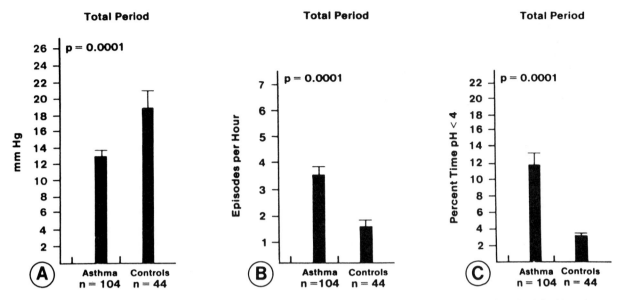

Fig. 31.14 Reflux parameters in asthmatic patients and controls. Compared with controls, asthmatic patients had significantly lower LOS pressures (left), more reflux episodes (centre), and more oesophageal acid contact time (right). Bars indicate mean ± SE. (Reprinted by permission from Sontag et al 1990.)

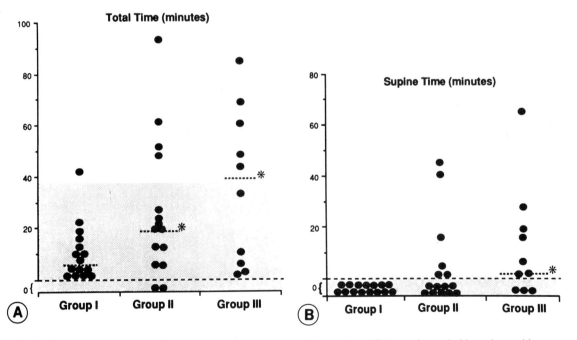

Fig. 31.15 Proximal oesophageal acid exposure during **A** the entire 24-h study and **B** the supine period in patients with GORD without laryngeal symptoms (group I) and patients with laryngeal symptoms (dysphagia, cough, globus, frequent throat clearing or sore throat) without (group II) or with (group III) laryngoscopic findings suggestive of GORD. Median proximal oesophageal acid exposure was significantly longer in II and III patients compared to control group. None of the group I patients showed any supine proximal acid reflux, but six of group II and seven of Group III patients did. (Reprinted by permission from Jacobs et al 1991.)

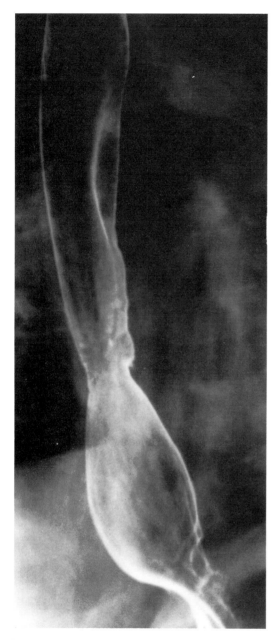

Fig. 31.16   Double-contrast barium oesophagram showing distal linear erosive oesophagitis, an oesophageal ulcer associated with a stricture and a large hiatus hernia. (X-ray courtesy of Robert Koehler MD.)

Table 31.2   Savary-Miller classification of reflux oesophagitis

Stage	Endoscopic findings
I	One or more supravestibular, non-confluent mucosal lesion accompanied by erythema, with or without exudate, or superficial erosions
II	Confluent erosive exudative lesions not covering the entire circumference
III	Erosive and exudative lesions covering the entire circumference leading to inflammatory infiltration of the wall without stricture
IV	Chronic mucosal lesions (ulcer, fibrosis, stricture, scarring with columnar epithelium)

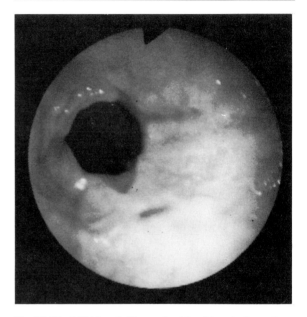

Fig. 31.17   Mild (grade I) oesophagitis with a single erosion without exudate extending from the oesophagogastric junction. (Picture courtesy of Guido Tytgat MD.)

jects, the absence of a radiographic hiatal hernia will exclude oesophagitis with 95% accuracy (Ott 1985).

Oesophagoscopy

In clinical practice, oesophagoscopy is generally the first procedure used for evaluating patients suspected of having GORD. Oesophageal endoscopy permits direct inspection and biopsy of the oesophageal mucosa facilitating detections of grade I or sometimes grade II oesophagitis which may not be apparent on X-ray examination. Unfortunately, there is no universally accepted classification system for staging reflux

(Hewson et al 1990). Lastly, the radiographic examination of the oesophagus can document the presence and size of an associated hiatus hernia. Although the hiatus hernia may be present in almost 40% of normal sub-

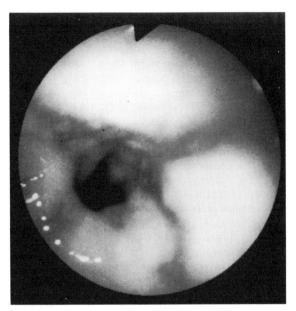

Fig. 31.18 Grade II oesophagitis with early confluent erosions covered by exudate. (Picture courtesy of Guido Tytgat MD.)

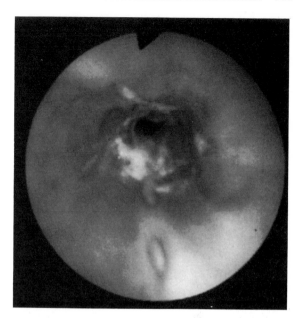

Fig. 31.20 Grade IV oesophagitis with stricture plus multiple proximal oesophageal erosions. (Picture courtesy of Guido Tytgat MD.)

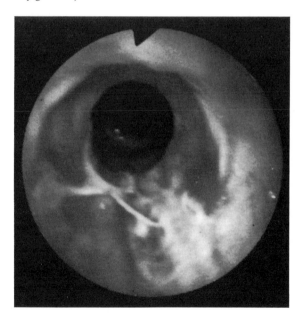

Fig. 31.19 Grade III oesophagitis with circumferential inflammation associated with oesophageal ulcers. (Picture courtesy of Guido Tytgat MD.)

oesophagitis, but the Savary–Miller classification (1978) is the most popular (Table 31.2, Figs 31.17–31.20). Macroscopic features of oesophagitis are variable ranging from friable, granular distal oesophageal

mucosa to mucosal erosions, ulcerations or stricture. When grade II oesophagitis is present, endoscopy has a specificity approaching 95% but a sensitivity of only 65% (Breen & Whelan 1978, Behar et al 1967). Inclusion of grade I lesions in the endoscopic diagnosis of oesophagitis has strikingly improved this test sensitivity (95%) but also markedly compromises the specificity (41%) (Breen & Whelan 1978, Kobayashi & Kasugai 1974). Markers of grade I oesophagitis include erythema, oedema of the mucosa with obliteration of the normal vascular pattern, mild friability and increased irregularity of the Z-line.

Mild changes of GORD are best diagnosed by histologic examination of the oesophageal mucosa. The classic histologic features of oesophagitis are epithelial erosion or ulceration accompanied by an inflammatory infiltrate consisting of neutrophils and/or eosinophils. Necrosis, pseudomembranes, or fibrosis generally identify patients with severe oesophagitis. More subtle reparative changes associated with reflux disease have been proposed by Ismail-Beigi et al (1970). They noted hyperplasia of epithelial basal cells and elongated dermal papillae in 85% of mild cases of GORD (Fig. 31.21). Weinstein et al (1975) later found that these histologic changes were only reliable if obtained 5 cm above the manometrically defined LOS. Unfortunately, the above data were generated using suction biopsies (seldom employed in clinical practice), rather

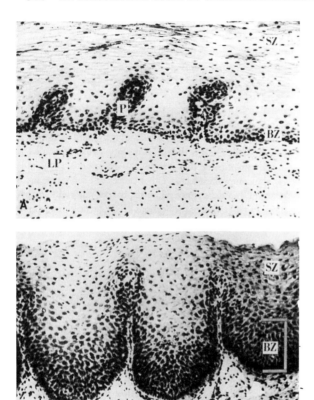

Fig. 31.21 Oesophageal mucosal biopsy by suction technique in a healthy control subject (**A**) and patient with reflux disease (**B**). In the reflux patient, the basal cell zone (**BZ**) is thickened and more than 15% of the overall mucosal thickness. Unlike the control subject, the dermal papillae (**P**) extend almost to the free surface. The lamina propria (**LP**) contain round cells in both subjects. **SZ**: squamous cell zone. (Reprinted by permission from Ismail-Beigi et al 1970.)

than endoscopic biopsies, which are significantly inferior in terms of size of specimen, depth of biopsy, appropriateness of orientation, and ease of interpretation. Unless a good pathologist is available and biopsies are oriented well, conventional endoscopic biopsies may add little to the diagnosis of GORD if the oesophageal mucosa appears normal visually.

The diagnosis of Barrett's oesophagus and its associated dysplasia or malignancy is made by biopsies. Barrett's epithelium comprises three types of mucosa: specialized columnar epithelium resembling intestinal mucosa; junctional-type epithelium resembling the epithelium of the gastric cardia; and gastric fundic-type epithelium which contains parietal cells. The specialized columnar epithelium is usually most proximal and

is the only type with a malignant potential (Spechler & Goyal 1986). Patients with Barrett's oesophagus and progressive degrees of dysplasia have an increased risk of developing adenocarcinoma. Despite disputes over nomenclature, mucosal biopsies with high-grade dysplasia predict carcinoma in oeophagectomy specimens of approximately 60% of cases (Palley et al 1989). There are several practical points that make cancer surveillance programme difficult in these patients. The areas of high-grade dysplasia and/or carcinoma may be patchy, therefore, multiple biopsies are required (Reid et al 1988). Active inflammation may impair the assessment for dysplasia and give false-positive interpretations of high-grade dysplasia. Thus, patients should undergo intensive medical therapy before entertaining a definite diagnosis of high-grade dysplasia. Finally, high-grade dysplasia does not always mean invasive cancer. The progression of cancer may take many years in some patients, will not occur in others, and may actually regress to mild degrees of dysplasia in others.

Oesophageal manometry

Oesophageal manometry was employed in the past primarily to assess LOS pressure. But whereas LOS pressure is a major determinant of GOR, it is now well established that an isolated measure of LOS pressure is not a useful diagnostic test. Depending on patient selection, only 25–50% of patients with GORD have low resting LOS pressures (e.g. less than 10 mmHg). Furthermore, an even smaller percentage have markedly low values (less than 6 mmHg) that separate abnormal from control values (Richter & Castell 1982). Therefore, manometry should be reserved for patients in whom another diagnosis is suspected (e.g. achalasia) and is a mandatory test before anti-reflux surgery. Non-specific motility disturbances, such as low-amplitude peristaltic contractions and intermittent simultaneous contractions, are not contraindications to anti-reflux surgery because these disorders are probably secondary to the reflux disease itself. On the other hand, it is very important to identify aperistalsis, be it a manifestation of achalasia, scleroderma, or severe instage reflux disease. If this abnormality is found, it may be best to avoid surgery or warn the surgeon to perform a 'loose' Nissen fundoplication or an incomplete wrap so as to prevent worsening of their dysphagia.

Bernstein tests

The acid perfusion, or Bernstein test, is a simple screening procedure for determining whether the patient's symptoms are related to acid reflux (Fig.

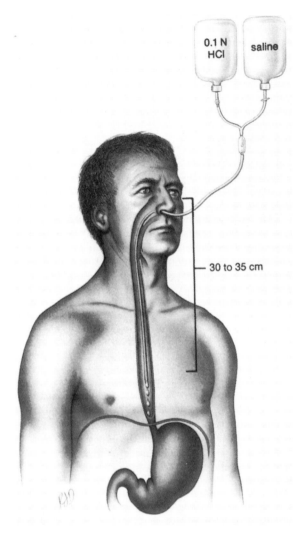

0.1 N
HCl

saline

30 to 35 cm

Fig. 31.22 Acid perfusion (Bernstein test). In the upright position, 0.1N HCl is infused by a nasogastric tube into the distal oesophagus at a minimum rate of 7 ml/min, using a saline infusion as the control. A positive test, suggesting acid sensitivity is defined as replication of the symptoms only during the acid perfusion.

31.22) (Bernstein & Baker 1958). Older studies suggested that intraluminal acid provoked heartburn by inducing non-peristaltic oesophageal activity; however, consensus now exists that acid induced heartburn results from the direct action of acid on damaged oesophageal epithelium. The test has a high predictive accuracy in the presence of endoscopic oesophagitis (about 80–90%) (Richter & Castell 1982). However, its use is superfluous in these patients. The major indication for Bernstein testing is for the evaluation of patients with non-cardiac chest pain and normal endoscopic or radiographic examinations of the oesophagus. Here the test has excellent specificity (90%) but poor sensitivity (36%) when compared to pH monitoring (Richter et al 1991). Thus a positive test is helpful but a negative test does not exclude acid reflux as a cause of symptoms.

Prolonged ambulatory oesophageal pH monitoring

Prolonged ambulatory monitoring of oesophageal pH is the most reliable means for diagnosing GORD. First described by Spencer in 1969 and popularized by Johnson and DeMeester (1974), prolonged monitoring of pH evolved from dissatisfaction with the previous tests for reflux. The test is remarkably well tolerated and involves the placement of a thin pH probe 5 cm above the manometrically determined LOS. Data are collected in a small lightweight box worn on a waist belt and the information analysed by computer. Studies are usually done as an outpatient with the individuals encouraged to ambulate and function in their normal environment. Patients are allowed to smoke and drink alcohol and most centres no longer restrict the pH of ingested foods.

Multiple variables can be measured during prolonged monitoring of oesophageal pH (Johnson & DeMeester 1974). Those used most often include the time pH is less than 4 in the upright, supine and combined positions, the number of reflux episodes lasting over 5 min, and the longest reflux episode. Large databases of normal values are now established using commercially available equipment adding to the accuracy of this test (Table 31.3) (Richter et al 1992). In everyday practice, the first three measurements of acid exposure time have a sensitivity of 85% and a specificity greater than 95% in defining GORD (Richter & Castell 1982). In general, subjects with reflux disease exhibit a higher rate of acid reflux (day, night or a combination) and increased oesophageal exposure to acid than do normal subjects (Fig. 31.23) (Johnson 1980). While prolonged pH monitoring detects and quanifies acid reflux, its greatest clinical utility may be in the correlation of symptoms with actual reflux events. Indeed, a symptom index has been developed to quantify the temporal relationship between reflux episodes and symptoms, most notably non-cardiac chest pain (Fig. 31.24) (Wiener et al 1988a).

Prolonged monitoring of oesophageal pH is moderately expensive, time consuming, and occasionally prone to technical problems. It should not be considered a perfect 'gold standard', but the test does have a concordance rate for the diagnosis of GORD

Table 31.3 24-hour oesophageal pH values for normal subjects *

	Median	Range	95th Percentile
Total time pH < 4 (%)	1.10	0–8.6	5.78
Upright time pH < 4 (%)	1.45	0–12.4	8.15
Supine time pH < 4 (%)	0.10	0–8.5	3.45
Total episodes (No.)	18.0	0–101	46
Episodes > 5 min (No.)	0	0–7	4
Longest episode (min)	3.0	0–46	18.5

Note: Based on studies of 110 healthy subjects (47 men, 63 women, mean age 38 years with a range of 20–84 years) From Richter et al 1992 with permission.

approximating 90% between studies (Wiener et al 1988b). The most common indications for prolonged oesophageal pH monitoring include non-cardiac chest pain, suspected pulmonary or ear, nose and throat complications of GORD, and intractable reflux symptoms associated with a negative work-up and not responding to medical therapy. Prolonged monitoring of pH should be conducted prior to antireflux surgery, if doubts exist about the diagnosis, as well as to assess the effectiveness of medical or surgical therapy in problem cases.

MANAGEMENT

The rationale for GORD therapy depends on a careful definition of specific goals. In patients without oesophagitis, the therapeutic goal is simply to relieve the acid-related symptoms. In patients with oesophagitis, the ultimate goal also is to heal the oesophagitis while attempting to prevent further complications such as strictures and Barrett's metaplasia. These goals are set against a complex background: GORD is a chronic condition that may wax and wane in intensity and relapses are common.

Natural history

Most patients found to have reflux oesophagitis report having symptoms lasting for 1–3 years before they seek medical help (Brunnen et al 1969). No clear relationship exists between symptoms and either the amount of reflux or the presence of oesophagitis. Furthermore, the frequency of symptomatic reflux as an acute self-limited disease versus a chronic relapsing disease is unknown. Thus remarkably little can be said of the natural history of GORD other than it has an excellent prognosis. In a 10-year study, approximately 80% of patients with non-inflammatory GORD were

found to have improved or became asymptomatic with medical treatment (Rex et al 1961). More is known about the natural history of patients with oesophagitis. After healing of oesophagitis with H_2 blockers or omeprazole, there is a disportionately high relapse rate after abrupt discontinuation of therapy (Sandmark et al 1988, Hetzel et al 1988). The type of drug therapy, dosing regimen, smoking and grade of oesophagitis at entry are not consistent predictors of relapse. On the other hand, a low LOS pressure and poor oesophageal clearance mechanisms, which are usually unchanged by any therapy, may be the best predictors of relapse (Lieberman 1987).

The major complications of oesophagitis are stricture formation, Barrett's epithelium and haemorrhage. Mortality associated with esophagitis is minimal with estimates of 0.1/100 000 being typical (Brunnen et al 1969). Prevalence of peptic strictures range from 8–20% of oesophagitis patients and ulceration is in (Wienbeck & Barnert 1989). Barrett's epithelium has been observed in 8–20% of patients with reflux oesophagitis and 44% of those with a peptic stricture (Spechler & Goyal 1986). Less than 2% of patients with oesophagitis develop significant gastrointestinal bleeding (Wienbeck & Barnert 1989). Unfortunately, we know very little about the efficacy of medical therapy in preventing these complications and maintaining oesophagitis in long-term remission. We assume that therapy prevents complications, but clinical experience suggests that most patients present initially with complications of GORD rather than developing them after onset of treatment.

Lifestyle modifications

Effective therapy for patients with minimally symptomatic heartburn is comprised of changes in lifestyle and antacids as needed. Cigarette smoking decreases LOS pressure, delays oesophageal acid clearance and increases distal oesophageal acid exposure (Dennish & Castell 1971). Hence, patients with GOR should stop smoking. Other adjustments concern diet modifications and changes in the volume and timing of meals. Liquids with a low pH or increased osmolality (i.e. citrus juices, tomato-based products, spices) can evoke heartburn in patients with an acid-sensitive oesophagus (Price et al 1978). Carminatives and ingredients found in certain foods (garlic, onions, peppermint and certain after-dinner liqueurs) lower LOS pressure and facilitate belching, often accompanied by reflux (Castell 1975). Foods high in fat content and chocolates decrease LOS pressure and delay gastric emptying. Patients should refrain from overeating, because

Physiologic Reflux Pattern

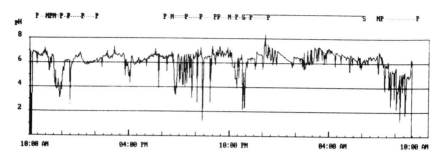

Upright Reflux Pattern

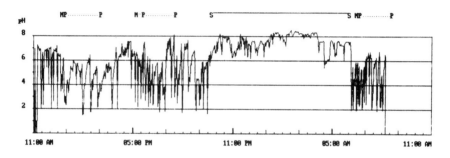

Combined Reflux Pattern

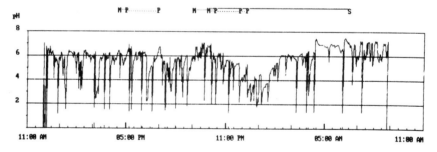

Fig. 31.23 Various patterns of GOR recorded by 24-h ambulatory oesophageal pH monitoring. pH is on the vertical axis and time on the horizontal axis. **M** = meal; **S** = sleep, and **P** = postprandial period. Upper graph: normal or 'physiologic' reflux pattern characterized by short, rapidly cleared acid reflux episodes after meals but not while asleep. Middle graph: 'upright reflux' pattern which primarily represents an exaggeration of the physiologic pattern without nocturnal reflux. These patients may have frequent symptoms but infrequently develop oesophagitis as the excess acid is rapidly cleared by gravity, peristalsis and saliva during the wakening hours. Lower graph: 'combined reflux' pattern with excessive acid reflux in both the upright and supine position. Note the prolonged acid exposure from 12:00 a.m. to 1:30 a.m. resulting from poor acid clearance. These patients frequently have severe symptoms, endoscopic evidence of oesophagitis and complications of GORD (stricture, ulcers, Barrett's oesophagus).

increased gastric volume increases the frequency of spontaneous transient LOS relaxations and associated reflux. For similar reasons, patients should not eat for several hours before retiring. Postural therapy (15–20

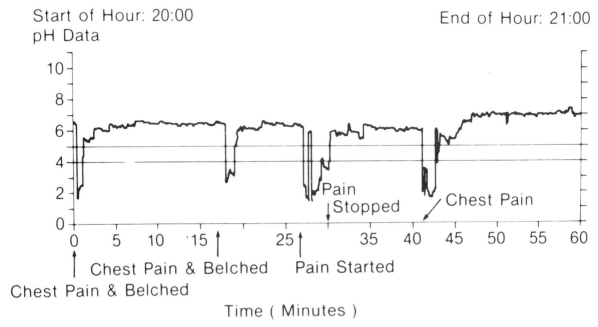

Fig. 31.24 A 1-h segment of ambulatory oesophageal pH tracing showing the association of chest pain and belching with acid reflux episode. Overall, the patient had a symptom index of 66% (symptom index = number of symptoms occurring with pH < 4 divided by total number of symptoms reported, multiplied by 100%).

cm bed blocks or a styrofoam wedge under the mattress) significantly reduces both oesophageal acid clearance time and acid exposure time. 15-cm blocks are nearly as effective as ranitidine (150 mg b.i.d.) in healing reflux oesophagitis (Harvey et al 1987). Avoidance of tight fitting garments and weight loss are interventions aimed at reducing the incidence of reflux by the 'abdominal stress' mechanism. Patients should also be carefully questioned about medications that lower LOS pressure and facilitate reflux (theophylline, progesterone, antidepressants, nitrates, calcium channel blockers) and those that can cause localized oesophagitis (quinidine, slow-release KCl, doxycycline, non-steroidal anti-inflammatory drugs).

Antacids and alginic acid

Antacids with or without alginic acid are useful for treating mild and infrequent reflux symptoms, especially when brought on by lifestyle indiscretions. Antacids work primarily by neutralizing acid, albeit for relatively short periods of time. Therefore, patients need to take these agents frequently, usually 1–3 h after meals and at bedtime, depending upon the severity of the symptoms. Gaviscon, containing alginic acid and antacids, mixes with saliva to form a highly viscous solution that floats on the surface of the gastric pool acting as a mechanical barrier. Recent studies confirm that Gaviscon effectively prevents episodes of upright acid reflux (Washington et al 1990). Neither antacids or Gaviscon have been shown to be superior to a white liquid placebo in controlling symptoms or healing oesophagitis (Fig. 31.25) (Graham & Patterson 1983). Nevertheless, in clinical practice, antacids and Gaviscon are useful for controlling mild to moderate symptoms of heartburn but have no role in treating oesophagitis.

Prokinetic drugs

The most studied prokinetic drugs for the treatment of GORD include bethanechol, metoclopramide and cisapride. Bethanechol, an acetylcholine (ACh) agonist, works by increasing LOS pressure, improving oesophageal peristalsis and increasing salivary flow which improves oesophageal acid clearance. Metoclopramide, a dopamine antagonist which also promotes the release of ACh, primarily works by improving gastric emptying. Multiple studies show that both drugs effectively relieve heartburn symptoms, but their efficacy in treating oesophagitis is equivocal (Ramirez & Richter 1993). At present, bethanechol and metoclopramide are best

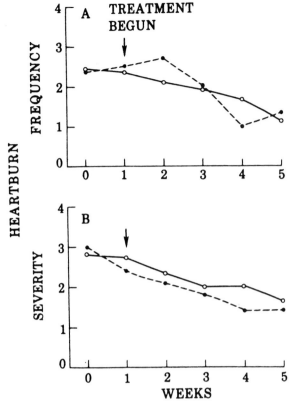

Fig. 31.25 Average frequency and severity of heartburn during a 5-week trial of antacid therapy (●) vs. placebo (○). There was no difference between the two regimens. (With permission from Graham & Patterson 1983.)

used as adjunctive therapy with H_2 antagonists when patients are not responding to acid inhibition alone. At a dose of 25 mg orally four times daily, bethanechol is well tolerated in all age groups. It is contraindicated in patients with bronchospastic lung disease and other side-effects include abdominal cramps, diarrhoea, urinary frequency and blurred vision. The most alarming feature of metoclopramide is its side-effect profile. Fatigue, lethargy, psychotropic and extrapyramidal problems have been reported in 10–30% of patients. These effects are reversible on cessation of drug therapy, although tardive dyskinesia may persist. The dopamine antagonist property of metoclopramide may also lead to hyperprolactinaemia and galactorrhoea. Metoclopramide is generally given in a dose of 10 mg before meals and at bedtime. It is possible to decrease the frequency of side-effects by decreasing the dose, giving a larger dose only before troubling meals (such as the largest meal of the day) or at bedtime or using a

sustained release tablet. Cisapride is the newest prokinetic agent that acts mainly by the release of ACh at the myenteric plexus. Studies have shown that it increases LOS pressure, improves peristaltic amplitude and accelerates gastric emptying. European studies have found cisapride (10 mg q.i.d.) to be more effective than placebo and equal to H_2 antagonists in controlling reflux symptoms and all grades of oesophagitis (Ramirez & Richter 1993). Unlike metoclopramide, cisapride is associated with minimal side-effects, the most common being abdominal cramps, borborygmi and diarrhoea.

Histamine$_2$ receptor antagonists

H_2 antagonists achieved the first real breakthrough in the treatment of GORD and have largely supplanted antacids for the relief of symptoms and healing of oesophagitis. Despite advertising to the contrary, all the H_2 antagonists are equally effective when used in proper doses; i.e. cimetidine 400 mg b.i.d., ranitidine 150 mg b.i.d., fanotidine 20 mg b.i.d. and nizatidine 150 mg b.i.d. It is important to remember that H_2 antagonist therapy for GORD differs from peptic ulcer disease in two ways: (1) a greater amount of acid suppression is required to control GORD; and (2) acid suppression is needed around the clock or at least during the periods of increased reflux. To keep acid reflux under control, short-acting H_2 antagonists are given four times a day while those with a longer half-life are given once or preferably twice a day. As shown in Figure 31.26, recent data on patterns of acid exposure show that the bulk of acid reflux occurs during the early evening hours after dinner and decreases markedly during the sleeping hours (Gudmundsson et al 1988). Therefore, it may be preferable to dose an H_2 antagonist 30 min after the evening meal rather than at bedtime.

Clinical GORD trials show that heartburn (both day and night) can be significantly decreased by H_2 antagonists when compared to placebo although symptoms are rarely abolished. Recent reviews find that overall oesophagitis healing rates with H_2 antagonists rarely exceed 60–75% even after 12 weeks of treatment (Fig. 31.27) (Koelz 1989, Sontag 1990). As a general rule, symptom resolution does not correlate well with mucosal healing and mucosal healing rates are directly proportional to the length of treatment. More frequent dosing with H_2 blockers is also more effective in healing oesophagitis than lower, less frequent dosing. Nevertheless, the most important factor in healing rates is the degree of oesophagitis before therapy: grade I and II oesophagitis heals in 75–90% of

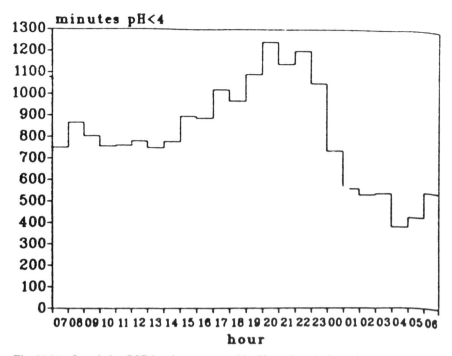

Fig. 31.26 Cumulative GOR in minutes spent with pH < 4, hour by hour, in 220 oesophagitis patients undergoing prolonged oesophageal pH monitoring. Note that the greatest amount of acid exposure is in the evening (16:00–23:00 h) usually after the last meal of the day. (With permission from Gudmundsson et al 1988.)

patients while grade III and IV only heals in 40–50% of patients.

For patients with severe reflux oesophagitis or intractable symptoms there are several options: (1) higher, more frequent doses of H$_2$ antagonists (Collen et al 1987); (2) adding a prokinetic agent to the H$_2$ antagonist (Lieberman & Keefe 1986); (3) switching to a more potent inhibitor of gastric acid secretion such as omeprazole; or (4) antireflux surgery. Although higher dose H$_2$ antagonist therapy improves the healing rates of severe oesophagitis, the expense and inconvenience may not be worth their minimal gain. For this reason, omeprazole has replaced the H$_2$ antagonists in treating more severe forms of GORD.

Omeprazole

Omeprazole, a substituted benzimidazole, is a potent and long-acting inhibitor of both basal and stimulated gastric acid secretion. It acts by selective, non-competitive inhibition of the H$^+$/K$^+$ ATPase enzyme located in the secretory membrane of the parietal cell. Omeprazole, 20–30 mg/day for one week, reduces acid secretion by more than 90% compared to 50% by cimetidine,

1000 mg/day, and 70% for ranitidine, 300 mg/day (Sharma et al 1984). Ambulatory oesophageal pH studies demonstrate almost complete disappearance of acid reflux episodes following treatment of oesophagitis patients with omeprazole 20 or 40 mg/day. Controlled studies show that omeprazole completely abolishes reflux symptoms in the majority of patients with severe GORD, usually within 1–2 weeks. Complete healing of oesophagitis occurs after 8 weeks in >80% of patients. Comparison studies consistently show that omeprazole is superior to ranitidine (150 mg) or cimetidine (800 mg) twice per day in relieving symptoms and healing oesophagitis (Fig. 31.28) (Sontag 1990, Maton 1991).

For short-term use, omeprazole has proven quite safe although it interacts with the cytochrome P-450 system in the liver sometimes necessitating dosage adjustment of warfarin, phenytoin and diazepam. The main concern with omeprazole is long-term safety. The profound hypoacidity produced by omeprazole stimulates gastrin release promoting the proliferation of enterochromaffin-like (ECL) cells in the gastric fundus. Prolonged high-dose omeprazole therapy caused a disturbingly high frequency of carcinoid

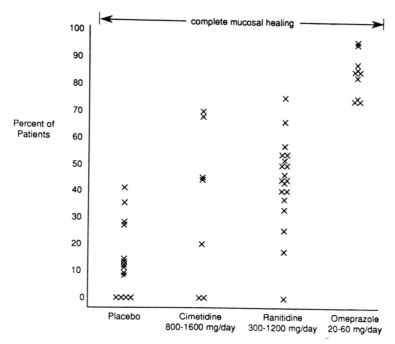

Fig. 31.27 Summary of clinical trials comparing placebo, cimetidine, ranitidine, and omeprazole in the healing of oesophagitis. Each **x** represents the percentage of patients healed in each treatment group of the clinical studies. (Reprinted with permission from Sontag 1990.)

tumours in rats with gastrin levels exceeding 1000 pg/ml, but not in similarly treated mice or dogs (Maton 1991). In humans, hypergastronaemia secondary to the achlorhydria of pernicious anaemia is associated with ECL proliferation but less than 5% of patients develop gastric carcinoid tumours. However, gastrin levels rarely exceed 500 pg/ml during routine omeprazole therapy (Sontag 1990). No patients with oesophagitis or ulcer disease have developed carcinoid tumours to date. Nevertheless, it is advisable that omeprazole should not be used for more than 8–12 weeks.

Maintenance medical therapy

Although we can virtually heal all cases of acute oesophagitis, keeping these patients in remission is a major problem as nearly 80% will relapse within 1 year of discontinuing therapy. Not surprisingly, the major predictors of relapse are a low LOS pressure as well as the initial severity of oesophagitis. Therefore, maintenance acid suppression is important and the doses required are similar to those needed for treating the acute disease. Data from 1-year maintenance studies with H_2 antagonists do not consistently show effective-

ness, even with full-dose therapy. A recent study from Europe (Tytgat et al 1992) suggests that the new prokinetic agent, cisapride, may be effective in preventing relapses in patients with mild oesophagitis. Only long-term maintenance therapy with omeprazole 10–20 mg daily can effectively prevent the relapse of all grades of oesophagitis, but this treatment probably should be reserved, at this time, for patients with severe oesophagitis who are not surgical candidates (Fig. 31.29) (Maton 1991).

Antireflux surgery

While most patients with GORD can be managed medically, approximately 10% will require antireflux surgery. In the past, the primary indication for surgery was failure of medical therapy. However, this is much less common with the availability of omeprazole, although surgery should still be considered in younger patients with severe GORD who otherwise would require lifelong medical therapy. Other indications for antireflux surgery include recurrent difficult-to-dilate strictures, non-healing ulcers, severe bleeding from oesophagitis, and reflux-related respiratory tract com-

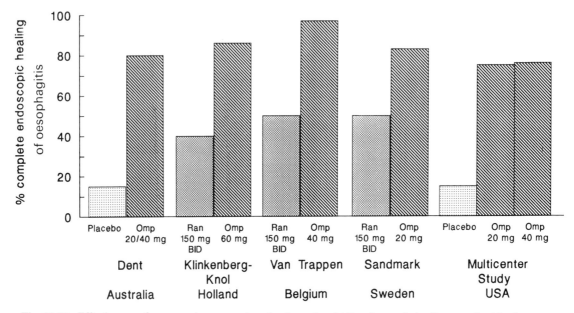

Fig. 31.28 Effectiveness of omeprazole compared to placebo and ranitidine therapy in healing oesophagitis after 8 weeks of therapy. Across these five studies from different countries, the omeprazole rates were consistently around 80%.

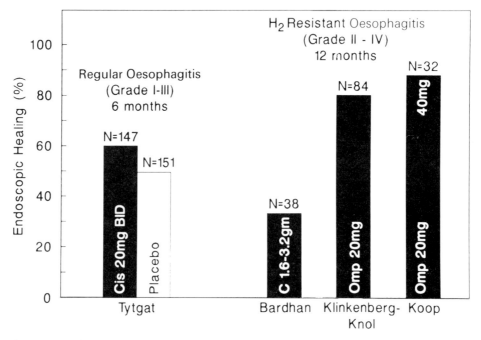

Fig. 31.29 Maintenance therapy studies for preventing the relapse of erosive oesophagitis. Cisapride 20 mg b.i.d. may be effective in preventing relapse of mild oesophagitis. Only long-term therapy with omeprazole can effectively prevent the relapse of severe grades of oesophagitis.

plications not responding to medical therapy. The presence of Barrett's oesophagus alone is not an indication for antireflux surgery. These procedures are cur-

rently performed through the abdomen and chest and all employ: (1) crural tightening after returning the hiatus hernia and oesophagogastric junction into the abdomen and anchoring it there; and (2) varying degrees of fundoplication. These operations include the Nissen (360°) and Belsey (270°) fundoplication and Hill gastropexy (DeMeester et al 1974). Paramount to successful antireflux surgery is a complete evaluation of oesophageal function prior to surgery and the skill and experience of the surgeon which generally is reflected by the frequency that this operation is performed. In the hands of an experienced surgeons with careful oesophageal preoperative testing, the result of these three operations are nearly equal; i.e. up to 80–90% of patients have a good long-term outcome (Siewert & Feussner 1987, DeMeester et al

1986). Surgical failures usually occur immediately after surgery or within the first 2 years from poor technique or excessive strain on the suture line by postoperative nausea and vomiting, excessive weight gain or isometric exercises. A cost-effective analysis between surgery and long-term medical therapy is lacking.

ACKNOWLEDGEMENT

The author thanks Mrs Linda Pugh for her excellent secretarial assistance in the preparation of this manuscript.

REFERENCES

Allison P R 1946 Peptic ulcer of the esophagus. J Thoracic Surg 308–312

Behar J, Biancani P, Sheahan D G 1967 Evaluation of esophageal tests in the diagnosis of reflux esophagitis. Gastroenterology 71: 9–15

Bernstein L M, Baker L A 1958 A clinical test for esophagitis. Gastroenterology 34: 760–778

Breen K J, Whelan G 1978 The diagnosis of reflux oesophagitis: an evaluation of five investigative procedures. Aust NZ J Surg 49: 156–161

Brunnen P L, Karmody A M, Needham C D 1969 Severe peptic oesophagus. Gut 10: 831–837

Castell D O 1975 The lower esophageal sphincter: physiologic and clinical aspects. Ann Int Med 83: 390–401

Castro L deP 1967 Reflux esophagitis as the cause of heartburn in pregnancy. Am J Obstet Gynecol 98: 1–10

Collen M J, Ciarleglio C A, Stanczak V J, et al 1987 Esophageal pH monitoring, gastric acid output, and gastric volume output in patients with GERD unresponsive to standard antisecretory therapy. Gastroenterology 92: 1350A

Collen M J, Lewis J H, Benjamin S B 1990 Gastric acid hypersecretion in refractory GERD. Gastroenterology 98: 654–661

DeMeester T R, Bonavina L, Albertucci M 1986 Nissen fundoplication for gastroesophageal reflux disease. Evaluation of primary repair in 100 consecutive patients. Ann Surg 204: 9–20

DeMeester T R, Johnson L F, Kent A H 1974 Evaluation of current operations for the prevention of gastroesophageal reflux. Ann Surg 180: 511–525

DeMeester T R, O'Sullivan G C, Bermudez G, Midell A I, Cimochowski G E, O'Drobiniak J O 1982 Esophageal function in patients with angina-type chest pain and normal coronary angiograms. Ann Surg 196: 488–498

DeMeester T R, Wang C I, Wernly J A et al 1980 Technique, indications, and clinical use of 24 hour esophageal pH monitoring. J Thorac Cardiovas Surg 79: 656–670

Dennish G W, Castell D O 1971 Inhibitory effect of smoking on the lower esophageal sphincter. N Engl J Med 284: 1136–1137

Dent J, Dodds W J, Friedman R M et al 1980 Mechanisms of GER in recumbent asymptomatic human subjects. J Clin Invest 65: 356–357

Dodds W J, Dent J, Hogan W J et al 1982 Mechanisms of GER in patients with reflux esophagitis. New Engl J Med 307: 1547–1552

Eckardt V F 1988 Does healing of esophagitis improve esophageal motor function? Dig Dis Sci 33: 161–165

Freidin N, Fisher M J, Taylor W et al 1991 Sleep and nocturnal acid reflux in normal subjects and patients with reflux oesophagitis. Gut 32: 1275–1279

Gallup (1988) Survey on heartburn across America. Gallup Organization, Princeton, New Jersey

Goldbert H I, Dodds W J, Gee S et al 1969 Role of acid and pepsin in acute experimental esophagitis. Gastroenterology 56: 223–230

Graham P Y, Patterson D J 1983 Double-blind comparison of liquid antacid and placebo in treatment of symptomatic reflux esophagitis. Dig Dis Sci 28: 559–566

Gudmundsson K, Johnsson F, Joelsson B 1988 The time pattern of gastroesophageal reflux. Scand J Gastroenterol 23: 75–79

Hamilton B H, Orlando R C 1989 In vivo alkaline secretion by mammalian esophagus. Gastroenterology 97: 640–648

Harvey R F, Gordon P C, Hadley N et al 1987 Effects of sleeping with the bed-head raised and of ranitidine in patients with severe peptic oesophagitis. Lancet 2: 1200–1203

Helm J F, Dodds W J, Hogan W J et al 1982 Acid neutralizing capacity of human saliva. Gastroenterology 83: 69–74

Helm J F, Dodds W J, Riedel D R et al 1983 Determinants of esophageal acid clearance in normal subjects. Gastroenterology 85: 607–612

Helm J R, Dodds W J, Pelc L R, Palmer D W, Hogan W J, Teeter B C 1984 Effect of esophageal emptying and saliva on clearance of acid from the esophagus. New Engl J Med 310: 284–288

Hetzel D J, Dent J, Reed W P et al 1988 Healing and relapse of severe peptic esophagitis after treatment with omeprazole. Gastroenterology 95: 903–912

Hewson E G, Ott D J, Dalton C B, Chen Y M, Wu W C, Richter J E 1990 Manometry and radiology: complementary studies in the assessment of esophageal motility disorders. Gastroenterology 98: 626–632

Hewson E G, Sinclair J W, Dalton C B, Richter J E 1991 Twenty-four-hour esophageal pH monitoring: the most useful test for evaluating noncardiac chest pain. Am J Med 90: 576–583

Hirschowitz B I 1991 A critical analysis, with appropriate controls, of gastric acid and pepsin secretion in clinical esophagitis. Gastroenterology 101: 1149–1158

Holloway R H, Hongo M, Berger K, McCallum R W 1985 Gastric distension: a mechanism for postprandial gastroesophageal reflux. Gastroenterology 89: 779–784

Holloway R H, Kocyan P, Dent J 1991 Provocation of transient lower esophageal sphincter relaxations by meals in patients with symptomatic gastroesophageal reflux. Dig Dis Sci 36: 1034–1039

Holloway R H, Wyman J B, Dent J 1989 Failure of transient lower oesophageal sphincter relaxation in response to gastric distension in patients with achalasia: Evidence for neural mediation of transient lower oesophageal sphincter relaxations. Gut 30: 762–767

Ismail-Beigi F, Horpon P F, Pope C E II 1970 Histological consequences of gastroesophageal reflux in man. Gastroenterology 58: 163–174

Jacobs P, Kahrilas P J, Herzon G 1991 Proximal esophageal pH-metry in patients with 'reflux laryngitis'. Gastroenterology 100: 305–310

Johnson D A, Winters C, Drane W E et al 1986 Solid-phase gastric emptying in patients with Barrett's esophagus. Dig Dis Sci 31: 1217–1220

Johnson L F 1980 24-hour pH monitoring in the study of gastroesophageal reflux. J Clin Gastroenterol 2: 387

Johnson L F, DeMeester T R 1974 Twenty-four hour pH monitoring of the distal esophagus: A quantitative measure of gastroesophageal reflux. Am J Gastroenterol 62: 325–332

Johnson L F, DeMeester T R 1981 Evaluation of elevation of the head of the bed, bethanechol and antacid foam tablets on GER. Dig Dis Sci 26: 673–680

Johnsson F, Joelsson B, Gudmundson K, Grieff L 1987 Symptoms and endoscopic findings in the diagnosis of gastroesophageal reflux disease. Scand J Gastroenterol 22: 714–719

Kahrilas P J, Dodds W J, Hogan W J et al 1986 Esophageal peristaltic dysfunction in peptic esophagitis. Gastroenterology 91: 897–904

Kahrilas P J, Gupta R R 1989 The effect of cigarette smoking on salivation and esophageal acid clearance. J Lab Clin Med 114: 431–438

Klinkenberg-Knol E C, Jansen J M B J, DeBruyne J W et al 1987 Long-term treatment with omeprazole (OME) in resistant reflux oesophagitis: effects on endoscopic healing and serum gastrin (G) levels. Gut 28: A1379

Kobayashi S, Kasugai T 1974 Endoscopic and biopsy criteria for the diagnosis of esophagitis with a fibreoptic esophagoscope. Dig Dis Sci 19: 345–352

Koelz H R 1989 Treatment of reflux esophagitis with H_2 blockers, antacids and prokinetic drugs. An analysis of randomized clinical trials. Scand J Gastroenterol 24 (suppl 156): 25–36

Korsten M A, Rosman A S, Fishbein S, Shlein R D, Goldberg H E, Beiner A 1991 Chronic xerostomai increases esophageal acid exposure and is associated with esophageal injury. Am J Med 90: 701–708

Lieberman D A 1987 Medical therapy for chronic reflux esophagitis. Long-term follow-up. Arch Int Med 147: 1717–1720

Lieberman D A, Keefe D B 1986 Treatment of severe reflux esophagitis with cimetidine and metoclopramide. Ann Int Med 104: 21–26

Lillemoe K D, Johnson L F, Harmon J W 1983 Alkaline esophagitis: a comparison of the ability of components of the gastroduodenal contents to injure the rabbit esophagus. Gastroenterology 85: 621–629

McCallum R W, Berkowitz D M, Lerner E 1981 Gastric emptying in patients with gastroesophageal reflux. Gastroenterology 80: 285–291

Maton P N 1991 Omeprazole. N Engl J Med 324: 965–975

Mittal R K, Lange R C, McCallum R W 1987 Identification and mechanism of delayed esophageal acid clearance in subjects with hiatus hernia. Gastroenterology 92: 130–135

Mittal R K, McCallum R W 1987 Characteristics of transient lower esophageal sphincter relaxation in humans. Am J Physiol 252: G636–G643

Mittal R K, Rochester D F, McCallum R W 1989 Sphincteric action of the diaphragm during a relaxed LES in humans. Am J Physiol 256: 6139–6144

Mittal R K, Stewart W R, Schirmer B 1990 Effect of a catheter in the pharynx on frequency of transient lower esopahgeal sphincter relaxation. Gastroenterology 98: 375 (abstract)

Mulholland M W, Reid B J, Levine D S et al 1989 Elevated gastric acid secretion in patients with Barrett's metaplastic epithelium. Dig Dis Sci 34: 1329–1335

Nebel O T, Fornes M F, Castell D O 1976 Symptomatic gastroesophageal reflux: incidence and precipitating factors. Dig Dis Sci 21: 953–956

Orlando R C 1986 Esophageal epithelial resistance. J Clin Gastroenterol Suppl 1: 12–16

Orr W C, Robinson M G, Johnson L F 1981 Acid clearance during sleep in the pathogenesis of reflux esophagitis. Dig Dis Sci 26: 423–427

Ott D J 1985 Barium esophagram in: Castell D O, Wu W C, Ott D J (eds) Gastroesophageal reflux disease: pathogenesis, diagnosis, therapy. Mt Future Kisco, New York pp 109–128

Ott D J, Wu W C, Gelfand D W 1981 Reflux esophagitis revisited: prospective analysis of radiologic accuracy. Gastrointest Radiol 6: 1–7

Palley S L, Sampliner R E, Garewal H S 1989 Management of high-grade dysplasia in Barrett's esophagus. J Clin Gastroenterol 11: 369–372

Price S F, Smithson K W, Castell D O 1978 Food sensitivity in reflux esophagitis. Gastroenterology 75: 240–243

Quigley E M, Turberg L A 1987 pH of the microclimate living human gastric and duodenal mucosa in vivo. Studies in control subjects and in duodenal ulcer patients. Gastroenterology 92: 1876–1884

Ramirez B, Richter J E 1993 Promotility drugs in the treatment of gastroesophageal reflux disease. Aliment Pharmacol Ther 2: 5–20

Reid B J, Winestine W B, Lewin K J et al 1988 Endoscopic biopsy can detect high grade dysplasia or early adenocarcinoma in Barrett's esophagus without grossly recognizable neoplastic lesions. Gastroenterology 94: 81–90

Rex J C, Andersen H A, Bartholomew L G, Cain J C 1961 Esophageal hiatal hernia – a 10 year study of medically treated cases. J Am Med Assoc 178: 117–122

Richter J E, Bradley L A, DeMeester T R, Wu W C 1992 Normal 24-hr ambulatory esophageal pH values. Influence of study center, pH electrode, age and gender. Dig Dis Sci 37: 849–856

Richter J E, Castell D O 1982 GE reflux: pathogenesis, diagnosis and therapy. Ann Int Med 97: 93–103

Richter J E, Hewson E G, Sinclair J W, Dalton C B 1991 Acid perfusion test and 24 hour esophageal pH monitoring with symptom index. Comparison of tests for esophageal acid sensitivity. Dig Dis Sci 36: 565–571

Sandmark S, Carlsson R, Fausa O, Lundell L 1988 Omeprazole or ranitidine in the treatment of reflux esophagitis. Scand J Gastroenterol 23: 625–632

Savary M, Miller G 1978 The esophagus in: Handbook and atlas of endoscopy. Gassman, Solothurn, Switzerland pp 135–139

Sharma B K, Walt R P, Pounder R E et al 1984 Optimal dose of oral omeprazole for maximal 24 hour decrease of intragastric acidity. Gut 25: 957–965

Shay S S, Eggli D, McDonald C, Johnson L F 1987 Gastric emptying of solid food in patients with GER. Gastroenterology 92: 459–465

Siewert J E, Feussner H 1987 Early and long-term results of anti-reflux surgery: a critical look in: Tytgat G N J (ed.) Bailliére's clinical gastroenterology. Bailliére Tindall, London, pp 821–842

Singh S, Bradley L A, Richter J E 1993 Determinants of oesophageal alkaline pH environment in controls and patients with gastroesophageal reflux. Gut 34: 309–316

Sonnenberg A, Steinkamp U, Weise A et al 1982 Salivary secretion in reflux esophagitis. Gastroenterology 83: 889–895

Sontag S J 1990 The medical management of reflux esophagitis. Role of antacids and acid inhibition. Gastroenterol Clin North Am 19: 683–712

Sontag S, O'Connell S, Khandelwal S et al 1990 Most asthmatics have gastroesophageal reflux with or without bronchodilator therapy. Gastroenterology 99: 613–620

Spechler S J, Goyal R K 1986 Barrett's esophagus. N Engl J Med 315: 362–371

Spencer J 1969 Prolonged pH recording in the study of gastro-oesophageal reflux. Br J Surg 56: 912–914

Tytgat G N J, Anker-Hansen O J, Carling L et al 1992 Effect of cisapride on relapse of reflux oesophagitis, healed with an antisecretory durg. Scand J Gastroenterol 27: 175–183

Washington N, Greaves J L, Wilson C G 1990 Effect of time of dosing relative to a meal on the raft formation of an anti-reflux agent. J Pharm Pharmacol 42: 50–53

Weinstein W M, Bogoch E R, Boyles K L 1975 The normal human esophageal mucosa: a histological reappraisal. Gastroenterology 68: 40–44

Wienbeck M, Barnert J 1989 Epidemiology of reflux disease and reflux esophagitis. Scand J Gastroenterol 24 (suppl 156): 7–13

Wiener G J, Richter J E, Copper J B, Wu W C, Castell D O 1988a The symptom index: a clinically important parameter of ambulatory 24-hour esophageal pH monitoring. Am J Gastroenterol 83: 358–361

Wiener G J, Morgan T M, Copper J B et al 1988b Ambulatory 24-hour esophageal pH monitoring: reproducibility and variability of pH parameters. Dig Dis Sci 33: 1127–1133

Winkelstein A 1935 Peptic esophagitis. A new clinical study. JAMA 104: 906.

Wolf R P, Mole P J, Rawlings J et al 1981 Comparison of the effect of ranitidine, cimetidine and placebo on the 24 hour intragastric acidity and noctural acid secretion in patients with duodenal ulcer. Gut 22: 49–55

32. Motility disorders of the stomach and duodenum

G. Stacher

INTRODUCTION

Symptoms of disordered gastroduodenal motor function are often non-specific and thus liable to be misinterpreted. Conversely, patients with a proven motor disorder may present with only minor complaints or be entirely symptom free. The net effect of impaired gastroduodenal motility, delayed or, in rare instances, accelerated gastric emptying of ingesta, may result from a decreased or increased tone of the fundus, an altered antral and pyloric contractile activity and an impaired gastroduodenal motor coordination. However, there is little information on the role such abnormalities play alone or in combination in specific disorders. Gastroduodenal motor abnormalities may be the result of a variety of processes, such as diseases or lesions affecting the extrinsic or intrinsic nervous structures controlling the contractile activity and its coordination, of diseases affecting the function of the smooth muscle, but also the result of drug and radiation therapy and of disordered eating behaviour or inadequate food intake leading to malnutrition. The more important of these processes and the results of pharmacotherapeutic interventions directed against their sequelae are reviewed here.

DISEASES AFFECTING THE NERVOUS CONTROL OF MOTILITY

Viral infection

Several viruses, such as the *Rotavirus*, the *Norwalk virus* and the enteric *Adenovirus*, have been revealed to cause diarrhoea, particularly in children. *Rotavirus* gastroenteritis is characterized by nausea, vomiting, dehydrating diarrhoea and a complete recovery without sequelae (Flewet 1982). Although there are no identifiable changes in the gastric mucosa (Widerlite et al 1974), gastric emptying was found, in 6–12-month-old children, to be markedly delayed during the acute stage of the infection (Bardhan et al 1992). Markedly delayed emptying has also been observed in adult volunteers who ingested the *Norwalk* and *Hawaii* viral agents (Meeroff et al 1980).

Of 15 patients with chronic idiopathic gastroparesis and alterations in gastroduodenal interdigestive motor activity but no illness known to impair gastrointestinal motility, 12 showed medium or highly positive antibody titres against *Cytomegalovirus*, but not against *Measles*, *Herpes simplex*, *Varicella zoster*, *Coxsackie* and *Adenoviruses* (Bortolotti et al 1987). By contrast, only three of 13 subjects with normal gastrointestinal motility had a medium antibody titre against the *Cytomegalovirus*. As the *Cytomegalovirus* tends to localize in the myenteric plexus (Press et al 1980), the impaired emptying may be due to a disordered nervous control.

Disordered gastrointestinal motor function has also been observed subsequent to infection with the *Herpes zoster* virus (Wyburn-Mason 1957) and in the Guillain-Barré syndrome (Susman & Maddox 1940).

Diabetes

Gastric retention of ingesta in patients with diabetes mellitus was described for the first time by Rundles (1945) as a late complication of the disease. Since the disorder has been found to affect about 50% of randomly selected patients with insulin-dependent (Keshavarzian et al 1987, Horowitz et al 1986a) and non-insulin-dependent diabetes (Horowitz et al 1989). In the antrum, reduced contractile activity has been found to prevail postprandially as well as during phase III of the interdigestive migrating motor complex (MMC) (Malagelada et al 1980). The pylorus was observed, in 14 of 24 diabetics with recurrent nausea or vomiting, to display tonic contractions (Mearin et al 1986). In the proximal small intestine, postprandial contractions were found to be non-propagated and decreased in number and often to occur in uncoordinated bursts (Camilleri & Malagelada 1984). As impaired gastric motor function makes the delivery of ingesta into the small intestine and the time of their absorption unpredictable, insulin may be administered at inappropriate times and poor glucose control ensues (Russell et al 1983a). It thus seems advisable to screen patients with poor glycaemic control for slow gastric emptying.

The fact that impaired gastric motor activity was found to be frequent in diabetic patients with severe autonomic neuropathy suggested that the former was a consequence of the latter (Hodges et al 1947, Kassander 1958, Buysschaert et al 1987). Polyneuropathy is present in practically all patients who suffer from diabetes for more than a few years, and its manifestations may range from subclinical alterations of nerve conduction to severe forms with life-threatening autonomic dysfunction (Said et al 1992). Despite reports that delayed gastric emptying occurred only in patients with severe autonomic neuropathy (Hongo et al 1986) and that there was an inverse relationship between the severity of neuropathy and the emptying rate (Keshavarzian et al 1987), there is no good evidence that autonomic neuropathy in fact is aetiologically related to the gastric motor impairment. In 16 patients with longstanding diabetes mellitus, of whom five were suffering from gastroparesis, no abnormalities of the neurons or axons in the myenteric plexus and the vagus nerve or of intestinal smooth muscle were found (Yoshida et al 1988b). No clear-cut relationships between the presence of autonomic or peripheral neuropathy on the one hand and the severity of gastric dysfunction on the other could be revealed also in other studies (Scarpello et al 1976, Kim et al 1991).

By contrast, a crucial role for the orderly motor function of the stomach seems to be played by the blood glucose concentration. In healthy human subjects, acute hyperglycaemia slows gastric emptying (Aylett 1962, McGregor et al 1976, Grainger et al 1983, Morgan et al 1988, Fraser et al 1990, Øster-Jørgensen et al 1990), reduces antral (Barnett & Owyang 1988, Fraser et al 1991) and stimulates pyloric contractile activity (Mearin et al 1986, Fraser et al 1989), the latter apparently by increasing the occurrence of isolated pyloric pressure waves (Fraser et al 1991). Acute hyperglycaemia further has been shown to reduce efferent activity in the vagal nerve (Hirano & Niijima 1980). Prolonged states of hyperglycaemia such as prevail in diabetes mellitus may not only reduce gastric motility and slow down emptying for extended periods, but also alter nerve metabolism (Greene et al 1987). The latter effect may result in a reduction of the density of myelinated and unmyelinated nerve fibres (Said et al 1992), in a length-related neuropathy of the dying-back type, i.e. the centripetal degeneration of peripheral axons (Said et al 1983, Said et al 1992)

and/or in multifocal ischaemic lesions mainly affecting microvessels (Johnson et al 1986, Dyck et al 1986). Thus, the abnormally slow gastric emptying in diabetic patients may result from prolonged hyperglycaemic states leading to neuropathy rather than from neuropathy as such. Conversely, there is growing evidence that good diabetic control and the absence of extended hyperglycaemic periods are associated with less frequent and less severe polyneuropathy (Dyck 1992).

The treatment of gastric stasis in patients with diabetes is, despite of the advent of potent prokinetic drugs, still unsatisfactory. Only a small number of studies have been undertaken, which evaluated the effects of such agents administered orally over longer periods of time (Table 32.1). Only three investigations of the latter type were carried out placebo controlled and under double-blind conditions. In one of these (Havelund et al 1987), cisapride 10 mg administered q.i.d. over 4 weeks was no more active than was a placebo. In another, neither cisapride 10 mg t.i.d. nor metoclopramide 10 mg t.i.d., each given over 8 weeks, accelerated emptying more than did a placebo; regarding symptom relief, however, there was a 'positive trend' in favour of the two agents in comparison with a placebo (DeCaestecker et al 1989). A parallel group study revealed that gastric emptying of solids as well as of liquids was significantly faster (Fig. 32.1) and symptoms alleviated significantly more after cisapride 10 mg q.i.d. for 4 weeks than after a placebo (Horowitz et al 1987b).

Open trials investigating the effects of the dopamine$_2$-receptor antagonist, domperidone, showed either no lasting effect of the drug (Horowitz et al 1985, Fig. 32.2) or an acceleration of emptying (Patterson et al 1991). A promising agent, whose prokinetic effects have only recently been discovered, is the macrolide antibiotic erythromycin, which presumably acts via a binding to motilin receptor sites on intestinal smooth muscle (Tomomasa et al 1986, Depoortere et al 1988). Erythromycin has been shown to accelerate gastric emptying in patients with diabetic gastroparesis not only after a single intravenous infusion, but also when given orally over a 4-week period (Janssens et al 1990). Motilin, when infused intravenously, accelerated emptying in patients with severe diabetic gastroparesis as well (Peeters et al 1992).

Amyloidosis

Amyloidosis can lead to gastrointestinal dysfunction by an infiltration of autonomic nervous structures and/or smooth muscle (Cohen 1967). Furthermore, the deposition of amyloid in blood vessels may result in intestinal infarction, perforation, bleeding and

Table 32.1 Effects of longer-lasting oral administration of prokinetic drugs on gastric emptying of a solid meal and on upper gastrointestinal symptoms in patients with diabetic gastroparesis

Authors	Patients	Drug and dosage	Treatment duration	Study design	Placebo control	Effects Emptying	Symptoms
Horowitz et al 1985	12	Domperidone 20 mg t.i.d.	35–51 d	Open	No	None	Less
Patterson et al 1991	14	Domperidone 20 mg q.i.d.	1 year	Open	No	Acceleration	Less
Havelund et al 1987	14	Cisapride 10 mg q.i.d.	28 d	Double-blind, crossover	Yes	None	None
Horowitz et al 1987b	10	Cisapride 10 mg q.i.d.	28 d	Double-blind, parallel group	Yes	Significant acceleration	Less
De Caestecker et al 1989	19	Cisapride 10 mg t.i.d.	56 d	Double-blind, crossover	Yes	None	'Positive trend'
		Metoclopramide 10 mg t.i.d.	56 d			None	'Positive trend'
Janssens et al 1990	10	Erythromycin 250 mg t.i.d.	28 d	Open	No	Significant acceleration	Less

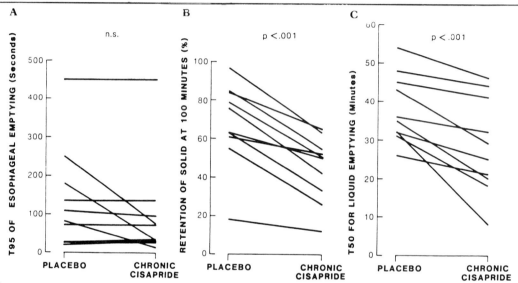

Fig. 32.1 Oesophageal emptying (**A**) and gastric emptying of solids (**B**) and liquids (**C**) after cisapride, 10 mg q.i.d. for 4 weeks, or placebo in patients with insulin-dependent diabetes. T50, 50% emptying time. (Reproduced with permission from Horowitz et al 1987b.)

malabsorption (Gilat & Spiro 1968, Gilat et al 1969, Kyle & Bayrd 1975). Reddy et al (1983) reported that metoclopramide, 10 mg intravenously, enhanced emptying in two patients with gastroparesis in spite of amyloid smooth muscle infiltration.

Neurofibromatosis

The gastrointestinal tract may be involved in as many as 10% of patients with von Recklinghausen's disease (Hochberg et al 1974). Neurofibromas or leiomyomas were found, mainly in the jejunum and stomach, in about 7% of patients. The disordered motor function results from a lesion of the myenteric plexus, manifested as angiomatosis, a plexiform pattern of the den-

dritic processes of the ganglion cells and neuronal dysplasia (Ternberg & Winters 1965, Phat et al 1980, Feinstat et al 1984).

Paraneoplastic neuropathy

In patients suffering from pulmonary carcinoma or carcinoid, disturbed gastrointestinal motor function may be due to paraneoplastic neuropathy. In seven patients, the myenteric plexus showed signs of degeneration, a diminution of neurons and axons, an infiltration by inflammatory cells and a proliferation of glial cells, whereas the submucosal plexus seemed unaffected (Chinn & Schuffler 1987). Six of the seven patients had gastroparesis, four oesophageal dysmotility and all had constipation.

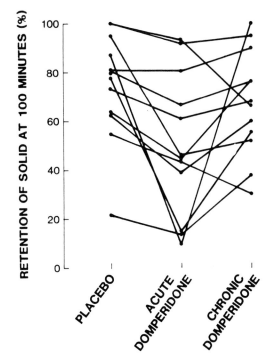

Fig. 32.2 Gastric emptying of a solid meal after placebo or a single dose of 40 mg dompertidone p.o., and 20 mg domperidone t.i.d. for 4 weeks in patients with diabetes mellitus. (Reproduced with permission from Horowitz et al 1985.)

Chronic idiopathic pseudo-obstruction

Gastric emptying can be delayed and antroduodenal motility disturbed in patients with both the myopathic and neuropathic forms of chronic idiopathic pseudo-obstruction (Mayer et al 1988).

Myotonic dystrophy

Myotonic dystrophy may be associated with a disordered motor function of parts or the whole of the gastrointestinal tract (Kuiper 1971, Lewis & Daniel 1981, Nowak et al 1982). Degenerative changes similar to the ones observed in striated muscle, with fatty infiltration and collagen formation, have been found in small intestinal and colonic smooth muscle cells (Nowak et al 1984) and a degenerative neuropathy of the myenteric plexus as underlying megacolon (Yoshida et al 1988a). Gastroparesis may be present in the congenital form of myotonia (Bodensteiner & Grunow 1984) and Kuiper (1971) found a gastric bezoar in a patient affected with the disease. Of 16 patients with dystrophia myotonica, 15 had a slower than normal rate of gastric emptying of solids as well as of liquids (Horowitz et al 1987a, (Fig. 32.3). In the latter patients, metoclopramide accelerated the evacuation of solids from the stomach in eight out of nine cases.

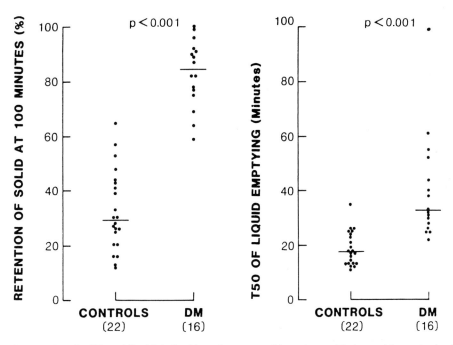

Fig. 32.3 Gastric emptying of solids and liquids in healthy volunteers and in patients with dystrophia myotonica (DM). Horizontal lines: median values; T50: 50% emptying time. (Reproduced with permission from Horowitz et al 1987a.)

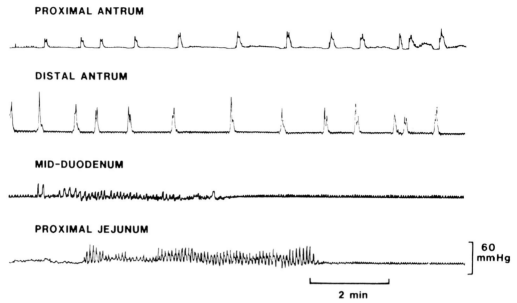

PROXIMAL ANTRUM

DISTAL ANTRUM

MID-DUODENUM

PROXIMAL JEJUNUM

60 mmHg

2 min

Fig. 32.4   Interdigestive antroduodenal motor activity in a patient 3 months after complete high-cord transection. Note the continuous antral phase II activity despite the migration of a phase III from the duodenum to the jejunum. (Reproduced with permission from Fealey et al 1984.)

Parkinson's disease

Gastric emptying has been found to be impaired in many patients with Parkinson's disease and accentuated by the medication of levodopa (Evans et al 1981).

Traumatic spinal cord transection

After spinal cord transection, gastric distension and ileus often pose major problems. In four out of five patients with complete interruption of the cord above T1, i.e. above the sympathetic outflow to the intestine, a dissociation between antral and duodenal interdigestive phase III activity and a reduced number of MMCs originating in the antrum was found (Fealey et al 1984, Fig. 32.4). No such disturbances were observed in three patients with transections at levels lower than T10. The postprandial interruption of the MMC was similar in both patient groups and did not differ from normal. In 11 quadruplegic and nine paraplegic patients with chronic spinal cord injury, gastric emptying was found to be delayed; after an intravenous dose of 10 mg metoclopramide, emptying was accelerated into the normal range (Segal et al 1987).

EATING DISORDERS

Primary anorexia nervosa and malnutrition

Gastric motor function is often severely impaired in primary anorexia nervosa. The disorder is diagnosed mainly in females during adolescence and young adulthood. The diagnostic criteria (American Psychiatric Association 1987) include a refusal to maintain body weight over a minimal weight for age and height, an intense fear of gaining weight or becoming fat, even though underweight, a disturbance in the way in which body weight, size or shape are experienced, and the absence of at least three consecutive menstrual cycles when otherwise expected to occur.

Gastrointestinal symptoms in patients with anorexia nervosa have long been noticed. Often, however, they are overlooked or misinterpreted and one of the most renowned researchers in the field stated: 'Anorexics will complain of feeling full after a few bites . . . One gains the impression that this sense of fullness is a phantom phenomenon, projection of formerly experienced sensations' (Bruch 1973). That sensations of that type are by no means phantom phenomena has been demonstrated in studies which established that gastric emptying is markedly delayed in a high proportion of patients (Dubois et al 1979, Holt et al 1981, McCallum et al 1985, Stacher et al 1986, 1987a, 1992, Abell et al 1987, Rigaud et al 1988, Robinson et al 1988) (Fig. 32.5).

The mechanisms underlying the delay in gastric emptying are still unclear. However, there is evidence to suggest that malnutrition plays a crucial role. In

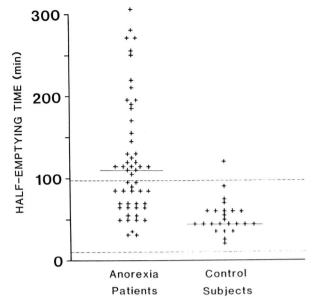

Fig. 32.5 Gastric half-emptying times of a semi-solid meal in 53 patients with primary anorexia nervosa and in 24 healthy subjects. Horizontal lines: median times; area between broken lines: mean half-emptying time ± SD in the 24 healthy subjects. (Reproduced with permission from Stacher et al 1992.)

depleted patients with anorexia, not only skeletal muscle fibre atrophy (Lindboe et al 1982, Sletterbø et al 1984, Alloway et al 1985), but also significant changes in muscle contraction–relaxation characteristics and fatigability properties have been observed. After refeeding and restoration of muscle electrolytes, features of the latter type all disappeared (Russell et al 1983b), as did gastrointestinal symptoms (Waldholtz & Andersen 1990, Stacher et al 1992). Similar effects might impair gastric smooth muscle function. In Indians with mixed deficiency diseases, muscular atrophies to the point that the stomach and the intestines appeared as 'tissue paper thin' have been described (Passmore 1947). Muscular atrophy may underlie the acute gastric distention observed to occur upon refeeding of patients with anorexia nervosa (Russell 1966, Scobie 1973, Jennings & Klidjian 1974) as well as in chronically starved prisoners of war (Markowski 1947), in neglected children (Gloebl et al 1976, Franken et al 1978) and in volunteers participating in starvation experiments (Keys et al 1950). With progressing gastric distention, venous occlusion, infarction and rupture may occur (Evans 1968, Saul et al 1981, Abdu et al 1987). However, disordered gastric motor function may also result from peripheral neuropathy as has been found to impair skeletal muscle function in

patients with anorexia and bulimia nervosa (Toifl et al 1984, Alloway et al 1985).

The contractile activity of the antrum, on which a normal rate of gastric emptying depends, is compromised in anorexia nervosa as well (Stacher et al 1987a, 1992): contraction amplitudes were found to be lower than in healthy individuals, and the postprandial increases in amplitude and decreases in contraction frequency, which normally coincide with the onset of emptying, were absent (Houghton et al 1988). In contrast to what has been reported previously (Abell et al 1987), patients with anorexia exhibited no heightened incidence of gastric dysrhythmia although their range of contraction frequencies was wider than in healthy individuals (Stacher et al 1987a, 1992).

It is important to note that, on primary evaluation, symptoms of vomiting and weight loss may be mistaken as indicating anorexia. This is suggested by the incidence of no less than 11 cases of achalasia among 124 patients referred to our institution from 1985 to 1990 under the diagnostic label of anorexia nervosa. In diagnosing anorexia at primary evaluation, the physicians may have been biased not only by the patients' emaciation but also by their young age and female sex, which led them to view certain aspects of history and behaviour as suggesting a pathological attitude towards eating and body weight. Another factor liable to contribute to misdiagnosis is that patients, who are, or have been, in psychiatric or psychosomatically oriented treatment, tend to learn 'their' psychiatric or psychosomatic history. They thus not only misinterpret their own symptoms but also mislead their physicians: nine of our 11 patients diagnosed primarily as having anorexia nervosa and later demonstrated to have achalasia were convinced that they were suffering from anorexia, that they had a distorted attitude towards eating and that they found their weight loss, at least subconsciously, desirable.

The delayed gastric emptying in patients with anorexia nervosa can readily be accelerated by cisapride (Fig. 32.6), which also increases the amplitude of antral contractions. Preliminary results suggest that the administration of cisapride over prolonged periods of time can, by accelerating emptying and thus reducing symptoms of gastric fullness, also contribute to an improved nutritional status (Stacher et al 1993a). The ultimate goal of therapy, the resumption of normal eating behaviour, can certainly not be achieved by prokinetic agents alone. Effects of other prokinetics have been evaluated in a small number of studies (McCallum et al 1985, Stacher et al 1986, 1993b). In a recent double-blind study we found that erythromycin, 200 mg infused intravenously, significantly enhanced

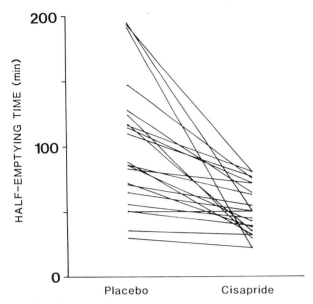

Fig. 32.6 Gastric emptying of a semi-solid meal in patients with anorexia nervosa after administration of placebo and 8 mg cisapride i.v. (Reproduced with permission from Stacher et al 1992.)

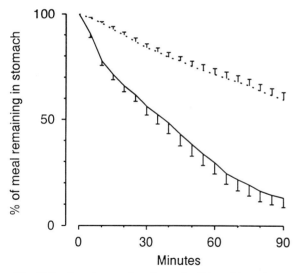

Fig. 32.7 Gastric emptying of a semi-solid meal in patients with primary anorexia nervosa after 200 mg erythromycin infused i.v. over 20 min (———) and placebo (· · · · ·). Vertical bars: SE. (Reproduced with permission from Stacher et al 1993b.)

emptying in all of 10 patients (Stacher et al 1993b, Fig. 32.7).

Bulimia nervosa

Bulimia nervosa is an eating disorder related to ano-

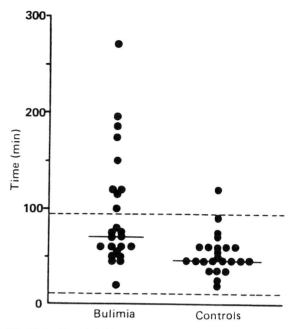

Fig. 32.8 Gastric half-emptying times of a semi-solid meal in 24 patients with bulimia nervosa and in 24 healthy subjects. Area between broken lines: mean half-emptying time ± SD in the healthy subjects. (Reproduced with permission from Kiss et al 1990.)

rexia nervosa, which has been reported as more and more prevalent on college campuses (Halmi et al 1981, Pyle et al 1986), although clinically significant bulimia seems to be rare (Schotte & Stunkard 1987, Connors & Johnson 1987). The diagnostic criteria require a minimum average of two binge eating episodes a week for at least 3 months and a persistent overconcern with body shape and weight (American Psychiatric Association 1987). Affected individuals sooner or later find out that the pain of abdominal distention during or after an eating binge can be counteracted by self-induced vomiting. Vomiting may lead to electrolyte imbalance and dehydration, especially when the patient also abuses laxatives or diuretics.

The functioning of organs likely to be affected by the bulimic behaviour, that is, the stomach and the oesophagus, has received little attention. This is all the more surprising, as symptoms such as postprandial fullness, early satiety, bloating and epigastric pain are encountered in a substantial proportion of patients (Abraham & Beumont 1982, Mitchell et al 1985, Chami et al 1991). In a study carried out on consecutive patients with bulimia in our institution (Kiss et al 1990), gastric emptying of a semi-solid meal was found to be grossly delayed in nine of 24 cases (Fig. 32.8). In addition, antral contraction amplitudes were markedly

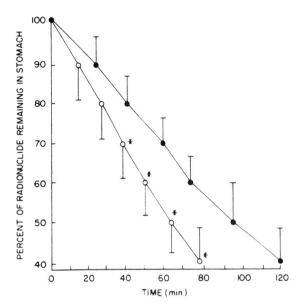

Fig. 32.9 Gastric emptying of a solid meal in obese (○) and non-obese (●) subjects. * = significant differences. (Reproduced with permission from Wright et al 1983.)

lower than in healthy individuals, and the normally occurring postprandial increase in amplitude was not present. In another study (Block et al 1990), the emptying of liquids was prolonged in 13 and that of solids in seven of 23 patients. Others found the emptying of a solid meal to be delayed in only one out of 10 patients (Robinson et al 1988) or even to be normal (Hutson et al 1988, Leventhal et al 1989). In one of the latter studies (Hutson et al 1988), however, emptying data of the bulimic patients were compared to those of a group of premenopausal women, which included individuals with morbid obesity and inflammatory bowel disease and whose gastric half-emptying times were highly scattered. Shih et al (1987) found gastric emptying of cream of wheat to be delayed in 12 of 20 patients, but to be rapid in the remaining eight. Rapid emptying has not been found in any of the patients of the above mentioned studies.

The factors contributing to the impaired gastric motor function in bulimia have not been fully elucidated. In our study (Kiss et al 1990), the absence or presence of a history of anorexia nervosa or of laxative abuse and the frequency of vomiting bore no relationship to the rate of gastric emptying. However, there was a significant inverse relationship between half-emptying times and serum-potassium levels, and a tendency of low percentages of desirable weight to be associated with slow emptying. As in depleted patients with anorexia nervosa, incidences of dilatation, infarc-

tion and rupture of the stomach upon the ingestion of large quantities of food have been recorded in patients with bulimia (Mitchell et al 1982, Abdu et al 1987, Petrin et al 1990). Smooth muscle atrophy caused by malnutrition and/or electrolyte depletion resulting from the self-induced vomiting may be a crucial factor.

Obesity

It has been suggested that one of the factors predisposing to obesity is a rapid gastric emptying, which would allow a high food intake (Hunt 1980). This hypothesis seemed to be supported by a study, in which 46 men and women with an average weight of 77% over ideal body weight were found to empty solid food significantly faster from their stomachs than 31 age-, sex- and race-matched non-obese individuals (Fig. 32.9); their emptying of liquids, however, was not accelerated (Wright et al 1983). By contrast, others found the emptying of solid meal components, due to a longer lag period, to be significantly slower in 15 obese than in 11 non-obese subjects; the duration of the lag period correlated with the excess body weight (Horowitz et al 1983). In a further study, very obese subjects tended to empty their stomachs more slowly than moderately obese individuals (Sasaki et al 1984). In view of the relatively small numbers of patients studied and the contradictory results reported, the questions, as to whether gastric emptying in the obese in fact differs systematically from emptying in non-obese subjects and whether or not the rate of gastric emptying contributes to the development of obesity, deserve further study.

PEPTIC ULCER DISEASE AND DYSPEPSIA

Duodenal ulcer

Increased gastric acid secretion has been considered of crucial importance in the development and the course of peptic ulcer disease. This belief was questioned by the fact that only a relatively small proportion of ulcer patients had higher levels of basal and stimulated acid secretion than healthy individuals. Thus it was hypothesized that the development of the ulcer resulted from prolonged contact of secretions with the mucosa due to a disordered gastroduodenal motor activity. This hypothesis seemed to be supported by the results of a study in 11 patients with an active and 10 with a healed duodenal ulcer as well as in 15 healthy subjects (Kerrigan et al 1991, Fig. 32.10). The patients with both active and healed ulcers had a similarly disordered motor activity: in the postprandial phase there was a

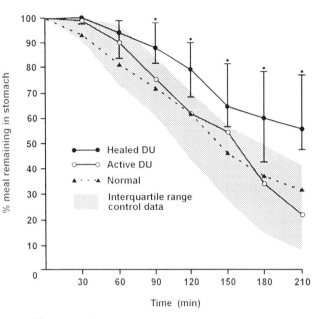

Fig. 32.10 Gastric emptying (median rates) in 10 patients with healed and 11 with active duodenal ulcer (DU) as well as in 15 healthy volunteers. Shaded area and horizontal bars: interquartile ranges (omitted for active DU); ★ = significant differences between patients with healed DU and healthy volunteers. (Reproduced with permission from Kerrigan et al 1991.)

decreased number of pressure waves sweeping aborally through the duodenum, and the incidence of retropulsive as well as atypical, complex forms of duodenal contractions was high throughout the study. The gastric emptying of solids was significantly slower in the patients with healed but not in those with active ulceration than in the healthy individuals. The results of this study, however, contradict those of earlier investigations, in which the emptying of solids did not differ in rate or pattern between duodenal ulcer patients and healthy individuals (Holt et al 1986a) or did not differ in its overall effect, although the lag phase was shorter and the linear emptying rate slower in ulcer patients (Maddern et al 1985).

Gastric ulcer

For patients with gastric ulcer as well, contradictory findings have been reported. Morguelan et al (1978) observed that gastric emptying was significantly slower in patients with an active ulcer in the corpus or proximal antrum as well as in patients with a gastric ulcer together with a duodenal ulcer or a scarred duodenal bulb than in healthy individuals, whereas emptying was significantly faster in patients with a prepyloric

ulcer. By contrast, patients with gastric ulcer but no pyloric obstruction (Holt et al 1986b) and Type I gastric ulcer (Müllner-Lissner et al 1983) were found not to differ in their emptying rate from healthy subjects. Patients with gastric ulcer have also been reported not to differ from healthy individuals with regard to duodenogastric reflux (Müllner-Lissner et al 1983, Schindlbeck et al 1987).

Effects of drugs reducing gastric acid secretion

Drugs reducing gastric acid secretion, which until recently have been the main remedies in the therapy of peptic ulcer, may alter gastroduodenal motor activity, but the pertinent information is far from unanimous. In healthy individuals, single oral doses of the histamine$_2$-receptor blockers cimetidine, 400 and 800 mg, and ranitidine, 300 mg, have been found to have no effect on gastric emptying (Houghton & Read 1987). 400 mg cimetidine given 60 min before an emptying study and 800 mg at the start of meal ingestion, however, resulted in a significant delay of the emptying of solids (Kerrigan et al 1989). By contrast, cimetidine, 1000–2000 mg per day administered to patients with duodenal ulcer for 4–8 weeks, significantly accelerated emptying (Forrest et al 1979). In rhesus monkeys, emptying was slowed by cimetidine and markedly accelerated by the specific histamine$_2$ receptor agonist, dimaprit (Dubois et al 1978). A dose of 20 mg omeprazole, which reduces gastric acid secretion by an inhibition of the proton pump in the parietal cell, was found to slow down the gastric emptying of six healthy subjects (Hongo et al 1989) although the difference was not significant.

Idiopathic dyspepsia

The symptoms of idiopathic dyspepsia, which are common in the general population (Jones et al 1990), have been assumed to be related, at least in part, to disordered gastroduodenal motor function resulting in either slow gastric emptying or increased duodenogastric reflux. Of 27 patients with chronic idiopathic dyspepsia, as defined by the presence of chronic unexplained symptoms suggestive of gastric stasis and directly related to food ingestion, 16 were found to have delayed gastric emptying, which was manifest with liquids more often than with solids (Jian et al 1989). The patients' symptoms, however, were of no predictive value for the presence of an emptying disorder. By contrast, Biliotti et al (1991) found that nausea, epigastric distention and pain were more frequently complained of by patients with idiopathic dyspepsia, who had delayed emptying.

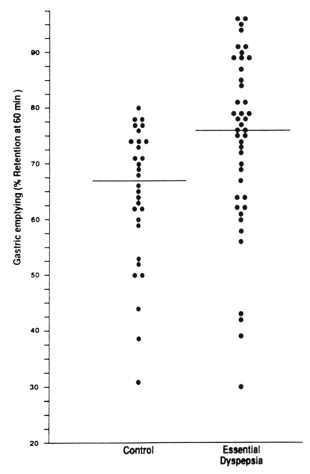

Fig. 32.11   Gastric emptying of solids in 30 symptom-free subjects and 43 patients with essential dyspepsia. Horizontal lines: median values. (Reproduced with permission from Wegener et al 1989.)

Wegener et al (1989) reported that 13 of 43 patients with idiopathic dyspepsia had emptying delayed beyond the values of 30 healthy subjects (Fig. 32.11). In these patients, the presence or absence of gastric *Helicobacter pylori* colonization was not associated with delayed emptying (Wegener et al 1988). In another study, emptying was slightly but significantly faster in 19 patients with idiopathic dyspepsia and *Helicobacter* infection than in non-infected individuals (Caldwell et al 1992).

Mearin et al (1990) found postprandial antral hypomotility to be present in 10 of 40 patients with moderate to severe upper abdominal pain, bloating, fullness, nausea and vomiting; duodenogastric reflux activity was not increased and not associated with antral hypo-

motility. On the basis of the pertinent findings it thus remains unclear whether a disordered gastric motor function underlies the symptoms of more than a subset of the patients with idiopathic dyspepsia.

Lémann et al (1991) studied the perception of visceral pain in response to gastric distention in consecutive patients with chronic idiopathic dyspepsia. They found that 13 of the 24 patients, but only one of 20 healthy subjects, experienced pain at distention volumes of greater than 400 ml of air, and that the perception of pain did not differ between patients with and without gastric stasis. However, the patients' enhanced perception of the distention as painful might well have been a reaction to the presence of their symptoms and the consecutive heightened attention to visceral sensations.

CONNECTIVE TISSUE DISEASES

Progressive systemic sclerosis (PSS)

In PSS, serious gastrointestinal involvement is frequent. The smooth muscle cells appear morphologically normal but are decreased in number. In some cases, collagen replaces the muscle fibres without reducing the overall thickness of the involved muscle layer, in others, the thickness of the fibrotic muscle is reduced; the myenteric plexus remains unaffected (Schuffler & Beegle 1979). In nine patients with PSS and evidence of small intestinal involvement, the overall motor activity of the antrum was significantly less than in six patients without intestinal involvement and in eight healthy subjects (Rees et al 1982). In another study (Maddern et al 1984), nine of 12 patients with PSS had their gastric emptying of solids delayed beyond the normal range (Fig. 32.12). Wegener et al (1991) found delayed emptying in seven of 13 patients with PSS. In eight PSS patients with delayed emptying, Horowitz et al (1987c) observed that emptying was accelerated and symptoms reduced by the administration of cisapride, 10 mg q.i.d. for 1 month.

Polymyositis and dermatomyositis

In polymyositis and dermatomyositis, weakness of, and inflammatory infiltrates within, skeletal muscles are the primary characteristics. The involvement of the striated muscle portion of the oesophagus is well documented, but the smooth muscle can be affected as well (Jacob et al 1986, Stacher et al 1987b). Little is known about the impact of the disease on gastric motor function (Kleckner 1970). Horowitz et al (1986b) found that the emptying of solids as well as of

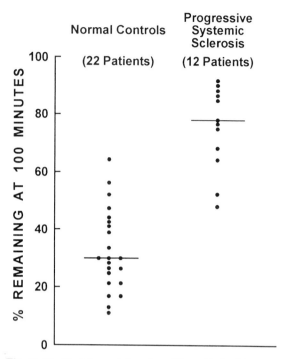

Fig. 32.12 Gastric emptying of a solid meal in healthy volunteers and in patients with progressive systemic sclerosis. Horizontal lines: median values. (Reproduced with permission from Maddern et al 1984.)

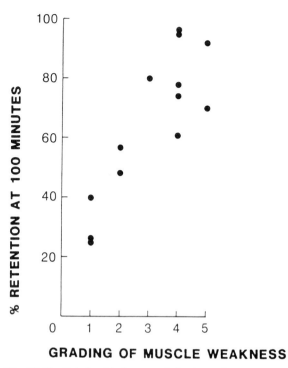

Fig. 32.13 Relationship between skeletal muscle weakness (grades 1 to 5) and the gastric emptying of solids in patients with polymyositis or dermatomyositis. (Reproduced with permission from Horowitz et al 1986b.)

liquids was slow, i.e. outside the normal range, in eight of 13 cases and that the presence of slow emptying was associated with skeletal muscle weakness (Fig. 32.13).

GASTRIC DYSFUNCTION INDUCED BY IRRADIATION AND CYTOTOXIC DRUGS

Severe and protracted nausea and vomiting are frequent concomitants of anti-cancer therapy and may induce malnutrition and electrolyte imbalance. The mechanisms eliciting these effects are poorly understood. The synthesis of prostanoids and lipoxygenase products of arachidonic acid has been shown to be increased, due to the generation of free radicals, by irradiation (Dean 1987), but to be blocked by the cytotoxic agents dactinomycin and cycloheximide (Fagan & Goldberg 1986). Thus, prostanoids do not seem to represent the sole agents involved. Irradiation yields an increased permeability of intestinal capillaries (Kingham & Loehry 1976), which may be responsible for a release of endotoxins into the circulation.

For some time, impairment of gastric functions has been regarded as of crucial importance for the develop-

ment of nausea and vomiting (Alphin et al 1986). In rhesus monkeys (Dorval et al 1985), radiation was found to lead to a transient suppression of gastric emptying (Fig. 32.14) and acid secretion, and emptying has been found to be suppressed also in dogs (Dubois et al 1984). Cisplatin has been shown to disrupt the normal gastric pacemaker activity in dogs and to initiate retroperistalsis that results in vomiting (Akwari 1983).

The observation that high doses of metoclopramide greatly reduced cisplatin-evoked emesis (Gralla et al 1981) seemed to point at a therapeutic role of dopamine$_2$-receptor antagonists. Later, however, it was found that the specific dopamine$_2$-antagonist domperidone could not prevent, even at high doses, cisplatin-induced emesis (Tonato et al 1985) and had no effect on the radiation-induced slow gastric emptying and vomiting (Dorval et al 1985). Subsequently it became clear that the anti-emetic effects of metoclopramide were due to an antagonism of 5-hydroxytryptamine$_3$ (5-HT$_3$) receptors and that these receptors mediated cytotoxic drug and radiation-evoked emesis (Miner et al 1987).

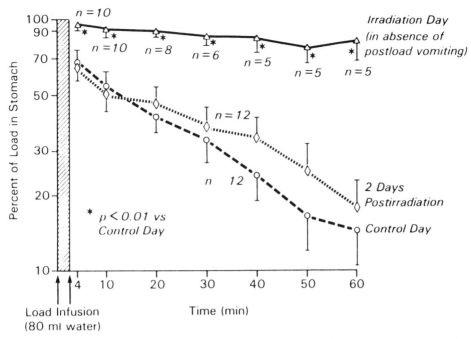

Fig. 32.14 Gastric emptying of a waterload before (control day), shortly after (irradiation day) and 2 days after 0.8 Gy whole body irradiation with cobalt 60 gamma-rays in rhesus monkeys. Values are means ± SE. (Reproduced with permission from Dorval et al 1985.)

Following this discovery, selective 5-HT$_3$ antagonists were developed. Of these, ondansetron (Kris et al 1988, Hesketh et al 1989) and granisetron (Chevallier 1990) were shown to yield high anti-emetic response rates in patients receiving cytotoxic therapy without causing more than mild side effects. As 5-HT$_3$ receptor antagonists do not accelerate delayed gastric emptying (Nielsen et al 1990, Stacher et al 1991), a disturbance of the latter type does not seem to be of major importance for the nausea and vomiting in patients undergoing anti-cancer therapy.

REFERENCES

Abdu R A, Garritano D, Culver O 1987 Acute gastric necrosis in anorexia nervosa and bulimia. Arch Surg 122: 830–832

Abell T L, Malagelada J-R, Lucas A R et al 1987 Gastric electromechanical and neurohormonal function in anorexia nervosa. Gastroenterology 93: 958–965

Abraham S F, Beumont P J V 1982 How patients describe bulimia or binge eating. Psychol Med 12: 625–635

Akwari O E 1983 The gastrointestinal tract in chemotherapy-induced emesis. A final common pathway. Drugs 25 (suppl 1): 18–34

Alloway R, Reynolds E H, Spargo E, Russell G F M 1985 Neuropathy and myopathy in two patients with anorexia and bulimia nervosa. J Neurol Neurosurg Psychiatry 48: 1015–1020

Alphin R S, Proakis A G, Leonard C A et al 1986 Antagonism of cisplatin-induced emesis by metoclopramide and dazopride through enhancement of gastric motility. Dig Dis Sci 31: 524–529

American Psychiatric Association 1987 Diagnostic and Statistical Manual of Mental Disorders, 3rd edn, revised. American Psychiatric Association, Washington, DC, pp 67–69

Aylett P 1962 Gastric emptying and change of blood glucose level as affected by glucagon and insulin. Clin Sci 22: 171–178

Bardhan P K, Salam M A, Molla A M 1992 Gastric emptying of liquid in children suffering from acute rotaviral gastroenteritis. Gut 33: 26–29

Barnett J L, Owyang C 1988 Serum glucose concentration as a modulator of interdigestive gastric motility. Gastroenterology 94: 739–744

Biliotti D, Pallotta N, Corazziari E, Torsoli A 1991 Delayed gastric emptying (GE) and its relationship with symptoms in idiopathic dyspepsia. Gastroenterology 100: A421

Block G D, Van Thiel D H, Brouillette D, Leventhal R, Kaye W, Hsu G 1990 Gastrointestinal dysmotility in bulimic non-pregnant females. Gastroenterology 98: A22

Bodensteiner J B, Grunow J E 1984 Gastroparesis in neonatal myotonic dystrophy. Muscle Nerve 7: 486–487

Bortolotti M, Bersani G, Labò G 1987 Association between chronic idiopathic gastroparesis and cytomegalovirus infection. Gastroenterology 92: 1324

Bruch H 1973 Anorexia nervosa In: Lindner A E (ed.), Emotional factors in gastrointestinal illness. Excerpta Medica, Amsterdam, pp 1–15

Buysschaert M, Moulart M, Urbain J L et al 1987 Impaired gastric emptying in diabetic patients with cardiac autonomic neuropathy. Diab Care 10: 448–452

Caldwell S H, Valenzuela G, Marshall B J et al 1992 Helicobacter pylori infection and gastric emptying of solids in humans. J Gastrointest Mot 4: 113–117

Camilleri M, Malagelada J-R 1984 Abnormal intestinal motility in diabetics with the gastroparesis syndrome. Eur J Clin Invest 14: 420–427

Chami T N, Andersen A E, Crowell M D, Schuster M M, Whitehead W E 1991 Gastrointestinal symptoms in bulimia nervosa: effects of treatment. Gastroenterology 100 (suppl): A427

Chevallier B on behalf of the Granisetron Study Group 1990 Efficacy and safety of granisetron compared with high-dose metoclopramide plus dexamethasone in patients receiving high-dose cisplatin in a single-blind study. Eur J Cancer Clin Oncol 26 (suppl 1): 533–536

Chinn J S, Schuffler M D 1987 Paraneoplastic visceral neuropathy is a cause of severe gastrointestinal motor dysfunction in patients with lung cancer. Gastroenterology 92: 1345

Cohen A S 1967 Amyloidosis. N Engl J Med 277: 522–583, 628–637

Connors M E, Johnson C L 1987 Epidemiology of bulimia and bulimic behaviors. Addict Behav 12: 165–179

De Caestecker J S, Ewing D J, Tothill P, Clarke B F, Heading R C 1989 Evaluation of oral cisapride and metoclopramide in diabetic autonomic neuropathy: an eight-week double-blind crossover study. Aliment Pharmacol Ther 3: 69–81

Dean R T 1987 Free radicals, membrane damage and cell-mediated cytolysis. Br J Cancer 55 (suppl VIII): 39–45

Depoortere I, Peeters T L, Matthijs G, Vantrappen G 1988 Macrolide antibiotics are motilin receptor agonists. Hepatogastroenterology 35: 198

Dorval E D, Mueller G P, Eng R R, Durakovic A, Conklin J J, Dubois A 1985 Effect of ionizing radiation on gastric secretion and gastric motility in monkeys. Gastroenterology 89: 374–380

Dubois A, Nompleggi D, Myers L, Castell D O 1978 Histamine H_2 receptor stimulation increases gastric emptying. Gastroenterology 74: 1028

Dubois A, Gross H A, Ebert M H, Castell D O 1979 Altered gastric emptying and secretion in primary anorexia nervosa. Gastroenterology 77: 319–323

Dubois A, Jacobus J P, Grissom M P, Eng R R, Conklin J J 1984 Altered gastric emptying and prevention of radiation-induced vomiting in dogs. Gastroenterology 86: 444–448

Dyck P J 1992 New understanding and treatment of diabetic neuropathy. N Engl J Med 326: 1287–1288

Dyck P J, Lais A, Karnes J L, O'Brien P, Rizza R 1986 Fiber loss is primary and multifocal in sural nerves in diabetic polyneuropathy. Ann Neurol 19: 425–439

Evans D S 1968 Acute dilatation and spontaneous rupture of the stomach. Br J Surg 55: 940–942

Evans M A, Broe G A, Triggs E J, Cheung M, Creasey H, Paull P D 1981 Gastric emptying rate and the systemic availability of levodopa in the elderly parkinsonian patient. Neurology 31: 1288–1294

Fagan J M, Goldberg A L 1986 Inhibitors of protein and RNA synthesis cause a rapid block in prostaglandin production at the prostaglandin synthase step. Proc Nat Acad Sci U S A 83: 2771–2775

Fealey R D, Szurszewski J H, Merritt J L, DiMagno E P 1984 Effect of traumatic spinal cord transection on human upper gastrointestinal motility and gastric emptying. Gastroenterology 87: 69–75

Feinstat T, Tesluk H, Schuffler M D et al 1984 Megacolon and neurofibromatosis: a neuronal intestinal dysplasia; case report and review of the literature. Gastroenterology 86: 1573–1579

Flewet T H 1982 Clinical features of rotavirus infection. In: Tyrell D A J, Kapikian A Z (eds) Virus infections of the gastrointestinal tract. Marcel Dekker, New York, pp 125–146

Forrest J A H, Fettes M R, McLoughlin G P, Heading R C 1979 Effect of long-term cimetidine on gastric acid secretion, serum gastrin, and gastric emptying. Gut 20: 404–407

Franken E A, Fox M, Smith J A, Smith W L 1978 Acute gastric dilatation in neglected children. Am J Roentgenol 130: 297–299

Fraser R, Horowitz M, Graham S, Dent J 1989 Acute hyperglycaemia and antropyloroduodenal motility in humans. Gastroenterology 96: A157

Fraser R J, Horowitz M, Maddox A F, Harding P E, Chatterton B E, Dent J 1990 Hyperglycaemia slows gastric emptying in Type 1 (insulin-dependent) diabetes mellitus. Diabetologia 33: 675–680

Fraser R, Horowitz M, Dent J 1991 Hyperglycaemia stimulates pyloric motility in normal subjects. Gut 32: 475–478

Gilat T, Revach M, Sohar E 1969 Deposition of amyloid in the gastrointestinal tract. Gut 10: 98–104

Gilat T, Spiro H M 1968 Amyloidosis and the gut. Am J Dig Dis 13: 619–633

Gloebl H J, Capitano M A, Kirkpatrick J A 1976 Radiographic findings in children with psychosocial dwarfism. Pediatr Radiol 4: 83–86

Grainger S L, Gaunt J I, Brown P M, Thompson R P H, Croft D N 1983 Gastric emptying in diabetes: relationship to blood glucose levels. Gut 24: A485

Gralla R J, Itri L M, Psiko S E et al 1981 Antiemetic efficacy of high-dose metoclopramide: randomized trials with placebo and prochlorperazine in patients with chemotherapy-induced nausea and vomiting. N Engl J Med 305: 905–909

Greene D A, Lattimer S A, Sima A A F 1987 Sorbitol, phosphoinositide, and sodium-potassium-ATPase in the pathogenesis of diabetic complications. N Engl J Med 316: 599–606

Halmi K A, Falk J R, Schwarz E 1981 Binge eating and vomiting: A survey of a college population. Psychol Med 11: 697–706

Havelund T, Øster-Jørgensen E, Eshoj O, Larsen M L, Lauritsen K 1987 Effects of cisapride on gastroparesis in patients with insulin-dependent diabetes mellitus. A double-blind controlled trial. Acta Med Scand 222: 339–343

Hesketh P J, Murphy W K, Lester E P et al 1989 GR 38032F (GR-C507/75): a novel compound effective in the prevention of acute cisplatin-induced emesis. J Clin Oncol 7: 700–705

Hirano T, Niijima A 1980 Effects of 2-deoxy-d-glucose, glucose and insulin on efferent activity in gastric vagus nerve. Experientia 36: 1197–1205

Hochberg F H, Dasilva A B, Galdabini J, Richardson E P Jr 1974 Gastrointestinal involvement in von Recklinghausen's neurofibromatosis. Neurology 24: 1144–1151

Hodges F J, Rundles R W, Hanelin J 1947 Roentgenologic study of small intestine. II. Dysfunction associated with neurologic diseases. Radiology 49: 659–673

Holt S, Ford M J, Grant S, Heading R C 1981 Abnormal gastric emptying in primary anorexia nervosa. Br J Psychiatry 39: 550–552

Holt S, Heading R C, Taylor T V, Forrest J A, Tothill P 1986a Is gastric emptying abnormal in duodenal ulcer? Dig Dis Sci 31: 685–692

Holt S, Lavery J, Miron S et al 1986b Is gastric emptying abnormal in gastric ulcer? Gastroenterology 90: 1464

Hongo M, Lin Y F, Satake K, Toyata T, Okuyama S, Goto Y 1986 Gastric emptying in patients with diabetes mellitus with and without autonomic neuropathy. Gastroenterology 90: 1464

Hongo M, Lin Y F, Ujiie H et al 1989 Acid suppression by omeprazole inhibits gastric emptying in normal subjects. Gastroenterology 96: A218

Horowitz M, Collins P J, Cook D J, Harding P E, Shearman D J C 1983 Abnormalities of gastric emptying in obese patients. Int J Obes 7: 415–421

Horowitz M, Harding P E, Chatterton B E, Collins P J, Shearman D J C 1985 Acute and chronic effects of domperidone on gastric emptying in diabetic autonomic neuropathy. Dig Dis Sci 30: 1–9

Horowitz M, Harding P E, Maddox A et al 1986a Gastric and oesophageal emptying in insulin-dependent diabetes mellitus. J Gastroenterol Hepatol 1: 97–113

Horowitz M, McNeil J D, Maddern G J, Collins P J, Shearman D J C 1986b Abnormalities of gastric and esophageal emptying in polymyositis and dermatomyositis. Gastroenterology 90: 434–439

Horowitz M, Maddox A, Maddern G J, Wishart J, Collins P J, Shearman D J C 1987a Gastric and esophageal emptying in dystrophia myotonica. Effect of metoclopramide. Gastroenterology 92: 570–577

Horowitz M, Maddox A, Harding P E et al 1987b Effect of cisapride on gastric and esophageal emptying in insulin-dependent diabetes mellitus. Gastroenterology 92: 1899–1907

Horowitz M, Maddern G J, Maddox A, Wishart J, Chatterton B E, Shearman D J C 1987c Effects of cisapride on gastric and esophageal emptying in progressive systemic sclerosis. Gastroenterology 93: 311–315

Horowitz M, Harding P E, Maddox A F et al 1989 Gastric and oesophageal emptying in patients with type 2 (non-insulin-dependent) diabetes mellitus. Diabetologia 32: 151–159

Houghton L A, Read N W 1987 A comparative study of the effect of cimetidine and ranitidine on the rate of gastric emptying of liquid and solid test meals in man. Aliment Pharmacol Ther 1: 401–408

Houghton L A, Read N W, Heddle R et al 1988 Relationship of the motor activity of the antrum, pylorus, and duodenum to gastric emptying of a solid-liquid mixed meal. Gastroenterology 94: 1285–1291

Hunt J N 1980 A possible relation between the regulation of gastric emptying and food intake. Am J Physiol 239: G1–G4

Hutson W, Wald A, Mooney J, Kane R, Kalla R 1988 Gastric emptying (GE) and antral motility (AM) in anorexia nervosa and bulimia. Gastroenterology 94: A198

Jacob H, Berkowitz D, McDonald E, Bernstein L H, Beneventano T 1986 The esophageal motility disorder of polymyositis. A prospective study. Arch Intern Med 143: 2262–2264

Janssens J, Peeters T L, Vantrappen G et al 1990 Improvement of gastric emptying in diabetic gastroparesis by erythromycin. Preliminary studies. N Engl J Med 322: 1028–1031

Jennings K P, Klidjian A M 1974 Acute gastric dilatation in anorexia nervosa. Br Med J 2: 477–478

Jian R, Ducrot F, Ruskone A et al 1989 Symptomatic, radionuclide and therapeutic assessment of chronic idiopathic dyspepsia. A double-blind placebo-controlled evaluation of cisapride. Dig Dis Sci 34: 657–664

Johnson P C, Doll S C, Cromey D W 1986 Pathogenesis of diabetic neuropathy. Ann Neurol 19: 450–457

Jones R H, Lydeard S E, Hobbs F D R et al 1990 Dyspepsia in England and Scotland. Gut 31: 401–405

Kassander P 1958 Asymptomatic gastric retention in diabetics (gastroparesis diabeticorum). Ann Intern Med 48: 797–812

Kerrigan D D, Mangnall Y F, Read N W, Johnson A G 1989 Cimetidine delays gastric emptying of solid food. Gastroenterology 96: A253

Kerrigan D D, Read N W, Houghton L A, Taylor M E, Johnson A G 1991 Disturbed gastro-duodenal motility in patients with active and healed duodenal ulceration. Gastroenterology 100: 892–900

Keshavarzian A, Iber F L, Vaeth J 1987 Gastric emptying in patients with insulin-requiring diabetes mellitus. Am J Gastroenterol 82: 29–35

Keys A, Brožek J, Henschel A, Michelsen O, Longstreet-Taylor H 1950 The biology of human starvation. University of Minnesota Press, Minneapolis, pp 587–600

Kim C H, Kennedy F P, Camilleri M, Zinsmeister A R, Ballard D J 1991 The relationship between clinical factors and gastrointestinal dysmotility in diabetes mellitus. J Gastrointest Mot 3: 268–272

Kingham J G C, Loehry C A 1976 Permeability of the small intestine after intra-arterial injection of histamine-type mediators and irradiation. Gut 17: 517–526

Kiss A, Bergmann H, Abatzi Th-A et al 1990 Oesophageal and gastric motor activity in patients with bulimia nervosa. Gut 31: 259–265

Kleckner F S 1970 Dermatomyositis and its manifestations in the gastrointestinal tract. Am J Gastroenterol 53: 141–146

Kris M G, Gralla R J, Clark R A, Tyson L B 1988 Dose-ranging evaluation of the serotonin antagonist GR-C507/75 (GR38032F) when used as an antiemetic in patients receiving anticancer chemotherapy. J Clin Oncol 6: 659–662

Kuiper D H 1971 Gastric bezoar in a patient with myotonic dystrophy. A review of the gastrointestinal complications of myotonic dystrophy. Am J Dig Dis 16: 529–534

Kyle R A, Bayrd E D 1975 Amyloidosis: review of 236 cases. Medicine 54: 271–299

Lémann M, Dederding J P, Flourié B, Franchisseur C,

Rambaud J C, Jian R 1991 Abnormal perception of visceral pain in response to gastric distension in chronic idiopathic dyspepsia. The irritable stomach syndrome. Dig Dis Sci 36: 1249–1254

Leventhal R I, Brouillette D, Cuellar R et al 1989 Gastric emptying in bulimia. Gastroenterology 96: A297

Lewis T D, Daniel E E 1981 Gastroduodenal motility in a case of dystrophia myotonica. Gastroenterology 81: 145–149

Lindboe C F, Askevold F, Sletterbø M 1982 Changes in skeletal muscles of young women with anorexia nervosa. An enzyme histochemical study. Acta Neuropathol 56: 299–302

McCallum R W, Grill B B, Lange R, Planky M, Glass E E, Greenfeld D G 1985 Definition of a gastric emptying abnormality in patients with anorexia nervosa. Dig Dis Sci 30: 713–722

MacGregor I L, Gueller R, Watts H D, Meyer J H 1976 The effect of acute hyperglycemia on gastric emptying in man. Gastroenterology 70: 190–196

Maddern G J, Horowitz M, Jamieson G G, Chatterton B E, Collins P J, Roberts-Thomson P 1984 Abnormalities of esophageal and gastric emptying in progressive systemic sclerosis. Gastroenterology 87: 922–926

Maddern G J, Horowitz M, Hetzel D J, Jamieson G G 1985 Altered solid and liquid gastric emptying in patients with duodenal ulcer disease. Gut 26: 689–693

Malagelada J-R, Rees W D W, Mazzotta L J, Go V L W 1980 Gastric motor abnormalities in diabetic and post-vagotomy gastroparesis: effect of metoclopramide and bethanechol. Gastroenterology 78: 286–292

Markowski B 1947 Acute dilation of the stomach. Br Med J 2: 128–130

Mayer E A, Elashoff J, Hawkins R, Berquist W, Taylor I L 1988 Gastric emptying of mixed solid-liquid meal in patients with intestinal pseudoobstruction. Dig Dis Sci 33: 10–18

Mearin F, Camilleri M, Malagelada J-R 1986 Pyloric dysfunction in diabetics with recurrent nausea and vomiting. Gastroenterology 90: 1919–1925

Mearin F, Rodriguez R, Cucala M, Malagelada J-R 1990 Is duodenogastric reflux a pathogenetic factor in chronic functional dyspepsia? Gastroenterology 98: A88

Meeroff J C, Schrieber D S, Trier J S, Blacklow N R 1980 Abnormal gastric motor function in viral gastroenteritis. Ann Intern Med 92: 470–413

Miner W D, Sanger G J, Turner D H 1987 Evidence that 5-hydroxytryptamine$_3$ receptors mediate cytotoxic drug and radiation-evoked emesis. Br J Cancer 56: 159–162

Mitchell J E, Pyle R L, Miner R A 1982 Gastric dilatation as a complication of bulimia. Psychosomatics 23: 96–97

Mitchell J E, Hatsukami D, Eckert E D, Pyle R L 1985 Characteristics of 275 patients with bulimia. Am J Psychiatry 142: 482–485

Morgan L M, Tredger J A Hampton S M, French A P, Peake J C, Marks V 1988 The effect of dietary modification and hyperglycaemia on gastric emptying and gastric inhibitory polypeptide (GIP) secretion. Br J Nutr 60: 29–37

Morguelan B, Ippoliti A, Sturdevant R 1978 Gastric emptying in patients with gastric ulcer (GU). Gastroenterology 74: 1070

Müller-Lissner S A, Fimmel C J, Sonnenberg A et al 1983 Novel approach to quantify duodenogastric reflux in healthy volunteers and in patients with type I gastric ulcer. Gut 24: 510–518

Nielsen O H, Hvid-Jacobsen K, Lund P, Langholz E 1990 Gastric emptying and subjective symptoms of nausea: lack of effects of a 5-hydroxytryptamine-3 antagonist ondansetron on gastric emptying in patients with gastric stasis syndrome. Digestion 46: 89–96

Nowak T V, Ionasescu V, Anuras S 1982 Gastrointestinal manifestations of the muscular dystrophies. Gastroenterology 82: 800–810

Nowak T V, Anuras S, Brown B P, Ionasescu V, Green J B 1984 Small intestinal motility in myotonic dystrophy patients. Gastroenterology 86: 808–813

Øster-Jørgensen E, Pedersen S A, Larsen M L 1990 The influence of induced hyperglycaemia on gastric emptying rate in healthy humans. Scand J Clin Lab Invest 50: 831–836

Passmore R 1947 Mixed deficiency diseases in India: a clinical description. Trans R Soc Trop Med Hyg 41: 189–206

Patterson D J, Botoman V A, Kozarek R A, Skinner S M 1991 Domperidone is effective long-term treatment for diabetic gastroparesis. Gastroenterology 100 (suppl): A137

Peeters T L, Muls E, Janssens J et al 1992 Effect of motilin on gastric emptying in patients with diabetic gastroparesis. Gastroenterology 102: 97–101

Petrin C, Tacchetti G, Preciso G, Gallo F, Bernardi S, Mion M 1990 Distension aigue suivie de rupture gastrique après un accès de boulimie. A propos d'un cas. J Chir 127: 213–215

Phat V N, Sezeur A, Danne M, Dupuis D, de La Vaissière G, Camilleri J-P 1980 Primary myenteric plexus alterations as a cause of megacolon in von Recklinghausen's disease. Pathol Biol 28: 585–588

Press M F, Riddell R H, Ringus J 1980 Cytomegalovirus inclusion disease. Its occurrence in the myenteric plexus of a renal transplant patient. Arch Pathol Lab Med 104: 580–583

Pyle R L, Halvorson P A, Neuman P A, Mitchell J E 1986 The increasing prevalence of bulimia in freshman college students. Int J Eating Dis 5: 631–647

Reddy A B, Wright R A, Wheeler G E, Nazer H 1983 Nonobstructive gastroparesis in amyloidosis improved with metoclopramide. Arch Intern Med 143: 247–248

Rees W D W, Leigh R J, Christofides N D, Bloom S R, Turnberg L A 1982 Interdigestive motor activity in patients with systemic sclerosis. Gastroenterology 83: 575–580

Rigaud D, Bedig G, Merrouche M, Vulpillat M, Bonfils S, Apfelbaum M 1988 Delayed gastric emptying in anorexia nervosa is improved by completion of renutrition program. Dig Dis Sci 33: 919–925

Robinson P H, Clarke M, Barrett J 1988 Determinants of delayed gastric emptying in anorexia nervosa and bulimia nervosa. Gut 29: 458–464

Rundles R W 1945 Diabetic neuropathy; general review with report of 125 cases. Medicine 24: 111–160

Russell C O H, Gannan R, Coatsworth J et al 1983a Relationship among esophageal dysfunction, diabetic gastroenteropathy and peripheral neuropathy. Dig Dis Sci 28: 289–293

Russell D McR, Prendergast P J, Darby P L, Garfinkel P E, Whitwell J, Jeejeebhoy K N 1983b A comparison between muscle function and body composition in anorexia nervosa:

the effect of refeeding. Am J Clin Nutr 38: 229–237

Russell G F M 1966 Acute dilatation of the stomach in a patient with anorexia nervosa. Br J Psychiatry 112: 203–207

Said G, Slama G, Selva J 1983 Progressive centripetal degeneration of axons in small fibre diabetic polyneuropathy. Brain 106: 791–807

Said G, Goulin-Goeau C, Slama G, Tchobroutsky G 1992 Severe early-onset polyneuropathy in insulin-dependent diabetes mellitus. A clinical and pathological study. N Engl J Med 326: 1257–1263

Sasaki H, Nagulesparan M, Dubois A et al 1984 Gastric function and obesity: gastric emptying, gastric acid secretion and plasma pepsinogen. Int J Obes 8: 183–190

Saul S H, Dekker A, Watson C G 1981 Acute gastric dilatation with infarction and perforation. Gut 22: 978–983

Scarpello J M B, Barber D C, Hague R V, Cullen D R, Sladen G E 1976 Gastric emptying of solid meals in diabetics. Br Med J 2: 671–673

Schindlbeck N E, Heinrich C, Stellaard F, Paumgartner G, Müller-Lissner S A 1987 Healthy controls have as much bile reflux as gastric ulcer patients. Gut 28: 1577–1583

Schotte D E, Stunkard A J 1987 Bulimia vs bulimic behaviors on a college campus. JAMA 258: 1213–1215

Schuffler M D, Beegle R G 1979 Progressive systemic sclerosis of the gastrointestinal tract and hereditary hollow visceral myopathy: two distinguishable disorders of the intestinal smooth muscle. Gastroenterology 77: 664–671

Scobie B A 1973 Acute gastric dilatation and duodenal ileus in anorexia nervosa. Med J Aust 2: 932–934

Segal J L, Milne N, Brunnemann S R, Lyons K P 1987 Metoclopramide-induced normalization of impaired gastric emptying in spinal cord injury. Am J Gastroenterol 82: 1143–1148

Shih W-J, Humphries L, Digenis G A, Castellanos F X, Domstad P A, DeLand F H 1987 Tc-99m labeled triethylene tetraamine polysterene resin gastric emptying studies in bulimia patients. Eur J Nucl Med 13: 192–196

Sletterbø M, Lindboe C F, Askevold F 1984 The neuromuscular system in patients with anorexia nervosa: electrophysiological and histologic studies. Clin Neuropathol 3: 217–224

Stacher G, Kiss A, Wiesnagrotzki S, Bergmann H, Höbart J, Schneider C 1986 Oesophageal and gastric motility disorders in patients categorised as having primary anorexia nervosa. Gut 27: 1120–1126

Stacher G, Bergmann H, Wiesnagrotzki S et al 1987a Intravenous cisapride accelerates delayed gastric emptying and increases antral contraction amplitude in patients with primary anorexia nervosa. Gastroenterology 92: 1000–1006

Stacher G, Schneider C, Smolen J, Schmierer G, Gaupmann G 1987b Oesophageal motor abnormalities in patients with connective tissue diseases in: Siewert J R, Hölscher A H (eds), Diseases of the esophagus. Springer, Berlin, pp 890–894

Stacher G, Bergmann H, Granser-Vacariu G V et al 1991 Lack of systematic effects of the 5-hydroxytryptamine$_3$ receptor antagonist ICS 205–930 on gastric emptying and antral motor activity in patients with primary anorexia nervosa. Br J Clin Pharmacol 32: 685–690

Stacher G, Bergmann H, Wiesnagrotzki S, Steiner-Mittelbach G, Kiss A, Abatzi Th-A 1992 Primary anorexia nervosa. Gastric emptying and antral motor activity in 53 patients. Int J Eating Dis 11: 163–172

Stacher G, Abatzi-Wenzel Th-A, Wiesnagrotzki S, Bergmann H, Schneider C, Gaupmann G 1993a Gastric emptying, body weight and symptoms in primary anorexia nervosa: long-term effects of cisapride. Br J Psychiatry 162: 398–402

Stacher G, Peeters T L, Bergmann H et al 1993b Erythromycin effects on gastric emptying, antral motor activity and plasma motilin and pancreatic polypeptide concentrations in anorexia nervosa. Gut 34: 166–172

Susman E, Maddox K 1940 The Guillain-Barré syndrome. Med J Aust 1: 158–162

Ternberg J L, Winters K 1965 Plexiform neurofibromatosis of the colon as a cause of congenital megacolon. Am J Surg 109: 663–665

Toifl K, Mamoli B, Neumann E 1984 Subklinische Polyneuropathien bei Anorexia nervosa in: Gerstenbrand F, Mamoli B, Sluga E (eds), Metabolische und entzündliche Polyneuropathien. Springer, Berlin, pp 57–62

Tomomasa T, Kuroume T, Arai H, Wakabayashi K, Itoh Z 1986 Erythromycin induces migrating motor complex in human gastrointestinal tract. Dig Dis Sci 31: 157–161

Tonato M, Roila F, Del Favero A, Tognoni G, Franzosis G, Pampalonas S 1985 A pilot study of high dose domperidone as an anti-emetic in patients treated with cis-platin. Eur J Cancer Clin Oncol 21:807

Waldholtz B D, Andersen A 1990 Gastrointestinal symptoms in anorexia nervosa. A prospective study. Gastroenterology 98: 1415–1419

Wegener M, Börsch G, Schaffstein J, Schulz-Flake C, Mai U, Leverkus F 1988 Are dyspeptic symptoms in patients with campylobacter pylori-associated type B gastritis linked to delayed gastric emptying? Am J Gastroenterol 83: 737–740

Wegener M, Börsch G, Schaffstein J, Reuter C, Leverkus F 1989 Frequency of idiopathic gastric stasis and intestinal transit disorders in essential dyspepsia. J Clin Gastroenterol 11: 163–168

Wegener M, Schaffstein J, Coenen C, Berger E, Schmidt G 1991 Gastrointestinal transit in progressive systemic sclerosis. Gastroenterology 100: A183

Widerlite L, Trier J S, Blacklow N R, Schriefer D S 1974 Structure of gastric mucosa in acute infectious non-bacterial gastroenteritis. J Infect Dis 129: 705–708

Wright R A, Krinsky S, Fleeman C, Trujillo J, Teague E 1983 Gastric emptying and obesity. Gastroenterology 84: 747–751

Wyburn-Mason R 1957 Visceral lesions in herpes zoster. Br Med J 1: 678–681

Yoshida M M, Krishnamurthy S, Wattchow D A, Furness J B, Schuffler M D 1988a Megacolon in myotonic dystrophy caused by a degenerative neuropathy of the myenteric plexus. Gastroenterology 95: 820–827

Yoshida M M, Schuffler M D, Sumi S M 1988b There are no morphologic abnormalities of the gastric wall or abdominal vagus in patients with diabetic gastroparesis. Gastroenterology 94: 907–914

33. Motor disorders of the biliary tract

J. Toouli

INTRODUCTION

Bile flows from the liver to the duodenum in a regulated fashion due to the combined effects of the hepatic secretory pressure, gallbladder contraction and sphincter of Oddi (SO) motility. The normal activity of the gallbladder and SO during the interdigestive period and after a meal has been described previously. Abnormalities in this orderly activity, either in the gallbladder or SO may give rise to clinical syndromes which mainly present as recurrent episodes of biliary or pancreatic type pain.

GALLBLADDER AND CYSTIC DUCT

Motility disorders of the gallbladder and cystic duct present with symptoms which suggest gallstone disease. However, investigations for gallstones are normal. In a subgroup of patients, 'sludge' may be found on ultrasound of the gallbladder (Bolondi et al 1984). This abnormality usually is associated with long term parenteral nutrition and may subsequently lead to gallstones (Lee et al 1988).

Gallbladder dyskinesia

The most common presentation for patients with gallbladder motility disorders (i.e. gallbladder dyskinesia) is recurrent biliary type pain. Most of the patients are female in the 35–55-year-old age group, however, the condition is diagnosed also in younger and older patients of either sex. Examination of the patient during an episode of pain reveals tenderness under the right costal margin and there may be localized guarding. The temperature is usually normal and there are no changes in the white cell count or in liver transaminases, bilirubin, alkaline phosphatase or serum amylase.

Investigation

Following presentation, a provisional diagnosis of biliary colic due to gallstones is usually made. However, biliary ultrasound and/or oral cholecystogram reveals a normal gallbladder and bile duct with no evidence of stones.

Further investigation will depend on the severity of symptoms, the number of previous episodes of pain and any serum biochemical anomalies. It is essential to rule out the possibility of other common upper abdominal conditions, such as gastric, duodenal and colonic disorders. In particular, non-ulcer dyspepsia, *Helicobacter pylori* gastritis, duodenal giardiasis and colonic irritable bowel syndrome should be considered and appropriate therapy given, as these conditions may closely mimic biliary tract symptoms.

ERCP

In patients in whom the suspicion of biliary tract disease remains strong, further investigation is warranted. Endoscopic retrograde cholangiopancreatography (ERCP) is an important investigation which provides structural definition of the biliary and pancreatic ducts. It is mandatory in any patient with associated liver enzyme, bilirubin, alkaline phosphatase or amylase change with episodes of pain. In such patients there is a strong possibility of identifying small stones in either the gallbladder or bile duct by careful screening of the biliary tract after controlled infusion of dilute contrast (Venu et al 1983). Furthermore, pancreatic pathology, sclerosing cholangitis, Caroli's disease or choledochal cyst can be excluded.

Cholesterol crystals

At the end of the endoscopic procedure, gallbladder contraction may be produced by intravenous injection of cholecystokinin octapeptide (CCK-OP) 40 ng/kg and gallbladder bile which flows into the duodenum aspirated through the ERCP catheter for examination to determine the presence of cholesterol crystals

(Freeman et al 1975). A finding of cholesterol crystals in gallbladder bile is strongly associated with the presence of small calculi in the gallbladder or cholesterolosis. This finding supports the diagnosis of early gallbladder stone disease and the patient should be treated by cholecystectomy.

CCK provocation test

Pain provocation tests have been used to select for treatment patients with suspected gallbladder motility disorders. The most common test uses a fixed bolus of CCK-OP and a positive response is taken as the subjective reproduction of the pain (Rhodes et al 1988). A radiological modification of this test is the 'CCK cholecystogram'. The gallbladder is opacified by oral cholecystography and the subject given an intravenous injection of CCK-OP (20 ng/kg). A positive response is when the patient's pain is reproduced and an exaggerated contraction is seen on X-ray (Dunn et al 1974). The specificity and sensitivity of these tests in selecting patients who will respond to treatment varies between studies. When gallbladder emptying is assessed in response to an IV bolus of CCK-OP, it has been shown that the reproducibility of gallbladder emptying is poor. Furthermore, bolus injections of CCK-OP not only stimulate the gallbladder but also the colon (Harvey & Read 1973), and pain may not necessarily arise from gallbladder contraction. Current data suggest that the CCK provocation test should not be used in selecting patients for treatment of gallbladder motility disorders.

Gallbladder scintigraphy

Currently, this is the most specific test using CCK-OP for diagnosis of possible gallbladder motility abnormalities. The gallbladder ejection fraction (GBEF) is determined as described previously. Using scintigraphy it has been shown that the normal gallbladder empties in excess of 50% of its volume in response to a standard meal or 45 min intravenous infusion of CCK-OP (20 ng/kg/h). One study (Kishk et al 1987) showed a significant difference in the GBEF of patients with gallstones when compared to controls. The gallbladder emptying in 14 of 20 patients with gallstones measured below 50% after ingestion of a corn oil meal. In another study, 24 patients with abnormal CCK-OP GBEF (< 40%) were identified and randomized half to cholecystectomy (Yap et al 1991). All but one of the patients having cholecystectomy were cured of biliary symptoms at 3-year followup. Histology of the removed gallbladders revealed increased gallbladder wall thickness and evidence of chronic cholecystitis. The patients not having cholecystectomy have continued with symptoms and indeed three have subsequently formed gallstones. Unlike CCK-OP provocation studies, none of the patients receiving an infusion of CCK experienced pain.

Treatment

The most appropriate treatment for patients with identified gallbladder motility disorder is cholecystectomy as it permanently eliminates the organ which produces the symptoms. In the 1990s, cholecystectomy would be achieved via the laparoscopic approach in the majority of patients. However, in certain individuals, cholecystectomy may be delayed as the motility disorder might be transient.

Decreased gallbladder contraction might be caused by (1) a primary abnormality of gallbladder muscle, (2) muscle disorder secondary to chronic cholecystitis or lithogenic bile (3) suboptimal hormonal or neural stimulation or (4) circulation of an inhibiting substance or hormone. A lithogenic diet given to prairie dogs or guinea pigs impairs gallbladder contractility and leads to gallstones. Patients with gallstones or on long-term parenteral nutrition have impaired gallbladder emptying; women in the second and third trimesters of pregnancy exhibit an abnormally high resting gallbladder volume and also impaired fractional emptying in response to a fatty meal (Everson et al 1982). In pregnancy or in patients on parenteral nutrition, gallbladder emptying disorders may be transient, hence treatment via non-operative means may alleviate and prevent subsequent disease.

In one study, the prokinetic substance cisapride (Marzio et al 1990) has been used to treat symptomatic patients with ultrasound-demonstrated gallbladder hypokinesia. Long-term treatment produced relief of symptoms and a reversal of the motility changes. This study suggests that in a small group of patients, prokinetic drugs may be useful in the treatment of gallbladder motility disorders. However in the majority of patients who normally present with longstanding symptoms remote from events such as pregnancy or parenteral nutrition, cholecystectomy is the most appropriate therapy.

In some patients the above investigations may not be conclusive for a gallbladder motility disorder and the possibility of a SO motility disorder may arise. Most data on SO dysfunction has been derived from patients after cholecystectomy. A small percentage of these patients may have had cholecystectomy for acalculous gallbladder disease. Such a finding suggests that the primary motility anomaly may be in the SO and not the gallbladder. In these patients, SO motility should be evaluated via endoscopic manometry.

SPHINCTER OF ODDI

Over the past decade, motility disorders of the SO have been described and have been associated with distinct clinical symptoms. Our understanding of SO motility disorders is based on improved knowledge of normal physiology of the SO and the ability to accurately record manometrically the sphincter's motor activity. Based on the manometric description of normal and abnormal activity, we suggested that abnormalities of SO motility be called 'SO dysfunction' (Toouli et al 1985a). This all-embracing term does away with terms such as stenosis, papillitis or Odditis which imply a pathological diagnosis, as pathological correlates are lacking in this condition. Furthermore, the term is specific to the sphincter as compared to the more general terms of 'post-cholecystectomy syndrome' or 'biliary dyskinesia/dyssynergia'.

SO dysfunction

Clinically patients who present with SO dysfunction divide into two broad groups. The majority of patients have symptoms which are mainly referable to the biliary tract, whilst a smaller group present with symptoms which are referable to the pancreas.

The majority of patients with SO dysfunction are 40–50-year-old females who often present with recurrent biliary type pain approximately 5 years after cholecystectomy. The operation has usually been done for symptomatic gallstones and resulted in cure. The patients experience a recurrence of the pain which is usually identified as being similar to that produced by gallstones (Bar-Meir 1984). The pain is situated in the epigastrium to right upper quadrant. It may radiate into the back and be associated with nausea plus vomiting in some patients. The pain generally occurs in episodes which last 3–4 h or until relieved by analgesics. These episodes of pain may occur at intervals of weeks or months. Some patients describe a background of a lesser more constant discomfort which is more frequent and may occur every day. The more acute episodes of pain occur over and above the more frequent background discomfort. In some patients, close questioning reveals symptoms consistent with irritable bowel disease, however the biliary like symptoms are usually described as distinct from these. Some patients describe that the pain may be produced on taking opiate containing medications and that they have learned to avoid such medication. The first episode of pain may have been experienced following opiate premedication, usually for an unrelated procedure.

Physical examination of a patient during an episode of pain reveals a distressed afebrile patient who is often moving on the examination couch in order to find the most comfortable position. Abdominal examination is usually non-contributory other than mild to moderate tenderness in the epigastrium to right upper quadrant. Signs of local or general peritonitis are not associated with this condition.

Blood screens reveal a normal white cell count, however, in some patients elevated serum liver transaminases may be found. The abnormality is often seen in a specimen of blood that is taken 3–4 h after the onset of pain. Occasionally bilirubin and liver alkaline phosphatase also may be elevated in conjunction with a pain episode. In a subgroup of patients the serum amylase may be elevated either solely or in conjunction with the liver enzymes changes. This group of patients often are given the clinical label of idiopathic recurrent pancreatitis. We have previously described SO manometric abnormalities in a group of patients with idiopathic recurrent pancreatitis (Toouli et al 1985b).

Initial treatment of patients presenting with the above clinical symptoms is directed at relief of pain which is usually achieved via administration of a systemic analgesic or buscopan. Pethidine (meperidine) is thought to be the most appropriate analgesic in patients with suspected SO dysfunction. In a recent study from our unit we have manometrically confirmed that this analgesic is less reactive on the SO when compared to morphine (Thune et al 1990).

Investigations

A number of investigations have evolved for the diagnosis of SO dysfunction. The most specific and sensitive is SO manometry. However, similar to other gastrointestinal motility disorders, diagnosis is often reached as a result of assessing a number of investigations and excluding structural abnormalities.

ERCP

Patients who present with significant post-cholecystectomy biliary or pancreatic type symptoms should have the biliary and pancreatic ducts visualised via ERCP. The majority of patients will have a cause other than SO dysfunction to explain their symptoms, hence ERCP is an important early investigation in these patients. In the performance of the ERCP it is important to correctly position the patient in order to adequately screen the bile and pancreatic ducts. Note should be made whether pain is produced on manipulating the SO with the ERCP catheter. In addition, the patient is positioned to evaluate drainage time of contrast from the bile duct. Both of these signs on their own are non-specific for SO dysfunction, however, taken with other symptoms and radiological signs such as duct dilatation may support a diagnosis of SO dysfunction. A number of studies have now shown that significant bile duct dilatation does not result following cholecystectomy (LeQuesne et al 1989, Hunt & Scott 1989) and the finding of a dilated bile duct suggests a relative stenosis of the SO. We have taken the corrected diameter of 12 mm as the upper limit of normal for the bile duct and diagnose duct dilatation if the maximum corrected diameter exceeds this value. Abnormal drainage is defined if contrast is present in the bile duct at 45 min following its introduction.

Morphine provocation test

The effect of opiates on SO contractility is well known. Furthermore, some patients with suspected SO dysfunction volunteer that the pain often is reproduced following morphine injection. Therefore, the morphine – neostigmine provocation test was devised in an attempt to identify patients with symptomatic SO dysfunction who may benefit from therapy on the sphincter. In its early usage, the test was applied to patients presenting with idiopathic recurrent pancreatitis (Nardi & Acosta 1966). A positive test comprised of reproduction of pain and a significant rise in serum amylase. In some centres the test proved useful in selecting patients who might benefit from surgical division of the sphincter, however, closer scrutiny showed that normal subjects also produced a positive result and hence the sensitivity and specificity of the investigation fell into disrepute (LoGiudice et al 1979).

The efficacy of the morphine – neostigmine test was re-evaluated for diagnosis of SO dysfunction after two changes. Firstly, the morphine and neostigmine were given according to unit per kilogram weight (in previous reports a fixed dose was used); secondly, changes in liver enzymes as well as amylase were assessed. In a group of patients with recurrent post-cholecystectomy pain thought to originate from SO dysfunction, the morphine – neostigmine test was significantly positive when compared to matched controls (Roberts-Thomson & Toouli 1985). However as in previous studies its specificity and sensitivity was poor. When compared with SO manometry, patients with a positive morphine

– neostigmine test had a greater incidence of sphincter stenosis when compared to patients with normal morphine – neostigmine test.

The role of the morphine provocation test in selecting patients who will benefit from therapy to the SO has not been clarified. One study concluded that it is poorly sensitive and a non-specific investigation for the selection of patients who will benefit from sphincterotomy (Geenen et al 1989). Its major role might be as a screening investigation which adds support to other clinical data towards the diagnosis of SO dysfunction. However, on its own it should not be used to select patients for division of the SO.

Ultrasonography

Two additional non-invasive investigations using ultrasonography may be used to indirectly assess SO function.

Fatty meal sonography is a 'real-time' ultrasound investigation designed to evaluate bile duct diameter following a standard fatty meal stimulus of 3.3 ml/kg corn oil (lipomul). Once in the duodenum the corn oil releases circulating CCK that normally causes SO relaxation. In normal circumstances the fall in SO resistance enhances bile flow into the duodenum and bile duct diameter either diminishes or remains unchanged. With a partial obstruction of the distal end of the bile duct, the diameter increases 1 mm or more, thus suggesting SO stenosis (Darweesh et al 1988). The test is sensitive where a structural obstruction to flow through the sphincter such as a stone or tumour is present. However, it is insensitive for diagnosing SO motility changes. A positive test suggests a possible motility disorder and the patient should be further assessed by manometric studies.

A similar investigation is used to evaluate the pancreatic portion of the SO in patients with suspected pancreatic SO dysfunction. The diameter of the pancreatic duct within the body of the pancreas is determined. Normally this diameter does not exceed 1 mm. Secretin (1 μ/kg) is intravenously infused over 15 min while the pancreatic duct diameter is monitored. As a result of increased flow of pancreatic juice, ductal diameter increases but rapidly returns to normal within 30 min. If the duct remains dilated (i.e. > 1.5 mm) at the 30-min time interval, it is thought to be as a result of increased resistance across the pancreatic sphincter, which is consistent with SO dysfunction (Bolondi et al 1984). The sensitivity and specificity of this test is undefined. However, in patients with idiopathic recurrent pancreatitis, the test may be used as a non-invasive screening investigation of SO function.

Table 33.1 Sphincter of Oddi pressures

	Median	Normal Range	Abnormal
Basal pressure (mmHg)	15	3–35	> 40
Amplitude (mmHg)	135	95–195	> 300
Frequency (n/min)	4	2–6	> 7
Sequences			
Antegrade %	80	12–100	
Simultaneous %	13	0–50	
Retrograde %	9	0–50	> 50
CCK 20ng/kg		Inhibits	Contracts

Table 33.2 Sphincter of Oddi dysfunction

Stenosis	● Basal pressure ≥ 40 mmHg
Dyskinesia	● Frequency ≥ 7 per min
	● Intermittent rise in basal pressure
	● Retrograde contractions ≥ 50%
	● Paradoxical CCK-OP response.

Cholescintigraphy

Flow across the SO may be evaluated in post-cholecystectomy subjects following injection of ^{99m}Tc DIDA which is excreted into bile from the liver (Roberts-Thomson et al 1986). This is a minimally invasive investigation which potentially may provide useful data regarding flow dynamics across the SO. Methodological difficulties relating to the position of the duodenum in relation to the bile duct, plus the error produced in dilated ducts make this investigation one of low sensitivity for SO dysfunction. However, delay in flow of radionuclide from the bile duct into the duodenum may represent a raised resistance to flow which may be due to SO dysfunction. Its major role is confined to screening of patients suspected of SO dysfunction.

SO manometry

Endoscopic SO manometry is the most objective of all available investigations in determining SO motility characteristics (Table 33.1). Furthermore, diagnosis made as a result of manometry is reproducible, and appears to identify normal from abnormally functioning sphincters (Thune et al 1992). Manometrically, the SO is characterized by regular phasic contractions which are superimposed on a modest basal pressure. The majority of the contractions appear to be orientated in an antegrade direction, however simultaneous and retrograde contractions are also recorded.

Manometric abnormalities have been identified in patients with clinically suspected SO dysfunction. Using the manometric findings, SO dysfunction may be considered in two major groups irrespective of whether the symptoms are primarily biliary or pancreatic (Table 33.2). This manometric division has allowed for targeting of specific therapy for patients in whom diagnosis of SO dysfunction is made. The two major groups are SO stenosis and SO dyskinesia (Toouli et al 1985a).

SO stenosis. Manometrically, it is characterized by abnormally elevated SO basal pressure which is defined as a basal pressure above 40 mmHg (Fig. 33.1). Stenosis may be produced by fibrosis of the sphincter or smooth muscle hypertrophy. The fibrotic changes may be secondary to trauma of the sphincter due to the passage of stones, or instruments during surgery. In addition, the fibrosis or hypertrophy may follow repeated episodes of local inflammation which may occur with the dyskinetic motility disorders, and may represent the most advanced of the changes in SO dysfunction. Histological correlation between manometric stenosis and fibrotic changes has been made in anectodal cases, but large series which attempt to correlate manometric with pathological changes do not exist.

Patients with manometric stenosis of the SO may have evidence on ERCP of a dilated bile duct and are noted to have abnormal elevation of liver enzymes during episodes of pain. However, the correlation is not strong, hence these signs cannot be used to predict which patients may have SO stenosis.

The finding of SO stenosis may be isolated to one or be in both bile and pancreatic duct sphincter. Stenosis in the pancreatic duct sphincter is associated with pancreatic SO dysfunction and treatment of these patients requires not only division of the bile duct portion of the SO, but also the septum between the bile duct and pancreatic duct.

SO dyskinesia. In this group are placed the other manometric abnormalities which have been described in patients with suspected SO dysfunction.

Rapid phasic contraction frequency. Spontaneously occurring bursts of rapid phasic contraction may be recorded. These episodes are distinct from activity fronts which relate to the migrating motor complex (MMC) (Worthley et al 1989) as they may extend for periods of time in excess of normal MMC activity. The patient may experience pain during these episodes. They have been likened to similar recordings which have been made in the stomach (tachygastria) and have been named tachy Oddia.

In order to make the diagnosis of tachy Oddia on manometry, recording should not commence until the

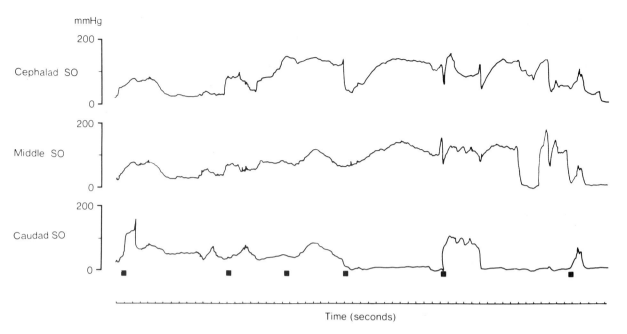

Fig. 33.1 Manometric tracings illustrating SO stenosis characterized by a high basal pressure. The black squares illustrate a stepwise withdrawal of the triple lumen catheter across a narrow stenosis.

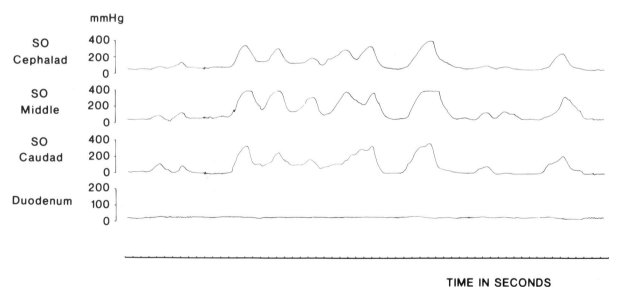

Fig. 33.2 Manometric tracing illustrating rapid SO contractions recorded in all three lumens. The duodenum is quiet.

initial artefact following the introduction of the catheter subsides. A sustained frequency in excess of 7 contractions per minute is considered abnormal (Fig. 33.2).

Intermittent episodes of elevated basal pressure. Similar to tachy Oddia and often in association, an intermittent elevation of the basal pressure may be noted. This is unlike the stenotic recordings in that the basal pressure returns to normal, and may respond to inhalation

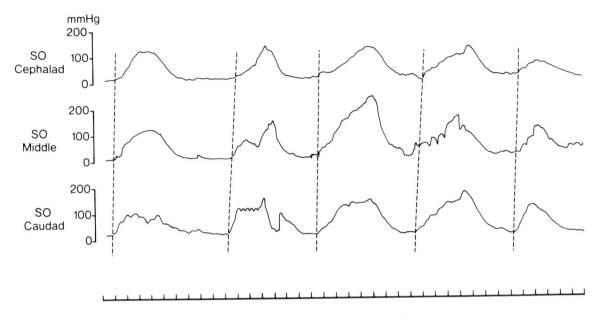

Fig. 33.3 Manometric tracing illustrating an excess of retrograde SO contraction. The dotted lines are drawn at the onset of each contraction and indicate the wave sequence.

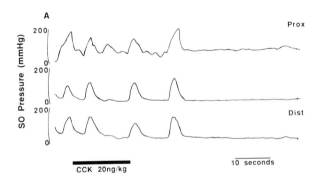

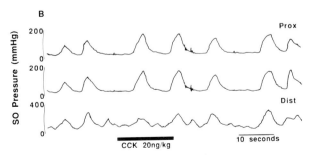

Fig. 33.4 Manometric tracing demonstrating a paradoxical response to CCK-OP. An increase in contraction frequency (**B**) is noted instead of the normal inhibition (**A**) (with permission).

of amyl nitrate. Both this and tachy Oddia reflect what is thought to be 'irritable' sphincter which appears to readily produce 'spasm', whether it be to the stimulus of a recording catheter or some other stimulus such as food in the duodenum or emotional stress.

Excessive retrograde contractions. In normal subjects the majority of SO contractions are orientated in an antegrade direction. However, an excess of simultaneous and retrograde contractions may reflect an abnormally functioning sphincter as this may produce relative retardation to flow (Fig. 33.3). This subtle manometric finding may be of low significance and its reproducibility is poor. Taken in isolation it should not be used to make a diagnosis of SO dysfunction.

Paradoxical response to CCK. The normal response of the human SO to the administration of CCK is that of inhibition of phasic contractions and a fall in basal pressure. A paradoxical response is recorded when CCK has no effect on the SO contractions or produces an increase in contraction frequency and/or a rise in basal pressure (Fig. 33.4). CCK produces its normal action on the sphincter by stimulation of non-adrenergic non-cholinergic inhibitory neurones. In patients exhibiting a paradoxical response to CCK, it is thought that the inhibitory nerves may be either damaged or absent and CCK has a direct effect on the smooth muscle to produce contraction.

Table 33.3   Sphincter of Oddi dysfunction groups

Groups	1	2	3
Pain	+	+	+
LFTs	+	±	−
Dilated CBD	+	±	−
Delay in duct emptying	+	±	−

Table 33.4   Endoscopic sphincterotomy (ES) and sphincter of Oddi dysfunction

	SO basal pressure < 40 mmHg		SO basal pressure > 40 mmHg	
	Sham	ES	Sham	ES
n	12	12	12	12
Improve	33%	42%	25%	91%
No change	67%	58%	75%	9%

Treatment

Until recently the treatment of SO dysfunction has been largely directed at the relief of symptoms by analgesics. However, recent studies suggest that for patients with manometrically defined SO stenosis division of the SO is associated with improvement in symptoms. For patients with biliary SO dysfunction, the results of treatment and correlation with investigations has led to the following recommendations for diagnosis and treatment (Dodds 1990). Patients may be divided into three groups and their management appropriately tailored (Table 33.3).

Patients in group 1 have biliary pain, abnormal liver enzymes associated with the pain episodes and a dilated bile duct on ERCP. Invariably most of these patients (> 70%) will have abnormal manometry. If manometry is not readily available, then it is appropriate to proceed to sphincterotomy.

Patients in group 2 have biliary pain and either abnormal liver enzymes or a dilated bile duct. Only 50% of these patients register abnormal manometry, suggesting that the disorder may not be as advanced as in group 1. Manometry should be done in this group of patients and treatment tailored according to the abnormality.

Patients in group 3 have biliary pain and no detectable abnormalities in liver enzyme or bile duct size. Manometry is mandatory in these patients prior to treatment.

In a prospective study patients with biliary-like pain of groups 1 and 2 were randomized into endoscopic sphincterotomy or sham procedure (Geenen et al 1989). Manometry was done but not used to determine therapy. The results of the manometry were correlated with the clinical outcome. After a 4-year follow-up, it was found that patients with SO stenosis characterized by a basal pressure > 40 mmHg showed improvement in symptoms (Table 33.4). The clinical improvement was significantly different when compared to patients who had the sham procedure. Patients with the manometric diagnosis of dyskinesia did not show a significant difference in clinical improvement between sphincterotomy and sham sphincterotomy. The results from this study led to the conclusion that patients with significant SO dysfunction as characterized by an elevated basal pressure (stenosis) should be treated by division of the SO.

In patients with idiopathic recurrent pancreatitis, division of the biliary sphincter by endoscopic sphincterotomy is not associated with relief of symptoms. Recording from the pancreatic duct sphincter revealed a group of patients with an abnormally elevated SO basal pressure. This was seen even in patients who have had a biliary sphincterotomy for the treatment of recurrent pancreatitis. This finding has led to the conclusion that stenosis of the pancreatic duct sphincter is associated with recurrent pancreatitis and treatment must include division of the pancreatic sphincter. Division of this sphincter is done via a transduodenal open operation, and the septum between the bile duct and pancreatic duct is divided so that a wide opening is made into the pancreatic duct as well as the bile duct.

The results of this operation in producing symptomatic relief in patients with recurrent pancreatitis depend on the selection of patients. Approximately 70% of patients with an abnormally elevated basal pressure improved following sphincteroplasty and pancreatic septoplasty. Lack of improvement may relate to the fact that many of these patients have been treated for many years with a variety of opiates for pain and a dependence to these medications has developed (Nardi et al 1983).

The role of pharmacotherapy in SO dysfunction is limited as there are no drugs which are specific, long acting and lack side-effects. Buscopan has been used to relieve acute episodes of pain. It is effective, however, its action is short-lived and cannot be taken prophylactically. The calcium channel blocker nifedipine has been used with some success in relieving pain. However, most patients experience cardiovascular side effects making prolonged use unacceptable (Guelrud et al 1988).

Possible candidates for future trials of efficacy are the new prokinetic drugs and the cerulitide type compounds. These may produce a decrease in SO contractility and thus prevent episodes of pain.

REFERENCES

Bar-Meir S 1984 Frequency of papillary dysfunction among cholecystectomized patients. Hepatology 4: 328–330

Bolondi L, Gaiani S, Gullo L, Labo G 1984 Secretin administration induces a dilatation of the main pancreatic duct. Dig Dis Sci 29: 802–808

Bolondi L, Gaiani S, Testa S, Labo G 1985 Gallbladder sludge formation during prolonged fasting after gastrointestinal surgery. Gut 26: 734–738

Darweesh R M A, Dodds W J, Hogan W J et al 1988 Efficacy of quantiative hepatobiliary scintigraphy and fatty meal sonography for evaluating patients with suspected partial common bile duct obstruction. Gastroenterology 94: 779–786

Dodds W J 1990 Biliary tract motility and its relationship to clinical disorders. AJR 155: 247–258

Dunn F H, Christensen E C, Reynold J et al 1974 Cholecystokinin cholecystectomy. J Am Med Assoc 22: 89–97

Everson G T, McKinley C, Lawson M, Johnson M, Kern F J R 1982 Gallbladder function in the human female: effect of the ovulatory cycle, pregnancy and contraceptive steroids. Gastroenterology 82: 711–719

Freeman J B, Cohen W N, Den Besten L 1975 Cholecystokinin cholangiography and analysis of duodenal bile in the investigation of pain in the right upper quadrant of the abdomen without gallstones. Surg Gynecol Obstet 140: 371–376

Geenen J E, Hogan W J, Dodds W J, Toouli J, Venu R P 1989 The efficacy of endoscopic sphincterotomy in post-cholecystectomy patients with sphincter of Oddi dysfunction. N Engl J Med 320: 82–87

Guelrud M, Mendoza S, Rossiter G, Ramirez L, Barkin J 1988 Effect of nifedipine on sphincter of Oddi motor activity: studies in healthy volunteers and patients with biliary dyskinesia. Gastroenterology 95: 1050–1055

Harvey R F, Read A E 1973 Effects of cholecystectomy on colonic motility and symptoms in patients with the irritable bowel syndrome. Lancet 1–3

Hunt D R, Scott A J 1989 Changes in bile duct diameter after cholecystectomy: 15 year perioperative study. Gastroenterology 97: 1485–1488

Kishk S M A, Darweesh R M A, Dodds W J et al 1987 Am J Roentgenol 148: 875–879

Le Quesne L P, Whiteside C G, Hand H T 1959 The common bile duct after cholecystectomy. Br Med J 1: 329–332

Lee S P, Maher K, Nicholls J F 1988 Origin and fate of biliary sludge. Gastroenterology 94: 170–176

LoGiudice J A, Geenen J E, Hogan W J, Dodds W J 1979 Efficacy of the morphine-rostigmin test for evaluating patients with suspected papillary stenosis. Dig Dis Sci 24: 455–458

Marzio L, Difelice F, Laico M G, Celiberti W, Gross L, Del Bianco R 1990 Gallbladder hypokinesia and normal gastric emptying of liquids in patients with dyspeptia symptoms: a double blind placebo controlled trial with cisapride. Gastroenterology A255

Nardi G L, Acosta J M 1966 Papillitis as a cause of pancreatitis and abdominal pain: role of evocative test operative pancreatography and histologic evaluation. Ann Surg 164: 611–621

Nardi G L, Michelassi F, Zannini P 1983 Transduodenal sphincteroplasty: 5–25 year follow-up of 89 patients. Ann Surg 198: 453–461

Rhodes M, Lennard T W J, Farndon J R, Taylor R M R 1988 Cholecystokinin (C C K) provocation test: Longterm followup after cholecystectomy. Br J Surg 75: 951–953

Roberts-Thomson I C, Toouli J 1985 Abnormal responses to morphine neostigmine in patients with undefined biliary type pain. Gut 26: 1367–1372

Roberts-Thomson I C, Toouli J, Blanchett W, Lichtenstein M, Andrews J T 1986 Assessment of bile flow by radioscintigraphy in patients with biliary type pain after cholecystectomy. ANZ J Med 16: 788–793

Thune A, Baker R A, Saccone G T P, Owen H, Toouli J 1990 Differing effects of pethidine and morphine on human sphincter of Oddi motility. Br J Surg 77: 992–995

Thune A, Scicchitano J, Roberts-Thomson I C, Toouli J 1991 Reproducibility of endoscopic sphincter of Oddi manometry. Dig Dis Sci 36: 1401–1405

Toouli J, Roberts-Thomson I C, Dent J, Lee J 1985a Manometric disorders in patients with suspected sphincter of Oddi dysfunction. Gastroenterology 88: 1243–1250

Toouli J, Roberts-Thomson I C, Dent J, Lee J 1985b Sphincter of Oddi manometric disorders in patients with idiopathic recurrent pancreatitis. Br J Surg 72: 859–863

Venu R P, Geenen J E, Toouli J, Stewart E T, Hogan W J 1983 ERCP diagnosis of cholelithiasis in patients with normal gallbladder X-rays and ultrasound studies. JAMA 249(6): 758–761

Worthley C S, Baker R A, Iannos J, Saccone G T P, Toouli J 1989 Humans fasting and post-prandial sphincter of Oddi motility. Br J Surg 76: 709–714

Yap L, McKenzie J, Wycherley A, Toouli J 1991 Gallbladder ejection fraction for acalculous gallbladder pain. Gastroenterology 101: 786–793

34. Ileus and mechanical obstruction

M. J. Benson   D. L. Wingate

INTRODUCTION

The terminology of ileus is confusing. Ileus, or adynamic ileus, is an adynamic state, in which there is partial or complete motor inertia of part or all – with the exception of the oesophagus – of the gastrointestinal tract. Two main types of adynamic ileus are recognized (Table 34.1) – postoperative and paralytic.

Postoperative ileus is a condition that is, by definition, entirely iatrogenic; it is an acute and usually self-limiting state that is a sequel of surgical trauma of the bowel, and, in man, appears to predominantly affect the stomach and colon. Paralytic ileus is a similar condition, but usually also involves the small bowel, and there are multiple causes. One cause of paralytic ileus is prolonged postoperative ileus, which suggests that postoperative ileus is no more than a less severe form of paralytic ileus. This is, however, not the case. Postoperative ileus has a specific local cause (a surgical procedure), whereas the causes of paralytic ileus are

Table 34.1 Classification of the causes of adynamic ileus in man

Type	Cause
Postoperative ileus	Following intra-abdominal surgery
	Following some types of extra-abdominal surgery
Paralytic ileus	Prolonged postoperative ileus
	Peritonitis (chemical or infective)
	Biliary and renal colic
	Pancreatitis
	Retroperitoneal haemorrhage
	Myocardial infarction
	Basal pneumonia
	Widespread trauma
	Metabolic disturbance (hypophosphataemia, hypokalaemia, acute anaemia, hypo-osmolality)
	Drugs (especially those with parasympatholytic action)
	Porphyria and heavy metal poisoning

more generalized, ranging from peritoneal irritation through metabolic imbalance to overwhelming infection. Abnormal prolongation of the postoperative ileus may produce the systemic changes that precipitate the paralytic state. Research protocols in animals have not always distinguished between 'postoperative' and 'paralytic' ileus; thus, while surgeons attempt to avoid peritoneal irritation when they perform a laparotomy, some research workers have deliberately induced peritoneal irritation in animals in an attempt to model postoperative ileus.

Mechanical obstruction of the gut due to a variety of conditions (Table 34.2) produces gradual motor failure of the regions proximal to the obstruction; while dissimilar in pathogenesis, prolongation of the obstruction, if untreated, may provoke generalized paralytic ileus.

The clinical manifestations of these conditions are similar, with abdominal distension, pain, nausea and vomiting, and inability to retain food or to expel flatus or faeces; all these patients are ill, in that they require urgent supportive treatment with fluid repletion, analgesia, and, where possible, decompression and relief of mechanical obstruction. Collectively, these conditions constitute the only reversible causes of motor failure of the gut, and are thus of considerable scientific interest. In practical terms, they are of considerable importance because they are potentially fatal conditions; their 'reversibility' may depend upon appropriate and timely therapeutic intervention.

Systematic study of motility is not easy in patients suffering acute discomfort and pain following surgery; the additional discomforts that can be imposed by research procedures, often run counter to the efforts of medical and nursing staff to alleviate suffering. Because of this, animal models have been much used to study the problem. Too often, however, the question of variation between species has been ignored. In the rat, for example, postoperative ileus is a transient state which is always self-limiting and is confined to an

Table 34.2   Classification of the causes of intestinal mechanical obstruction in man

Obturation of the intestinal lumen	Intrinsic bowel lesions	Extrinsic bowel lesions
Intussusceptum	Congenital (atresia, stenosis, duplication)	Adhesions
Faeces	Neoplasm	External hernias
Meconium	Crohn's stricture	Extrinsic masses (e.g. abscess, neoplasm)
Bezoars	Post-radiation therapy stricture	Volvulus

hour or two, whereas in the horse, in contrast, postoperative ileus is severe, prolonged, and a major cause of mortality (approximately 30%; Gerring, personal communication) following major abdominal surgery.

POSTOPERATIVE ILEUS

Introduction

Although ileus may occur following extra-abdominal operations, it is most pronounced and almost inevitable following intra-abdominal and retroperitoneal operations. Suppression of gastrointestinal motor activity following laparotomy was first described at the turn of the century (Bayliss & Starling 1899), but it is only relatively recently that improvements in technology have allowed accurate qualitative and quantitative assessment of these changes.

Regional involvement

Stomach

Gastric emptying is delayed in both the rat (Dubois et al 1973a, Ruwart et al 1979) and dog (Baker & Webster 1968, Dubois et al 1973b, Smith et al 1977) following celiotomy. In dogs, emptying of a 500 ml nutrient liquid meal is impaired for about 24 h (Dubois et al 1973b), while 7 mm indigestible spheres are retained for 60 h (Smith et al 1977). In man, radiological observations of a small bolus of liquid barium given a few hours after surgery, showed that, following non-gastric intra-abdominal surgery, emptying is delayed for approximately 24 h or even longer (Rothnie et al 1963, Wells et al 1964, Nachlas et al 1972); this is probably the cause of the nausea and vomiting experienced by patients after oral feeding in the immediate postoperative period. It is not known when the normal gastric emptying response to nutrient is restored following surgery or whether the duration of impairment varies with the type of operation.

Celiotomy results in little change in antral slow wave activity in the dog (Smith et al 1977). Dauchel et al (1976) reported that, after cholecystectomy, human

gastric electrical activity was markedly disorganized, but these findings were not confirmed by others (Coelho et al 1990, Waldenhausen et al 1990). It is thus unlikely that myogenic incoordination is the cause of the postoperative delay in gastric emptying. Woods et al (1978) and Graber et al (1982) reported that antral contractile activity in monkeys returned to normal within 2–3 h after celiotomy. In the canine stomach, irregular antral spike activity, was present immediately following surgery, although the incidence was diminished for the first postoperative day (Brolin et al 1985), while the incidence of aborally propagated short bursts and more prolonged bursts (phase III) of spike activity was greatly reduced during the first 24 h (Smith et al 1977). The return of this activity is consistent with the return of normal gastric emptying of a nutrient liquid meal in the dog (Dubois et al 1973b), and antral postprandial spike activity in the dog which returned to normal after 24 h (Brolin et al 1985). A similar depression of antral phasic activity has been reported in man. By 12–24 h after operation, the frequency of antral spike activity (Dauchel et al 1976, Waldenhausen et al 1990) or its mechanical equivalent, recorded by intraluminal manometry (Goodall 1964, Ingram & Catchpole 1981) was not significantly different from control values. As in the canine stomach, phase III activity was either absent or very much reduced during the first 24 h (Ingram & Catchpole 1981, Waldenhausen et al 1990).

Small intestine

Gas does not tend to accumulate in the small bowel, as it does in the colon and stomach, during postoperative ileus (Wells et al 1961, Rothnie et al 1963, Nachlas et al 1972, Wilson 1975), and investigators have recorded phasic bursts of phase III-like activity in the small bowel within a few hours of surgery. However Smith et al (1977) demonstrated that the transit of indigestible spheres through the canine small bowel was markedly delayed after celiotomy, requiring a mean of 23 h compared to 2 h in controls. Postoperative small bowel transit was also prolonged in the rat (Dubois et al

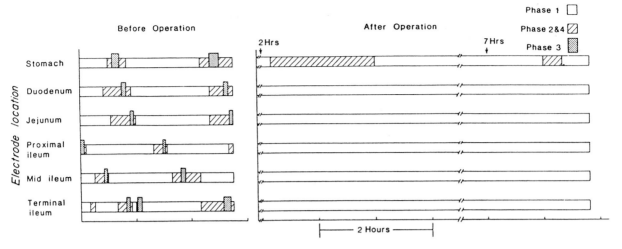

Fig. 34.1 Abolition (right) of normal canine fasting gastric and small bowel myoelectric activity after experimental trauma to the bowel. (Reproduced with permission from Smith et al 1977.)

1973a, Ruwart et al 1979), although Nilsson and Jung (1973) were unable to confirm these findings. In man, while Wells et al (1961) found no impairment of the small bowel transit of liquid barium, several studies (Wells et al 1964, Noer 1967, Nachlas et al 1972, Dauchel et al 1976) have shown that small bowel transit of barium is prolonged, requiring up to 24–36 h to reach the ileocaecum. Thus the postoperative small bowel is capable of propulsive activity, but it should not be assumed that it is normal either in the immediate post operative period or even 24 h later.

As in the stomach, there is little or no disorganization of the small intestinal slow wave during the postoperative period in either dogs (Smith et al 1977, Carmichael et al 1977) or in man (Stoddard et al 1978, Coelho et al 1990, Waldenhausen et al 1990), but there are conflicting data on the return of phase III activity in both animals and man. In the dog, celiotomy abolished spike activity but it returned to normal by 24 h (Bueno et al 1978a, Brolin et al 1985). Phase III activity that was either abolished or markedly attenuated during the first 24–48 h after surgery, gradually increasing over the next 3–7 to days to normal, has also been observed (Smith et al 1977, Morris et al 1983) (Fig. 34.1). In contrast, both Mishra et al (1975) and Carmichael et al (1977) reported only a minimal decrease or no change, respectively, in canine small bowel spike activity following laparotomy.

In man, the early return of phase III activity reported by some groups (Catchpole & Duthie 1978, Stoddard et al 1978, Sarna 1985, Waldenhausen et al 1990, Benson et al 1992) is in direct contrast to the findings of others (Dauchel et al 1976, Soper et al 1990, Schippers et al 1991) who reported spike activity and/or the presence of phase III activity to be markedly reduced or absent, during the first 24 h. While some of the change in phase III activity may be an effect of opiate analgesia, Benson et al (1992), demonstrated that in the early postoperative phase, the migrating motor complex (MMC) period is significantly less than when the identical dose of opiate is given to healthy individuals. In man (Schippers et al 1991, Benson et al 1992) as in the dog (Carmichael et al 1977), the MMC period lengthens with time after the operation, returning to normal in 24–60 h (Fig. 34.2) However, the early presence of phase III activity does not signify the presence of normal motility. Little is known about whether phasic activity is normally propagated activity or is lumen-occlusive. Absent or uncoordinated distal migration of phase III activity has been reported until the second to third postoperative day in dogs (Smith et al 1977) and during the first 24 h in man (Stoddard et al 1978, Benson et al 1992) (Fig. 34.3.) Continuous intraluminal recordings from the human jejunum have shown that the mean amplitude of phasic pressure change in phase III may be significantly reduced for up to 72 h after surgery (Benson et al 1992) (Fig. 34.4) While passive dilatation of the small bowel by gas is a possible cause, gaseous distension is uncommon, and contractions may be non-occlusive due to a postoperative loss of non-electrogenic tone.

Absence or marked reduction of phase II activity, which is known to be important for the propulsion of

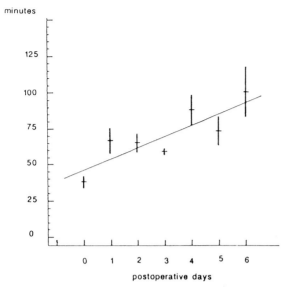

Fig. 34.2 Increase in interval between human small bowel MMCs on successive days following surgery. Each point represents mean ± one standard error (*n* = 13) for 5-h daily recording period. (Reproduced with permission from Schippers et al 1991.)

intraluminal content (Summers et al 1975), has been observed in both dogs (Smith et al 1977) and man (Stoddard et al 1978, Benson et al 1992) in the postoperative period. The return of phase II may be a consequence of the increasing period of the MMC cycle with time after the operation. Sarna (1985) has proposed that phase III, is followed by a refractory state of inhibition decays into a relatively refractory state (phase II). Early in the postoperative period, when the intervals between phase III are short (15–20 min);

phase III may recur at the end of the absolute refractory period, and thus it is not until the MMC period increases in duration that phase II activity is possible; thus, the reappearance of phase II may be a secondary phenomenon dependent upon the lengthening of the MMC period.

Colon

In a radiographic study of patients following intraabdominal surgery, Wells et al (1964) noted that intestinal gas tended to accumulate mainly within the colon; similar findings were reported by others (Rothnie et al 1963, Nachlas et al 1972 and Wilson 1975). The presence of a distended and dilated colon several days after surgery, with normal gas shadowing within the stomach and small bowel led to the hypothesis that the inhibition of colonic motor activity after surgery is more prolonged than elsewhere in the gastrointestinal tract. Woods et al (1978) used implanted electrodes and strain-gauge transducers, to record contractile activity from both the ascending and sigmoid colon in monkeys following celiotomy. The frequency of contractile activity in the colon was reduced for a much longer period of time than in either the stomach or small bowel (Figs 34.5a, 34.5b). The contractile incidence returned to control levels in the right colon after the first postoperative day, but was delayed until the third day in the sigmoid colon. A similar more prolonged reduction of the contractile activity recorded from the left colon as compared to the right, was reported by Graber et al (1982). Morris et al (1984), using an impedance technique in the dog, found that movement in the descending colon was present on the first postoperative day, although clearly reduced for the first 3 days.

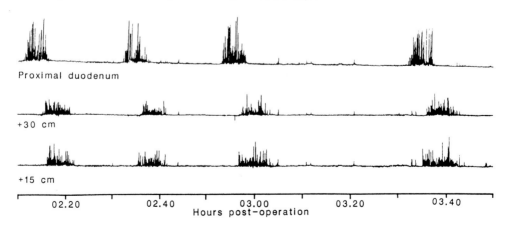

Fig. 34.3 Human small bowel motility in the early postoperative period. Note that phase II is absent, and that propagation in the jejunum (lower traces) is abnormal.

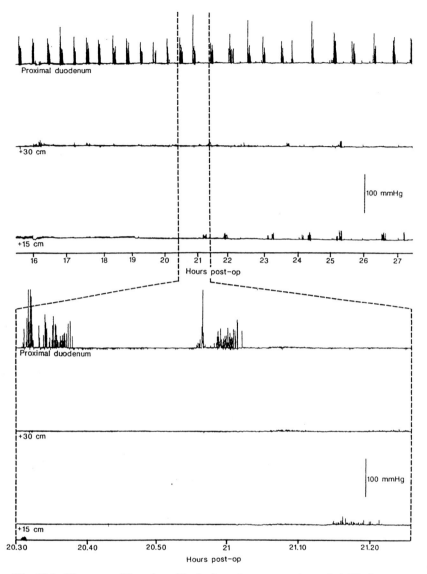

Fig. 34.4 Human small bowel motility in the early postoperative period. The lower three traces represent an expanded portion of the upper three traces. Note that the amplitude of phase III contractions at the distal sensors is very low, suggesting that these contractions are not lumen-occlusive.

There are only a few published studies of human colonic motor activity during postoperative ileus. Wilson (1975) used a single radiotelemetry capsule to measure intraluminal pressures from the proximal ascending colon. He reported that colonic phasic pressure activity was inhibited for approximately 2 days after surgery. Condon et al (1986) recorded spike activity from bipolar electrodes sutured to the ascending and descending colon, following a variety of different operations, ranging from laparotomy to gastrectomy. Although slow waves were omnipresent, Fourier analysis revealed a bimodal frequency distribution (lower range 2–9 cpm, higher range 9–14 cpm) in the ascending colon (Fig. 34.6). There was a shift from the higher to the lower dominant frequency with time after surgery; although this was highly variable, and was absent in 40% of the patients. There was less variability in the descending colon, with persistent

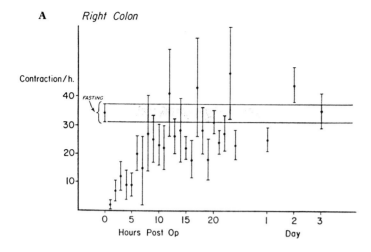

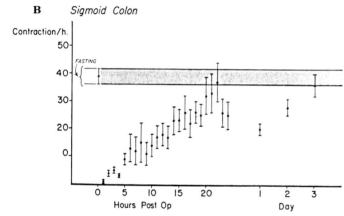

Fig. 34.5 Response of monkey right colon (**A**) and sigmoid colon (**B**) to celiotomy. The shaded region represents the mean ± one standard error (SE) of fasting contractile incidence in non-operated (control) state. Each point represents mean ± 1 SE for pooled data (*n* = 11) for 1-h recording epochs. Note the more marked delay in the return of contractile incidence in the sigmoid colon. (Reproduced with permission from Woods et al 1978.)

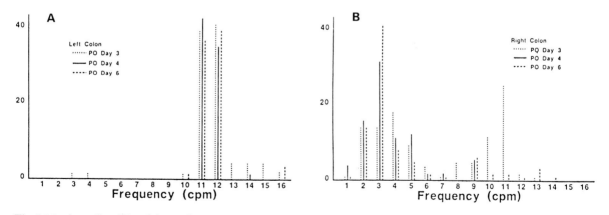

Fig. 34.6 Ascending (**A**) and descending (**B**) human colonic slow wave frequencies following laparotomy. The y-axis represents the relative power spectrum incidence of the various slow wave frequencies. Note shifting dominant slow wave frequency with time following operation in the ascending colon. (Reproduced with permission from Condon et al 1986.)

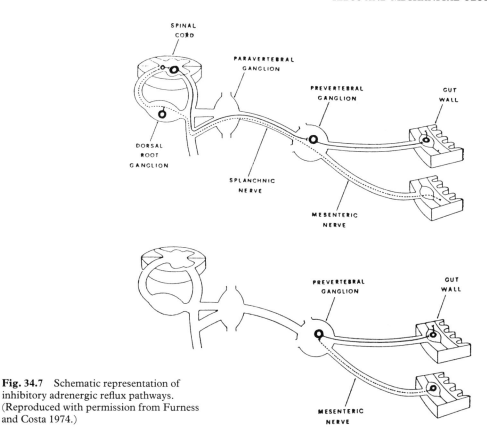

Fig. 34.7 Schematic representation of inhibitory adrenergic reflux pathways. (Reproduced with permission from Furness and Costa 1974.)

dominance of the higher frequency. Non-propagated random bursts of discrete spike activity were present on the first post-operative day while propagated bursts were absent until the second to third post-operative day, with occasional bidirectional propagation in the descending colon. Aborally propagated long spike bursts were present as early as day 3 and were associated with either the passage of flatus or stool. In a similar study, Waldenhausen et al (1990) reported three slow wave frequency ranges (2–3 cpm, 9–14 cpm and 20–28 cpm): the mid-range frequencies predominated during the first 48 h after surgery with the higher frequency becoming prevalent thereafter. Short spike bursts were absent for the first 24 h and, again, the appearance of long spike bursts was delayed, until the end of the fifth postoperative day. After surgery, phasic motor activity is suppressed longer in the colon than in either the small bowel or the stomach, but our knowledge of colonic motor activity during postoperative ileus is still fragmentary, since recordings have not been continuous but have been confined to relatively brief and discontinuous periods.

Aetiopathogenesis

Neuromuscular mechanisms

Sympathetic activity. A schematic representation of the intestinal sympathetic inhibitory reflex pathways is shown in Figure 34.7. The spinal reflex pathway can be abolished by splanchnic nerve or dorsal root section, and by crushing or anaesthesia of the spinal cord. The peripheral reflex is abolished by the removal of the prevertebral ganglia, but is unaffected by blockade of more central pathways. Both pathways are abolished by adrenergic antagonists. Cannon and Murphy (1907) noted that localized ileus of the feline small bowel produced by extra-abdominal trauma, could be prevented by prior section of the splanchnic nerves. This classic study suggested that a spinal reflex pathway was involved, and splanchnic section was subsequently shown to prevent ileus due to peritoneal irritation (Arai 1922) or even simple laparotomy (Markowitz & Campbell 1927). Olivecrona (1927), however, found that inhibition induced by the handling of the intestines was not prevented by section of the splanchnic

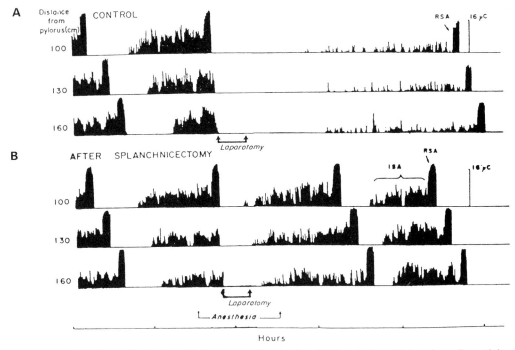

Fig. 34.8 Inhibition of both phase II (irregular spike activity, ISA) and phase II (regular spike activity, RSA) activity in the canine jejunum following celiotomy (**A**). Following splanchnicectomy a normal fasting pattern returns immediately after surgery (**B**). (Reproduced with permission from Bueno et al 1978a.)

nerves but could be by removal of the coeliaco-mesenteric plexus. Bueno et al (1978a) found that the complete inhibition of small bowel spike activity in the dog could be abolished by splanchnicectomy (Fig. 34.8). The same group showed that, in the rat, the inhibition of small bowel spike activity could be reduced by spinal cord demedullation and, again, abolished by splanchnicectomy, while transection of the spinal cord and vagotomy were without effect (Bueno et al 1978b). These findings suggest that inhibition following intestinal handling is effected through the high-threshold reflex pathways that relay in the prevertebral ganglia.

David and Loring (1930) found that the more severe the intraperitoneal insult, the less effective was splanchnic anaesthesia in preventing ileus. It has been suggested that the source and intensity of the stimulus determine whether the sympathetic reflexes are restricted to spinal pathways (Furness & Costa 1974).

Data from pharmacological studies support the concept of increased sympathetic activity in ileus. Destruction of sympathetic nerve endings by pretreatment with 6-hydroxydopamine prevented the reduction of gastric emptying and the decrease in intestinal transit time observed in the rat following abdominal surgery (Dubois et al 1973a) (Fig. 34.9). There is increased synthesis and release of noradrenaline (NA) from the wall of rat stomach, small bowel and colon in the immediate postoperative period (Dubois et al 1973a, Dubois et al 1974) (Fig. 34.10). Administration of the adrenergic blocker, bretyllium, while without significant effect on emptying of unoperated canine stomach, prevented the impairment of emptying following operation (Dubois et al 1973b) (Fig. 34.11). In the rat, impaired gastric emptying, small bowel transit and colonic transit following celiotomy, could be restored by alpha-adrenergic blockade but not by beta-blockade (Ruwart et al 1980a). Capsaicin produces a reduction in ileus similar in magnitude to the protection by alpha- and beta-blockade (Holzer et al 1986). In dogs, adrenergic receptor blockade prevents the inhibition of gastric phase III activity, but is without effect on small intestinal spike activity or either gastric emptying and small bowel transit (Smith et al 1977). It would appear that ileus is not due solely to the increased release of NA from reflexly activated sympathetic nerves, but that other mediators are involved.

Non-adrenergic non-cholinergic [NANC] activity. Abrahamson et al (1979) and Glise and Abrahamson (1980) have shown that following laparotomy

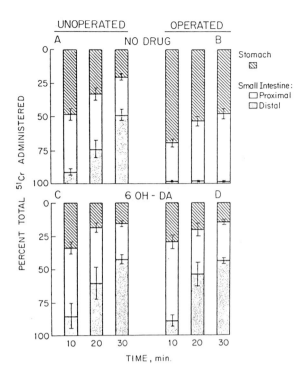

Fig. 34.9 Upper gastrointestinal transit assessed by distribution of ^{51}Cr-labelled test meal in operated (**A** and **C**) and non-operated (**B** and **D**) rats. Animals were sacrificed at 10, 20 and 30 min after the ingestion of the test meal. Note that chemical sympathectomy abolished the impairment of transit observed following laparotomy. (Reproduced with permission from Dubois et al 1973a.)

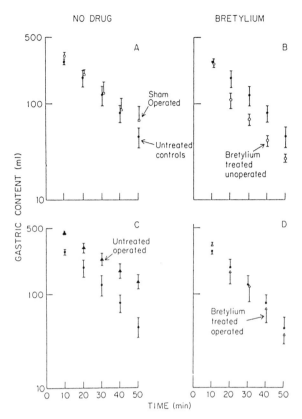

Fig. 34.11 Gastric emptying of 500 ml test meal in non-operated (**A** and **B**) and operated (**C** and **D**) dogs. Treatment with bretylium appeared to prolong the period of rapid gastric emptying in non-operated dogs (**B**). Celiotomy impaired gastric emptying, while pretreatment with bretylium abolished this effect. (Reproduced with permission from Dubois et al 1973b.)

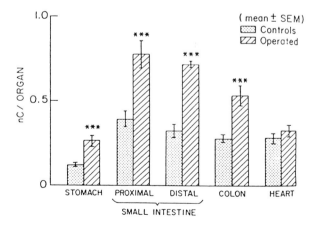

Fig. 34.10 Increased synthesis of noradrenaline in the stomach, small bowel and colon following operation in the rat. The relative synthesis of noradrenaline is unchanged in cardiac tissue.

in the cat, stimulation of intra-abdominal nociceptors, in addition to causing sympathetic adrenergic inhibition, induces marked vagally-mediated NANC reflex inhibition of gastric motility. The afferents to the spinal cord for these two reflexes are essentially the same. These observations suggest that NANC reflex inhibitory activity may be involved in postoperative ileus.

Local factors

Duration and extent of surgery. Following simple cholecystectomy or appendicectomy, a liquid diet within 24 h of surgery is usually well tolerated, while after major surgery, such as colectomy, it will usually induce nausea, vomiting and abdominal distension. This suggests that the extent of disruption of normal motor activity following abdominal surgery varies according to the type of operation. In support of this, Schippers et al (1991) has reported that the inhibition of phase III activity in the small bowel varied with the type of surgical procedure, returning far sooner after cholecystectomy than after colectomy. However, this is in direct conflict with some published reports. Studies in both animals (Woods et al 1978, Graber et al 1982) and man (Wilson 1975, Condon et al 1986) suggest that the clinical duration of ileus is independent of both the extent and duration of the operation. In addition to the stimulation of nociceptors by surgical manipulation, continuing activation of these receptors may conceivably occur after abdominal closure due to intraperitoneal irritation. Chemical irritation of the peritoneum has been shown to abolish small intestinal activity in rats (Enochsson et al 1987) and dogs (Mishra et al 1975).

Circulating catecholamines. Adrenalin, which unlike NA is not released from sympathetic nerve terminals, is released from the adrenal glands during stress. However, Smith et al (1977) demonstrated only a transient elevation in plasma adrenalin together with a more prolonged elevation of NA following laparotomy in the dog (Fig. 34.12); plasma adrenalin levels returned to control levels while postoperative ileus persisted. These findings indicate that adrenal catecholamines do not contribute to postoperative ileus, and this is supported by the observation that adrenalectomy does not alter the duration of postoperative ileus (Douglas & Mann 1941, Dubois et al 1975) and that paralytic ileus is very uncommon in patients with phaeochromocytoma (Cruz & Cowell 1972).

Drugs. Anaesthetic agents can alter gastrointestinal motor activity, the effect differing between agents (Wright et al 1982). Halothane anaesthesia has been variously reported to inhibit gastric (Marshall et al 1961) and small intestinal activity (Marshall et al 1961, Tinckler 1965) or to have no effect on either (Smith et al 1977); both halothane (Marshall et al 1961, Condon et al 1987) and enflurane (Condon et al 1987) depressed colonic phasic activity. The effects of volatile inhalational anaesthetic agents are dose-dependent and motility returns to normal by the time the patient regains consciousness. Thus these agents are unlikely themselves to be responsible for or significantly contribute to postoperative ileus (Aitkenhead 1988). Pentobarbitone does not alter canine small intestinal spike activity (Bueno et al 1978b) while in the rat (Bueno et al 1978b) it induces a slight increase in spiking activity with irregular transient disruption of the MMC, that reverts to normal before the animal recovers from the anaesthesia. Thiopentone slows phase III migration velocity in the rat (Bueno et al 1978a) while it stimulates electrical and mechanical activity in the canine

small bowel (Healy et al 1981). Recent experience with laparoscopic surgery, where postoperative ileus is not a problem, would suggest that anaesthesia is indeed unimportant.

Analgesia is a different matter. Nitrous oxide has no inhibitory action on gastrointestinal motor activity (Tinckler 1965, Condon et al 1987) but, in man, opiates are routinely administered intraoperatively and postoperatively for pain control, and may also be part of a premedication regime. Systemic administration of opiates causes characteristic changes in gastrointestinal motility. In most species, including man, opiates delay gastric emptying and prolong small intestinal and colonic transit (Miller and Hirning 1989). Opiates do not, however, paralyse the gut in dogs, monkeys and man; despite an overall reduction in intestinal transit, opiates increase the proportion of segmenting, nonpropulsive contractile activity. In contrast, as has been outlined above, phasic segmenting activity in both the small and large intestine during the early postoperative period is either greatly diminished or absent, Frantzides et al (1992) has reported that intravenous. or intramuscular morphine, from the third postoperative day onwards, induces non-migrating spike activity in the human colon and appeared to diminish propagated activity.

Treatment

Supportive

The loss of effective peristaltic activity of the gastrointestinal tract leads to distension of the bowel with fluid and gas. Since its introduction some 50 years ago, the mainstay of treatment remains nasogastric intubation (Wangensteen 1931) and fluid replacement, with the correction of any electrolyte imbalance. However, this only permits decompression and drainage of gastric secretion as impairment of gastric motility during ileus means that the tip of the tube rarely passes through the pylorus. Patient discomfort is increased by nasogastric intubation; this has stimulated interest in more effective methods of non-invasive treatment.

Therapeutic manipulation

Sympatholytics and cholinomimetics. Despite the sound theoretical rationale, the effectiveness of sympatholytic drugs in the clinical treatment of ileus has not been unequivocally established and the reported benefits must be considered in relation to the frequent systemic side-effects. Alpha-blockade with neuroleptics (chlorpromazine or trifluperidol) has been

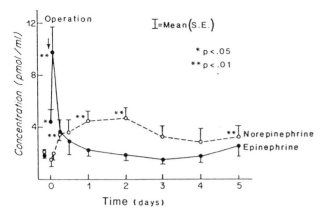

Fig. 34.12 The effect of celiotomy on plasma concentrations of adrenaline (epinephrine) and noradrenaline (norepinephrine) in the dog. There is a significant but transient increase in plasma adrenaline, with a more prolonged increase in noradrenaline. Values marked with asterisks differ significantly from preoperation levels as shown. (Reproduced with permission from Smith et al 1977.)

reported to diminish the duration of postoperative ileus (Petri et al 1971). Altaparmakov et al (1984) reported that dihydroergotamine, an alpha-adrenergic blocker, stimulated upper gastrointestinal motility and reduced the duration of clinical postoperative ileus following cholecystectomy, as assessed by the passage of stool, but another study failed to demonstrate any benefit (Thorup et al 1983). Beta-adrenoceptor antagonists have been reported to reduce the clinical duration of ileus following colonic surgery (Hallerbäck et al 1987). Rada et al (1979) failed to show any significant reduction by alpha and beta blockers in the duration of clinical ileus. Pantothenic acid, which increases the synthesis of acetylcholine (ACh), reduced the duration of postoperative ileus in dogs (Polacek et al 1960), but two controlled trials in man showed no benefit (Garvey & Wilson 1961, Wayne et al 1962). Although there is a rationale for using cholinomimetics to stimulate the release of ACh, such agents (e.g. bethanechol and neostigmine) have not been used in isolation in an attempt to stimulate activity during postoperative ileus, because of their systemic side-effects. They have however been used in combination with sympatholytics. In an uncontrolled study in patients with paralytic ileus, treatment with either an alpha-blocker (phentolamine) or an adrenergic neurone blocker (guanethidine) and a cholinomimetic (neostigmine or bethanechol) shortened the duration of clinical ileus (Catchpole 1969, Neely & Catchpole 1971). This impression of a beneficial effect was not confirmed in a placebo controlled study using a similar drug regimen (Heimbach & Crout 1971).

Epidural analgesia. Epidural analgesia exerts sympatholytic effects by blocking both spinal sympathetic afferent and efferent activity. Following colonic surgery continuous epidural analgesia with bupivicaine significantly reduced both small intestinal (Ahn et al 1988) and colonic transit time (Ahn et al 1988, Scheinin et al 1987) compared with untreated controls. A similar effect on colonic transit has been reported following hysterectomy (Wattwil et al 1989) but not after cholecystectomy (Wallin et al 1986). Epidurally administered opiates have an inhibitory effect on gastrointestinal motility, as they do when given systemically (Bardon & Ruckebusch 1985, Thorén & Wattwil 1988), presumably via opiate receptors within the spinal cord. The apparent beneficial effects of epidural anaesthesia maintained with local anaesthetic are lost if it is combined with or replaced by opioids (Hjortsø et al 1985, Scheinin et al 1987, Thorén et al 1989).

Prokinetic agents. An alternative approach to the use of sympatholytic agents is the use of 'prokinetic' drugs to stimulate gut motility and accelerate transit. These include substituted benzamides such as metoclopramide and cisapride, and analogues of cholecystokinin (CCK). Intravenous cisapride has been reported to hasten the passage of flatus in the postoperative period compared to controls (Boghaert et al 1987, Pescatori 1987, Verlinden et al 1987, van Rooy et al 1988), but others have not found any significant difference (von Ritter 1987, Clevers et al 1988). Intravenous cisapride given regularly throughout the postoperative period promotes an earlier return of propulsive activity, as assessed by the movement of markers, in all regions of the colon (Tollesson et al 1991) and an increase in left colonic pressure activity (Clevers et al 1988) when compared to untreated controls. Metoclopramide has proved to be ineffective in reducing the period of ileus, as assessed by the passage of flatus (Breivik & Lind 1971, Davidson et al 1979, Jepsen et al 1986). Ceruletide, the synthetic analogue of the decapeptide caerulein, is pharmacodynamically similar to the gastrointestinal hormone CCK, and has been shown to stimulate gastrointestinal motility in dogs (Mantovani et al 1969) and man (Bertaccini & Agosti 1971). In uncontrolled studies in patients with both postoperative and paralytic ileus, caerulin caused stimulation of gastrointestinal motor activity, as assessed by return of bowel sounds and passage of flatus and stool (Agosti et al 1971, Montero et al 1980). In the patients studied by Agosti et al (1971), treatment with neostigmine had proved ineffective, and those patients with paralytic ileus had a faster and more prolonged response than patients with postoperative ileus. Controlled trials of ceruletide given either intramuscularly

8-hourly (Madsen et al 1983) or as a single intravenous bolus (Sadek et al 1988) reduced the clinical duration of postoperative ileus, allowing significantly earlier resumption of oral alimentation (Sadek et al 1988). Schippers et al (1991) found that an intravenous infusion of ceruletide induced a marked increase in contractile activity, which closely resembled postprandial activity, but the response rapidly diminished after cessation of the infusion. It did not reduce the clinical duration of ileus.

Prostaglandins. Prostaglandins are thought to play an important modulatory role in the regulation of digestive tract motor activity (Demol 1988, Burakoff & Percy 1992). The possible therapeutic role of prostaglandins (PGs) in the treatment of ileus has received little attention to date. Infusion of PGE improved gastric emptying and small and large bowel transit in postoperative rats (Gromljez et al 1977, Ruwart et al 1980b). Therapeutic trials in man have not been reported.

Electrical pacing. The slow waves of gut muscle coordinate and organize the occurrence of spike bursts which are the myoelectric correlates of contractions. The canine small intestinal slow wave can be controlled by direct electrical pacing (Sarna & Daniel 1975, Akwari et al 1975) which in turn can stimulate propulsion of intraluminal content (Kelly & Code 1977, Sarr & Kelly 1981). In an uncontrolled trial in man, Bilgutay et al (1963) reported that electrical pacing of the small bowel may have a beneficial effect in reducing the duration of postoperative ileus. These observations were not confirmed in subsequent controlled trials (Quast et al 1965, Berger et al 1966, Soper et al 1990). Stimulation of contractile activity using pulsed radiofrequency has also failed to reduce significantly the duration of postoperative ileus (Barker et al 1984). It has to be remembered, however, that it is not slow wave activity that is disorganized after surgery but spike bursts; their incidence will not be altered by artificial modulation of the slow wave frequency (which is, in effect, what is achieved by pacing).

Physiological stimulation. Food induces a motor response in the stomach, small bowel and colon that is characterized by a marked increase in the incidence of contractile activity. Enteral nutrition during ileus has been advocated, on the basis that either the nutrition itself or the associated stimulation of gastrointestinal motor activity will induce a reduction in the duration of ileus. An uncontrolled study of early postoperative feeding via a nasoduodenal tube following cholecystectomy appeared to reduce the duration of ileus (Moss et al 1986). This was not confirmed in a placebo-controlled trial on a similar group of patients (Frankel &

Horowitz 1989). Clinical ileus following cholecystectomy is less prolonged when compared to that after major intra-abdominal surgery and any benefit might be expected to be small. This may not be the case following major intra-abdominal surgery and warrants further study.

Physical exercise appears to stimulate gastrointestinal contractile activity, for instance in the colon as well as increasing activity, it reduces transit time (Sarna 1991). After surgery, patients are usually confined to bed and it is possible that this enforced immobility may contribute to reduced contractile activity recorded after surgery. This hypothesis was tested by Waldenhausen and Schirmer (1990). Their results indicated that early ambulation had no significant effect on either gastric, jejunal or colonic electromyographic activity.

PARALYTIC ILEUS

Compared with postoperative ileus, paralytic ileus is even less amenable to systematic study, not least since in man it is a an uncommon phenomenon and its occurrence in a given clinical situation is difficult to predict. Only a relatively few animal studies of nonoperative or paralytic ileus have been published. These have been restricted to observations of motility following peritoneal irritation.

Arai (1922) demonstrated that an intraperitoneal injection of iodine or pathogenic bacteria decreased the movement of barium throughout the gastrointestinal tract and found that section of the splanchnic nerves prevented the inhibitory effects of peritoneal irritation. Studies of small intestinal motor activity have shown that stimulation of peritoneal nociceptors by intraperitoneal injection of a chemical irritant (iodine or hydrochloric acid), inhibited small intestinal transit (Holzer et al 1986) and motility in rats (Enochsson et al 1987), and dogs (Mishra et al 1975). In rats, the period of inhibition lasted several hours; Mishra et al (1975) reported that canine small intestinal motility had returned to normal by 24 h. Holtzer et al (1986) showed that in rats treated with capsaicin, iodine-induced peritonitis caused significantly less impairment of small intestinal transit than in untreated rats, although the absolute improvement was small. Alpha- and beta-blockade reduced small intestinal transit in non-capsaicin treated rats by the same degree as treatment with capsaicin. In capsaicin-treated rats, alpha- and beta-blockade was without effect. As in post-operative ileus, these data suggest that other mediators apart from sympathetic reflex hyperactivity may be involved. Whether such animal studies are a valid models for 'paralytic' ileus in man is not clear.

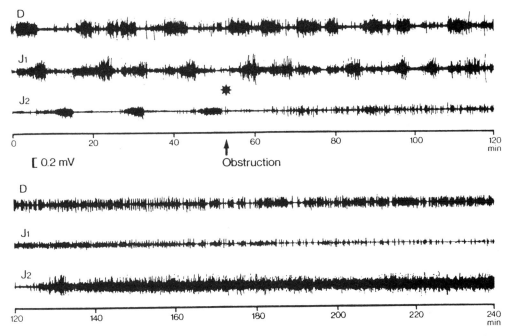

Fig. 34.13 Onset of mechanical obstruction between the two jejunal recording sites (J_1 and J_2) abolished phase III activity distal to the obstruction. Initially regular phase III activity continued in the proximal segment but was later replaced by rapidly migrating clusters of spike activity. (Reproduced with permission from Enochsson et al 1987.)

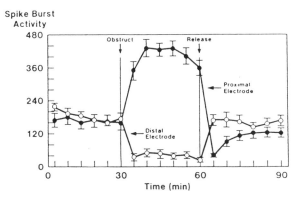

Fig. 34.14 The effect of balloon obstruction on canine small bowel spike activity in the fed state. Points represent mean ± 1 SE of pooled data ($n = 12$) for 5-min epochs. All points proximal and distal to the obstruction are significantly different from pre-obstruction control values. (Reproduced with permission from Summers et al 1983a.)

MECHANICAL OBSTRUCTION

The causes of mechanical obstruction are summarized in Table 34.2. Mechanical obstruction of the small bowel causes the accumulation of fluid and gas (primarily nitrogen from swallowed air) proximal to the obstruction, producing distension of the bowel. In large bowel obstruction, there is much less fluid secretion into the lumen and if the ileocaecal valve is competent, there may be little or no accompanying small bowel distention. Early observations on animals showed that intestinal contractile activity, increased proximal (Antoncic & Lawson 1941) and decreased distal to an obstruction (Carlson & Wangensteen 1930). Electromyography has not established whether electrical coupling of small intestinal smooth muscle is altered during acute obstruction. Summers et al (1983a) found that slow waves were unaltered in dogs, but Lausen et al (1988) reported the slow wave frequency to be significantly reduced proximal to an obstruction in the rabbit small bowel. Acute obstruction of the rat small bowel (Enochsson et al 1987), initially has no effect on interdigestive spike activity proximal to the obstruction while distally this activity is replaced by intense irregular activity (Fig. 34.13). With an increasing period of obstruction, the pattern of proximal motor activity becomes abnormal: the MMC cycle being replaced with discrete caudally propagated clusters of spike activity. In dogs, acute obstruction has no effect on the the MMC cycle, which is maintained both proximal and distal to the obstruction (Summers et al

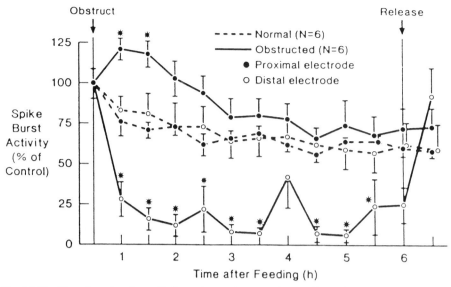

Fig. 34.15   The effect of prolonged balloon obstruction on canine small bowel spike activity in the fed state. Points represent mean ± 1 SE of pooled data ($n = 6$) for 5-min. * represent $p < 0.05$ compared to non-obstructed values. Distal inhibition of spike activity persists, while spike activity proximal to the obstruction normalizes with time. See text for explanation. (Reproduced with permission from Summers et al 1983a.)

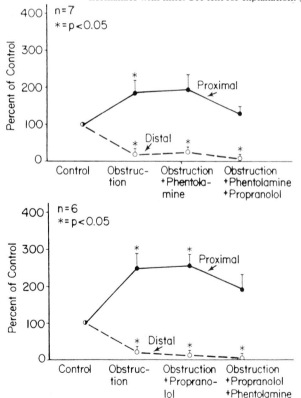

Fig. 34.16   Alpha- and beta-adrenoceptor antagonists are ineffective in reducing inhibition in small bowel distal to the site of balloon obstruction. (Reproduced with permission from Prihoda et al 1984.)

1983a). However the postprandial response is abnormal, being significantly reduced in the segment distal to the obstruction and significantly increased in the proximal segment (Summers et al 1983a, Prihoda et al 1984) (Fig. 34.14). With more prolonged obstruction, activity distal to the obstruction continues to be diminished, whilst the pattern of proximal activity changes to periods of predominantly aborally propagated spike activity separated by periods of motor quiescence (Summers et al 1983a). The duration of the periods of quiescence lengthens as the period of obstruction is prolonged, with the result that overall spike activity decreases with time (Fig. 34.15). Propagated clustered activity has been shown to be highly propulsive (Summers & Dusdieker 1981), and these changes in motor activity may therefore represent an attempt to overcome the obstruction to the normal aboral flow.

The increase in proximal activity is potentiated by neostigmine and decreased by atropine, suggesting that activation of cholinergic pathways may be involved in the proximal response (Prihoda et al 1984). The reduction of distal activity is, in part, due both to the absence of chyme in the distal segment and to an inhibitory intestino-intestinal reflex evoked by stimulation of mechanoreceptors in the distended region immediately proximal to the obstruction (Prihoda et al 1984). As in paralytic ileus, this reflex is probably mediated via sympathetic efferents, relaying either in the spinal cord or the prevertebral ganglia. Distal inhibition is not abolished by either alpha or beta sympatholytic agents (Prihoda et al 1984) suggesting that NANC

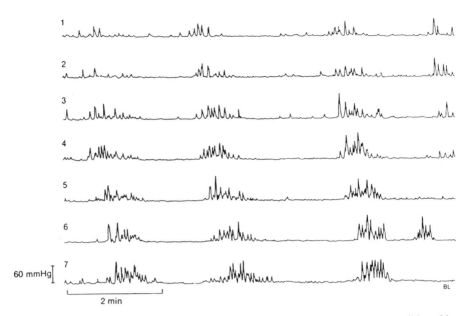

Fig. 34.17   An example of multiple propagated clustered contractions in proximal small bowel in a patient with mechanical obstruction, after a meal. (Reproduced with permission from Summers et al 1983b.)

neurones may be involved (Fig. 34.16). Chronic obstruction of the monkey distal colon results in a decreased spike activity in the right colon, an increase in the region immediately proximal to the obstruction and no change distally (Frazer et al 1980, Frazer et al 1981). Simultaneous contraction or distension events also occur, suggesting that the proximal colon becomes a common cavity filled with gas and fluid content (Frazer et al 1980).

Summers et al (1983b) reported that in patients with subacute obstruction the fasting motor activity of the small bowel is unaltered. However, the postprandial pattern is abnormal, being characterized by aborally propagated clustered contractions, which are not found in health (Fig. 34.17). The contractile frequency was significantly reduced, probably reflecting increasingly prolonged periods of quiescence separating clusters of contractions (Fig. 34.18). This abnormality of the fed motor pattern may be abolished by surgical correction of the obstruction (Fig. 34.19). In addition to postprandial clustered activity, Camilleri (1989) noted the presence of simultaneous prolonged single contractions (duration 15 s) in both the fed and fasted states (Fig. 34.20). Similar propagated pressure events have been recorded from the jejunum in patients following procto-colectomy and ileal pouch-anal anastomosis (Stryker et al 1985), and they may reflect an adaptive response to ileal distension.

Diagnosis of patients with acute obstruction of the bowel is largely clinical and usually confirmed by X-ray. In subacute obstruction, there seem to be reproducible abnormal motor patterns at least in the proximal small bowel. Whether manometric study will prove to be a useful diagnostic adjunct to radiological techniques needs to be established in a prospective study. It may prove useful in assessing the degree of dysfunction, and in minimizing the radiation exposure that is associated with the management of chronic inflammatory bowel disease.

CONCLUSION

Two aspects of the problem of ileus – one biological and the other clinical – deserve further comment.

Even though the pattern of ileus varies according to the cause and to the species affected, it is clear that it is a condition that affects the entire digestive tube, with one notable exception. The oesophagus is the only section of the gut that exhibits unmodified peristalsis; in the absence of disease, a contraction at the proximal end moves at a predictable speed to the distal end. Yet it is the only portion of the gut that is unaffected by ileus. This suggests that ileus is a condition that does not affect the physiological components of peristalsis – muscle function and the neural components of the peristaltic reflex – but rather the complex neural control circuitry of the stomach and bowel.

Compared with many other less common motor dysfunctions, ileus has been little studied, even though it is the only type of acute motor failure that demands urgent clinical intervention. It has been argued that ileus is an almost inevitable consequence of surgery that responds to standard supportive therapy. For the future, the problem of ileus seems to have been substantially diminished by the introduction of laparascopic abdominal surgery, where ileus seems to present a much smaller problem than following open laparotomy. However, the patients at greatest risk from ileus are those undergoing major surgical procedures involving extensive manipulation, such as the excision of tumours or reconstructive procedures, that require open rather than endoscopic surgery. In these patients, the diminution or abolition of ileus not only decreases postoperative suffering but reduces hospital stay, and even marginal reductions in high-dependency care can have considerable impact on the demands for health care resources. The unfilled need for effective therapies for ileus, is thus more than a matter of academic interest.

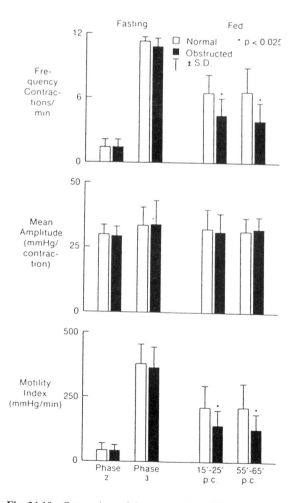

Fig. 34.18 Comparison of the contractile incidence, mean contractile amplitude and motility index in normals and obstructed patients for phase II, phase III, and 15–25 min and 55–65 min after a standard meal. See text for explanation. (Reproduced with permission from Summers et al 1983b.)

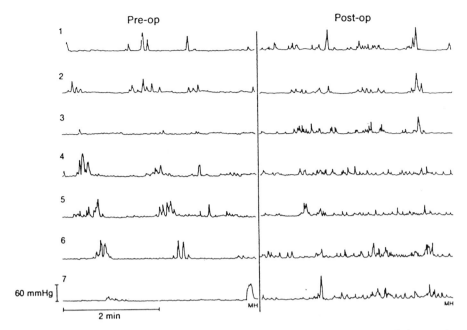

Fig. 34.19 Resolution of propagated clustered activity after feeding, following surgical correction of obstructive lesion. (Reproduced with permission from Summer et al 1983b.)

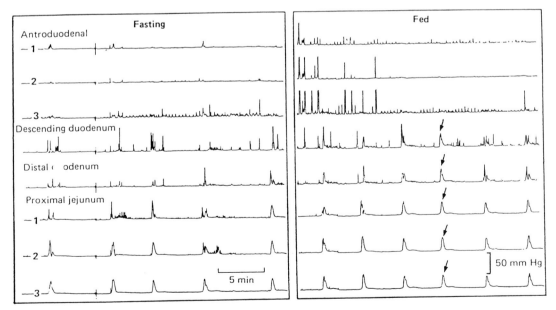

Fig. 34.20 Fasting and fed proximal small bowel motor activity in a patient with a distal ileal radiation stricture. Note the occurrence of simultaneous prolonged contractions (arrowed) in the small bowel proximal to the obstruction. (Reproduced with permission from Camilleri 1989.)

REFERENCES

Abrahamson H, Glise H, Glise K 1979 Reflex suppression of gastric motility during laparotomy and gastroduodenal nociceptive stimulation. Scand J Gastroenterol 14: 101–106

Agosti A, Bertaccini G, Paulucci R, Zanella E 1971 Cærulin treatment for paralytic ileus. Lancet i: 395

Ahn H, Bronge A, Johansson K, Ygge H, Lindhagen J 1988 Effect of continuous postoperative epidural analgesia on intestinal motility. Br J Surg 75: 1176–1178

Aitkenhead A R 1988 Anaesthesia and the gastrointestinal system. Eur J Anaesthiol 5: 73–112

Akwari O E, Kelly K A, Steinbach J H, Code C F 1975 Electrical pacing of the intact and transected canine small intestine and its computer model. Am J Physiol 229: 1188–1197

Altaparmakov I, Erckenbrecht J F, Weinbeck M 1984 Modulation of the adrenergic system in the treatment of postoperative bowel atonia. Scand J Gastroenterol 19: 1104–1106

Antoncic R F, Lawson H 1941 The muscular activity of the small intestine, in the dog, during acute obstruction. Ann Surg 114: 415–423

Arai K 1922 Experimentelle unterschungen über die Magendarm-bewegungen bei akuter peritonitis. Arch Exp Path Pharmakol 94: 149–189

Baker L W, Webster D R 1968 Postoperative intestinal motility. An experimental study in dogs. Br J Surg 55: 374–378

Bardon T, Ruckebusch Y 1985 Comparative effects of opiate agonists on proximal and distal colonic motility in dogs. Eur J Pharmacol 110: 329–334

Barker P, Allcutt D, McCollum C N 1984 Pulsed electromagnetic energy fails to prevent postoperative ileus. J R Coll Surg Edinburgh 29: 147–150

Bayliss W M, Starling E H 1899 The movements and innervation of the small intestine. J Physiol 24: 99–143

Benson M J, Roberts J, Wingate D L, Rogers J, Castillo F D, Williams N S 1992 Small bowel motility following major bowel trauma. Gastroenterology 102: Abstract 424

Berger T, Kewenter J, Kock N G 1966 Response to gastrointestinal pacing: antral, duodenal and jejunal motility in control and postoperative patients. Ann Surg 164: 139–144

Bertaccini G, Agosti A 1971 Action of caerulein on intestinal motility in man. Gastroenterology 60: 55–63

Bilgutay A M, Wingrove R, Griffen W O, Bonnabeau R C, Lillehei C W 1963 Gastro-intestinal pacing: a new concept in the treatment of ileus. Ann Surg 158: 338–347

Boghaert A, Haesaert G, Mourisse P, Verlinden M 1987 Placebo-controlled trial of cisapride in postoperative ileus. Acta Anaesth Belg 38: 195–199

Breivik H, Lind B 1971 Anti-emetic and propulsive peristaltic properties of metoclopramide. Br J Anaesth 43: 400–402

Brolin R E, Reddell M T, Thompson D A 1985 Intestinal myoelectric activity in fasting and non-fasting canine models of ileus. Arch Surg 120: 417–423

Bueno L, Fioramonti J, Ruckebusch Y 1978a Postoperative intestinal motility in dogs and sheep. Dig Dis 23: 682–689

Bueno L, Ferre J-P, Ruckebusch Y 1978b Effects of anaesthesia and surgical procedures on intestinal myoelectric activity in rats. Dig Dis 23: 690–695

Burakoff R, Percy W H 1992 Studies in vivo and in vitro on the effects of PGE2 on colonic motility in rabbits. Am J Physiol 262: G23–G29

Camilleri M 1989 Jejunal manometry in distal subacute mechanical obstruction: significance of prolonged simutaneous contractions. Gut 30: 468–475

Cannon W B, Murphy F T 1907 Physiologic observations on experimentally produced ileus. JAMA 840–843

Carlson R S, Wangensteen O H 1930 Motor activity of the distal bowel in intestinal obstruction. Proc Soc Exp Biol Med 27: 676–681

Carmichael M J, Weisbrodt N W, Copeland E M 1977 Effect of abdominal surgery on myoelectric activity in the dog. Am J Surg 133: 34–38

Catchpole B N 1969 Ileus: use of sympathetic blocking agents in its treatment. Surgery 66: 811–820

Catchpole B N, Duthie H L 1978 Postoperative gastrointestinal complexes in: Duthie H L (ed.) Gastrointestinal motility in health and disease. MTP Press, Lancaster pp 33–41

Clevers G J, Smout A J P M, Akkermans L M A, Wittebol P 1988 Restoration of gastrointestinal transit and colonic motility after major abdominal surgery; effects of cisapride. Sur Res Comm 4: 205–213

Coelho J C U, Gouma D J, Moody F G, Li Y F, Senninger N 1986 Gastrointestinal motility following small bowel obstruction in the opossum. J Surg Res 41: 274–278

Coelho J C U, Pupo C A, Campos A C L, Moss A A 1990 Electromyographic activity of the gastrointestinal tract following cholecystectomy. World J Surg 14: 523–528

Condon R E, Cowles V E, Schulte W J, Frantzides C T, Mahoney J L, Sarna S K 1986 Resolution of postoperative ileus in humans. Ann Surg 203: 574–581

Condon R E, Cowles V, Ekboum G A, Schulte W J, Hess G 1987 Effects of halothane, enflurane, and nitrous oxide on colon motility. Surgery 101: 81–85

Cruz S R, Colwell L J A 1972 Pheochromocytoma and ileus. JAMA 219: 155–158

Da Cunja Melo J, Summers R W, Yanda R, Wingate D L 1981 Effects of intestinal secretagogues and distension on the small bowel myoelectric activity in fasted and fed conscious dogs. J Physiol 321: 483–494

Dauchel J, Schang J C, Kachelhoffer J, Eloy R, Grehier J F 1976 Gastrointestinal myoelectric activity during post-operative period in man. Digestion 14: 293–303

David V C, Loring M 1930 Splanchnic anaesthesia in the treatement of paralytic ileus. Ann Surg 92: 721–725

Davidson E D, Hersh T, Brinner R A, Barnett S M, Boyle L P 1979 The effects of metoclopramide on postoperative ileus. A randomised double-blind study. Ann Surg 190: 27–30

Demol P 1988 Effect of prostaglandins on the motility of the digestive tract in: Domsche W, Damman H G (eds), Prostaglandins and leukotrienes in gastrointestinal disease. Springer-Verlag, Berlin, pp 90–106

Douglas D M, Mann F C 1941 The effect of peritoneal irritation on the activity of the intestine. Br Med J 15: 227–231

Dubois A, Weise V K, Kopin I J 1973a Postoperative ileus in the rat: physiopathology, etiology and treatment. Ann Surg 178: 781–786

Dubois A, Watanabe A M, Kopin I J 1973b Postoperative gastric ileus. Dig Dis 18: 39–42

Dubois A, Kopin I J, Pettigrew K D, Jacobowitz D M 1974 Chemical and histochemical studies of post-operative sympathetic activity in the digestive tract in rats. Gastroenterology 66: 403–407

Dubois A, Henry D P, Kopin I J 1975 Plasma catecholamines and postoperative gastric emptying and small intestinal propulsion in the rat. Gastroenterology 68: 466–469

Enochsson L, Hellström P M, Nylander G, Johansson C 1987 Myoelectric motility patterns during mechanical obstruction and paralysis of the small intestine in the rat. Scand J Gastroenterol 22: 969–974

Frankel A M, Horowitz G D 1989 Nasoduodenal tubes in short-stay cholecystecomy. Surg Gynecol Obstet 168: 433–436

Frantzides C T, Cowles V, Salaymeh B, Tekin E, Condon R E 1992 Morphine effects on human colonic myoelectric activity in the postoperative period. Am J Surgery 163: 144–149

Fraser I D, Condon R E, Schulte W J, DeCosse J J, Cowles V E 1980 Intestinal motility changes in experimental large bowel obstruction. Surgery 87: 677–682

Fraser I D, Condon R E, Schulte W J, DeCosse J J, Cowles V E 1981 Bowel motility after primary resection for colonic obstruction. Br J Surg 68: 113–116

Furness J B, Costa M 1974 Adynamic ileus, its pathogenesis and treatment. Med Biol 52: 82–89

Garvey R F, Wilson B J 1961 Clinical appraisal of D-pantothenyl alcohol in postoperative ileus: A double blind study. Arch Surg 83: 916–920

Glise H, Abrahamson H 1980 Spino-vagal nonadrenergic inhibition of gastric motility elicited by abdominal nociceptive stimulation in the cat. Scand J Gastroenterol 15: 665–672

Goodall P 1964 Early gastroduodenal motility following operation. Br J Surg 51: 864–867

Graber J N, Schulte W J, Condon R E, Cowles V E 1982 Relationship of duration of postoperative ileus to extent and site of operative dissection. Surgery 92: 87–92

Gromljez P F, Kaminski D L, Willman V L 1977 The effects of prostaglandins on experimental postoperative ileus. Surg Forum 26: 400

Hallerbäck B, Carlsen E, Carlsson K et al 1987 Beta-adrenoceptor blockade in the treatment of postoperative adynamic ileus. Scand J Gastroenterol 22: 149–155

Healy T E J, Foster G E, Evans D F, Syed A 1981 Effects of some i.v. anaesthetic agents on canine gastrointestinal motility. Br J Anaesth 53: 229–233

Heimbach D M, Crout J R 1971 Treatment of paralytic ileus with adrenergic neuronal blocking drugs. Surgery 69: 582–587

Hjortsø N C, Neumann P, Frøig F 1985 A controlled trial of the effect of epidural analgesia with local anaesthetics and morphine on the morbidity after abdominal surgery. Acta Anesthiol Scand 29: 790–796

Holzer P, Lippe I T, Holzer-Petsche U 1986 Inhibition of gastrointestinal transit due to surgical trauma or peritoneal irritation is reduced in capsaicin-treated rats. Gastroenterology 91: 360–363

Ingram D M, Catchpole B N 1981 Effect of opiates on gastroduodenal motility following surgical operation. Dig Dis Sci 26: 989–992

Jepsen S, Klærke, Neilson P H, Simonsen O 1986 Negative effect of metoclopramide in postoperative ileus. A prospective adynamic ileus. A prospective, randomized, double blind study. Br J Surg 73: 290–291

Kelly K A, Code C F 1977 Duodenal-gastric reflux and slowed gastric emptying by electrical pacing of the canine duodenal pacesetter potential. Gastroenterology 72: 429–433

Kruis W, Azpiroz F, Phillips S F 1985 Contractile patterns and transit of fluid in the canine terminal ileum. Am J Physiol 87: G857–G866

Lausen M, Reichenbacher D, Ruf G, Schöffel U, Pelz K 1988 Myoelecric activity of the small bowel in mechanical obstruction and intra-abdominal bacterial contamination. Eur Surg Res 20: 304–309

Madsen P V, Lykkegaard-Neilsen M 1983 Ceruletide reduces postoperative intestinal paralysis: A double-blind placebo-controlled trial. Dis Colon Rectum 26: 159–160

Mantovani P, Piccinin G L, Bertaccini G 1969 Activity ratio between intestinal and cardiovascular actions of caerulin and related substances in the anesthetized dog. Pharmacol Res Comm 1: 172–174

Marshall F N, Pittinger C B, Long J P 1961 Effects of halothane on gastrointestinal motility. Anesthesiology 22: 363–366

Miller R J, Hirning L D 1989 Opioid peptides and the gut in: Schultz S G (ed.) Handbook of physiology. section VI The Gastrointestinal System, vol II, American Physiological Society Bethesda, Maryland pp 631–660

Mishra N K, Appert H E, Howard J M 1975 Studies of paralytic ileus. Effects of intraperitoneal injury on motility of the canine small intestine. Am J Surg 129: 559–563

Montero V F, Laganga A M, Garcia E A 1980 Usefulness of caerulin in the treatment of postoperative intestinal atony. J Int Med Res 8: 98–104

Morris I R, Darby C F, Hammond P, Taylor I 1983 Changes in small bowel myoelectrical activity following laparotomy. Br J Surg 70: 547–548

Morris I R, Darby C F, Hammond P, Taylor I 1984 Colonic motility in the postoperative period. Digestion 30: 204–210

Moss G, Regal M E, Lichtig L 1986 Reducing postoperative pain, narcotics, and length of hospitalization. Surgery 99: 206–210

Nachlas M M, Younis M T, Pio Roda C, Wityk J J 1972 Gastrointestinal motility studies as a guide to postoperative management. Ann Surg 175: 510–522

Neely J, Catchpole B 1971 Ileus: the restoration of alimentary tract motility by pharmacological means. Br J Surg 58: 21–28

Nilsson F, Jung B 1973 Gastric evacuation and small bowel propulsion after laparotomy. Acta Chir Scand 139: 724–730

Noer T 1967 Radiological transit time through the small intestine in the immediate postoperative period. Acta Chir Scand 124: 557–580

Olivecrona H 1927 An experimental and clinical study of the postoperative, so-called paralytic ileus. Acta Chir Scand 61: 485–534

Pescatori M 1987 Effect of cisapride on clinical parameters of postoperative ileus. Prog Med 43: 111–114

Petri G, Szenohradszky J, Pórszász-Gibiszer K 1971 Sympatholytic treatment of 'paralytic' ileus. Surgery 70: 359–367

Prihoda M, Flatt A, Summers R W 1984 Mechanisms of motility changes during acute intestinal obstruction in the dog. Am J Physiol 247: G37–G42

Polacek M A, Close A S, Ellison E H 1960 Double blind study of the effect of d-Pantothenyl alcohol on experimental postoperative ileus. Surg Forum 11: 325–327

Quast D C, Beall A C, DeBakey M E 1965 Clinical evaluation of the gastrointestinal pacer. Surg Gynecol Obstet 120: 35–37

Rada O, Stoicu G, Russo I 1979 Influence of alpha and beta receptor blocking agents on the recovery of intestinal transit and postoperative complications in aged patients. Rev Chir 27: 71–77

Rothnie N G, Harper R A, Catchpole B N 1963 Early postoperative gastrointestinal activity. Lancet 2: 64–67

Ruwart M J, Klepper M S, Rush B D 1979 Carbacol stimulation of gastrointestinal transit in the postoperative ileus rat. J Surg Res 26: 18–26

Ruwart M J, Klepper M S, Rush B S 1980a Adrenergic and cholinergic contributions to decreased gastric emptying, small intestinal transit in the post-operative rat. J Surg Res 29: 126–134

Ruwart M J, Klepper M S, Rush B D 1980b Prostaglandin stimulation of gastrointestinal transit in post-operative ileus rats. Prostaglandins 19: 415–427

Sadek S A, Cranford C, Eriksen C, et al 1988 Pharmacological manipulation of adynamic ileus: controlled randomised double-blind study of ceruletide on intestinal motor activity after elective abdominal surgery. Aliment Pharmacol Ther 2: 47–54

Sarna S K 1985 Cyclic motor activity; Migrating Motor Complex: 1985. Gastroenterology 89: 894–913

Sarna S K 1991 Physiology and pathophysiology of colonic motor activity. Dig Dis Sci 36: 998–1018

Sarna S K, Daniel E E 1975 Electrical stimulation of small intestinal electrical control activity. Gastroenterology 69: 660–669

Sarna S K, Daniel E E, Kingma Y J 1971 Stimulation of the electrical control activity of stomach by an array of relaxation oscillators. Am J Dig Dis 17: 299–310

Sarr M G, Kelly K A 1981 Myoelectric activity of the autotransplanted canine jejunoileum. Gastroenterology 81: 303–310

Scheinin B, Asantila R, Orko R 1987 The effect of bupivicaine and morphine on pain and bowel function after colonic surgery. Acta Anaesthesiol Scand 31: 161–164

Schippers E, Hölscher A H, Bollschweiler E, Siewert J R 1991 Return of the inter-digestive motor complex after abdominal surgery: end of postoperative ileus? Dig Dis Sci 36: 621–626

Smith J, Kelly K, Weinshilboum R M 1977 Pathophysiology of postoperative ileus. Arch Surg 122: 203–209

Soper N J, Sarr M G, Kelly K A 1990 Human duodenal myoelectric activity after operation and with pacing. Surgery: 63–68

Stoddard C J, Smallwood R H, Duthie H L 1978 Migrating myoelectrical complexes in man in: Duthie H L (ed.) Gastrointestinal motility in health and disease. MTP Press, Lancaster pp. 9–15

Stryker S J, Borody T J, Phillips S F, Kelly K A, Dozois R R, Beart R W 1985 Motility of the small intestine after proctocolectomy and ileal pouch-anal anastomosis. Ann Surg 1985 351–356

Summers R W, Dusdieker N S 1981 Patterns of spike burst spread and flow in the canine small intestine. Gastroenterology 81: 742–750

Summers R W, Helm J, Christiansen J 1975 Intestinal propulsion in the dog: its relation to food intake and the migratory myoelectric complex. Gastroenterology 70: 753–758

Summers R W, Yanda R, Prihoda M, Flatt A 1983a Acute intestinal obstruction: an electromyographic study in dogs. Gastroenterology 85: 1301–1306

Summers R W, Anuras S, Green J 1983b Jejunal manometry patterns in health, partial intestinal obstruction, and pseudoobstruction. Gastroenterology 85: 1290–1300

Thorén T, Wattwil M 1988 Effects on gastric emptying of thoracic epidural analgesia with morphine or bupivicaine. Anest Analg 67: 687–694

Thorén T, Sundberg A, Wattwil M, Garvill J-E, Jürgensen U 1989 Effects of epidural bupivicaine and epidural morphine on bowel function and pain after hysterectomy. Acta Anaesthesiol Scand 33: 181–185

Thorup J, Will-Jørgensen P, Jørgensen T, J Kjærgaard 1983 Dihydroergotamine in postoperative ileus. Clin Pharm Ther 34: 54–55

Tinckler L F 1965 Surgery and intestinal motility. Br J Surg 52: 140–150

Tollesson P O, Cassuto J, Rimbäck G, Faxén A, Bergman L, Mattsson E 1991 Treatment of postoperative paralytic ileus with cisapride. Scand J Gastroenterol 26: 477–482

Van Rooy F, Creve U, Verlinden M, Hubens A 1988 Effect of cisapride on the post-cholecystectomy upper gastrointestinal transit time. Int J Clin Pharmacol Ther Tox 26: 265–268

Verlinden M, Michiels G, Boghaert A, de Coster M, Dehertog P 1987 Treatment of postoperative gastrointestinal atony. Br J Surg 74: 614–617

Von Ritter C, Hunter S, Hinder R A 1987 Cisapride does not reduce postoperative paralytic ileus. S Afr J Surg 25: 19–21

Waldenhausen J H T, Schirmer B D 1990 The effect of ambulation on recovery from postoperative ileus. Ann Surg 212: 671–677

Waldenhausen J H T, Shaffrey M E, Skenderis II B S, Jones R S, Schirmer B D 1990 Gastrointestinal myoelectric and clinical patterns of recovery after laparotomy. Ann Surg 211: 777–785

Wallin G, Cassuto J, Högström S, Rimbäck G, Faxén A, Tollesson P O 1986 Failure of epidural anesthesia to prevent postoperative paralytic ileus. Anesthesiology 65: 292–297

Wangensteen O H 1931 The early diagnosis of acute intestinal obstruction with comments on pathology and treatment with a report of successful decompression of three cases of mechanical bowel obstruction by nasal catheter suction siphonage. West J Surg Obstet Gynecol 40: 1–17

Wattwil M 1988 Postoperative pain relief and gastrointestinal motility. Acta Chir Scand Suppl 550: 140–145

Wattwil M, Thorén T, Hennerdal S, Garvill J-E 1989 Epidural analgesia with bupivicaine reduces postoperative paralytic ileus after hysterectomy. Anesth Analg 68: 353–358

Wayne A L, Mendoza C, Rosen R, Nadler S, Case R 1962 The role of dexpanthenol in postoperative ileus. JAMA 181: 827–830

Wells C, Rawlinson K, Tinckler L, Jones H, Saunders J 1961 Ileus and post-operative motility. Lancet ii: 136–137

Wells C, Tinckler L, Rawlinson K, Jones H, Saunders J 1964 Post-operative gastointestinal motiliy. Lancet i: 4

Wilson J P 1975 Postoperative motility of the large intestine in man. Gut 1975 16: 689–692

Woods J H, Erickson L W, Condon R E, Schulte W J, Sillin L F 1978 Postoperative ileus: a colonic problem? Surgery 84: 527–533

Wright J W, Healy T E J, Balfour T W, Hardcastle J D 1982 Effects of inhalational anesthetic agents on the electrical and mechanical activity of the rat duodenum. Br J Anaesth 54: 1223–1229

35. Chronic pseudo-obstruction

J. Christensen   K. Orvar

INTRODUCTION

Sometimes patients seem to suffer from an obstruction to flow in a gastrointestinal viscus even though no mechanical obstruction exists. The term *pseudo-obstruction* refers to this situation.

The term had occasional use after its introduction (Dudley et al 1958), but it received more currency 20 years later after a comprehensive review article on the subject (Faulk et al 1978a). The 1978 popularization of the term came at a time when the study of the processes involved in gastrointestinal flow had suddenly revived after decades of relative torpor, and so it found an audience newly prepared to think about the causes of disordered gastrointestinal flow.

Like 'malabsorption syndrome', the term has found considerable use to describe a general clinical situation which, also like 'malabsorption syndrome', has many causes. But some physicians now use it incorrectly as a specific diagnostic term when, in fact, it only describes a clinical picture. Those who use it to denote a specific diagnosis thereby tend to abandon the consideration of causes. Such a loose usage hinders constructive thought about the complex processes that govern gastrointestinal flow.

If the term received the usage intended by its originators, it could provide a framework that would allow categorization of all the various disorders in which the mechanisms that generate gastrointestinal flow fail. In *mechanical obstruction* forces generating flow fail to overcome the heightened resistance to flow even though they may undergo compensatory modifications. In *pseudo-obstruction* the forces fail primarily, while resistances remain normal. That, the intended meaning of the term upon its introduction, constitutes the meaning it receives in this review and the meaning it should retain.

Our understanding of the ways in which the motions of gastrointestinal muscle regulate or generate gastrointestinal flow has advanced a great deal in the past three decades, so that pseudo-obstruction represents disturbed processes which we can now actually describe, in some cases, at least. Many review articles have appeared and continue to appear, illustrating the rapid advance in understanding of these disorders (Anuras 1988), Anuras & Christensen 1983, Anuras et al 1978, Colemont & Camilleri 1989, Faulk et al 1978a, Faulk et al 1978b, Franken et al 1987, Isaacson et al 1985, Nowak et al 1982, Schuffler et al 1981, Smith 1983, Vanek & Al-Salti 1986, Wegener & Borsch 1987). Furthermore, pathologists have now defined the pathology in some instances, so that these constitute morphologically-defined disorders rather than 'functional' disorders.

Some forms in children are different from those seen in adults (Byrne et al 1977, Faber et al 1987, Glassman et al 1989, Greenall & Gough 1983, Hyman et al 1988, Kaschula et al 1987, Reinarz et al 1985, Schuffler et al 1988, Shaw et al 1979, Vargas et al 1988, Yamigawa et al 1988).

As these nosological entities become better known and better characterized, they themselves should become the diagnostic terms and the use of 'pseudo-obstruction' as a diagnosis should tend to disappear.

A complete review of the recent literature appeared recently (Christensen et al 1990).

THE CLINICAL PICTURE THAT SHOULD SUGGEST PSEUDO-OBSTRUCTION

As the term indicates, the clinical picture generally resembles that of mechanical obstruction of the gastrointestinal viscera (Table 35.1). Pseudo-obstruction should come to mind only when mechanical obstruction comes to mind. The term applies to any of the viscera, though pseudo-obstruction of the small intestine gets the most attention. Most of the processes that produce pseudo-obstruction affect more than one viscus and so the clinical picture often suggests trouble in more than a single organ.

Table 35.1   The symptoms to suggest pseudo-obstruction in various organs of the gastrointestinal tract

Oesophagus	Stomach	Small intestine	Colon
Dysphagia	Nausea	Nausea	Abdominal distension
Regurgitation of ingesta	Sensation of gastric fullness	Bloating or abdominal distension	Constipation
Chest pain	Bloating or abdominal distension	Vomiting	
	Vomiting	Generalized abdominal pain	
	Epigastric pain	Constipation and/or diarrhoea	

Entering into the differential diagnosis of suspected mechanical obstruction, pseudo-obstruction usually manifests itself as nausea, vomiting, and cramping abdominal pain. Experienced clinicians know that lesser degrees of mechanical obstruction produce lesser symptoms than complete mechanical obstruction, and they realize that relatively small degrees of obstruction may indeed produce quite minor or intermittent episodes of obstructive symptoms. The various causes of pseudo-obstruction rarely mimic a complete obstruction. Rather, the confusion occurs with minor, incomplete, or intermittent mechanical obstruction.

In such cases, the clinician must search diligently for incomplete obstructions. This search usually takes the form of radiographic studies seeking at least dilatation of a viscus. The finding of such dilatation may prompt thought of endoscopic or surgical exploration for an obstruction. When studies have gone this far without the clear demonstration of a mechanical obstruction, the possibility of pseudo-obstruction arises.

THE PATHOGENESIS OF PSEUDO-OBSTRUCTION

The disordered motility that prevents normal antegrade flow in the gut could reflect several kinds of muscular dysfunction (Table 35.2). Simple *weakness* of the smooth muscle, a reduced force of contraction, can arise from several abnormalities, and weakness of contractions underlies many causes. *Dysrhythmia*, analogous to cardiac dysrhythmias, certainly can occur as well. *Vector disturbances* for peristalsis probably also occur, but they evade ready detection by current means: one can only speculate that retrograde peristalsis occurs in some forms of pseudo-obstruction. Similarly, *defective tonus mechanisms* may occur, but no reasonable way exists to detect them in the clinic.

It probably makes little difference whether muscle weakness, dysrhythmia, vector disturbances, or defective tonus mechanisms dominate in any single case because they all could well occur together, given the sorts of factors that underly pseudo-obstruction.

Pseudo-obstruction reflects dysfunction of the neuromuscular apparatus of the gut, and that dysfunction may manifest itself in any of several kinds of disturbances of the operation of the apparatus.

The pathogenesis of pseudo-obstruction, then, lies in the disruption of any of the functions of the enteric nerves and gastrointestinal smooth muscle. A complete understanding of pathogenesis requires a complete knowledge of those structures and functions, a state of understanding which remains to be achieved.

THE ENTERIC NERVOUS SYSTEM (ENS)

Another chapter of this book treats the enteric nerves from the morphologic point of view. These nerves function, in large part, in independence of the central nervous system (CNS) and even of the other parts of the autonomic system. And yet, as an integrated nervous system, the ENS shares the features of nerves everywhere. Thus, as terminally-differentiated cells, enteric nerve cells cannot reproduce. They show resistance to radiation damage and susceptibility to hypoxia. And, especially, all noxious influences which can damage the CNS can also damage the enteric nerves. The enteric nerves are not absolutely unique. Thus, certain disorders normally considered to be disorders of the CNS can also produce pseudo-obstruction through disturbances they produce in the operation of the ENS.

Recent work has greatly advanced our understanding of the ENS (Furness & Costa 1987), and that current understanding depicts a system that rivals the brain itself in complexity. Neurological disorders specific to the ENS do occur. Some take the form of developmental diseases where the migration and implantation of precursor nerve cells from the neural crest fails completion (as in Hirschsprung's disease and probably hypertrophic pyloric stenosis). Others seem to be acquired, perhaps as infections with neurotropic viruses. But the complexity of the ENS allows for a great many other neural disease processes that could interfere with gut muscle function.

Table 35.2 Four specific kinds of muscular dysfunction that can occur in pseudo-obstruction

Muscular dysfunction	Cause
Weakness of rhythmic contractions	Weakness due to a deficit in the contractile process in the smooth muscle itself
	Weakness due to insufficient excitation of muscle by nerves
Dysrhythmia	Tachyarrhythmia, e.g. 'tachygastria'
	Bradyarrhythmia, e.g. 'bradygastria'
Vector disturbances	'Antiperistalsis'
Defective tonus mechanisms	Defective neurogenic relaxation of tonus at sphincters, as in achalasia.
	Defective maintenance of myogenic tonus in maintenance of sphincter closure, as occurs in scleroderma of the oesophagus to foster regurgitation.

GASTROINTESTINAL SMOOTH MUSCLE

Smooth muscle, once considered 'primitive' as compared to somatic muscle, in fact exhibits its own special complexities. Furthermore, it varies qualitatively from one tissue to another. The long-standing oversimplification of smooth muscle as a subject for serious study has led to a comparative ignorance of the ways in which it can go wrong. Pseudo-obstruction commonly results from smooth muscle disease which reflects sometimes a disease of all kinds of muscle, sometimes a disease only of smooth muscle, and sometimes a disease only of gastrointestinal smooth muscle.

A smooth muscle cell is a complicated structure (Fig. 35.1). The activation of a muscle cell to contract or to relax involves a sequence of causally-related events: (1) activation of a membrane receptor to an extrinsic substance, a nerve or hormone, (2) opening (or closing) of ion-specific channels in the membrane, (3) release of 'second messengers' inside the cell membrane, (4) release of calcium from inactive stores in the muscle itself, and (5) activation of the sliding filament-mechanism to induce alterations in the length of the muscle cell. The integration of contractions or relaxations of all cells throughout a tissue, so that they all work together, depends in part upon physiological communications between adjacent muscle cells through cell-to-cell junctions. Mechanical linkages between cells also occur through connective tissue bands that create a three-dimensional mesh of considerable complexity and regularity, a system that transfers tension changes uniformly throughout the tissue. With such a complex physiological and mechanical arrangement, quite clearly a great many sorts of processes can fail that would interfere with the normal operation of gut smooth muscle.

THE WAYS IN WHICH CHRONIC PSEUDO-OBSTRUCTION CAN OCCUR

Normal propulsive movements of the gut wall require the smooth muscle itself to contract and to relax normally. They also require the control systems that establish the patterns of contraction and relaxation to operate normally. Thus, disordered propulsion can represent dysfunction of either or both the muscle (the effector system) or the enteric nerves (the major control system). In both cases, the dysfunction may be irreversible or reversible.

In most instances, the causes of pseudo-obstruction lie outside the gut itself, in a disease that is recognized therefore as systemic or generalized. Although primary enteric neuropathies and myopathies (in which the disease process appears to be confined to the gut) seem to exist, that impression may only mean that the expression of these diseases in non-enteric nerve and muscle is inapparent.

THE CLINICAL CLASSIFICATION OF THE FORMS OF PSEUDO-OBSTRUCTION

Conventional classifications group the causes of pseudo-obstruction into 'primary' forms (those where the disorder, of unknown cause, seems to be confined to the gut and related viscera) and 'secondary' forms (where the pseudo-obstruction develops as part of a recognized disease, as part of a more widespread disorder). Such a classification emphasizes the many clinical situations in which pseudo-obstruction can occur, but it also tends to give as much weight to the very rare as to the very common. The classification given here (Table 35.3) encompasses the whole list of causes. The more common forms of the disorder receive further discussion in subsequent sections of this chapter.

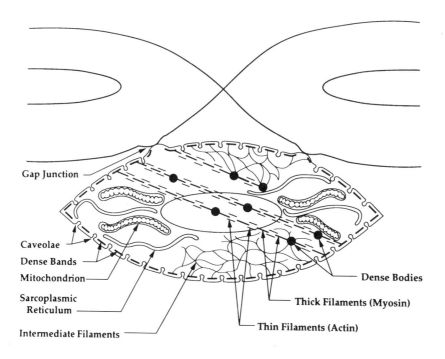

Fig. 35.1 A diagram of a smooth muscle cell. (From Christensen J in Kumar D, Waldron D J, Williams N S (eds) Clinical Measurement in Coloproctology. Copyright 1991 by Springer-Verlag London Limited. (Reprinted with permission.)

Table 35.3 The causes of chronic pseudo-obstruction

Visceral myopathy	Visceral neuropathy	Drug-related pseudo-obstruction	Metabolic dysfunctions	Miscellaneous/ unclassifiable causes
Primary visceral myopathies	Primary visceral	Well-established causative	Endocrine	Postoperative pseudo-
Familial visceral myopathy	neuropathy	drugs	disorders	obstruction
Non-familial visceral	Familial visceral	Opiates and anti	Hypothyroidism	Jejunoileal bypass
myopathy	neuropathy	cholinergic agents	Hypoparathyroidism	operations
Connective tissue diseases	Non-familial visceral	Cytotoxic agents used in	Pheochromocytoma	Organ transplant
Scleroderma or CREST	neuropathy	cancer chemotherapy	Metabolic intoxica	Paraneoplastic pseudo-
syndrome	Achalasia	Probable contributory drugs	tions	obstruction
Dermatomyositis/	Hirschsprung's	Antidepressants or anti-	Uraemia	Small-cell carcinoma
polymyositis	disease	anxiety agents	Porphyria	of the lung
Lupus erythematosus	Hypertrophic	Anti-parkinsonian agents		Radiation injury
Muscular dystrophies	pyloric stenosis	Cathartics, especially		
Myotonic dystrophy	Diffuse visceral	anthraquinones		
Other muscular	neuropathy			
dystrophies	Generalized nervous			
Infiltrative diseases	system disease			
Amyloidosis	Parkinson's disease			
Ceroidosis	Diabetic			
Lymphoid infiltration of	polyneuropathy			
the intestine	Primary autonomic			
	dysfunction			
	Post-viral pseudo-			
	obstruction			
	Disease largely confined			
	to the autonomic			
	nervous system			
	Chagas' disease			

A COMMENTARY ON TABLE 35.3

The visceral myopathies

More cases of pseudo-obstruction arise from visceral myopathies than from visceral neuropathies. The myopathy accompanying scleroderma arises far more often than the others.

Scleroderma myopathy

This occurs more often with the CREST syndrome than with the other forms of this cluster of diseases. It seems never to occur with localized scleroderma, or morphea. CREST, an acronym, comes from the association of **Ca**lcinosis, **Re**ynaud's phenomenon, **E**sophageal symptoms, **S**clerodactyly and **T**elangiectasia. As the acronym implies, the myopathy involves especially the oesophageal musculature, producing dysphagia and (because of failure of the lower oesophageal sphincter, LOS) chronic gastro-oesophageal reflux, with consequent oesophagitis and stricture formation. The myopathy affects other viscera as well so that delayed gastric emptying and dilation of the small intestine and colon frequently occur, accompanied by chronic obstructive symptoms and, often, intermittent diarrhoea from small intestinal bacterial overgrowth. The pathologist sees degeneration of the smooth muscle with collagen replacement in both muscle layers in the affected organs (Fig. 35.2). The patchy nature of the lesion produces areas where the replacement is complete which are interspersed with less-affected or even unaffected muscle. In the colon, the intraluminal pressure may force some of these patches formed wholly of collagen to protrude outward, to produce the characteristic large and wide-mouthed diverticula.

Myotonic dystrophy

This is probably a primary nerve disorder rather than a primary muscle dystrophy, and commonly gives rise to visceral obstructive symptoms, though they rarely achieve the severity that characterizes such symptoms in the other visceral myopathies. This familial disorder, an autosomal dominant, produces a familiar cluster of signs, including slowness of relaxation of somatic muscle, somatic muscle weakness, premature balding, cataracts, and testicular atrophy. Visceral muscle involvement rather infrequently brings patients to the gastroenterologist because patients often accept and tolerate the symptoms as relatively trivial or inconsequential. The disease usually affects the oesophagus and stomach much more prominently than other regions, although constipation from colonic dysfunction occasionally becomes a major problem. The histopathology of the visceral myopathy remains to be comletely described.

Primary visceral myopathies

These have received a disproportionate degree of attention partly because of their mysterious origin and partly because it was the modern awareness of these particular disorders that gave rise especially to the concept of pseudo-obstruction as a syndrome. Although some careful family studies have clearly established the heritable nature of some forms of primary visceral myopathy, acquired forms must exist as well since some cases clearly lack evidence of a genetic cause when there has been a search of relatives. Both dominant and recessive patterns of inheritance exist, and so the familial visceral myopathies constitute several distinct disorders (Figs 35.3 & 35.4). Some are dominant, others recessive. Some are generalized, other more local. In some forms, the pathologic process affects other organs as well, notably the urinary bladder, the uterus, and the extraocular muscles. The histopathology of the affected gut muscle resembles that of scleroderma, with degeneration of the smooth muscle and collagen replacement. The fibrosis can affect any of the muscle layers, usually as a diffuse lesion rather than the patchy lesion seen in scleroderma. The characterization of the individual forms of the familial visceral myopathies relies more fully upon the pattern of inheritance and the pattern of organ involvement than it does upon the histopathology. The most fully characterized form of familial visceral myopathy, an autosomal dominant, produces duodenal involvement most conspicuously. The frequency of essentially asymptomatic cases in families with this well-defined entity speaks for the likelihood that the disorder commonly goes unrecognized as such, or often earns only descriptive (nonhistopathologic) terms like 'idiopathic megaduodenum' or 'superior mesenteric artery syndrome'. Another well-characterized form, an autosomal recessive, produces external ophthalmoplegia and multiple small intestinal diverticula.

Infiltration of the smooth muscle

This rarely appears as a cause of pseudo-obstruction. Although *amyloidosis* certainly can do so, this is a rare manifestation of a rare disease. *Ceroidosis*, a rare histopathological entity in which a brown pigment, ceroid, infiltrates the gut wall, signifies chronic wasting illness of any sort, and its association with pseudo-obstruction may only mean that the wasting illness itself has produced visceral muscle dysfunction and, therefore, pseudo-obstruction.

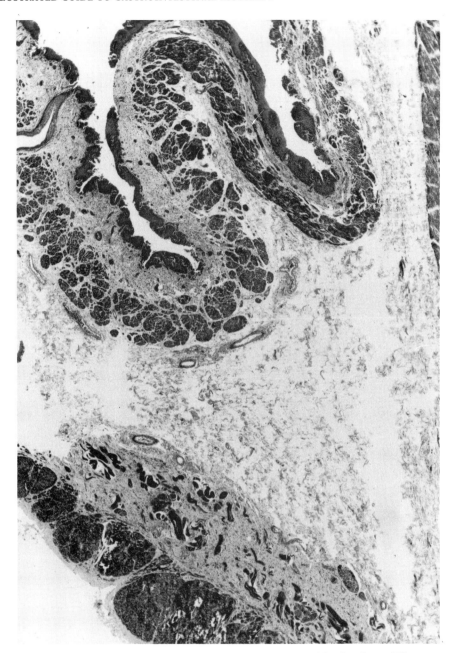

Fig. 35.2   Histological section from mid oesophagus in a patient with scleroderma. Fibrous tissue has almost completely replaced the circular smooth muscle layer. (From Mitros F A in Ming S and Goldman H (eds) Pathology of the Gastrointestinal Tract. Copyright 1992 by W. B. Saunders Company. Reprinted with permission.)

The visceral neuropathies

Achalasia

The classic *acquired* visceral neuropathy, achalasia, rep-

resents a well-defined neuropathic pseudo-obstruction. Death or dysfunction of the enteric nerves in the oesophagus leads to the failure of the LOS to relax and the failure of the smooth-muscle part of the oesopha-

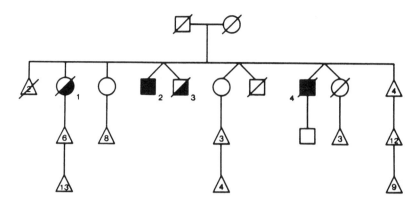

Fig. 35.3 Pedigree table of a family with visceral myopathy. Squares denote males, circles females. Slashes across squares of circles are deceased family members. Completely dark squares or circles are affected family members. Numbers in triangles denote numbers in groups of persons. The fact that the four patients with the disease are all in the second generation suggests an autosomal recessive transmission. (From Anuras S, Mitros F A, Milano A et al 1986. A Familial Visceral Myopathy with Dilatation of the Entire Gastrointestinal Tract. Gastroenterology 90: 385. Copyright 1986 by the American Gastroenterological Association. Reprinted with permission.)

geal body to contract in response to swallowing. The idea that this is a purely neuropathic disorder arose from physiological studies before anatomic evidence confirmed the concept. The disorder seems virtually never to extend to other organs. The reason for the selectivity of the neuropathy for the oesophagus re-

mains mysterious. Not all cases behave in exactly the same way: some develop massive dilatation of the oesophageal body (Figs 35.5 & 35.6) while others do not, the oesophageal body being spastic. Very rarely, cases revert to normal function after a time. Thus, some variations within this clinical entity occur, but it

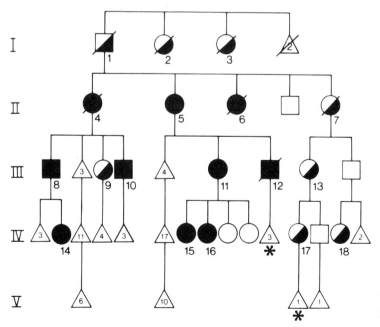

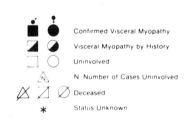

Fig. 35.4 Pedigree table of a family with familial visceral myopathy. The mode of inheritance is either autosomal dominant or sex-linked dominant. The Roman numerals specify the generations. The numbers outside symbols specify individual persons described in the reference. (From Faulk D L, Anuras S, Gardner G D et al 1978. A Familial Visceral Myopathy. Ann Intern Med 89: 600. Copyright 1978 by the American College of Physicians. Reprinted with permission.)

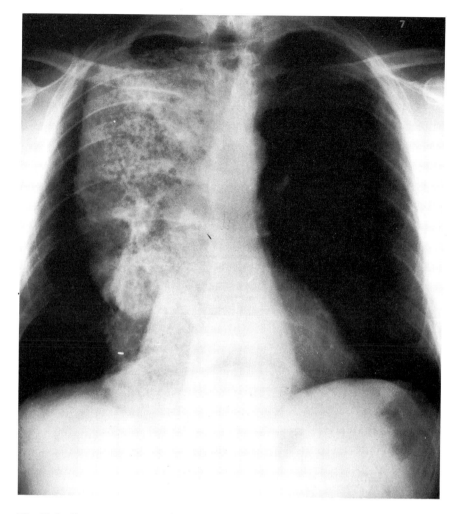

Fig. 35.5   Chest roentgenogram demonstrating massively dilated oesophagus filled with food.

remains a reasonably distinct and well-defined neuropathic disease.

Hirschsprung's disease

This the classic *congenital* visceral neuropathy, resembles achalasia only in that strong evidence supports the wholly neuropathic nature of the disorder. In contrast, it affects only the caudal end of the gastrointestinal tract, the denervated segment of rectum or distal colon exhibiting spastic contraction, (Fig 35.7) while the more proximal (and histologically normal) parts of the colon become dilated passively from obstruction (Fig 35.8). Where the pathogenesis of achalasia still eludes explanation, that of Hirschsprung's disease lies in the demonstration of a defective migration of neural crest

cells to the distal colon in embryogenesis, at least as shown in an animal model of the disease.

Hypertrophic pyloric stenosis

On recent evidence, this also reflects neuropathy, with a deficiency of ganglion cells and axons in the pylorus causing a sustained contraction, just as the deficit in Hirschsprung's disease makes for sustained contraction in the rectoanal segment. As a congenital disorder, hypertrophic pyloric stenosis seems to reflect a developmental defect like that of Hirschsprung's disease. Unlike Hirschsprung's disease, hypertrophic pyloric stenosis, untreated, tends to correct itself with maturation of the infant.

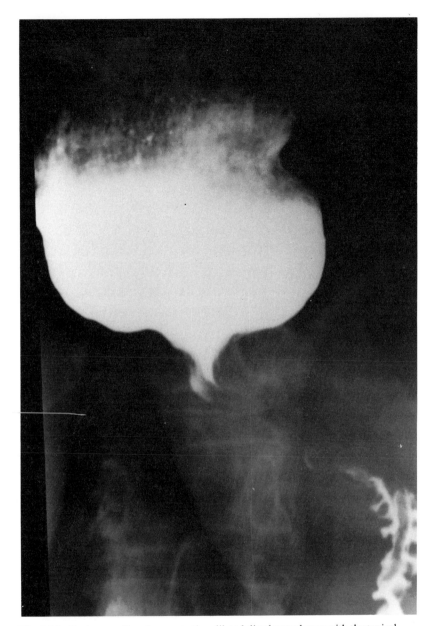

Fig. 35.6   Barium swallow demonstrating dilated distal oesophagus with the typical beak in a patient with achalasia.

Other forms of primary visceral neuropathy

These seem to reflect neurotropic virus infections or hereditary disorders of unknown nature (Fig. 35.9). The familial or hereditary neuropathic disorders, less common than the myopathies, await full characterization in epidemiological, histopathological and clinical terms.

Diabetic polyneuropathy

By all odds, this accounts for more cases of neuropathic pseudo-obstruction than all other causes combined. The same fundamental neuropathic process that accounts for the somatic neuropathies of diabetes apparently also affect the ENS, according to current views, but the fact that enteric nerve involvement develops

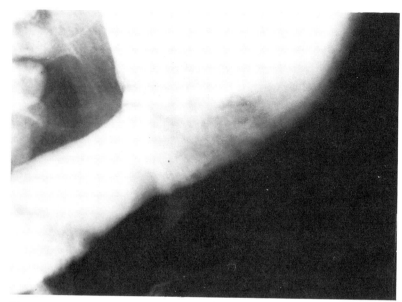

Fig. 35.7 A narrowed segment of distal colon typical of aganglionosis in Hirsch-sprung's disease.

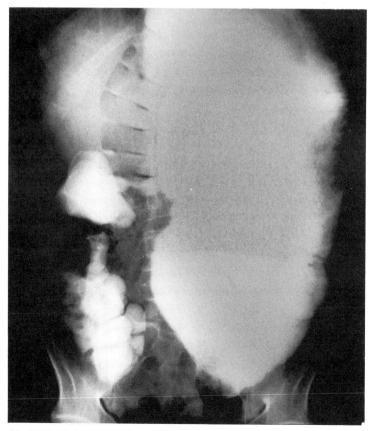

Fig. 35.8 Barium enema in a patient with Hirschprung's disease demonstrating markedly dilated left colon.

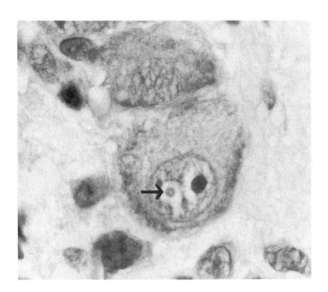

Fig. 35.9 Neuronal pseudo-obstruction; note the intranuclear inclusion (arrow) adjacent to the nucleolus in this colonic submucosal ganglion cell (H + E, × 250). (Courtesy of Frank Mitros, M.D.)

later, and usually in a setting of long-standing poor control of the diabetes, suggests that the enteric nerves resist the process better than the somatic nerves. Diabetic enteroneuropathy can affect all the gastrointestinal viscera from the distal oesophagus to the colon, to produce any of the symptoms of pseudo-obstruction. The oesophageal involvement rarely produces anything more than mild dysphagia, but the gastric involvement commonly creates a severe problem in nutrition and so it complicates the control of the diabetes itself. Small intestinal involvement most commonly takes the form of bacterial overgrowth with diarrhoea, while colonic involvement accounts for the severe constipation which troubles many such patients. Considering the incidence of diabetic enteroneuropathy and the management problems it produces, the clinical problem has called forth surprisingly little basic science study. No histopathological definition exists, nor has any full explanation emerged that accounts for the features of diabetic enteroneuropathy or that allows a rational treatment to be designed.

Parkinson's disease

The idea that Parkinson's disease involves the ENS developed rather late in the history of the understanding of that illness. One cannot yet be certain that the pseudo-obstruction which commonly develops in patients with Parkinson's disease arises in the neurological disease itself rather than from the drugs usually used to treat the disease, for many such drugs affect autonomic nerve function. Still, recent evidence strongly implicates the disease itself. The symptoms indicate involvement of any or all the gastrointestinal viscera. The histopathology remains to be fully examined in the gut.

Chagas' disease

Very rarely encountered in North America, Chagas' disease destroys the enteric nerves in all parts of the gut, but often affects the oesophagus to produce a megaoesophagus that resembles that of achalasia. The full pathogenesis remains unknown.

Drug-related pseudo-obstruction

Opiates and anticholinergic agents

These drugs, which have held a place in therapeutics for a very long time, depress gastrointestinal motor functions to some degree in normal doses, but especially so in large doses. They seem to spare the oesophagus relative to the stomach and colon. One would think that all physicians would recognize such effects as a part of the actions of such drugs, but gastroenterologists not rarely are called upon to explain gastric distension or megacolon in patients where the use or abuse of such drugs provides the whole explanation.

Cytotoxic drugs

Some cytotoxic drugs used in cancer chemotherapy, especially adriamycin, seem to depress nerve function enough to produce pseudo-obstruction. Of course, pseudo-obstruction developing in such critically-ill patients could have other explanations as well in the inevitable setting of polypharmacy, sepsis and metabolic derangements, but most students of the subject attribute at least some of the pseudo-obstruction to the cytotoxic agents themselves.

Agents to treat depression, anxiety and hypertension

Modern pharmacology has produced a great many neurotropic agents to treat depression, anxiety and hypertension. That these can also affect gastrointestinal motor functions should surprise no one. Occasionally, especially in large dosages, they can create disturbances suggestive of obstruction in the gut. The same can be said of some of the agents used to treat Parkinson's disease, many of them anticholinergics. *Cathartic* abuse, specifically of the anthraquinones, may produce pseudo-obstruction mainly of the colon. Much remains to be learned of the mechanism of this effect.

Metabolic dysfunctions

Clinical wisdom has long taught that *hypothyroidism* can cause a clinical picture closely resembling bowel obstruction, so-called myxedema ileus. At one time, surgeons occasionally fell into the trap of abdominal exploration in such cases, but that seems no longer to occur. As for *hypoparathyroidism* and *pheochromocytoma*, pseudo-obstruction seems a very rare manifestation, described only in isolated case reports.

The dilated bowel and nausea of advanced *uraemia*, once so very common, rarely occurs in this era of renal transplantation and dialysis, but those who have seen it know how strongly the picture can resemble bowel obstruction. Pseudo-obstruction also certainly occurs as an occasional manifestation of *acute intermittent porphyria*. Given that an acute neuropathy so frequently develops in exacerbations of porphyria, an enteric neuropathy seems the most likely explanation for the intestinal pseudo-obstruction that sometimes occurs.

Unclassifiable causes

The causes listed in Table 35.3 as *miscellaneous* or *unclassifiable* principally reflect single case reports or a very limited experience, so that they can all be considered unproved. The one exception, *paraneoplastic pseudo-obstruction*, also rare but well-established, has reflected, in all reported cases, a small-cell carcinoma of the lung. No one knows which of the several endocrine substances such tumours can produce accounts for the pseudo-obstruction.

PSEUDO-OBSTRUCTION AS A FORM OF FUNCTIONAL BOWEL SYNDROME

'Functional bowel syndrome', or 'irritable bowel syndrome', terms current for about 50 years, still find a use in categorizing patients with any combination of long-standing gastrointestinal symptoms that include nausea, vomiting, altered bowel-habit, abdominal pain, gas, bloating, and feelings of incomplete rectal evacuation which defy explanation after investigation for organic disease. The idea that the symptoms reflect altered gastrointestinal motility persists, despite the fact that it never had convincing support, and emotional disease has often received the blame for the presumed abnormal motility. With the modern development of methods to measure gastrointestinal motility precisely, repeatedly and safely, patients thought to have the functional bowel syndrome have come under new scrutiny.

The discovery of an objectively demonstrable abnormality in a patient with the functional bowel syndrome would seem to remove him or her from the category of the functional bowel syndrome, where the absence of objectively demonstrable pathology constitutes a part of the definition. When the study of such a patient reveals actual disease, the physician has a new term for the malady.

This has happened before, for example, with the discovery of lactase deficiency and of microscopic (collagenous and lymphocytic) colitis. And it has happened again. This time, it happened with the application of jejunal manometry to patients with the functional bowel syndrome. When jejunal manometry revealed abnormal patterns of motility (not detectable in other ways) in such patients (Fig. 35.10), they received the 'diagnosis' of pseudo-obstruction syndrome, apparently to distinguish them from those with the functional bowel syndrome. Thus, a special category of pseudo-obstruction now exists which does not fit the classification given in Table 35.3 because no one has any suggestion as to cause. It is a duodenojejunal dysrhythmia.

THE DIAGNOSTIC APPROACH TO PSEUDO-OBSTRUCTION

Methods

As in all aspects of medicine, a thoughtful and rational analysis of the symptoms, their clinical setting, and the physical findings must precede 'investigations' in pseudo-obstruction. Commonly, such a symptom-analysis, along with a review of the full circumstances of the patient – put simply, the taking and interpreting of a complete history and physical examination – provides nearly all the evidence needed to explain the symptoms in pseudo-obstruction. In the process of getting and interpreting the history and physical findings, physicians must keep Table 35.3 in mind in order that they will know what points

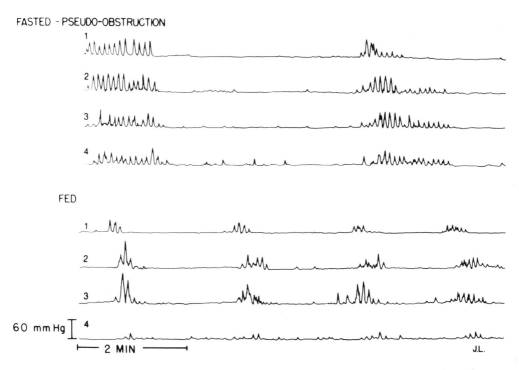

FASTED - PSEUDO-OBSTRUCTION

FED

60 mm Hg

2 MIN

J.L.

Fig. 35.10 Jejunal manometry tracings from a patient with pseudo-obstruction demonstrating intermittent high-amplitude clustered contractions both before and after a meal. (From Summers R W, Anuras S, Green J 1983 Jejunal manometry patterns in health, partial intestinal obstruction, and pseudo-obstruction. Gastroenterology 85: 1290. Copyright 1983 by the American Gastroenterological Association. Reprinted with permission.)

to think about. If they think to look for the connective tissue diseases, neurological disease, myxedema, and the use of neurotropic drugs, they will discover most causes.

In any case, the physician often uses diagnostic techniques designed for the study of gastrointestinal motility, either to find (or to rule out) mechanical obstruction or to document and measure the abnormality in motor function. Such diagnostic techniques constitute (1) the use of radiographic methods, including scintigraphy, (2) tracer studies, (3) the direct measurement of contractions by manometry or kymography, and (4) histopathology.

Radiography

This with the use of barium sulphate or other contrast media, finds use mainly to exclude mechanical obstruction. The finding of a dilated organ without a point of stenosis suggests defective motility.

Scintigraphy

Scintigraphy has its principal application in the measurement of gastric emptying where the incorporation of an isotope into a physiologically 'normal' meal avoids the problems intrinsic in the use of barium sulphate or other contrast meals which can themselves abnormally affect the appearance of gastric emptying. Scintigraphy, moreover, works well in the stomach where the area of the gastric silhouette fairly accurately reflects the volume of the reservoir and the stomach maintains a reasonably constant position. Scintigraphy finds far less use in measuring oesophageal, intestinal and colonic transit, for various reasons.

Tracer studies

Once common, tracer studies have fallen from use with only a few exceptions. One technique makes use of ingested radiopaque markers whose course through the gut is followed by fluoroscopy. The wide variations in normal values limit the usefulness of this method to study gastric and intestinal flows, but it survives as the best way to measure colonic transit in constipation. Serial abdominal films taken at fixed intervals of days can distinguish 'slow transit' constipation (motor dysfunction of the right colon) from constipation that is related to anorectal and pelvic floor dysfunction. Other tracer techniques, useful for the gut above the colon, involve the ingestion of substances which, when they reach the caecum, feed the colonic bacteria who convert them to gases detectable in the breath. Thus, non-absorbed carbohydrate becomes hydrogen when it reaches the caecum, and the time for breath hydrogen concentrations to rise after the ingestion of a load of such a carbohydrate measures mouth-to-caecum transit. Bacterial overgrowth in the small intestine, which can occur both in mechanical obstruction and in pseudo-obstruction, makes the technique useless.

Manometry

The measurement of intraluminal pressures from tubes has become the standard means to measure the characteristics of oesophageal peristalsis, and it has more recently found use in assessing duodeno-jejunal motility. Here, its capacity to delineate the timing of the phases of the fasted pattern of motility has proved particularly useful. Disorders in this pattern characterize several forms of pseudo-obstruction.

Histopathology

Despite the fact that it could so obviously clarify understanding of motor disorders, histopathology remains poorly used except in certain instances. Histopathology, of course, requires a generous and full-thickness biopsy to show the muscle and nerve adequately. The deficit in the application of histopathology mainly arises not from defective histopathological techniques but from inadequate utilization, by surgeons, of opportunities for generous biopsies at the operations which patients with pseudo-obstruction frequently undergo.

Strategy

The first step, in any case of suspected obstruction or pseudo-obstruction, requires the careful analysis of the complaints and their course, and of the physical findings, with special reference to the causes of pseudo-obstruction that appear in Table 35.3. The importance of this frame of reference cannot be over-emphasized.

In the absence of mechanical obstruction, the second step involves the application of methods to show, objectively, the nature and degree of any abnormalities in gastrointestinal motor function that may exist. The symptoms of pseudo-obstruction seem to be much the same no matter which organ is mainly involved, and, in any case, the motor disorder rarely confines itself to a single organ. Thus, in this step, we suggest a standard battery of tests, those for which the techniques and values find widespread acceptance: (1) oesophageal manometry, (2) the scintigraphic measurement of gastric emptying, (3) duodenojejunal manometry, (4) a colonic marker transit study.

The use of the methods and strategy

The methods and strategy set forth above help principally in two ways: (1) to better define a motor disturbance or to follow the progress of a motor disturbance that has already made itself quite clear, and (2) to allow the consultant to say that the most precise testing has failed to demonstrate a motor abnormality. The second use arises more often, consultants finding themselves doing these tests mainly in order to be able to say that even the most subtle motor disorder cannot be found.

Two examples may help to illustrate our meaning:

One of us (J.C.) recently saw a 20-year-old man whose persistent vomiting and sharp upper abdominal pain raised the possibility of pseudo-obstruction. As a type I diabetic, rather poorly controlled, and a victim of schizophrenia, he presented two reasons for his physician to suspect pseudo-obstruction, in the form of possible diabetic enteroneuropathy and in the several psychotropic drugs which he took regularly. Contrast X-rays of the gastrointestinal tract had shown no abnormality, and so the referring physician asked me to consider the possibility of a motor abnormality. After a complete blood count and a panel of blood chemistries, which were normal, I chose to examine the upper gastrointestinal tract endoscopically, knowing that nausea and sharp upper abdominal pain can reflect mucosal inflammation not detected by contrast radiography. The endoscopy revealed the absence of obstruction but the presence of mild diffuse mucosal inflammation in the stomach which proved, on testing, to be due to *Helicobacter pylori*. After 2 weeks of appropriate antibiotic treatment, the patient reported complete relief of his symptoms, but his physician still pressed me to investigate further to rule out a motor dysfunction. An oesophageal manometry, a scintigraphic study of gastric emptying, and a duodenojejunal manometric study all gave completely normal results. These permitted me to respond to the referring physician that the most sophisticated tests showed that neither his diabetes nor his psychotropic drugs affected his gastrointestinal motor function detectably, leaving the *Helicobacter* gastritis as the sole and sufficient explanation of his symptoms.

Also, I recently saw a 13-year-old boy, entirely healthy except for persistent daily vomiting for several months which led to such weight loss that he had required central venous nutrition. Although contrast radiography had shown no obstruction in the upper gastrointestinal tract, his physicians performed a laparotomy at which they found and lysed adhesions. The operation made no difference. The persistent vomiting resulted in his being brought to me to be investigated for pseudo-obstruction. Careful questioning and direct observation established that the patient regurgitated rather than vomited, the food returning to the mouth within 1 or 2 after a swallow, and the act being neither preceded nor followed by any sensation of nausea. Likewise, the patient acknowledged a good appetite and normal feelings of hunger. I ordered a barium swallow and performed upper gastrointestinal endoscopy, both examinations showing no abnormalities. Because the symptom seemed so clearly oesophageal in origin, I performed oesophageal manometry twice and found, both times as the sole abnormality, a LOS which failed to relax with swallowing. This suggested a neurological defect in the inhibitory innervation of the sphincter. The boy seemed to have achalasia without paralysis of the oesophageal body, the other feature of classical achalasia. A diagnosis of incipient achalasia seemed appropriate, and a pneumatic dilation of the LOS produced complete and lasting abatement of the regurgitation.

THE MANAGEMENT OF PSEUDO-OBSTRUCTION

Although we and others have written in scholarly fashion before on the general approach to management of pseudo-obstruction, such a discussion cannot escape sounding diffuse, fatuous, or even absurd in light of the many different disease processes that can cause or contribute to defective gastrointestinal motility. The management of each situation depends wholly upon the cause. The most effective management requires the most specific diagnosis as to cause, and hence the first rule in management: *make as precise a diagnosis as possible*. Once the cause has become clear, the available means to ameliorate the symptoms become evident.

In many cases of defective gastrointestinal motility, more than one factor contributes to the abnormality. Hence, the second rule in management: *do not stop at one cause but seek out all other reasonable factors that occur to you*, because you only need to be able to find one that is amenable to treatment in order to offer your patient some relief.

As for the further rules of management, they mostly amount to common sense:

1. Correct blood electrolyte disturbances, if present.
2. Treat endocrine diseases appropriately.
3. Reduce dosages of any drugs that may be contributing, making substitutions with other drugs or eliminating the drugs if possible.
4. If diarrhoea occurs because of small bowel bacterial overgrowth, treat it aggressively with antibiotics.
5. Maintain nutritional support by whatever means possible.
6. Restrict operations to those which bypass dysfunctional segments if they exist.

REFERENCES

Anuras S 1988 Intestinal pseudo-obstruction syndrome. Ann Rev Med 39: 1–15
Anuras S, Christensen J 1983 Primary (or idiopathic) chronic intestinal pseudo-obstruction. Prog Gastroenterol 4: 269–281
Anuras S, Crane S A, Faulk D L et al 1978 Intestinal pseudoobstruction. Gastroenterology 74: 1318–1324
Byrne W J, Cipel L, Euler A R et al 1977 Chronic idiopathic intestinal pseudo-obstruction syndrome in children – clinical characteristics and prognosis. J Pediatr 90: 585–589
Christensen J, Dent J, Malagelada J-R et al 1990 Pseudo-obstruction. Gastroenterol Int 3: 107–119
Colemont L J, Camilleri M 1989 Chronic intestinal pseudo-obstruction: diagnosis and treatment. Mayo Clin Proc 64: 60–70
Dudley H A F, Sinclair I S R, McLaren I F et al 1958 Intestinal pseudo-obstruction. J R Coll Surg Edin 3: 206–217
Faber J, Fich A, Steinberg A et al 1987 Familial intestinal pseudoobstruction dominated by a progressive neurologic disease at a young age. Gastroenterology 92: 786–790
Faulk D L, Anuras S, Christensen J 1978a Chronic intestinal pseudoobstruction. Gastroenterology 74: 922–931
Faulk D L, Anuras S, Freeman J B 1978b Idiopathic chronic intestinal pseudo-obstruction. JAMA 240: 2075–2076
Franken E A Jr, Smith W L, Frey E E et al 1987 Intestinal motility disorders of infants and children: classification, clinical manifestations and roentgenology. CRC Crit Rev in Diagn Imaging 27: 203–236

Furness J B, Costa M 1987 The enteric nervous system. Churchill Livingstone, Edinburgh

Glassman M, Spivak W, Mininberg D et al 1989 Chronic idiopathic intestinal pseudoobstruction: a commonly misdiagnosed disease in infants and children. Pediatrics 83: 603–608

Greenall M J, Gough M H 1983 Chronic idiopathic intestinal pseudo-obstruction in infancy and its successful treatment with parenteral feeding. Dis Colon Rectum 26: 53–54

Hyman P E, McDiarmid S V, Napolitano J et al 1988 Antroduodenal motility in children with chronic intestinal pseudo-obstruction. J Pediatr 112: 899–905

Isaacson C, Wainwright H C, Hamilton D G et al 1985 Hollow visceral myopathy in black South Africans. A report of 14 cases. S Afr Med J 67: 1015–1017

Kaschula R O C, Cywes S, Katz A et al 1987 Degenerative leiomyopathy with massive megacolon. Perspect Pediatr Pathol 11: 193–213

Nowak T V, Ionasescu V V, Anuras S 1982 Gastrointestinal manifestations of the muscular dystrophies. Gastroenterology 82: 800–810

Reinarz S, Smith W L, Franken E A Jr et al 1985 Splenic flexure volvulus: a complication of pseudoobstruction in infancy. AJR 145: 1303–1304

Schuffler M D, Rohrmann C A, Chaffee R A et al 1981 Chronic intestinal pseudo-obstruction. Medicine 60: 173–196

Schuffler M D, Pagon R A, Schwartz R et al 1988 Visceral myopathy of the gastrointestinal and genitourinary tracts in infants. Gastroenterology 94: 892–898

Shaw A, Shaffer H, Teja K et al 1979 A perspective for pediatric surgeons: chronic idiopathic intestinal pseudo-obstruction. J Pediatr Surg 14: 719–727

Smith B 1983 The neuropathology of intestinal pseudo-obstruction in: Chey W H (ed) Functional disorders of the gastrointestinal tract. Raven Press, New York pp 231–236

Vanek V W, Al-Salti M 1986 Acute pseudo-obstruction of the colon (Ogilvie's syndrome): an analysis of 400 cases. Dis Colon Rectum 29: 203–210

Vargas J H, Sachs P, Ament M E 1988 Chronic intestinal pseudo-obstruction syndrome in pediatrics. Results of a national survey by members of the North American Society of Pediatric Gastroenterology and Nutrition. J Pediatr Gastroenterol Nutr 7: 323–332

Wegener M, Borsch G 1987 Acute colonic pseudo-obstruction (Ogilvie's syndrome). Presentation of 14 of our own cases and analysis of 1027 cases reported in the literature. Surg Endosc 1: 1269–174

Yamagiwa I, Ohta M, Obata K et al 1988 Intestinal pseudoobstruction in a neonate caused by idiopathic muscular hypertrophy of the entire small intestine. J Pediatr Surg 23: 866–869

36. The irritable bowel syndrome

D. L. Wingate

INTRODUCTION

There can be few clinicians who have not, at some time during their undergraduate training or postgraduate experience, encountered patients with the 'irritable bowel syndrome' (IBS). Recognition of the challenge of the irritable bowel does not, however, confer understanding of the underlying problem, and, until recently, clear agreement on how the syndrome might be defined was lacking. IBS is one of the 'functional disorders' of the gastrointestinal tract; these are disorders of function that do not appear to be the result of verifiable disease processes, and that therefore cannot be attributed to a distinct pathophysiology. IBS thus presents a paradox; in operational terms, it is convenient to assume that it is a diagnostic entity, but when subjected to rigorous scrutiny, difficulties in defining the entity have caused some (Christensen 1990) to speculate that it is non-existent.

In considering the problem in relation to gastrointestinal motor function, two related questions must be addressed. First, what is IBS, and can it be defined? If so, is IBS a disturbance of *motor* function? For many years, it has been difficult to answer the second question because of failure to achieve general agreement on the first question. This problem has confounded the interpretation of much published work on the topic because the entry criteria for patients undergoing functional studies reflected the opinions of individual investigators rather than a generally agreed definition, and thus patient cohorts have not been strictly comparable.

WHAT IS IBS?

IBS has a long history (Thompson 1979) under various names, such as 'mucous colitis', 'irritable colon' and 'spastic colon'. These names reflect the judgment of many physicians that disorders of defaecation are manifestations of colonic dysfunction. Clearly this is not invariably the case, since the disturbed defaecation of coeliac disease is due to pathology in the proximal small bowel, but it has to be remembered that the irritable colon was recognized as a disorder long before the discovery of Crohn's disease or gluten enteropathy. The positive evidence for IBS as a colonic disorder was based upon somewhat anecdotal evidence such as the radiological sign of colonic spasm during a barium enema or the brisk contraction of the rectum on air insufflation during proctosigmoidoscopy. Even though the argument was less than overwhelming, it was generally accepted not only by clinicians, but also by the pharmaceutical industry; most, if not all, medications recommended for the relief of IBS have been intended to relieve 'colonic spasm'.

The first step towards a more rigorous definition of IBS was achieved by Manning et al (1978), who postulated that the term should only be used to describe disordered defaecation with associated abdominal pain. Several subsequent studies (Kruis et al 1984, Mazumdar et al 1988) showed that use of the 'Manning criteria' could clearly differentiate between patients with organic bowel pathology and those with only a disorder of function. Finally, a consensus on the definition of IBS was achieved by a group of gastroenterologists meeting in Rome (Thompson et al 1989); since then, the 'Rome criteria' (Table 36.1) have replaced the 'Manning criteria' as the 'best fit' definition of IBS.

The Rome criteria serve to distinguish between syndromes that had previously been grouped together, such as (Table 36.2) chronic constipation and chronic intractable abdominal pain. Chronic constipation is characterized by a bowel habit that is invariably, if not treated, infrequent; discomfort and distension are usually mild and sometimes absent, and actual pain is often anal in origin due to the passage of inspissated faeces. In IBS the bowel habit is above all erratic and often unpredictable and defaecation is associated with subumbilical abdominal pain. Psychiatric morbidity, originally considered to be a dominant feature of the

Table 36.1   Required symptoms for the diagnosis of IBS

Abdominal pain, relieved by defaecation, or associated with changes of frequency or consistency of stool

and/or

Disturbed defaecation (two or more of):
● Altered stool frequency
● Altered stool form (hard or loose/watery)
● Altered stool passage (straining, urgency, feeling of incomplete evacuation)
● Passage of mucus

usually with

Bloating or feeling of abdominal distension

Table 36.2   IBS and related functional disorders

	Erratic defaecation	Constant defaecation	Pain	Bloating	Psycho pathology
Irritable bowel	+ +	−	+	+ +	−
Chronic constipation	−	+	+	±	−
Chronic abdominal pain	−	+	+ +	−	+

irritable bowel (Hislop 1971) is not a specific feature of IBS when carefully defined (Smith et al 1990), but is frequently associated (Klein 1990) with chronic intractable abdominal pain, a syndrome in which defaecation is usually normal.

IS IBS A MOTOR DISORDER?

Since IBS as now defined requires defaecation to be disordered, and since defaecation is a motor function, it is clear that at least in this sense, IBS is a motor abnormality. However, since defaecation is a motor behaviour under voluntary control, it can be argued that the disturbance of defaecation may not be due to disturbed *enteric* motor activity. It could be due to an abnormal behaviour pattern, or, if there is a sensory disturbance in IBS, the result of an urge to defaecate in response to misleading sensory information; for example, symptoms of rectal discomfort when the rectum has not filled will lead to strenuous attempts to void a rectum that contains little or no stool. Thus the analysis of symptoms points in several different directions, and the question can only be settled by the systematic study of enteric motor activity and visceral sensation.

The literature on gut motility in IBS may be broadly divided into two categories. On the one hand are studies that show that some aspect of motor activity in *groups* of IBS patients differs significantly from the activity in a *group* of 'healthy controls' but the overlap between the two groups does not allow an *individual* to be clearly identified as IBS or non-IBS; earlier work on the colon falls into this category. On the other hand, some studies have demonstrated a specific motor abnormality that is found in a majority of IBS patients, but is absent in 'healthy controls'; these abnormalities can therefore – in theory, at least – serve as *positive diagnostic tests* in clinical practice. Paradoxically for a disorder ascribed to colonic dysfunction, allegedly specific motor markers of IBS have been reported only in the small intestine, but this may be no more than a reflection of the fact that progress in defining normal colonic motility has been slow.

The colon

Abnormal movements of the colon in IBS have been noted by clinicians for many years; these include excessive haustration or constriction during barium contrast fluoroscopy, and 'the winking rectum' (recurrent rectal contractions during proctosigmoidoscopy). Such observations have to be regarded as anecdotal, since the patients in whom they have been seen have not been carefully defined, and the observations have not been made systematically.

Objective studies of colonic motor activity in IBS have not been frequently reported, nor have they proved to be useful for the evaluation of patients. In the 1970s, abnormalities of rectosigmoid myoelectrical activity in IBS were reported by groups in Philadelphia and Liverpool, but the observations could not be confirmed by others (Latimer et al 1981). A more promising study by Bueno et al (1980) studying the left colon, showed differences in the incidence of long and short spike burst activity between healthy controls, and patients with either constipation and abdominal pain or diarrhoea (Fig. 36.1). It is not, however, clear, whether the entry criteria for patients in this study conformed with the current criteria for defining IBS (Table 36.1), and these observations remain to be confirmed by others.

An overview of the published literature on colonic motor activity in IBS leads to two conclusions:

1. When colonic motor activity in groups of IBS patients is compared with that found in healthy controls, statistically significant differences in group

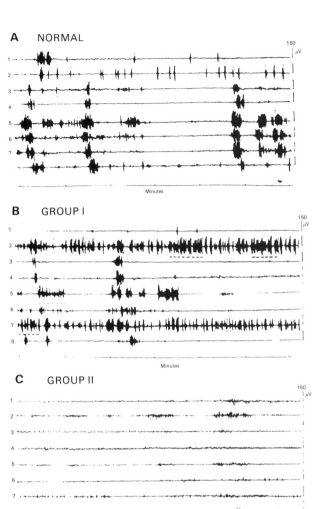

A NORMAL

150 | μV

Minutes

B GROUP I

150 | μV

Minutes

C GROUP II

150 | μV

Minutes

Fig. 36.1 Colonic myoelectrical activity recorded in a healthy person (**A**), a patient suffering from painful constipation (**B**) and a patient suffering from diarrhoea (**C**). The normal pattern shows a mixture of short and long spike bursts. In the constipated patient, there is a marked increase in short spike bursts, whereas in the patient with diarrhoea these are absent. (Reprinted with permission from Bueno et al 1980.)

means may be found under defined circumstances, such as following a mixed meal or during stress. *But*
2. There is, as yet, *no* specific feature of colonic motor activity that can be regarded, in an individual patient, as diagnostic of, or specific to IBS.

The small intestine

More than 30 years have passed since Horowitz and

Farrar (1962) reported abnormal proximal small bowel motility in patients with 'functional gastrointestinal disorders', but systematic evidence in support of this observation has been accumulated only slowly and relatively recently. The Horowitz and Farrar study preceded the description of the human migrating motor complex (MMC) by Vantrappen et al (1977); it is possible that some of the 'abnormalities' may have been no more than normal phase III episodes. and it is not clear whether these patients were all suffering from what is now defined as IBS. The first study in the 'post-MMC' era of the small bowel in IBS in which it was recognized that the slow biorhythm of the bowel required prolonged recording periods for the detection of abnormalities, was a single case report by Thompson et al (1979). In this instance, there was no doubt that the patient would have conformed with the 'Rome criteria' (Table 36.1), but the severity of his symptoms (at the time of study, he was under investigation as a tertiary referral) was atypical for IBS. A prospective study of patients with 'functional abdominal pain' by Kingham et al (1984) revealed no abnormality, but the technology available at that time allowed no more than the analysis of phase III incidence; again, it is not clear how many of these patients might have conformed to the current diagnosis of IBS.

A prospective study of small bowel motility in response to stress in healthy volunteers, and in patients with IBS or inflammatory bowel disease by Kumar and Wingate (1985) antedated the publication of the 'Manning criteria' (see above), but the clinical data published make it clear that 21 of the 22 patients would now be diagnosed as IBS, the exception being a patient with painless constipation. In 18 of the 22 patients, abnormal sequences of clustered contractions were seen, mostly during exposure to stress (Fig. 36.2), and most of these episodes were accompanied by abdominal discomfort (Fig. 36.3). In addition, in several patients, phase III episodes were not seen during stress, but this did not happen with subjects in the other groups.

The 'minute rhythm' of clustered contractions in IBS patients was confirmed in two subsequent studies. Using prolonged perfused tube manometry – of itself, a somewhat stressful procedure – Kellow and Phillips (1987) recorded prolonged sequences of discrete clustered contractions in the proximal jejunum of IBS patients (Fig. 36.4) that were often accompanied by discomfort. Some of these episodes were spontaneous, and others were provoked by cholecystokinin (CCK) or bethanechol. The provocation with CCK echoed an earlier study by Harvey and Read (1973). Kellow and

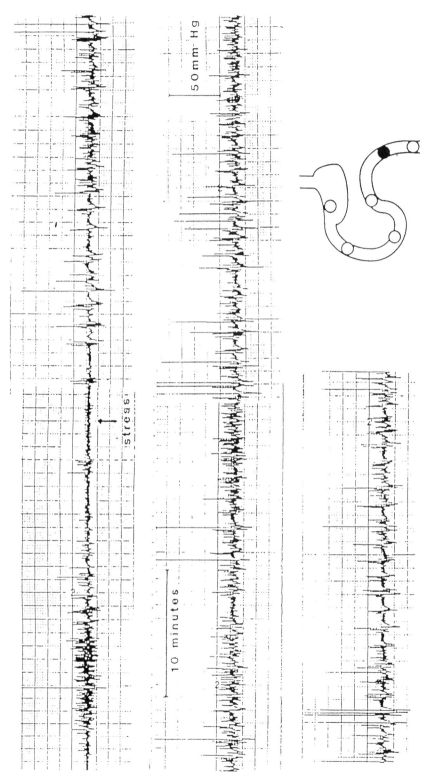

Fig. 36.2 Continuous recording from a single radiotelemetric pressure sensitive capsule, located in the proximal jejunum of a patient with IBS, during exposure to stress. The location of the capsule is indicated in the diagram inset (bottom right). At the beginning of the recording, one episode of phase III activity is seen. Shortly after the exposure to the stressor is started, clustered contractions begin and continue without interruption throughout. The large deflections are pressure changes due to body movements. The pressure changes appear to be biphasic because the recording was played back through an active bandpass filter to eliminate shifts in the baseline. (Reprinted by kind permission of Mr Devinder Kumar.)

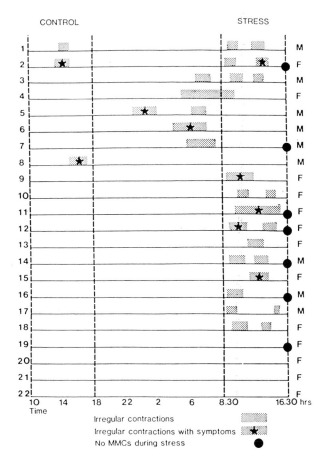

Fig. 36.3 Incidence of motor abnormalities in 22 patients suffering from IBS during a 30.5 h continuous ambulant recording of proximal small bowel motility. Each line indicates an individual patient. In the first part of the recording (control) patients rested undisturbed but fasting in the clinical laboratory for 8 h. On the following day, in the third part of the recording (stress) patients carried out stressful tasks while fasting during an 8-h period. It will be noted that 19 of 22 patients had either abnormal clustered contractions or abolition of phase III during stress or both. (Reprinted with kind permission from Kumar and Wingate 1985.)

Phillips also noted, in some of these patients, an exaggerated motor response to a meal (Fig. 36.5), although it was not possible to quantify this as a specific motor abnormality. The latter finding was consistent with the ileal arrest of radiolabelled bran in bloated patients recorded by Trotman and Price (1986).

The second study to confirm the presence of clustered contractions was reported by Kellow et al (1990). They used prolonged ambulant manometry in patients who continued their normal activities at work and at home during the 72 h of the study. Abnormal runs of clustered contractions were detected in 11 of 12 patients, but in no controls (Figs 36.6, 36.7). One interesting point about this study is that in contrast to the studies of Kumar and Wingate (1985), and Kellow and Phillips (1987), subjects were not subjected to either provocative stress or stress due to prolonged immobilization, but only to the stress of their own habitat.

Opinion is divided as to the significance of the clustered contractions. No-one has claimed that IBS is predominantly a disorder of the proximal jejunum; the latter merely happens to be a convenient recording site which yields consistent results in normal individuals (Kellow et al 1986). But, on the one hand, it has been proposed that these clustered contractions are a relatively specific marker for IBS and suggests that IBS affects the small as well as the large intestine. While on the other hand, doubts have been expressed as to whether these are a consistent finding in IBS and Quigley (1992) has pointed out that sequences of clusters during phase II of the MMC are seen in healthy individuals.

It is indeed true that sequences of clusters occur in healthy individuals, but Kellow et al (1990) were careful to point out that these are indicative of IBS only when continuous sequences exceed 10 min in length, and the data of Quigley et al (1992) show that these did not occur in their healthy control subjects. Neither, however. were they a feature of the 5 h of study in their IBS patients.

The answer to this conundrum is that the clustered contractions appear to be 'protocol-specific'. This is best illustrated by analysing the study of Kumar and Wingate (1985) as though it consisted of three separate studies (Fig. 36.8). In the first study period, subjects were at rest, fasting, in a laboratory environment, conditions not dissimilar to the average perfused tube study. Only three of 22 showed clustered contractions under these conditions. The second study period was normal overnight sleep; five of 22 IBS patients woke during the night with clustered contractions and, in two cases, abdominal discomfort; these were similar to the patient reported by Thompson et al (1979). In the third study period of 8 h of fasting, subjects were required to perform stressful tasks, and this provoked clusters in 14 of 22 patients. One patient only had clusters on the first (rest) day, one other patient did not have any clusters, but exhibited complete suppression of phase III under stress. However, when the three periods are aggregated, 18 of 22 patients showed cluster sequences, and this proportion is similar to the 11 of 12 patients showing cluster sequences in the study by Kellow et al (1990). Thus it would appear that prolonged ambulant manometry reproduces the

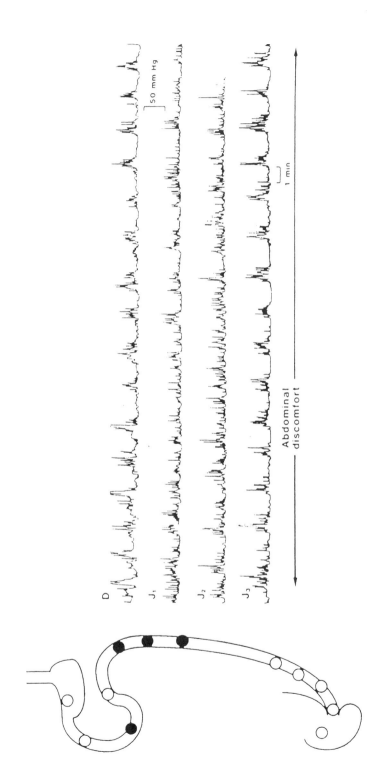

Fig. 36.4 Clustered contractions recorded using multi-lumen perfused tube manometry. ● represent positions at which presented traces (D, J_1–J_3) were recorded. D = duodenum; J_{1-3} = jejenum. (Reprinted with kind permission from Kellow and Phillips 1987.)

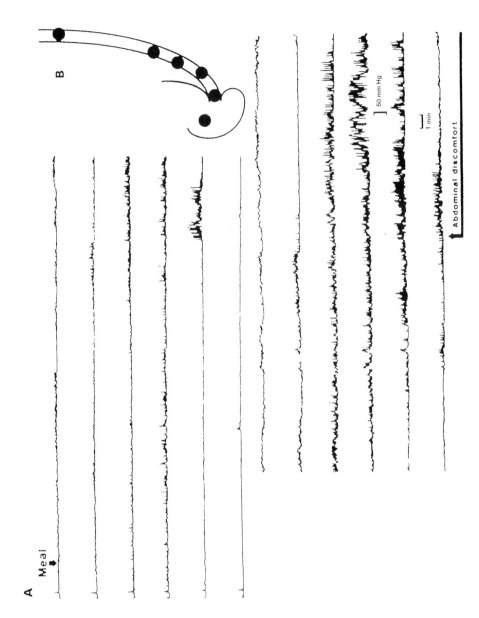

Fig. 36.5 Ileocaecal motor activity recorded with multi-lumen perfused tube manometry from an IBS patient following a meal. The location of the recording sites is indicated in **B**. Note that the excessive motor response towards the end of the recording was accompanied by abdominal discomfort. (Adapted with kind permission from Kellow and Phillips 1987.)

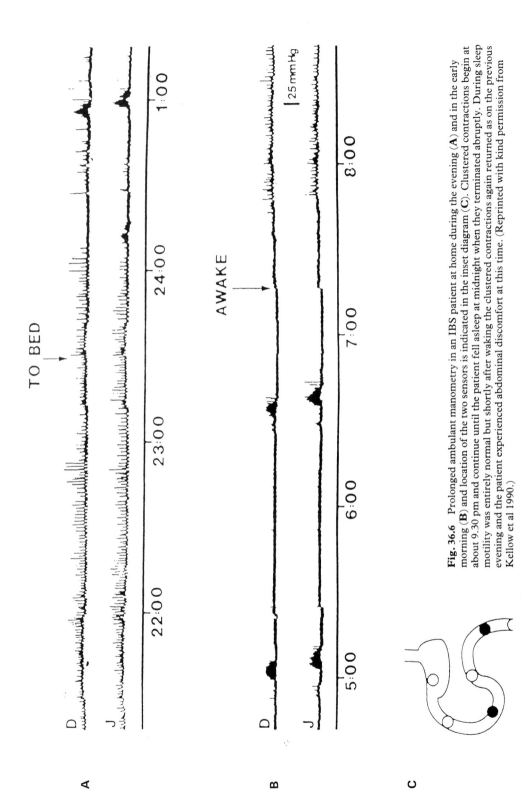

Fig. 36.6 Prolonged ambulant manometry in an IBS patient at home during the evening (**A**) and in the early morning (**B**) and location of the two sensors is indicated in the inset diagram (**C**). Clustered contractions begin at about 9.30 pm and continue until the patient fell asleep at midnight when they terminated abruptly. During sleep motility was entirely normal but shortly after waking the clustered contractions again returned as on the previous evening and the patient experienced abdominal discomfort at this time. (Reprinted with kind permission from Kellow et al 1990.)

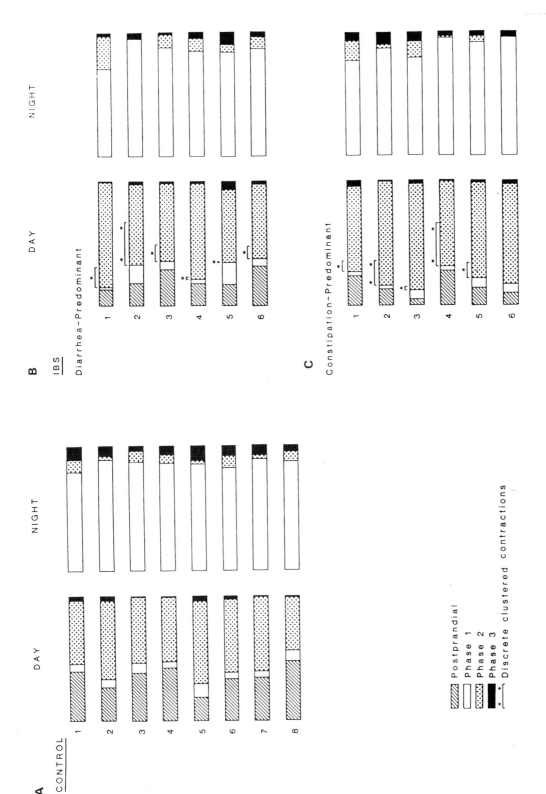

Fig. 36.7 Summary of motor patterns in the proximal jejunum over 72 h of recording from eight healthy subjects (**A**) and 12 patients with IBS (**B**, **C**). During the study, patients slept at home and were free to pursue normal daytime activities and to eat and drink as they wished. Comparison of the daytime and night time recordings show that during the day, phase II was the dominant pattern with relatively small amounts of phase I and phase III activity. During the night, phase I was dominant. There was no important difference between controls and patients with respect to these motor patterns, but in 11 of the 12 patients there were varying amounts of sequences of clustered contractions. In two of these patients, clustered contractions were seen at night. (Adapted with kind permission from Kellow et al 1990.)

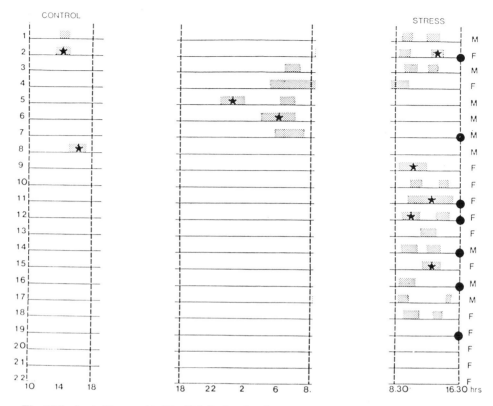

Fig. 36.8   Study illustrated in Fig. 36.3 displayed as three separate studies. For explanation see text.

provocative conditions of the laboratory, and is more effective than the deliberate application of artificial stressors to patients (a practice which, as Valori (1993) has pointed out, is both arbitrary and somewhat absurd).

ARE MOTILITY STUDIES OF CLINICAL VALUE FOR IBS PATIENTS?

Even though studies of motility in IBS may have failed to reveal diagnostic abnormalities, they can be useful in the prosecution of research into the pathophysiology and therapeutics of IBS, but that is of little benefit to the individual patient. Can they be useful in the diagnosis and management of IBS?

From what has already been pointed out above, it is clear that rectosigmoid or colonic motility studies have, at the moment, no place in clinical practice, since they do not produce answers to pertinent clinical questions. For the small bowel, the answer – from this author – is somewhat different. For the experienced clinician, the diagnosis of IBS presents no great problem, and is almost always possible on the basis of a careful history

supplemented, as appropriate, by tests to eliminate other relevant diagnoses (for example, screening for colon cancer is important in a 50-year-old patient with a recent change in bowel habit, but not in a 28-year-old patient with an 8-year history of irregular defaecation). There remain, however, two groups of patients in whom prolonged ambulant manometry can be helpful:

1. Patients with atypical IBS symptoms in whom subacute mechanical obstruction due to adhesions, or chronic pseudo-obstruction, cannot be eliminated either on the basis of the history, or by conventional radiography;
2. Patients who are unwilling to accept the diagnosis of IBS and who believe, in the absence of evidence to the contrary, that they are suffering from a more serious organic – and hitherto undetected – disease.

These two groups are essentially the same: patients in whom there is diagnostic doubt. In the former, the doubt is in the mind of the physician, whereas, for the latter, it is the conviction of the patient.

In these patients, prolonged ambulant manometry is

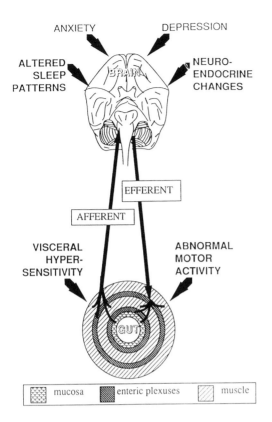

ANXIETY

DEPRESSION

ALTERED
SLEEP
PATTERNS

NEURO-
ENDOCRINE
CHANGES

BRAIN

EFFERENT

AFFERENT

VISCERAL
HYPER-
SENSITIVITY

ABNORMAL
MOTOR
ACTIVITY

GUT

| mucosa | enteric plexuses | muscle |

Fig. 36.9 Three-component model of the IBS.

now a practical, and not especially expensive, procedure. It should be carried out over not less than 24 h, and include a period of diurnal fasting, one or more mixed meals, and a restful overnight sleep, preferably at home. IBS may be confirmed by the presence of sequences of contraction clusters at regular intervals of

1–1.5 min during phase II, or for much longer periods following a mixed meal, but it is clear that these will not be found in every IBS patient. For the exclusion of pseudo-obstruction and mechanical obstruction, motor activity during sleep should be entirely normal, and there should be an active motor response to food. Clusters of contractions recurring less frequently (5–20 min) are suggestive of mechanical or pseudo-obstruction, and, if present during sleep, eliminate the diagnosis of IBS. Such recordings, particularly when clustered contractions are associated with abdominal discomfort, can be invaluable in reassuring the sceptical patient.

It seems reasonable to predict that motility tests will assume a prevalence and significance in IBS comparable to the place of oesophageal manometry in gastro-oesophageal reflux disease, being needed for only a small proportion of the patient population, but important where there is diagnostic doubt. Whether or not colonic motility tests will replace upper small bowel manometry in this context remains a matter for speculation.

CONCLUSION

The contribution of disordered motility to the pathophysiology of IBS remains uncertain. It is clear that there are other components to the syndrome. Visceral hypersensitivity is an important element (Whitehead et al 1990), and recent sleep studies suggest a CNS abnormality (Kumar et al 1992). Thus the best fit model in the present state of knowledge appears to be a three-component model (Fig. 36.9) in which, in a syndrome that is not well-defined (Christensen 1990), it is the motor component that is the least shrouded in ignorance.

REFERENCES

Bueno L, Fioramonti J, Ruckebusch Y, Frexinos J, Coulom P 1980 Evaluation of colonic myoelectrical activity in health and functional disorders. Gut 21: 480–485

Christensen J 1990 Heraclides or the physician. Gastroenterol Int 3: 45–48

Harvey R F, Read A E 1973 Effect of cholecystokinin on colonic motility and symptoms in patients with the irritable bowel syndrome. Lancet 1: 1–3

Hislop I G 1971 Psychological significance of the irritable bowel syndrome. Gut 12: 452–457

Horowitz L, Farrar J T 1962 Intraluminal small intestinal

pressures in normal patients and in patients with functional gastrointestinal disease. Gastroenterology 42: 455–464

Kellow J E, Borody T J, Phillips S F, Tucker R L, Haddad A C 1986 Human interdigestive motility: variations in patterns from oesophagus to colon. Gastroenterology 91: 386–395

Kellow J E, Gill R C, Wingate D L 1990 Prolonged ambulant recordings of small bowel motility demonstrate abnormalities in the irritable bowel syndrome. Gastroenterology 98: 1208–1218

Kellow J E, Phillips S F 1987 Altered small bowel motility is correlated with symptoms in irritable bowel syndrome. Gastroenterology 92: 1885–1893

Kingham J G C, Brown R, Colson R, Clark M L 1984 Jejunal motility in patients with functional abdominal pain. Gut 25: 375–380

Klein K B 1990 Chronic intractable abdominal pain. Sem Gastrointest Dis 1: 43–56

Kruis W, Thieme C H, Weinzierl M et al 1984 A diagnostic score for the irritable bowel syndrome: its value in the exclusion of organic disease. Gastroenterology 87: 1–7

Kumar D, Thompson P D, Wingate D L, Vesselinova-Jenkins G, Libby G 1992 Abnormal R E M sleep in the irritable bowel syndrome. Gastroenterology 103: 12–17

Kumar D, Wingate D L 1985 The irritable bowel syndrome: a paroxysmal motor disorder. Lancet ii: 973–977

Latimer P, Sarna S, Campbell D, Latimer M, Waterfall W, Daniel E E 1981 Colonic motor and myoelectrical activity: a comparative study of normal subjects, psychoneurotic patients, and patients with the irritable bowel syndrome. Gastroenterology 80: 893–901

Manning A P, Thompson W G, Heaton K W, Morris A F 1978 Towards positive diagnosis of the irritable bowel. Br Med J 2: 653–654

Mazumdar T N L, Prasad K V S, Bhat P V 1988 Formulation of a scoring chart for irritable bowel syndrome: a prospective study. Indian J Gastroenterol 7: 101–102

Quigley E M M 1992 Intestinal manometry – technical advances, clinical limitations. Dig Dis Sci 37: 10–13

Quigley E M M, Donovan J P, Lane M J, Gallagher T F 1992 Antroduodenal manometry: limitations and usefulness as an outpatient study. Dig Dis Sci 37: 20–28

Smith R C, Greenbaum D S, Vancouver J B et al 1990 Psychosocial factors are associated with health care seeking rather than diagnosis in irritable bowel syndrome. Gastroenterology 98: 293–301

Thompson D G, Laidlaw J M, Wingate D L 1979 Abnormal small bowel motility demonstrated by radiotelemetry in a patient with irritable colon. Lancet ii: 321–323

Thompson W G 1979 The irritable gut: functional disorders of the alimentary canal. University Park Press, Baltimore

Thompson W G, Dotevall G, Drossman D A, Heaton K W, Kruis W 1989 Irritable bowel syndrome: guidelines for the diagnosis. Gastroenterol Int 2: 92–95

Trotman I F, Price C C 1986 Bloated irritable bowel defined by dynamic ^{99m}Tc bran scan. Lancet ii: 364–366

Valori R 1993 Lines written on reading another review article about the irritable bowel syndrome. 1: 36–37

Vantrappen G, Janssens J, Hellemans J, Ghoos Y 1977 The interdigestive motor complex of normal subjects and patients with bacterial overgrowth of the small intestine. J Clin Invest 59: 1158–1166

Whitehead W E, Holtkotter B, Enck P et al 1990 Tolerance for rectosigmoid distention in the irritable bowel syndrome. Gastroenterology 98: 1187–1192

37. Constipation

G. Devroede

SEMANTICS

Constipation is not a disease, nor a sign. As a symptom, it may be indicative of many diseases, and the differential diagnosis covers as wide a spectrum as for abdominal pain. A symptom is the experience of a sign by a patient: not only is the subjective appreciation highly variable from patient to patient, but, also, previous unpleasant experiences of the same nature, both physical and emotional, interfere with the perception of the present experience. Dismissing the symptom as unimportant as compared with the sign, and dismissing the emotions as marginally relevant, is bound to lead to an oversimplified approach to constipation. This textbook is an illustrated guide to gastrointestinal motility, and the reader must constantly remain aware that any kind of recording from any part of the gastrointestinal tract only reflects aspects of the signs of constipation. Knowledge derived from motility recordings is more scientific but provides at best limited and partial information. Moreover, our understanding of the mechanisms of constipation and our approach to treatment is plagued by the fact that variable definitions of constipation are used in different studies.

A thorough review of constipation is beyond the scope of this publication, and has been published elsewhere (Devroede 1993a).

THE NATURE OF CONSTIPATION

The meaning of constipation varies according to what patients view as a 'normal' pattern of defaecation.

What are normal bowel habits?

Faecal output differs markedly throughout the world, and not only because of racial factors. Blacks are more constipated than whites (Everhart et al 1989; Sandler & Drossman 1987) in North America, but are less so in South Africa (Walker et al 1982). In Senegal, people

defaecate morning and evening, and consider themselves constipated if they only have one stool per day (Epelboin 1982). In the western world, wide variations in faecal measurements and gastrointestinal transit times occur, not only between individuals but on repeated measurements within the same individual (Wyman et al 1978).

It is more difficult for normal subjects to defaecate a 1.8 cm incompressible sphere than a 50 ml deformable balloon: presumably this applies to the expulsion of rabbit-size small stool pellets by constipated patients (Bannister et al 1987).

90% of healthy subjects empty their rectum only when they defaecate, while the other 10% evacuate the entire length of bowel at once, from the splenic flexure to the anus (Halls 1965), producing a much longer stool. The relevance of this to constipation is not known.

The 'normal' range of stool weight varies from 35–450 g per stool in males and 5–335 g in females (Davies et al 1986; Wyman et al 1978; Rendtorff & Kashgarian 1967). Stool weight averages 100 g in the UK and the USA, but averages 300 g in India and 500 g in Uganda (Glober et al 1977; Burkitt et al 1972). There is also a large variation from one stool to another, in a given individual, and from individual to individual. Mean daily faecal weight is uninfluenced by exercise, provided the diet remains constant (Bingham & Cummings 1989), but is markedly influenced by personality attributes, regardless of their dietary intake: people who are extroverted and have a high self-esteem have heavier stools (Tucker et al 1981).

Stool consistency can be measured objectively, but available techniques have little practical clinical applicability.

Stool frequency is the easiest parameter of stool output to quantify and thus use clinically. However, a stool of 10 g evacuated from the distal part of the rectum does not result from the same physiological mechanisms as one of 300 g that was harboured in the

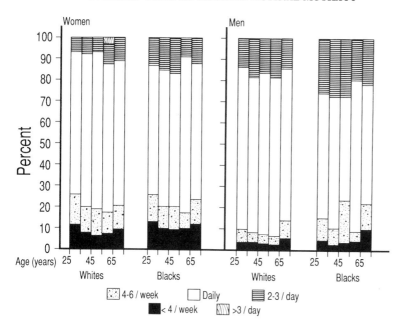

Fig. 37.1 Self-reported stool frequency in the USA, n = 14407. Stool frequency is unaffected by age. The figure also shows that the overwhelming majority of people defaecate everyday (Everhart 1989).

distal bowel from the splenic flexure to the anus. Thus, recording stool frequency, although popular in scientific studies of constipation, does not reflect adequately stool output, which is the product of *both* stool frequency and stool weight, is better correlated to colorectal transit times (Davies et al 1986), and remains an imperfect indicator of constipation. Old surveys have shown that 95% of adult subjects have between three and 21 bowel movements per week (Rendtorff & Kashgarian 1967; Connell et al 1965). This is still the justification why many clinicians and researchers do not consider patients having more than three stools per week as constipated. In fact, most subjects in large samples of the general population defaecate every day (Everhart et al 1989; Martelli et al 1978a; Dent et al 1986) (Fig. 37.1), and no healthy subject has less than five stools per week (Sandler & Drossman 1987). The complaint of constipation increases markedly with age, regardless of sex and race (Fig. 37.2), but without accompanying decrease in stool frequency (Everhart et al 1989; Dent et al 1986; Milne & Williamson 1972; Donald et al 1985) (Fig. 37.1). Women have been reported to pass less frequent (Fig. 37.3), harder, more formed and less heavy stools (Davies et al 1986; Sandler & Drossman 1987), and to complain more often of constipation than men, regardless of race (Everhart et al 1989; Sandler & Drossman 1987); but psychosocial variables, such as fewer years

of education, low physical activity and symptoms of depression, are associated independent risk factors (Everhart et al 1989). Some studies have not found any sex-related differences in physical characteristics of stools (Wyman et al 1978). There are no sex-related differences in colorectal transit times, when subjects claim that stress does not modify their bowel habits and does not trigger abdominal pain (Verduron et al 1988), nor in frequency of bowel movement within an apparently well population (Dent et al 1986). In constipated subjects, recorded stool frequency is greater than recalled frequency (Verduron et al 1988; Manning et al 1976; Corazziari et al 1987). This may be due to the emphasis of a symptom over a 'hidden agenda', as a way to attract attention, and to the difference between disease and illness, secondary gains being obtained from a sick role. It may also reflect the impact of a good doctor–patient relationship on bodily function through transferential mechanisms.

The feeling of incomplete evacuation cannot be used for diagnosis, because most normal subjects who refrain from defaecating have no rectal sensation, yet can defaecate at will stools that remain in the rectum (Edwards & Beck 1971). Difficulties in expelling stools can now be measured by defaecometry, where the pressure within a rectal balloon is recorded throughout its expulsion. The curve which is recorded reflects a workload composed of duration of expulsion and pres-

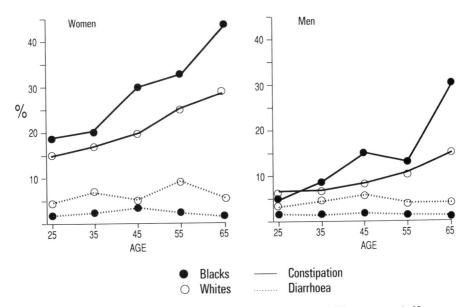

Fig. 37.2 Self-reported disturbed bowel habits in USA, n = 14407. The symptom (self-reported) of constipation increases with age in males and females both in blacks and whites (Everhart 1989).

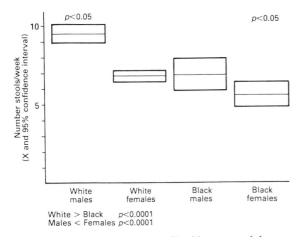

Fig. 37.3 Normal bowel habits of healthy young adults (Sandler & Drossman 1987). On the basis of this study, physicians concluded that people who have more than five stools per week are not constipated.

sure within the anal barrier (Lestar et al 1989). Little data are available in constipation.

Although there is a correlation between the severity of constipation and the frequency of laxative ingestion (Corazziari et al 1987), many people use them even if they do not report constipation, infrequent defaecation or hard stools (Everhart et al 1989; Corazziari et al 1987). Elderly people are prone to consume more

laxatives (Dent et al 1986; Corazziara et al 1987). Moreover, there is no relationship between laxative intake and more objective parameters of constipation, such as bowel frequency recorded prospectively in a diary, gastrointestinal transit time or segmental colorectal transit time (Corazziari et al 1987). Thus, laxative consumption is largely a part of the culture, and has staggering economic implications (Glaser & Chi 1983; IMS America Canadian Drugstore and Hospital Purchases Audit 1986–1990).

Although the amount of fibre intake does not influence self-reported bowel habits (Everhart et al 1989), nor any of the symptoms of constipation (Cummings 1984), vegetarians have a greater frequency of defaecation (Davies et al 1986; Goldberg et al 1977; Kuhnlein et al 1981), pass larger amounts of faeces (Davies et al 1986; Miettinen & Tarpila 1978), have softer stools (Davies et al 1986), and, in both sexes, tend to have shorter bowel transit times (Gear et al 1981). Dietary fibre accelerates colorectal transit time and increases stool weight and frequency (Tucker et al 1981; Cummings 1984), but stool frequency may also be influenced by other variables in the environment. Elderly people at home defaecate more often than those in a geriatric day hospital of the same area (Donald et al 1985). Sedentarity is probably not an important variable per se, because stool frequency is not influenced by exercise (Bingham & Cummings 1989). Personality

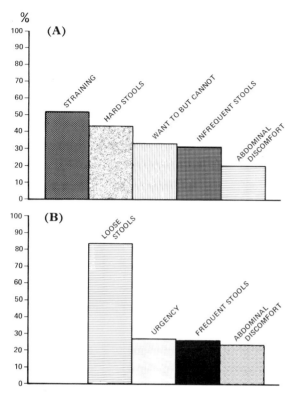

Fig. 37.4 Perception of constipation (**A**) and diarrhoea (**B**). Straining, hard stools and impossibility to defaecate at will are more worrisome to ordinary people than a number of stools less than a predetermined epidemiological range (Sandler & Drossman 1987).

features have as much impact on stool frequency as they have on stool weight: extroverted people who like themselves defaecate more often (Tucker et al 1981).

Overall, what can be safely said is that the overwhelming majority of people have at least one stool per day. For the rest, data are so confusing that no patient complaining of disturbed bowel habit should be dismissed as normal: what needs to be done is to place in perspective the subjective complaint and the objective measurements. Frequency per se is not of much concern to people, who worry more about efforts to defaecate, excessive stool consistency and incapacity to defaecate at will (Sandler & Drossman 1987) (Fig. 37.4).

EPIDEMIOLOGY OF CONSTIPATION

Self-reported constipation is commonly used as a selection criterium in epidemiologic research; but it is unreli-

able to study constipation because it does not reflect any scientific criterium used to define either its clinical aspects or its mechanisms. Despite this limitation, various national surveys have confirmed that blacks and women (Fig. 37.5) are constipation prone (Sonnenberg & Koch 1989a; Johanson et al 1989; Sonnenberg & Koch 1989b; Sandler et al 1990). Constipation is the most common digestive complaint, being found in four million people in the USA. The complaint – but not incidence – of low stool frequency markedly increases after age 60, (Fig. 37.5), varies according to geographical areas (for instance, it is more common in the Southern part of the USA) and is more prevalent in families with low income and brief education (Sonnenberg & Koch 1989a, b; Sandler et al 1990b) (Fig. 37.6). Constipation is more often reported among subjects with little physical activity (Sandler et al 1990). It accounts, in the USA, for 13.7 million days per year of restricted activity (Collins 1986).

The inadequacy of available surveys of the epidemiology of constipation is exemplified by data obtained in a USA randomized survey, searching for the prevalence of functional gastrointestinal disorders on the basis of research diagnostic criteria (Drossman et al in press). At 69%, they are epidemic. One must thus question the nature of these symptoms: body clues to disease or really indicative of disease? There is a marked overlap between syndromes, and therefore studies of constipation may for instance resemble those of the irritable bowel syndrome. The female preponderance is found only for defined syndromes, and not all of them vary according to income: poorer people suffer more often from dyschezia – a pelvic outlet problem – but not from functional constipation. This is interesting because psychoanalysts find symbolic links between faeces and money (Borneman). Finally, there are many more people suffering from defined syndromes, than there are who consult for them (Fig. 37.7).

Only 12% of patients with chronic idiopathic constipation do not take laxatives and 30% do not defaecate if they do not take them continuously; but there is no correlation between laxative intake and observed bowel frequency after laxatives have been withdrawn (Corazziari et al 1987).

The ratio of females to males varies along the lifespan. Little boys are more often constiped than little girls (Davidson et al 1963; Loening-Baucke & Cruickshank 1986; Martelli et al 1978b; Wald 1986; Watier et al 1985; Ducrotte et al 1985), but a reversal of the ratio occurs later in life, women becoming much more often constipated than men (Martelli et al 1978b; Wald 1986). Towards the end of life there is a tendency

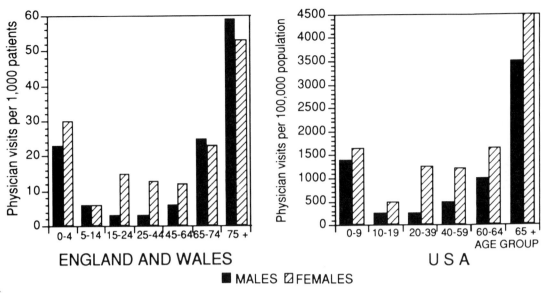

Fig. 37.5 Epidemiology of constipation. Consulting for constipation is found more often among women, children and the elderly (Johanson et al 1989, Sonnenberg & Koch 1989b).

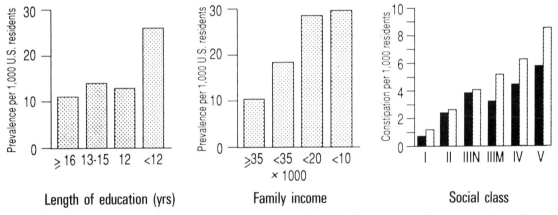

Fig. 37.6 Social aspects of constipation. The fact that constipation is found more commonly in poor uneducated people is clear evidence it is not a simple organic disease (Johanson et al 1989).

to return to a 1:1 ratio. We have too few data available to compare this to the first week of life (Fig. 37.8). The sex ratio in constipation also depends on which physiological criterium is used to define it. When constipation is defined as delayed transit in the ascending colon, it is an overwhelming problem of women (Watier et al 1985), in contrast to when colorectal transit is normal (Bouchoucha et al 1992). All constipated patients with a normal size colon at barium enema are women, but this is not so in patients with megarectum (Verduron et al 1988) or megacolon (Preston et al 1984b). The female to male ratio also varies according to anorectal function. It is 6:1 among patients with normal motility, 3:1 among those with anal hypertonicity, and 2:1 among those with a rectoanal inhibitory reflex that is of less than normal amplitude (Ducrotte et al 1985).

Up to one-third of elderly people complain of constipation (Donald et al 1985; Whitehead et al 1989; Hale et al 1986; Talley et al 1992), but this is not reflected by their bowel physiology: 95% defaecate between three times a day and three times a week (Donald et al 1985; Whitehead et al 1989; Hale et al 1986; Milne & Williamson 1972), and have normal whole gut transit times

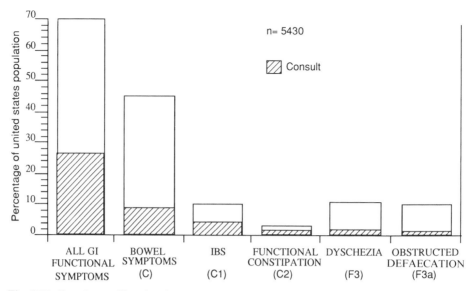

Fig. 37.7   Prevalence of functional large bowel symptoms. It is only a fraction of constipated people who consult. Why? (Drossman et al in press.)

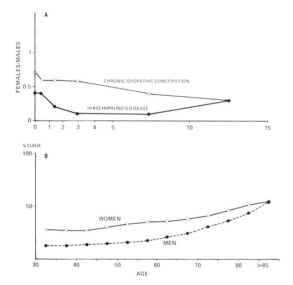

Fig. 37.8   Sex ratio in constipated children. Constipation: a little boy's problem (**A**), an adult woman's problem (**B**), a non-sexist elderly problem (**B**). What's this all about? (Devroede 1993a, Hammond 1964.)

(Eatwood 1972). The primary symptom, which they use to define constipation, is having to strain in order to defaecate (Donald et al 1985; Whitehead et al 1989) and this correlates well to radiological findings (Donald et al 1985). Self-report of constipation also correlates to a number of psychological symptoms in older women, including depression (Donald et al 1985;

Whitehead et al 1989). Lack of mobility (Donald et al 1985), chronic illnesses, and the use of non-laxative medication in women (Whitehead et al 1989) are also associated to constipation.

The natural history of constipation is not known. Prognosis is generally poor: only one out of 34 constipated patients is symptom free at 2 years' follow-up (Bleijenberg & Kuijpers 1987). Constipation may be learned: male volunteers who voluntarily suppress defaecation have decreased stool weight and frequency, and prolonged segmental transit times in the right colon and the rectosigmoid (Klauser et al 1990) (Fig. 37.9). Longitudinal studies should be undertaken to see what happens to constipated people over a lifespan.

Operational definitions of sub-groups of functional gastrointestinal disorders have been obtained, by consensus of an international panel of clinical investigators, in order to standardize criteria for research purposes and compare data from study to study. Functional constipation may be considered as separate from irritable bowel syndrome if the symptoms are not associated with an alternative bowel pattern. It may or may not coexist with abdominal pain (Drossman et al 1990). There is no generally accepted definition of constipation and there are limitations to the three kinds of operational definitions in use.

1. Undefined self-reported symptoms may differ in meaning according to different subjects.

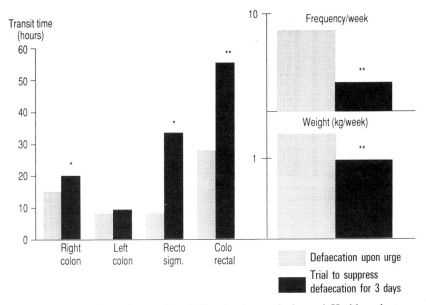

Fig. 37.9 Learning to be constipated. Constipation can be learned. Healthy volunteers who repress defaecation will have not only decreased stool frequency but decreased stool weight, not only rectal stasis but delayed transit in the ascending colon. What is learned can be unlearned. (Klauser et al 1990.)

2. It is not possible to speak of the prevalence of constipation on the basis of stool frequency because it is defined a priori to be about 2%, and because the threshold has been selected arbitrarily and without reference to any standard of clinical significance.
3. The upper limit of 'normal' whole gut transit time has also been arbitrarily defined and, as with stool frequency, the prevalence of clinically significant constipation cannot be determined by this criterion.

Because of these limitations, the definition should be based on self-report (Whitehead et al 1991).

RELATED CONDITIONS

Faecal incontinence as presenting symptoms of constipation

Involuntary passage of faeces by children may result from constipation. For the sake of clarity, the term 'faecal incontinence' should be reserved to indicate the leakage of small amounts of liquid, soft or formed stool. The term 'encopresis', as originally coined, should only designate the passage of an *entire* stool, in the underwear, or an abnormal place, on an involuntary psychogenic basis or on the basis of a clear organic lesion such as myelomeningocele. Although no good data

are available to distinguish 'faecal incontinence' from 'encopresis', the latter, as defined above, is probably not related to constipation. In large series of incontinent children, constipation is present most of the time in patients who defaecate enormous-calibre stools that need to be mechanically broken up prior to flushing the toilet (Levine 1975), in those who have their rectum loaded with faeces (Bellman 1966), and those who have intervals of 4 days or longer between bowel movements (Davidson et al 1963). It is not unusual to see constipated patients, presenting for faecal incontinence, with a history of antidiarrhoeic drugs prescription.

The relationship between constipation and the irritable bowel syndrome (IBS)

Patients with constipation may or may not have abdominal pain (Drossman et al 1990) and the presence of pain is associated with shorter transit times (Lanfranchi et al 1984) (Fig. 37.10). Constipation and abdominal pain are two features found in patients with IBS. Abdominal bloating, simulating pregnancy because of bowel distention, lumbar lordosis, and forward tipping of the pelvis, are often found, together with other symptoms among patients with IBS, but they are also found in patients with colonic inertia

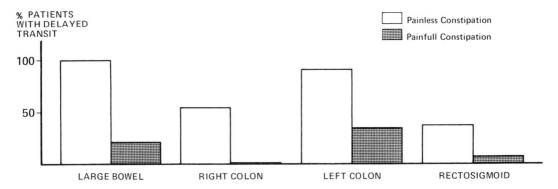

Fig. 37.10 Colonic transit time in chronic idiopathic constipation. Patients with painless constipation have a greater derangement of the large bowel than those who complain of abdominal pain (Lanfranchi et al 1984).

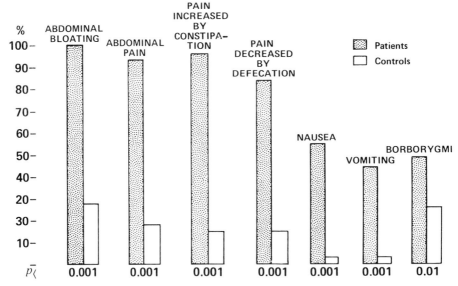

Fig. 37.11 Colonic inertia: abdominal symptoms. Symptoms found in patients with colonic inertia (Watier et al 1985) have abdominal symptoms quite like those found in patients with IBS (original data).

(Figs. 37.11, 37.12) or slow-transit constipation (Preston & Lennard-Jones 1986) (Fig. 37.13). Straining and the use of fingers to assist defaecation point to a strong 'willpower' mechanism at work in some constipated subjects, in lieu of the normal physiological mechanisms. Practically all constipated subjects have symptoms suggestive of IBS, and the prevalence and severity of symptoms fall markedly with effective laxative treatment; conversely, normal subjects made constipated with loperamide develop one or more symptoms of IBS (Marcus & Heaton 1987). Epidemiologic research has found an independent constipation category, however, which includes self-reported constipation, straining at defaecation, feeling of incomplete evacua-

tion and rectal bleeding, apart from IBS (Whitehead et al 1990). This is now referred to as obstructed defaecation as opposed to functional constipation.

At this stage of our knowledge, we do not exactly know the link between constipation and IBS. We do not know either the difference between a 'physiologic' defaecation (a call to stool occurs when faeces enter the rectum, the subject responds quickly, relaxes the pelvic floor and the entire hindgut empties) and 'sociologic' defaecation (the call to stool is refrained and replaced by a command to defaecate at another time, but the pelvic floor becomes 'disobedient' and this can be counteracted by finger manoeuvres or all sorts of other technical means such as suppositories, enemas and

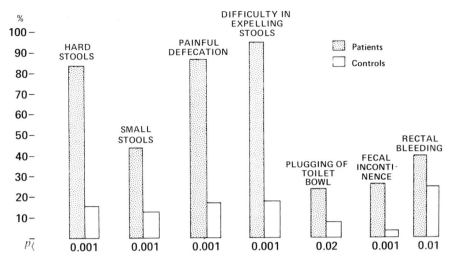

Fig. 37.12 Colonic inertia: symptoms and signs related to defaecation. Patients with colonic inertia (Watier et al 1985) have symptoms and signs akin to those found in the IBS and obstructed defaecation (original data).

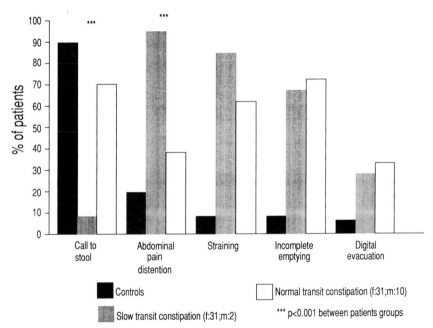

Fig. 37.13 Symptoms in intractable constipation. Patients with slow transit constipation have less urge to defaecate, and more abdominal pain and distension, than patients who complain of constipation but have normal colorectal transit times. As such, they resemble patients with colonic inertia shown on Fig. 37.20. However, they do not strain more; they have a feeling of incomplete evacuation and they often use their fingers to assist defaecation – as much as constipated patients with normal transit. It is thus difficult to differentiate the various syndromes from IBS (Roe et al 1986).

laxatives; additionally variable amounts of spasms and other motor disturbances can occur at a more proximal level in the colon and may reflect of more unconscious mechanisms).

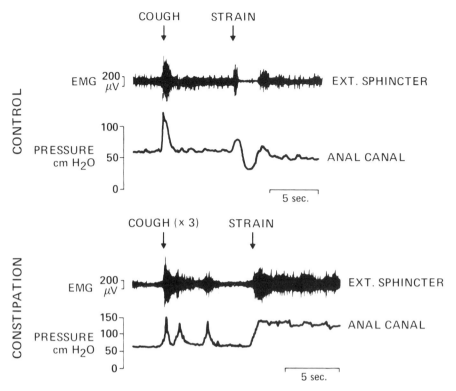

Fig. 37.14 Anismus. Patients with this erroneous reflex (it is not a disease, has never been cured by surgery or medication, but is correctable by biofeedback) contract their pelvic floor during straining, instead of normally relaxing it to let the stool go through (Preston & Lennard-Jones 1985b).

Sexual abuse, anismus and constipation

50% of women with functional gastrointestinal disorders are victims of sexual abuse, and this is known to the gastroenterologist in charge in less than one-fifth of the cases (Drossman et al 1990; Leroi et al submitted). This provides some enlightenment to anecdotal reports, where cure from constipation occurred synchronous to release of emotions related to an abuse (Devroede 1990; Devroede et al 1989; Drossman et al in press; De San Lazaro 1989). In fact, 20% of children, who have been sexually abused, present to the emergency room not for this reason, but for abdominal pain or constipation (Seidel et al 1986); and somatic reactions to sexual abuse, particularly of prolonged duration, include abdominal pain, constipation and appetite disturbance (Rimsza et al 1988).

Medical problems of adults who were sexually abused in childhood have barely begun to be investigated (Arnold et al 1990). Abused patients are more likely than non-abused patients to report pelvic pain,

multiple somatic symptoms and particularly more lifetime surgeries (Drossman et al 1990). Patients with functional upper gastrointestinal disorders are much less likely to have a history of sexual abuse than those with lower gastrointestinal disorders, and, among the latter, constipation, diarrhoea and abdominal pain are the most common presenting complaints (Leroi et al submitted). Women victims of full coitus during childhood or adolescence frequently see gastroenterologists and surgeons in consultation and are submitted during their lifetime to eight operations on average, 70% of them without any pathological findings (Arnold et al 1990). Among these procedures (Arnold et al 1990), laparotomy, ileostomy and proctocolectomy have been performed on constipated patients.

Anismus (Fig. 37.14), or rectosphincteric dyssnergia, where the patients contracts the pelvic floor during straining to defaecate, instead of normally relaxing it, has been found in all but one of 40 women, victims of incest or rape, and seen consecutively in a gastroenterology service, where they consulted not for the abuse

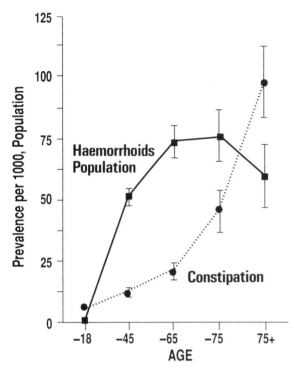

Fig. 37.15 Haemorrhoids are not caused by constipation. If haemorrhoids were caused by constipation, their prevalence rate would follow the same curve (Johanson & Sonnenberg 1990).

but constipation and abdominal pain (Denis et al 1992); it is more common among victims of abuse than non-victims (Leroi et al submitted).

THE NUISANCE OF CONSTIPATION

Genitourinary system

Urinary tract dysfunctions commonly disappear after recovery from constipation (Neumann et al 1973). Constipation is associated with many urinary tract symptoms, bladder calculi and dysfunction, and dilatation of the upper renal tract (Preston & Lennard-Jones 1986; Loening-Baucke 1990; Bannister et al 1986; Shopfner 1968; O'Regan & Yazbeck 1985; O'Regan et al 1985). Constipation and abnormal accommodation properties of the rectum are associated with uninhibited bladder contractions; rectometrograms have patterns similar to cystometrograms. The response of the bladder to bethanechol is faster and stronger in constipated patients who have a delayed transit time through the entire colon (Watier et al 1985).

The pelvic floor is a neuromuscular unit, traversed by the urinary, genital and intestinal tracts. Prostatorrhoea (involuntary emission of prostatic fluid secretions) is associated with constipation and haemorrhoids. Puborectalis strength is related to both orgasmic response and bladder function (Meier 1977). Anismus is associated with an increased capacity and reduced sensitivity in both rectum and bladder. For a given volume, both rectal and bladder pressures are similar in patients and controls, suggesting that the primary abnormality is not an increase in capacity, but blunting of sensation without difference in compliance (Bannister et al 1988). Women complaining of constipation, and found at anorectal manometry to have a rectoanal inhibitory reflex of decreased amplitude, all complain of vaginismus, while half of those with anal hypertony and ultraslow waves complain of frigidity and lack of orgasm (Weber et al 1987b).

Digestive system

Constipation is often diagnosed among obese subjects (Percora et al 1981) but body mass index is similar, regardless of age and sex, in people who do or do not report constipation (Sandler et al 1990).

Stercoraceous perforation is a lethal consequence of prolonged storage of hard faeces (Gekas & Schuster 1981), but only 21 cases per year are reported in the USA with constipation being listed as the primary cause of death (Sonnenberg & Koch 1989a,b).

Several studies established a link between cancer of the large bowel and constipation, particularly in women, but the magnitude of risk for a given patient is not known. Men are at risk of distal cancer, while women are at risk of a more proximal cancer (Higginson 1966; Wynder & Shigematsu 1967). Differences are small and other associated variables, such as obesity (Wynder & Shigematsu 1967), or dietary factors (Kune et al 1988) may be responsible. What definition of constipation has been used to study the question is an important variable: having only three stools per week for a long period of time is a risk factor for large bowel cancer, but self-reported constipation is not (Vobecky et al 1983). In addition, low prevalence of cancer of the large bowel is associated to greater stool weight but not with differences in rates of transit (Glober et al 1977).

Chronic straining with perineal descent will stretch the pudendal nerves and result in a weak and lax pelvic floor, with denervated striated muscles (Kiff et al 1984). This is conducive to faecal incontinence.

Haemorrhoids are not caused by constipation. Their prevalence differs markedly (Fig. 37.15), and, in a prospective case-control study, diarrhoea but not

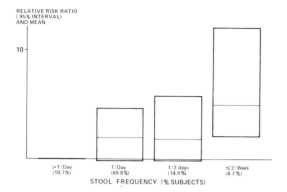

Fig. 37.16   Stool frequency and breast epithelial dyplasia in women. Women who defaecate less often have more breast epithelial dysplasia (Petrakis & King 1981). Not surprisingly, they run a higher risk of breast cancer. This does not mean a cause to effect relationship, but is a simple correlation.

constipation was found to be a risk factor for haemorrhoids (Johanson & Sonnenberg 1990; Johanson & Sonnenberg 1991). Stool consistency and frequency, and ease of defaecation are independent of the presence of haemorrhoids, and patients with haemorrhoids are not necessarily constipated, even if they have a tighter and longer anal canal (Gibbons et al 1988).

Breast disease

There is an increased risk of breast cancer in women with decreased stool frequency and firm consistency of stools; laxative use or self-reported constipation, as expected, have no predictive value (Micozzi et al 1989). In support of this, the incidence of epithelial dysplasia in mammary secretions was found to be in reverse correlation with stool frequency (Petrakis and King 1981) (Fig. 37.16).

Medicalization and unnecessary surgery

Constipation is associated with numerous digestive and extradigestive unpleasant symptoms (Martelli et al 1978b). Each of those, taken individually, may trigger consultation: for instance, up to 50% of women seen by gynaecologists in fact suffer from IBS and undergo more surgery than necessary for abdominal pain (Prior et al 1989; Longstreth et al 1990). Thus, constipated patients are at high risk for unnecessary surgery (Preston & Lennard-Jones 1986; Chaudhary & Truelove 1962; Fielding 1983). Acute abdominal pain in a patient with a long-standing history of constipation should not, without associated symptoms and signs, be used as an indication for surgery.

Many physicians are unaware that psychiatric illness, in particular hysteria, is often present in subjects with IBS, and seldom recognized by internists (Young et al 1976). Yet, hysteria is a polysymptomatic illness, where unnecessary surgery is often performed (Young et al 1976; Purtell et al 1951) and excess medications and hospitalization prescribed (Young et al 1976).

Medicalization is a distorted way to practice medicine, where a suffering human being is fragmented into a number of sick organs each of which is being taken care of by a physician, and no one having an eagle view of the entire person or relating to the patient.

THE AETIOLOGY AND MECHANISMS OF CONSTIPATION

Aetiology

There are many specific causes to constipation that have to be searched for before resigning oneself to a diagnosis of chronic idiopathic constipation. Drugs, metabolic and endocrine abnormalities, congenital and acquired causes of neurological lesions, both central and peripheral, and of muscular lesions along the gastrointestinal tract, may all interfere with normal transit throughout the gastrointestinal tract and must be looked for with great care.

This is not a textbook of gastroenterology on how to make a diagnosis of constipation secondary to a specific aetiology. The reader is referred to an extensive review of the question in another textbook, dealing not only with mechanisms but also with aetiologies (Devroede 1993a).

Mechanisms of constipation secondary to an organic disease

Endocrine abnormalities

Gastrointestinal transit time, from mouth to caecum, is prolonged in the second and third trimesters of pregnancy (Wald et al 1982; Lawson et al 1985). In patients with hypothyroidism, transit time to the caecum decreases after adequate treatment (Shafer et al 1984). The normal postprandial increase in motor activity of the sigmoid colon does not occur in diabetic patients who complain of severe constipation, presumably because of autonomic neuropathy (Battle et al 1980). Those with mild constipation have a postprandial increase in motor activity of the sigmoid colon but it is delayed.

Neurological abnormalities

When the frontal lobe area is injured, constipation may occur; abnormalities include rectal hypoesthesia

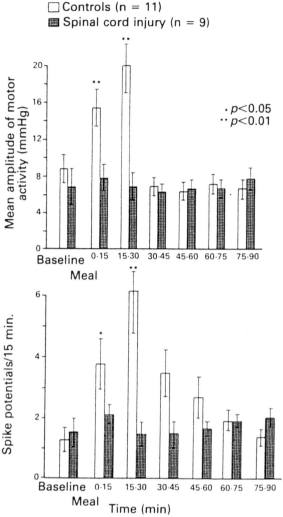

Fig. 37.17   Colonic dysfunction in male patients with complete thoracic spinal cord injury. In male patients with complete thoracic spinal cord injury, the ingestion of a meal does not increase the number of spike potentials in the large bowel. The intraluminal pressure, accordingly, does not change either (Glick et al 1984).

and spontaneous contractions, absence of rectoanal inhibitory reflex and weak voluntary contraction of the anal canal with hypertonicity at rest (Weber et al 1990). In anterior lesions to the pons, transit through the ascending colon is delayed, the rectoanal inhibitory reflex absent, and bladder function abnormal; in posterior lesions, it is the transit in the left colon which is prolonged, with normal anorectal and bladder function, but poor oesophageal coordination (Weber et al 1985). These two studies provide convincing evi-

dence for supraspinal control of colonic and rectoanal motility.

In patients with traumatic transection of the spinal cord above the level of the first lumbar vertebra, there is no colonic response to a meal (Fig. 37.17), while good response to neostigmine (Fig. 37.18) indicates the muscle itself is normal. Colonic compliance and tolerance to fluid filling are markedly reduced (Glick et al 1984). The reverse occurs in patients with lower lesions of the spinal cord and destruction of the cauda

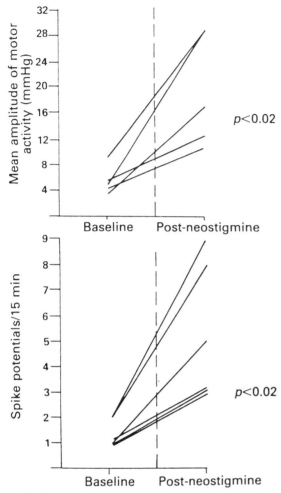

Fig. 37.18 Colonic response to neostigmine in male patients with complete thoracic spinal cord injury. In contrast to what is seen in Fig. 37.17, neostigmine evokes a normal response of the large bowel in male patients with complete thoracic spinal cord injury. Thus, the muscle itself is normal and the lack of response to a meal means that the response is modulated by extrinsic innervation (Glick et al 1984).

equina: pressure–volume curves within the colon are flat during filling and the compliance markedly enhanced (White et al 1940; Scott & Cantelli 1949). Neither right nor left colon transit is abnormal in these patients, regardless of the level of spinal cord injury, but rectosigmoid transit time is prolonged in cases of complete transection of the spinal cord below the level of the ninth thoracic vertebra, accounting for the delayed total large bowel transit time (Beuret-Blanquart et al 1990). The rectoanal inhibitory reflex is present in all patients with spinal cord injury. There is no correlation between level of rectal distension and configuration of the reflex. When transection involves the second, third and fourth sacral vertebrae, this is associated with anal hypertonicity (Devroede et al 1979; Beuret-Blanquart et al 1990).

Colonic compliance of patients with multiple sclerosis is also decreased (Glick et al 1982), and transit through the colon delayed (Weber et al 1987a). Colonic motor activity, at rest, is decreased, and there is no postprandial increase in motility (Glick et al 1982). Some patients have spontaneous rectal contractions and many manometric abnormalities in the anorectal area suggestive of outlet obstruction: hypertonicity of the anal canal, unstable anal canal pressure, or decreased amplitude of the rectoanal inhibitory reflex. The activity of the striated pelvic floor is also impaired (Weber et al 1987a).

Although it is classically said that sympathectomy exerts no influence on colonic, rectal and anal motility, this really has not been studied adequately. In contrast, parasympathetic innervation has, repeatedly, been found essential (Kettlewell 1972; Devroede & Lamarche 1974; Devroede et al 1979): trauma or resection of the nervi erigentes leads to obstipation, loss of rectal sensation and delayed transit through the large bowel. Rectal sensation is lost and rectal capacity to distension increases after bilateral but not after unilateral sacrifice of sacral nerves (Gunterberg et al 1976). The loss of rectal sensation may be neurogenic, through damage of the afferent nerves, but could simply be due to a loss of rectal muscle tone. Bypass of the hindgut restores transit, suggesting that sacral parasympathetic outflow exerts no influence on the ascending colon. Pathologic evaluation of the resected specimen of distal colon demonstrates neuronal loss, decrease in size of remaining neurons, and focal Schwann cell hyperplasia (Devroede & Lamarche 1974). Transit time is prolonged in the large bowel and the anal canal becomes hypertonic. The rectoanal contractile reflex of the external anal sphincter is much weaker than normal (Devroede et al 1979). An internal anal sphincter relaxing in the presence of minimal rectal distension, and associated with a poorly functioning external anal sphincter, of course offers little protection against faecal incontinence if laxatives or enemas are used to overcome constipation.

Mechanisms of constipation in IBS

Patients with constipation-predominant IBS have been found to tolerate a significantly greater (Prior et al 1990a), or smaller (Varma & Smith 1984), volume during balloon distension of the rectum before they have discomfort: this is ample evidence that this diagno-

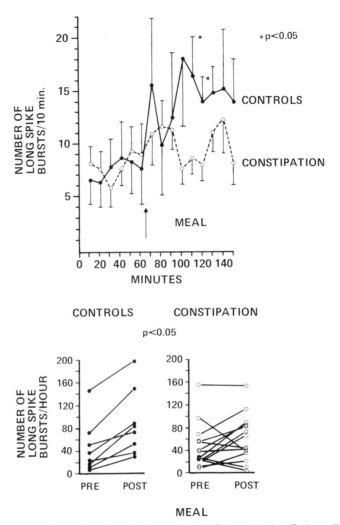

Fig. 37.19 Electrical activity in the colon of patients with painful constipation. Patients diagnosed as suffering from IBS, with a second selection criterion of having less than three stools per week, have little postprandial increase in colonic motor activity (Dapoigny et al 1985).

sis encompasses a very inhomogeneous group of patients in terms of pathophysiology, with no relationship between subjective complaints and objective measurements (Oettle & Heaton 1987).

The time taken for a solid meal to pass through the stomach, small intestine and colon is prolonged in both small and large bowel in patients with IBS complaining mainly of constipation, and their average daily stool weight is less than normal (Cann et al 1983). Prolonged ambulant monitoring of proximal bowel motor activity has demonstrated striking abnormalities (Kellow et al 1990; Kellow et al 1992; Kellow & Phillips 1987). The duration of postprandial activity in the duodenojejunum is shorter than normal; propagated and non-propagated clusters of contraction may

also occur during daytime. Migrating motor complexes (MMCs) cycle length is much prolonged, and this does not change at night; the amplitude of phase III is less than normal and this is found day and night. Compared to patients with IBS who complain mainly of diarrhoea, there are fewer changes from day to night in those who complain of constipation: this indicates that central nervous system mechanisms have a much less direct and immediate impact in this condition. In the colon, patients with a constipation-type IBS have fewer high-amplitude caudally propagated contractions and non-propagated contractions than normal (Crowell et al 1989; Dapoigny et al 1985) (Fig. 37.19). They also have little response to meal (Dapoigny et al 1985). Similar abnormalities have been

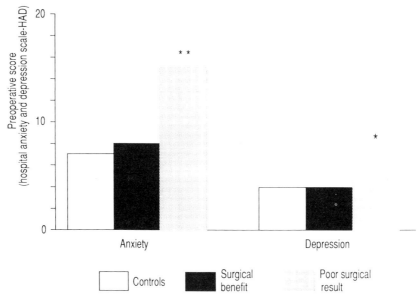

Fig. 37.20   Psychological aspects of patients treated surgically for chronic idiopathic constipation. Patients who are treated surgically for constipation and are anxious or depressed before the operation fare poorly subsequently (Fisher et al 1989).

recorded in patients with severe constipation, showing clearly an overlap between 'constipation' and 'IBS' which may reflect selection criteria of patients rather than real difference (Loening-Baucke & Anuras 1986).

Mechanisms of chronic idiopathic constipation

Constipation as a body clue: disease of the person

That emotions, personality and bowel habits are interrelated was already discussed over 50 years ago by Groddeck (Groddeck 1926), and there is some support for the idea that a conflict between parent and child may modify bowel habits (Pinkerton 1958). There is a relationship between stool output and personality. Healthy volunteers, self-selected because accepting to have a chaperon constantly and to refrain from sexual activity for 6 months, tend to produce more frequent and heavier stools if they display a greater degree of self-esteem and are more outgoing (Tucker et al 1981). Constipated patients found to have normal colorectal transit times have significantly more psychopathology than those with delayed transit, where the pathophysiological sign is coherent with the symptom of constipation (Wald 1986; Wald et al 1989). Clinicians who rely upon scientific measurements only will fall into the

trap of not recognizing the 'hidden agenda' of the patient, cannot help him/her, and so expose themselves to litigation. Not surprisingly, constipated patients fare poorly after surgery for their symptom if they are anxious or depressed (Fisher et al 1989) (Fig. 37.20). Constipated patients with severe constipation and delayed transit through the ascending colon have high scores on several scales of the Minnesota Multiphasic Personality Inventory (MMPI): hypochondria, hysteria, control and low back pain. They score lower on the MF scale, which means they are more feminine, whatever arbitrary value is attributed to 'being feminine' (Devroede et al 1989a, b). High scores of hypochondria and hysteria with lower scores of depression in between provide a profile known as the 'pschosomatic V' or 'conversion valley': this means patients are protected from depression by their symptoms. Constipated and arthritic patients are so different in personality profile that they can be differentiated by discriminant analysis: use of the MMPI data alone yields 83% correct answers; addition of age raises this to 97% (Fig. 37.21)! This means the computer can recognize a constipated patient versus an arthritic one just with personality and age, regardless of medical investigation! To understand if changes in personality are antecedent, synchronous or consequent to motor dysfunc-

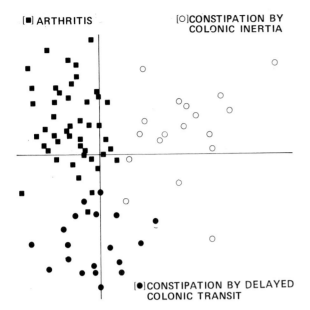

[■] ARTHRITIS [O] CONSTIPATION BY COLONIC INERTIA

[●] CONSTIPATION BY DELAYED COLONIC TRANSIT

Fig. 37.21 Discriminant analysis of constipated and arthritic women (MMPI data and age). Constipated women with delayed transit in the ascending colon is so different from an arthritic control in terms of personality, that they can be differentiated just with items of the Minnesota Multiphasic Personality Inventory and age, regardless of more 'medical' data (Devroede et al 1989). Colonic inertia refers to a situation where there is stagnation in the ascending colon; while constipation by delayed colonic transit is a more active phenomenon where faeces progress little overall because they move back and forth between right and left colon (Watier et al 1985, Likongo et al 1986).

tion, long-term studies of single patients are needed but anecdotal evidence exists of a change in personality during psychotherapy before constipation disappears (Fig. 37.22) (Devroede et al 1989a). Megacolon is found in psychotic patients (Ehrentheil & Wells 1955; Watkins & Oliver 1965), and this also suggests the possibility of a link between mind and body. Acutely ill paranoid hallucinating schizophrenics appear to be particularly at risk; similarly, in patients with constipation by colonic inertia, transit time in the ascending colon correlates with the level of paranoia (Devroede et al 1989).

There is a very close relationship between levels of anxiety and transit time in the ascending colon of patients with constipation by delayed colonic transit who have some evidence of motor activity in the large bowel (Devroede et al 1989b). This means constipation is literally part of their personality, and protects them from anxiety.

Constipated patients have a high incidence of a disturbed childhood, psychosexual problems, and personality difficulties (Preston et al 1984). Adult subjects who consult for IBS have a recollection of more painful childhood events, but separate analysis for constipation has not been done. It is essential to take in perspective the fact that memory is coloured by intervening events and also that what matters really is not the event itself, but its meaningfulness (Lowan et al 1987).

Numerous behaviour problems are reported, on parental ratings of a checklist, in children with faecal incontinence and constipation, but the severity of the problems is less than in children referred for mental services (Gabel et al 1986; Loening-Baucke et al 1987a). Social withdrawal behaviour increases with age, perhaps because of peer and adult rejection. Affective–dependent behaviour is also markedly abnormal, but does not increase with age, reflecting signs of depression, affective lability and anxiety. Those abnormalities disappear with recovery from encopresis (Levine et al 1980). Constipated boys with incontinence are more obsessive–compulsive if they are found not to be able to defaecate rectal balloons full of water. They are more delinquent and less anxious if they have abdominal pain. Girls unable to defaecate these balloons are less competent socially, and those with pain are more aggressive and cruel (Loening-Baucke et al 1987a). The link between pain, constipation and aggressiveness is logical since anger makes the colon contract (Welgan et al 1988). Children do not differ, after treatment, in terms of social competence or behaviour, whether they recover or not (Loening-Baucke et al 1987a). Those that do not recover were initially more aggressive and more socially withdrawn: despite the fact they remain encopretic, they make substantial gains in social adaptation (Levine et al 1980).

Available data thus concur on the need to include an appraisal of psychological elements in the medical management of patients with chronic idiopathic constipation.

Can chronic idiopathic constipation be ascribed to a single pathophysiological mechanism?

No single mechanism can be held responsible for chronic idiopathic constipation. The more functional tests are performed, the more some abnormalities are found in almost all patients (Meunier et al 1984; Shouler & Keighley 1986) (Fig. 37.23). In addition, abnormal mechanisms are common to apparently very different groups of constipated patients (Barnes & Lennard-Jones 1985).

Stomach and small bowel function. An abnor-

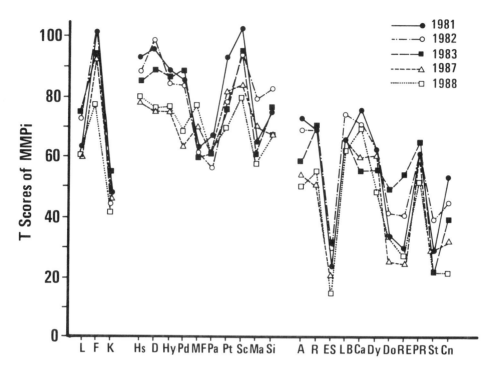

Fig. 37.22 Changes in personality profile of a patient with severe chronic idiopathic constipation. This patient had a depression of almost psychotic nature, when she consulted for severe constipation (one stool per 2 months). She cured overnight when her father, who raped her at 16, died. The figure shows clear evidence of progressive improvement over the year in personality profile, particularly on the hypochondria, depression, hysteria and psychopathy scales. Before the death of her father, depression was higher but afterwards there was a vague configuration in psychosomatic valley (see text), with depression lesser than hysteria and hypochondria. For details of this case report see Devroede 1989.

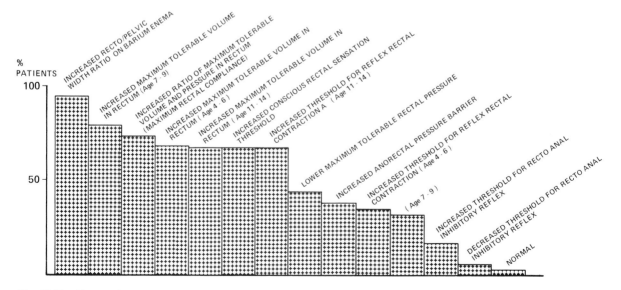

Fig. 37.23 Abnormal anorectal motility in children with chronic idiopathic constipation. Very few patients with chronic idiopathic constipation have no functional recordable abnormality (see right of figure) (Meunier et al 1984).

mally long transit to the caecum in patients with constipation is corrected by treatment (Marzio et al 1989; Bassotti et al 1987). The delay is not of major clinical importance: if, within 24 h, swallowed radiopaque markers are not in the large bowel (Arhan et al 1981), an organic lesion or chronic idiopathic pseudo-obstruction should be suspected.

Phase II of the MMC cycle is prolonged in patients with chronic idiopathic constipation, persists at night and there are abnormal clusters of contractions. Postprandial activity is shorter. If this is found in a given patient, colectomy should be avoided to prevent postoperative persistent symptomatology (Panaganuwa et al 1991).

Large bowel absorption. The contribution of the colonic mucosa to constipation is minimal and purely induced by delayed transit and prolonged storage (Devroede & Soffie 1973). Increasing stool consistency, however, compounds a colonic motor problem.

COLORECTAL TRANSIT STUDIES

Mechanisms of constipation can be approached in two different ways: following the progress of faeces along the large bowel, or evaluating bowel wall muscular activity and tone. The first method provides an estimate of the end results induced by abnormalities demonstrated by the second method.

On the basis of radiopaque marker studies, patients with constipation may be divided into three different groups. In the first, there is delay in the colon (Martelli et al 1978b; Watier et al 1985). In the second, faeces pass normally along the colon but are stored too long in the rectum (Verduron et al 1988; Hinton & Lennard-Jones 1968). In the third, transit time of the radiopaque markers is normal.

The incidence of patients with delayed transit in the ascending colon is only 15% of a cohort complaining of constipation, but up to 41% of those found to have delayed colorectal transit. Right colonic stasis is very seldom limited to that site and practically always associated with overall colorectal delayed transit (Wald 1986; Watier et al 1985; Chaussade et al 1989; Ducrotte et al 1986).

Patients with hindgut dysfunction have normal right colon transit and distal delay. 33% of patients with less than two stools per week have such a pattern and are subdivided roughly in half with delay in the left colon and rectosigmoid area, and another half with functional outlet obstruction only (Wald 1986). Isolated stasis in the left colon occurs in 15% of a constipated cohort, or 36% of those found to have delayed overall large bowel transit (Chaussade et al 1989).

Some patients have normal colonic function but rectal stasis; they suffer from functional outlet obstruction (Verduron et al 1988; Martelli et al 1978b). This occurs in only 13% of a constipated cohort, but 31% of those found to have delayed overall large bowel transit (Chaussade et al 1989).

29% of patients with less than *two* stools per week, but 50% of those with less than *three* stools per week have 'normal' transit in the large bowel (Wald 1986; Schang 1985). This indicates the influence of diagnostic criteria used by clinicians on pathophysiologic evaluation. Patients with 'normal' transit may have isolated delay segmental transit in the descending colon, and some may have 'normal' segmental transit times with overall delayed transit (Wald 1986; Chaussade et al 1989; Schang 1985). Only one-third of patients with 'normal' colorectal transit also have 'normal' segmental transit time (Kuijpers 1990) (Fig. 37.24), and in only four out of 61 patients were both anorectal manometry *and* studies of colorectal transit times 'normal' (Ducrotte et al 1986). Thus, great care should be used before dismissing a patient as being 'normal'.

The complaint of constipation is confirmed by the physiopathological finding of a delayed transit more often in women, than it is in men (Bouchoucha et al 1992; Chaussade et al 1989). This, and the joint analysis of colonic transit time with clinical signs, suggests that data collected during patient interview have little usefulness in distinguishing the different subsets of transit disturbance. For instance, the use of digital pressure to assist defaecation (Preston & Lennard-Jones 1986), although relevant, does not differentiate right colonic from rectosigmoid stasis (Chaussade et al 1989); but low stool frequency and abdominal distension may occur more frequently when colorectal transit time is prolonged (Ducrotte et al 1986).

Colonic constipation

Patients with slow-transit constipation have a large bowel of normal size and configuration, in contrast to those with colonic inertia. Markers stagnate along the entire large intestine in both groups, almost exclusively of the female sex (Watier et al 1985; Preston & Lennard-Jones 1986). Delayed transit in the ascending colon may be merely secondary to a distal obstacle, as for instance in hindgut dysgenesis (Likongo et al 1986). Retrograde movement of faeces may be shown with radiopaque markers, which travel back and forth from right to left colon, and disappear, in a bumpy fashion from the ascending colon (Devroede et al 1989a). Reflux

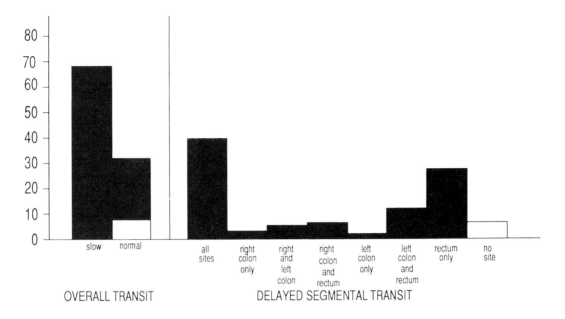

Fig. 37.24   Slow transit vs segmental constipation. This figure shows that only a small proportion of constipated patients, with 'normal' large bowel transit time, remain classified as 'normal', if a delayed segmental transit time in the different areas of the colon is also taken as evidence of functional derangement (Kuijpers 1990).

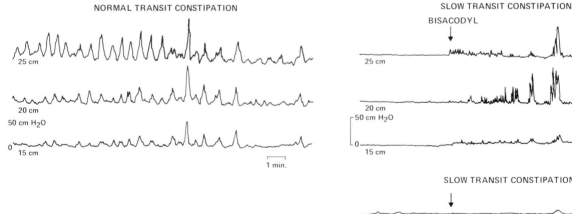

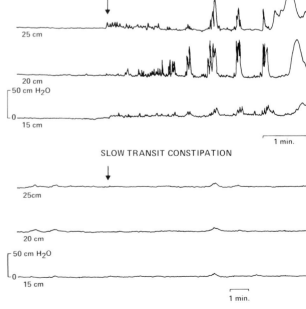

Fig. 37.25   Rectosigmoid pressure in constipation. The colon of some patients with slow transit constipation does not contract in response to bisacodyl (Preston & Lennard-Jones 1985a).

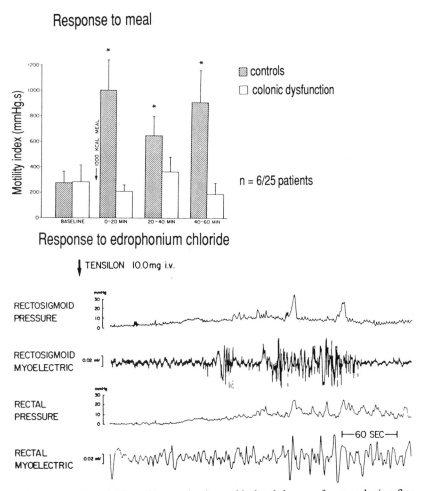

Fig. 37.26 Chronic idiopathic constipation and isolated absence of gastrocolonic reflex. The colon of some constipated patients does not react more to meal than it does to bisacodyl, yet is responsive to edrophonium (Reynolds et al 1987).

of markers is associated with retrograde, orally directed, propagated electrical activity (Schang et al 1985). The term 'colonic inertia' should probably be reserved for the situation in which transit time in the ascending colon is prolonged and no reflux of markers from the left colon is demonstrated, because there is little or no colonic motor activity. There is thus some evidence that two distinct patterns of colonic motor activity may be found in patients with constipation: some are hypomotor, with little movement and progression of faeces from the caecum, while others are normo, or hypermotor, with a pattern resembling that of normal subjects and responding to a number of stimuli (Bazzocchi et al 1990; Kamm

et al 1988). Bisacodyl stimulates the appearance of powerful peristaltic waves in the distal colon of normal subjects, but not in 50% of patients with slow-transit constipation (Preston & Lennard-Jones 1985b) (Fig. 37.25). After meals, some constipated patients have no postprandial increase in distal colonic motility (Fig. 37.26), and others have a postprandial increase in motor activity, with retrograde and antegrade movement: colonic scintigraphy is able to distinguish these two patterns of motor activity (Bazzocchi et al 1990) (Fig. 37.27). Patients with painless constipation have higher levels of rectal sensation, urge to defaecate, and rectal pain at distension, while those with painful constipation

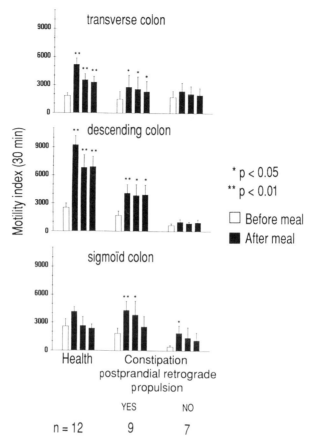

Fig. 37.27 Postprandial motor activity in health and chronic idiopathic constipation. Colonic scintigraphy permits identification of two types of motor activity in patients with chronic idiopathic constipation. When there is postprandial retrograde propulsion of the material, there is an increase in motility after meal similar to that which occurs in health; when there is none, there is no effect of meal (Bazzocchi et al 1990).

have lower ones; the latter group complains more often of abdominal distension, and has feelings of incomplete evacuation, thus resembling patients diagnosed as having IBS (Lanfranchi et al 1984). The response or no-response of colonic motility to bisacodyl, food or edrophonium chloride may perhaps help in the future to recognize patients who have an inert colonic musculature.

In patients with prolonged colonic transit time, the number of propagating electrical potentials is significantly decreased in fasting conditions, and little postprandial increase is observed (Schang 1985; Schang et al 1985; Dapoigny et al 1985) (Figs 37.19, 37.28). As re-

corded by manometry, colonic mass movements are much less frequent, shorter (Fig. 37.29) and are totally absent over 24 h in one-third of patients (Bassotti et al 1988). Isolated chronic colonic pseudo-obstruction may be a label given to some patients with colonic inertia or slow-transit constipation: most have severe constipation and very few unequivocal abnormalities in either muscular or neural structures. Motor activity is less than normal in fasting conditions. Amplitude of contractions in the distal large bowel is lower after a meal, and the rectal wall is much more inelastic (flaccid) (Loening-Baucke et al 1987a). Abdominal catastrophes, often ascribed to pseudo-obstruction are

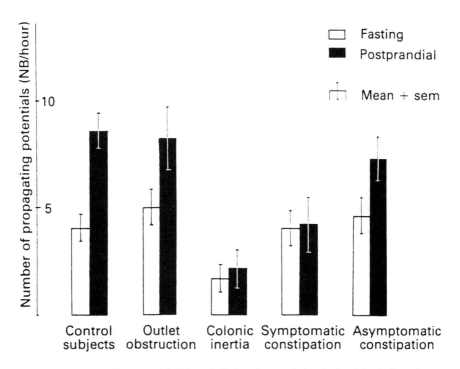

Fig. 37.28 Propagating potentials. There is little propagated electrical activity in the colon of patients with colonic inertia, and, in contrast to other normal subjects or constipated patients, it does not increase after meal (Schang 1985). Compare this figure with Fig. 37.19, where postprandial colonic response is also impaired. Selection criterium here, however, was a delayed transit of radio-opaque markers through the ascending colon as a prerequisite to making a diagnosis of colonic inertia; in contrast, in Fig. 37.19, clinical criteria were used. This is good evidence that there is a lot of overlap in the literature on constipation, depending on selection criteria.

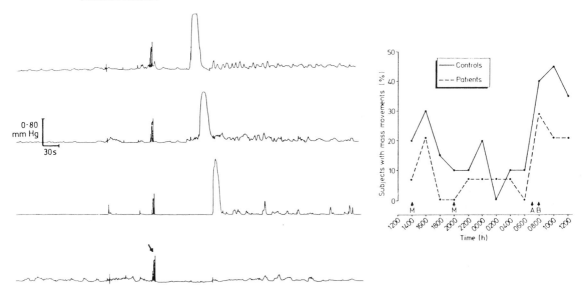

Fig. 37.29 Colonic mass movements in idiopathic chronic constipation. Colonic mass movements, an example of which is shown on the left, where a high amplitude contraction wave is seen to propagate from proximal (top) to distal (bottom) colon, occur much less often in constipated patients (right of figure) (Bassotti et al 1988).

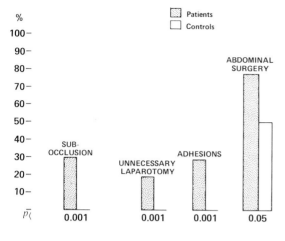

Fig. 37.30   Colonic inertia: abdominal catastrophes. Abdominal catastrophes occur often in patients with colonic inertia (Watier et al 1985).

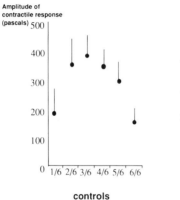
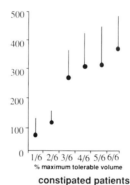

Fig. 37.31   Sigmoid response to distension. While in health, optimal contractile response of the sigmoid colon is reached at half the maximum tolerable volume, in constipated patients, this occurs only at maximum distension. It indicates an overstretch of the muscle in constipation, and poor contractile possibilities (Chevalier et al 1989).

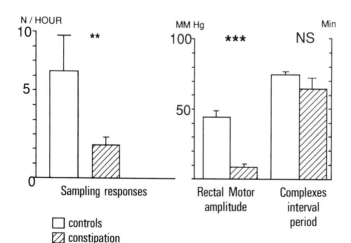
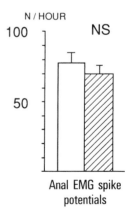

Fig. 37.32   Nyctemeral anorectal motor activity in chronic intractable constipation. In patients with chronic intractable constipation, transit of faeces is reduced through the rectum: rectal motor complexes have a decreased amplitude, and sampling responses in the anal canal are less frequent (Waldron et al 1990).

also found in patients with colonic inertia (Fig. 37.30).

The elastic properties of the sigmoid colon differ from health in constipated patients who have delayed left colonic transit. There is decreased compliance of the bowel wall. Contractile activity, in health, reaches a peak at half the maximum tolerable volume, and then decreases because of muscle overstretch; in constipation, the maximum activity is reached at maximum distension (Chevalier et al 1989) (Fig. 37.31). In patients with slow-transit constipation, there is decreased motor activity and impaired response both to feeding and awakening, not only in the sigmoid colon but also in the rectum and anal canal (Read et al 1985). Higher volumes of rectal distension are required to generate rectal contractions in elderly patients admitted with faecal impaction (Read et al 1985) and in chronically constipated children with incontinence (Loening-Baucke 1990; Loening-Baucke 1991).

Rectal motor complexes occur as often in patients with slow-transit constipation without anismus as they do in controls, but with markedly reduced amplitude. This, and the less frequent occurrence of sampling reflexes (spontaneous fall of anal sphincter pressure of less than 1 min duration), indicative of rectal filling, support the concept of reduced transit of faeces to the rectum from the colon (Waldron et al 1990) (Fig. 37.32).

Are colonic inertia and slow-transit constipation diseases of the large bowel only? Dysphagia and gastro-oesophageal reflux are associated with hypertonic pharyngo-oesophageal and weak gastro-oesophageal sphincter in patients with colonic inertia (Fig. 37.33). They also have a high incidence of simultaneous contractions of the oesophagus (tertiary contractions) (Watier et al 1985) (Fig. 37.34).. Gastric emptying is delayed and so is the orocaecal transit (Coremans et al 1991). They have many urinary symptoms, residual urine, abnormal urodynamic studies and hypersensitivity of the bladder to bethanechol (Watier et al 1985; Preston & Lennard-Jones 1986). The rectum is also hypersensitive to bethanechol, contracting more and faster than in controls (Abdel-Rahman et al 1981), and the anus is hypertonic (Watier et al 1985). Thus, there is evidence for abnormal function of the oesophagus, stomach, small and large bowel, anus and bladder in these patients. Orthostatic hypotension is common (Watier et al 1985). Finally, there is a high incidence of galactorrhoea with normal prolactin levels (Watier et al 1985; Preston & Lennard-Jones 1986). This all points to a systemic disease or disorder.

Constipation by outlet obstruction

There are several mechanisms for outlet obstruction.

Hyperactive rectosigmoid junction

A zone of complex wave activity, is found 9–15 cm from the anal margin in constipated patients. Neither secretin nor cholecystokinin influence the wave activity of the hyperactive segment, but atropine and glucagon inhibit the motility of this segment, suggesting overactivity of the muscarinic effector cells (Dinoso et al 1983).

Abnormal anorectal motility

Resting pressure in the anal canal of patients with chronic idiopathic constipation may be increased, normal or decreased (Devroede 1993a), depending on patient selection and modalities of recording. Pressure in a sphincter only reflects its resistance to distension. Water perfusion systems, for instance, produce errors because the rate of perfusion influences recording: it is the pressure within the artificially produced water-filled compartment that is measured. In addition, leaking of fluid modifies external anal sphincter activity, and can even abolish the presence of a normal rectoanal inhibitory reflex because of reflex pelvic contraction to prevent incontinence (Devroede and Hémond 1990). As for patient selection, elderly constipated patients may (Varma et al 1988) or may not have a hypotonic anal canal, whether they have faecal impaction (Read et al 1985) or not (Varma et al 1988). Similarly, the anal canal of constipated patients who have abdominal pain is hypertonic, but it is not if they don't (Lanfranchi et al 1984) (Fig. 37.35).

Normally, anal pressure is higher in the upper anal canal than in the lower anal canal (Martelli et al 1978a), but in one-fifth of constipated patients an inverted profile may be recognized (Veyrac et al 1988). The length of the anal canal is longer in constipated children, presumably because of greater activity of the external anal sphincter (Kaya et al 1988).

Instability of the anal pressure in constipation may take the appearance of ultra-slow waves of low frequency and high amplitude, or of slow waves of higher frequency and lower amplitude, which may, or may not be associated with a higher than normal level of resting pressure (Ducrotte et al 1985; Arhan et al 1983).

The amplitude of the rectoanal inhibitory reflex

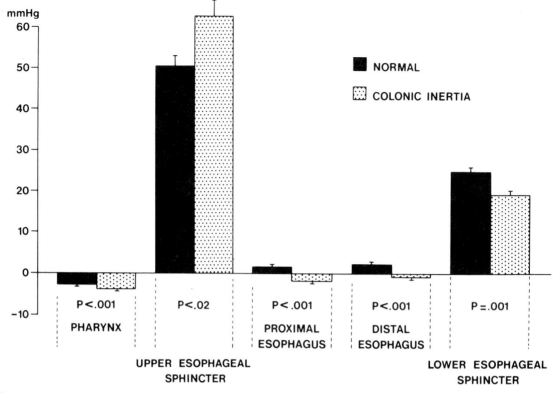

Fig. 37.33 Resting pressure. Patients with colonic inertia have a hypertonic pharyngo-oesophageal sphincter, and a hypotonic gastro-oesophageal sphincter (Watier et al 1985).

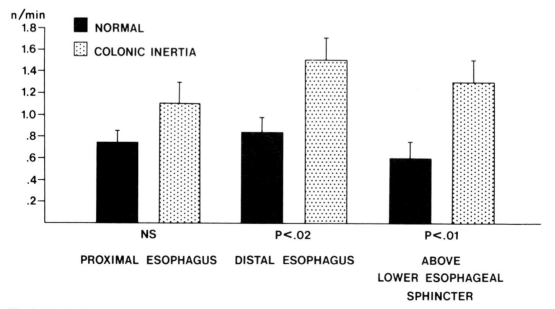

Fig. 37.34 Incidence of spontaneous tertiary contractions. Tertiary contractions of the oesophagus are common in patients with colonic inertia (Watier et al 1985).

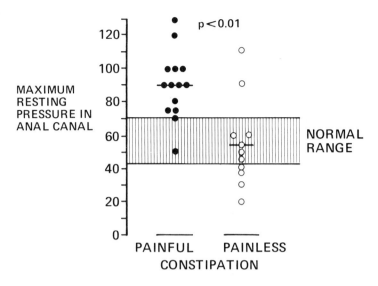

Fig. 37.35 Anal canal pressure in chronic idiopathic constipation. Patients with painful constipation have a hypertonic anal canal; those with painless constipation don't (Lanfranchi et al 1984).

may be normal, decreased or increased (Devroede 1993a). Higher levels of residual pressure during the rectoanal inhibitory reflex (Lester et al 1991) may be found. Patient's selection is surely one of the factors which explain these differences: for instance, patients with painful constipation have a rectoanal inhibitory reflex of greater amplitude than those with painless constipation (Lanfranchi et al 1984). An increase in threshold of the rectoanal inhibitory reflex has also been recognized (Loening-Baucke & Cruickshank 1986; Arhan et al 1983; Meunier et al 1979; Reboa et al 1984). The electrical stimulus of the rectal mucosa necessary to achieve maximum relaxation of the internal anal sphincter is greater in constipation, suggesting abnormal intrinsic innervation (Kamm & Lennard-Jones 1990). In some constipated patients the duration of the reflex does not increase with increasing levels of rectal distension (Veyrac et al 1988), and in others, found to have a rectoanal inhibitory reflex of lesser than normal amplitude, the amplitude of the reflex decreases with progressive rectal distension and increasing rectal wall tension, in contrast to normal subjects Ducrotte et al 1985).

Anismus

Anismus is a common mechanism of outlet obstruction

(Preston & Lennard-Jones 1990). The term is synonymous to various other designations: spastic pelvic floor syndrome, sphincteric disobedience syndrome, paradoxical external sphincter contraction or function, rectoanal dyssynergia, abdomino-levator incoordination, abdominopelvic asynchronism, abnormal defaecation dynamics or pattern, and abnormal anorectal expulsion dynamics. Normally, during defaecation, the pelvic floor, which at rest is in a state of constant activity and contraction, relaxes completely (Parks et al 1962). Some constipated patients contract the external anal sphincter (Fig. 37.14) and/or the puborectalis muscle during straining to defaecate (Veyrac et al 1988; Kerrigan et al 1989; Wald et al 1986).

Anismus, although common in constipated women, is also found in men, in patients with normal colorectal transit times (Barnes & Lennard-Jones 1988; Kuijpers & Bleijenberg 1985; Kuijpers et al 1986), and in those with a colon and rectum of abnormal size (Barnes & Lennard-Jones 1988). Its cause is unknown. Malfunction of the anorectal structure, on an organic basis, is highly unlikely because surgical attempts to correct the dysfunction has failed (Kuijpers et al 1986; Barnes et al 1985). A focal dystonic phenomenon has been considered because it may be found in some patients with Parkinson's disease (Mathers et al 1989), but the association of the disease and constipation does not

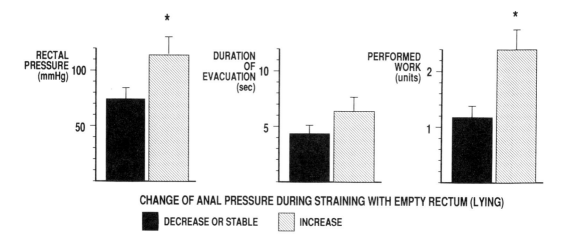

Fig. 37.36   Rectosphincteric dyssynergia at defaecometry (sitting). Anismus is not 'normal': healthy subjects who increase anal pressure ($\bar{X}$ + SE) during straining must exert a greater effort during defaecation, as exemplified by increased intrarectal pressure, and greater work to perform at defaecometry (Lestar et al 1989).

imply a cause to effect relationship, and the dyssynergia might be either a chance finding, a simple correlation, or the result of the burden of the main disease. The only successful treatment found to date for this has been biofeedback, and this suggests the nature of it is an abnormal learning process rather than a disease. Moreover, many constipated children strain when asked to squeeze, squeeze when asked to strain, or to do both and reverse the command: hence the labelling of a sphincteric disobedience syndrome (Hero et al 1985). Also it is not known why anismus is predominantly a problem of little boys, and why it is found mainly in adult women. A final argument against anismus being an organic disease is that it is commonly found in patients who have been sexually abused (Denis et al 1992; Leroi et al submitted).

Anismus is also found in patients with the solitary rectal ulcer syndrome and those with the descending perineum syndrome (Rutter 1974; Jones et al 1987; Kuijpers et al 1986). Patients with the solitary rectal ulcer syndrome have an internal rectal prolapse and complain of obstructed defaecation while patients with the descending perineum syndrome have a weak pelvic floor: both groups are constipated. Although anismus is found in 95% of patients unable to expel a water-filled rectal balloon (Barnes & Lennard-Jones 1988), it is also in 50% of patients with idiopathic perineal pain (Jones et al 1987). In some studies, up to one-third of 'normal' subjects have anismus (Barnes & Lennard-

Jones 1988), while other authors report very few (Barnes & Lennard-Jones 1988) or claim they never found anismus during defaecation trials in healthy controls (Loening-Baucke & Cruikshank 1986; Lestar et al 1991). This all might suggest anismus is a nonspecific finding but 'normal' subjects, who do not relax their pelvic floor during straining, must perform a greater amount of work in order to defaecate, placing them perhaps at risk for prolapse and descent (Lestar et al 1989) (Fig. 37.36). Patients with anismus able to evacuate a simulated stool need, nevertheless, significantly more time and have to perform more work to defaecate than controls (Lestar et al 1991). Thus, anismus is not always the sole cause of constipation, but is never innocuous. Its presence creates an obstacle to defaecation and presumably, to a complaint of constipation.

The puborectalis muscle is innervated in part by a branch of the sacral nerve that lies above the pelvic floor; the pudendal nerve supplies only the ipsilateral external anal sphincter muscle (Percy et al 1981; Hamel-Roy 1984). Not surprisingly, patients may have anismus limited to the puborectalis muscle, or to the external anal sphincter, even if both muscles are involved in the overwhelming majority of patients (Lebel and Grand-Maison 1988).

The term anismus is quite appropriate because of its analogy with vaginismus, where a spasm of the pelvic floor muscle also occurs, but as a resistance to penetra-

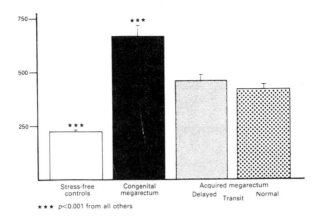

750 —

500 —

250 —

***

***

| Stress-free controls | Congenital megarectum | Acquired megarectum |
| | | Delayed   Transit   Normal |

*** *p*<0.001 from all others

Fig. 37.37   Maximum tolerable volume in megarectum ($\bar{X}$ + SE). As defined by rectometrogram, patients with megarectum may be classified into a group, where constipation began at birth, and another one, where it was acquired later in life. The latter group is subdivided into a group, where colorectal transit time is normal and another one where it is slow, suggesting that constipation and megarectum links are complex (Verduron et al 1988).

tion instead of expulsion. A similar pathology exists in the anterior part of the pelvic floor. Vesicourethral dyssynergia is conducive to bladder retention and infection: patients contract the external urethral sphincter when they try to void (Pavlakis et al 1986). Not surprisingly, patients with anismus have more frequent urinary symptoms (Veyrac et al 1988). Chronic pelvic tensions have been said to result from psychologic conflicts during childhood and lead to urinary control problems and diminished orgasmic response (Lowen 1967): the contractile strength of the pelvic floor muscles is related to both urinary control and orgasmic response (Meier 1977). Therefore, the pelvic floor should be treated as a neuromuscular unit, taking into account the functions of all orifices.

The demonstration of anismus may be done in several ways. At defaecography the anorectal angle is narrow and does not open during straining to defaecate; on rare occasions it becomes more narrow during straining. Electromyographic evidence of pelvic floor contraction may be found during attempted defaecation. Another way to search for anismus is to record at anorectal manometry the anal resting pressure during a Valsalva manoeuvre. An abnormality associated with anismus is related not to straining but to rectal distension: occasionally, in the midst of the

rectoanal inhibitory reflex it is possible to record an external anal sphincteric contraction (Devroede 1985). This is found in 45% of encopretic children who exhibit external anal sphincter contraction during expulsion, and this, of course, is thought to contribute to faecal retention (Wald et al 1986). A final and clinical way to detect anismus is to ask the ptient to strain while doing a rectal examination.

Descending perineum syndrome

In some constipated patients, the perineum descends during straining, and this can be measured by defaecography. Although anismus may be present (Rutter 1974; Kuijpers et al 1986), in about half of the patients there is prolonged inhibition of the pelvic floor muscles (Rutter 1974; Bartolo et al 1985); mean motor unit potential duration is prolonged, indicating neuropathic changes (Bartolo et al 1985). It is possible that the descending perineum syndrome is the consequence of anismus, and that the long-term result of denervation (Bartolo et al 1985; Bartolo et al 1983; Kiff et al 1984) abolishes the pelvic floor muscle activity, but this has not been studied longitudinally to learn the natural history of anismus and the descending perineum syndrome.

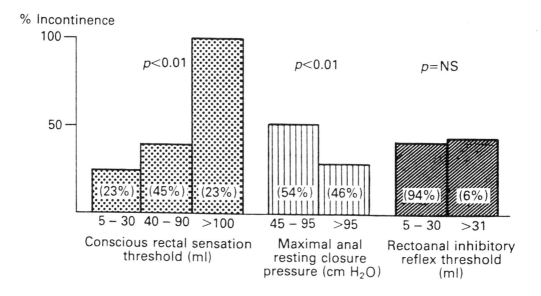

Fig. 37.38 Faecal incontinence in chronically constipated (< 3 stools/week) children (% subjects with abnormality). This figure suggests that the incidence of faecal incontinence increases as the level of constant rectal sensation rises, and might imply a sensory problem in the rectal wall. Yet, as seen in patients with megarectum (Verduron et al 1988), the same would occur in case of a hypotonic bowel wall, regardless of sensory mechanisms (Meunier et al 1976).

Megarectum

In patients with megarectum (Fig. 37.37), the rectal wall has little elasticity (Verduron et al 1988). Although impaired rectal sensation has been reported (Meunier et al 1976) (Fig. 37.38), the level of pressure at which sensation occurs is the same regardless of rectal volume, suggesting the nature of the problem being not impaired rectal sensation but inelasticity of the musculature (Verduron et al 1988). The rectoanal inhibitory reflex is also impaired, since it is triggered by rectal accommodation (Arhan et al 1979); its amplitude is lesser than normal, and the reflex can even be abolished at low levels of distention, mimicking Hirschsprung's disease. Patients with constipation from birth, found to have megarectum, differ from those who become constipated later in life: colonic transit is normal and storage exists exclusively in the rectum, which accommodates huge volumes (Fig. 37.39). They are all incontinent and, predominantly, males. In patients with late-onset megarectum (predominantly females) a greater recorded as compared with recalled stool frequency, clinical improvement by vastly different treatment modalities such as surgery or psychotherapy, delayed transit at the colonic as well as rectal level, and absence of

correlation between colonic transit and rectal capacity (Fig. 37.40) all point to a functional problem (Verduron et al 1988). Only half of these patients have faecal incontinence unrelated to stool frequency.

The diagnosis of megarectum may be made on barium enema (Preston et al 1985) or from rectometrographic studies (Verduron et al 1988). There is a correlation between them which justifies the repetitive use of rectal accommodation studies as index of quality control during follow-up (Bouchoucha et al 1989) (Fig. 37.41). Simply measuring the recto-pelvic ratio, or rectal diameter, is a poor reflection of the elastic properties of the rectum (Meunier et al 1984). Thus, in many studies of patients with constipation, patients with megarectum are mixed with others who don't have any, and this explains why an increase in rectal compliance is not always found (Loening-Baucke 1990; Meunier et al 1984; Loening-Baucke 1991; Varma & Smith 1988). Technical modalities are also crucial: a decreased compliance, sometimes found in constipation (Roe et al 1986), may be due to faster rates of rectal infusion, which render the rectum more resistant to distension (Sun et al 1990) (Fig. 37.42) and decrease (Fig. 37.43) the reproducibility (Fig. 37.44) of rectometrographic studies (Kendall et al 1990).

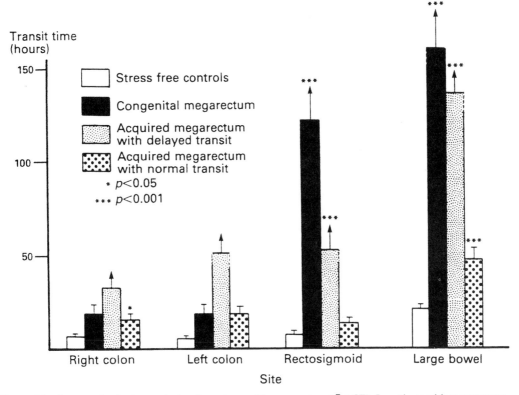

Fig. 37.39 Segmental colonic transit time in patients with megerectum ($\bar{X}$ + SE). In patients with megerectum who were constipated at birth, colonic transit is near normal and thus there is outlet obstruction (Verduron et al 1988).

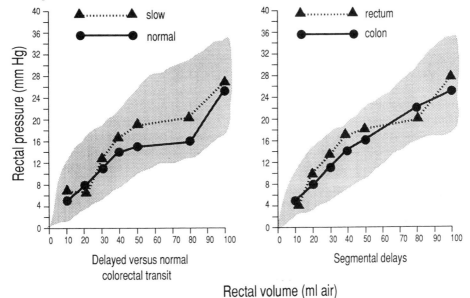

Fig. 37.40 Rectal elasticity does not correlate with colorectal transit times in chronic constipation. The rectometrogram does not differ, whether colorectal transit is normal or slow, and if slow, whether there is colonic or rectal delay. This is ample evidence that ascribing constipation to rectal accommodation abnormalities only is simplistic (De Medicis et al 1989).

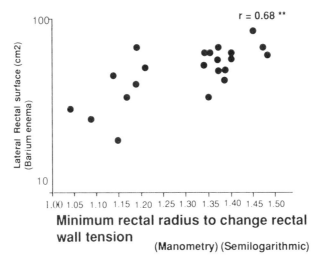

Fig. 37.41   Correlation between rectal surface and accommodation. Rectal surface on barium enema correlates well (p less than 0.01) to the minimal rectal radius necessary during rectal accommodation studies to trigger a change in rectal wall tension. Thus, the rectometrogram, without radiation, may be used in lieu of the barium enema during the follow up of patients with rectal accommodation disorders (Bouchoucha et al 1989).

The relationship between anismus and megarectum is not well known. Constipated children who have faecal incontinence, often have anismus (Wald et al 1986) and greater rectal compliance than those who don't (Cucchiara et al 1984). Conversely, constipated patients with anismus have increased rectal compliance at the level of constant sensation (Lestar et al 1991) (Fig. 37.45). Thus, it is possible that megarectum and faecal soiling in children are the consequence of anismus. No specific study of anismus, however, has been done in patients with megarectum. There is anecdotal observation of their association, as demonstrated by electromyography (Jennings 1967), and this is also found in chronically constipated children with encopresis who pass episodically very large amounts of stools, sufficient to clog the toilet, and are thus likely to have a megarectum (Loening-Baucke & Cruikshank 1986). Also, patients with constipation and megarectum tend to increase anal pressure to greater extent during straining than those who have normal barium enema (Barnes & Lennard-Jones 1988) (Fig. 37.46). No prospective study of rectal accommodation in patients who initially have anismus and normal rectal compliance has been done, and this is what is needed before concluding that anismus produces megarectum. Conversely, recovery from anismus through biofeedback with synchronous recovery of normal rectal compliance (unpublished obervation) provides no definitive answer because biofeedback therapy is multifactorial in elements including some working through the psyche. There is not even a single study evaluating together clinical symptoms, colorectal transit times, rectal accommodation and pelvic floor dyssynergia. Thus, there are two distinct possibilities: (1) megarectum may coexist with anismus but be independent; and (b) megarectum is the consequence of anismus.

What is the link between megarectum and faecal impaction in the elderly? There is little, if any, change in large bowel function, with age, in healthy subjects (Varma & Smith 1984), and the elasticity of the rectal wall of constipated patients does not change (Bouchoucha et al 1989; Devroede et al 1982 (Fig. 37.47) with aging despite marked morphological differences. Faecal impaction occurs in half of elderly patients and they have reduced rectal sensitivity (Read et al 1985). Conversely, some elderly constipated patients who have a megarectum present with faecal impaction, but most have decreased rectal compliance (Varma et al 1988) (Fig. 37.48). Patients with lack of sensation, in fact, have a megarectum, the decreasing compliance accounting for the lack of sensation (Fig. 37.49). Constipated patients may be subdivided into those with hypo-

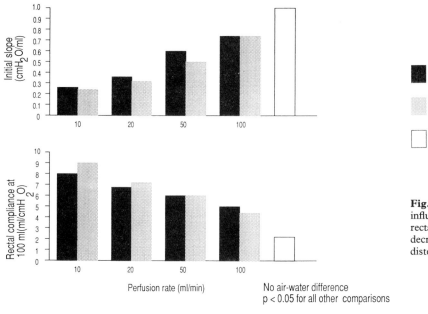

Water inflation

Air inflation

Intermittent rapid distension

Perfusion rate (ml/min)

No air-water difference
$p < 0.05$ for all other comparisons

Fig. 37.42 Rectal accommodation is influenced by technical modalities of rectal distension. Rectal compliance decreases with increasing rate of rectal distension (Sun et al 1990).

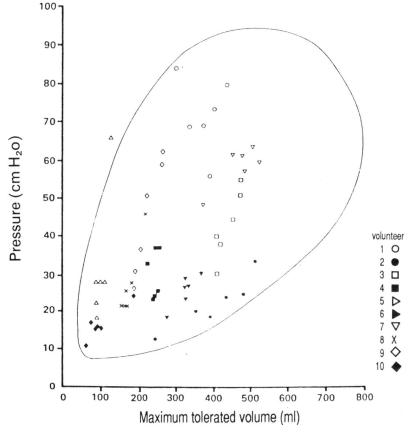

volunteer
1 ○
2 ●
3 □
4 ■
5 ▷
6 ▶
7 ▽
8 ✕
9 ◇
10 ◆

Fig. 37.43 The rectum of a human being is not an inflatable balloon. If the rectum is treated as a child's balloon and quickly (in this case: 150 ml/min!) distended as if it was inert material, wide dispersion of data are to be expected, presumably because of individual sensitivites (Kendall et al 1990).

(95% bivariate confidence)

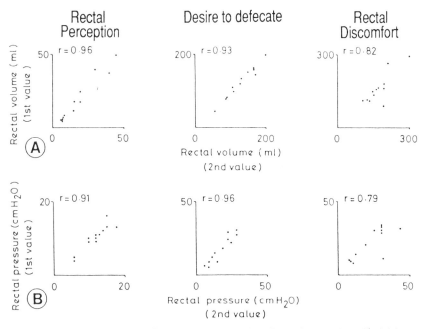

Fig. 37.44 Reproducibility of rectometrogram at slow distension rate (20 ml/min) in healthy males. When properly done, rectometrographic studies are highly reproducible (Sun et al 1990).

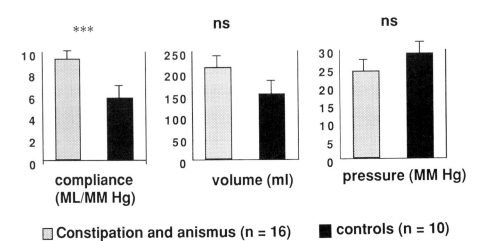

Fig. 37.45 Anismus and rectal compliance. Patients, who are constipated and have anismus, have a greater rectal compliance at the level of constant sensation, either as a consequence, or simply in association. To distinguish the two possibilities, prospective studies of rectal compliance in subjects who develop anismus should be done but are hardly conceivable. Two other ways of investigation are to follow up rectal accommodation after correction of anismus, and do case control studies, matching carefully constipated patients with anismus to constipated patients with similar motor dysfunctions except anismus, and compare their rectal compliance (Lestar et al 1991).

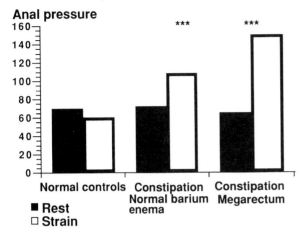

Fig. 37.46 Megarectum and anismus. In this study, all constipated patients increase anal pressure during straining rather than relaxing it, but those with megarectum do it to a greater extent (Barnes & Lennard-Jones 1988).

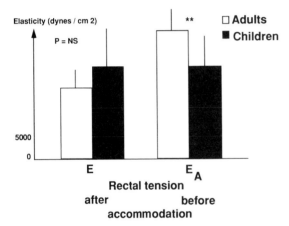

Fig. 37.47 Effects of age on rectal elasticity. Although adults react to sudden rectal distension by a greater increase in rectal wall tension (E_A), once accommodation has settled, the elasticity (E) is similar to that in children (Bouchoucha et al 1989).

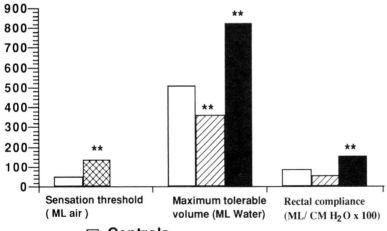

Fig. 37.48 Rectal accommodation in elderly constipated patients. In this study, elderly constipated patients may have either a megarectum or one of lesser capacity than normal (Varma et al 1988).

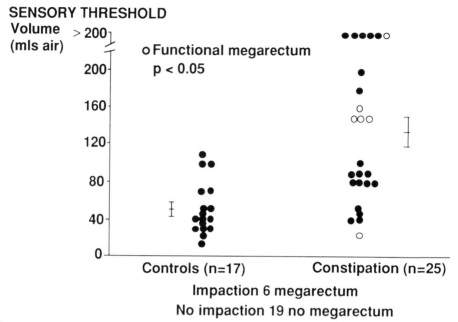

Fig. 37.49 Rectal sensation in elderly constipated patients. Compare this figure with Fig. 37.48. It is clear that half of patients with decreased rectal sensation also have a megarectum, and the lack of tone in the bowel wall by itself may explain the blunting of sensation (Varma et al 1988).

motor activity of the large bowel, hypermotile or normal activity (Fig. 37.50) (Meunier et al 1979). It appears that children and the elderly tend to have a hypotonic rectum, but the natural history of these motor patterns is unknown. Factors other than age may have an impact. For instance, in patients where intractable constipation develops after hysterectomy, there may be increased rectal volumes and compliance, with accompanying deficit of rectal sensory function. This decreased motor activity of the distal large bowel is accompanied by a pressure profile against propulsion of faeces following neostigmine stimulation, and an exacerbated response to carbachol (Fig. 37.51) (Smith et al 1990); in another study, however, no difference from patients with de novo constipation was found (Roe et al 1988).

Children with constipation and encopresis produce methane much more often than those who are constipated but without encopresis, or controls, and most stop producing methane when constipation is treated successfully (Fiedorek et al 1990). Breath methane analysis is thus a useful indirect tool to assess the interaction of constipation and intracolonic bacterial metabolism.

Anorectal structures during defaecation

To evaluate anorectal structures during defaecation, defaecography has proved very disappointing for two main reasons. First, in normal subjects without defaecatory disturbance, there is a high incidence of mucosal prolapse, intussusception and rectocele, even with barium entrapment after the examination, and broad ranges of anorectal angle and pelvic floor descent overlap with reported pathological states (Shorvon et al 1989; Wald et al 1990; Berretta et al 1990; Bartram et al in press). Second, there is marked observer variation in the radiological measurement of the anorectal angle (Penninckx et al 1990).

Rectal sensation

Rectal sensation is often decreased in constipation (Devroede 1993a). It is more severely reduced in patients with objective evidence of prolonged gastrointestinal transit time (Fig. 37.52) and, among them, those with slow transit in the rectum (De Medicis et al 1989) (Fig. 37.53), but this is disputed (Wald et al 1989). Impaired rectal sensation is not related to the capacity to defaecate balloons placed in the rectum (Loening-Baucke & Cruikshank 1986), rectal compliance, or threshold for internal sphincter relaxation (Wald 1986; Wald et al 1989). In patients with megarectum, sensation occurs at a given level of rectal pressure, regardless of rectal volume; this suggests that hypoesthesia is entirely secondary to inelasticity of the rectum (Verduron et al 1988). The subject of rectal sensation is an open field for research.

Sacral reflex function

Electrical stimulation of the dorsogenital nerve may, on occasion, fail to elicit an evoked reflex activity in the external anal and urethral sphincters in some constipated women (Kerrigan et al 1989; Varma & Smith 1988; Varma et al 1988). This suggests impairment of the integration of sensory information, or nerve damage to the efferent side of the reflex.

Constipation with normal transit times

Many constipated patients have normal gastrointestinal transit times, but this depends on the selection modalities (Devroede 1993a). For instance, most patients with painful constipation have normal transit, but not those with painless constipation (Lanfranchi et al 1984). Normal transit may be found in patients who defaecate less than twice a week (Wald 1986) as well as in those with megarectum (Verduron et al 1988). It also depends on the definition of normality: transit is faster in controls whose bowel habits are not modified by stress (Verduron et al 1988; Bouchoucha et al 1992; Schang et al 1985).

Patients with normal transit times often take psychotropic agents, particularly antidepressants, receive psychiatric counselling and are involved in litigation, in contrast to what is observed in patients with delayed transit (Wald 1986). They have more psychopathology (Wald et al 1983). Some – but not all – of them clearly deny they defaecate: markers disappear from plain films of their abdomen, while they fail to report any stool (Hinton & Lennard-Jones 1968; Preston et al 1984b; Devroede 1989). The diagnosis is that of Münchausen's syndrome if the pseudo-diagnosis of constipation leads to unnecessary surgery (Devroede 1989), or pseudologia fantastica if it only implies the clinician's puzzling frustration.

Prognosis varies according to mechanisms of constipation. Even if subjective improvement occurs in up to 40% of all groups of patients during medical treatment, objective evaluation confirms this only in patients with constipation by hindgut dysfunction or outlet obstruction. Only 17% of patients with colonic inertia and 10% of those with normal transit constipation improve during follow-up (Wald 1986; Heywood et al 1991). In children, the presence of abdominal pain is an indicator of a successful treatment for chronic constipation (Fig. 37.54). As time goes by without success, the outcome becomes poorer. Even if they are continent, the prognosis is far from perfect (Abrahamian & Lloyd-Still 1984).

THE APPROACH TO A CONSTIPATED PATIENT

Organic evaluation

Constipation is a problem of little boys, and adult women. There is a sexist element that cannot be avoided and is unexplained. Functional disorders in other systems are often present and should not be forgotten by focusing in a simplistic fashion on a target organ (Fig. 37.55).

The key question to ask at first visit is about the onset of constipation. Most patients who have Hirschsprung's disease or myelomeningocele, have had difficulties with their bowel habits from birth. Later in life, constipation of recent onset is frequently due to significant pathology. The most important disease to rule out is, of course, colonic malignancy. A history of 2 years or more is a safe cut-off point (Kruis et al 1984).

Faecal impaction should be looked for in patients with constipation, but also in those with faecal incontinence: up to 20% of children, where incontinence is associated with faecal impaction, are treated with anti-diarrhoeal drugs (Cucchiara et al 1984).

Absence of cutaneous sensations around the anus may indicate the level of neurological lesions. Anal canal tone at rest, evaluated digitally, correlates fairly well with the incidence of incontinence (Stewart & Dodds 1979). Gaping of the anal canal, when the puborectalis muscle is grasped by the examining finger and pulled posteriorly, is not normal. In cervical transection, the anus remains closed and a balloon can be retained in the rectum, whereas in low lesions of the medulla, the anus is patulous and unable to contract to prevent extrusion of the balloon (Connell et al 1963). Buggery in young children, including infants and toddlers, is a serious, common and under-reported type of child abuse (Hobbs & Wynne 1986). Since

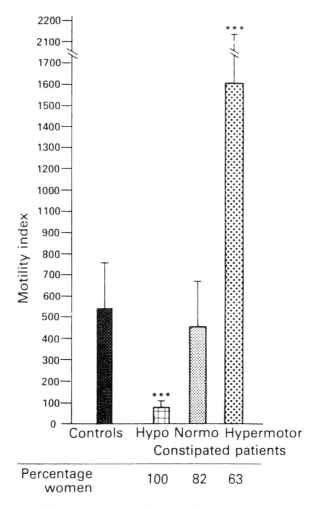

Fig. 37.50 Motor activity of the sigmoid colon in patients with chronic idiopathic constipation (< 3 stools/week). The motor response of the sigmoid colon to a meal makes it possible to distinguish different types of constipation (Meunier et al 1979).

constipation is associated with sexual abuse (Drossman et al 1990; Devroede 1990; Devroede et al 1989a; Drossman in press; De San Lazaro 1989; Rimsza et al 1988; Arnold et al 1990; Denis et al 1992; Leroi et al submitted), signs of anal abuse should be looked for. These include: shortening or eversion of the anal canal and proximation of the anorectal junction to the external orifice, i.e. the anal canal is laid open; single or multiple anal fissures not only seen posteriorly but in other segments of the anus; external blue discoloration, venous swelling and haematomas; and swelling of the perianal tissue (Hobbs & Wynne 1986; Hobbs & Wynne 1989). However, it is unsafe to diagnose sexual abuse on the basis of anal dilatation only in a child who is grossly constipated (Clayden 1988; Agnarrson et al 1990; McCann et al 1989; Cannon et al 1988; Priestley & Taitz 1989). Anismus can be appreciated grossly during rectal examination. The patient is asked to strain, while the clinician keeps his or her finger in the rectum. Patients with anismus will squeeze. Descent of the perineum is also easy to recognize and is often associated with a rectocele.

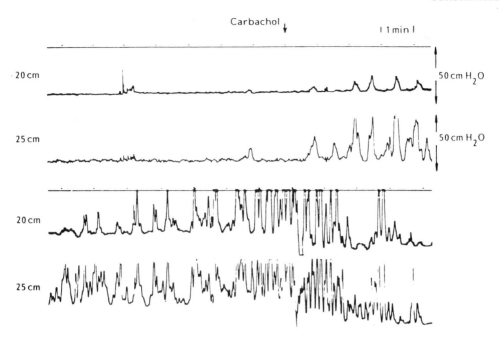

Fig. 37.51 Hypersensitive response to carbachol. The colon of this hysterectomized patient, who developed severe constipation after surgery, reacts markedly to carbachol injection (Smith et al 1990).

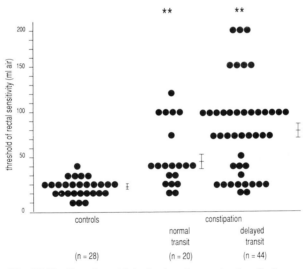

Fig. 37.52 Rectal sensitivity in chronic constipation. Patients with slow-transit constipation tend to have blunted rectal sensation (De Medicis et al 1989).

of the perineum is also easy to recognize and is often associated with a rectocele.

Tests to be performed will vary according to the clinical evaluation (Devroede 1993a).

Endoscopy, with flexible instruments, will help rule out organic lesions. It is also useful to appreciate the degree of bowel spasticity. Melanosis coli is a term used to describe the appearance of the colonic mucosa after abuse of mainly, but exclusively anthracene laxatives (Badioli et al 1985).

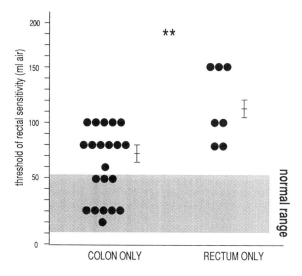

Fig. 37.53   Rectal sensitivity in chronic constipation with delayed transit. Among patients with slow-transit constipation, those with rectal stasis only have decreased rectal sensation as compared to those with colonic stasis only (De Medicis et al 1989).

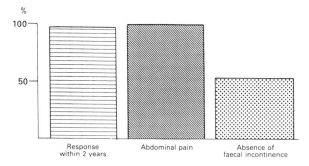

Fig. 37.54   Prognostic factors in chronic childhood constipation. Constipated children with abdominal pain will all eventually be cured. The response should be expected in a reasonably short period of time. In contrast, it is more difficult to help constipated children who are also faecally incontinent: faecal incontinence is present in 53% of children who will be cured from their constipation, while it is present in 89% of those who will not (Abrahamian & Lloyd-Still 1984).

In constipation of recent origin, a barium enema is mandatory to rule out organic disease, particularly carcinoma. In chronic constipation, the size of the distal bowel is greater than normal, but on a single examination the radiologist is unable to distinguish constipated from non-constipated patients, and the change in bowel size after treatment does not correlate well with its outcome (Patriquin et al 1978). A useful measure to remember is 6.5 cm, the upper limit of normal rectosigmoid width on lateral view at the pelvic brim (Preston et al 1985). In patients with long-segment Hirschprung's disease, a narrow rectum can be demonstrated at barium enema. However, in short-segment disease, and in total aganglianosis there is no narrow segment.

Ultrasound examination of the abdomen should be performed to detect dilatation of the renal collecting system often present in severe constipation (Herbetko & Hyde 1990).

The absence of neurons in a rectal suction biopsy specimen, taken at least 25 mm above the distal edge of the internal sphincter, is suggestive of Hirschprung's

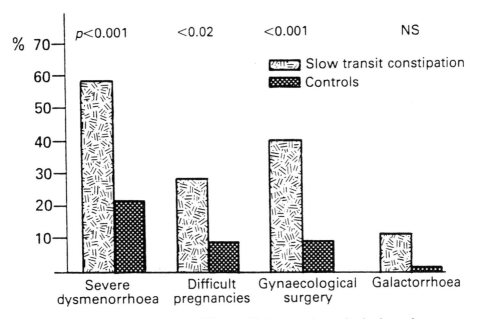

Fig. 37.55 Constipation and femininity. Women with slow-transit constipation have other complaints related to the fact of being female (Preston & Lennard-Jones 1986).

disease. Cholinesterase activity evaluation is the most sensitive way to make the diagnosis (Watier et al in press).

Functional evaluation

The technique of measurement of colonic transit times is simple, reproducible (Bouchoucha et al 1992), and can be done in any radiology department. The subject ingests radiopaque markers, remains on a high-residue diet, and refrains from laxatives, enemas and all non-essential drugs. The markets are commercially available (SITZMARKS R, Konsyl Pharmaceutical Inc, Fort Worth, Texas 76109) or simply cut from a radio-paque nasogastric tube. Stools may be visualized radio-graphically or, to distinguish between the different types of constipation, the progression of markers along the colon may be followed by daily radiographs of the abdomen. Films are taken until total expulsion of mark-ers, for a maximum of 7 days after ingestion. On plain films of the abdomen, constipation may be diagnosed if eight or more markers are retained 3 days after ingestion of 20 radiopaque markers (Bouchoucha et al 1992). To calculate segmental transit times, markers are counted in the right colon, left colon and rectosig-moid area by using the bony landmarks of the spine and pelvic contours. A simplified formula can be used if the patient swallows 20 markers and a film is ob-tained every 24 h: markers are counted in each colon segment, each day, until disappearance, numbers are added and the sum multiplied by 1.2 (Bouchoucha et al 1992; Arhan et al 1981). To minimize radiation, markers may be ingested repetitively instead of once, after which a single X-ray of the abdomen is taken following a variable length of time (Bouchoucha et al 1992; Chaussade et al 1989; Chaussade et al 1986; Metcalf et al 1987; Fotherby & Hunter 1987; Metcalf 1990). It should be clearly understood, however, that this technique does not measure mean transit time of a single marker, as the original technique did, but mean of mean transit times, presuming they do not change from day to day, which they do (Metcalf et al 1987). Moreover, the technique requires the establishment of steady-state conditions, and requires longer periods of ingestion as the severity of constipation increases. Markers should be ingested at least for 1 week in patients with normal transit constipation, 2 weeks in those with left colon dysfunction, and 4 weeks in those with colonic inertia (Bouchoucha et al 1989). As can be seen in table 37.1, there are important variations in upper limits of normal values found in different cen-tres. In some studies there are also gender differences (Metcalf et al 1987), while in others there are none (Chaussade et al 1990; Bouchoucha et al 1992; Hinds et al 1989). In subjects who do not react to stress, transit times are much shorter and there is also no difference between men and women (Bouchoucha et al

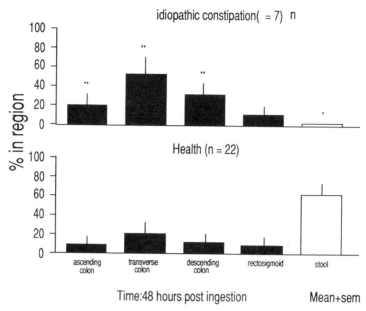

Fig. 37.56 Scintigraphic measurement of regional colonic transit in idiopathic constipation. Transit of radioactive material throughout the colon is delayed in patients with idiopathic constipation (Stivland et al 1991).

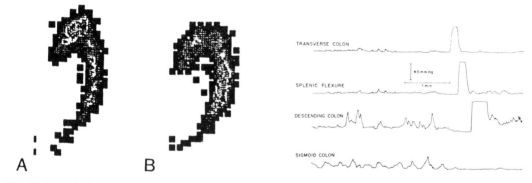

Fig. 37.57 Scintigraphic assessment of colonic propagating contraction. To the right of the figure, a high-amplitude colonic propagating contraction is shown. The scintigraphic counterpart to the left shows movement of bowel content (Bazzocchi et al 1990).

1992). With the single-ingestion multiple-X-rays technique, there were segmental differences between adults and children, but no overall difference was found in the entire large bowel (Arhan et al 1991); with the multiple-ingestion single-X-ray technique, this information is not available. It appears that children (Bautista et al 1991) resemble adults who claim stress does not modify their bowel habits nor trigger abdominal pain (Bouchoucha et al 1992) (Table 37.1). Markers can also be counted in stools, to evaluate mouth to anus transit time, but not segmental abnormalities along the gastrointestinal tract. The first marker should

be excreted by the end of the third day after ingestion, and 80% within 5 days (Hinton & Lennard-Jones 1968).

Colonic scintigraphy is a technique which may help recognize delayed colorectal transit in chronic idiopathic constipation (Fig. 37.56). Ingestion of a long peroral tube (Krevsky et al 1989; Kamm et al 1988) and instillation at the splenic flexure (Bazzocchi et al 1990) although useful (Figs. 37.57, 37.58, 37.59) will probably not become popular clinically. [111]In incorporated in non-digestible (Stubbs et al 1991) or coated capsules that disperse in the ileocaecal region (Stivland et al 1991), or Iodine-131-cellulose (McClean et al

Table 37.1 Maximum 'normal' transit time through the large bowel

Adults	(Mean + 2 S.D., in hours)[*]						
	Chaussade 1986	Chaussade 1990	Metcalf 1990	Arhan 1981	Hinds 1989	Bouchoucha 1992	Bouchoucha 1992[**]
Right colon	24	24	32	38	24	37	20
Left colon	30	31	39	37	32	26	14[a]
Rectosigmoid	44	33	36	34	45	41	25
Colon and rectum (total)	67	67	68	93	76	88	43[a]
Markers technique	Multiple ingestion			Single ingestion			

Children	Arhan 1981 (single ingestion)	Bautista 1991 (multiple ingestion)
Right colon	18	18
Left colon	20	18
Rectosigmoid	34	19
Colon and rectum (total)	62	50

[*] Except for data from Arhan's study, which are not calculated from a gaussian curve but are the maximal experimental values
[**] Stress-free controls
a $p < 0.01$, as compared to other controls

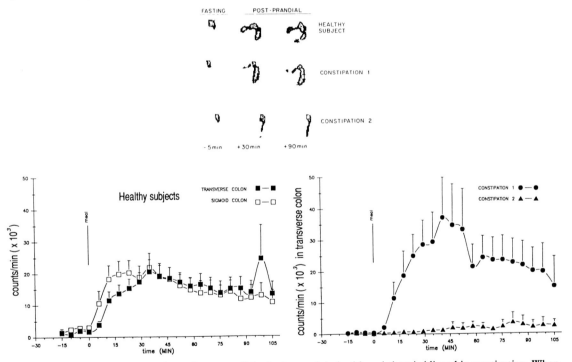

Fig. 37.58 Scintigraphic assessment of postprandial colonic transit in health and chronic idiopathic constipation. When radioactive material is placed at the splenic flexure and the subject eats, there is, normally (left of the figure), an increase in counts in the transverse and sigmoid colon, indicative of retrograde and antegrade propulsion. In constipation (right of the figure), using retrograde movement to the transverse colon, as an index, one of two patterns can be observed: a hypomotile situation with no change in counts proximal to the splenic flexure, and a normal pattern (Bazzocchi et al 1990).

1990), provide non-invasive technique. When the bolus of isotope is liberated into the caecum, calculation of transit time in the distal sites is markedly dependent on what occurs more proximally, creating a source of

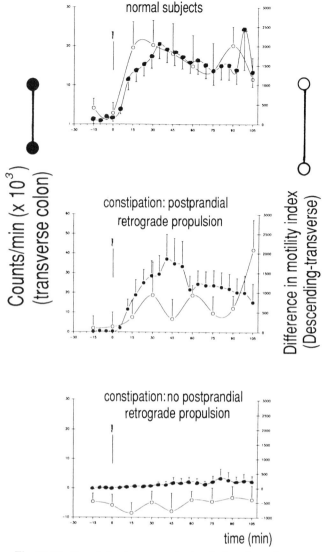

Fig. 37.59 Correlation between colonic scintigraphy and intraluminal pressure. Meal has been used in this study as a colonic stimulus. It triggers similar changes in scintigraphy and intraluminal pressure recording (see Fig. 37.58 to understand the three groups of subject) (Bazzocchi et al 1990).

error (Arhan et al 1981). Transits of radiopaque markers appear to be faster than those obtained by scintigraphy (Stivland et al 1991; Proano et al 1990): the relative importance of particle size on transit (Tomlin & Read 1988), particularly in the liquid milieu of the ascending colon, and that of methodology are unknown. For instance, ingesting markers for 3 days in a row in a constipated patient (Stivland et al 1991) is insufficient to reach steady-state conditions (Bouchoucha et al 1992). Dynamic scanning of the large

bowel with either food (Bazzocchi et al 1990) or bisacodyl (Kamm et al 1988) (Fig. 37.60) stimulation will most likely become essential to distinguish patients with slow-transit constipation who have a hypomotile colon from those who have a hypermotile colon.

Recording electrical activity in the large bowel may occasionally be a key element to dictate conduct (Likongo et al 1986). Sporadic spike bursts, particularly when propagating, are associated with both intraluminal pressure waves and significant propulsion of

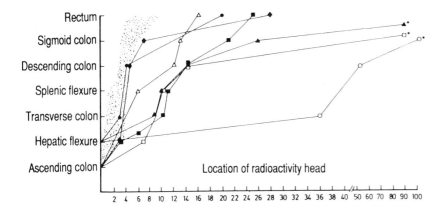

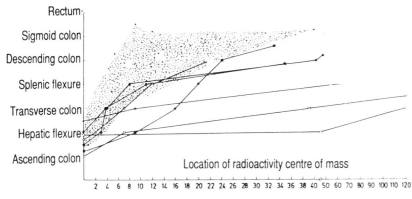

Fig. 37.60 Dynamic scanning in health and constipation. In this scintigraphic study, radioactive material has been placed in the caecum, and followed by bisacodyl infusion in the same site. It can be clearly seen that it takes longer in constipation for the material to reach the rectum, with evidence for a group where patients are almost similar to healthy subjects, material reaching the rectum within 24 h, and three other patients where it trails in the colon (Kamm et al 1988).

bowel content; rhythmic bursts, on the other hand, do not seem to be involved in colonic propulsive activity (Schang et al 1986).

The usefulness of anorectal manometry on a single patient is limited at present to the diagnosis of Hirschsprung's disease, where there is no rectoanal inhibitory reflex (Watier et al in press) (Fig. 37.61), and that of anismus (Meunier 1991) (Fig. 37.14). Studies of the elastic properties of the rectum permit it to distinguish outlet obstruction by hypo- or hypertonic rectum from simple anal achalasia (Fig. 37.62). Viscous properties (evaluated through rapid air distension) reflect accommodation of the rectum to distension, and elastic properties (evaluated through slow water distension) the residual tension after accommodation. Injection of 10 ml of water within 5 s every 30 s provides reliable and reproducible measurements.

The search for anismus has provided some impetus to more routine performance of electromyography of the external anal sphincter and the puborectalis muscle, with needles or less invasive plug electrodes (Fig. 37.14).

Balloon defaecation is used to investigate rectoanal dynamics during defaecation (Loening-Baucke & Cruikshank 1986; Barnes & Lennard-Jones 1985). The ballon proctogram also permits evaluation of the anorectal angle and its relationship with the pubococcygeal level (Preston et al 1984). Balloon topography, in addition to this, yields opening pressures of the anal canal during distension, and anal canal length (Lahr et al 1986). Defaecometry is a promising technique, which records the pressure within a balloon, over time, as it is defaecated. This is the only technique capable of detecting the amount of work performed during defaecation (Lestar et al 1989).

Defaecography, performed with a barium paste that

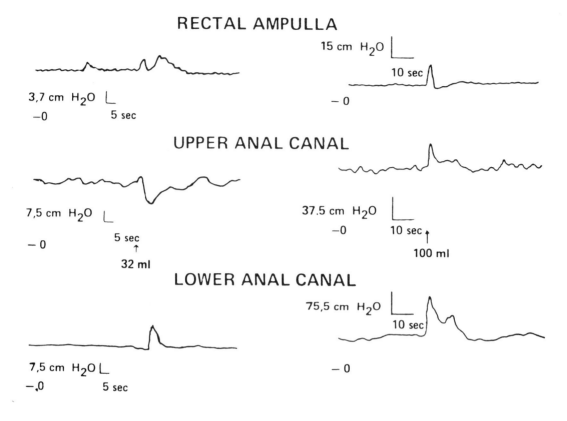

RECTAL AMPULLA

15 cm H$_2$O

10 sec

— 0

3,7 cm H$_2$O

—0   5 sec

UPPER ANAL CANAL

7,5 cm H$_2$O

— 0   5 sec

↑

32 ml

37.5 cm H$_2$O

—0   10 sec ↑

100 ml

LOWER ANAL CANAL

75,5 cm H$_2$O

10 sec

7,5 cm H$_2$O

—,0   5 sec

— 0

Fig. 37.61   To the left of the figure, is a normal recording of anorectal motility before and after sudden and short lived (5 s) rectal distension. A normal rectoanal inhibitory reflex is seen in the upper anal canal (middle line). In contrast, to the right of the figure, this patient has no reflex even after 10 s rectal distension with 100 ml: he has Hirschsprung's disease (original recording).

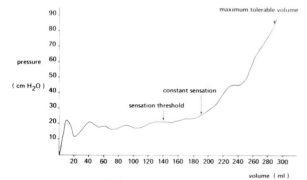

pressure
(cm H$_2$O)

maximum tolerable volume

constant sensation

sensation threshold

20 40 60 80 100 120 140 160 180 200 220 240 260 280 300

volume (ml)

Fig. 37.62   Elastic properties of the human rectum. A normal rectometrogram (original data).

reproduces stool consistency (Mahieu et al 1984), is useful to confirm the existence of a complete rectal prolapse, or a rectocele (Fig. 37.63), and to put some light on other data obtained during the investigation.

The rectum is composed of three different functional zones (Figs. 37.64, 37.65). Digital substraction recording (Fig. 37.66) will probably change our views about anal and rectal function (Lesaffer 1990; Costalat et al 1989; Garrigues et al 1989).

Who is that constipated person? Constipation is not only the passage of hard and infrequent stools via different investigable mechanisms, but what this does subjectively to the patient. Recording a life history as well as a case history is essential. An interview reviewing in-depth major life experiences serves this purpose (Devroede 1985; Devroede 1993b). A cruder approach is to use the MMPI or another psychological test and relate the findings and profile interpretation to the patient. The existence of a sexual abuse in the past history must be recognized. Disclosure of the trauma, particularly if it is accompanied with emotional release, may suddenly cure constipation associated with what has been labelled the pathogenic secret. Anxiety is

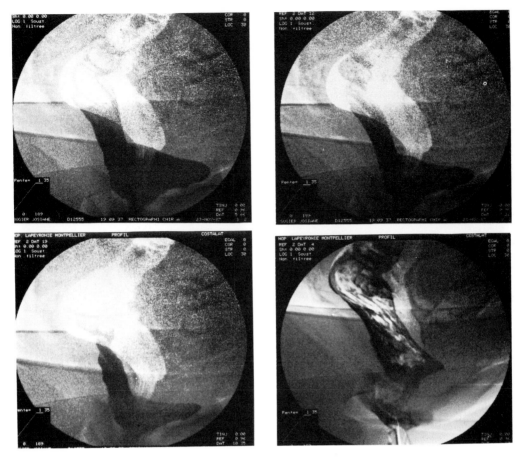

Fig. 37.63 Digital superposition of lateral X-ray of the rectum at rest (white) and during straining (black) provides clear evidence of a rectocele in this patient. Progression is top to bottom, left to right (courtesy of doctor J. M. Garrigues) (Garrigues et al 1989; Costalat et al 1989).

replaced by constipation in some patients (Fig. 37.67): disappearance of constipation may enhance anxiety, much more easy to handle with words and thus cure the somatization.

Treatment

Staying in a spa station brings a significant but very short-lived reduction in transit time (Nisard et al 1982) (Fig. 37.68); but in patients who are clinically improved, functional disorders persist over long periods of time (Loening-Baucke 1984) (Fig. 37.69). These observations must be kept in mind to critically evaluate all available data on the treatment of constipation. No random study of any kind of treatment has ever been done which takes into account the natural history of constipation: out of 200 patients with functional abdominal complaints, 34 were found to suffer from

constipation and only one had become asymptomatic at follow-up 2 years later (Bleijenberg & Kuijpers 1987). Displacement of symptoms into another system is also a possibility. Long-term results with evaluation of the total person are needed.

A critical evaluation of the treatment of constipation may be found elsewhere (Devroede 1993a). The following is a brief review of what can be tried when no specific aetiology has been found to be responsible for the constipation.

The quality of the doctor–patient relationship is a determinant for outcome in the field of constipation. Patients are often dismissed – with a high level of frustration – as 'not sick' or 'sick in their head', or told that 'nothing can be done': functional disorders are not synonymous with no disorders. Making a positive diagnosis that there is something wrong and relating the findings of the functional evaluation of constipation

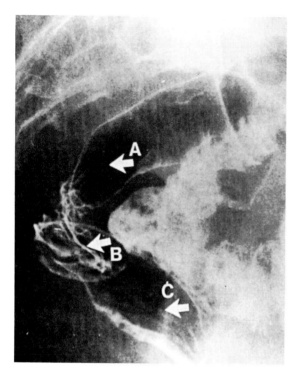

Fig. 37.64   As seen on this lateral air-contrast film of the rectum, there are three components: the sacral portion of rectum (A), the ampullary portion of the rectum (C), and their transitional zone, the sacculum recti, where the Houston valves create transverse folds (B). (Courtesy of doctor Luc Lesaffer) (Lesaffer 1990).

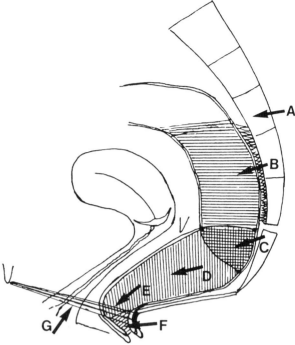

Fig. 37.65   A schematic illustration of Fig. 37.64, showing the functional zones of the anorectum: A: sacrum; B: sacral portion of the rectum; C: transitional zone; D: ampullary portion of rectum; E: anorectal junction (hiatus); F: anal canal; G: puborectalis muscle (Courtesy of doctor Luc Lesaffer) (Lesaffer 1990).

serves an important purpose to establish a therapeutic alliance with the patient. When a trust is present, it becomes easier to relate the message that the basis for functional abnormality is not necessarily organic.

Personality differences exert as much influence on stool output as dietary fibre (Tucker et al 1981). This casts a shadow on data available with regard to the effects of dietary fibres on bowel function. They increase stool weight, frequency and water content (Cummings 1984), but have the least effect when patients are constipated, with low stool output and slow transit (Muller-Lissner 1988). Moreover, there is a strong placebo effect to dietary fibre (Ornstein et al 1981; Soltolt et al 1976). The increase in stool weight correlates with increased intake of pentose-containing polymers present in the fibre; fibres that take up most water in vitro have the least effects on bowel habit, while the most effective faecal bulkers, such as bran, hold very little water on a weight to weight basis (Cummings 1984). Faecal microbial mass increases when dietary fibre is fed, and this correlates with

faster transits (Cummings 1984; Cummings 1983). A trial with a high-fibre diet should be done prior to any investigation, in patients with chronic idiopathic constipation, and a diary kept prospectively. A difference between recalled and recorded stool frequency may result from diet, unconscious or conscious exaggeration of the problem, or transferential mechanisms, and is important information to obtain.

Faecal impactions should be treated as soon as recognized, with multiple enemas and laxatives.

Spending time on the toilet at regular intervals, is seldom prescribed as a sole treatment, but is as effective as prescribing laxatives (Nolan et al 1991).

Laxatives or enemas may be used to reinstate normal bowel habits. This brings a 50–75% cure rate over long-term periods (Davidson et al 1963; Cucchiara et al 1984; Sarahan et al 1982; Lowery et al 1985). There are some limitations to this simple approach. The success rate is much lower in constipated children without faecal soiling than in those with, despite similarly prolonged colorectal transit times (Cucchiara et

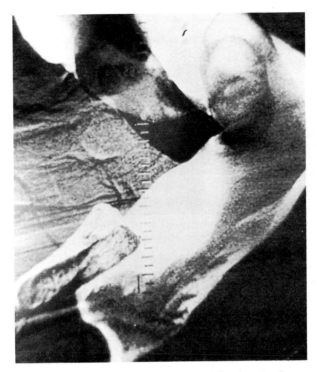

Fig. 37.66 A normal digital substraction defaecography. In white, film taken 4 s after onset of straining. In black, image is taken at end of defaecation while still straining (courtesy of doctor Luc Lesaffer) (Lesaffer 1990).

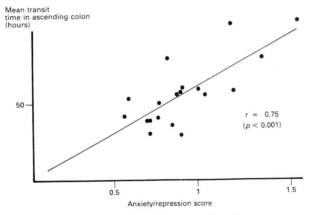

Fig. 37.67 Constipation as a mirror of anxiety. In some chronically constipated subjects anxiety correlates to transit time in the ascending colon. The scores of anxiety and repression were measured with the Minnesota Multiphasic Personality Inventory (Devroede et al 1989).

al 1984). There is a 30% drop-out rate from treatment (Cucchiara et al 1984; Lowery et al 1985) in children and 50% in adults (Eshchar & Cohen 1981).

Finally, one child in four substitutes one or more entirely new symptoms to constipation (Levine et al 1980).

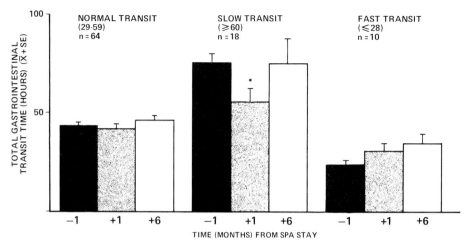

Fig. 37.68 Effect of a stay in a spa station on intestinal transit time of patients with IBS. Holidays improve constipation (Nisard et al 1982).

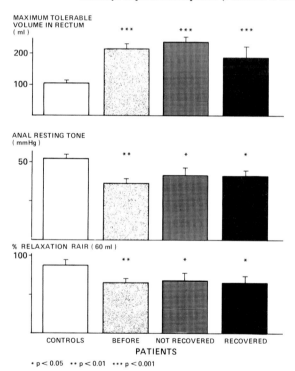

Fig. 37.69 Long-term persistence (3 years) of abnormal anorectal motility in children with severe chronic constipation and encopresis ($\bar{X}$ + SE). Anorectal motility may remain persistently abnormal despite clinical improvement (Loening-Baucke 1984).

There is no good study on the effect of exercise, swimming and massages on constipation. Exercise per se does not modify bowel function in health.

Numerous studies provide evidence that biofeedback may correct anismus, if not constipation (Devroede 1993a). Pending questions are to know why and how this occurs, and in whom. All modalities of treatment aim at teaching subjects to relax the pelvic floor during straining, instead of contracting it (Fig. 37.70), but in most studies other variables are always associated. It would also be simplistic to reduce the approach of a psychofunctional abnormality to the correction of its manometric component (Denis et al 1990). Patients forget the technical act, complain spontaneously of sexual problems (Weber et al 1987b) and unleash emotions when the body is worked upon (Denis et al 1990); women with pelvic floor dysfunction who have been sexually abused refuse to go into psychotherapy, but accept biofeedback where they react a lot, interfering with the re-education process (Denis et al 1992). The technical act then becomes secondary and the technician, most of the time untrained for this, must listen to the patient's life history (Devroede 1993b). Thus, biofeedback therapy for anismus has been evaluated in randomized studies. As compared to ingestion of mineral oil therapy, in encopretic children also instructed to attempt defaecation each day after breakfast and dinner, there was a non-significant trend for superiority of biofeedback only in patients anismus (Wald et al 1987). A second controlled study compared biofeedback plus milk of magnesia therapy to milk of magnesia therapy alone, in a large group of children with anismus. Biofeedback was superior, but the cure rate in the group of patients randomized to milk of magnesia alone was only 15%, much lower than expected (Loening-Baucke 1990). Roughly one-third of

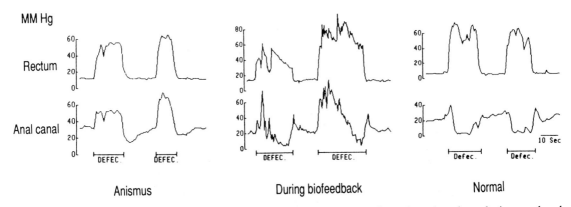

Fig. 37.70 Biofeedback correction of anismus. To the left, the patient squeezes the anal canal, as shown by increased anal canal pressure, when straining, as shown by increased rectal pressure. To the right, he still strains well, but relaxes the anal canal (Keren et al 1988).

patients cannot learn to relax the external anal sphincter, one-third can but do not recover from constipation, and the last third are cured from both anismus and constipation (Loening-Baucke 1991) (Fig. 37.71), with evidence of a learning curve (Fig. 37.72).

Psychotherapy improves symptoms of IBS, except constipation (Guthrie et al 1991). However, many of these patients are depressed or anxious (Guthrie et al 1991), and patients with slow-transit constipation have a lot of psychopathology, including a high level of self-control (Devroede et al 1989a; Devroede et al 1989b). It is probably unrealistic to expect benefits from psychotherapy within 3 months: a woman defaecating once every 2 months and raped at adolescence by her father, cured suddenly by putting a long letter in his coffin at his death; repeatedly prolonged colorectal transit times became suddenly normal permanently; this occurred after 50 visits over 5 years (Devroede et al 1989a). Group therapy reduces constipation in only 15% of subjects with severe symptoms but results in marked psychometric improvement on several dimensions (Wise et al 1982).

Hypnotherapy is superior to psychotherapy, in patients with severe refractory IBS, to reduce abdominal pain and distention, and improving bowel habits (Prior et al 1990b; Whorwell et al 1984; Whorwell et al 1987; Harvey et al 1989). Hypnosis is a learning process and, since constipation may be learned (Klauser et al 1990), it is logical to believe that it may be unlearned. The exact mechanisms by which hypnotherapy is effective are unclear, and no study has been done to see its effects on the individual founding symptoms, including constipation, but changes in rectal sensitivity occur during and after hypnotherapy (Prior et al 1990b).

In children, constipation may be part of a constellation of familial difficulties. They may be symptom free in the hospital, but constipated at home. Treatment includes convincing the parents that what they regard most of the time as physical disorder is in fact of emotional origin. Parents, because they feel implicated, tend to react with frank incredulity or hostile resistance (Pinkerton 1958). Play therapy with sand-trays (Pinkerton 1958), drawings (Pinkerton 1958; Trent 1992), plastic dough or ceramics (Huschka 1942; Feldman et al 1993), and releasing anger through competitive sports or with a device known as the aggression board (Pinkerton 1958) are useful. This approach alone, without any medical treatment, may cure for years two-thirds of constipated children (Pinkerton 1958) and, in particular, those refractory to all treatments (Feldman et al 1993).

Cisapride, a gastrointestinal prokinetic drug without antidopaminergic or direct cholinomimetic effects, is useful in constipation, but results depend on whether they are evaluated by patients or doctors, and it slows down normal transit. Rectal sensation improves with cisapride, but may also improve with other less specific therapeutic modalities (Devroede 1993a). Trimebutine interacts with opiate receptors in the intestine, and is useful in constipated patients who have evidence of delayed colonic transit, probably by stimulation of propagated electrical activity: proper selection of patients must include functional evaluation to appreciate the effects of a drug (Schang et al in press).

There is no place for surgery as long as there is anismus, and there is mounting evidence that surgery for chronic idiopathic constipation is a placebo procedure merely palliative in nature. Total colectomy with ileorectal anastomosis has not been the subject of

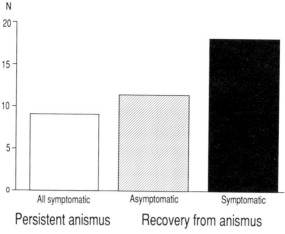

Fig. 37.71 Biofeedback training in children with severe constipation, encopresis and anismus. Children may recover from anismus and still be constipated (in black). This is ample evidence that constipation is often multifactorial in origin. For instance, many adult patients have both IBS – not expected to disappear simply by biofeedback reeducation of the pelvic floor – and anismus (Loening-Baucke 1991).

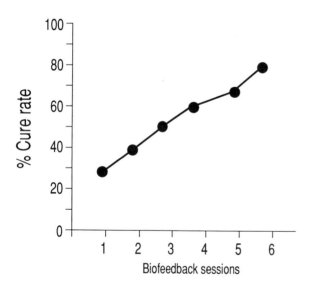

Fig. 37.72 Biofeedback therapy for anismus induces a learning process. There is evidence of a learning curve in biofeedback treatment of anismus. This is education, and not merely technique: all factors influencing education are at work (Loening-Baucke 1991).

a randomized study, should be performed only in the absence of oesophageal, gastric and small intestine motor dysfunction, and should only be considered in patients with severe complaints, and after extensive physiological and psychological evaluation (Rex et al 1992; Devroede 1992; Wald 1990; Fisher et al 1989).

When definitive therapy cannot be offered, laxatives may be prescribed. This has enormous economic impli-cations. Almost half a billion dollars worth of laxatives are sold annually in the USA. In Canada, at constant dollar value, laxative consumption has increased by 14% between 1986 and 1990. Consumption of bulk producing laxatives has increased by 38%, irritant stimulating laxatives by 17% and saline laxatives by 25%; in contrast, enemas have decreased by 9% and emollient laxatives by 10% (IMS Canada 1992).

REFERENCES

Abdel-Rahman M, Toppercer A, Duguay C et al 1981 Urorectodynamics in patients with colonic inertia. Urology 18: (4): 428–432

Abrahamian F P, Lloyd-Still J D 1984 Chronic constipation in childhood: a longitudinal study of 186 patients. J Pediatr Gastroenterol Nutr 3: 460–467

Agnarrson U, Warde C, McCarthy G, Evans N 1990 Perianal appearances associated with constipation. Arch Dis Child 65 (11): 1231–1234

Arhan P, Devroede G, Persoz B, Faverdin C, Dornic C, Pellerin D 1979 Response of the anal canal to repeated distension of the rectum. Clin Invest Med 2: 83–88

Arhan P, Devroede G, Jehannin B et al 1981 Segmental colonic transit time. Dis Colon Rectum 24: 625–629

Arhan P, Devroede G, Jehannin B et al 1983 Idiopathic disorders of faecal continence in children. Pediatrics 71: 774–779

Arnold R P, Rogers D, Cook D A G 1990 Medical problems of adults who were sexually abused in childhood. Br Med J 300: 705–708

Badioli D, Marcheggiano A, Pallone F et al 1985 Melanosis of the rectum in patients with chronic constipation. Dis Colon Rectum 28: 241–245

Bannister J J, Timms J M, Barfield L J, Donnelly T C, Read N W 1986 Physiological studies in young women with chronic constipation. Int J Colorect Dis 1: 175–182

Bannister J J, Davison P, Timms J M, Gibbons C, Read N W 1987 Effect of stool size and consistency on defecation. Gut 28: 1246–1250

Bannister J J, Lawrence W T, Smith A, Thomas D G, Read N W 1988 Urological abnormalities in young women with severe constipation. Gut 29: 17–20

Barnes P R H, Lennard-Jones J E 1985 Balloon expulsion from the rectum in constipation of different types. Gut 26: 1049

Barnes P R H, Hawley P R, Preston D M, Lennard-Jones J E 1985 Experience of posterior division of the puborectalis muscle in the management of chronic constipation. Br J Surg 72: 475

Barnes P R, Lennard-Jones J E 1988 Function of the striated anal sphincter during straining in control subjects and constipated patients with a radiologically normal rectum or idiopathic megacolon. Int J Colorectal Dis 3: 207–209

Bassotti G, Gaburri M, Clausi G G, Pelli M A, Morelli A 1987 Can idiopathic megacolon cause functional motor abnormalities in the upper gastrointestinal tract? Hepatogastroenterology 34: 186–189

Bassotti G, Gaburri M, Imbimbo B P et al 1988 Colonic mass movements in idiopathic chronic constipation. Gut 29: 1173–1179

Bartolo D C C, Read N W, Jarratt J A, Read M G, Donnelly T C, Johnson A G 1983 Differences in anal sphincter function and clinical presentation in patients with pelvic floor descent. Gastroenterology 85: 68

Bartolo D C C, Roe A M, Virjee J, Mortensen N J 1985 Evacuation proctography in obstructed defecation and rectal intussuception. Br J Surg 72: S111

Bartram C I, Turnbull G K, Lennard-Jones J E Evacuation proctography – a study of 20 subjects without defaecation disturbance. Gastrointest Radiol (in press)

Battle W M, Snape W J Jr, Alair A, Cohen S, Braunstein S 1980 Colonic dysfunction in diabetes mellitus. Gastroenterology 79: 1217

Bautista C A, Varela C A, Villanueva J, Castro-Gago M, Cadranel S, Tojo Sierra R 1991 Measurement of colonic transit time in children. J Pediatr Gastroenterol Nutr 13: 42–45

Bazzocchi J, Ellis J, Villanueva-Meyer J, Jing J, Reddy S N, Mena I, Snape W J Jr 1990 Postprandial colonic transit and motor activity in chronic constipation. Gastroenterology 98: 686–693

Beuret-Blanquart F, Weber J, Gouverneur J P, Demangeon S, Denis P 1990 Colonic transit time and anorectal manometric anomalies in 19 patients with complete transsection of the spinal cord. J Auton Nerv Syst 30: 199–208

Bellman M 1966 Studies on encopresis. Acta Paediatr Scand Suppl 170

Berretta A O, Chaussade S, Coquet M, Couturier D, Bonnin A, Guerre J 1990 Technique simplifiée de défécographie. Description et résultats. Presse Méd 19 (33): 1533–1537

Bingham S, Cummings J H 1989 Effect of exercise and physical fitness on large intestine function. Gastroeterology 97: 1389–1399

Bleijenberg G, Kuijpers H C 1987 Treatment of the spastic pelvic floor syndrome with biofeedback. Dis Colon Rectum 30: 108

Borneman E Psychanalyse de l'argent. Dunod, Paris

Bouchoucha M, Denis P, Arhan P et al 1989 Morphology and rheology of the rectum in patients with chronic idiopathic constipation. Dis Col Rectum 32: 788–792

Bouchoucha M, Devroede G, Arhan P et al 1992 What is the meaning of colorectal transit time measurement? Dis Colon Rectum 35: 773–782

Burkitt D P, Walker A R P, Painter N S 1972 Effect of dietary fibre on stools and transit times, and its role in the causation of disease. Lancet ii: 1408

Cann P A, Read N W, Brown C, Hobson N, Holdsworth C D 1983 Irritable bowel syndrome: relationship of disorders in the transit of a single solid meal to symptom patterns. Gut 24: 405–411

Cannon A F, Davidson G P, Moore D J 1988 Anal size in constipated and non-constipated children. Lancet Oct 15: 899

Chaudhary N A, Truelove S C 1962 The irritable colon syndrome. A study of clinical features, predisposing causes, and prognosis in 130 cases. Q J Med 31: 307

Chaussade S, Roche H, Khyari A, Couturier D, Guerre J 1986 Mesure du temps de transit colique (TTC): description et validation d'une nouvelle technique. Gastroenterol Clin Biol 10: 385–389

Chaussade S, Khyari A, Roche H et al 1989 Determination of total and segmental colonic transit time in constipated patients. Results in 91 patients with a new simplified method. Dig Dis Sci 34 (8): 1168–1172

Chaussade S, Gosselin A, Hostein J, Leman M, Ponsot P 1990, Détermination du temps de transit colique (TTC) global et segmentaire dans une population de 96 sujets volontaires sains. Gastroenterol Clin Biol 14: 95–97

Chevalier T, Arhan P, Bouchoucha M et al 1989 Etude de la motricité sigmoïdienne stimulée par la distension luminale. Modification de la réponse motrice dans la constipation par ralentissement du transit colique gauche. Gastroenterol Clin Biol 13: 245–249

Collins J G 1986 Prevalence of selected chronic digestive conditions, United States – 1979–1981. US Public Health

Service (Vital and Health Statistics; series 10, no. 155). Hyattsville, Maryland, National Center for Health Statistics, July 1986

Connell A M, Frankel H, Guttman L 1963 The motility of the pelvic colon following complete lesions of the spinal cord. Paraplegia 1: 98

Connell A M, Hilton C, Irvine G, Lennard-Jones J E, Misiewicz J J 1965 Variation of bowel habit in two population samples. Br Med J 2: 1095–1099

Corazziari E, Materia E, Baurano G et al 1987 Laxative consumption in chronic non organic constipation. J Clin Gastroenterol 9 (4): 427–430

Coremans G, Vergauwe P, Vantrappen G, Van Cutsen E 1991 Is severe chronic idiopathic constipation part of the clinical spectrum of chronic idiopathic intestinal pseudo-obstruction? Gastroenterology 100 (5 part 2): A433 (abst)

Costalat G, Garrigues J M, Dravet F, Noel P, Lopez P, Veyrac M, Vernhet J 1989 Rectopexie antéro-postérieure pour troubles de la statique rectale: résultats cliniques et radiologiques. Intérêt de la rectographie dynamique numérisée. A propos de trente cas. Ann Chir 9: 733–743

Crowell M D, Whitehead W E, Cheskin L J, Schuster M M 1989 Twenty four hour ambulatory monitoring of peristaltic activity from the colon in normals and constipation-predominant IBS patients. Gastroenterology 96: A103

Cucchiara S, Coremans G, Staiano A et al 1984 Gastrointestinal transit time and anorectal manometry in children with fecal soiling. J Pediatr Gastroenterol Nutr 3: 545–550

Cummings J H 1983 Fermentation in the human large intestine: evidence and implications for health. Lancet 1: 1206

Cummings J H 1984 Constipation, dietary fibre and the control of large bowel function. Postgrad Med J 60: 811–819

Dapoigny M, Tournut D, Trolese J F, Bommelaer G, Tournut R 1985 Activité myoélectrique colique à jeûn et en période post-prandiale chez le sujet sain et chez le colopathe. Gastroenterol Clin Biol 9: 223

Davies G J, Crowder M, Reid B, Dickerson J W T 1986 Bowel function measurements of individuals with different eating patterns. Gut 27: 164–169

Davidson M, Kugler M M, Bauer C H 1963 Diagnosis and management in children with severe and protracted constipation and obstipation. J Pediatr 62: 261

De Medicis A, Badioli D, Corazziari E, Bausano G, Anzini F 1989 Rectal sensitivity in chronic constipation. Dig Dis Sci 34 (5): 747–753

Denis Ph, Dewe C, Dorival M P et al 1990 Expérience des problèmes soulevés par le biofeedback au sein d'une équipe hospitalière. Gastroenterol Clin Biol 14: 5–7

Denis P, Duval V, Roussignol C, Weber J 1992 Anisme et agression sexuelle. Gastroenterol Clin Biol 16: A106

Dent O F, Goulston K J, Zubrzycki J, Chapuis P H 1986 Bowel symptoms in an apparently well population. Dis Colon Rectum 29: 243–247

De San Lazaro C 1989 Reflex anal dilatation and sexual abuse. Arch Dis Child 64: 303–304

Devroede G 1985 La constipation: du symptôme à la personne. Psychol Med 17: 1515–1524

Devroede G 1989 Obstipation: What is the appropiate therapeutic approach? in: Barkin J S, Rogers A I (eds)

Difficult decisions in digestive diseases. Year Book Medical Publishers, pp 458–484

Devroede G 1990 Constipation and sexuality. Med Aspects Hum Sexuality Feb: 40–46

Devroede G 1992 Constipation – a sign of a disease to be treated surgically, or a symptom to be deciphered as nonverbal communication? (Editorial) J Clin Gastroenterol 15 (3) 189–191

Devroede G 1993a Constipation. In: Sleisenger M H, Fordtran J S (eds) 5th edn. W B Saunders, Philadelphia

Devroede G 1993b Psychophysiological assessment of patients with pelvic floor dysfunction. Pain Research and Clinical Management Series. Elsevier

Devroede G, Soffie M 1973 Colonic absorption in idiopathic constipation. Gastroenterology 64: 552–561

Devroede G, Lamarche J 1974 Functional importance of extrinsic parasympathetic innervation to the distal colon and rectum in man. Gastroenterology 66: 273–280

Devroede G, Arhan P, Duguay C, Tetreault L, Akoury H, Perey B 1979 Traumatic constipation. Gastroenterology 77: 1258–1267

Devroede G, Vobecky S, Masse S et al 1982 Ischemic fecal incontinence and rectal angina. Gastroenterology 83 (5): 970–980

Devroede G, Bouchoucha M, Girard G 1989a Constipation, anxiety and personality: what comes first? in: Bueno L, Collins S, Junior J L (eds) Stress and digestive motility. John Libbey eurotext, London pp. 55–60

Devroede G, Roy T, Bouchoucha M et al 1989b Idiopathic constipation by colonic dysfunction: relationship with personality and anxiety. Dig Dis Sci 34 (9): 1428–1433

Devroede G, Hemond M 1990 Anorectal manometry: small balloon tube in: Smith L E (ed) Practical guide to anorectal testing. Igaku-Shoin Medical Publishers, New York pp 55–64

Dinoso V P Jr, Murphy S N S, Goldstein J, Rosner B 1983 Basal motor activity of the distal colon: a reappraisal. Gastroenterology 85: 637

Donald I P, Smith R G, Cruikshank J G, Elton R A, Stoddart M E 1985 A study of constipation in the elderly living at home. Gerontology 31: 112–118

Drossman D A, Thompson W G, Talley N J, Funch-Jensen P, Janssens J, Whitehead W E 1990 Identification of sub-groups of functional gastrointestinal disorders. Gastroenterol Int 3 (4): 159–172

Drossman D A, Leserman J, Nachman G et al 1990 Sexual and physical abuse in women with functional or organic gastrointestinal disorders. Ann Intern Med 113: 828–833

Drossman D A, Li Z, Andruzzi E et al A randomized survey of functional gastrointestinal symptoms in the United States: the 'Rome' multinational diagnostic criteria (in press)

Drossman D A Sexual and physical abuse and gastrointestinal disorders in women: what is the link? Med Aspects Hum Sexuality (in press)

Ducrotte P, Denis P, Galmiche J P et al 1985 Motricité anorectale dans la constipation idiopathique. Etude de 200 patients consécutifs. Gastroenterol Clin Biol 9: 10

Ducrotte P, Rodomanska B, Weber J et al 1986 Colonic transit time of radiopaque markers and rectoanal manometry in patients complaining of constipation. Dis Colon Rectum 29: 630–634

Eastwood H D H 1972 Bowel transit studies in the elderly: radiopaque markers in the investigation of constipation. Gerontol Clin 14: 154

Edwards D A W, Beck E R 1971 Movement of radiopacified faeces during defecation. Am J Dig Dis 16: 709

Ehrentheil O F, Wells E P 1955 Megacolon in psychotic patients. A clinical entity. Gastroenterology 29: 285

Epelboin A 1981–1982 Selles et urines chez les Fulbes Bande du Sénégal Oriental. Un aspect particulier de l'ethnomédicine. Cah ORSTOM, Ser Sci Hum 18 (4): 515–530

Eshchar J, Cohen L 1981 Reeducation of constipation patients. A non medicinal treatment. Am J Proctol Gastroenterol Colon Rectal Surg 32: 16

Everhart J E, Go V L, Johannes R S, Fitzsimmons S C, Roth H P, White L R 1989 A longitudinal survey of self-reported bowel habits in the United States. Dig Dis Sci 34: 1153–1162

Feldman P, Villanueva S, Lanne V I, Devroede G 1993 Use of play with clay to treat children with intractable encopresis. J Pediatrics 3: 483–487

Fielding J F 1983 Surgery and the irritable bowel syndrome: the singer as well as the song. Irish Med J 1: 33

Fiedorek S C, Pumphrey C L, Casteel H B 1990, Breath methane production in children with constipation and encopresis. J Pediatr Gastroenterol Nutr 10: 473–477

Fisher S E, Breckon K, Andrews H A, Keighley M R B 1989 Psychiatric screening for patients with faecal incontinence on chronic constipation referred for surgical treatment. Br J Surg 76: 352–355

Fotherby K J, Hunter J P 1987 Idiopathic slow transit constipation: whole gut transit times, measured by a new simplified method, are not shortened by opioid antagonist. Aliment Pharmacol Therap 1: 331–338

Gabel S, Hegedus A M, Wald A, Chandra R, Chiponis D 1986 Prevalence of behavior problems and mental health utilization among encopretic children: implications for behaviour pediatrics. Dev Behav Pediatr 7 (5): 293–297

Garrigues J M, Costalat G, Lopez P, Lamarque J L 1989 La rectographie numérisée. Ann Gastroenterol Hepatol 25: 174

Gear J S S, Brodribb A J M, Ware A M, Mann J I 1981 Fibre and bowel transit times. Br J Nutr 45: 77–82

Gekas P, Schuster M M 1981 Stercoral perforation of the colon: case report and review of the literature. Gastroenterology 80: 1054

Gibbons C P, Bannister J J, Read N W 1988 Role of constipation and anal hypertonia in the pathogenesis of hemorrhoids. Br J Surg 75: 656–660

Glaser M, Chi J 1983 Thirty-fifth annual report on consumer spending. Drug Topics Jul 4: 18–20

Glick M E, Meshkinpour H, Haldeman S, Bhatia N N, Bradley W E 1982 Colonic dysfunction in multiple sclerosis. Gastroenterology 83: 1002

Glick M E, Meshkinpour H, Haldeman S, Hoehler F, Downey N, Bradley W E 1984 Colonic dysfunction in patients with thoracic spinal cord injury. Gastroenterology 86: 287

Glober G A, Nomura A, Kamiyama S, Shimada A, Abba B C 1977 Bowel transit-time and stool weight in populations with different colon–cancer risks. Lancet ii: 110

Goldberg M J, Smith J W, Nichols R L 1977 Comparison of the faecal microflora of Seventh-Day Adventists with individuals consuming a general diet. Ann Surg 186: 97–100

Groddeck G 1926 Verstopfung als Typus des Widerstands. Die Arche No 8/9

Gunterberg B, Kewenter J, Petersen I, Stener B 1976 Anorectal function after major resections of the sacrum with bilateral or unilateral sacrifice of sacral nerves. Br J Surgery 63: 546

Guthrie E, Creed F, Dawson D, Torrenson B 1991 A controlled trial of psychological treatment for the irritable bowel syndrome. Gastroenterology 100: 450–457

Hale W E, Perkins L L, May F E, Marks R G, Stewart R B 1986 Symptom prevalence in the elderly. An evaluation of age, sex, disease and medication use. JAGS 34: 333–340

Halls J 1965 Bowel content shift during normal defaecation. Proc R Soc Med 58: 859–860

Hamel-Roy J, Devroede G, Arhan P, Tetreault J P, Lemieux B, Scott H 1984 Functional abnormalities of the anal sphincters in patients with myotonic dystrophy. Gastroenterology 86: 1469

Hammond E C 1964 Some preliminary findings on physical complaints from a prospective study of 1 054 004 men and women. Am J Public Health 54: 11

Harvey R F, Hinton R A, Gunary R M, Barry R E 1989 Individual and group hypnotherapy in treatment of refractory irritable bowel syndrome. Lancet Feb 25: 424–425

Herbetko J, Hyde I 1990 Urinary tract dilatation in constipated children. Br J Radiol 63: 855–857

Hero M, Arhan P, Devroede G et al 1985 Measuring the anorectal angle. J Biomed Eng 7: 321–325

Heywood T, Holeva K, Morandi C, Wald A 1991 Prognosis of chronic idiopathic constipation associated with normal and slow colonic transit. Gastroenterology 100 (5 part 2) A449 (abst)

Higginson J 1966 Etiological factors in gastrointestinal cancer in man. J Natl Cancer Inst 37: 527

Hinds J P, Stoney B, Wald A 1989 Does gender or the menstrual cycle affect colonic transit? Am J Gastroenterol 84 (2): 123–126

Hinton J M, Lennard-Jones J E 1968 Constipation: definition and classification. Postgrad Med J 44: 720

Hobbs C J, Wynne J M 1986 Buggery in childhood – a common syndrome of child abuse. Lancet Oct 4: 792–796

Hobbs J C J, Wynne J M 1989 Sexual abuse of English boys and girls: the importance of anal examination. Child Abuse Negl 13: 195–210

Huschka M 1942 The child's response to coercive bowel training. Psychosom Med 2: 301–308

IMS America Canadian Drugstore and Hospital Purchases Audit 1986–1990. IMS CANADA, Ontario

Jennings P J 1967 Megarectum and megacolon in adolescents and young adults: result of treatment at St Mark's Hospital. Proc R Soc Med 60: 805

Johanson J F, Sonnenberg A 1990 The prevalence of haemorrhoids and chronic constipation. An epidemiologic study. Gastroenterology 98: 380–386

Johanson J F, Sonnenberg A 1991 Diarrhea but not constipation is a risk factor for haemorrhoids. Gastroenterology 100 (5 part 2): A9 (abst)

Johanson J F, Sonnenberg A, Kock T R 1989 Clinical epidemiology of chronic constipation. J Clin Gastroenterol 11 (5): 525–536

Jones P N, Lubowski D Z, Swash M, Henry M M 1987 Is paradoxical contraction of puborectalis muscle of functional importance? Dis Col Rect 30: 667–670

Kamm M A, Lennard-Jones J E 1990 Rectal mucosal electrosensory testing – evidence for a rectal sensory neuropathy in idiopathic constipation. Dis Col Rect 33: 419–423

Kamm M A, Lennard-Jones J E, Thompson D G, Sobnack R, Garvie N W, Granowska M 1988 Dynamic scanning defines a colonic defect in severe idiopathic constipation. Gut 29: 1085–1092

Kaya I S, Dilmen U, Ceyhan M, Saglam R 1988 Rectal and anal pressure profile in constipated children. Lancet Nov 29: 1198–1199

Kettlewell M G W 1972 Surgical management of the bowel in cauda equina lesions. Proc R Soc Med 65: 69

Kellow J E, Phillips S F 1987 Altered small bowel motility in irritable bowel syndrome is correlated with symptoms. Gastroenterology 92: 1885–1893

Kellow J E, Gill R C, Wingate D L 1990 Prolonged ambulant recordings of small bowel motility demonstrate abnormalities in the irritable bowel syndrome. Gastroenterology 98: 1208–1218

Kellow J E, Eckersley G M, Jones M 1992 Enteric and central contributions to intestinal dysmotility in irritable bowel syndrome. Dig Dis Sci 37 (2): 168–174

Kendall G P N, Thompson D G, Day S J, Lennard-Jones J E 1990 Inter- and intra-individual variation in pressure–volume relations of the rectum in normal subjects and patients with the irritable bowel syndrome. Gut 31: 1062–1068

Keren S, Wagner Y, Heldenberg D, Golan M 1988 Studies of manometric abnormalities of the rectoanal region during defaecation in constipated and soiling children: modification through biofeedback therapy. Am J Gastroenterol 83 (8) 827–831

Kerrigan D D, Lucas M G, Sun W M, Donnelly T C, Read N W 1989 Idiopathic constipation associated with impaired urethrovesical and secral reflex function. Br J Surg 76: 748–751

Kiff E S, Barnes P R H, Swash M 1984 Evidence of pudendal neuropathy in patients with perineal descent and chronic straining at stool. Gut 25: 1279

Klauser A G, Voderholzer W A, Heinrich C A, Schindlbeck N E, Muller-Lissner S A 1990 Behavioural modification of colonic function. Can constipation be learned? Dig Dis Sci 35 (10): 1271–1275

Krevsky B, Maurer A H, Fisher R S 1989 Patterns of colonic transit in chronic idiopathic constipation. Am J Gastroenterol 84: 127–132

Kune G A, Kune S, Field B, Watson L F 1988 The role of chronic constipation, diarrhoea and laxative use in the etiology of large bowel cancer: Data from the Melbourne Colorectal Cancer Study. Dis Col Rect 31: 507–512

Kuhnlein O, Bergstrom D, Kuhnlein H 1981 Mutagens in faeces from vegetarians and non-vegetarians. Mutat Res 85: 1–12

Kuijpers H C 1990 Application of the colorectal laboratory in diagnosis and treatment of functional constipation. Dis Col Rect 33: 35–39

Kuijpers H C, Bleijenberg G 1985 The spastic pelvic floor syndrome. A cause of constipation. Dis Col Rect 28: 669

Kuijpers H C, Bleijenberg G, De Morree H 1986 The spastic pelvic floor syndrome. Large bowel outlet obstruction caused by pelvic floor dysfunction: a radiological study. Int J Colorect Dis 1: 44

Kruis W, Thieme C, Weinzierl M, Schussles P, Holl J, Paulus W 1984 A diagnosis score for the irritable bowel syndrome. Its value in the exclusion of organic disease. Gastroenterology 87: 1

Lahr C J, Rothenberger D A, Jensen L L, Goldberg S M 1986 Balloon topography. A simple method of evaluating anal function. Dis Col Rect 29: 1

Lanfranchi G, Bazzoichi A, Brignola C, Campieri M, Labo G 1984 Different patterns of intestinal transit time and anorectal motility in painful and painless chronic constipation. Gut 25: 1352

Lawson M, Kern F Jr, Everson G T 1989 Gastrointestinal transit time in human pregnancy: prolongation in the second and third trimesters followed by post-partum normalization. Gastroenterology 89: 996

Lebel M L, Grand'Maison F 1988 Etude électromyographique dynamique du plancher pelvien dans la constipation: importance de l'EMG à l'aiguille. Can J Neurological Sciences 15 (2): 212–213

Leroi A-M, Bernier C, Watier A, Goupil G, Black R, Devroede G Sexual abuse, anismus and constipation. Gastroenterology (submitted)

Lesaffer L P A 1990 Digital subtraction defecography. In: Smith L E (ed) Practical guide to anorectal testing. Igaku-Shoin, New York pp 127–134

Lestar B, Penninckx F M, Kerremans R P 1989 Defecometry. A new method for determining the parameters of rectal evacuation. Dis Col Rect 32: 197–201

Lestar B, Penninckx F, Kerremans R 1991 Biofeedback defaecation training for anismus. Int J Colorect Dis 6: 202–207

Levine M D 1975 Children with encopresis: a descriptive analysis. Pediatrics 56: 412

Levine M D, Mazonson P, Barkow H 1980 Behavioural symptom substitution in children cured of encopresis. Am J Dis Child 134: 663–667

Likongo Y, Devroede G, Schang J C et al 1986 Hindgut dysgenesis as a cause of constipation with delayed colonic transit. Dig Dis Sci 31: 993–1003

Loening-Baucke V A 1984 Abnormal rectoanal function in children recovered from chronic constipation and encopresis. Gastroenterology 87: 1299

Loening-Baucke V 1990 Modulation of abnormal defecation dynamics by biofeedback treatment in chronically constipated chilren with encopresis. J Pediatr 116: 214–222

Loening-Baucke V 1991 Persistence of chronic constipation in children after biofeedback treatment. Dig Dis Sci 36 (2): 153–160

Loening-Baucke V, Anuras S 1986 Jejunal and colonic motility in patients with severe constipation. Gastroenterology 91: 1060

Loening-Baucke V A, Cruikshank B M 1986 Abnormal defaecation dynamics in chronically constipated children with encopresis. J Pediatr 108: 562

Loening-Baucke V A, Anuras S, Mitros F A 1987a Changes in colorectal function in patients with chronic colonic pseudoobstruction. Dig Dis Sci 32 (10): 1104–1112

Loening-Baucke V, Cruikshank B, Savage C 1987b Defecation dynamics and behaviour profiles in encopretic children. Pediatrics 80 (5): 672–679

Longstreth G F, Preskill D B, Youketes L 1990 Irritable bowel syndrome in women having diagnostic laparoscopy or hysterectomy. Relation to gynaecologic features and outcome. Dig Dis Sci 35 (10): 1285–1290

Lowen A 1967 Love and orgasm. New American Library, New York

Lowery S P, Snour J W, Whitehead W E, Schuster M M 1985 Habit training as treatment of encopresis secondary to chronic constipation. J Pediatr Gastroenterol Nutr 4: 397–401

Lowman B C, Drossman D A, Cramer E M, McKee D C 1987 Recollection of childhood events in adults with irritable bowel syndrome. J Clin Gastroenterol 9 (3): 324–330

Mahieu P, Pringot J, Bodart P 1984 Defecography. I. Description of a new procedure and results in normal patients. Gastrointest Radiol 9: 247

Manning A P, Wyman J B, Heaton K W 1976 How trustworthy are bowel histories? Comparison of recalled and recorded information. Br Med J 2: 213–214

Marcus S N, Heaton K W 1987 Irritable bowel-type symptoms in spontaneous and induced constipation. Gut 28: 156–159

Martelli H, Devroede G, Arhan P, Duguay C, Dornic C, Faverdin C 1978a Some parameters of large bowel motility in normal man. Gastroenterology 75: 612–618

Martelli H, Devroede G, Arhan P, Duguay C 1978b Mechanisms of idiopathic constipation: outlet obstruction. Gastroenterology 75: 623–631

Mathers J E, Kempster P A, Law P J et al 1989 Anal sphincter dysfunction in Parkinson's disease. Arch Neurol 46: 1061–1064

Marzio L, Del Bianco R, Delle Donne M, Pieramico O, Cuccurullo F 1989 Mouth-to-cecum transit time in patients affected by chronic constipation: effect of glucomannan. Am J Gastroenterol 84 (8): 888–891

Meier E 1977 Pubococcygeal strength: relationship to urinary control problems and to female orgasmic response. PhD thesis. California School of Professional Psychology: Ann Arbor, MI, University Microfilms International.

Metcalf A 1990 Transit time in: Smith L E (ed) Practical guide to anorectal testing. Igaku-Shoin, New York pp 17–22

Metcalf A M, Phillips S F, Zinsmeister A R, MacCarty R L, Beart B W, Wolff B C 1987 Simplified assessment of segmental colonic transit time. Gastroenterology 92: 40–47

Meunier P 1991 Anorectal manometry. A collective international experience. Gastroenterol Clin Biol 15: 697–702

Meunier P, Mollard P, Marechal J-M 1976 Physiopathology of megarectum: the association of megarectum with encopresis. Gut 17: 224

Meunier P, Marechal J M, Joubert De Beaujeu M 1979 Rectoanal pressures and rectal sensitivity studies in chronic childhood constipation. Gastroenterology 77: 330

Meunier P, Louis D, Jaubert De Beaujeu M 1984 Physiologic investigation of primary chronic constipation in children: comparison with the barium enema study. Gastroenterology 87: 1351

Micozzi M S, Carter C L, Albanes D, Taylor P R, Licitra L M 1989 Bowel function and breast cancer in US women. Am J Pub Health 79 (1): 73–75

Miettinen T A, Tarpila S 1978 Fecal beta-sitosterol in patients with diverticular disease of the colon and in vegetarians. Scand J Gastroenterol 13: 573–576

Milne J S, Williamson J 1972 Bowel habits in older people. Gerontol Clin 14: 56–60

Muller-Lissner S A 1988 Effect of wheat bran as weight of stool and gastrointestinal transit time: a meta analysis. Br Med J 296: 615–617

McCann J, Voris J, Simon M, Wells R 1989 Perianal findings in prepubertal children selected for non abuse: a descriptive study. Child Abuse Negl 13: 179–193

McLean R G, Smart R C, Gaston-Parry D et al 1990 Colon transit scintigraphy in health and constipation using oral iodine-131-cellulose. J Nucl Med 31: 985–989

Neumann P A, De Domenico I J, Nogrady M B 1973 Constipation and urinary tract infection. Pediatrics 52: 241

Nisard A, Jian R, Chevalier J, Lefrant L 1982 Effet d'une cure thermale à Châtel-Guyon sur le temps de transit intestinal total de patients atteints de colopathie fonctionnelle. Rev Fr de Gastroenterol 175: 5

Nolan T, Debelle G, Oberklaid F, Coffey C 1991 Randomized trial of laxatives in treatment of childhood encopresis. Lancet 338: 523–527

O'Regan S, Yazbeck S 1985 Constipation: a cause of enuresis, urinary tract infection and vesico-ureteral reflux in children. Med Hypotheses 17: 409

O'Regan S, Yazbeck S, Schick E 1985 Constipation, bladder instability, urinary tract infection syndrome. Clin Nephrol 23: 152

Oettle G J, Heaton K W 1987 Is there a relationship between symptoms of the irritable bowel syndrome and objective measurements of large bowel function? A longitudinal study. Gut 28: 146–149

Ornstein M H, Littlewood E R, Baird I M, Fowler J, North W R S, Cox A G 1981 Are fibre supplements really necessary in diverticular disease of the colon? A controlled clinical trial. Br Med J 282: 1353

Panaganuwa B, Kumar D, Keighley M R B, Ortiz J 1991 Motor abnormalities in the terminal ileum in patients with chronic idiopathic constipation. Gastroenterology 100 (5 Part 2) A479 (abst)

Parks A G, Porter N H, Melzack J 1962 Experimental study of the reflex mechanism controlling the muscles of the pelvic floor. Dis Colon Rectum 5: 407

Patriquin H, Martelli H, Devroede G 1978 Barium enema in chronic constipation: is it meaningful? Gastroenterology 75: 619–622

Pavlakis A, Wheeler J S Jr, Krane R J, Siroky M B 1986 Functional voiding disorders in females. Neurourol Urodynam 5: 145

Penninckx F, Debruyne C, Lestar B, Kerremans R 1990 Observer variation in the radiological measurement of the anorectal angle. Int J Colorectal Dis 5: 94–97

Percora P, Suraci C, Antonelli M, De Maria S, Marrocco W 1981 Constipation and obesity: a statistical analysis. Bull Soc It Biol Sper 57: 2384

Percy J P, Swash M, Neill M E, Parks A G 1981 Electrophysiological study of motor nerve supply of pelvic floor. Lancet 1: 16

Petrakis N L, King E B 1981 Cytological abnormalities in nipple aspirates of breast fluid from women with severe constipation. Lancet ii: 1203

Pinkerton P 1958 Psychogenic megacolon in children: the implications of bowel negativism. Arch Dis Child 33: 371

Preston J E, Lennard-Jones J E 1985a Pelvic motility and response to intraluminal bisacodyl in slow transit constipation. Dig Dis Sci 30: 289

Preston D M, Lennard-Jones J E 1985b Anismus in chronic constipation. Dig Dis Sci 30: 413

Preston D M, Lennard-Jones J E 1986 Severe chronic constipation in young women: idiopathic slow transit constipation. Gut 27: 41

Preston D M, Lennard-Jones J E, Thomas B M 1984a The balloon proctogram. Br J Surg 17: 29

Preston D M, Pfeffer J M, Lennard-Jones J E 1984b Psychiatric assessment of patients with severe constipation. Gut 25: A582–A583

Preston D M, Lennard-Jones J E, Thomas B M 1985, Toward a radiologic definition of idiopathic megacolon. Gastrointest Radiol 10: 167

Prior A, Wilson K, Whorwell P J, Faragher E B 1989 Irritable bowel syndrome in the gynecological clinic. Survey of 798 new referrals. Dig Dis Sci 34 (12): 1820–1824

Prior A, Maxton D G, Whorwell P J 1990a Anorectal manometry in irritable bowel syndrome: differences between diarrhoea and constipation predominant subjects. Gut 31 (4): 458–462

Prior A, Colgan S M, Whorwell P J 1990b Changes in rectal sensitivity after hypnotherapy in patients with irritable bowel syndrome. Gut 31: 896–898

Purtell J J, Robins E, Cohen M E 1951 Observations on clinical aspects of hysteria: a quantitative study of 50 hysteria patients and 156 control subjects. JAMA 146: 902

Priestley B L, Taitz L S 1989 Reflex anal dilatation associated with severe chronic constipation. Arch Dis Child 64: 302–303

Proano M, Camilleri M, Phillips S F, Brown M L, Thomforde G M 1990 Transit of solids through the human colon: regional quantification in the unprepared bowel. Am J Physiol 258: G856–G862

Read N W, Abouzekry L, Read M G et al 1985 Anorectal function in elderly patients with faecal impaction. Gastroenterology 89: 959–966

Reboa G, Arnulfo G, Frascio M, Di Somma C, Pitto G, Berti-Riboli E 1984 Colon motility and coloanal reflexes in chronic idiopathic constipation. Effects of a novel enterokinetic agent cisapride. Eur J Clin Pharmacol 26: 745

Rendtorff R C, Kashgarian M 1967 Stool patterns of healthy adult males. Dis Colon Rectum 10: 222–228

Rex D K, Lappas J C, Goulet R C, Madura J A 1992 Selection of constipated patients as subtotal colectomy candidate. J Clin Gastroenterol 15: 212–217

Reynolds J C, Ouyang A, Lee C A, Baker L, Sunshine A G, Cohen S 1987 Chronic severe constipation. Prospective motility studies in 25 consecutive patients. Gastroenterology 92: 414–420

Rimsza M E, Berg R A, Locke C 1988 Sexual abuse: somatic and emotional reactions. Child Abuse Negl 12: 201–208

Roe A M, Bartolo D C C, Mortensen N J McC 1986 Diagnosis and surgical management of intractable constipation. Br J Surg 73: 854–861

Roe A M, Bartolo D C C, Mortensen N J McC 1988 Slow transit constipation. Comparison between patients with and without previous hysterectomy. Dig Dis Sci 33: 1159–1163

Rutter K R P 1974 Electromyographic changes in certain pelvic floor abnormalities. Proc R Soc Med 67: 53

Sandler R S, Drossman D A 1987 Bowel habits in young adults not seeking health care. Dig Dis Sci 32: 841–845

Sandler R S, Jordan M C, Shelton B J 1990 Demographic and dietary determinants of constipation in the US population. AJPH 80 (2): 185–189

Sarahan T, Weintraub W H, Coran A G, Wesley J R 1982 The successful management of chronic constipation in infants and children. J Pediatr Surg 17: 171

Scott H W Jr, Cantrell J R 1949 Colonmetrographic studies of the effects of section of the parasympathetic nerves of the colon. Bull Johns Hopkins Hosp 85: 310

Schang J C 1985 Colonic motility in subgroups of patients with the irritable bowel syndrome in: Poitras P (ed) Proceedings of the first international symposium on small intestinal and colonic motility. Centre de Recherches Cliniques, Hôpital Saint-Luc, and Jouveinal Laboratoires/laboratories, Montreal pp. 101–112

Schang J C, Devroede G, Duguay C, Hemond M, Hebert M 1985 Constipation par inertie colique et obstruction distale: étude électromyographique. Gastroenterol Clin Biol 9: 480

Schang J C, Hemond M, Hebert M, Pilote M 1986 Myoelectrical activity and intraluminal flow in human sigmoid colon. Dig Dis Sci 31: 1331

Schang J C, Devroede G, Pilote M Effects of trimebutine on colonic function in patients with chronic idiopathic constipation: evidence for the need of a physiological rather than clinical selection. Dis Col Rect (in press)

Seidel J S, Elvik S L, Berkowitz C D et al 1986 Presentation and evaluation of sexual misuse in the emergency department. Pediatr Emerg Care 2: 157

Shafer R B, Prentiss R A, Bond J H 1984 Gastrointestinal transit in thyroid disease. Gastroenterology 86: 852

Shopfner C E 1968 Urinary tract pathology associated with constipation. Radiology 90: 865

Shorvon P J, McHugh S, Diamant N E, Somers S, Stevenson G W 1989 Defecography in normal volunteers: results and impaction. Gut 30: 1737–1749

Shouler P, Keighley M R B 1986 Changes in colorectal function in severe idiopathic constipation. Gastroenterology 90: 414

Smith A N, Varma J S, Binnic N R, Papachrysostomou M 1990 Disordered colorectal motility in intractable constipation following hysterectomy. Br J Surg 77: 1361-1366

Soltolt J, Gudmand-Hayes F, Krag B, Kirstensen F, Wulfe M R 1976 A double-blind trial of the effect of wheat bran on symptoms of irritable bowel syndrome. Lancet i: 270

Sonnenberg A, Koch T R 1989a Epidemiology of constipation in the United States. Dis Col Rect 32: 1–8

Sonnenberg A, Koch T R 1989b Physician visits in the United States for constipation: 1958 to 1986. Dig Dis Sci 34 (4): 606–611

Stewart E T, Dodds W J 1979 Predictability of rectal incontinence on barium enema examination. AJR 132: 197

Stivland T, Camilleri M, Vassallo M et al 1991 Scintigraphic measurement of regional gut transit in idiopathic constipation. Gastroenterology 101: 107–115

Stubbs J B, Valenzuela G A, Stubbs C C et al 1991 A non invasive scintigraphic assessment of the colonic transit of non digestible solids in man. J Nutr Med 32: 1375–1381

Sun W M, Read N W, Prior A, Daly J A, Cheah S K, Grundy D 1990 Sensory and motor responses to rectal distension vary according to rate and pattern of balloon inflation. Gastroenterology 99: 1008–1015

Talley N J, O'Keefe E A, Zinsmeister A R, Melton III L J 1992 Prevalence of gastrointestinal symptoms in the elderly: a population-based study. Gastroenterology 102: 895–901

Tomlin J, Read N W 1988 Laxative properties of indigestible plastic particles. Br Med J 297: 1175–1176

Trent B 1992 Art therapy can show a light into the dark history of a child's sexual abuse. Can Med Assoc J 146 (8): 1412–1422

Tucker D M, Sandstead H H, Logan G M Jr et al 1981 Dietary fibre and personality factors as determinants of stool output. Gastroenterology 81: 879–883

Varma J S, Smith A N 1984 Abnormalities of rectal distensibility in the irritable bowel syndrome. Gut 25: A1169

Varma J S, Smith A M 1988, Neurophysiological dysfunction in young women with intractable constipation. Gut 29: 963–968

Varma J S, Bradnock J, Smith R G, Smith A N 1988 Constipation in the elderly. A physiologic study. Dis Col Rect 31: 111–115

Verduron A, Devroede G, Bouchoucha M et al 1988 Megarectum. Dig Dis Sci 33 (9): 1164–1174

Veyrac M, Parelon G, Daures J P, Bories P, Michel H 1988 Une cause de constipation terminale: l'hypertonie de la musculature striée pelvienne. Intérêt des explorations complémentaires. Gastroenterol Clin Biol 12: 931–934

Vobecky J, Caro J, Devroede G 1983 A case control study of risk factors for large bowel carcinoma. Cancer 51: 1958–1963

Wald A, Van Thiel D H, Hoechstetter L et al 1982 Effect of pregnancy on gastrointestinal transit. Dig Dis Sci 27: 1015

Wald A, Hinds J P, Caruana B J 1983 Psychological and physiological characteristics of patients with severe idiopathic constipation. Gastroenterology 97: 932–937

Wald A, Chandra R, Chiponis D, Gabel S 1986 Anorectal function and continence mechanisms in childhood encopresis. J Pediatr Gastroenterol Nutr 5: 346–351

Wald A 1986 Colonic transit and anorectal manometry in chronic idiopathic constipation. Arch Intern Med 146: 1713

Wald A 1990 Surgical treatment for refractory constipation – more hard data about hard stools? Am J Gastroenterol 85 (6): 759–760

Wald A, Chandra R, Gabel J, Chiponis D 1987 Evaluation of biofeedback in childhood encopresis. J Pediatr Gastroenterol Nutr 6: 554–558

Wald A, Hinds J P, Carvana B J 1989 Psychological and physiological characteristics of patients with severe idiopathic constipation. Gastroenterology 97: 932–937

Wald A, Caruana B J, Freimanis M G, Bauman D H, Hinds J P 1990 Contributions of evacuation proctography and anorectal manometry to evaluation of adults with constipation and defaecatory difficulty. Dig Dis Sci 35 (4): 481–487

Waldron D J, Kumar D, Hallan R I, Wingate D L, Williams N S 1990 Evidence for motor neuropathy and reduced filling of the rectum in chronic intractable constipation. Gut 31 (11): 1284–1288

Walker A R P, Walker B F, Bhamjee D, Walker E J, Ncongwane J, Segal I 1982 Defaecation frequencies in Black, Indian, Coloured and White populations – what do they signify. S Afr Med J 62: 195–199

Watier A, Devroede G, Duranceau A et al 1985 Constipation with colonic inertia. A manifestation of systemic disease? Dig Dis Sci 28: 1025–1033

Watier A, Feldman P, Martelli H, Arhan P, Devroede G Hirschsprung's disease in: Bockus gastroenterology, 5th edn (in press)

Watkins G L, Oliver G A 1965 Giant megacolon in the insane: further observations in patients treated by subtotal colectomy. Gastroenterology 48: 718

Weber J, Denis P, Mihout B et al 1985 Effect of brain stem lesion on colonic and anorectal motility. Study of three patients. Dig Dis Sci 30 (5): 419–425

Weber J, Grise P, Roquebert M et al 1987a Radio-opaque markers transit and anorectal manometry in 16 patients with multiple sclerosis and urinary bladder dysfunction. Dis Col Rect 30: 95

Weber J, Ducrotte Ph, Touchais J Y, Roussignol C, Denis Ph 1987b Biofeedback training for constipation in adults and children. Dis Col Rect 30: 844–846

Weber J, Delangre T, Hannekin D, Beuret-Blanquart F, Denis P 1990 Anorectal manometric anomalies in seven patients with frontal lobe brain damage. Dig Dis Sci 35 (2): 225–230

Welgan P, Meshkinpour H, Beeler M 1988 Effect of anger on colon motor and myoelectric activity in irritable bowel syndrome. Gastroenterology 94: 1150–1156

White J C, Verlot M G, Ehrentheil O 1940 Neurogenic disturbances of the colon and their investigation by the colonmetrogram. Ann Surg 112: 1042

Whitehead W E, Drinkwater D, Cheskin L J, Heller B R, Schuster M M 1989 Constipation in the elderly living at home. Definition, prevalence, and relationship to lifestyle and health status. JAGS 37: 423–429

Whitehead W E, Crowell M D, Bosmajian L et al 1990 Existence of irritable bowel syndrome supported by factor analysis of symptoms in two community samples. Gastroenterology 98: 336–340

Whitehead W E, Chaussade S, Corazziari E, Kumar D 1991 Report of an international workshop on management of constipation. Gastroenterol Int 4 (3): 99–113

Whorwell P J, Prior A, Faragher E B 1984 Controlled trial of hypnotherapy in the treatment of severe refractory irritable-bowel syndrome. Lancet ii: 1232

Whorwell P J, Prior A, Colgan S M 1987 Hypnotherapy in severe irritable bowel syndrome: further experience. Gut 28: 423–425

Wise T N, Cooper J N, Ahmed S 1982 The efficacy of group therapy for patients with irritable bowel syndrome. Psychosomatics 23: 465

Wyman J B, Heaton K W, Manning A P, Wicks A C B 1978 Variability of colonic function in healthy subjects. Gut 19: 146–150

Wynder E L, Shigematsu T 1967 Environmental factors of cancer of the colon and rectum. Cancer 20: 1520

Young S J, Alpers D H, Norland C C, Woodruff R A Jr 1976 Psychiatric illness and the irritable bowel syndrome. Practical implications for the primary physician. Gastroenterology 70: 162

38. Abnormalities of anorectal function

R. L. Grotz   J. H. Pemberton

INTRODUCTION

The anorectum maintains enteric continence and facilitates defaecation. Anorectal disorders result in sensorimotor dysfunction, which is characterized clinically as either incontinence or disordered defaecation. The aim of this chapter is to describe the present understanding of the pathophysiology, diagnostic approaches and available therapeutic interventions for anorectal dysfunction.

DISORDERED DEFAECATION

Patients with disorders of defaecation present with a long history of constipation or straining at defaecation. The aetiology is unknown but is probably a heterogenous group of disorders (Fig. 38.1). Symptoms include infrequent evacuation of stool, prolonged or painful defaecation, the need for manual disimpaction or assuming contorted postures for defaecation, and passing 'hard' stools. A sensation of pelvic pressure or 'blockage' in the anus or rectum with incomplete evacuation implies pelvic floor dysfunction. Chronic, protracted straining is an early sign of obstructed defaecation yet, if evaluation is deferred, these patients may ultimately present with faecal incontinence (Fig. 38.2).

Anismus

Anismus is defined as failure of the striated pelvic muscles to relax upon straining (Preston & Lennard-Jones 1985). The aetiology is unknown but psychologic factors may play a role (Kuijpers & Bleijenberg 1985). Difficulties with childhood toilet training or traumatic events in the past may contribute to these factors.

On physical examination, an unyielding posterior bar of puborectalis muscle which does not relax on straining may be indicative of anismus. Defaecography demonstrates a non-relaxing puborectalis muscle with incomplete rectal evacuation, an anorectal angle which remains acute and an immobile pelvic floor which fails to descend with straining (Fig. 38.3). In some patients, electromyographic (EMG) studies of the puborectalis muscle show paradoxically increased electrical activity (Fig. 38.4); however, this is a finding in some healthy subjects without constipation (Jones et al 1987). In these patients a colonic transit study is indicated to exclude slow transit constipation.

The balloon expulsion test evaluates overall function of the pelvic floor. Healthy subjects voluntarily expel a balloon filled with 50 ml of water or after placement of up to 150 gm of weight has been added to the opposite end of the balloon. In contrast, patients with anismus are unable to pass the balloon spontaneously or until large amounts of weight are added (sometimes greater than 500 gm) (Pezim et al 1987a).

Scintigraphic assessment during defaecation quantitates the efficiency of evacuation of an artificial stool infused into the rectum. If anismus is present, poor dynamic emptying with evacuation of less artificial stool is evident compared to that seen in healthy controls (Pezim et al 1987a).

Treatment of anismus with laxatives, suppositories and enemas usually has little impact. Surgical treatment has also had limited success. Barnes et al (1985) divided the puborectalis muscle in nine patients with anismus. Two patients improved yet five developed incontinence. Thus, the mainstay of treatment is not surgery, but pelvic floor retraining with biofeedback techniques. The patient is conditioned by visual reinforcement to reduce the electrical activity of the puborectalis muscle while straining, thus allowing the pelvic floor to relax during defaecation. The overall successful response rate is 70–90% (Bleijenberg & Kuijpers 1987, Loening-Baucke 1990, Fleshman et al 1992, Wexner et al 1992).

If the patient has a combination of slow transit constipation, defined by marker or scintigraphic studies, *and* pelvic floor obstruction, pelvic floor retraining with biofeedback techniques is indicated first. If

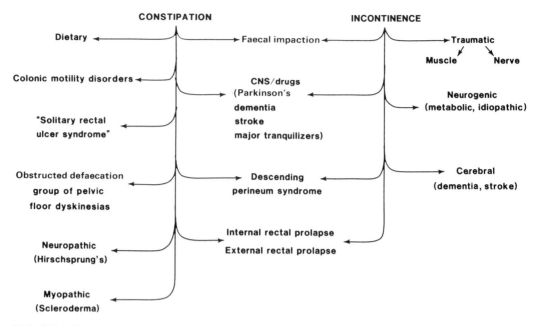

Fig. 38.1 Pelvic floor syndromes are classified according to the dominant symptom of incontinence or constipation. (Reprinted with permission of publisher. From: Perry R E, Pemberton J H 1990. The pelvic floor syndromes in: Postgraduate advances in colorectal surgery. Forum Medicum Publishers, Berryville, VA, pp 1–19.)

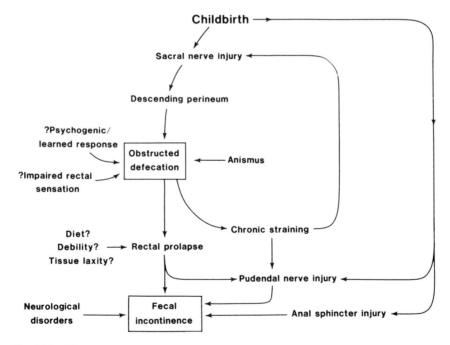

Fig. 38.2 There are complex interrelationships among the pelvic floor disorders. An abnormality in one component of the continence mechanism may cause a second abnormality in another component. (Reprinted with permission of publisher. From: Perry R E, Pemberton J H 1990. The pelvic floor syndromes in: Postgraduate advances in colorectal surgery. Forum Medicum Publishers, Berryville, VA, pp. 1–19.)

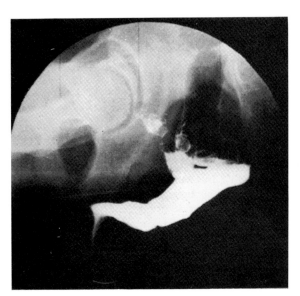
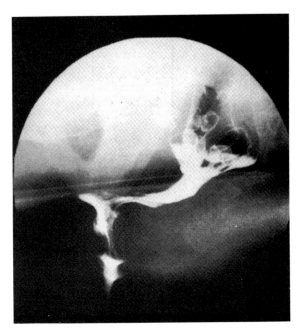

Fig. 38.3 Series of defaecating proctograms demonstrating failure of the anorectal angle to widen in response to straining (anismus). (Reprinted with permission of publisher. From: Bartolo D C C 1988. Pelvic floor disorders in: Schrock T R (ed.) Perspectives in colon and rectal surgery vol 1. Quality Medical Publishing, St Louis, pp. 1–24.)

A   **B**

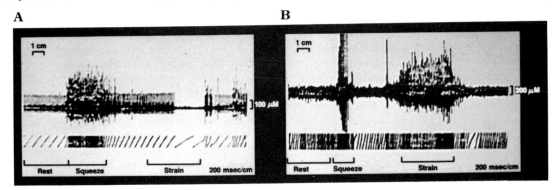

Fig. 38.4 Puborectalis muscle electromyogram. **A** Normal tracing. During squeeze, the muscle increases its firing rate: and during straining, it silences. **B** Abnormal tracing. During straining, a paradoxical increase in puborectalis muscle firing rate is illustrated. (Reprinted with permission from publisher. From: Snooks S J, Swash M 1985. Electromyography of pelvic floor disorders in: Henry M M, Swash S J (eds) Coloproctology and the pelvic floor pathophysiology and management. Butterworths, London, pp. 88–103.)

retraining is successful, the colonic transit study is repeated. In only a few patients will the transit time return to normal. In most, slow transit persists and a subtotal colectomy with ileorectostomy is indicated *if symptoms are disabling* (Pemberton et al 1991).

Disturbed rectal sensation

If rectal sensation is impaired, constipated patients fail to appreciate rectal distension until large volumes are attained (Miller et al 1989a). The cause of impaired sensation is unclear. Although the internal sphincter may relax, rectal filling is frequently not sensed and stool accumulates. It is not known whether the easily demonstrable anatomic abnormality of megarectum is caused by a disorder of rectal muscular compliance, by an abnormality of innervation, or from sphincter dysfunction. Additionally, a behavioural problem from neglecting the call to stool is a possible explanation.

Protracted, forceful straining is probably responsible for many secondary effects of impaired rectal sensation. Many patients with faecal incontinence have a history of constipation and excessive straining at stool (Kiff & Swash 1984a). Repeated stretching of the pudendal nerve during forceful straining causes a neuropraxia. The end result is pudendal neuropathy and progressive denervation of the external sphincter leading to faecal incontinence (Bartolo et al 1983a). The longer the history of straining, the more severe the EMG findings of pudendal neuropathy (Kiff et al 1984). These abnormalities are similar to those found in patients with faecal incontinence but to a lesser degree (Snooks et al 1985a).

Megarectum

Megarectum is diagnosed with radiocontrast studies which includes a lateral view of the pelvis to rule out a narrow distal segment of aganglionosis (Hirschsprung's disease). Moreover, anorectal manometry demonstrates an intact rectal–anal sphincter inhibitory response. The caliber of the proximal colon should also be examined for coexisting megacolon. Colonic transit studies are necessary to exclude a pancolonic dysmotility disorder.

Treatment is initiated by clearing the rectum of faecal material and establishing a regular bowel regimen. Pelvic floor retraining assists some patients in achieving normal bowel habits. Patients with intractable symptoms from megarectum may be improved with a rectal bypass (Duhamel) procedure (Stabile et al 1991), proctectomy and coloanal anastomosis (Stabile et al 1990), or a colectomy and ileal pouch–anal anastomosis (Hosie et al 1990).

Descending perineum syndrome

Descending perineum syndrome results from injury to the innervation of the levator ani, puborectalis and external anal sphincter (EAS) muscles, injury to the muscles themselves during childbirth, or from excessive straining during defaecation (Kiff & Swash 1984a). The lack of support of the pelvic floor muscles and perirectal tissues is reflected by perineal bulging upon straining. Further increases in intra-abdominal pressure do not propel the faecal bolus aborally. Once the pelvic floor is weakened, any straining causes significant descent. Rectal fullness is perceived, however, as the rectum descends and invaginates and the cycle of straining is initiated. Interestingly, an abnormal degree of perineal descent occurs in a high percentage of patients with constipation and chronic straining at

stool (Parks et al 1966). Conversely, most patients with perineal descent give a long history of straining at a defaecation (Parks et al 1966).

Pelvic floor descent is measured on dynamic proctography as the perpendicular distance between the anorectal junction to a line connecting the coccygeal tip and the pubic bone (Parks et al 1966). At rest, the anorectal junction is located within 1 cm of this line; on straining, the pelvic floor descends between 1–4 cm below the line (Fig. 38.5) (Bartram et al 1988).

Excessive pelvic floor descent stretches the pudendal nerve distal to its fixed point in the pudendal canal causing weakness in the external sphincter (Neill et al 1981). In healthy subjects, the pudendal nerve terminal motor latency (PNTML) is reversibly increased following straining; conversely, in patients with abnormal perineal descent, the degree of perineal descent is directly related to prolongation of the PNTML. Miller et al (1989b) found impaired mucosal electrosensitivity and thermal sensitivity in patients with excessive perineal descent compared to controls.

Bartolo et al (1983b) found similar impairment of the rectoanal inhibitory reflex (RAIR), changes in the anorectal angle, and EMG abnormalities confirming denervation in continent and incontinent patients with descending perineum syndrome; however, resting anal canal pressures were higher in the continent patients. Thus, preservation of continence in patients with descending perineum syndrome relies on the ability of the anal sphincters to maintain anal canal pressures.

Patients with profound perineal descent and obstructed defaecation are candidates for biofeedback. At the present time, no surgical procedures are available to treat descending perineum syndrome reliably.

Hirschsprung's disease

A short aganglionic segment at the anorectal junction is a rare cause of obstructed defaecation in adults. If the RAIR is repeatedly absent on manometric testing, a diagnosis of Hirschsprung's disease is likely and a full-thickness rectal biopsy is indicated. This diagnosis is difficult to establish in view of the wide variation in density of ganglion cells at the level of the anorectal junction in normal subjects (Aldridge & Campbell 1968, Weinberg 1970). Treatment of short segment Hirschsprung's disease with anorectal myomectomy is frequently successful. For long aganglionic segments, good long-term functional results are achieved with the Soave endorectal pull-through or the Duhamel bypass procedure (Wheatley et al 1990).

A

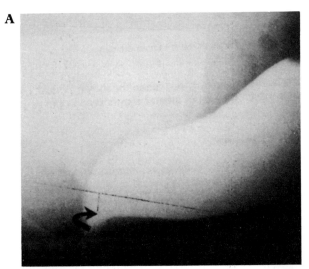

B

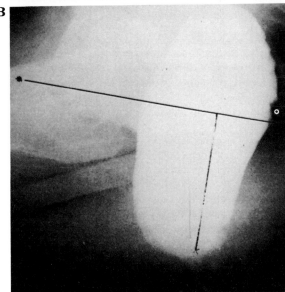

Fig. 38.5 Defaecating proctogram. **A** Normal position of the rectum, anorectal angle and anal canal. **B** Gross perineal descent. (Reproduced with permission of the publisher. From: Barthram C I, Makieu P H G 1985. Radiology and the pelvic floor in: Henry M M, Swash M (eds) Coloproctology and the pelvic floor. Pathophysiology and management. Butterworths, London, pp. 141–186.)

Complete rectal prolapse

Rectal prolapse is associated with profoundly abnormal defaecation (Fig. 38.6). Faecal incontinence is associated with rectal prolapse in 63–81% of patients (Madden et al 1992, Morgan et al 1972, Penfold & Hawley

1972, Keighley & Fielding 1983). It seems that all patients with rectal prolapse will inevitably develop faecal incontinence from repeated traction on the pudendal nerve, abnormal perineal descent, and progressive anal dilatation (Kiff et al 1984, Neill et al 1981, Snooks et al 1984). Constipation, on the other hand, is the predominant symptom in 19–65% of patients with rectal prolapse (Morgan et al 1972, Sayfan et al 1990, Mann & Hoffmann 1988). A cause and effect relationship between pelvic floor laxity and rectal prolapse has yet to be substantiated. However, rectal prolapse precedes overt faecal incontinence for months to years suggesting prolapse is responsible for the incontinence.

Incontinent patients with rectal prolapse will have low resting pressures; in contrast, continent patients have normal pressures (Bartolo 1988). Impairment of the internal anal sphincter (IAS) is related to chronic stretch injury to the sphincter, activation of the RAIR from the advancing prolapsed segment (Holmstrom et al 1986), and disturbed anorectal sensation (Ihre & Seligson 1975).

Maximum voluntary contraction in patients with rectal prolapse is reduced suggesting denervation of the external sphincter (Williams et al 1991a, Metcalf & Loening-Baucke 1988). Histological (Parks et al 1977) and EMG (Neill et al 1981) evidence of a denervation and reinnervation pattern have been identified in the external sphincter.

The majority of patients are best treated by an abdominal approach whereby the rectum is completely mobilized and the sigmoid colon resected. Rectopexy to the sacrum is optional. *Perineal* rectosigmoidectomy is reserved for frail or debilitated patients. About 50% of patients with preoperative incontinence will improve following repair (Schlinkert et al 1985, Duthie & Bartolo 1992, Williams et al 1991a). However, constipation may be more frequent following rectopexy (Mann & Hoffmann 1988).

Nonetheless, inducing constipation does *not* seem to be the method by which continence is restored after operations for rectal prolapse. Rather, restoration of sphincter function is probably the most important factor. Although an increase in anal pressures has not been correlated with improved clinical outcome by some authors (Madden et al 1992, Ihre & Seligson 1975, Sayfan et al 1990), others have reported improved continence only in patients with increased resting anal canal tone (Duthie & Bartolo 1992, Broden et al 1988). Upper anal canal sensation improves following repair presumably from relocation of the upper anal canal to its normal position (Duthie & Bartolo 1992). These findings suggest that multiple factors are important in the restoration of continence.

Occult rectal prolapse

Occult rectal prolapse results from rectal intussusception in response to prolonged increases in intra-abdominal pressure. There appears to be an association between anterior mucosal prolapse, internal intussusception, solitary rectal ulcer and abnormal perineal descent (Sun et al 1989a). After 5 years, 30% of patients presenting with anterior rectal prolapse and abnormal perineal descent are incontinent and 20% have developed complete rectal prolapse (Allen-Mersch et al 1987). About one-third of patients with occult rectal prolapse are incontinent of stool (Bartolo 1988). These patients usually have higher anal canal pressures than incontinent patients with complete rectal prolapse (Bartolo 1988).

Occult rectal prolapse is sometimes palpable when the patient strains while sitting on a commode. Defaecography demonstrates the anatomical abnormality reliably (Fig. 38.7). Interpretation of the results must be made with great caution since 50–60% of healthy subjects without constipation may show signs of occult rectal prolapse during this examination (Shorvon et al 1989).

Occult rectal prolapse is managed by bowel retraining with avoidance of straining during defaecation. Results of surgical treatment are disappointing. Bartolo (1988) reported poor results in 75% of patients undergoing surgical repair of symptomatic occult rectal prolapse.

Solitary rectal ulcer syndrome

Solitary rectal ulcer is an uncommon chronic ulceration most often located in the anterior rectum. The aetiology is unknown but a strong association with descending perineum syndrome (Snooks et al 1985b) and rectal prolapse (Kuijpers et al 1986) has been identified. Ulceration may arise from trauma to leading edge of the intussusceptum caused by forceful straining against an immobile pelvic floor. Womack et al (1987) demonstrated during dynamic assessment of rectal emptying in patients with solitary ulcer syndrome that occult prolapse was present in the majority. Moreover, upon straining, the anal sphincters failed to relax. Others have noted a non-relaxing puborectalis muscle during straining (Snooks et al 1985b, Mackle & Parks 1990). Treatment is directed toward correcting the rectal intussusception and bowel training to avoid straining during defaecation.

Rectocele

Rectoceles can be demonstrated in up to 77% of healthy women evaluated with defaecography (Shorvon et al 1989). Ihre and Seligson (1975) used rectal scintigraphy to demonstrate preferential filling of the rectocele instead of being evacuated in some women with obstructed defaecation. To counteract filling of the rectocele, some patients place a finger in the vagina and push toward the rectum, or on the perineum and push upward during straining. Other patients must extract the stool digitally.

Posterior rectal hernias have also been described. Upon straining, the posterior rectal wall bulges backwards and downwards to the levator muscles (Fig. 38.8). Repair of symptomatic rectoceles located in the low- to mid-rectum is possible through transanal, transperineal or transvaginal approaches.

FAECAL INCONTINENCE

Many patients with faecal incontinence will not volunteer a history of this embarrassing symptom unless specifically questioned (Read et al 1979, Leigh & Turnberg 1982). Important points to ascertain include the need to wear a pad or change undergarments, and the reluctance to leave home or travel far from a toilet. A history of vaginal deliveries, previous episiotomies or perineal tears, forceps deliveries, prolonged labour or large birthweight babies should be elicited (Table 38.1).

Important physical signs are a perianal scar from a previous obstetrical tear or anorectal procedure, patulous anus, weak resting or squeeze anal tone, shortened anal canal, perineal effacement with straining, and occult or complete rectal prolapse. Mechanical disorders, including anorectal neoplasms, inflammatory bowel disease, anal fissures, fistula-in-ano or faecal impaction are excluded by careful inspection and rigid proctoscopic examination.

Striated sphincter dysfunction

A history of sphincter tear during childbirth or following anorectal surgery is present in a minority of incontinent patients. However, a very recent report using endoanal ultrasound documented *occult* anal sphincter injury in one-third of women after a vaginal delivery (Sultan et al 1992). Moreover, neurological impairment of the pelvic floor is the most frequent cause of striated muscle dysfunction (Snooks et al 1984).

Manometric studies in incontinent patients usually demonstrate reduced maximum resting and squeeze

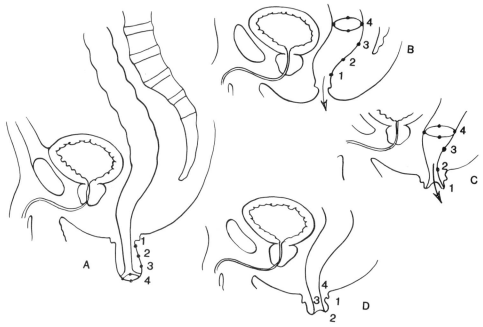

Fig. 38.6   Cause of rectal prolapse is intussusception of the rectum. **A** Radiopaque beads are clipped to the prolapse in positions 1 to 4. **B** The prolapse is reduced. **C** The patient strains. Bead at position 1 appears first. **D** Continued straining. Bead at position 2 appears next, followed by bead at position 3, and then those at position 4. (Reproduced with permission of publisher. From: Theuerkauf F J, Beahrs O H, Hill J R 1970. Rectal prolapse: causation and surgical treatment. Ann Surg 171: 819–835.)

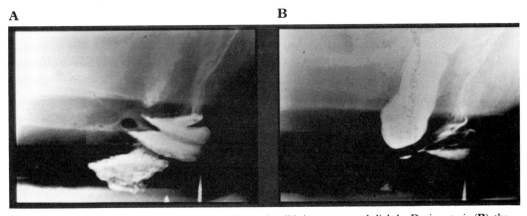

Fig. 38.7   Defaecating proctogram. At rest (**A**), the rectal wall is intussuscepted slightly. During strain (**B**), the sigmoid colon descends low into the pouch of Douglas obstructing the outflow of barium. (Reproduced with permission of publisher. From: Pemberton J H 1990. The clinical value of anorectal motility. Surg Annu 22: 185–214.)

pressures compared to controls (Matheson & Keighley 1981, McHugh & Diamant 1987). Interestingly, 35–40% of patients with faecal incontinence have normal resting and squeeze pressures (McHugh & Diamant 1987, Rasmussen et al 1992). However, in comparing healthy and incontinent patients with normal manometric pa-

rameters, Rasmussen et al (1992) found that the anorectal pressure gradient at rest and during maximal squeeze effort was considerably lower in incontinent patients.

Progressive neuropathic damage to the striated musculature of the pelvic floor is the most frequent finding

A

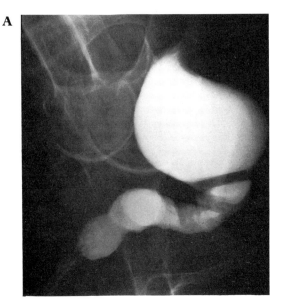

B

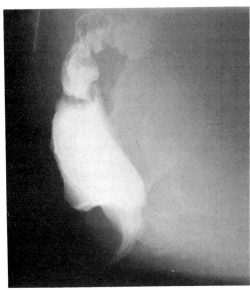

Fig. 38.8   Defaecating proctograms showing 'herniation' of the rectum into the pelvic floor posteriorly at rest (**A**) and with straining (**B**). (Reproduced with permission of publisher. From: Pemberton J H 1991. Anatomy and physiology of the anus and rectum in: Zuidema G D (ed.) Shackelford's surgery of the alimentary tract 3rd edn W B Saunders, Philadelphia, vol. IV pp. 242–274.

Table 38.1   Possible aetiologies for faecal incontinence

Anal canal high pressure zone	Trauma, surgery, prolapse, neurological disorder, Crohn's disease, congenital anomaly
Anorectal angle	Surgery (infection), 'high' fistulotomy, neurological disorder, congenital anomaly
Sensation and reflex	Age, prolapse, impaction, surgery, learned behaviour
Rectal capacity, compliance	Surgery, radiation, carcinoma, prolapse, IBD
Anal canal motility	Tumour, prolapse, Crohn's disease, surgery, neurological disorder
Colon transit	Resection, IBS, IBD
Stool volume and consistency	Diet, diarrhoea (IBS, IBD, infection)

IBD = inflammatory bowel disease
IBS = irritable bowel syndrome

spinal cord differentiates between a lesion in the cauda equina (incredibly rare) and stretch injury to the pudendal nerve (incredibly common). Most patients with neuropathic faecal incontinence, therefore, have a distal conduction delay (Fig. 38.9) (Kiff & Swash 1984b).

EMG abnormalities of the EAS are characterized by decreased activity with motor unit potentials of larger amplitude and longer duration. These findings are consistent with a denervation/reinnervation pattern. Histological studies of the external sphincter in patients with neurogenic incontinence confirm denervation of the pelvic striated muscles (Kiff & Swash 1984b, Parks et al 1977). Physiological studies before and after parturition for forceps and breech deliveries have shown increased external sphincter fibre density and prolonged pudendal nerve terminal motor latency (Snooks et al 1984). These findings are more pronounced in multiparous than primiparous women and were more likely to persist at 2 months postpartum in the multiparous women suggesting a cumulative injury with increasing number of vaginal deliveries. In women who underwent a caesarean section, no physiological abnormalities were identified.

Endoanal sonography is useful for detecting sphincter defects in incontinent patients (Burnett et al 1991). Interestingly, sphincter defects are also visible sonographically in *continent* patients following primary repair of obstetrical tears (Nielsen et al 1992). Whether these patients are able to compensate for the external

in patients with faecal incontinence (Womack et al 1986). Conduction in the distal portion of the pudendal nerve, demonstrated by pudendal nerve terminal motor latency, is prolonged from a stretch injury (Swash et al 1985). As a result, resting and squeeze pressures are reduced. Transcutaneous electrical stimulation of the

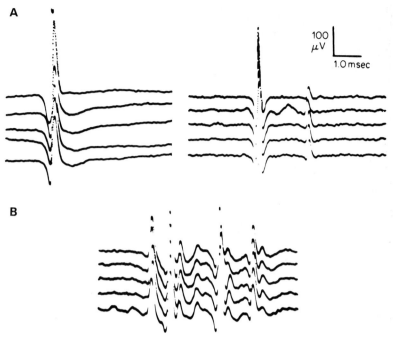

Fig. 38.9 Single fibre EMG of EAS muscle. **A** normal units consisting of one or two spike components. **B** polyphasic units of increased duration from a patient with neurogenic stress faecal incontinence. (Reproduced with permission of publisher. From: Swash M, Snooks S J 1985. Electromyography in pelvic floor disorders in: Henry M M, Swash M (eds) Coloproctology and the pelvic floor. Pathophysiology and management. Butterworths, London pp. 88–103.)

sphincter defect by using other pelvic floor muscles remains incompletely understood.

Internal sphincter dysfunction

Internal sphincter dysfunction is a cause of faecal incontinence in about 25% of patients (Sun et al 1989b). Prolonged ambulatory recordings in incontinent patients have demonstrated spontaneous relaxations in resting anal canal pressure which are longer lasting and more frequent compared to healthy controls (Kumar et al 1989). In fact, in incontinent patients, frequent anal canal relaxations are associated with lower trough pressure levels and reduced rectal volumes to induce sphincter relaxation (Sun et al 1990a). Moreover, protective increases in external sphincter activity during spontaneous sphincter relaxation are not generated reliably in incontinent patients.

EMG studies of the internal sphincter in incontinent patients using bipolar wire electrodes have demonstrated a reduced frequency of slow wave activity (Duthie et al 1990). Using surface electrode techniques, slow wave activity was frequently not recordable (Lubowski et al 1988). The latter authors used electron microscopy to identify ultrastructural abnormalities in the internal sphincter in six incontinent patients. Pharmacological studies of the internal sphincter demonstrate a reduced sensitivity to noradrenaline and to electrical field stimulation (Speakman et al 1990). These findings suggest that denervation may also be responsible for internal sphincter dysfunction. Recently, Speakman et al (1992) found the intrinsic innervation of the IAS to be normal in patients with neurogenic incontinence, thus, implicating abnormal *extrinsic* innervation as a cause of inappropriate IAS relaxations.

Endoanal ultrasound has shown a correlation between internal sphincter thickness and resting anal pressure (Law et al 1991). Incontinent patients with low resting anal canal pressures had reduced thickness of the internal sphincter compared to healthy subjects. Furthermore, unsuspected defects in the EAS were also identified.

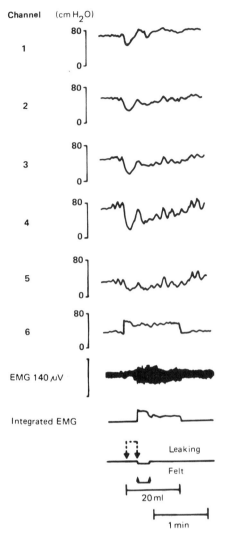

Fig. 38.10 Recordings of anorectal pressures at ports situated 0.5, 1.0, 1.5, 2.0, 2.5 and 4.5 cm from the anal margin (channels 1 to 6) and the EMG activity of the external sphincter during distension of a rectal balloon with 20 ml of air in a patient with impaired rectal sensation. Note that the rectal distension elicits a phasic rectal contraction and internal anal sphincter relaxation. The rectal pressure is higher than the residual anal pressure at the beginning of the distension and leakage occurs. This stops once the subject feels the rectal sensation, which triggers the EAS activity increasing the anal pressure to a value higher than the rectal pressure. (Reproduced with permission of the publisher. From: Sun W M, Read, N W, Miner P B 1990. Relation between rectal sensation and anal function in normal subjects and patients with faecal incontinence. Gut 31: 1056–1061.)

Both continent and incontinent patients with abnormal perineal descent have similar EMG changes and impairment in squeeze pressure suggesting striated muscle denervation (Womack et al 1986). However, continent patients have normal resting pressures implying that the internal sphincter is impaired in the incontinent patients.

Impaired anorectal sensation

Patients with faecal incontinence need less rectal volume to elicit faecal urgency and have lower maximum tolerable rectal volumes compared to controls (Rasmussen et al 1990, Read et al 1983). Furthermore, reflex contraction of the external sphincter is delayed when attempting to prevent release of faeces (Fig. 38.10).

Gunterberg et al (1976) studied patients following major resections of the sacrum and found that discrimination of anorectal contents was disturbed if the sacral nerves are sacrificed bilaterally. In contrast, unilateral sacral nerve resection did not disturb anal canal sensation. Similarly, continence to intrarectal saline infusion is not impaired following topical anal canal anesthesia (Read & Read 1982).

Central neurological lesions lead to an inability of patients to sense rectal distension. In low spinal lesions, the external sphincter response to rectal distension is delayed and weak (Sun et al 1990b). In high spinal lesions, rectal sensation and conscious control of the external sphincter are absent. Faecal incontinence from systemic disorders such as diabetes mellitus and multiple sclerosis are likely due to a combined sensorimotor defect (Caruana et al 1991).

Reduced rectal compliance

Rasmussen et al (1990) reported reduced rectal compliance and maximum tolerable volume, and increased faecal urgency in patients with idiopathic faecal incontinence compared to controls. On the other hand, an intact sensation of rectal distension in incontinent patients has been demonstrated by Ferguson et al (1989).

A rectal aetiology for faecal incontinence has also been attributed to a reduced sensory threshold from chronic radiation injury (Varma et al 1985), and diminished rectal compliance following low anterior resection (Pederson et al 1986). Patients with active chronic ulcerative colitis have increased stool frequency, urgency, tenesmus, and episodes of soilage caused by loss of rectal wall compliance. Abnormally elevated rectal pressures occasionally exceed anal pressures causing leakage (Read et al 1983). Although impaired anal sphincter function is the most common cause of faecal incontinence, a reduction in rectal compliance aggravates the incontinence by increasing the frequency of defaecation. Importantly, large volumes of liquid stool emptied rapidly into the rectum may overcome the sphincter mechanism causing faecal incontinence even in healthy subjects (Read et al 1979).

Treatment of faecal incontinence

Figure 38.11 depicts an algorithm for evaluation and management of patients with pelvic floor dysfunction. Many patients with incontinence will improve symptomatically with diet modifications, constipating or stool bulking agents, and pelvic floor exercises. Biofeedback will improve 70–90% of patients with faecal incontinence (Miner et al 1990, McHugh et al 1988, MacLeod 1987, Riboli et al 1988), although no randomized study has been performed showing a benefit compared to surgical repair. Surgery is suitable for patients for complete loss of faecal control. The postanal repair has traditionally been offered to patients with neurogenical faecal incontinence with an overall long-term success rate of about 60% (Miller et al 1988, Henry & Simson 1985, Orrom et al 1991, Keighley 1984). Anterior sphincteroplasty, used commonly for traumatic sphincter injuries, has comparable results to the postanal repair (Jacobs et al 1990, Pezim et al 1987b, Wexner et al 1991, Laurberg et al 1988). In highly motivated patients who have failed previous attempts at sphincter repair or lack sufficient sphincter muscle for reconstruction, muscle transpositions using the gracilis or gluteus maximus muscles may be attempted. The electrically stimulated modification of the gracilis muscle transposition procedure may prevent muscle fatigue, thus possibly adding dynamic features to the neosphincter (Williams et al 1991b). Finally, of course, a completely diverting colostomy is a viable option in patients with debilitating incontinence who have failed other treatment modalities.

PROCTALGIA FUGAX

Proctalgia fugax is a disorder of severe, intermittent rectal pain, occurring most commonly at night, which resolves spontaneously without residual symptoms. The aetiology is unclear but spasm of the levator ani muscle has been implicated. Intraluminal pressure measurements during episodes of rectal pain have demonstrated increased sigmoid contractility suggesting the pain is referred to the rectum rather than from actual spasm of the pelvic floor muscles (Harvey 1979). More recently, Kamm et al (1991) described functional and structural abnormalities in the internal sphincter consistent with a localized myopathy in three related

patients with proctalgia fugax. Importantly, other functional gastrointestinal disorders are common in patients with proctalgia fugax. Local measures using sitz baths and heat application provide some relief.

IRRITABLE BOWEL SYNDROME (IBS)

Patients with IBS have been found to have a 'hypertonic' rectum and sigmoid colon, associated with hypersensitivity and increased contractility (Ritchie 1973, Whitehead et al 1980). Although the anal sphincter mechanism is normal, inappropriate rectoanal inhibition occurs at lower rectal volumes and is sustained for long periods (Sun & Read 1988). In addition, there is an enhanced colonic response to meals, stress and luminal distension (Preston & Lennard-Jones 1986).

ANAL FISSURE

Anal canal ultraslow waves are recorded in up to 80% of patients with fissure-in-ano but their significance is unknown (Hancock 1977). Impaired mucosal sensitivity has also been described (Roe et al 1986). Resting pressures are high compared to controls but squeeze pressures are usually normal (Hancock 1977, Gibbons & Read 1986). When eliciting the rectoanal inhibitory response, a large rebound contraction occurs immediately after normal internal sphincter relaxation (Martelli et al 1978). However, these findings are also seen in some patients with obstructed defaecation. Whether the elevated resting pressures are a cause or result of the fissure remains unclear. Following lateral internal sphincterotomy, resting anal canal pressures decline to normal levels within 1 week (Cerdan et al 1982).

HAEMORRHOIDS

Higher resting anal canal pressures have been demonstrated in some but not all patients with haemorrhoids: the reason for this finding is unclear. Dysfunction of the IAS has been suggested as a cause of submucosal venous stasis and impaired emptying of the internal haemorrhoidal plexus (Thompson 1975). The threshold of mucosal sensitivity is elevated in patients with haemorrhoids (Roe et al 1986). Additionally, ultraslow waves have been documented in 50% of patients with haemorrhoids compared to 5% of healthy subjects (Hancock & Smith 1975). The normal frequency gradient for intraluminal contractile activity increases distally in the anal canal but this is lost in patients with haemorrhoids.

Read et al (1989) measured vascular pressures within haemorrhoidal tissues in symptomatic patients and

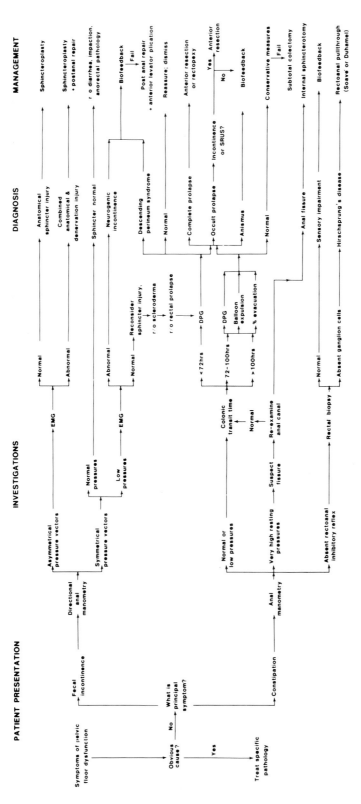

Fig. 38.11 Flow diagram for the evaluation and management of patients presenting with symptoms of pelvic floor dysfunction. (Reproduced with permission of the publisher. From: Perry R E, Pemberton J H 1990, The pelvic floor syndromes in: Postgraduate advances in colorectal surgery. Forum Medicum Publishers, Berryville, VA, pp. 1–19.)

found intravascular pressure to rise dramatically during straining. Following haemorrhoidectomy, Roe et al (1987) noted a reduction in anal canal pressure and suggested that the haemorrhoidal tissue was responsible for the elevated anal pressures.

PRURITIS ANI

Pruritis ani is associated with leakage of stool in about 50% of patients (Smith et al 1982). Local (i.e. anorectal) or systemic diseases (i.e. diarrhoea, dermatitis) predispose to soiling and increased perianal sensitivity. Most patients with pruritis ani have normal resting anal pressures but an exaggerated RAIR (Allan et al 1987,

Eyers & Thomson 1979). Management is directed at correcting the underlying disorder, improving hygiene, and avoiding foods which exacerbate symptoms.

SUMMARY

The pathophysiology of motility disorders of the anorectum remains incompletely understood. It is important to remember there is considerable overlap in the aetiologies and presenting symptoms of pelvic floor disorders. A comprehensive stepwise approach to evaluation will differentiate between aetiologies of incontinence and constipation.

REFERENCES

Aldridge R T, Campbell P E 1968 Ganglion cell distribution in the normal rectum and anal canal: a basis for the diagnosis of Hirchsprung's disease by anorectal biopsy. J Pediatr Surg 3: 475–490

Allan A, Ambrose N S, Silverman S, et al 1987 Physiological study of pruritis ani. Br J Surg 74: 576–579

Allen-Mersch T G, Henry M M, Nicholls R J 1987 Natural history of anterior muscosal prolapse. Br J Surg 74: 679–682

Barnes P R H, Hawley P R, Preston D M 1985 Experience of posterior division of the puborectalis muscle in the management of chronic constipation. Br J Surg 72: 475–477

Bartolo D C C 1988 Pelvic floor disorders. Incontinence, constipation, and obstructed defecation. Perspect Colon Rectal Surg 1: 1–24

Bartolo D C C, Jarratt J A, Read M G, et al 1983a The role of partial denervation of the puborectalis in idiopathic faecal incontinence. Br J Surg 70: 664–667

Bartolo D C C, Read N W, Jarratt J A et al 1983b Differences in anal sphincter function and clinical presentation in patients with pelvic floor descent. Gastroenterology 85: 68–75

Bartram C I, Turnbull G K, Lennard-Jones J E 1988 Evacuation proctography: an investigation of rectal expulsion in 20 subjects without defecatory disturbance. Gastrointest Radiol 13: 72–80

Bleijenberg G, Kuijpers H C 1987 Treatment of the spastic pelvic floor syndrome with biofeedback. Dis Colon Rectum 30: 108–111

Broden G, Dolk A, Holmstrom B 1988 Recovery of internal anal sphincter following rectopexy: a possible explanation for continence improvement. Int J Colorectal Dis 3: 23–28

Burnett S J D, Speakman C T M, Kamm M A et al 1991 Confirmation of endosonographic detection of external sphincter defects by simultaneous electromyographic mapping. Br J Surg 78: 448–450

Caruana B J, Wald A, Hinds J P et al 1991 Anorectal sensory and motor function in neurogenic fecal incontinence. Gastroenterology 100: 465–470

Cerdan F J, Ruiz de Leon A, Azpiroz F et al 1982 Anal sphincteric pressure in fissure-in-ano before and after

lateral internal sphincterotomy. Dis Colon Rectum 25: 198–201

Duthie G S, Bartolo D C C 1992 Abdominal rectopexy for rectal prolapse: a comparison of techniques. Br J Surg 79: 107–113

Duthie G S, Miller R, Bartolo D C C 1990 Internal anal sphincter electromyographic frequency is related to anal canal resting pressure. Both are reduced in idiopathic faecal incontinence. Gut 31: A619

Eyers A A, Thomson J P 1979 Pruritis ani: is anal sphincter dysfunction important in aetiology? Br Med J 2: 1549–1551

Ferguson G H, Redford J, Barrett J A et al 1989 The appreciation of rectal distension in fecal incontinence. Dis Colon Rectum 32: 964–967

Fleshman J W, Dreznik Z, Meyer K et al 1992 Outpatient protocol for biofeedback therapy of pelvic floor outlet obstruction. Dis Colon Rectum 35: 1–7

Gibbons C P, Read N W 1986 Anal hypertonia and fissures: cause or effect? Br J Surg 73: 443–445

Gunterberg B, Kewenter J, Petersen I et al 1976 Anorectal function after major resections of the sacrum with bilateral or unilateral sacrifice of sacral nerves. Br J Surg 63: 546–554

Hancock B D 1977 The internal anal sphincter and anal fissure. Br J Surg 64: 92–95

Hancock B D, Smith K 1975 The internal sphincter and Lord's procedure for haemorrhoids. Br J Surg 62: 833–836

Harvey R F 1979 Colonic motility in proctalgia fugax. Lancet 2: 713–714

Henry M M, Simson J N L 1985 Results of postanal repair: a retrospective study. Br J Surg 72 (suppl): S17–S19

Holmstrom B, Broden G, Dolk A et al 1986 Increased anal resting pressure following the Ripstein operation: a contribution to continence? Dis Colon Rectum 29: 485–487

Hosie K B, Kmiot W A, Keighley M R B 1990 Constipation: another indication for restorative proctocolectomy. Br J Surg 77: 801–802

Ihre T, Seligson U 1975 Intussusception of the rectum — internal procidentia: treatment and results in 90 patients. Dis Colon Rectum 11: 391–396

Jacobs P P M, Scheuer M, Kuijpers H C et al 1990 Obstetric fecal incontinence. Role of pelvic floor denervation and results of delayed sphincter repair. Dis Colon Rectum 33: 494–497

Jones P N, Lubowski D Z, Swash M et al 1987 Is paradoxical contraction of puborectalis muscle of functional importance? Dis Colon Rectum 30: 667–670

Kamm M A, Hoyle C H V, Burleigh D E et al 1991 Hereditary internal anal sphincter myopathy causing proctalgia fugax and constipation. Gastroenterology 100: 805–810

Keighley M R B 1984 Postanal repair for faecal incontinence. J R Soc Med 77: 285–288

Keighley M R, Fielding J W 1983 Results of Marlex Mesh abdominal rectopexy for rectal prolapse in 100 consecutive patients. Br J Surg 70: 229–232

Kiff E S, Barnes P R H, Swash M 1984 Evidence of pudendal neuropathy in patients with perineal descent and chronic straining at stool. Gut 25: 1279–1282

Kiff E S, Swash M 1984a Slowed conduction in the pudendal nerves in idiopathic (neurogenic) faecal incontinence. Br J Surg 71: 614–616

Kiff E S, Swash M 1984b Normal proximal and delayed distal conduction in the pudendal nerves of patients with idiopathic (neurogenic) faecal incontinence. J Neurol Neurosurg Psych 47: 820–823

Kuijpers H C, Beijenberg G 1985 The spastic pelvic floor syndrome: a cause of constipation. Dis Colon Rectum 28: 669–672

Kuijpers H C, Schreve R H, Hoedemakers H T C 1986 Diagnosis of functional disorders of defecation causing solitary rectal ulcer syndrome. Dis Colon Rectum 29: 126–129

Kumar D, Waldron D L, Williams N S 1989 Home assessment of anorectal motility and external sphincter EMG in idiopathic faecal incontinence. Br J Surg 76: 635–636

Laurberg S, Swash M, Henry M M 1988 Delayed external sphincter repair for obstetrical injury. Br J Surg 75: 786–788

Law P J, Kamm M A, Bartram C I 1991 Anal endosonography in the investigation of faecal incontinence. Br J Surg 78: 312–314

Leigh R J, Turnberg L A 1982 Faecal incontinence: the unvoiced symptom. Lancet 1: 1349–1351

Loening-Baucke V 1990 Modulation of abnormal defecation dynamics by biofeedback treatment in chronically constipated children with encopresis. J Pediatr 116: 214–222

Lubowski D Z, Nicholls R J, Burleigh D E et al 1988 Internal anal sphincter in neurogenic fecal incontinence. Gastroenterology 95: 997–1002

McHugh S M, Diamant N E 1987 Effect of age, gender, and parity on anal canal pressures. Dig Dis Sci 32: 726–736

McHugh S, Kersey K, Diamant N E 1988 Biofeedback training for fecal incontinence. Outcome according to physiological parameters. Gastroenterology 94: A295

MacLeod J H 1987 Management of anal incontinence by biofeedback. Gastroenterology 93: 291–294

Mackle E J, Parks T G 1990 Solitary rectal ulcer syndrome. Aetiology, investigation and management. Dig Dis Sci 8: 294–304

Madden M V, Kamm M A, Nicholls R J et al 1992 Abdominal rectopexy for complete prolapse: prospective study evaluationg changes in symptoms and anorectal function. Dis Colon Rectum 35: 48–55

Mann C V, Hoffmann C 1988 Complete rectal prolapse: the anatomical and functional results of treatment by an extended abdominal rectopexy. Br J Surg 75: 34–37

Martelli H, Devroede G, Arhan P et al 1978 Mechanisms of idiopathic constipation: outlet obstruction. Gastroenterology 75: 623–631

Matheson D M, Keighley M R B 1981 Manometric evaluation of rectal prolapse and fecal incontinence. Gut 22: 126–129

Metcalf A M, Loening-Baucke V 1988 Anorectal function and defecation in patients with rectal prolapse. Am J Surg 155: 206–210

Miller R, Bartolo D C C, James D et al 1989a Air-filled microballoon manometry for use in anorectal physiology. Br J Surg 76: 72–75

Miller R, Bartolo D C C, Cervero F et al 1989b Differences in anal sensation in continent and incontinent patients with perineal descent. Int J Colorectal Dis 4: 45–49

Miller R, Bartolo D C C, Locke-Edmunds J C et al 1988 A prospective study of conservative and operative treatment for faecal incontinence. Br J Surg 75: 101–105

Miner P B, Donnelly T C, Read N W 1990 Investigation of mode of action of biofeedback in treatment of fecal incontinence. Dig Dis Sci 35: 1291–1298

Morgan C N, Porter N H, Klugman D J 1972 Ivalon (polyvinyl alcohol) sponge in the repair of complete rectal prolapse. Br J Surg 59: 841–846

Neill M E, Parks A G, Swash M 1981 Physiological studies of the anal sphincter musculature in faecal incontinence and rectal prolapse. Br J Surg 68: 531–536

Nielsen M B, Hauge C, Rasmussen O O et al 1992 Anal endosonographic findings in the follow-up of primarily sutured sphincteric ruptures. Br J Surg 79: 104–106

Orrom W J, Miller R, Cornes H et al 1991 Comparison of anterior sphincteroplasty and postanal repair in the treatment of idiopatic fecal incontinence. Dis Colon Rectum 34: 305–310

Parks A G, Porter N H, Hardcastle J 1966 The syndrome of the descending perineum. Proc R Soc Med 59: 477–482

Parks A G, Swash M, Urich H 1977 Sphincter denervation in anorectal incontinence and rectal prolapse. Gut 18: 656–665

Pederson I K, Christiansen J, Hint K et al 1986 Anorectal function after low anterior resection for carcinoma. Ann Surg 204: 133–135

Pemberton J H, Rath D M, Ilstrup D M 1991 Evaluation and surgical treatment of severe chronic constipation. Ann Surg 214: 403–413

Penfold J C, Hawley P R 1972 Experiences with Ivalon-sponge implant for complete rectal prolapse at St. Mark's Hospital, 1960–70. Br J Surg 59: 846–848

Pezim M, Pemberton J H, Phillips S F 1987a The immobile perineum: pathophysiologic implications in severe constipation. Dig Dis Sci 32: A924

Pezim M E, Spencer R J, Stanhope C R et al 1987b Sphincter repair for fecal incontinence after obstetrical or iatrogenic injury. Dis Colon Rectum 30: 521–525

Preston D M, Lennard-Jones J E 1985 Anismus in chronic constipation. Dig Dis Sci 30: 413–418

Preston D M, Lennard-Jones J E 1986 Severe constipation of young women: idiopathic slow transit constipation. Gut 27: 41–48

Rasmussen O O, Christensen B, Sorensen M et al 1990

Rectal compliance in the assessment of patients with faecal incontinence. Dis Colon Rectum 33: 650–653

Rasmussen O O, Sorensen M, Tetzschner T et al 1992 Anorectal pressure gradient in patients with anal incontinence. Dis Colon Rectum 35: 8–11

Read N W, Harford W V, Schmulen A C et al 1979 A clinical study of patients with fecal incontinence and diarrhea. Gastroenterology 76: 747–756

Read N W, Haynes N W, Bartolo D C C et al 1983 Use of anorectal manometry during rectal infusion of saline to investigate sphincter function in incontinent patients. Gastroenterology 85: 105–113

Read M G, Read N W 1982 Role of anorectal sensation in preserving continence. Gut 23: 345–347

Read N W, Sun W M, Weston-Davies W H 1989 Haemorrhoids, constipation and hypertensive anal cushions. Lancet 1: 610

Riboli E B, Frascio M, Pitto G et al 1988 Biofeedback conditioning for fecal incontinence. Arch Phys Med Rehabil 69: 29–31

Ritchie J 1973 Pain from distension of the pelvic colon by inflating a balloon in the irritable colon syndrome. Gut 14: 125–132

Roe A M, Bartolo D C C, Mortensen N J McC 1986 New method for assessment of anal sensation in various anorectal disorders. Br J Surg 73: 310–312

Roe A M, Bartolo D C C, Vellacott K D et al 1987 Submucosal versus ligation excision hemorrhoidectomy: a comparison of anal sensation, anal sphincter manometry and postoperative pain and function. Br J Surg 74: 948–951

Sayfan J, Pinho M, Alexander-Williams J et al 1990 Sutured posterior abdominal rectopexy with sigmoidectomy compared with Marlex rectopexy for rectal prolapse. Br J Surg 77: 143–145

Schlinkert R T, Beart R W Jr, Wolff B G et al 1985 Anterior resection for complete rectal prolapse. Dis Colon Rectum 28: 409–412

Shorvon P J, McHugh S, Diamant N E et al 1989 Defaecography in normal volunteers: results and implications. Gut 30: 1737–1749

Smith L E, Henrichs D, McCullah R D 1982 Prospective studies on the etiology and treatment of pruritis ani. Dis Colon Rectum 25: 358–363

Snooks S J, Barnes P R H, Swash M et al 1985a Damage to innervation of the pelvic floor musculature in chronic constipation. Gastroenterology 89: 977–981

Snooks S J, Nicholls R J, Henry M M et al 1985b Electrophysiological and manometric assessment of the pelvic floor in the solitary rectal ulcer syndrome. Br J Surg 72: 131–133

Snooks S J, Setchell M, Swash M et al 1984 Injury to innervation of pelvic floor sphincter musculature in childbirth. Lancet 2: 546–550

Speakman C T M, Hoyle C H V, Kamm M A et al 1990 Adrenergic control of the internal anal sphincter is abnormal in patients with idiopathic faecal incontinence. Br J Surg 77: 134–144

Speakman C T M, Kamm M A 1992 Rectal sensation, compliance and internal sphincter innervation in neurogenic faecal incontinence. Gastroenterology 102: A518

Stabile G, Kamm M A, Lennard-Jones J E et al 1990 Idiopathic megarectum and megacolon: which operation offers the best results? Gut 31: A1172

Stabile G, Kamm M A, Hawley P R et al 1991 Results of the Duhamel operation in the treatment of idiopathic megarectum and megacolon. Br J Surg 78: 661–663

Sultan A H, Kamm M A, Hudson C N et al 1992 Vaginal delivery causes anal sphincter disruption in 37% of patients (prospective ultrasound study) – a major determinant for development of faecal incontinence. Gastroenterology 102: A522

Sun W M, Read N W 1988 Anorectal manometry and rectal sensation in patients with irritable bowel syndrome. Gut 27: 283–287

Sun W M, Read N W, Donnelly T C et al 1989a A common pathophysiology for full-thickness rectal prolapse, anterior mucosal prolapse and solitary rectal ulcer. Br J Surg 76: 290–295

Sun W M, Read N W, Donnelly T C 1989b Impaired internal anal sphincter in a subgroup of patients with idiopathic fecal incontinence. Gastroenterology 97: 130–135

Sun W M, Read N W, Miner P B et al 1990a The role of transient internal sphincter relaxation in faecal incontinence. Int J Colorectal Dis 5: 31–36

Sun W M, Read N W, Donnelly T C 1990b Anorectal function in incontinent patients with spinal disease. Gastroenterology 99: 1372–1379

Swash M, Snooks S J, Henry M M 1985 A unifying concept of pelvic floor disorders and incontinence. J R Soc Med 78: 906–911

Thompson W H F 1975 The nature of haemorrhoids. Br J Surg 62: 833–836

Varma J S, Smith A N, Bussutil A 1985 Correlation and manometric abnormalities of rectal function following chronic radiation injury. Br J Surg 72: 875–878

Weinberg A G 1970 The anorectal myenteric plexus: its relationship to hyperganglionosis of the colon. Am J Clin Pathol 54: 637–642

Wexner S D, Cheape J D, Jorge J M N et al 1992 Prospective assessment of biofeedback for the treatment of paradoxical puborectalis contraction. Dis Colon Rectum 35: 145–150

Wexner S D, Marchetti F, Jagelman D G 1991 The role of sphincteroplasty for faecal incontinence reevaluated: a prospective physiologic and functional review. Dis Colon Rectum 34: 22–30

Wheatley M J, Wesley J R, Coran A G et al 1990 Hirschsprung's disease in adolescents and adults. Dis Colon Rectum 33: 622–629

Whitehead W E, Engel B T, Schuster M M 1980 Irritable bowel syndrome: physiological and psychological differences between diarrhea predominate and constipation predominate patients. Dig Dis Sci 25: 404–413

Williams J G, Wong W D, Jensen L et al 1991a Incontinence and rectal prolapse: a prospectric manometric study. Dis Colon Rectum 34: 209–216

Williams N S, Patel J, George B D et al 1991b Development of an electrically stimulated neoanal sphincter. Lancet 338: 1166–1169

Womack N R, Morrison J F B, Williams N S 1986 The role of pelvic floor denervation in the aetiology of idiopathic faecal incontinence. Br J Surg 73: 404–407

Womack N R, Williams N S, Mist J H H et al 1987 Anorectal function in the solitary rectal ulcer syndrome. Dis Colon Rectum 30: 319–323

Effects of surgery

39. Post-surgical motility disorders

F. Moody   N. Weisbrodt

INTRODUCTION

The effects of disease states on the propulsive function of the gastrointestinal tract have been extensively studied and reported upon. There is less knowledge however about the disturbances in gastric and intestinal motility that accompany the surgical treatment of the diseases that afflict these organs which are so essential to normal digestion. As a first principle, it must be recognized that the activity of the digestive system, as is true of organ systems in general, has a large functional reserve and the ability to adapt (Papasova & Atanassova 1989). In fact, it is remarkable how well the gastrointestinal tract can accommodate to division, shortening, denervation, and bypass or ablation of the sphincters which circumscribe the limits of its areas of specialized function.

In this chapter, we will discuss briefly the normal motor function of the gastrointestinal system. Then we will discuss the motility changes induced by surgical manipulation of the digestive system in normal animals. Finally, we will use this background to discuss some of the major clinical problems that derive from disturbances in motor function which follow operations performed upon the gastrointestinal tract for relatively common disease entities. Although the motility disturbances associated with inflammatory bowel disease will be discussed elsewhere, the clinical liabilities associated with an ileostomy and ileal-pouch–anal anastomosis will be considered below in detail. The motor disturbances associated with small bowel transplantation, an area of increasing interest, are covered in Chapter 40.

NORMAL GASTROINTESTINAL MOTOR FUNCTION IN THE SURGICAL PATIENT

The ingestion, digestion and absorption of nutrients, and the elimination of wastes from the gastrointestinal tract require a carefully timed movement of liquids and solids down its lumen. The process begins with activity of the mouth, pharynx, and esophagus (Weisbrodt 1991a). Little digestion and absorption take place in these organs. They are almost totally involved with motility. Once swallowing begins, peristaltic contractions of the pharynx and oesophagus quickly move contents from the mouth to the stomach. In addition, sphincters at both ends of the oesophagus prevent the entry of air from above and of gastric contents from below.

The normal motor functions of the stomach during the ingestion of a meal have been well characterized and include accommodation of the ingestant through receptive relaxation and its fragmentation and mixing with the digestive enzymes within the gastric juice through antral peristaltic contractions (Moody et al 1988, Weisbrodt 1991b). The content when reduced into particulate size is then delivered into the duodenum in a rhythmic fashion. The pyloric sphincter in part regulates the emptying of solid particles by their size and prevents the regurgitation of duodenal contents into the stomach during periods of vigorous mixing that occurs in this segment of the small intestine. Osmotically and chemically sensitive receptors in the small intestine set into motion patterns of motility of the stomach, pylorus, and duodenum that then further modulate the flow of contents from the stomach. In addition, the duodenum serves as a mixing chamber for the gastric chyme and the alkaline secretions of bile and pancreatic juice.

The motor functions of the gastrointestinal tract are complex and consist not only of accommodation and fragmentation of solid ingestates and their mixing with secretions within the stomach and duodenum, but also accomplish presentation of the digestant, intestinal chyme, to the enterocytes that line the intestinal lumen (Weisbrodt 1991c). The muscular layer of the small intestine therefore provides for further mixing through localized contractions of its circular muscle layer. The segmentation that occurs increases the residence time of the well mixed succus and by intermittent

A

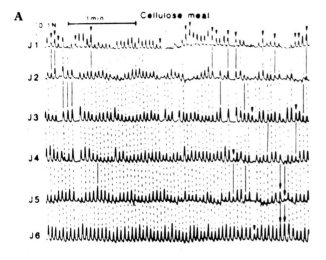

B

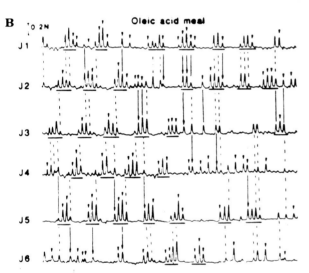

Fig. 39.1 Intestinal contractions recorded from the dog jejunum after intragastric instillation of a meal consisting of cellulose (**A**) and of a meal of cellulose plus oleic acid (**B**). Contractions were monitored at sites 4 cm apart. Dashed lines indicate propagative contractions. Note that there are fewer contractions overall and fewer propagative contractions when oleic acid is part of the meal. (Adapted from Schemann & Ehrlein 1986 with permission.)

contraction and relaxation induces a caudad movement of the contents within its lumen. The actual number and pattern of these contractions is a function of the volume and chemical composition of the chyme (Fig. 39.1).

The ileal segment of the gut has receptors that when activated alter the motility of the stomach and upper small bowel to slow emptying and transit (Welch et al 1988, Soper et al 1990). The ileum also exhibits pat-

terns of contractions not normally seen in more proximal regions. These contractions are coordinated with relaxations of the ileocaecal sphincter and contractions of the colon to effect the movement of chyme from the small intestine to the large intestine (Fig. 39.2). It appears that the ileocaecal valve offers little resistance to the movement of small intestinal contents into the colon (Neri et al 1991), but serves primarily to prevent the regurgitation of colonic contents into the ileum (Köhler et al 1991).

Colonic motility is quite distinct from that which is exhibited by the small intestine (Christensen 1989, Weisbrodt 1991d). The faecal bulk is moved from the right to the left colon by a series of massive contraction waves, and the colon evacuates its contents by a similar type of contraction as the anal sphincters relax. Segmentation, as evidenced by haustral markings on barium radiographs, is a prominent feature of circular muscle activity in the colon and may serve the same function as the non-peristaltic contractions that are associated with mixing in the small intestine. The ability to retain the faecal mass for long periods of time within the left and sigmoid colon is a unique feature of colonic function. The periodic and usually well-timed evacuation of the colon is also a remarkably integrated motor event that depends upon neurally generated signals from the anorectal mucosa and pressure sensors within the wall of the rectum and anus.

The above brief description of the normal motor functions of the stomach and intestines provides a background for considering how surgical procedures upon the gastrointestinal tract might alter this important activity. It must be recognized that even at rest or during interdigestive intervals, the gastrointestinal tract is actively moving its contents towards the colon. It does so by eliciting so-called migrating complexes of contractile and myoelectric activity fronts that occur about every 100 min between meals, and are designed to move air, residual food particles, secretions, desquamated cells and bacteria down the gut (Fig. 39.3). Less frequent but more powerful ileal contractions have also been described that are apparently also designed to clear material from the ileum into the colon (Quigley et al 1984).

MOTILITY EFFECTS OF SURGICAL MANIPULATION – PHYSIOLOGICAL BASES

There have been numerous studies performed on experimental animals in which surgical manipulations were involved. Although most of these studies were designed to investigate mechanisms that regulate motility, results from these studies make it possible to

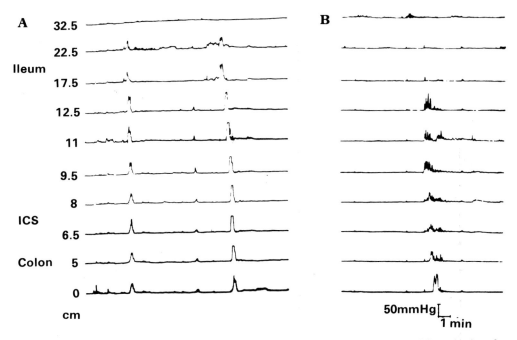

Fig. 39.2 Recordings of intraluminal pressure from the ileum, ileocaecal sphincter (ICS), and colon of a healthy human. Note the large single, phasic contractions that last 20–40 sec and that appear to propagate rapidly aborally (**A**). Also note the short bursts of contractions that also appear to migrate aborally (**B**). (Reproduced with permission from Quigley et al 1984.)

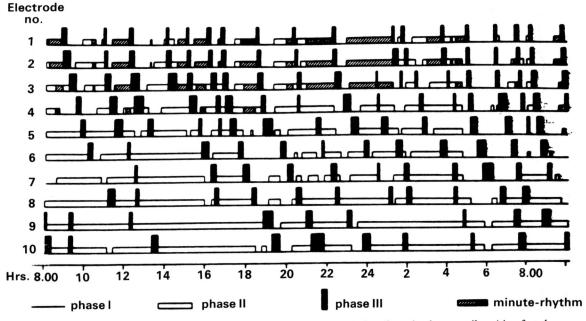

Fig. 39.3 Temporal distribution of spike potentials, hence contractions, at 10 sites (from duodenum to ileum) in a fasted human. The various phases of the MMC that occurred at each site over a 24-h period are shown. Note how the complexes recurred at each site and how many of the complexes appeared to migrate aborally. (Reproduced with permission from Fleckenstein & Oigaard 1978.)

predict to a certain degree the effect that surgical procedures in patients might have on motility. As mentioned above, it is surprising that major segments of the stomach and intestine can be manipulated or removed with little noticeable effect. One must remember, however, that this unfortunately is not always the case in patients who are ill. Some patients suffer serious consequences when even relatively minor procedures are performed upon their stomach or intestinal tract. This may be the result of the combination of the disease process and the manipulation. For this reason and for reasons of species variation, one cannot always predict patient outcome based on studies conducted in healthy animals.

Motility patterns of the various organs of the digestive tract differ in their sensitivities to manipulations. As a general rule, motility of the small intestine is the least sensitive. This is followed by the colon and stomach. The reasons for the differences in sensitivity are not known.

A major consideration in evaluating the effects of surgery of intestinal motility is the concomitant use of pharmacological agents. Indeed, certain anesthetics alone have been shown to alter patterns of small intestinal contractions. For example, in the rat, diethyl ether and pentobarbital both inhibit the fasting pattern of motility. On the other hand, halothane and thiopental have less of an effect (Bueno et al 1978). Furthermore, many of the drugs used postoperatively, such as the opioids, markedly alter gastric emptying as well as small and large intestinal transit (Burks 1987).

Any procedure that results in transection of the muscular layers of the gut wall would be expected to alter motility. In the stomach, small bowel and colon, the smooth muscle cells of the muscularis externa are electrically coupled to one another. Signals (often called slow waves) are generated within the muscular wall of the stomach, small intestine, and colon and then spread in such a way that they coordinate contractile activities at adjacent sites within the organs. Because muscle cell-to-muscle cell connections are required for optimal coordination, a complete circumferential transection should be avoided. Contractions will still occur if all pathways are transected because slow waves are generated at all levels of the gut; however, a loss of coordination across the transection will occur. Although true for all levels of the gastrointestinal tract, the significance of this coordinating mechanism is perhaps best exemplified in the stomach where a pacemaker has been localized in the mid-stomach (Fig. 39.4). Unless a pathway from the mid-to distal stomach is maintained, peristaltic contractions and thus emptying will be altered. Transection appears to cause less of an effect in the bowel. This may be because most of the contractions are segmental and can be supported by local activities of the muscle cells and intrinsic nerves. Exactly how propulsive contractions are altered after transection is not known; however, transit does not appear to be significantly altered.

Transection of the bowel wall does more than just interrupt muscular continuity. It also disrupts enteric nerves. As mentioned above, this 'little brain' is extremely important in coordinating patterns of contractions in the bowel. For example, transection of the small intestine will disrupt the migration of the migrating motor complex (MMC) down the bowel. MMCs will still occur above and below the transection; however, coordination of the various phases across the transection is lost, at least temporarily (Hocking et al 1990, Sarr et al 1990, Arnold et al 1991). Fortunately, this does not appear to have major significant effects on intestinal transit. Less is known about the effects of transection of the colon. In the stomach, it is difficult to separate the effects of transection of the enteric nerves from those of transection of the muscle. However, as discussed above, the effects can be major.

Although transection of the small bowel does not have a major effect on transit, the reversal of a segment of bowel to form an antiperistaltic loop does. Both the spread of intestinal slow waves and the projections of the enteric nerves have polarity that is maintained even after operation. Thus, loops will always maintain the tendency to propel contents in what was originally their aboral direction. If a loop of bowel is reversed, it then will propel contents in an oral direction and if the loop is long enough, it will form an obstruction (Grivel & Ruckebusch 1977).

The effects of extrinsic denervation vary remarkably from one organ to another. Complete extrinsic denervation of the mid portion of the small intestine in the dog appears to induce only subtle changes, the significance of which are not known (Sarr et al 1990). All phases of the MMC still occur (Fig. 39.5) and the pattern of motility still changes with ingestion of a meal although a larger meal is required. Although a major pathway for external influences to affect the gut is lost, how this ultimately affects overall motility is not known. In contrast to the small intestine, extrinsic denervation of the stomach has major effects. Division of the vagus nerve innervating the antrum causes a marked delay in gastric emptying of solids (Baxter et al 1987). Denervation of the cardia and fundus results in a loss of receptive relaxation (Fig. 39.6). Effects on the colon are less clear. However, spinal injury and section of the sacral nerves leads to a loss of forceful migrating contractions, constipation, and alteration of the rectosphincteric reflex (Krier 1989).

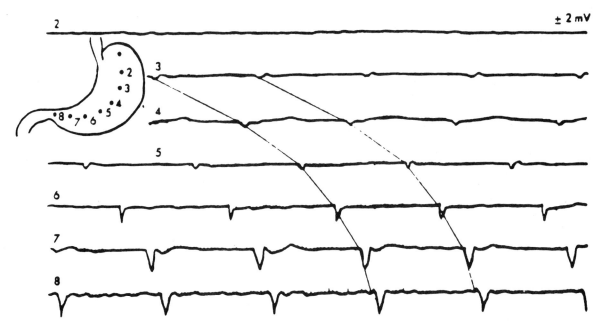

Fig. 39.4 Electrical activity of smooth muscle cells of the stomach. Electrodes placed on the serosal surface record no fluctuations in potential from the orad region. In the mid-region, however, slow waves occur continuously at intervals of 12–20 s. Slow waves give the appearance of moving caudad at increasing velocities. (Reproduced with permission from Kelly et al 1969.)

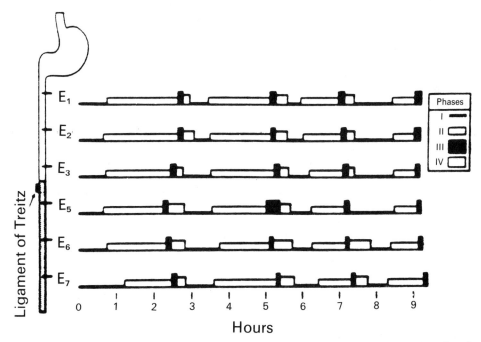

Fig. 39.5 Temporal distribution of spike potential, hence contractions, recorded from the intestine of a fasted dog. The shaded area below the ligament of Treitz had been extrinsically denervated. Note that the various phases of the MMC in the extrinsically denervated area are coordinated with those in the innervated area. (Reproduced with permission from Sarr et al 1990.)

A   cm H$_2$O

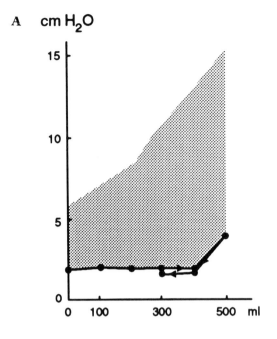

B   cm H$_2$O

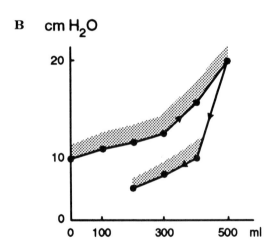

Fig. 39.6   Volume/pressure relationship of the stomach of a human before (**A**) and after (**B**) truncal vagotomy. Note that higher pressures are recorded at the same volumes after vagotomy. (Reproduced with permission from Stadaas & Aune 1970.)

The following discussion will consider some of the more common clinical syndromes that accompany surgical procedures upon the digestive system, and explanations will be put forth that relate to our current understanding of the motility of the gastrointestinal tract.

CLINICAL OUTCOME

Oesophageal operations

The mouth, pharynx, and oesophagus, the normal portal for the entry of nutrients, is often bypassed in the surgically treated or injured patient. The delivery of nutrients directly into the stomach or small intestine appears to have no significant effects on gastrointestinal motility, providing allowances are made for rate of delivery and osmotic load. This suggests that the removal of the pharynx or the oesophagus is not associated with discernible disturbances in gastrointestinal motility providing an appropriate conduit is available for the delivery of nutrients into the gastrointestinal tract. Ablation of the lower oesophageal sphincter (LOS) is quite another matter. This incurs a high degree of gastroesophageal reflux and the unpleasant sequelae of heartburn and regurgitation of gastric contents and ingestates. The motor abnormalities associated with diseases and operations upon the lower oesophagus and its sphincter are discussed in detail in Chapter 30. It should be emphasized here however that disturbances in gastric emptying may not only aggravate but may in themselves be sources of gastrooesophageal reflux.

Gastric operations – historical perspectives

The surgical approach to peptic ulcer disease has undergone remarkable changes during the past two decades, not only as a consequence of the development of potent antisecretory agents but also in recognition of the serious sequelae that may follow surgical intervention for this disease (Moody & McGreevy 1990, Moody et al 1988). A variety of unpleasant and occasionally incapacitating side-effects may follow even a minimally invasive procedure such as a proximal gastric vagotomy which is designed to avoid the major complications of the older and arguably more effective operations. The procedures that were performed frequently in the past are shown schematically in Figure 39.7.

Gastroenterostomy without vagal interruption, used extensively at the turn of the century, was associated with remarkably few unpleasant sequelae. Unfortunately, the incidence of recurrent ulceration at the site of gastrojejunal anastomosis increased as a function of the length of follow-up.

Gastrectomy emerged as a more effective treatment of the complications of peptic ulcer. It was recognized early in the experience with gastrectomy that some patients had significant digestive complaints after removal of even only the distal portion of the stomach (partial gastrectomy) which was the preferred treat-

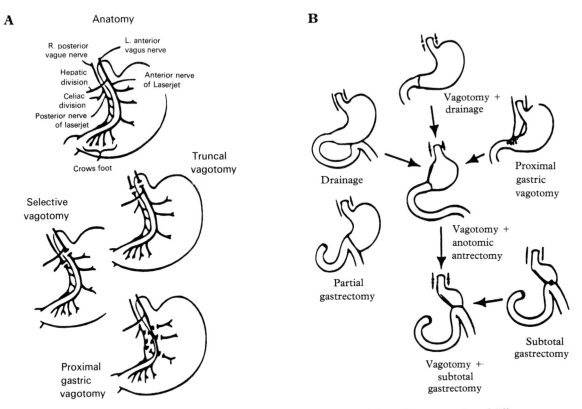

Fig. 39.7 A Schematic representation of different types of vagotomy. **B** Schematic representation of different procedures for the treatment of peptic ulcer disease. (Reproduced with permission from Fromm 1985, 1990.)

ment in patients with benign gastric ulceration. Subtotal gastrectomy, in which not only the antrum but also a large portion of the parietal cell mass was removed, emerged as an effective operation for duodenal ulcer. There was a direct, inverse correlation between the extent of stomach removed and the incidence of recurrence. Subtotal gastrectomy was adopted for the treatment of common manifestations of duodenal ulcer including intractable pain, and total gastrectomy was required for the control of ulceration associated with gastrinoma, the so-called Zollinger–Ellison Syndrome.

Truncal vagotomy (Fig. 39.7), also an effective way to control ulcer symptoms, enjoyed a brief period of popularity. The problems with gastric emptying and ulceration of the stomach led to the use of a drainage procedure when this type of vagotomy was employed. Pyloroplasty emerged as the procedure of choice for gastric drainage, although truncal vagotomy with gastroenterostomy appeared to be equally effective. The stage was set for a period of assessment of the efficacy and safety of these procedures for the treatment of

duodenal ulcer (Johnston & Blackett 1988, Hoffmann et al 1989, Koruth et al 1990). Truncal vagotomy with drainage and truncal vagotomy with subtotal gastrectomy were carefully assessed. The detailed follow-up and analysis offered by randomized trials provided not only an accurate estimation of the safety and efficacy of these procedures, but also produced a comparison of the late postoperative sequelae which followed their application to the treatment of ulcer disease.

Although most patients derived benefit from an operative approach to their ulcer problems, some developed digestive symptoms that were far worse than the periodic pain they experienced from their disease. These symptoms have been generally categorized (Moody 1985) into postgastrectomy syndromes as listed below:

- Small capacity
- Delayed emptying
- Rapid emptying (dumping)
- Postvagotomy diarrhoea

- Bile gastritis
- Malnutrition
- Metabolic bone disease
- Anaemia

Postgastrectomy syndromes

Small capacity

It is understandable why a subtotal gastrectomy whereby less than 25% of the stomach remains should produce early satiety in a patient so treated. This radical operation for peptic ulcer reduces the ability of the stomach to accommodate a large ingestate. Obviously, receptive relaxation, an essential component of accommodation, also is ablated. The patient, following this procedure, is relegated to a lifetime of small frequent meals and in many instances long-term sequelae of chronic malnutrition. Unfortunately, patients who have undergone subtotal gastrectomy may, in addition, experience all the other manifestations of the postgastrectomy syndrome as described in detail below. In fact, even delayed emptying from the small gastric remnant may occur.

Delayed gastric emptying

Most patients are relatively asymptomatic after operation for peptic ulcer, even during their early phases of recovery. This is somewhat surprising since vagotomy, gastrectomy, and drainage procedures of all types are associated with a remarkable array of physiologic changes in gastrointestinal functions. Apparently, an equally responsive array of adaptive processes is instigated by these interventions (Geldof et al 1990, Mistiaen et al 1990, Hartley & Mackie 1991). Unfortunately, these processes do not always function in a way to leave the patient symptom-free and capable of normal digestion (Raimes et al 1986, Calabuig et al 1988, Parr et al 1988, Hom et al 1989, Fich et al 1990, Gortz et al 1990). Although some failures in gastric function may be due to mechanical factors following a poorly constructed gastrointestinal anastomosis or an obstruction in intestine below a drainage procedure, most often delayed or rapid emptying of a gastric remnant is unexplained. A group of patients who are at high risk for motility disturbances after gastric surgery has been identified. These include patients with diabetes mellitus, pancreatitis, pancreatic neoplasm, gastric outlet obstruction, and patients who have had a Roux limb reconstruction after gastrectomy in order to prevent postgastrectomy sequelae (Moody & McGreevy 1990).

Delayed gastric emptying in diabetics is thought to

be a manifestation of the generalized neuropathy that accompanies this disease (Brown & Khanderia 1990). It primarily is expressed in the type I diabetic where other neuropathic disorders such as renal disease are already present. The motility defect is believed to be due primarily to altered intrinsic nerves as part of an overall autonomic neuropathy. Indeed, some of the more promising prokinetic agents for possible use to speed emptying act by enhancing transmission within these nerves (Reynolds 1989) and by stimulating receptors on smooth muscle (Peeters et al 1992). However, since insulin is an important peptide for smooth muscle cell nutrition, it is possible that the perceived defect in gastric motility is in fact primarily a consequence of a generalized smooth muscle defect. Patients who undergo vagotomy and pyloroplasty appear to be especially susceptible to this perplexing complication that may persist for several weeks following operation. This may be because a mechanical disruption of the intrinsic nerves and muscle is being added to the underlying metabolic disruption.

Pancreatitis and pancreatic neoplasms are disease states that are associated with a high incidence of delayed gastric emptying. Although the reasons for this are poorly understood, one possibility is purely mechanical. The enlarged head of the pancreas may interfere with passage of gastric content into and through the duodenum. Unfortunately, even a gastrojejunostomy in an attempt to bypass the duodenum may not improve gastric emptying. Thus, more than just mechanical factors appear to be involved. Possible humoral candidates are the cytokines. Several cytokines have been shown to depress smooth muscle function (Beasley et al 1989). Thus, cytokines such as those associated with inflammation in the case of pancreatitis (interleukins 1 and 6) and tumour necrosis factor in the presence of pancreatic cancer may have a deleterious effect on gastric smooth muscle.

Reparation for delayed gastric emptying following operation for peptic ulcer or for gastric outlet obstruction is associated with a high risk for gastric stasis. Possibly in such patients the delayed emptying is a part of the ulcer disease that remains undetected or untreatable. While one would anticipate a re-establishment of gastric motor function after operation for gastric outlet obstruction, it is surprising how well these patients respond to simple gastroenterostomy with or without vagotomy. The remarkably enlarged and presumably decompensated stomach rapidly achieves its normal function once the obstruction has been relieved. This is an excellent example of the gut's ability to adapt (Moody et al 1962).

A large body of knowledge has rapidly accumulated

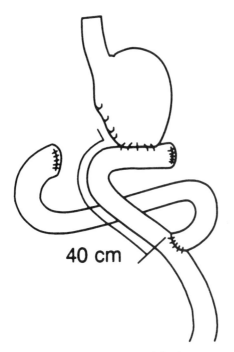

40 cm

Fig. 39.8 Schematic representation of distal gastrectomy and end-to-side isoperistaltic Roux-Y gastrojejunostomy. (Reproduced with permission from Miedema & Kelly 1991.)

as to why patients who undergo a Roux-limb reconstruction have delayed gastric emptying (Fig. 39.8). It appears that the Roux jejunal limb itself undergoes a change in motility in which retrograde contractions retard the movement of gastric contents into its lumen (Fig. 39.9). This pathophysiological disturbance is of distinct advantage in those in whom the gastric contents enter the intestine too rapidly; but in some, the delay leads to gastric stasis, nausea, vomiting and an inability to maintain nutrition. The reason(s) for the retrograde contractions may be a combination of extrinsic denervation as well as section of the enteric nerves and muscle between the duodenum and the section of jejunum that makes up the Roux limb. Slow wave frequency of the limb decreases; and perhaps more importantly, the spread of the slow waves changes periodically to an orad direction. This plus the demonstration that antiperistaltic contractions independent of slow waves can occur in this region of the intestine and may explain the retrograde contractions (Stewart et al 1977). Studies in animals have shown that maintenance of muscular continuity of the Roux limb with the duodenum will prevent the decrease in slow wave frequency and the periodic reversal of slow wave

spread (Miedema & Kelly 1992). Similar maintenance of normal slow wave activity also has been maintained experimentally by electrical pacing of the Roux limb (Morrison et al 1990). When successfully paced, gastric emptying appears to be closer to normal (Karlstrom & Kelly 1989). Whether either maintenance of muscular continuity or pacing proves clinically feasible and/or effective remains to be seen (Miedema et al 1992).

Alkaline gastritis

A relatively large number of patients following gastrectomy or a drainage procedure develop a vague generalized abdominal pain and dyspeptic symptoms following gastric operations for peptic ulcer (Sawyers 1990, Burden et al 1991). Imaging studies may reveal delayed gastric emptying or an excess of refluxed bile into the stomach or gastric remnant. Upper endoscopy often will reveal superficial gastric ulceration and large volumes of bile within the stomach. Biopsy of the mucosa, especially at sites of erosion, provides histologic evidence of inflammation. This entity, alkaline reflux gastritis, is unfortunately unpredictable in its occurrence but is effectively treated by a Roux jejunal limb in which bile is excluded from the stomach (Miedema & Kelly 1991). This clinical outcome suggests that bile is deleterious to the motor function of the stomach. It is unlikely that bile is the sole cause of the syndrome. Residual acid secretion may possibly also play a role at least in the vague pain associated with the syndrome. Patients who are post-cholecystectomy or who undergo cholecystectomy after gastric procedures are especially susceptible to this troublesome complication. Although the Roux limb conversion may relieve the painful aspect of the syndrome, it may also aggravate the gastric stasis that is a prominent and permanent feature of alkaline gastritis in some patients.

Dumping syndrome

Rapid emptying of gastric contents of high osmolality leads to a well characterized cluster of symptoms that include light headedness, palpations, sweating, crampy abdominal pain and diarrhoea (Snook et al 1989, Miholic et al 1990). These symptoms usually have their onset shortly after the ingestion of a meal. Approximately 20% of patients after gastric procedures will experience these symptoms to some degree. Even pyloroplasty and vagotomy is associated with these symptoms. In 1% of patients, the symptoms persist and are incapacitating even when low-carbohydrate dry meals are substituted. Fortunately, a more intimate understanding of neurohumoral aetiologic mechanisms

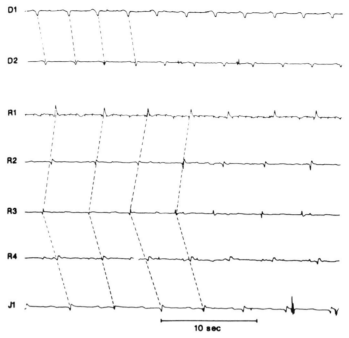

Fig. 39.9 Myoelectric recordings from the duodenum (D1 & D2), Roux limb (R1, R2 & R3), and jejunum (J1) of a dog with Roux-en-Y gastrojejunostomy. Note the abnormal, orad propagation of slow waves in the proximal Roux limb. (Reproduced with permission from Harrison et al 1990.)

responsible for the syndrome has led to an effective pharmacologic treatment for patients with severe dumping syndrome (Geer et al 1990, Richards et al 1990, Gray et al 1991, Miller 1991). Many of the symptoms are due to the release of vasoactive chemicals from the intestinal mucosa in response to the osmotic insult, a response that is suppressed by somatostatin. Somatostatin may also act in part by delaying gastric emptying and intestinal transit. Octreotide acetate, a more metabolically stable form of somatostatin in a dosage of 100 μg, has provided remarkable relief for these unfortunate patients. Smaller numbers of patients have a delayed onset of similar but milder symptoms several hours after eating. Diarrhoea is usually not a prominent feature of their illness. The mechanism of their problem relates to hypoglycaemia secondary to insulin release in response to the rapid absorption of sugar. Their symptoms can usually be managed by dietary adjustment.

Since rapid gastric emptying initiates the dumping syndrome, its restriction by a Roux jejunal interposition has emerged as an effective surgical remedy (Vogel et al 1988, Miedema & Kelly 1991). In fact, many patients with post-gastrectomy sequelae will have nu-

merous digestive complaints including dumping. It is for this reason that a Roux-limb construction has emerged as a preferred operation for the treatment of post-gastrectomy complaints.

Post-vagotomy diarrhoea

Intermittent episodic diarrhoea not associated with eating or dumping symptoms is one of the most perplexing and devastating complications of truncal vagotomy (Raimes et al 1986, Parr et al 1988). For unknown reasons, females are more prone to develop this inconvenient, sometimes embarrassing, but rarely incapacitating problem. It is presumed that patients with this problem have lost cholinergic autonomic control over intestinal motility, although this explanation lacks not only experimental proof, but also clinical validity. If autonomic nerve disruption were the case, all patients with truncal vagotomy should have the problem to some degree. Severe malnutrition characterized by extensive weight loss attributed to post-vagotomy diarrhoea has been successfully treated by the reversal of a 10-cm segment of intestine within the mid-portion of the small intestine (Eagon et al 1992). This outcome suggests that the major problem in such cases is rapid intestinal transit.

Afferent and efferent loop syndromes

Gastrointestinal anastomosis in the form of a gastrojejunostomy may be associated with either obstruction of the limb coming towards (afferent) or leaving (efferent) the stomach. Although each is associated with bilious vomiting, the latter is usually also associated with the presence of undigested food either with or prior to the ejection of bile. Both of these complications are due to mechanical factors at the anastomosis and are not secondary to motor defects from the operative procedure or surgical correction.

Therapeutic strategies

The frequency and severity of post-gastrectomy syndromes have been greatly reduced by the development of an effective medical therapy for peptic ulcer. The H_2 receptor antagonists and proton pump blockers have incurred a dramatic reduction in gastric procedures. Furthermore, the introduction of proximal gastric vagotomy for the treatment of the complications of peptic ulcer has decreased the side-effects of surgical treatment to a surprisingly low rate. The low frequency of ulcer surgery and the low rate of sequelae that follows its current surgical approach have made the post-gastrectomy patient a nearly extinct species. This is fortunate, since the reasons for their adverse outcome in the past remains obscure.

Gastric operations for neoplasms

Gastric operations for malignant neoplasms usually require an extensive resection of the stomach with removal of adjacent lymph bearing tissue or organs such as the spleen, tail of the pancreas or the transverse colon. It is curious that subtotal and even total gastrectomy in this situation is not associated with as many late digestive symptoms as similar procedures for peptic ulcer. Possibly this relates to the short survival experienced by most patients with gastric cancer. However, even when the stomach is removed for benign disease such as Menetrier's gastropathy or Zollinger–Ellison syndrome, unpleasant sequelae or malnutrition is unusual. It is for this reason that near total or total gastrectomy has been recommended for patients with intractable post-gastrectomy symptoms where the very presence of a residual gastric remnant incurs a high liability.

Duodenectomy

Incision into the duodenum (duodenotomy) or resection of accessible segments for benign disease or trauma does not appear to be associated with significant disturbances in its motor or digestive function. Recent data indicate that transection near the pylorus could affect gastric emptying due to the loss of feedback inhibition of emptying from the duodenum (Treacy et al 1992). Whether this is important in humans and whether it is of clinical significance remains to be investigated.

It is difficult to clinically assess removal of the duodenum as an independent event, since it has such an intimate relationship to the pancreas and the biliary tree. The most frequent indication for removal of the duodenum, radical pancreaticoduodenectomy (Whipple Procedure) (Fig. 39.10), requires the simultaneous removal of the head of the pancreas and the distal bile duct as well as cholecystectomy. The original operation, as described by Whipple, also involved removal of the lower half of the stomach and in selected cases, truncal vagotomy. The reconstruction consists of anastomosing the pancreatic remnant, bile duct, and gastric remnant to the jejunum which has been transected several centimetres beyond the ligament of Treitz. It is surprising how well patients function once they recover from this extensive procedure. Although they usually lose several pounds in weight, some will regain the weight lost during the early phases of their illness. In fact, weight loss after full recovery is usually a sign of recurrence of cancer. Pancreatic exocrine deficiency in the form of steatorrhoea or malnutrition is also an unusual clinical outcome, although insulin-requiring diabetes is uniform after total pancreatectomy and also common years after the Whipple procedure. It is not surprising that ablation of duodenal function by its removal is so well tolerated, since bypass by gastrojejunostomy is not usually associated with significant clinical side-effects in patients without peptic ulcer disease.

More recently, efforts have been made to reduce the post-gastrectomy side-effects of the Whipple procedure. The so-called pylorus-sparing Whipple procedure (Fig. 39.10) has in fact been associated with a decrease in dumping symptoms, a more normal dietary intake, and a decrease in faecal fat loss. This improved late outcome, however, is associated with a higher incidence of prolonged gastric stasis and a lower survival rate when employed in surgical treatment of patients with large pancreatic cancers (Roder et al 1992). This major advantage would appear to apply in patients who have undergone resection of the pancreatic head for benign disease or low-grade duodenal neoplasms.

A

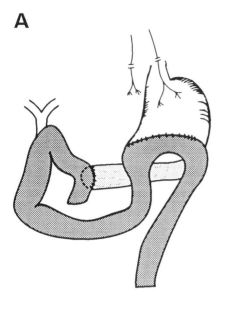

B

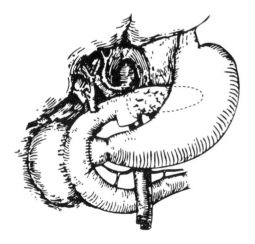

Fig. 39.10 Reconstruction after Whipple procedures. **A** End-to-end pancreatic jejunostomy, **B** Pyloric-preserving. (Modified from Wahlstrom & Moossa 1990 with permission.)

Small bowel operations

Transection

Simple enterotomy or transection and reanastomosis of the small intestine appears to have no discernible clinical consequences with regard to either the motor or absorptive capacity of the gut. A small decrease in the frequency of slow wave activity distal to a point of transection has been shown in both animals (Sarna 1989) and humans, but this occurs without clinically significant influence on propulsive activities of the gut. As discussed above, migration of the MMC across a complete transection is disrupted; however, MMCs do occur below the transection at about the same or higher frequency as those above and they do migrate along the remainder of the small intestine. This may explain the lack of clinical significance. Also, there are data in animals to indicate that if the anastomosis is made end-to-end, migration across the area of transection returns (Fig. 39.11). This could be due to re-establishment of neural and/or muscular continuity.

Resection and bypass

The intestine has a remarkable functional reserve, thereby allowing a marked reduction in its length, either by resection or bypass if the ileum is preserved. A complete removal of the jejunum can be carried out without clinical manifestations of maldigestion or absorption. Resection of the ileum, however, is associated with difficult-to-manage diarrhoea. Surgeons are well aware of this undesirable side-effect and, therefore, spare as much ileum as possible during intestinal operations. An attempt is also made to retain the ileocaecal valve when surgically treating small bowel disease. It is not known precisely how much small bowel including the ileum is required to avoid the manifestations of diarrhoea and malnutrition, the hallmarks of the short gut syndrome. About 30 cm of ileum and 15 cm of jejunum are sufficient when the ileocaecal valve is intact, although 120 cm of ileum and 60 cm of jejunum is more predictably associated with normal alimentation. In fact, it is best to preserve as much small bowel as possible when confronted with adhesive small bowel obstruction, volvulus, Crohn's disease, or penetrating injury. Vascular occlusive disease with acute infarction requires a great deal of surgical judgment as to the extent of resection. It is probably best to err on the side of leaving questionable bowel with a plan of re-exploration in 24 h rather than leaving the patient with such a small amount of bowel that a short gut syndrome will most surely follow. The mesenteric in-flow

A

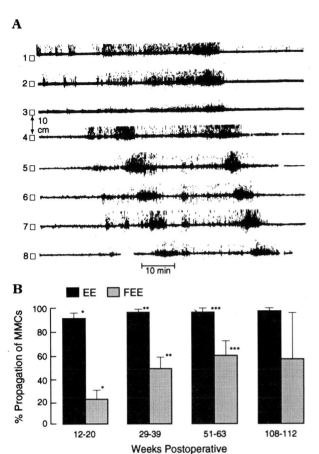

B

Fig. 39.11   **A** Myoelectric activity recorded from the jejunum of a dog with a functional end-to-end anastomosis (side-to-side) between electrodes 3 and 4 and a true end-to-end anastomosis between electrodes 6 and 7. Note the additional phase III of the MMC that begins at electrode 4. Also note that both phase IIIs migrate normally between electrodes 6 and 7. **B** The percentage of pahse IIIs of the MMC that migrate across the end-to-end (EE) and the functional end-to-end (FEE) anastomoses at various times after operation. (Reproduced with permission from Hocking et al 1990.)

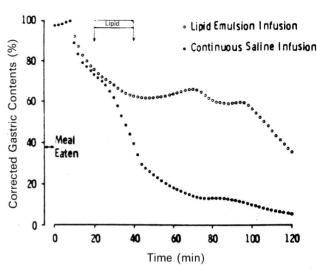

Fig. 39.12   Gastric emptying of a solid meal in a human during the ileal infusion of saline or of a lipid emulsion. Note the slowing effect of lipid infusion. (Reproduced with permission from Welch et al 1988.)

should be reconstructed whenever possible in order to gain as much viable small intestine as possible. Even several centimetres may make a difference with regard to whether the patient will be able to enjoy normal alimentation.

Few studies exist as to the extent of gut adaptation in response to resection (see below), although it is known that the mucosa as well as the muscularis of the residual gut increases several-fold in thickness and most likely in function. It is also known that reversal of segments of short gut will slow intestinal transit and improve its absorptive efficiency. Unfortunately, reverse intestinal pacing is not effective in this regard,

even though transit can be slowed by this technique (O'Connell & Kelly 1987, Hoepfner et al 1988).

There are several possible reasons why the ileum is so important to orderly and controlled transit of nutrients, fluids and electrolytes. First and possibly of prime importance is the specialized function of ileal bile salt reabsorption. Bile salts are known to be a cathartic when they gain entrance to the colon. This cathartic action neutralizes the backup capacity of the colon to reabsorb the excess water delivered to it by the shortened small intestine. A second potentially important factor is loss of the modulating effect of the ileal brake on gastrointestinal transit. It has recently been shown that nutrients instilled into the ileum slow gastric emptying (Fig. 39.12) and gastrointestinal transit, thereby enhancing intestinal absorption. Removal of the resistance of the ileocaecal valve might further contribute to the rate of delivery of fluid and electrolytes to the colon and thereby hasten the passage of liquid stool to the rectum. Under normal conditions, resection of the ileocaecal valve as a component of chronic resection is not associated with diarrhoea if the ileum is left intact and re-anastomosed to the colon at a point even as low as the rectosigmoid junction (Drapanos et al 1973). This arrangement may lead to an increase in bowel evacuation from one to up to two or three movements per day, but usually the stools are soft but not of a watery inconsistency in this situation. This observation suggests that the ileum is a critical segment in the aboral movement and absorption of fluids, electrolytes and nutrients.

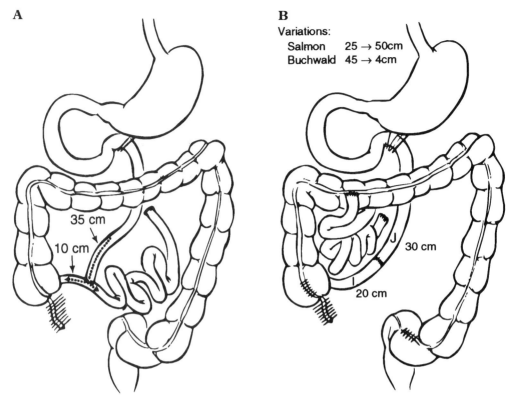

Fig. 39.13 Schematic of jejunoileal bypass procedures for treatment of the morbidly obese patient. **A** End-to-side jejunoileostomy popularized by Payne. **B** End-to-end jejunoileostomy with draining of bypassed bowel into the colon popularized by Scott. (Modified from Deitel 1989 with permission.)

The importance of the ileum is highlighted by the extensive experience with jejunal ileal bypass (Fig. 39.13) in the treatment of chronic morbid obesity. This operation which reduces the small intestinal functional unit to 45–50 cm is associated with a remarkable degree of weight loss from malabsorption. Unfortunately, there is troublesome diarrhoea with acute metabolic imbalance and fluid and electrolyte losses, a complication that has required a re-establishment of intestinal continuity in a large number of patients. Approximately 50 cm of ileum is required for the normal absorption of gastrointestinal secretion and ingested nutrients. In rats, if approximately the same percentage of ileum is maintained after jejunal-ileal bypass, some diarrhoea and weight loss occurs immediately after operation; but then weight gain ensues (Nemeth et al 1981). In these animals, transit through the functioning small intestine is rapid initially during the fed state. Within a few weeks, however, transit through the shortened small intestine takes as long as transit through the entire small intestine of a normal animal. This slowing of transit is accompanied by an early increase in mass of the smooth muscle of the remaining gut, especially the ileum, and in the mRNA levels that code for one of the contractile proteins in that muscle (Bowers et al 1986, Lai et al 1990, Weisbrodt et al 1985).

Colectomy

It is surprising that the majority of the colon can be removed without significant clinical manifestations from loss of its fluid absorption, waste storage and disposal function. This is further evidence of the remarkable redundancy of the functional aspects of the digestive system. Coloproctectomy does not influence gastric emptying but markedly reduces the rate of intestinal transit (Soper et al 1989). It was learned early in the experience with cutaneous ileostomies that its ejectate would have less fluid as a function of time, but not to a point where it receives a solid stool.

The development of the ileal pouch (Fig. 39.14) provided for an even longer residence time for intestinal chyme and a more concentrated ileal content that

A

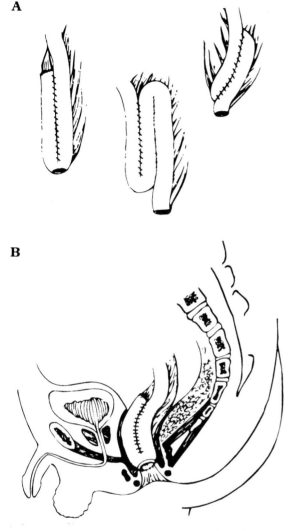

B

Fig. 39.14 **A** Schematic of ileal pouch configurations in patients undergoing endorectal ileoanal anastomosis. **B** Schematic of ileal 'J' pouch–anal anastomosis. (Modified from Becker & Moody 1991 with permission.)

could be accommodated for several hours prior to evacuation. An ileostomy without a pouch has minimal influence on intestinal transit or the motility characteristics of the small intestine. A pouch as expected incurs large contraction waves (Fig. 39.15), characteristic of the obstructed small intestine. Again, time favours an adaptation that allows an increase in pouch capacity, thereby preventing the crampy abdominal pain associated with intestinal obstruction.

Total coloproctectomy for ulcerative colitis and familial polyposis has offered a unique opportunity for

study of gastrointestinal motility. Kelly and his associates at the Mayo Clinic have carried out a large number of informative studies, many of which have previously been reviewed. Their efforts to develop a normal route and pattern for defaecation after total coloproctectomy have contributed a vast fund of knowledge of anal sphincter function and small bowel physiology. The ileal-pouch–anal anastomosis has provided a unique opportunity to study mechanisms of faecal storage and anal evacuation of contents after colectomy. The features of the reconstruction are shown Figure 39.15. Their general agreement is that the J-pouch configuration provides the best functional reservoir. It is easy to construct and fits well in the pelvis. Most pouches can hold about 300–350 ml of a semi-solid faecal waste before the sensation for the evacuation occurs. Most patients will have six to seven stools per day and infrequent nocturnal seepage. Daytime incontinence is rare when the pouch and ileoanal anastomosis have been properly constructed.

Gastrointestinal transit after ileal-pouch-anal reconstruction has been carefully studied and compared to normal in patients with standard Brooke ileostomies. Utilizing a dual isotope technique, Soper and his colleagues (Soper et al 1989) at the Mayo Clinic found that gastric emptying was similar in each group, but that intestinal transit was prolonged in patients with ileal-pouch-anal anastomosis (178 ± 26 min) compared to patients with a Brooke ileostomy (80 ± 32 min) or control (75 ± 15 min). Stool frequency, however, did not correlate with the rate of intestinal transit. Several factors placed stress upon the anal sphincter after ileal-pouch-anal anastomosis. Pouch capacitance, the volume of stool delivered per unit time, and incomplete emptying of the pouch are major determinants in the frequency of stooling and the incidence of incontinence. Kelly and his associates at the Mayo Clinic (O'Connell et al 1987) have demonstrated that the capacity and distensibility of an ileal-pouch of the J-type is equal to that of the normal rectum. Patients with a good result revealed a higher pouch capacity (409 ± 33 ml) than those with a poor result (290 ± 27 ml). Distensibility, however, did not correlate with the clinical outcome.

Enteral bacteriology has been shown to play an important role in patients who experience excessive stooling. The Mayo group has shown that patients with a poor result in this regard have an aerobic as well as anaerobic overgrowth within their jejunums (O'Connell et al 1986). There was no correlation in stool frequency with bacterial overgrowth or histological evidence of inflammation of the ileal pouch (pouchitis), a uniform finding.

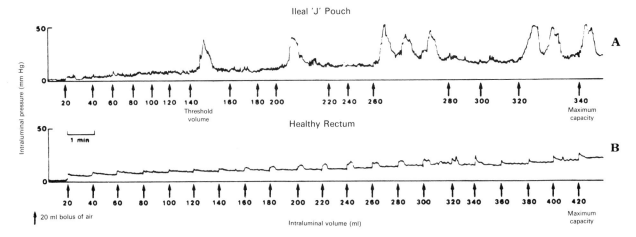

Fig. 39.15   Intraluminal pressure response to distension of an ileal 'J' pouch (**A**) and healthy rectum (**B**). Note the large pressure waves in the pouch in response to distension at volumes larger than 140 ml. (Reproduced with permission from O'Connell et al 1987.)

The anorectal angle, an important determinant to defaecation in the normal, has also been studied in patients with ileal-pouch-anal anastomosis. Surprisingly, the angle in the pouch of patients is similar to unoperated controls. Elevation of the pelvic floor with gluteal squeeze, however, was decreased in the ileal pouch group (Barkel et al 1988). Apparently, the decreased mobility of the pelvic floor in the latter did not influence pouch evacuation in an adverse fashion, since about 95% of patients have a relatively normal capacity to completely evacuate their pouch, and about 85% have excellent faecal continence. O'Connell and associates at the Mayo Clinic (O'Connell et al 1988) have shown that patients with episodic incontinence have a lower transanal sphincter pressure than those with perfect continence. Although the frequency of anal slow waves is decreased following mucosectomy and ileal-pouch–anal anastomosis, there is no correlation between anal myoelectric activity and the incidence of incontinence.

Perioperative complications in the form of perianal abscess, perianal sinuses and fistulae, intra-abdominal abscesses, and anastomotic strictures represent a major source of pouch dysfunction. The Mayo group has reported that 20% of 114 patients who had such complications eventually required removal of their pouches and construction of an abdominal wall ileostomy stoma (Galandiuk et al 1990).

REFERENCES

Arnold J H, Alevizatos C A, Cox S F, Richards W O 1991 Propagation of small bowel migrating motor complex activity fronts varies with anastomosis type. J Surg Res 51: 506–511

Barkel D C, Pemberton J H, Pezim M E et al 1988 Scintigraphic assessment of the anorectal angle in health and after ileal pouch-anal anastomosis. Ann Surg 208: 42–49

Baxter J N, Grime J S, Critchley M et al 1987 Relationship between gastric emptying of a solid meal and emptying of the gall bladder before and after vagotomy. Gut 28: 855–863

Beasley D B, Cohen R A, Levinsky N G 1989 Interleukin 1 inhibits contraction of vascular smooth muscle. J Clin Invest 83: 331–335

Becker J M, Moody F G 1991 Ulcerative colitis in: Sabiston D C Jr (ed.) Textbook of surgery. W B Saunders, Philadelphia pp 927–940

Bowers R L, Eeekhout C, Weisbrodt N W 1986 Actomyosin, collagen, and cell hypertrophy in intestinal muscle after jejunoileal bypass. Am J Physiol 250: G70–G75

Brown C K, Khanderia U 1990 Use of metoclopramide, domperidone, and cisapride in the management of diabetic gastroparesis. Clin Pharm 9: 357–365

Bueno L, Ferre J-P, Ruckebusch Y 1978 Effects of anesthesia and surgical procedures on intestinal myoelectric activity in rats. Am J Dig Dis 23: 690–695

Burden W R, Hodges R P, Hsu M, O'Leary J P 1991 Alkaline reflux gastritis. Surg Clin North Am 71: 33–44

Burks T F 1987 Actions of drugs on gastrointestinal motility in: Johnson L R, Christensen J, Jackson M J, Jacobson E D, Walsh J H (eds) Physiology of the gastrointestinal tract, 2nd edn. Raven Press, New York pp 723–744

Calabuig R, Carrió I, Monés J et al 1988 Gastric emptying after truncal vagotomy and pyloroplasty. Scand J Gastroenterol 23: 659–664

Christensen J 1989 Colonic motility in: Schultz S G, Wood J

D, Rauner B B (eds) Handbook of physiology, section 6: The gastrointestinal system, volume 1. Motility and circulation. American Physiological Society, Bethesda, Maryland pp 939–974

Deitel M 1989 Jejunocolic and jejunoileal bypass: an historical perspective in: Deitel M (ed.) Surgery for the morbidly obese patient. Lea and Febiger, Philadelphia pp 81–90

Drapanos T, Pennington D G, Kappelmen M, Lindsey E S 1973 Emergency subtotal colectomy: preference approach to management of massively bleeding diverticular disease. Ann Surg 177: 519–526

Eagon J C, Miedema B W, Kelly K A 1992 Postgastrectomy syndromes. Surg Clin North Am 72: 445–465

Fich A, Neri M, Camilleri M et al 1990 Stasis syndromes following gastric surgery: clinical and motility features of 60 symptomatic patients. J Clin Gastroenterol 12: 505–512

Fleckenstein P, Oigaard A 1978 Electrical spike activity in the human small intestine. Am J Dig Dis 23: 776–780

Fromm D 1985 Ulceration of the stomach and duodenum in: Fromm D (ed.) Gastrointestinal Surgery vol 1. Churchill Livingstone Inc, New York, pp 233–323

Fromm D 1990 Duodenal ulcer in: Moody F G (ed.) Surgical treatment of digestive disease. Year Book Medical Publishers, Chicago pp 197–211

Galandiuk S, Scott N A, Dozois R R et al 1990 Ileal pouch – anal anastomosis. Ann Surg 212: 446–454

Geer R J, Richards W O, O'Dorisio T M 1990 Efficacy of octreotide acetate in treatment of severe postgastrectomy dumping syndrome. Ann Surg 212: 678–687

Geldof H, Van der Schee E J, Van Blankenstein M et al 1990 Effects of highly selective vagotomy on gastric myoelectrical activity. Dig Dis Sci 35: 969–975

Gortz L, Björkman A-C, Andersson H, Kral J G 1990 Truncal vagotomy reduces food and liquid intake in man. Physiol Behav 48: 779–781

Gray J L, Debas H T, Mulvihill S J 1991 Control of dumping symptoms of somatostatin analogue in patients after gastric surgery. Arch Surg 126: 1231–1236

Grivel M L, Ruckebush Y 1977 A study in the dog and cat of the electrical activity of the small intestine some months after transection and transplantation. Life Sci 10: 241–250

Harrison W D, Hocking M P, Vogel S B 1990 Gastric emptying and myoelectric activity following Roux-en-Y gastrojejunostomy. J Surg Res 49: 385–389

Hartley M N, Mackie C R 1991 Gastric adaptive relaxation and symptoms after vagotomy. Br J Surg 78: 24–27

Hocking M P, Carlson R G, Courington K R, Bland K I 1990 Altered motility and bacterial flora after functional end-to-end anastomosis. Surgery 108: 384–392

Hoepfner M T, Kelly K A, Sarr M G 1988 Pacing the canine ileostomy. Surgery 104: 476–481

Hoffmann J, Jensen H-E, Christiansen J et al 1989 Prospective controlled vagotomy trial for duodenal ulcer. Ann Surg 209: 40–45

Hom S, Sarr M G, Kelly K A, Hench V 1989 Postoperative gastric atony after vagotomy for obstructing peptic ulcer. Am J Surg 157: 282–286

Johnston D, Blackett R L 1988 A new look at selective vagotomies. Am J Surg 156: 416–427

Kelly K A, Code C F, Elveback L R 1969 Patterns of canine gastric electrical activity. Am J Physiol 217: 461–470

Köhler L W, Heddle R, Miedema B W et al 1991 Response

of canine ileocolonic sphincter of intraluminal acetic acid and colonic distension. Dig Dis Sci 36: 194

Koruth N M, Dua K S, Brunt P W, Matheson N A 1990 Comparison of highly selective vagotomy with truncal vagotomy and pyloroplasty: results at 8–15 years. Br J Surg 77: 70–72

Krier J 1989 Motor function of anorectum and pelvic floor musculature in: Schultz S G, Wood J D, Rauner B B (eds) Handbook of Physiology, Section 6: The Gastrointestinal System, Volume 1. Motility and Circulation. American Physiological Society, Bethesda, MD pp 1025–1053

Lai M, Thomason D B, Weisbrodt N W 1990 Effect of intestinal bypass on the expression of actin mRNA in ileal smooth muscle. Am J Physiol 258: R39–R43

Miedema B W, Kelly K A 1991 The Roux operation for postgastrectomy syndromes. Am J Surg 161: 256–261

Miedema B W, Kelly K A 1992 The Roux stasis syndrome. Arch Surg 127: 295–300

Miedema B W, Sarr M G, Kelly K A 1992 Pacing the human stomach. Surgery 111: 143–150.

Miholic J, Reilmann L, Meyer H-J et al 1990 Extracellular space, blood volume, and the early dumping syndrome after total gastrectomy. Gastroenterology 99: 923–929

Miller T A 1991 Treatment of severe postgastrectomy dumping with a long-acting somatostatin analog: is effective management finally available? Gastroenterology 101: 1129–1130

Mistiaen W, Van Hee R, Block P, Hubens A 1990 Gastric emptying for solids in patients with duodenal ulcer before and after highly selective vagotomy. Dig Dis Sci 35: 310–316

Moody F G 1985 Stomach and duodenum in: Beahrs O H, Beart R W (eds) General surgery – therapy update service. Berwal Publishing Media, PA, pp 7–21

Moody F G, Cornell G N, Beal J M 1962 Pyloric obstruction complicating peptic ulcer disease. Arch Surg 84: 462–466

Moody F G, McGreevy J M 1990 Complications of gastric surgery in: Littlefield L J (ed.) Complications in surgery and trauma. J B Lippincott, Philadelphia pp 449–470

Moody F G, McGreevy J M, Miller T A 1988 Stomach in: Schwartz S I, Shires G T, Spencer F C (eds) Principles of surgery. McGraw-Hill, New York pp 1157–1188

Morrison P, Miedema B W, Kohler L, Kelly K A 1990 Electrical dysrhythmias in the Roux jejunal limb: cause and treatment. Am J Surg 160: 252–256

Nemeth P R, Kwee D J, Weisbrodt N W 1981 Adaptation of intestinal muscle in continuity after jejunoileal bypass in the rat. Am J Physiol 241: G259–G263

Neri M, Phillips S F, Fich A, Haddad A C 1991 Canine ileocolonic sphincter: flow, transit, and motility before and after sphincterotomy. Am J Physiol 260: G284–G289

O'Connell P R, Kelly K A 1987 Enteric transit and absorption after canine ileostomy. Arch Surg 122: 1011–1017

O'Connell P R, Pemberton J H, Brown M L, Kelly K A 1987 Determinants of stool frequency after ileal pouch–anal anastomosis. Am J Surg 153: 157–164

O'Connell P R, Rankin D R, Weiland L H, Kelly K A 1986 Enteric bacteriology, absorption, morphology and emptying after ileal pouch–anal anastomosis. Br J Surg 1986 73: 909–914

O'Connell P R, Stryker S J, Metcalf A M et al 1988 Anal

canal pressure and motility after ileoanal anastomosis. Surg Gynecol Obstet 166: 47–54

Pappasova M, Atanassova E 1989 Adaptation to surgical perturbations. In: Schultz S G, Wood J D, Rauner B B (eds) Handbook of Physiology, Section 6: The Gastrointestinal System, Volume 1. Motility and Circulation. American Physiological Society, Bethesda, MD pp 1199–1224

Parr N J, Grime S, Brownless S et al 1988 Relationship between gastric emptying of liquid and postvagotomy diarrhoea. Br J Surg 75: 279–282

Peeters T L, Muls E, Janssens, J et al 1992 Effect of motilin on gastric emptying in patients with diabetic gastroparesis. Gastroenterology 102: 97–101

Quigley E M M, Borody T J, Phillips S F et al 1984 Motility of the terminal ileum and ileocecal sphincter in healthy human. Gastroenterology 87: 857–866

Raimes S A, Smirniotis V, Wheldon E J et al 1986 Postvagotomy diarrhoea put into perspective. Lancet iv: 851–853

Reynolds J C 1989 Prokinetic agents: a key in the future of gastroenterology. Gastroenterol Clin North Am 18: 437–457

Richards W O, Geer R, ODorisio T M et al. 1990 Octreotide acetate induces fasting small bowel motility in patients with dumping syndrome. J Surg Res 49: 483–487

Roder J D, Stein H J, Hüttl W, Siewert J R 1992 Pylorus-preserving versus standard pancreaticoduodenectomy: an analysis of 110 pancreatic and periampullary carcinomas. Br J Surg 79: 152–155

Sarna S K 1989 In vivo myoelectric activity: methods, analysis, and interpretation in: Schultz S G, Wood J D, Rauner B B (eds) Handbook of physiology, section 6: The gastrointestinal system, volume 1. Motility and circulation. American Physiological Society, Bethesda, Maryland pp 817–864

Sarr M G, Duenes J A, Zinsmeister A R 1990 Factors in the control of interdigestive and postprandial myoelectric patterns of canine jejunoileum: role of extrinsic and intrinsic nerves. J Gastrointest Mot 2: 247–257

Sawyers J L 1990 Management of postgastrectomy syndromes. Am J Surg 159: 8–14

Schemann M, Ehrlein H J 1986 Postprandial patterns of canine jejunal motility and transit of luminal content. Gastroenterology 90: 991–1000

Snook J A, Wells A D, Prytherch D R et al 1989 Studies on the pathogenesis of the early dumping syndrome induced by intraduodenal instillation of hypertonic glucose. Gut 30: 1716–1720

Soper N J, Chapman N J, Kelly K A et al 1990 The 'ileal brake' after ileal pouch–anal anastomosis. Gastroenterology 98: 111–116

Soper N J, Orkin B A, Kelly K A et al 1989 Gastrointestinal transit after proctocolectomy with ileal pouch–anal anastomosis or ileostomy. J Surg Res 46: 300–305

Stadaas J, Aune S 1970 Intragastric pressure/volume relationship before and after vagotomy. Acta Chir Scand 136: 611–615

Stewart J J, Burks T F, Weisbrodt N W 1977 Intestinal myoelectric activity after activation of central emetic mechanism. Am J Physiol 233: E131–E137

Treacy P J, Jamieson G G, Dent J et al 1992 Duodenal intramural nerves in control of pyloric motility and gastric emptying. Am J Physiol 263: G1–G5

Vogel S B, Hocking M P, Woodward E R 1988 Clinical and radionuclide evaluation of Roux-Y diversion for postgastrectomy dumping. Am J Surg 155: 57–62

Wahlstrom H E, Moossa A R 1990 The pancreas, pt. 2 Neoplastic diseases in: Nora P F (ed.) Operative surgery. W B Saunders, Philadelphia pp 760–781

Weisbrodt N W 1991a Swallowing in: Johnson L R (ed.) Gastrointestinal physiology, 4th edition. Mosby-Year Book, St Louis, Missouri pp 23–31

Weisbrodt N W 1991b Gastric emptying in: Johnson L R (ed.) Gastrointestinal physiology, 4th edn. Mosby-Year Book, St Louis, Missouri pp 32–41

Weisbrodt N W 1991c Motility of the small intestine in: Johnson L R (ed.) Gastrointestinal physiology, 4th edn. Mosby-Year Book, St Louis, Missouri pp 42–49

Weisbrodt N W 1991d Motility of the large intestine in: Johnson L R (ed.) Gastrointestinal physiology, 4th edn. Mosby-Year Book, St Louis, Missouri pp 50–56

Weisbrodt N W, Nemeth P R, Bowers R L, Weems W A 1985 Functional and structural changes in intestinal smooth muscle after jejunoileal bypass in rats. Gastroenterology 88: 958–963

Welch I McL, Cunningham K M, Read N W 1988 Regulation of gastric emptying by ileal nutrients in humans. Gastroenterology 94: 401–404

40. The effects of resection, restorative procedures and transplantation on intestinal motility

E. M. M. Quigley

Given the important role of motor activity in intestinal homeostasis in health and disease (Quigley 1987), it comes as somewhat of a surprise to find that little is known of the effects of even the most radical surgical procedures on intestinal motility. Studies of their

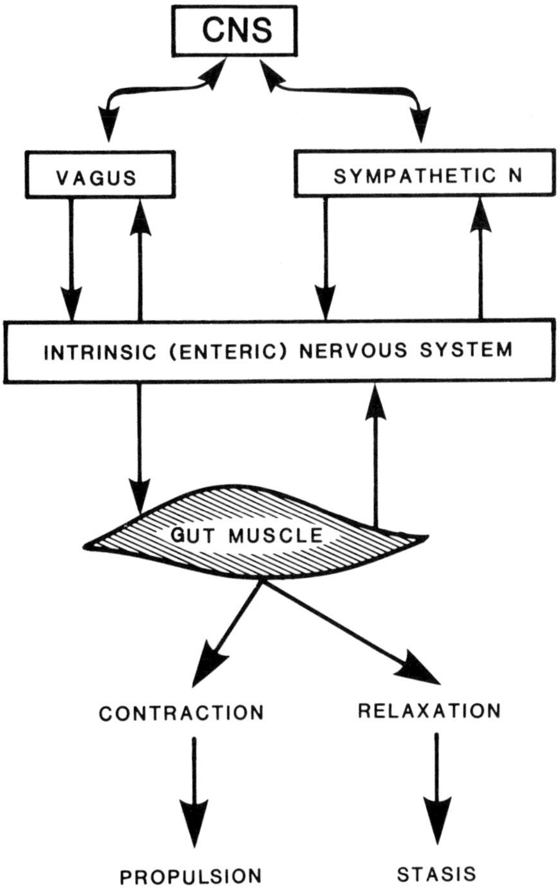

Fig. 40.1 The levels of control of intestinal motor activity. (Reproduced with permission from Quigley 1987.)

motor effects in man are indeed few and far between; most available information being derived from animal models.

A PHYSIOLOGICAL BASIS FOR THE EFFECTS OF INTESTINAL SURGERY

Before going on to describe the motor consequences of such procedures as intestinal resection, the creation of artificial valves and intestinal transplantation a brief review of the levels at which such disruption might occur seems appropriate.

The apparatus which generates the motor patterns of the intestine consists of the smooth muscle of the gut wall and the neural, hormonal and peptidergic control mechanisms which regulate and integrate its activity. Gut motor activity can be modulated, and therefore disrupted at any one of a number of closely integrated levels (Fig. 40.1). At the most fundamental level is the smooth muscle cell, additional tiers of control being provided by the interconnections between individual muscle cells, the intrinsic nerves of the gut (the enteric nervous system, ENS), the extrinsic autonomic nerves and, at the highest level, the central nervous system (CNS).

A unique property of the membrane potential of gastrointestinal smooth muscle cells, and one fundamental to the genesis of motility, is its ability to undergo spontaneous, slow, transient depolarization to a level which, though below that which triggers an action potential, results in the generation of a slow wave (Szurszewski 1986) (Fig. 40.2). These slow waves are an omnipresent phenomenon throughout the small intestine (Fig. 40.3). While slow waves do not in themselves lead to contractions, they do regulate contractile activity. Thus spikes (or action potentials), the electrical events which generate contractions, occur only on the crest of slow waves. In this manner, the occurrence of spikes and therefore contractions are phase locked to slow waves. The maximum frequency of contractile

691

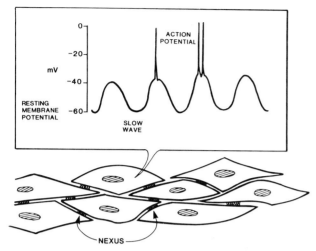

Fig. 40.2   The electrophysiological basis of intestinal motility. Inset represents recording of intracellular electrical activity from a single smooth muscle cell.
Note: (1) resting membrane potential of − 60 mV which regularly undergoes spontaneous depolarization to − 40 mV to produce rhythmic slow waves; (2) action (or spike) potentials occur only on the summit of slow waves and result in muscle contraction; (3) nexuses permit propagation of electrical signals between individual cells. (Reproduced with permission from Quigley 1987.)

activity at a given site in the small intestine is thereby directly related to the slow wave frequency of that region. Given this background, it is easy to understand how hypoxia (Szurszewski & Steggerda 1968a, b, Kyi & Daniel 1970) or manoeuvres, such as intestinal cooling, which may affect slow wave activity can have such profound effects on motor function.

In the small intestine, slow waves are thought to originate in the interstitial cells of Cajal located on the serosal edge of Auerbach's plexus (Daniel & Berezin 1992). The transmission of electrical signals between smooth muscle cells is facilitated by areas of close contact (nexuses) (Fig. 40.2). Groups of smooth muscle cells thereby come to function as an integrated unit or syncytium – the dimensions of this unit being directly related to the degree of electrical coupling between cells. By virtue of these syncytial properties, slow waves can propagate through the muscle layers in both longitudinal and circumferential directions. As a consequence, the duodenum, as the region of the small intestine with the fastest intrinsic slow wave frequency, comes to act as the pacemaker for the entire small intestine (Duthie et al 1971). Conversely, surgical insults, such as transection, which disrupt these interconnections will interrupt myogenic transmission.

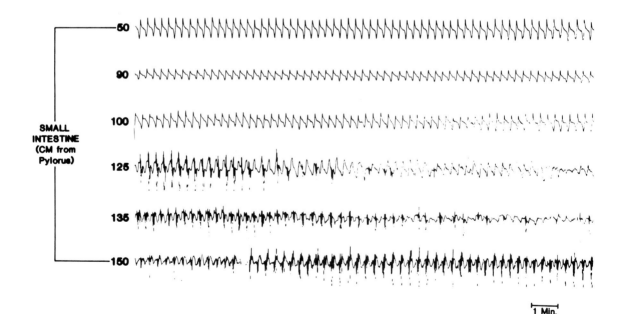

Fig. 40.3   In vivo myoelectrical activity (recorded from canine duodenum and jejunum in fasted state).
Note: (1) Omnipresent, regular slow wave at all sites; (2) Spikes occur only on plateau of slow waves; (3) phase I of MMC in proximal electrodes – no spike activity, slow waves alone recorded; (4) phase III of MMC traverses distal electrodes – defined by presence of intense spike activity on sequential slow waves.

One of the most significant recent advances in gastrointestinal physiology has been in our understanding of the intrinsic nerves of the gut. It is now appreciated that the nerve plexi of the gut wall together with their interconnecting neurons play an extremely important role in processing and integrating afferent signals and in coordinating and directing efferent responses. While its complexity continues to be unravelled, it is clear that the ENS exerts a considerable degree of autonomy and truly behaves as a 'mini brain' within the gut. Neurons of the ENS can project over considerable distances, both longitudinally and circumferentially. Based upon these interconnections and by drawing upon its impressive armamentarium of inhibitory and excitatory neurotransmitters and neuromodulatory peptides the ENS can generate complex and coordinated motor responses to incoming stimuli from the muscularis and mucosa. The ENS can independently generate and propagate such complex contractile events as the migrating motor complex (Sarna 1985, Sarna et al 1981, 1983). The extent to which a given intervention interferes with ENS function will, therefore, determine, in large part, its motor effects.

In the light of these new neuroanatomical and neurophysiological concepts it would appear that the extrinsic autonomic nerves, should be viewed as further levels of control above the ENS, capable of modifying enteric neural activity. Among their roles are the mediation of such 'long' reflexes as the intestino-intestinal or enterogastric reflexes and the relaying of intestinal information between the gut and higher centres (Wingate 1985, Thompson 1988). Surgical transection of these nerves would lead, therefore, to both the 'isolation' of the intestine from central input as well as to the loss of regulatory feedback mechanisms between distant parts of the intestine.

Surgical injury at any one or a number of these levels will achieve clinical expression through its effects on those various patterns of intestinal motor activity which can be recorded in vivo.

Slow waves

Interventions could affect their frequency and propagation.

The migrating motor complex (MMC)

This motor pattern, described in detail elsewhere in this book, dominates small intestinal motor activity in the fasted state (Wingate 1981, 1983, Sarna 1985, Quigley 1987, 1992b). It consists of three distinct phases which occur in sequence and migrate slowly along the length of the small intestine (Fig. 40.4a & 40.4b). In man, individual cycles last between 1 and 2 h and continue to recur as long as the subject remains fasted. In man, the majority of MMCs originate in the proximal small intestine and migrate aborally; the velocity of propagation slowing as they progress distally. Several aspects of the MMC are subject to disruption and include MMC frequency, the interval (or period) between MMC cycles, the duration of its constituent phases (I, II and III), the site of origin and extent of MMC propagation and the migration velocity of the most distinctive phase – phase III. Indeed, MMC effects are often the focus of studies of the motor consequences of various interventions.

Other interdigestive patterns

Distinctive motor patterns in the fasted state, other than the MMC, are, as described by Drs Basilisco and Phillips in Chapter 27, best characterized in the ileocolonic junctional region (Phillips et al 1988, Quigley 1988, Quigley et al 1984a,b, 1985) (Fig. 40.5). These include recurrent discrete bursts of rhythmic activity (termed discrete clustered contractions – DCCs) (Fig. 40.5b), and high-amplitude rapidly-propagated phasic waves (prolonged propagated contractions – PPCs) (Fig. 40.5c) which are, though infrequent, highly propulsive. In the ileocolonic junctional region DCCs replace the more irregular contractile activity typical of phase II of the MMC in the proximal intestine. These patterns appear to be of primary importance both in the regulation of ileocolonic transit and the clearance of refluxed colonic contents from the distal ileum (Kruis et al 1985, 1987). The regulation of these patterns is poorly understood but available evidence suggests that their generation may be intrinsic to the gut. Their appearance in the more proximal intestine has also been associated with alterations in the luminal milieu (Sarna 1987).

Post-prandial motility – the fed motor response

Under normal circumstances food administration has two important and related consequences: the abolition of MMC cycling and the induction of the 'fed' pattern (Figs 40.6a and 40.6b). This pattern which features apparently random contractions can last, in man, from as little as 2.5 h to over 8 h at which time MMC cycling resumes, assuming, of course, that no further meals have been taken in the interim. Effects of surgery on postprandial motility could thus include the failure of food ingestion either to disrupt MMC cycling or to generate the fed pattern.

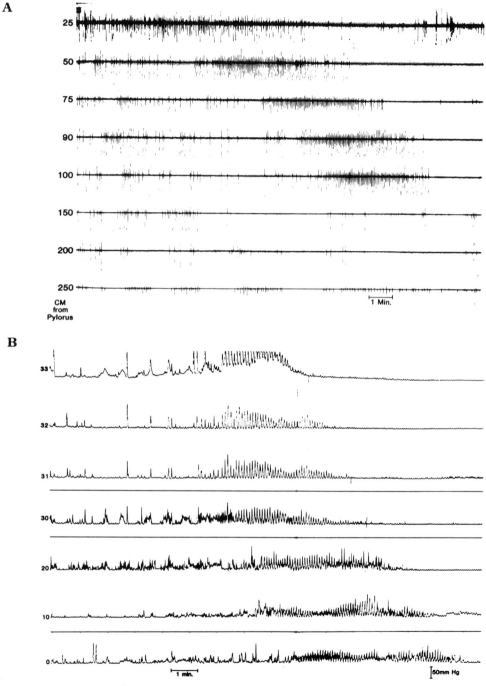

Fig. 40.4   The migrating motor complex (MMC). **A** Myoelectrical equivalent (dog); irregular activity (phase II) on left is followed by intense band of uninterrupted spikes (phase III) which migrates slowly along small intestine; quiescence (phase I) of next cycle follows. **B** Motor equivalent (man); irregular contractile activity (phase II) followed by band of rhythmic contractions (phase III) which migrates slowly through proximal jejunum; motor quiescence (phase I) follows (distances in cm from catheter tip). (Reproduced with permission from Quigley 1992b.)

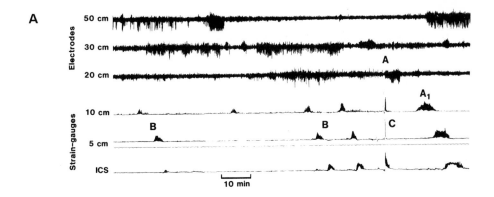

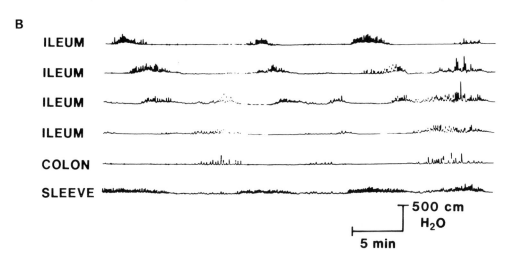

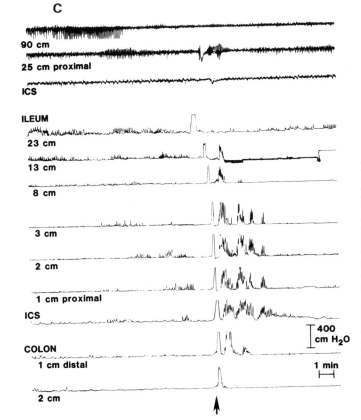

Fig. 40.5 Motor patterns of the distal ileum **A** Slow sweep speed recording illustrates dominant motor patterns in ileocolonic junction. Phase III of MMC migrates from more proximal electrodes (**A**) to strain gauges in distal ileum and at ileocolonic sphincter (**A₁**); recurrent clusters of rhythmic contractions (discrete clustered contractions – DCCs) (**B**) slowly migrate through region; rapidly propagated high-amplitude wave (**C**) (prolonged propagated contraction – PPC) sweeps through region. (Reproduced with permission from Quigley et al 1984.) **B** Discrete clustered contractions (DCCs) migrate slowly through distal ileum into proximal colon (sleeve at ileocolonic sphincter). (Reproduced with permission from Quigley et al 1984.) **C** Prolonged propagated contraction (PPC) sweeps through ileocolonic junction. (Reproduced with permission from Quigley et al 1984.)

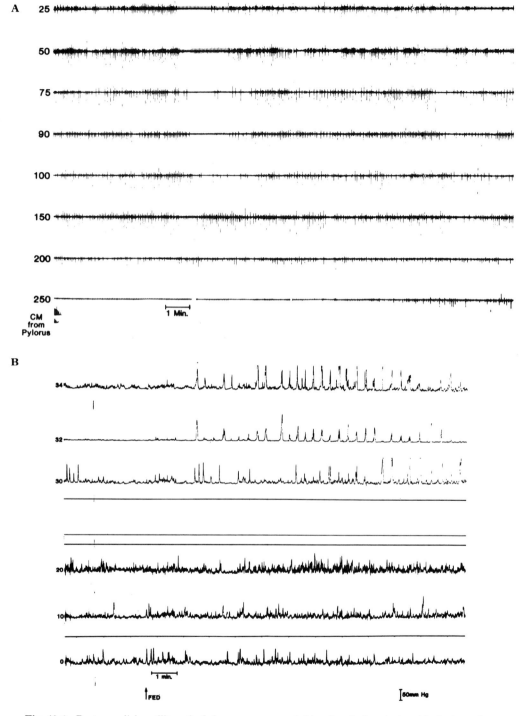

Fig. 40.6   Post-prandial motility – the fed motor response. **A** Myoelectrical equivalent (dog) – irregular spike activity throughout small intestine. **B** motor equivalent (man) – simultaneous recordings from antrum (top 3 traces) and duodenum (lower 3 traces) illustrating onset of irregular, intense contractions at all sites following a meal (arrow) (distances in cm from catheter tip). (Reproduced with permission from Quigley 1992b.)

Finally, it should be stressed that these various procedures may not only disrupt normal motility patterns but may also lead to the appearance of abnormal patterns. The definition of what is truly abnormal in the human small intestine, in particular, is still in its infancy and the status of the various abnormal patterns reported in these and other circumstances remains controversial (Quigley 1992a,b).

Changes in these motor patterns, interesting though they may be, will achieve clinical relevance only through their impact on transit, digestion and absorption. Studies of intestinal transit provide, therefore, important insights into the motor consequences of a given procedure and correlations between motility, transit and absorption would greatly enhance the interpretation of motor effects. Such an integrated approach is, unfortunately, all too rare and therefore will continue to limit the extrapolation of these experimental observations to the clinical arena.

THE MOTOR CONSEQUENCES OF INTESTINAL RESECTION

The pathophysiology of the motor response to intestinal resection is complex and may include the effects of transection/anastomosis, those related to the removal of a part of the intestine and those consequent upon any resultant changes in the intraluminal milieu.

The effects of transection/re-anastomosis

The resection of any part of the intestine necessitates its transection and, in most instances, subsequent re-anastomosis. Before discussing the effects of resection per se the consequences of intestinal transection and anastomosis deserve, therefore, some consideration.

Available evidence suggests that a complete transection alone exerts significant effects on motility. Thus, neither a lateral enterotomy (Thompson & Quigley 1991) (Fig. 40.7) or a transection, complete but for the retention of a bridge of muscularis (Fig. 40.8) (Collin et al 1979, Sarr & Kelly 1980, Quigley et al 1983, Jacobs et al 1990), interferes with either the coordination of slow wave or MMC activity or the nature of the fed pattern on either side of the defect. Following a complete transection, in contrast, obvious changes occur and result from the interruption of myogenic and neurogenic transmission.

Slow wave frequency drops sharply in the intestine distal to the transection – loss of entrainment with the proximal duodenal pacemaker resulting in the 'appearance' of the lower intrinsic slow wave frequency of that region (Diamant & Bortoff 1969a, b). An increased incidence of retrograde propagation of slow waves has also been reported, in the dog (Tanner et al 1978). In man, however, where the slow wave frequency gradient is less steep than in the dog, for example, the reduction in slow wave frequency distal to a transection is far less dramatic (Reiser et al 1991).

Whether myogenic transmission can recover remains uncertain. While large animal studies have, in general, failed to detect any evidence of recovery of transmission, a recent study in the guinea pig, and in which meticulous attention was paid to the approximation of the various layers of the intestine, reported the growth of muscle cells across an anastomosis (Galligan et al 1989); under less precise, but perhaps more clinically relevant, conditions the interposition of a fibrotic scar may form a permanent barrier to the recovery of myogenic transmission.

Transection and re-anastomosis may also disrupt MMC activity (Bueno et al 1979, Sarna et al 1981, 1983, Quigley et al 1989) (Fig. 40.9). Sarna and his colleagues (1983) noted that during the first 30–40 days following intestinal transection and reanastomosis, MMCs did not propagate across the anastomosis but cycled independently in segments on either side. By 98–108 days MMC propagation across all transection sites had recovered completely. This observation has been confirmed by others (Wittmann et al 1986, Galligan et al 1989) and a direct relationship between this restoration of coordinated MMC activity and growth of intrinsic nerves across the anastomotic site described (Galligan et al 1989). Caution needs to be exercised, however, in defining relationships between MMC activity on either side of an anastomosis. Because the intrinsic frequency of MMC cycling in separate intestinal segments may be very similar, MMCs may appear to propagate when, in fact, they are cycling independently (Sarna et al 1983, Galligan et al 1989).

The anastomotic technique may also influence MMC propagation as demonstrated in a recent comparison of the motor effects of conventional end-to-end and stapled side-to-side anastomoses on motility (Hocking et al 1990). By 12–20 weeks after operation, 91% of MMCs crossed the end-to-end anastomosis but only 22% traversed the side-to-side anastomosis. Even after 2 years only 56% of MMCs crossed the stapled anastomosis.

By disrupting longitudinal projections of enteric neurons, transection of the intestine could also alter interrelationships between adjacent parts of the intestine. Thus, some, albeit limited, data suggests that transection may affect motor activity in the distal intestine – increased spike activity, MMC cycling and phase III duration being reported distal to the site of transection and re-anastomosis (Bueno et al 1979, Sarna et al

A

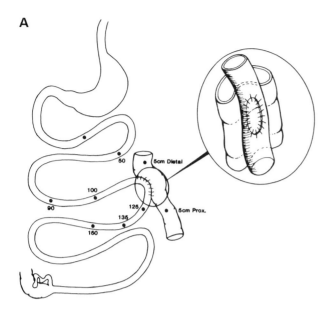

Fig. 40.7 Effects of a lateral enterotomy on motor activity. **A** serosal patch (lateral enterotomy) experimental model. Defect created in jejunum 105 cm from pylorus and closed by suturing margins to the serosal surface of ascending colon (● marks location of serosal electrodes). (Reproduced with permission from Thompson and Quigley 1991.) **B** Myoelectrical recording illustrating normal migration of MMC across area of lateral enterotomy (patch). Note also slow wave frequency unaffected by patch.

B

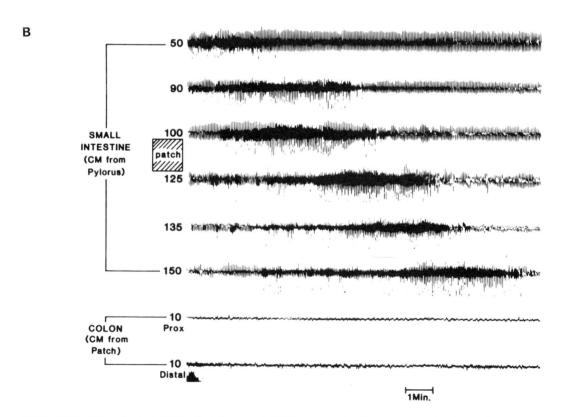

1981, 1983, Heppel et al 1983, Quigley et al 1989, Thompson & Quigley 1991). These changes have been interpreted to represent the 'release' of the distal intestine from proximal inhibition. Changes in motility proximal to a transection have also been reported suggesting that inhibitory effects may be bidirectional (Quigley et al 1989).

In contrast to these various effects on the slow wave

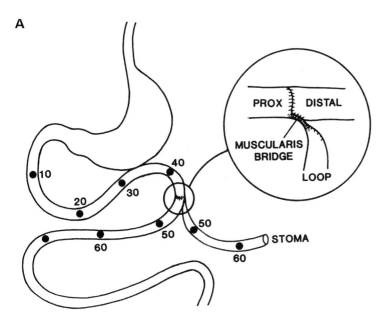

Fig. 40.8 Effects of incomplete intestinal transection on MMC activity. **A** bridged loop/transection model – luminally isolated loop maintains myoneural continuity with the proximal intestine through retention of a bridge of tunica muscularis (i.e. *incomplete* transection) (reproduced with permission from Jacobs et al 1990). **B** Recording of myoelectrical activity; note normal propagation of phase III of MMC through proximal intestine into loop.

and MMC, transection and re-anastomosis appear to have little influence on the fed pattern (Quigley et al 1989). This is consistent with the concept of both MMC disruption and the induction of the fed response being generated by extrinsic autonomic nerves and/or circulating hormones.

Ultrastructural changes have also been described in relation to an intestinal transection and re-anastomosis. In his studies in the rat, Nygaard (1967a) noted an increased thickness of the muscle coat following transection and re-anastomosis of either the jejunum or ileum. Though confined to its immediate vicinity, this hypertrophy was evident on both sides of the anastomosis. In an extension of these studies Weisbrodt and his

A

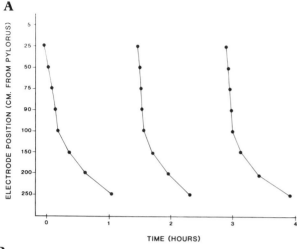

B

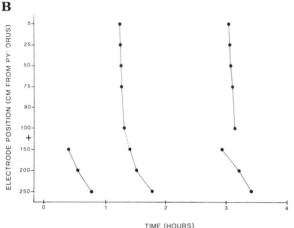

Fig. 40.9 Effects of intestinal transection and re-anastomosis on MMC. **A** recording from control animal – orderly migration of regularly recurring phase III bursts along canine small intestine. Note normal slowing of phase III migration velocity in distal small intestine. **B** Recording from animal following transection and re-anastomosis of jejunum 110 cm from pylorus. Note: (1) 'ectopic' MMCs arising distal to anastomosis; (2) 'apparent' migration of second MMC across anastomosis – this may simply represent the coincidence of independent cycles. (On these plots each • represents an MMC phase III.)

colleagues (1985) confirmed thickening of the circular muscle layer distal to an anastomosis and demonstrated that this was associated with the generation of increased active stress in muscle strips.

What are the effects of these changes on intestinal function? Given the proposed role for the MMC in the prevention of bacterial overgrowth one could predict, for example, some alterations in intestinal flora (Vantrappen et al 1977); evidence for these or other functional changes is, at present, scanty.

Nonetheless, there is a suggestion that transection and reanastomosis may affect transit – Gustavsson (1979), for example, reporting delayed transit and increased mixing of luminal contents in a bowel segment between two end-to-end anastomoses. Simultaneous motility recordings were not performed thus precluding direct motility-transit correlations. In rats subjected to a resection of the proximal half of the jejunum, Nygaard (1967d) reported effects on transit in the proximal intestine which appeared to be dependent on the anastomotic technique – both gastric emptying and transit in the proximal remnant being delayed in those animals with side-to-side but not in those with either end-to-side or end-to-end anastomoses. If one assumes that regrowth of enteric nerves is most likely to occur across an end-to-end anastomosis, these observations provide circumstantial evidence to support a role for the return of MMC coordination in the functional consequences of a transection and re-anastomosis. These changes may, indeed, translate into effects on bacterial flora; overgrowth in the remaining intestine following a proximal resection being most striking when intestinal continuity had been restored by the side-to-side technique (Nygaard 1967c).

The effects of removal of a segment of intestine

While transection may disrupt the longitudinal transmission of ascending and descending inhibition mediated via the ENS a similar release of proximal or distal inhibition could result from the removal of an intestinal segment which possesses a distinctive peptidergic or neural mechanism, a specialized sensory apparatus or unique homeostatic functions. The distal ileum serves as a good example.

In contrast to the more proximal intestine, levels of neurotensin (Polak et al 1977), enteroglucagon (Ferri et al 1983), vasoactive intestinal peptide (VIP) (Ferri et al 1983), peptide YY (Taylor 1985) and enkephalin (Ferri et al 1987) are particularly high in the distal ileum and important roles for these various agents both as traditional hormones and enteric neurotransmitters have been postulated and, in some cases, demonstrated. Evidence for morphological and functional specialization of enteric neurons and ganglia in this region also exists (Christensen et al 1983, Llewellyn-Smith et al 1984). Together these factors may well be fundamental to the unique ability of this part of the intestine to generate its distinctive motor properties in response to various intraluminal stimuli. The extent to which these motor functions, which serve to regulate colonic filling and prevent coloileal reflux, can be assumed by the more proximal intestine following ileal resection remains largely unknown but could well be central to the overall adaptive response.

A unique ileal 'sensing' function is illustrated by the phenomenon referred to as the 'ileal brake'; the instillation of fat solutions directly into the ileum resulting in a slowing of gastric emptying and small intestinal transit (Spiller et al 1984, Read et al 1984, Holgate & Read 1985, Soper et al 1990). This response may represent an attempt by the intestine to conserve fat in conditions of fat maldigestion and/or malabsorption. The loss of this mechanism following ileocolonic resection could well contribute to the steatorrhea so frequently observed in such patients. Nylander (1967) has indeed supplied some experimental evidence to support this concept. In a comparison of the effects of a 15% resection of either the proximal jejunum or the distal ileum in the rat, he noted that both gastric emptying and small bowel transit were accelerated following the ileal resection. Gastric emptying was, in contrast, not affected by the jejunal resection which slowed rather than accelerated intestinal transit.

The effects of an altered luminal milieu

Intestinal resection can also result in changes in the intraluminal milieu (Nygaard 1967c) and thereby, in turn, influence motor patterns. The terminal ileum serves, again, as an excellent and clinically relevant example. Following extensive distal small bowel resections, and related perhaps to the loss of both the ileocaecal valve and the unique propulsive properties of the distal ileum, the intestinal remnant is now exposed to a luminal milieu populated by a colonic bacterial flora. While the motor effects of the normal colonic flora in the small intestine have not been directly examined, several lines of evidence indicate that bacteria may have a significant impact on motility. Mathias and his associates have, for example, demonstrated a characteristic motor response in the rabbit and rat intestine following the instillation of pathogenic bacteria and their toxins (Mathias et al 1976, 1980, Justus et al 1981, Koch et al 1983). Furthermore, volatile fatty acids, products of bacterial fermentation, can induce a dramatic motor response (Kamath et al 1987, 1988, Kamath & Phillips 1988, Fich et al 1989). The pathophysiology of this motor response to bacteria is undoubtedly complex and could include the direct effects of toxin on muscle or nerve (Gilbert et al 1989 a,b), effects mediated by other structural components of the organism, as well as those induced by inflammatory mediators released in reaction to the presence of the bacterium or its toxins and the effects of bacterial products such as volatile fatty acids and deconjugated bile salts (Kruis et al 1986).

Given the important role of the distal ileum in the absorption of bile salts and, thus, in fat digestion, its resection will result in the accumulation of unabsorbed bile salts and fat; both exerting significant motor effects. Most recently, it has been suggested that an intact enterohepatic circulation is essential for the regular cycling of the duodenal MMC (Ozeki et al 1992) – yet another example of interrelationships between distant parts of the small intestine.

Despite these many theoretical considerations and in contrast to the vast literature relating to morphological and biochemical adaptation, (Dowling & Booth 1966, Compston & Creamer 1977, Williamson 1978a, b, Besterman et al 1982, Lilja et al 1983, Murphy et al 1985, Ulrich-Baker et al 1986, Adrian et al 1987) the motor consequences of intestinal resection have received scant attention. Nevertheless, available data strongly indicates a major role for motility in the intestinal response to resection.

Following jejunal, but not ileal resection in the rat, intestinal transit is slowed and gastric emptying delayed (Nygaard 1967b, Nylander 1967, Wittmann et al 1986). Myoelectric recordings in a rat model demonstrated that removal of the proximal 50% of the small intestine resulted in a prolongation of individual MMC cycles, a reduction in the duration of phase I and an increase in the duration of phase II (Wittmann et al 1985, 1986); the net result being the generation of MMC cycles akin to those recorded in the intact distal ileum. The resection of a similar length of the distal intestine was accompanied by only transient effects on the MMC and surgical bypass of the jejunum had little effect on motor patterns (Schang et al 1982, Wittmann et al 1985, 1986). Wittmann and colleagues (1988) also studied the effects of resection and bypass on postprandial motility. Following jejunal resection or bypass, the duration of the postprandial inhibition of the MMC was prolonged – a change that should promote digestion and absorption. While not associated with any delay in the return of the MMC the intensity of postprandial spike activity was significantly suppressed throughout the remaining small intestine following ileal resection; a motor perturbation which might slow transit and thus also promote digestion and absorption.

It would appear, therefore, that, as in the case of mucosal function, motor adaptation is more likely and more effective following resection of the proximal intestine. Indeed, some limited morphological studies suggest that an adaptive hypertrophy of the muscle layer occurs only following resection of the proximal intestine (Nygaard 1967a).

We have recently examined, in the dog, the effects

75% RESECTION

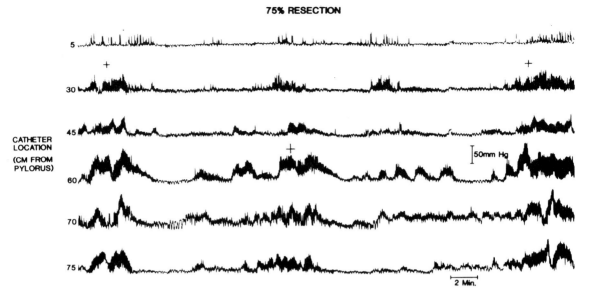

Fig. 40.10   The motor response to massive intestinal resection. Recurrent clusters of rhythmic contractions dominate motor activity in the remaining duodenum and jejunum. Note intense phasic contractions with associated elevations in basal tone.

of distal resections of varying extent on the motor function of the remaining proximal intestine (Quigley & Thompson 1990). We prepared four groups of animals: control animals, and animals who had undergone either a 25%, 50% or 75% resection. The ileocaecal sphincter was retained in all. Fasting and postprandial recordings of intraluminal pressure events along the length of the intestinal remnant were performed at intervals over a 3-month study period. As expected, a 75% resection was accompanied by the development of the clinical features of the short bowel syndrome which included weight loss, malnutrition, diarrhoea and steatorrhoea. While resection did not appear to exert any significant influence on either the frequency of MMC cycling or the maximal frequency of phasic pressure activity along the remnant other patterns showed striking changes. Most characteristic was the development of prominent cluster activity during phase II in the distal parts of the remnant in the 50% and 25% resection groups and throughout the entire remnant in the 75% resection animals. In this latter group, clusters were especially dominant being a persistent and consistent feature of both fasting and postprandial activity and often featuring both sustained elevations of basal tone and intense high amplitude phasic activity (Fig. 40.10). In contrast to those clustered contractions which are a normal feature of distal ileal motility (Quigley et al 1984a,b, 1985, 1987);

clusters in the resection animals were poorly coordinated and propagation was seldom obvious.

One could reasonably speculate that this intense activity may be associated with symptoms, disordered transit and impaired digestion and absorption and that these motor effects could play an important role in the pathogenesis of the early clinical manifestations of the short bowel syndrome. In these relatively short term studies there was also some evidence of 'motor' adaptation – the migration velocity of phase III of the MMC slowing in the distal reaches of the remnant, to approximate that seen in the intact distal ileum, and transit within the remnant slowing significantly with time.

Taken together with the appearance of prominent cluster activity, these observations suggest that following resection motility in the distal remnant become 'ilealized'. The factors which might mediate these changes are unknown but may include the effects of altered intraluminal contents as well as those of enteric peptides and hormones.

To date only one study has evaluated motility in the short bowel syndrome in man, Remington and her colleagues (1983) reporting an increased rate of MMC cycling and a shortening of MMC phase II in a relatively small group of patients (Fig. 40.11). Postprandial motor activity was identical in patients and controls. As the interval from resection to study was not stated, comparisons with animal data are not possible and it

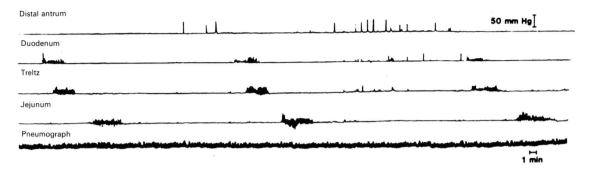

Fig. 40.11   MMC activity in patient with short-bowel syndrome. Recording of proximal intestinal motility in the fasted state from patient with short bowel syndrome demonstrating frequent MMCs and relative disappearance of phase II activity (reproduced with permission from Remington et al 1983).

remains to be determined whether, for example, these changes simply represent another example of release of distal inhibition or rather reflect a true adaptive response.

MOTILITY AND INTESTINAL BYPASS

Surgical procedures which result in a segment of intestine being bypassed and thereby isolated from the intestinal stream are commonly associated with the development of bacterial overgrowth. While changes in intestinal smooth muscle morphology and in vitro function have been demonstrated in the bypassed intestine (Weisbrodt et al 1985); the role of altered motility in the pathogenesis of this complication remains, largely, to be defined. Surprisingly, available data suggests little impact for bypass on the motility of either the bypassed segment or the rest of the intestine (Nygaard 1967c,d, Wittmann et al 1986, 1988).

MOTILITY AND RESTORATIVE SURGICAL PROCEDURES

Surgical procedures designed to ameliorate the short bowel syndrome aim either to retard the transit of intestinal contents through the remaining intestine or to increase its absorptive surface area (Mitchell et al 1984, Thompson 1985, 1988, Thompson & Rikkers 1987, Vanderhoof et al 1992).

Procedures designed to slow transit

These include the construction of artificial sphincters or valves, the interposition of antiperistaltic, colonic and recirculating segments and intestinal pacing. Of these artificial sphincters and antiperistaltic segments appear to offer greatest promise for use in man.

Sphincter substitutes

The use of sphincter substitutes (Glassman 1942, Gazet & Kopp 1964, Stahlgren et al 1964, Lopez-Perez et al 1965, Schiller et al 1967, Griffen et al 1971, Richardson & Griffen 1972, Grier et al 1971, Hidalgo et al 1973, Grosfeld et al 1974, Reid 1975, Caresky et al 1981, Ricotta et al 1981, Diego et al 1982, Stacchini et al 1982, Grieco et al 1983, Myrvold et al 1984, Vinograd et al 1984, Stacchini et al 1986) (Fig. 40.12) is based upon the recognition that retention of the native ileocaecal sphincter at the time of intestinal resection exerts a significant positive impact on nutritional outcome (Gazet & Kopp 1964, Singleton et al 1969, Richardson 1970, Wilmore 1972, Reid 1975, Cosnes et al 1978, Husemann et al 1979). These techniques do not, of course, allow for the possibility that the function of the ileocolonic junctional region, in man, in particular, may owe at least as much to distal ileal motility as to the presence of a sphincter (Phillips et al 1988, Quigley 1988, Fich et al 1992). Furthermore, these substitutes cannot mimic the action of a true sphincter but operate perhaps solely as a low-grade obstruction.

While, in animal studies (Stahlgren et al 1964, Caresky et al 1981, Grieco et al 1983, Stacchini et al 1986), as well as in some very limited reports in man (Waddell et al 1970), prolongation of transit time, increased absorption and improved survival have been reported following the creation of sphincter substitutes, their long-term technical and functional viability remains unclear. Furthermore, little attempt has been

A

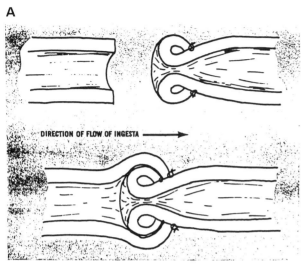

B

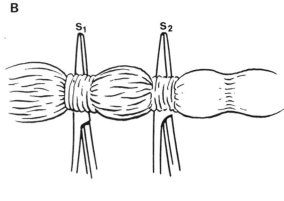

C

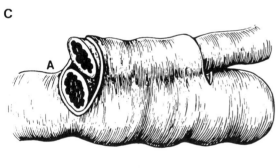

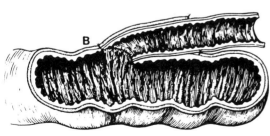

D

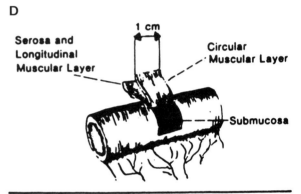

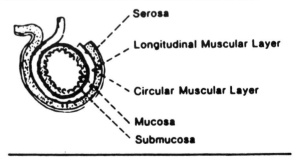

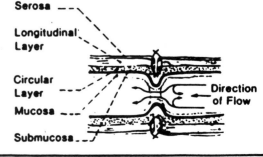

Fig. 40.12   Various models of sphincter substitutes. **A** Inverted nipple valve (reproduced with permission from Grier et al 1971). **B** Ablation of longitudinal muscle layer (reproduced with permission from Stacchini et al 1986). **C** Submucosal tunnelled valve (**A** external aspect showing small intestine tunnelled through colonic submucosal tunnel; **B** internal aspect) (reproduced with permission from Vinograd et al 1984). **D** mucosal/submucosa invagination (reproduced with permission from Diego et al 1982).

made to compare the relative effectiveness of various sphincter models and little is known of their effects on motility.

We studied the effects of an ileocolonic sphincter substitute on canine small intestinal motor activity (Quigley et al 1989). For these experiments, an inverted nipple valve (as in Fig. 40.12a) was fashioned in the mid-jejunum and its effects on motility in the intestine on either side evaluated. Several motility changes were noted in the jejunum proximal to the valve: the frequency of MMC phase III complexes was suppressed and recurring bursts of propagated spike clusters dominated during fasting (Fig. 40.13). From time to time striking and very prolonged spike bursts were recorded from electrodes proximal to the sphincter substitute. Postprandial myoelectrical patterns were unchanged. While these observed motility patterns most likely reflected a response to a low-grade obstruction, none of these animals exhibited overt clinical, radiographic or autopsy evidence of intestinal obstruction.

Placement of a sphincter substitute, of a type advocated for replacement of the ileocolonic sphincter, results, therefore, in the proximal disruption of interdigestive motor activity. The motor patterns recorded from the jejunum proximal to the substitute were somewhat reminiscent of those normally seen in the distal ileum. We speculated that, whether through an increase in intraluminal pressure or by promoting stasis and thereby increased exposure to certain luminal contents, a sphincter substitute promotes the development of ileal-type motor activity and thereby may improve absorptive function.

This concept was supported by subsequent studies in which we assessed the influence of a sphincter substitute on both the motor and nutritional effects of a 75% distal small intestinal resection (Quigley et al 1991). The creation of a sphincter substitute at the time of resection not only lessened the deleterious nutritional impact of this subtotal intestinal resection, but also slowed transit within the remnant and was associated with a reduced incidence of clustered contractions.

Reversed segments

The use of reversed intestinal segments is based upon the assumption that orad-directed motor events within a segment would act to delay transit and thereby promote absorption (Stahlgren et al 1962, Keller et al 1965, Baldwin-Price et al 1965, Venables et al 1966, Fink and Olson 1967, Trinkle & Bryant 1967, Vayre et al 1967, Wilmore & Johnson 1968, Delaney et al 1970, O'Reilly 1971, Hutcher et al 1973, Pertsemlidis &

Kark 1974, Hutcher & Salzberg 1971, Lloyd 1978, Warden & Wesley 1978, Tanner et al 1978, Barros D'Sa 1979, Gustavsson 1979, Lloyd 1981, Garcia et al 1981, Sidhu et al 1985). While these concepts have been verified in experimental animals, this technique has not enjoyed widespread application in man due to continuing difficulties in defining precisely that length of bowel which, when reversed, will produce effective slowing of transit without causing obstruction (Tanner et al 1978, Gustavsson 1979, Carner & Raju 1981, Sidhu et al 1985).

Tanner and his colleagues (1978) demonstrated not only that the majority of slow waves propagated in an aboral direction within a 10-cm long reversed jejunal segment (Fig. 40.14) but also that retrograde propagation was predominant in the distal intestine. While a slowing of transit has been confirmed (Gustavsson 1979, Sidhu et al 1985) other mechanisms to explain the beneficial effects of these reversed segments have been proposed. Thus, Mitchell and colleagues (1983) by demonstrating a suppression of myoelectrical spike activity, coupled with slower transit and increased absorption of water, glucose and electrolytes with retrograde perfusion of a jejunal loop raised the possibility that this mechanism, an inevitable consequence of bowel reversal, may also be operative. Others have proposed hormonal effects (Barros D'Sa et al 1976).

Pacing

A similar concept underlies attempts to slow transit by the retrograde pacing of segments of intestine. In most animal models, duodenal transection is a prerequisite for successful pacing (Sarna & Daniel 1975, Akwari et al 1975, Collin et al 1978, 1979, Gladen & Kelly 1981a,b). By isolating the rest of the small bowel from the duodenal pacemaker, a lower, intrinsic frequency is revealed and can then be driven to pre-transection levels (Fig. 40.15). While this has been shown to be feasible in a dog model and indeed to result in slowed transit and improved absorption within the paced segment, progress in man has been hampered by the technical difficulties of attempting to capture the human intestinal slow wave (Richter & Kelly 1986). In man, the slow wave gradient along the intestine is far less steep than in the dog making it difficult to 'drive' slow waves. Thus, Richter and Kelly (1986) found that there was a drop of only 0.3 cpm across a jejunal transection rendering the frequency range for capture prohibitively low; not surprisingly, the slow wave was captured in only one of nine subjects studied.

Pacing may, however, have effects other than those based upon slow wave capture – animal studies demon-

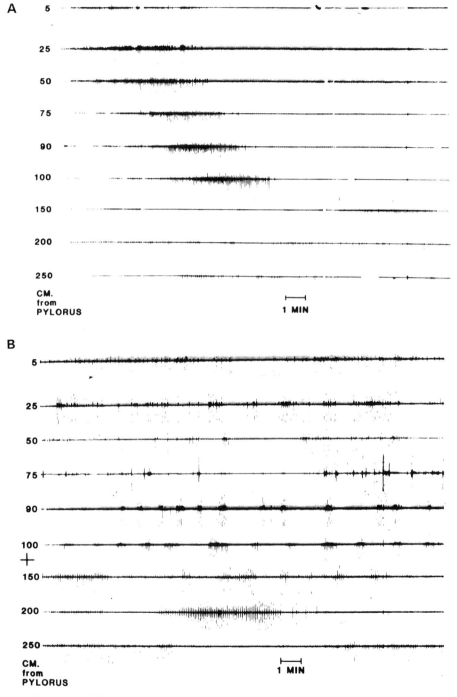

Fig. 40.13 Effects of a sphincter substitute on fasting intestinal motor activity. **A** Control animal – normal MMC. **B** Animal with sphincter substitute fashioned 110 cm from pylorus. Note: (1) normal MMC distal to sphincter substitute; (2) myoelectrical activity in proximal intestine dominated by 'clusters' of spikes (reproduced with permission from Quigley et al 1989).

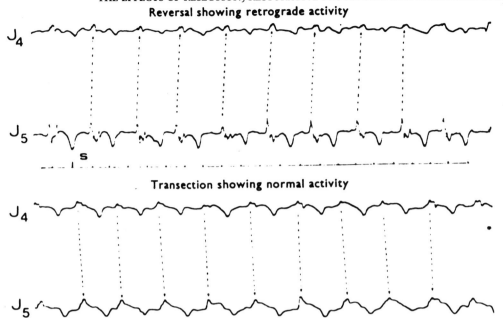

Fig. 40.14 Electrical activity in reversed bowel segment. Recordings from 10 cm long reversed jejunal segment (**A**) and jejunum distal to transection and anastomosis (**B**) illustrating reversal of slow wave propagation in reversed loop (reproduced with permission from Tanner et al 1978).

strating a suppression of motility and an enhancement of absorption in the intact bowel on pacing an excluded loop (Bjorck et al 1987, Reiser et al 1989, 1991). This effect, potentially beneficial in the short bowel syndrome, could not be achieved by pacing the intact bowel (Reiser et al 1991).

Increasing the effective absorptive area

The other major surgical strategy to ameliorate the short bowel syndrome attempts to increase the effective absorptive surface area of the remnant.

Serosal patching

One such approach takes advantage of the clinical and experimental observation that full thickness intestinal defects sealed by opposition to the serosal surface of adjacent bowel will eventually become epithelialized by lateral ingrowth of mucosa from the intact intestine at the edge of the defect (Wolfman et al 1964, Jones et al 1973). The leading edge of growth consists of a thin layer of columnar epithelial cells. Eventually, the defect becomes completely covered with mature intestinal villi and muscularis mucosa. This phenomenon of intestinal regeneration to seal a defect has been termed neomucosal growth (Binnington et al 1975, Gaton et al 1980, Lillemoe et al 1982, Thompson et al 1984, 1986,

1988). Though neomucosa has been shown, both in vivo and in vitro, to exhibit normal absorptive function (Binnington et al 1974, Lillemoe et al 1982, Thompson et al 1985a, 1987, 1988), the overall nutritional impact of serosal patching in experimental models of the short bowel syndrome has been disappointing, the net increase in absorptive surface area provided by neomucosa being limited by marked contraction of the defect. Most disturbing has been the observation that intestinal patching of dogs with the short bowel syndrome actually exacerbated weight loss and malabsorption (Thompson et al 1988). The pathophysiology of this deleterious effect is uncertain but does not appear to be related to motor disruption (Thompson & Quigley 1991). In the dog serosal patching does not alter either fasting (Fig. 40.7) or postprandial myoelectrical patterns in the small intestine; neither does it disrupt motor activity in the colon to which it is 'patched'.

Intestinal tapering and lengthening

The motor response to other restorative procedures such as the technique of first tapering and then lengthening a dilated intestinal remnant (the Bianchi procedure), though reported to be of clinical benefit in man has, as yet, not been studied (Bianchi 1980, Boekman & Traylor 1981, Weber et al 1982, Thompson et

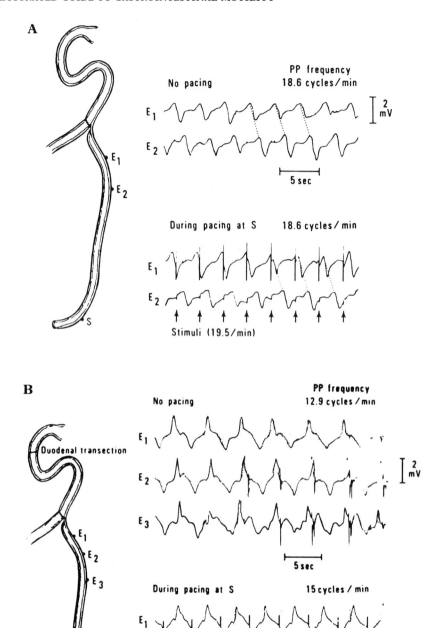

Fig. 40.15 Retrograde pacing. **A** without duodenal transection pacing at the stimulating electrode (S) fails to capture. **B** Following duodenal transection pacing captures slow wave and results in increased slow wave frequency and retrograde propagation of slow wave (reproduced with permission from Collin et al 1979).

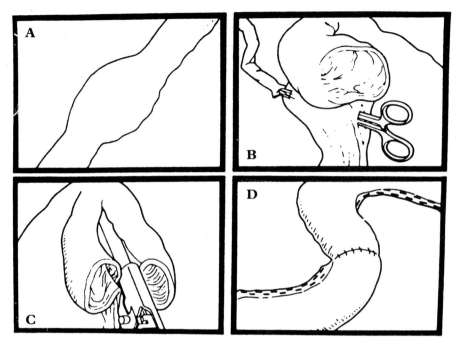

Fig. 40.16 Tapering and lengthening procedure. **A** dilated intestinal segment. **B** dissection of vessels along the mesenteric border. **C** longitudinal division of bowel with staples. **D** end-to-end anastomosis of divided segments (reproduced with permission from Thompson et al 1985b).

al 1985b). This procedure involves the longitudinal division of the remnant to create two intestinal 'tubes' which are then anastomosed end-to-end, thus potentially interfering with circumferential, rather than longitudinal, transmission of motor signals (Fig. 40.16).

MOTILITY AND INTESTINAL TRANSPLANTATION

Recent improvements in immunosuppression have renewed enthusiasm for intestinal transplantation as a means of increasing intestinal surface area in the short bowel syndrome (Grant et al 1990, Hoffman et al 1990, Quigley 1992c, Starzl et al 1992, Todo et al 1992). Although the immunologic aspects of intestinal transplantation have received considerable attention, the motor and absorptive function of the transplanted gut has been investigated less thoroughly.

In animal models, malabsorption and persistent nutritional defects have been described after allotransplantation (Cohen et al 1969, Holmes et al 1970, Ruiz et al 1972, Stamford & Hardy 1974, Reznick et al 1982, Diliz-Perez et al 1984, Schraut et al 1987, Schroeder et al 1987, Watson et al 1988, Quigley et al 1992, Thomp-

son et al 1992). While these may be related, in large part, to graft rejection, several other factors may be operative. It is difficult, however, to separate their possible contributions from those of rejection in an allograft model.

The technique of small intestinal autotransplantation provides a model for the study of these non-rejection-related consequences of allotransplantation. These non-immune-mediated phenomena include the effects of total extrinsic denervation, lymphatic disruption, ischaemic and re-perfusion injury and the temporary loss of stimulation from luminal nutrients and other substances. Given that it involves the complete transection of all extrinsic sympathetic and parasympathetic fibres to the autotransplanted gut, this model can provide insights into the role of extrinsic nerves in the control of intestinal function and has thus contributed to our understanding of the pathophysiology of the gastrointestinal manifestations of autonomic neuropathies. Such studies have, for example, advanced our understanding of the regulation of fasting and postprandial motility, of the role of extrinsic nerves in various secretory events and of extrinsic neural contributions to peptide release and interactions between intestinal organs (Sarr & Kelly 1981, Tanaka & Sarr 1988,

A

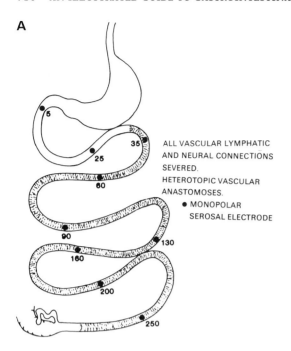

ALL VASCULAR LYMPHATIC
AND NEURAL CONNECTIONS
SEVERED.
HETEROTOPIC VASCULAR
ANASTOMOSES.
● MONOPOLAR
   SEROSAL ELECTRODE

Fig. 40.17 Motor activity in the autotransplanted intestine. **A** animal model. **B** disrupted fasting activity illustrated in graphic summary of recording obtained 6 weeks postoperatively. Note irregular MMC activity – complexes migrate over short distances only; prominent cluster activity. **C** normal MMC activity within autotransplanted jejunoileum 16 weeks postoperatively. Note regularly-recurring MMCs which migrate through autotransplanted intestine. No evidence of coordination with phase III activity in duodenum (reproduced with permission from Quigley et al 1990).

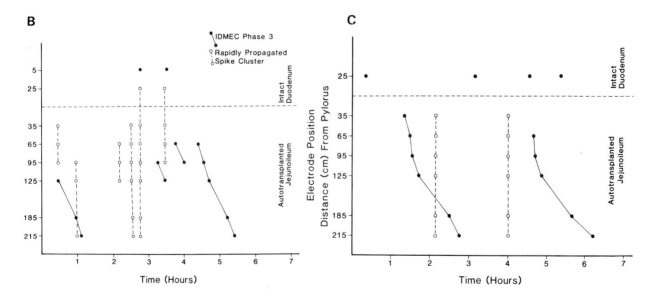

Hakim et al 1989, Sarr et al 1989, 1990, Spencer et al 1989, Quigley et al 1990, Nelson et al 1991, Soper et al 1991). These important physiological studies are beyond the scope of this chapter.

Our focus has been to examine, as a prelude to allotransplantation, the long-term effects of total jejunoileal autotransplantation on motility and absorption (Quigley et al 1990, Adrian et al 1991a, b, Rose et al 1991, Quigley et al 1992, Thompson et al 1992) (Fig.

40.17). Although initially disrupted, interdigestive motor activity demonstrated progressive organization in our animals (Quigley et al 1990) (Fig. 40.17b & 40.17c). Thus, in animals studied between 12 and 20 months following autotransplantation, 88% of MMCs demonstrated each phase in normal sequence. Longitudinal studies of several parameters of myoelectrical activity provided further evidence of progressive organization and entrainment of motor functions within

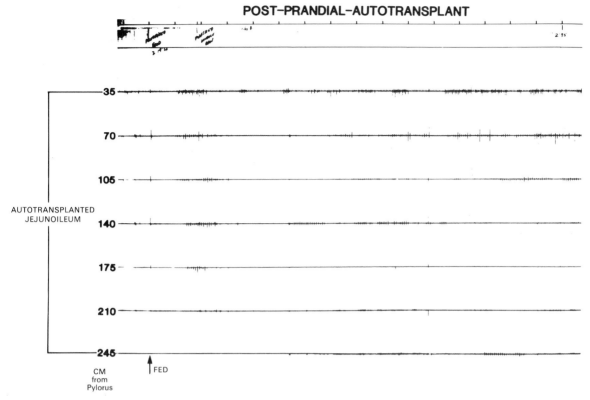

Fig. 40.18 Absent postprandial motor response in autotransplanted intestine. No evidence of myoelectrical equivalent of fed response following food administration (arrow).

the denervated intestine. Coordination with the proximal intact intestine did not, however, recover and a number of abnormal patterns were recorded within the autotransplanted segment during fasting. These included rapidly-propagated spike clusters, prolonged bursts of uninterrupted (phase III-like) activity and bursts of uninterrupted spike activity. Anoxic and cooling damage to enteric nerves and muscle incurred during the autotransplantation procedure may explain the abnormal patterns observed.

In contrast to the preservation of fasting motor patterns, the major component of the myoelectric response to feeding was permanently impaired, with a delayed onset and shortened duration of the fed response (Fig. 40.18).

We concluded that the extrinsically denervated intestine recovered the ability to generate and organize all phases of the MMC but that it demonstrated a permanent impairment of the major motor response to food. These findings are entirely consistent with current thoughts with regard to the relative roles of extrinsic and intrinsic neurons in the regulation of fasting and postprandial motor patterns.

Although body weight and serum albumin levels remained stable in these animals following autotransplantation and initial diarrhoea improved, stool moisture content was persistently elevated and late defects in fat and D-xylose absorption were observed (Quigley et al 1992, Thompson et al 1992). Others have also demonstrated a persistent secretory state; its pathophysiology remains, however, uncertain (Sarr et al 1991). Furthermore, in comparison with control animals, autotransplanted dogs demonstrated a significant overgrowth of faecal flora in the jejunum and ileum. These delayed defects in intestinal absorption of fat and D-xylose occurred more than 12 months following autotransplantation and did not appear to be related to alterations in intestinal structure but may well have been a consequence of some of the motor abnormalities observed, thus serving to underline the importance of the motor effects of the procedure (Quigley et al 1992, Thompson et al 1992).

To date motility in the allotransplanted intestine in either animal models or human patients has not been reported in any detail and several questions remain, therefore, unanswered. Will the long-term, and perhaps motility-related, changes in absorption observed in the autotransplant animals translate into significant clinical problems in patients who have undergone allografts? Could motor changes serve as sensitive indicators of graft rejection or dysfunction?

CONCLUSIONS

Despite the fundamental role of motility in gut homeostasis, our understanding of the motor consequences of these various surgical procedures remains in its infancy, and most available information has been derived exclusively from animal models. Available evidence suggests, nonetheless, that extensive intestinal resection results in a major disruption of motility in the remnant which may be relevant to the clinical features of the short bowel syndrome. There is also a suggestion that motor adaptation may be an important phenomenon. Some, at least, of those restorative surgical procedures developed to ameliorate the short bowel syndrome may also exert significant motor effects. Data from autotransplant studies indicate that motor changes may also contribute significantly to the function of intestinal allografts – the motility of human allografts and its relationship to overall graft function remain, however, to be defined.

REFERENCES

Adrian T E, Savage A P, Fuessl H S, et al 1987 Release of peptide YY (PYY) after resection of small bowel, colon, or pancreas in man. Surgery 101: 715–719

Adrian T E, Marsh J M, Herrington M K, et al 1991a Gastrointestinal hormone responses following extrinsic denervation of the small bowel. Gastroenterology 100: A413

Adrian T E, Marsh J M, Herrington M K, et al 1991b Effects of extrinsic denervation of the small intestine on enteric neuropeptides. Gastroenterology 100: A413

Akwari O E, Kelly K A, Steinbach J H, et al 1975 Electrical pacing of intact and transected canine small intestine and its computer model. Am J Physiol 229: 1188–1197

Baldwin-Price H K, Copp D, Singleton A O 1965 Reversed intestinal segments in the management of anenteric malabsorption syndrome. Ann Surg 161: 225–230

Barros D'Sa A A B 1979 An experimental evaluation of the segmental reversal after massive small bowel resection. Br J Surg 66: 493–500

Barros D'Sa A A B, Parks T G, Kennedy T L, et al 1976 Hormonal alterations caused by segmental reversal after massive small bowel resection. Eur Surg Res 8 (suppl): 3–4

Besterman H S, Adrian T E, Mallinson C N, et al 1982 Gut hormone release after intestinal resection. Gut 23: 854–861

Bianchi A 1980 Intestinal loop lengthening – a technique for increasing small intestinal length. J Pediatr Surg 15: 145–151

Binnington H B, Sumner H, Lesker P, Alpers D A et al 1974 Functional characteristics of surgically induced jejunal neomucosa. Surgery 75: 805–810

Binnington H B, Tumbleson M E, Ternberg J L 1975 Use of jejunal neomucosa in the treatment of the short gut syndrome in pigs. J Pediatr Surg 10: 617–621

Bjorck S, Kelly K A, Phillips S F 1987 Mechanisms of enhanced canine enteric absorption with intestinal pacing. Am J Physiol 252: G548–G553

Boeckman C R, Traylor R 1981 Bowel lengthening for short gut syndrome. J Pediatr Surg 16: 996–997

Bueno L, Pradduade F, Ruckebusch Y 1979 Propagation of electrical spiking activity along the small intestine: intrinsic versus extrinsic neural influences. J Physiol 292: 15–26

Caresky J, Weber T R, Grosfeld J L 1981 Ileocecal valve replacement. Its effect on transit time, survival and weight change after massive intestinal resection. Arch Surg 116: 618–622

Carner D V, Raju S 1981 Failure of anti-peristaltic colon interposition to ameliorate short-bowel syndrome. Am Surgeon 47: 538–540

Christensen J, Rick G A, Robinson B A, et al 1983 Arrangement of the myenteric plexus throughout the gastrointestinal tract of the opossum. Gastroenterology 85: 890–899

Cohen W B, Hardy M A, Quint J et al 1969 Absorptive function in canine jejunal autografts and allografts. Surgery 65: 440–446

Collin J, Kelly K A, Phillips S F 1978 Increased canine jejunal absorption of water, glucose and sodium with intestinal pacing. Dig Dis Sci 23: 1121–1126

Collin J, Kelly K A and Phillips S F 1979 Enhancement of absorption from the intact and transected canine small intestine by electrical pacing. Gastroenterology 76: 1422–1428

Compston J E, Creamer B 1977 The consequences of small intestinal resection. Q J Med 46: 485–497

Cosnes J, Gendre J P, LeQuintrec Y 1978 Role of the ileocaecal valve and site of intestinal resection in malabsorption after extensive small bowel resection. Digestion 18: 329–336

Daniel E E, Berezin I 1992 Interstitial cells of Cajal: are they major players in control of gastrointestinal motility? J Gastrointest Mot 4: 1–24

Delaney H M, Parker J G, Gliedman M L 1970 Experimental massive intestinal resection: comparison of surgical measures and spontaneous adaption. Arch Surg 101: 599–604

Diamant N E, Bortoff A 1969a Nature of the intestinal slow-wave frequency gradient. Am J Physiol 216: 301–307

Diamant N E, Bortoff A 1969b Effects of transection on the intestinal slow-wave frequency gradient. Am J Physiol 216: 734–743

Diego M D, de Miguel E, Lucea C M, et al 1982 Short-gut syndrome. A new surgical technique and ultrastructural study of the liver and pancreas. Arch Surg 117: 789–795

Diliz-Perez H S, McClure J, Bedetti C, et al 1984 Successful small bowel allotransplantation in dogs with cyclosporine and prednisone. Transplantation 37: 126–129

Dowling R H, Booth C C 1966 Functional compensation after small-bowel resection in man. Lancet 2: 146–147

Duthie H L, Kwong N K, Brown B H, et al 1971 Pacesetter

potentials of the human gastroduodenal junction. Gut 12: 250–256

Ferri G-L, Adrian T E, Ghatei I O, O'Shaughnessy D T, et al 1983 Tissue localizations and relative distribution of regulatory peptides in separated layers from the human bowel. Gastroenterology 84: 777–786

Ferri G-L, Morreale R A, Soimero L, et al 1987 Intraluminal distribution of met⁵-enkephalin-Arg⁶-gly⁷-leu⁸ in sphincter regions of the human gut. Neuroscience Letters: 306–308

Fich A, Phillips S F, Hakim N S, et al 1989 Stimulation of ileal emptying by short chain fatty acids. Dig Dis Sci 34: 1516–1520

Fich A, Steadman C J, Phillips S F et al 1992 Ileocolonic transit does not change after right hemicolectomy. Gastroenterology 103: 794–799

Fink W J, Olson J D 1967 The massive bowel resection syndrome: Treatment with reversed intestinal segments. Arch Surg 94: 700–706

Galligan J J, Furness J B, Costa M 1989 Migration of the myoelectric complex after interruption of the myenteric plexus: intestinal transection and regneration of enteric nerves in the guinea pig. Gastroenterology 97: 1135–1146

Garcia V F, Templeton J M, Eichelberger M R et al 1981 Colon interposition for the short bowel syndrome. J Pediatr Surg 16: 994–995

Gaton E, Czernobilsky B, Krans L et al 1980 The neomucosa and its surroundings after jejunoserosal patching in dogs. J Surg Res 29: 451–465

Gazet J C, Kopp J 1964 The surgical significance of the ileocecal junction. Surgery 56: 565–573

Gilbert R J, Triadafilopoulos G, Pothoulakis C, et al 1989a Effect of purified *Clostridium difficile* toxins on intestinal smooth muscle. I. Toxin A. Am J Physiol 256: G759–G766

Gilbert R J, Pothoulakis C, LaMont J T 1989b Effect of purified *Clostridium difficile* toxins on intestinal smooth muscle. II Toxin B. Am J Physiol 256: G767–G772

Gladen H E, Kelly K A 1981a Enhancing absorption in the canine short bowel by intestinal pacing. Surgery 88: 281–286

Gladen H E, Kelly K A 1981b Electrical pacing for the short bowel syndrome. Surg Gynecol Obstet 153: 697–700

Glassman J A 1942 An artificial ileocecal valve. Surg Gynecol Obstet 74: 92–98

Grant D, Wall W, Mimeault R, et al 1990 Successful small bowel/liver transplantation. Lancet 335: 181–194

Grieco G A, Reyes H M, Ostrovsky E 1983 The role of a modified intussusception jejunocolic valve in short-bowel syndrome. J Pediatr Surg 18: 354–359

Grier R L, Nelson A W, Lumb W V 1971 Experimental sphincter for short-bowel syndrome. Arch Surg 102: 203–208

Griffen W O, Richardson J D, Medley ES 1971 Prevention of small bowel contamination by ileocecal valve. Southern Med J 64: 1056–1058

Grosfeld J L, Cooney D R, Jesseph J E 1974 Experimental ileocecal valve replacement in puppies. Surg Forum 25: 364–365

Gustavsson S 1979 Transport of small bowel contents after interposition of an antiperistaltic jejunal segment in the rat. Eur Surg Res 11: 381–391

Hakim N S, Sarr M S, Spencer M P 1989 Postprandial disruption of migrating myoelectric complex in dogs: hormonal versus extrinsic nervous factors. Dig Dis Sci 34: 257–263

Heppel J, Kelly K A, Sarr M G 1983 Neural control of canine small intestinal interdigestive myoelectric complexes. Am J Physiol 244: G95–G100

Hidalgo F, Cortes M L, Salas S J, Zavala J 1973 Intestinal muscle layer ablation in short bowel syndrome. Arch Surg 106: 188–190

Hocking M P, Carlson R G, Courington K R, et al 1990 Altered motility and bacterial flora after functional end-to-end anastomosis. Surgery 108: 384–392

Hoffman A L, Makowka L, Banner B et al 1990 The use of FK-506 for small intestine allotransplantation. Transplantation 49: 483–490

Holgate A M, Read N W 1985 Effect of ileal infusion of intralipid on gastrointestinal transit, ileal flow rate, and carbohydrate absorption in humans after ingestion of a liquid meal. Gastroenterology 88: 1005–1011

Holmes S T, Yeh S D J, Winawer S J et al 1970 New concepts in structure and function of dog jejunal allografts. Surg Forum 21: 334–336

Husemann B, Schuck R, Schulz H P 1979 Resection of the valvula Bauhini and its effect on the metabolism. An experimental study in animals. Langenbecks Arch Clin 383: 183–190

Hutcher M E, Salzberg A M 1971 Pre-ileal transposition of colon to prevent the development of short bowel syndrome in puppies with 90 percent small intestine resection. Surgery 70: 189–197

Hutcher M E, Mendez-Picon G, Salzberg A M 1973 Pre-jejunal transportation of colon to prevent the development of short bowel syndrome in puppies with 90 percent small intestine resection. J Pediatr Surg 8: 771–777

Jacobs D L, Lof J, Quigley E M M et al 1990. The effect of mesenteric venous hypertension on gut motility and absorption. J Surg Res 48: 562–567

Jones S A, Gazzaniga A B, Keller T B 1973 The serosal patch: a surgical parachute. Am J Surg 126: 186–196

Justus P G, Mathias J R, Martin J L et al 1981 Myoelectric activity in the small intestine in response to *Clostridium perfringens* enterotoxin: correlation with histologic findings in an in vitro rabbit model. Gastroenterology 80: 902–906

Kamath P S, Phillips S F 1988 Initiation of motility in canine ileum by short chain fatty acids and inhibition by pharmacological agents. Gut 29: 941–948

Kamath P S, Hoepfner M T, Phillips S 1987 Short chain fatty acids stimulate motility of the canine ileum. Am J Physiol 16: G427–G433

Kamath P S, Phillips S F, Zinmeister AR 1988 Short chain fatty acids stimulate ileal motility in humans. Gastroenterology 95: 1496–1502

Keller T W, Stewart W R C, Westerheide R et al 1965 Prolonged survival with paired reversed segment after massive intestinal resection. Arch Surg 91: 174–179

Koch K L, Martin J L, Mathias J R 1983 Migrating action-potential complexes in vitro in cholera-exposed rabbit ileum. Am J Physiol 244: G291–G294

Kruis W J, Azpiroz F, Phillips S F 1985 Contractile patterns and transit of fluid in canine terminal ileum. Am J Physiol 249: G264–G270

Kruis W, Haddad A, Phillips S F 1986 Chenodeoxycholic and ursodeoxycholic acids alter motility and fluid transit in the canine ileum. Digestion 34: 185–194

Kruis W, Phillips S F, Zinmeister A R 1987 Flow across the canine ileocolonic junction: role of the ileocolonic sphincter. Am J Physiol 252: G13–G18

Kyi K K J, Daniel E E 1970 The effects of ischemia on intestinal nerves and electrical slow waves. Am J Dig Dis 15: 959–981

Lilja P, Wiener I, Inoue K et al 1983 Changes in circulating levels of cholecystokinin, gastrin and pancreatic polypeptide after small bowel resection in dogs. Am J Surg 145: 157–163

Lillemoe K D, Berry W R, Harmon J W et al 1982 Use of vascularized abdominal wall pedicle flaps to grow small bowel neomucosa. Surgery 91: 292–300

Llewellyn-Smith I J, Furness J B, O'Brien P E et al 1984 Noradrenergic nerves in human small intestine. Distribution and ultrastructure. Gastroenterology 87: 513–529

Lloyd P A 1978 Colonic interposition between the jejunum and ileum after massive small bowel resection in rats. Prog Pediatr Surg 12: 51–106

Lloyd P A 1981 Antiperistaltic colonic interposition following massive small bowel resection in rats. J Pediatr Surg 16: 64–69

Lopez-Perez, Martinez A J, Machusa J 1965 Experimental anti-reflux intestinal valve. Am J Surg 109: 32–38

Mathias J R, Carlson G M, DiMarino A J et al 1976 Intestinal myoelectric activity in response to live *Vibrio cholerae* and cholera enterotoxin. J Clin Invest 58: 91–96

Mathias J R, Carlson G M, Martin J L et al 1980 *Shigella dysenteriae* I enterotoxin: proposed role in the pathogenesis of shigellosis. Am J Physiol 239: G382–G386

Mitchell A, Collin J, Denton T G 1983 Effects of retrograde luminal perfusion of the canine jejunum on intestinal absorption and myoelectrical activity. Eur J Clin Invest 13: 245–254

Mitchell A, Watkins R M, Collin J 1984 Surgical treatment of the short bowel syndrome. Br J Surg 71: 329–333

Murphy R F, Chen M-H, Herlin P M et al 1985 Glucagon, secretin and vasoactive intestinal polypeptide immunoreactivities in rat gut after jejuno-ileal bypass and resection. Digestion 32: 106–113

Myrvold H, Tindel M S, Isenberg H D et al 1984 The nipple valve as a sphincter substitute for the ileocecal valve: prevention of bacterial overgrowth in the small bowel. Surgery 96: 42–47

Nelson D K, Sarr M G, Bailey J E et al 1991 Intestinal transplantation: effect of gut neuropeptides. Gut 32: 1336–1341

Nygaard K 1967a Resection of the small intestine in rats. III morphological changes in the intestinal tract. Acta Chir Scand 133: 233–248

Nygaard K 1967b Resection of the small intestine in rats. Adaptation of gastrointestinal motility. Acta Chir Scand 133: 407–416

Nygaard K 1967c Changes in the intestinal flora after resections and bypass-operations on the small intestine in rats. The effect of different types of anastomoses. Acta Chir Scand 133: 569–583

Nygaard K 1967d Gastrointestinal motility after resections and bypass operation on the small intestine in rats. The effect of different types of anastomosis. Acta Chir Scand 133: 653–663

Nylander G 1967 Gastric evacuation and propulsive intestinal motility following resection of the small intestine in the rat. Acta Chir Scand 133: 131–138

O'Reilly K 1971 Ileal reversal to compensate for the loss of the ileocaecal valve. Med J Aust 1: 805–806

Ozeki K, Sarna S K, Condon R E et al 1992 Enterohepatic circulation is essential for regular cycling of duodenal migrating motor complexes in dogs. Gastroenterology 103: 759–767

Pertsemlidis D, Kark A E 1974 Anti-peristaltic segments for the treatment of short bowel syndrome. Am J Gastroenterol 62: 526–530

Phillips S F, Quigley E M M, Kumar D et al 1988 Motility of the ileocolonic junction. Gut 29: 390–406

Polak J, Sullivan S N, Bloom S R et al 1977 Specific localization of neurotensin to the N cell in human intestine by radioimmunoassay and immunocytochemistry. Nature 270: 183–184

Quigley E M M 1987 Small intestinal motor activity – its role in gut homeostasis in health and disease. Q J Med 65: 799–810

Quigley E M M 1988 Motor activity of the distal ileum and ileocecal sphincter and its relation to the region's function. Dig Dis 6: 229–241

Quigley E M M 1992a Intestinal manometry – technical advances; clinical limitations. Dig Dis Sci 37: 10–13

Quigley E M M 1992b Antroduodenal manometry in: Hinder R A (ed.) Problems in general surgery: tests of foregut function. Lippincott, Philadelphia pp 152–171

Quigley E M M 1992c Small bowel transplantation – progress and problems. Gastrointest Journal Club 1: 11–12

Quigley E M M, Thompson J S 1990 The motor response to intestinal resection. Gastroenterology 98: A382

Quigley E M M, Phillips S F, Dent J et al 1983 Myoelectrical activity and intraluminal pressure of the canine ileocecal sphincter. Gastroenterology 95: 1054–1062

Quigley E M M, Phillips S F, Dent J 1984a Distinctive patterns of interdigestive motility at the canine ileocolonic junction. Gastroenterology 87: 836–844

Quigley E M M, Borody T J, Phillips S F et al 1984b Motility of the terminal ileum and ileocecal sphincter in healthy man. Gastroenterology 87: 857–866

Quigley E M M, Phillips S F, Cranley B et al 1985 Tonic pressures at the canine ileocolonic junction: topography and relationship to phasic motor activity. Am J Physiol 249: G350–G357

Quigley E M M, Dent J, Phillips S F 1987 Manometry of the canine ileocecal sphincter: comparison of the sleeve method to point sensors. Am J Physiol 252: G585–G591

Quigley E M M, Thompson J S, Lof J 1989 Disruption of jejunal interdigestive myoelectrical activity by an artificial ileocecal sphincter. Studies of the intestinal motor response to a surgically-fashioned sphincter substitute. Dig Dis Sci 34: 1434–1442

Quigley E M M, Spanta A D, Rose S G et al 1990 Long-term effects of jejunoileal autotransplantation on myoelectrical activity in the canine small intestine. Dig Dis Sci 35: 1505–1517

Quigley E M M, Thompson J S, Lof J et al 1991 Effects of a sphincter substitute on canine small intestinal motor activity and absorptive function in the small bowel syndrome. Gastroenterology 100: A241

Quigley E M M, Thompson J S, Rose S G 1992 The long-term function of canine jejuno-ileal autotransplants – insights into allo-graft physiology. Transplant Proc 24: 1105–1106

Read N W, McFarlane A, Kinsman R I et al 1984 Effect of infusion of nutrient solutions into the ileum on gastrointestinal transit and plasma levels of neurotensin and enteroglucagon. Gastroenterology 86: 274–280

Reid I S 1975 The significance of the ileocecal valve in massive resection of the gut in puppies. J Pediatr Surg 10: 507–510

Reiser S B, Weiser H F, Schuszdziarra V et al 1989 Effect of pacing on small intestinal motor activity and hormonal response in dogs. Dig Dis Sci 34: 579–584

Reiser S B, Schuszdziarra V, Bollschweiler E et al 1991 Effect of enteric pacing on intestinal motility and hormone secretion in dogs with short bowel. Gastroenterology 101: 100–106

Remington M, Malagelada J-R, Zinsmeister A R et al 1983 Abnormalities in gastrointestinal motor activity in patients with short bowels: effect of a synthetic opiate. Gastroenterology 85: 29–36

Reznick R K, Craddock G N, Langer B et al 1982 Structure and function of small bowel allografts in the dog: immunosuppression with cyclosporine A. Can J Surg 75: 51–55

Richardson J D 1970 The importance of the ileocecal valve in intestinal absorption. Texas Rep Biol Med 28: 408–409

Richardson J D, Griffen W O 1972 Ileocecal valve substitutes as bacteriologic barriers. Am J Surg 123: 149–153

Richter H M III, Kelly K A 1986 Effect of transection and pacing on human jejunal pacesetter potentials. Gastroenterology 91: 1380–1385

Ricotta J, Zuidema G D, Gadacz T R et al 1981 Construction of an ileocecal valve and its role in massive resection of the small intestine. Surg Gynecol Obstet 152: 310–314

Rose S G, Thompson J S, Spanta A D et al 1991 The effect of intestinal autotransplantation on serum diamine oxidase activity. J Surg Res 50: 223–227

Ruiz J O, Uchida H, Schultz L S et al 1972 Problems in absorption and immunosuppression after entire intestinal allotransplantation. Am J Surg 123: 297–303

Sarna S K 1985 Cyclic motor activity. Migrating motor complex: 1985. Gastroenterology 89: 894–913

Sarna S K 1987 Giant migrating contractions and their myoelectric correlates in the small intestine. Am J Physiol 253: G697–G705

Sarna S K, Daniel E E 1975 Electrical stimulation of small intestinal electrical motor activity. Gastroenterology 69: 660–667

Sarna S, Stoddard C, Belbeck L et al 1981 Intrinsic nervous control of migrating myoelectric complexes. Am J Physiol 241: G16–G23

Sarna S, Condon R E, Cowles V 1983 Enteric mechanisms of initiation of migrating myoelectric complexes in dogs. Gastroenterology 84: 814–822

Sarr M G, Kelly K A 1980 Patterns of movement of liquids and solids through canine jejunum. Am J Physiol 239: G497–G503

Sarr M G, Kelly K A 1981 Myoelectric activity of the autotransplanted canine jejunoileum. Gastroenterology 81: 303–310

Sarr M G, Duenes J M, Tanaka M 1989 A model of jejunoileal in vivo neural isolation of the entire jejunoileum: transplantation and the effects on intestinal motility. J Surg Res 47: 266–272

Sarr M G, Duenes J A, Zinsmeister AR 1990 Factors in the control of interdigestive and postprandial myoelectric patterns of canine jejunoileum: role of extrinsic and intrinsic nerves. J Gastrointest Mot 2: 247–257

Sarr M G, Duenes J A, Walters A M 1991 Jejunal and ileal absorptive function after a model of canine jejunoileal autotransplantation. J Surg Res 51: 223–239

Schang J C, Sauchel J, Marescaux J et al 1982 Importance de l'ileon dans l'adaptation motrice de l'intestin apres courtcircuit jejuno-ileal. Gastroenterol Clin Biol 2: 373–382

Schiller W R, Di Dio L J A, Anderson M C 1967 Production of artificial sphincters: ablation of the longitudinal layer of the intestine. Arch Surg 95: 436–442

Schraut W H, Lee K K W, Sitrin M 1987 Recipient growth and nutritional status following transplantation of segmental small bowel allografts. J Surg Res 43 : 1–9

Schroeder P, Deltz E, Sanfort F et al 1987 Absorptive capacity of the transplanted small bowel. Gut 28: 275–279

Sidhu G S, Narasimharao K L, Rani V U et al 1985 Absorption studies after massive small bowel resection and anti-peristaltic colon interposition in rhesus monkeys. Dig Dis Sci 30: 483–488

Singleton A O, Redmond D C, McMurray J E 1969 Ileocecal resection and small bowel transit and absorption. Ann Surg 159: 690–694

Soper N J, Chapman M J, Kelly K A et al 1990 The 'ileal brake' after ileal pouch-anal anastomosis. Gastroenterology 98: 111–116

Soper N J, Sarr M G, DiMagno E P et al 1991 Influence of in situ neural isolation of jejunoileum on postprandial pancreaticobiliary secretion and gastric emptying. Dig Dis Sci 36: 880–887

Spencer M P, Sarr M G, Hakim M S et al 1989 Interdigestive gastric motility patterns: the role of vagal and non-vagal extrinsic innervation. Surgery 106: 185–194

Spiller R C, Trotman I F, Higgins B E et al 1984 The ileal brake-inhibition of jejunal motility after ileal fat perfusion in man. Gut 25: 365–374

Stacchini A, Di Dio L J, Primo M L et al 1982 Artificial sphincter as surgical treatment of experimental massive resection of small intestine. Am J Surg 143: 721–726

Stacchini A, Di Dio L J A, Christoforidis A J et al 1986 Intestinal transit time is delayed by artificial sphincters after massive enterectomy in dogs. Am J Surg 151: 480–483

Stahlgren L H, Umana G, Roy R et al 1962 A study of intestinal absorption in dogs following massive small intestinal resection and insertion of an anti-peristaltic segment. Ann Surg 156: 483–492

Stahlgren L M, Roy R, Umana G 1964 A mechanical impediment to intestinal flow: physiological effects on intestinal absorption. JAMA 187: 141–144

Stamford W P, Hardy M A 1974 Fatty acid absorption in jejunal autograft and allograft. Surgery 75: 496–502

Starzl T E, Todo S, Tzakis A et al 1992 Multivisceral and intestinal transplantation. Transplant Proc 24: 1217–1223

Szurszewski J H 1986 Electrophysiological basis of gastrointestinal motility in: Johnson L R (ed.) Physiology of the Gastrointestinal Tract, 2nd ed. New York, Raven Press pp 383–422

Szurszewski J, Steggerda F R 1968a The effect of hypoxia on the electrical slow wave of the canine small intestine. Am J Dig Dis 13: 168–177

Szurszweski J, Steggerda F R 1968b The effect of hypoxia on the mechanical activity of the canine small intestine. Am J Dig Dis 13: 178–185

Tanaka M, Sarr M G 1988 The role of the duodenum in the

control of canine gastrointestinal motility. Gastroenterology 94: 622–629

Tanner W A, O'Leary J F, Byrne P J 1978 The effect of reversed jejunal segments on the myoelectrical activity of the small bowel. Br J Surg 65: 567–571

Taylor I 1985 Distribution and release of peptide YY in dog measured by specific radioimmunoassay. Gastroenterology 88: 731–737

Thompson D G 1988 Central control of human gastrointestinal function. Bailliere's Clinical Gastroenterology 2: 107–112

Thompson J S 1985 Surgical therapy for the short bowel syndrome. J Surg Res 39: 81–91

Thompson J S 1988 Surgical treatment of the short bowel syndrome. Pediatr Surg Int 3: 303–311

Thompson J S, Quigley E M M 1991 Effects of small intestinal serosal patch on small intestinal and colonic motor activity: the effects of a lateral enterotomy on small intestinal myoelectrical activity. J Invest Surg 4: 203–215

Thompson J S, Rikkers L F 1987 Surgical alternatives for the short bowel syndrome. Am J Gastroenterol 82: 97–106

Thompson J S, Vanderhoof J A, Antonson D L et al 1984 Comparison of techniques for growing small bowel neomucosa. J Surg Res 36: 401–406

Thompson J S, Vanderhoof J A, Davis S J et al 1985a Effect of intestinal location on growth and function of neomucosa. J Surg Res 39: 68–75

Thompson J S, Vanderhoof J A, Antonson D L 1985b Intestinal tapering and lengthening for short bowel syndrome. J Pediatr Gastroenterol Nutr 4: 495–497

Thompson J S, Kampfe P W, Newland J R et al 1986 Growth of intestinal neomucosa on prosthetic materials. J Surg Res 41: 484–492

Thompson J S, Moessner S P, Hollingsed T 1987 In vivo glucose absorption by neomucosa. Surgery 101: 297–303

Thompson J S, Harty R J, Saigh J A et al 1986 Morphologic and nutritional response to intestinal patching following intestinal resection. Surgery 103: 79–86

Thompson J S, Rose S G, Spanta A D et al 1992 The long term effects of jejunoileal autotransplantation on intestinal function. Surgery 111: 62–68

Todo S, Tzakis A G, Abu-Elmagd K et al 1992 Cadaveric small bowel and small bowel-liver transplantation in humans. Transplantation 53: 369–376

Trinkle J K, Bryant L R 1967 Reversed colon segment in an infant with massive small bowel resection. A case report. J Ky Med Assoc 65: 1090–1091

Ulrich-Baker M G, Hollwarth M E, Kvietys P R et al 1986 Blood flow responses to small bowel resection. Am J Physiol 251: G815–G822

Vanderhoof J A, Langnas A M, Pinch L W et al 1992 Short bowel syndrome and intestinal transplantation. J Pediatr Gastroenterol Nutr 14: 359–370

Vantrappen G, Janssens J, Hellemans J et al 1977 The interdigestive motor complex of normal subjects and patients with bacterial overgrowth of the small intestine. J

Clin Invest 59: 1158–1166

Vayre P, Hurean J, Soyer R 1967 Use of anti-peristaltic colon segment interposition on lower small bowel motility following extensive resection. Ann Clin 21: 521

Venables C W, Ellis H, Smith A D M 1966 Anti-peristaltic segments after massive intestinal resection. Lancet 2: 1390–1394

Vinograd I, Merguerian P, Udassin R et al 1984 An experimental model of a submucosally tunnelled valve for the replacement of the ileocecal valve. J Pediatr Surg 19: 726–731

Waddell W R, Kern F, Halgrimson C G et al 1970 A simple jejunocolic 'valve'. Arch Surg 100: 438–444

Warden M J, Wesley J R 1978 Small bowel reversal procedure for treatment of the short gut baby. J Pediatr Surg 13: 321–323

Watson A J M, Lear P A, Montgomery A et al 1988 Water, electrolyte, glucose and glycine absorption in rat small intestinal transplants. Gastroenterology 94: 863–869

Weber T R, Vane D W, Grosfeld J L 1982 Tapering enteroplasty in infants with bowel atresia and short gut. Arch Surg 117: 684–688

Weisbrodt N W, Nemeth P R, Bowers R L et al 1985 Functional and structural changes in intestinal smooth muscle after a jejunoileal bypass in rats. Gastroenterology 88: 958–963

Williamson R C N 1978a Intestinal adaptation. Structural, functional and cytokinetic changes. New Engl J Med 298: 1393–1402

Williamson R C N 1978b Intestinal adaptation. Mechanisms of control. New Engl J Med 298: 1444–1450

Wilmore D W 1972 Factors correlating with a successful outcome following extensive intestinal resection in new-born infants. J Pediatr 80: 88–95

Wilmore D W, Johnson D J 1968 Metabolic effects of small bowel reversal in treatment of the short bowel syndrome. Arch Surg 97: 784–791

Wingate D L 1981 Backwards and forwards with the migrating complex. Dig Dis Sci 26: 641–664

Wingate D L 1983 Complex clocks. Dig Dis Sci 28: 1133–1140

Wingate D L 1985 The brain-gut link. Viewpoints on Digestive Diseases 17: 17–20

Wittmann T, Crenner F, Pousse A et al 1985 Changes in motility after jejunal and ileal resection: electromyographic study in rats. Digestion 32: 114–123

Wittman T, Crenner F, Grenier J F 1986 Cyclic motor activity and trophicity after jejunal resection and bypass in rats. Dig Dis Sci 31: 65–72

Wittman T, Crenner F, Koenig M et al 1988 Adaptive changes in postprandial motility after intestinal resection and bypass. Electromyographic study in rats. Dig Dis Sci 33: 1370–1376

Wolfman E F, Trevino G, Heaps D K et al 1964 An operative technique for the management of acute and chronic lateral duodenal fistulas. Ann Surg 159: 563–569

Index

Abdominal pain, 192
Abdominal region, electrical impedance measurements, 279–280
Acetylcholine (ACh), 25, 78, 83, 123, 148–151, 153, 155, 158, 377, 378, 451, 557
Acetylcholinesterase inhibitors, 151–152
Acetylcholinesterase stains, 30
Achalasia, 475–482, 572–574
  EMG in, 481
  LOS, 368–370
  motility changes in, 477–480
  pathophysiology, 477
  pharmacologic agents for treatment of, 482–483
  striated muscle activity in, 479
  syndromes resembling, 480–481
  treatment, 482–483
  UOS, 360
Acid-peptic disease, 119
Acid perfusion test, 510
ACTH, 80, 112
Actin filaments, 40
Action potentials, 410–411
Adenine nucleotides, 25
Adenoviruses, 522
Adenosine triphosphate (ATP), 147, 443, 451
Adenylate cyclase, 146
Adrenalin, 556
Adrenergic drugs, 153–154
Adrenergic nerves, 23
Adrenergic receptor agonists and antagonists, 153
β-adrenergic receptors, 147, 153
Adriamycin, 577
Afferent loop syndrome, 683
Agonists, 147
Alginic acid in GORD, 514
Alkaline gastritis, 681
Allotransplanted intestine, 711
Alpha-actinin, 36
Alpha cortical rhythms, 52
Ambulant manometry, 200–210, 461–463
  background, 200

catheter placement, 200–201
equipment, 200
future directions, 208–209
intestinal, 201–206
pharyngo-oesophageal, 364
protocol for, 201
small bowel motility patterns, 201
solid state recorders, 200
use in research, 207–208
vs stationary, 201–206
Ambulatory recording, 194, 332, 461–463
Amphetamine, 154
Amyloidosis, 523–524, 571
Anal canal, 9, 449–450
  innervation, 450–451
  pressure, 451–453
Anal fissure, 665
Anal sensitivity, 459
Anal sphincter, 9
Analogue-to-digital (A/D) converters, 319, 320, 333
Anismus, 618–623, 644, 655–657
  and constipation, 604
Ano-coccygeus muscle, 43
Anoderm, 9
Anorectal angle, 459, 687
Anorectal continence, 458
Anorectal disorders, 655–669
Anorectal function, 457
Anorectal motility
  abnormal, 619–621
  ambulatory monitoring, 461–463
  in children with chronic idiopathic constipation, 612
Anorectal sensation impairment, 664
Anorectal structures during defaecation, 630
Anorectum, 8–9, 449–470
  anatomical considerations, 449
  clinical measurement of function, 457
  electromyography, 458
  innervation, 450–451
  physiological considerations, 451–457
Anorexia nervosa, 304
Antacids in GORD, 514

Antagonists, 147–148
Anti-adrenergic drugs, 153–154
Antidiarrhoeal drugs, 154, 158
Antiemetic drugs, 156
Antimony radiocapsule, 213
Antral circumference, 248–251
Antral contractions, 294
  ultrasound, 248
Antral distension, 249
Antral emptying
  radioscintigraphy, 231–232
  ultrasound, 247
Antral excursion, 249
  excursion/distension ratio, 249–250
  vs distension, 249
Antral filling, ultrasound, 247
Antral motor functions, ultrasound, 246–247
Antral peristalsis, 174
Antral peristaltic rhythmicity, ultrasound, 247
Antro-pyloric-duodenal tract, 174
Antroduodenal contractions, 285
Antroduodenal coordination, ultrasound, 250–251
Antrum, 4–5
  lateral movement after feeding, 251–252
Anxiety, 577–578
Apomorphine, 156
Applied potential tomography (APT), 281–282
Atropine, 152, 156
Autonomic nervous system (ANS), 10, 64, 70–73, 145, 379, 410, 451
Autotransplantation, 709–712
Axon terminals, 23

Barium studies, 181, 359–360, 506, 575
Barostat
  for reflex motor function of proximal stomach, 194
  in colonic manometry, 195–196
  technique, 437–438
Barrett's epithelium, 512
Barrett's oesophagus, 503, 506, 518

717

Basal myoelectrical activity (BMA), 436
Bernstein tests, 510
Bethanechol, 149–150, 155, 491, 514, 557, 619
Bicarbonate test Zeit, 213
Bile ducts, anatomy, 399
Biliary system
    anatomy, 399
    dynamics, radioscintigraphy, 232–235
    embryology, 399
    morphology, 399
    normal motility, 406–407
Biliary tract, 393–409
    anatomy, 393
    blood supply, 402
    electromyography, 397
    extrinsic innervation, 401
    fluorescence immunohistochemistry, 393
    in vitro techniques, 394
    intramural nerves, 19
    intrinsic innervation, 401
    isotope studies, 398
    motility studies, 394–398, 402–407
    motor disorders, 538–546
    resin casting techniques, 393
    study techniques, 393–398
    ultrasonography, 398–399
Billroth I and II, 304
Biofeedback therapy, 644, 646
Biorhythm interactions, 98–102
Bisacodyl, 614
Bolus feed, 60, 61
Bombesin, 158, 159, 377
Bombesin/gastrin releasing peptide (GRP)
    peptide structure, 87–88
    precursors localization, 87–88
    sites and mechanisms of enteric actions, 88
Bowel habits, 595–598
Bradygastrias, 304–305
Brain, 145
Brain tumours, 192
Brain-gut axis, 73–76
Brain-gut interactions, 76
Breast disease and constipation, 606
Breath hydrogen test, 309–316
    animal studies, 310
    clinical application, 316
    comparison with sulphasalazine method, 317
    contaminated small bowel syndrome, 313
    correlation with other methods, 314–316
    early peak and how to reduce it, 311
    failure to produce hydrogen, 313
    false high breath hydrogen due to smoking, 313
    high basal breath hydrogen, 313
    ileal emptying as cause of early rise in breath hydrogen, 311

measurement techniques, 311–313
non-absorbable carbohydrate, 314
oral fermentation, 311
performance procedure, 313–314
problems in performing test and how to avoid them, 311
reproducibility, 314–316
research application, 316
sampling method, 309–310
Bulimia nervosa, 528–529
Burst pattern neurons, 25
Buscopan, 540, 545

Caecum, 7, 33, 428, 432, 433
    breath hydrogen test, 309
    hypertrophy, 45
    ultrasound, 254
Calcitonin, 139
Calcitonin gene related peptide (CGRP)
    enteric actions, sites and mechanisms, 89
    peptide structure, precursors, localization, receptor subtypes, 89
cAMP, 147
Catecholamine fluorescence, 30
Catecholamines, 151, 556
Caveolae, 33, 45
Cell hypertrophy, 45
Cell-to-stroma junctions, 38
Central nervous system (CNS), 10, 27, 28, 52–53, 64, 70–73, 138, 139, 379, 389, 390, 443, 568, 691
    electrical activity in, 59
    maturation of, 53
    neurological development, 54
Ceroidosis, 571
Cerulitide, 545
Chagas' disease, 45, 481, 577
Chest pain, 485
Chlorisondamine, 153
Chlornaltrexamine, 148
Chlorpromazine, 556
Cholecystectomy, 235, 539
Cholecystitis
    acute, 233–234
    chronic, 234–235
Cholecystokinin (CCK), 53, 67, 80, 89–91, 134, 137–139, 141, 158–159, 233–235, 377, 388, 398, 406, 442, 443, 557, 585
    endogenous effects, 90
    exogenous effects, 90
    paradoxical response to, 544
    peptide structure, precursors, localization, receptor subtypes, 90
    provocation test, 539
    sites and mechanisms of enteric actions, 90–91
Cholecystokinin octapeptide, 158, 538–539
Cholescintigraphy, sphincter of Oddi, 542

Cholesterol crystals, 538
Cholinergic agents, 155
Cholinergic antagonists, 152
Cholinergic drugs, 148–153
Cholinergic nerves, 23, 123
Cholinesterase activity, evaluation, 635
Cholinomimetics, 556
Chronic idiopathic pseudo-obstruction, 191, 525
    see also Pseudo-obstruction
Cimetidine, 530
Cinedefaecography, 459–460
Cinefluorography, 165
Cineradiography, 404
Cisapride, 155, 156, 303, 524, 527, 539, 645
    in GORD, 514
Cisplatin, 532
Clonidine, 154
Clustered phasic activity, 59
Colectomy, 686–688
Colitis, 126
Collagen, 33, 40–41, 44, 120
Colon, 7–8, 33
    anatomical aspects, 427–428
    anatomical differences in various species, 427
    electromyography, 268–272
    in IBS, 584–585
    intramural nerves, 18–19
    longitudinal muscle, 42
    main functions of, 427
    peristalsis, 175
    postoperative ileus, 548–558
    pressure measurement, 217–219
    segmenting contraction, 173
    ultrasound, 254
Colonic constipation, 613–619
Colonic inertia, 601–603, 615–619
Colonic manometry, 194–196, 429–430
    ambulatory recordings, 196
    barostat in, 195–196
    comparison with other methods, 195
    future refinements, 195–196
    optimal recording, 195
    placement of manometric tubes into lower digestive tract, 195
Colonic motility, 133, 427–448, 674
    and physical exercise, 442
    diurnal changes, 437–438
    methods for studying, 428–437
    peptides in regulation of, 443, 445
    physiological control, 443
    physiological regulation, 437–443
Colonic motor activity, 62, 438
    in IBS, 584
Colonic myoelectrical activity, 430–436
Colonic response to eating (CRE), 440–442
    EMG, 440
    manometry, 440
    mechanisms of, 441–442
    modulation of, 441
Colonic scintigraphic studies, 440
Colonic smooth muscle, slow waves, 430

Colonic tone
  measurement of, 438
  physiological regulation of, 443
Colonic transit, radioscintigraphy, 235–237
Colonic transit time, 428–429
  spiking activity, 137
Coloproctectomy, 686, 687
Colorectal transit studies, 613–630
Colour Doppler ultrasonography, 244, 251, 253
Common bile duct (CBD), 399, 403
Complete rectal prolapse, 659
Computed tomography (CT), ultra-fast, 196–197, 474
Computerized data analysis, 319–333
  future directions, 333
Concentric needle EMG, 458
Conduction, 278–279
Conductivity, 276–278
Conjoined longitudinal muscle, 450
Connective tissue diseases, 483–485, 531
Connexin-43, 37
Connexons, 37
Constipation, 181, 595–654
  aetiology, 606
  and anismus, 604
  and breast disease, 606
  and digestive system, 605–606
  and irritable bowel syndrome (IBS), 601–603
  and personality profile, 612
  and sexual abuse, 604, 632
  as body clue, 610–611
  by outlet obstruction, 616–628
  chronic idiopathic, 610–613
  clinical evaluation, 633
  definition, 600
  epidemiology, 598–601
  functional evaluation, 635–641
  hidden agenda of the patient, 610
  mechanisms in IBS, 608–610
  mechanisms of chronic idiopathic, 610–613
  mechanisms secondary to organic disease, 606–608
  medicalization, 606
  nature of, 595–598
  nuisance of, 605–606
  onset of, 630
  operational definitions, 600–601
  organic evaluation, 630–635
  primary symptom, 600
  rectosigmoid pressure in, 615
  related conditions, 601–605
  semantics, 595
  sex ratio in children, 600
  slow transit vs segmental, 614
  social aspects, 599
  treatment, 641–646
  unnecessary surgery, 606
  with normal transit times, 628–630
Contaminated small bowel syndrome, 313

Continence
  mechanism, 456
  theories, 456–457
Continuous electrical response activity (CERA), 436
Contractile activity, electrical impedance measurements, 284–287
Contractile electrical complex (CEC), 436
Contraction abnormalities
  associated with pain and/or dysphagia, 485–493
  diagnosis, 489–492
  in pain/dysphagia, 488
  of oesophageal body, 487–493
  treatment, 492–493
Contractions
  analysis of, 322–328
  classifying into categories, 328
  coordination or propagation of, 411–412
  mechanism, 43–44
Contrast material, 337
Corticotrophin-releasing factor (CRF), 105, 138, 139
Coxsackie virus, 522
Craniosacral pathways, 11
CREST syndrome, 571
Cricopharyngeal achalasia, 475
Cricopharyngeal dysfunction, 168
Cricopharyngeal impression, 360
Cricopharyngeal myotomy, 357, 365, 475
Crohn's disease, 120, 121, 127
Cyclic adenosine monophosphate (cAMP), 80, 146
Cyclic guanosine monophosphate (cGMP), 146
Cycloheximide, 532
Cystic duct, 403, 538
Cytomegalovirus, 522
Cytotoxic drugs, 532–533, 577

Dactinomycin, 532
DAGO, 157
Dale's principle, 78
Data acquisition, 319–322
Data analysis see Computerized data analysis
Data filtering, 322
Data visualization, 322
Defaecating proctograms, 660–662
Defaecation
  anorectal structures during, 630
  evaluation of, 166–170
  mechanism of, 166–170
  normal pattern of, 595
  normal radiological sequence of, 169
  scintigraphic defaecography, 237–239
Defaecation disorders, 655
  radiology, 459
Defaecography, 168

Deglutition
  evaluation of, 165–166
  mechanism of, 165–166
Denonvilliers fascia, 8
Dense bands, 33–36, 45
Depression, 577
Dermatomyositis, 531
Descending perineum syndrome, 623, 658
Devazepide, 159
Diabetes, 522–523
Diabetes mellitus, 206, 523
Diabetic gastroparesis, 299, 523
Diabetic polyneuropathy, 575–577
Diacylglycerol, 147
Diaphragmatic hiatus, 4
Dicyclomine, 482
Dielectric dispersion for complex biological material, 277–278
Diffuse spasm, diagnostic criteria, 486
Digesta, flow of, 133
Digestive motility
  and nutrient absorption, 140–141
  and nutrition, 139
Digestive status
  large intestine, 131–133
  small intestine, 130–131
  stomach, 130
Digestive system, and constipation, 605–606
Digestive tract, 130
Dihydroergotamine, 557
Diltiazem, 492
Diphenoxylate, 158
Discrete clustered contractions (DCCs), 693
Displacement currents, 278–279
Distal ileum, motor patterns of, 695
Distension, 192
Domperidone, 155, 156, 523, 525
Dopamine antagonists, 155–156
Dopamine receptors, 153
Dopamine$_2$-receptor antagonists, 532
Dorsal root ganglion neurons, 48
Dorsal vagal complex (DVC), 72, 73
DPDPE, 157
Drug-induced tachygastrias, 304
Drugs, 144–161
  actions of, 148–159
  characteristics of, 147–148
  indirectly acting, 148
  inhibitory, 144
  mechanisms of actions, 144–148
  receptor systems, 146–147
  sites of action, 144
  stimulatory, 144
  ultrasound studies, 253
  see also specific drugs
Dumping syndrome, 681–682
Duodenal glucose perfusion (GLU), 73, 74
Duodenal motility and glucose absorption, 140
Duodenal peristalsis, 174
Duodenal ulcer, 529–530

Duodenectomy, 683–684
Duodenojejunal flexure, 6
Duodenum, 6
    functional morphology, 375
    motility disorders, 522–537
    peristalsis, 175
    pressure generated in, 59
    schematic diagram, 373
    segmenting contraction, 172
Dynorphin, 81
Dysphagia of oesophageal origin, 485
Dystrophia myotonica, 525

Eating disorders, 526–529
Edrophonium, 491
Effective dose equivalent (EDE), 228–229
Efferent loop syndrome, 683
Elastic fibres, 43
Electrical equivalent circuit for
        biological tissue, 279
Electrical impedance measurements,
        276–289
    abdominal region, 279–280
    applications, 280–288
    background, 276
    compliance measurement, 287–288
    contractile activity, 284–287
    gastric emptying, 280–283
        sources of errors, 282–283
    oesophagus, 285
Electrical pacing, 558
Electroencephalographic activity, 52
Electrogastrogram (EGG), 107, 290–307
    analysis of, 293–294
    external, 292
    internal, 292
    methods of recording, 291–293
Electrogastrography, 276, 290–307,
        328–332
    abnormal rhythms of the stomach,
        296–305
    electrodes, 293
    fasting conditions, 294–296
    normal activity of the stomach, 294–296
    postprandial patterns, 296
Electromyographic probe, 432, 433
Electromyography (EMG), 256–275,
        655, 658, 662–664
    achalasia, 481
    ambulatory recording, 461–463
    anorectum, 458
    biliary tract, 397
    colon, 268–272
    colonic response to eating, 439
    EAS, 455–456
    electrodes, 256–257, 260–262, 265–266, 268, 271–272
    gallbladder, 397
    gastrointestinal tract, 257–258
    history, 256
    intraluminal recordings of

    myoelectric activity in man,
        258–262
    oesophagus, 262–265, 338
    problems associated with, 259
    small intestine, 266–268
    smooth muscle electrical activity
        recording, 256–257
    sphincter of Oddi, 397
    stomach, 265
Endoanal sonography, 662
Endoanal ultrasound, 461
Endocrine abnormalities in
        constipation, 606
Endocrine cells, 53
Endoradiosondes, 211
Endoscopic retrograde
        cholangiopancreatography
        (ERCP), 538, 540–542, 545
Endoscopic sphincterotomy (ES),
        sphincter of Oddi dysfunction,
        545
Endoscopy, 207
Enemas, 642
Enflurane, 556
Enkephalins (ENK), 401, 402, 700
Enprostil, 253
Enteral bacteriology, 687
Enteral feed, 60, 61
Enteral nutrition, 53
Enteric ganglia, 48
Enteric nerves, from inflamed gut,
        120–121
Enteric nervous system (ENS), 10–31,
        64, 70–73, 145, 150, 191, 377,
        389, 390, 403, 406, 410, 412,
        416, 568, 691, 693
    development of, 52
    electrical activity in, 59
    function of, 65
    inhibitory networks in, 59
    maturation of, 53
    neurological development, 54
    ontogeny, 52
    relationship to CNS, 10
Enteric neurons
    morphology, 19–23
    transmitter substances of, 25
    Type 1 and Type 2, 23
Enterogastric reflux, radioscintigraphy,
        232–233
Enteroglucagon, 700
Ephedrine, 154
Epidural analgesia, 557
Epigastric impedance, 287
Epigastrography, 280–281
Ergonovine, 491
Erythromycin, 156–157, 446, 523, 527,
        528
    acting at motilin receptors, 83
Eserine, 151
Excessive retrograde contractions, 544
Excitatory postsynaptic potentials
        (EPSPs), 25–27
External anal sphincter (EAS), 450,
        451, 453, 455–456, 658, 662

Extrinsic denervation effects, 676
Extrinsic innervation, 70–73, 693
    functional role of, 73
Extrinsic neural control, classical
        concept, 64

Faecal incontinence, 601, 660
    treatment of, 665
Fast Fourier Transform (FFT)
        analysis, 320, 328, 430, 440
Fasting activity, 57–60, 130, 131, 192
    electrogastrography, 294–296
    patterns of, 57–60, 191
Fasting state, 95–97
Fed motor response, 693, 696
Feeding, 130, 132
Fetal motor activity, 53
Fibroblasts, 40
Flap-valve theory, 456–457, 460
Fluorescence immunohistochemistry
        techniques, biliary tract, 393
Fluoroscopic images, 165
Flutter valve theory, 456
Food, 130–143
    abnormal hypoactive response to, 204
    digestion and dispersion, 381–382
    hormonal influence of components
        on digestive motility, 139–140
    ingestion of, 204
Functional bowel syndrome, 578
Functional disorders, and stress, 104
Functional dyspepsia, 303
Fundal emptying, radioscintigraphy,
        231–232

G proteins, 146, 147
Galanin, 86–87, 401
    enteric actions, sites and
        mechanisms, 86
    peptide structure, precursors and
        localization, 86
Gallbladder, 83, 235, 538
    anatomy, 399
    electromyography, 397
    isotope studies, 398
    manometry, 394–397
    motility, 402–403, 406
    motor function, 398
    scintigraphy, 539
    ultrasonography, 398
Gallbladder disease, 234
Gallbladder dyskinesia, 538
Gallbladder ejection fraction (GBEF),
        398
Gallstones, 83
Gamma-aminobutyric acid, 25
Gamma cameras, 228
Ganglion, 12, 13, 15, 16, 18, 23, 145
Ganglion blocking drugs, 153
Gap junctions, 37–38, 45, 52
Gastrectomy, 678
Gastric acid secretion, effects of drugs
        reducing, 530

Gastric antrum
  pressure generated in, 59
  ultrasonsic appearance, 246
Gastric arrhythmias, 305
Gastric contractility, 294
Gastric digestion, 380–390
Gastric dysfunction induced by
    irradiation and cytotoxic drugs,
    532–533
Gastric dysrhythmias, 298, 303
Gastric emptying, 380–390
  delayed, 680–681
  effect of ileal infusion of lipid, 388–
    389
  effect of nutrients, 388
  effects of prokinetic drugs on, 524
  electrical impedance measurements,
    280–283
    sources of errors, 282–283
  forces promoting, 386
  liquids, 382–384
  paracetamol in, 308
  particulate solids, 382–384
  radioscintigraphy, 230–232
  reflex control of, 19
  solid meal, 383
  ultrasonography, 243
  ultrasound, 244, 247
Gastric factors in GORD, 502
Gastric inhibitory polypeptide (GIP),
    85
Gastric outflow resistance, 386–388
Gastric pacesetter potential, 375–377
Gastric pressure measurement, 217
Gastric smooth muscle, 375–377
Gastric surgery see Surgical procedures
Gastric ulcers, 303, 530
Gastrin, 67, 89–91, 134, 141, 159, 377,
    406
  endogenous effects, 90
  exogenous effects, 90
  peptide structure, precursors,
    localization and receptor
    subtypes, 90
  sites and mechanisms of enteric
    actions, 90–91
Gastrin releasing peptide (GRP), 85,
    159, 401, 402
  see also Bombesin
Gastroduodenal contractile pressure
    activity, 389
Gastroduodenal reflux, ultrasound,
    250–251
Gastroduodenojejunal manometry, 183
  future refinements, 193–194
  indication for, 192
  optimal recording, 185
  pitfalls in application of, 193
  placement of manometric tubes into
    upper digestive tract, 185
  practical significance of, 192
  sleeve methodology, 193–194
Gastroduodenojejunal pressure
    measurements, future
    directions, 196

Gastroenterostomy, 678
Gastrointestinal anastomosis, 683
Gastrointestinal motor activity in the
    human infant, 53
Gastrointestinal polypeptide
    hormones, 53
Gastrointestinal pressure
    measurement, future directions,
    208–209
Gastrointestinal system, normal motor
    function, 673
Gastrointestinal tract
  electromyography, 257–258
  gross morphology, 3–9
  motor functions, 673
  nerve supply, 3
  pH measurement, 221–222
Gastrojejunostomy, 683
Gastro-oesophageal junction, 4
  anatomy of, 55
Gastro-oesophageal reflux disease
    (GORD), 215, 221, 364, 369–
    371, 496–521
  antireflux surgery, 517–519
  atypical presentations, 505–506
  classic presentations, 505
  clinical presentation, 505–506
  diagnosis, 506–512
  epidemiology, 496
  gastric factors in, 502
  lifestyle modifications, 512–514
  maintenance medical therapy,
    517
  management, 512
  natural history, 512
  oesophagoscopy, 508–510
  pathophysiology, 496–505
  radiology, 506–508
  radioscintigraphy, 230
  treatment, 502
Gastroparesis, 201, 299–302
Gastroversion, 300
General adaptation syndrome, 112
Gizzard, musculature, 46
Glass pH-sensitive capsules, 213
Glucagon, 134, 141, 147, 406, 444
Glucose absorption and duodenal
    motility, 140
Golgi apparatus, 17
Growth hormone-releasing factor
    (GHRF), 85, 139
Guanethidine, 557
Guanosine monophosphate (cGMP),
    80
Guanosine triphosphate (GTP), 146
Guanylate cyclase, 146
Guillain-Barré syndrome, 522
Gut
  centres involved in motility, 28
  complex anatomy, 51
  extrinsic nerves, 10
  hormones, 64, 67–70
  inflamed or sensitized, 118–121
  innervation, 3
  intramural nerves, 23–27

methods to study morphology of
    nerves, 28–30
  motor behaviour of, 10
  sensory functions, 19

Haemorrhoids, 605, 665–667
Halothane, 556
Heidelberg capsule, 213, 221
Henle's plexus, 18, 19
Herpes simplex, 522
Herpes zoster virus, 522
Hexamethonium, 153
Hiatus hernia, 503–505
High-amplitude propagated
    contractions (HAPCs), 430
Hirschsprung's disease, 45, 180, 574,
    631, 634–635, 658
Histamine, 406
Histamine₂ receptor
  agonist, 530
  antagonists, 683
  in GORD, 515–516
Histopathology, pseudo-obstruction,
    580
Hollow visceral myopathy, 188
Hormones
  control of postprandial pattern, 133–
    139
  gut, 64, 67–70
  influence of food components on
    digestive motility, 139–140
  release in feeding, 134–137
Human infant, gastrointestinal motor
    activity in, 53
Human recombinant interleukin-1β
    (hrIL-1β), 124
Humoral system, 53
Hydralazine, 492
Hydrochloric acid, 491
Hydrogen ion-sensitive glass electrode,
    213
Hydrostats, 44
5-hydroxytryptamine (5-HT), 52, 127,
    155, 532, 533
  agonists and antagonists, 156
Hyoscyamine, 492
Hyperactive rectosigmoid junction,
    619
Hyperemesis gravidarum, 303
Hypertension, 577
Hypertrophic pyloric stenosis, 574
Hypnosis in constipation, 645
Hypnotherapy in constipation, 645
Hypoparathyroidism, 578
Hypothyroidism, 578

Idiopathic dyspepsia, 530–531
Idiopathic gastroparesis, 299, 304
Idiopathic inflammatory bowel disease
    (IBD), 119–121
Idiopathic intestinal pseudo-
    obstruction, 205
Ileal motility, 416–418

Ileal pouch, 686
Ileal-pouch-anal anastomosis, 688
Ileal-pouch-anal reconstruction, 687
Ileocaecal junction, 6–7
Ileocaecal region, 410–426
Ileocolonic junction (ICJ), 420–423
Ileocolonic sphincter (ICS), 421
Ileum, 6
    circular muscle, 36
    resection of, 684–686
Ileus, 547–559
    classification of causes, 547
    clinical manifestations, 547
    neuromuscular mechanisms, 553–555
    paralytic, 547, 558–559
    postoperative, 547–558
        aetiopathogenesis, 553–556
        and duration and extent of surgery, 555–556
        drug effects, 556
        local factors, 555–556
        regional involvement, 548–553
        therapeutic manipulation, 556–558
        treatment, 556–558
    sympathetic activity, 553–554
    terminology, 547
Image intensifier systems, 165
Imminodiacetic acid (HIDA), 232, 233
Immune system, 118–129
    animal studies, 121–127
    interaction with physiological systems, 118
Immunohistochemical stains, 28, 30
Impedance plethysmograph, 287
Independent effector, 43
Inflammation
    intestine, 121–123
    local and systemic effects, 125–126
    muscle responses to different inflammatory stimuli, 126
    of gut, 118–121
    regional differences in muscle responses to, 126
Inhibitory adrenergic reflux pathways, 553
Inhibitory postsynaptic potentials (IPSPs), 25–27
Inositol-1,4,5-trisphosphate (IP$_3$), 147
Insulin, 134
Interdigestive cycle, variations on, 414–416
Interdigestive motility, 412–419
Interdigestive myoelectrical complex (IDMEC), 413–414
Interdigestive period, flow and transit of contents in, 419
Interganglionic fascicles, 13
Interleukins (ILs)
    IL-1, 124, 125, 139
    IL-1β, 123–125
    IL-6, 124
Intermediate filaments, 40
Intermediate junctions, 36–37
Intermesenteric nerve (IMN), 75

Intermittent episodes of elevated basal pressure, 543
Internal anal sphincter (IAS), 450, 451, 453–455, 457, 663–664
    dysfunction, 663–664
    reflex relaxation of, 19
Interstitial cells of Cajal, 13–15, 40, 52
Intestinal bypass, 703
Intestinal manometry
    clinical value of, 208
    equipment fidelity, 207
    length of recording sessions, 206–207
    logistics, 207
    stationary or ambulatory, 201–206
Intestinal motility
    clinical value of, 208
    effects of surgery, 676
Intestinal motor activity, ontogeny of, 51–63
Intestinal musculature, 33
Intestinal resection
    effects of altered luminal milieu, 701–703
    effects of removal of segment of intestine, 700–701
    effects of transection/re-anastomosis, 697–700
    motor consequences of, 697–703
Intestinal tapering and lengthening, 707–709
Intestinal transplantation, 709–712
Intestine
    musculature, 32–33
    peristaltic reflex of, 19
Intraluminal pressure, 287
    analysis of, 430
Intramural nerves
    biliary tract, 19
    colon, 18–19
    general arrangement, 12
    histology, 12
    morphology, 12
    oesophagus, 15–17
    small intestine, 17–18
    synaptic transmission in, 25
Intrinsic innervation, 65–67, 693
Intrinsic neural elements, 52
Intussusception, 171
Irradiation, gastric dysfunction induced by, 532–533
Irritable bowel syndrome (IBS), 101–102, 109–112, 127, 191, 578, 583–594, 665
    and constipation, 601–603
    as motor disorder, 584
    constipation-predominant, 608–610
    definition of, 583
    diagnosis of, 584
    history, 583
    Manning criteria, 583
    minute rhythm of clustered contractions, 585–587
    motility studies, 592–593
    related functional disorders, 584

Rome criteria, 583, 585
    terminology, 583
    three component model, 593
Ischaemic gastroparesis, 299
Isometric contraction, 43
Isoproterenol, 154
Isosorbide, 482, 492
Isotonic contraction, 43–44
Isotope studies
    biliary tract, 398
    gallbladder, 398

Jejunum, 6, 132
    circular muscle, 39

L-364718, 159
Large bowel
    segmental transit time, 176–178
    stress, 109–112
Large intestine, 7–8
    digestive status, 131–133
    propulsion of digesta, 133
    segmenting activity, 173
Laxatives, 597, 642, 646
Levator ani, 8, 450
Lidamidine, 154
Long chain triglyceride (LCT), 56
Long spike bursts (LSBs), 434–436, 440
Loperamide, 158, 602
Lower anal canal (LAC), 450, 451
Lower oesophageal sphincter (LOS), 55, 118, 221, 265, 337, 338, 473, 477, 478, 483, 497–500
    ablation of, 678
    achalasia, 368–370
    anatomy, 55, 365–367
    as anti-reflux barrier, 370
    'at rest' motility, 339–343
    function, 55–56
    innervation of, 56
    manometry, 367–368
    motility after swallowing, 350–355
    muscle mass of, 56
    physiology, 365–367
    relaxation of, 54
    transient relaxations, 370–371
Lumen, dilatation, 182
Luminal flow, 252
    ultrasound, 250–251
Luminal milieu effects in intestinal resection, 701–703

Magnetic resonance imaging (MRI), 196–197
Malignant neoplasms, gastric operations for, 683
Malnutrition, 526–528
Manofluorometry, UOS, 362–364
Manometric catheter, 57
Manometry
    ambulatory see Ambulant manometry

animal studies, 396
anorectum, 457–458
colonic, 429–430
CRE, 440
gallbladder, 394–397
LOS, 367–368
oesophagus, 337, 510
pseudo-obstruction, 580
scleroderma, 485
sphincter of Oddi, 394–397, 403–406, 542–544
UOS, 360–361
Mast cells, 127
Mastocytosis, 127
Measles, 522
Measurement of motility see specific techniques
Mecamylamine, 153
Mechanical obstruction, 188, 189, 192, 559–563, 567
classification of causes, 548
clinical manifestations, 547
Mechanically-induced pattern neurons
'on' or 'on-off response' pattern, 25
sustained response pattern, 25
tonic response pattern, 25
Medelec Mystro, 458
Medium chain triglyceride (MCT), 56
Megacolon, 181
in Hirschsprung's disease, 180
Mega-oesophagus, 178, 179
Megarectum, 181, 623–627, 658
Meissner's plexus, 18, 19
Melanosis coli, 633
Menetrier's gastropathy, 683
Meperidine, 158
Metabolic dysfunctions, 578
Metachromatic stains, 28
Methantheline, 152
Metoclopramide, 155–156, 300, 483, 524, 532
in GORD, 514, 515
Microballoon catheters, 457
Microtransducers, 458
Migrating action potential complex (MAPC), 258
Migrating long spike bursts (MLSBs), 436, 438, 440
Migrating motor complexes (MMCs), 54, 59, 65, 98, 105, 130–134, 137–139, 258, 379, 559, 676, 684
fasting, 192
in intestinal resection, 697–702
low amplitude, 205
periodicity of, 76
phase I, 57, 66–67, 95, 133, 201, 203, 414, 694
phase II, 57, 67, 95–97, 109, 133, 141, 201, 414, 416, 550, 613, 693, 694, 702
phase III, 57, 66–67, 69, 83, 96, 98, 99, 101, 133, 140, 158, 193, 201, 205, 206, 258, 268, 339, 402, 405, 414, 416, 522, 526, 550, 609, 694, 702, 710

phase IV, 414
surgical intervention, 693
Minnesota Multiphasic Personality Inventory (MMPI), 610
Mitochondria, 45
Mitotic muscle cells, 45
Mixed connective tissue disease (MCTD), 483–484
Morphine, 157, 158, 556
Morphine provocation test, 541
Motilides, 82–83
Motilin, 82–83, 159, 445
agonists, 156–157
enteric actions, delivery, release, sites, mechanisms, 83
intravenous infusions, 83
peptide structure, precursors, localization, receptors, 82
sequence of events at neural receptors, 83
Motility measurement see specific techniques
Motility reponses, 29
Motion sickness, 304
Motor control systems and their development, 51–52
Mouth–caecum transit
breath hydrogen test for, 309–316
vs other methods, 314–316
calculation of time, 314
measurement using sulphasalazine, 317
Muscarinic cholinergic agonists, 150
Muscarinic cholinergic receptors, 147, 151
Muscarinic cholinergic transmission, 443
Muscarinic receptor antagonists, 153
Muscarinic receptors, 150
Muscle coats, 32, 51–52
Muscularis externa, 32
Myelomeningocele, 631
Myeloperoxidase (MPO), 122
Myenteric neurons, 48
Myenteric plexus, 13, 15, 16, 22, 26
Myenteric plexus neurons, 24
Myoelectric analysis, 328
Myoelectrical activity
colonic, 431
in vivo, 692
Myosin filaments, 40
Myotonic dystrophy, 525, 571

NADH stain, 30
Nausea, 192
of pregnancy, 303
Neonatal motor activity, 53
Neostigmine, 152, 155, 444, 557, 607, 608
Nerve–nerve synapses, 23, 78
Neural function in inflamed intestine, 123–125
Neurofibromatosis, 524
Neurohumoral transmitters, 25, 30

Neurokinins, 84, 159
neurokinin alpha see Substance P
neurokinin beta, 159
Neurological abnormalities in constipation, 606–608
Neuromedin see Substance P
Neuromedin K see Neurokinins, neurokinin beta
Neuromodulators, 78
Neuromsclular pharyngeal disease, 475
Neuromuscular tissues, 118
Neurons, functional specialization, 25
Neuropeptides, 79
neuropeptide Y (NPY), 401, 402, 451
enteric actions, sites, mechanisms, 88
peptide structure, precursors, localization, receptors, 88
Neurotensin, 134, 139, 377, 443, 700
peptide structure, precursors, localization, receptors, 87
sites and mechanisms of actions, 87
Neurotransmitters, action of, 78
Neutral endopeptidase (NEP), 121
Nicotine, 152
Nicotinic cholinergic receptors, 150–151
Nifedipine, 482, 492, 545
Nissl stains, 28–30
Nitric oxide, 27, 78, 147, 451
Nitroglycerin, 482, 492
Nitrous oxide, 556
Non-adrenergic non-cholinergic (NANC) neurotransmitters, 64, 83, 86
activity, 554–555
system, 451
transmission, 443
Noncardiac chest pain (NCCP), 505
Non-REM sleep, 95, 98, 101
Noradrenaline (NA), 25, 147, 148, 154, 377
Norwalk virus, 522
Nuclear medicine, 228
Nucleus of the tractus solitarius (NTS), 72
Nucleus of the vagus nerve (DVN), 72
Nutrients
absorption and hormonal control of digestive motility, 140–141
effect on gastric emptying, 388
Nutrition and digestive motility, 139
Nyctemeral anorectal motor activity, 618

Obesity, 529
Obstructive gastroparesis, 299
Occult rectal prolapse, 660
Octapeptide, 398
Oesophageal body
'at rest' motility, 339
contraction abnormalities, 487–493
motility after swallowing, 347

Oesophageal clearance, 500–503
Oesophageal epithelial resistance, 503
Oesophageal manometry, 510
Oesophageal pressure sensing, 216–217
Oesophageal transit, 179
  radioscintigraphy, 229
Oesophagogastric junction, 3
Oesophago-pharyngeal reflux, 364
Oesophagoscopy, GORD, 508–510
Oesophagus, 3–4, 337–356
  electrical impedance measurements, 285
  electromyography, 262–265, 338
  examination techniques, 337–338
  innervation of, 56
  intramural nerves, 15–17
  lower, 3, 4
  manometry, 337
  motor disorders, 473–495
  motor nerve supply, 4
  peristalsis, 173
  pH measurement, 221
  radiology with contrast material, 337
  scintiscanning, 338
  segmenting contractions, 170
  stress, 104
  structure, 3
  surgical procedures, 678
Omeprazole in GORD, 516–517
Ondansetron, 156
Onuf's nucleus, 451
Opiates, 80–82
  endogenous, 81
  enteric actions, sites, mechanisms, 81–82
  exogenous, 81
  receptor subtypes, 81
Opioids, 138, 157–158
Opium, 157
Organic diseases, diagnosis of, 192
Orocaecal transit time, 308
Osmic acid–zinc iodide stain, 28

Pacemaker region, 290, 292
Pain/dysphagia in contraction abnormalities, 488
Pain provocation tests, 539
Pancreatic duct
  anatomy, 399
  ultrasonography, 398–399
Pancreatic polypeptide (PP)
  enteric actions, sites, mechanisms, 88
  peptide structure, precursors, localization, receptors, 88
Pantothenic acid, 557
Paracetamol in gastric emptying, 308
Parafascicular ganglia, 15
Paraneoplastic neuropathy, 192, 524
Parasympathetic integration, 27–28
Parenteral nutrition, 205
Parkinson's disease, 526, 577
Passive contraction, 44

Peak finding algorithm, 325, 328
Pelvic floor, 8, 11, 450
  dysfunction, 665, 666
Pelvic nerves, 11
Pentagastrin, 491
Pentobarbitone, 556
Peptic oesophagitis, 118
Peptic ulcer disease, 529–531
  medical therapy, 683
  surgical approach, 678
Peptidases, 78
Peptidergic innervation, 52
Peptides, 78–92, 138, 139, 157–159, 401
  colocalization, 78–79
  co-released, 79
  degradation-resistant, 78
  families and modes of action, 78
  immunohistochemical demonstration of, 30
  in regulation of colonic motility, 446
  peptide HI (PHI), 79, 85, 86
  peptide HM (PHM), 79, 85, 86
  peptide YY (PYY), 388, 700
    enteric actions, sites, mechanisms, 88
    peptide structure, precursors, localization, receptors, 88
  receptors, 80
  release, 78–79
  second messengers, 80
  sites and mechanism of action, 80
  storage, 78–79
  structure, precursors, localization, 80–81
  synthesis, 78–79
Perfused catheters, 457
Perfused tube manometry, 183–199
  differentiation from normal patterns, 188
  disease identification by, 188–191
  equipment, 183–185
  manometric studies following, 192
  mechanical obstruction patterns, 188
  pathophysiologic processes identified by, 188–191
  practical advantages, 187–188
  see also Gastroduodenojejunal manometry
Peripheral nerve pathways, 29
Peristalsis, 173–176
  ultrasound, 246
Peristaltic dysfunction, 500
Peristaltic oesophageal motor activity, 500
Peristaltic reflex of intestine, 19
Peritoneum, 8
Permittivity, 276–278
Pethidine, 540
Peyer's patches, 6
pH monitoring, 511
pH sensing applications, 221–225
pH-sensitive radiotelemetry capsules, 213
Pharmacological agents see Drugs

Pharyngeal-oesophageal body disorders, 473–475
Pharyngo-oesophageal dual probe pH-metry, 364
Pharynx
  'at rest' motility, 338
  motility after swallowing, 345
Phenoxybenzamine, 148
Phentolamine, 154, 557
Phenylephrine, 154
Pheochromocytoma, 578
PHI/PHM see Peptides
Phosphatidylinositol 4,5-biphosphate, 147
Phospholipase C, 147
Phrenic ampulla, 365
Physiological stimulation, 558
Physostigmine, 151
PLO17, 157
Pneumohydraulic perfusion, 183
Polyethylene glycol (PEG), 309–316
Polymyositis, 531
Polypeptide hormones, 53
Portable data loggers, 332
Post-cholecystectomy, 304
Post-ganglionic neurones, 64
Post-gastrectomy syndromes, 679–683
  therapeutic strategies, 683
Post-operative ileus, 303
Post-prandial activity, 60–62, 100
  correlation of variables with length of, 62
Post-prandial antral hypomotility, 191, 192
Post-prandial motility, 419–420, 693, 696
Post-prandial motor activity, 616, 617
Post-prandial patterns
  electrogastrography, 296
  hormonal control, 133–139
Post-prandial state, 97–98, 130–131
Post-surgical motility, 673–690
Post-vagotomy antral hypomobility, 192
Post-vagotomy diarrhoea, 682
Pregnancy, nausea of, 303
Premature infants, 304
Pressure inversion point (PIP), 342
Pressure recording, 322–325
Pressure-sensitive radiocapsules, 212–213
Prevertebral ganglia, 27, 75
  functional organization, 27
  transmission in, 27
Prevertebral ganglion cells, efferent projections, 27
Prevertebral ganglion neurons, 48
Primary anorexia nervosa, 526–528
Primary plexus, 13
Primary visceral myopathies, 571
Proctalgia fugax, 665
Proctography, 170
Proenkephalin A, 80
Progresive systemic sclerosis (PSS), 188, 531

Prokinetic drugs, 155, 557–558
  in GORD, 514
Prolonged ambulatory oesophageal pH
    monitoring, 511
Prolonged propagated contractions
    (PPCs), 418, 693
Prostaglandin E$_2$ (PGE$_2$), 377
Prostaglandins, 126, 138, 558
Proton pump blockers, 683
Pruritis ani, 667
Pseudo-achalasia, 369, 480–481
Pseudo-obstruction, 258, 302
  as form of functional bowel
      syndrome, 578
  causes of, 569, 570
  clinical classification, 569
  clinical picture, 567
  diagnostic methods, strategy, 578–
      581
  drug-related, 577–578
  histopathology, 580
  management of, 581
  manometry, 580
  muscular dysfunction in, 569
  pathogenesis, 568
  radiography, 579
  scintigraphy, 579
  tracer studies, 579–580
  unclassifiable causes, 578
  use of term, 567
Psychotherapy in constipation, 645
Puborectalis muscle, 621, 655
Pudendal nerve terminal motor latency
    (PNTML), 658
Pudendal nerves, 11
  assessment, 458–459
Pyloric contractility, sleeve
    methodology, 193–194
Pylorus, 5
  structure and closure, 374–375

Quinacrine fluorescence, 30

Radioactive tracers, 228
Radiocapsules see Radiotelemetry
Radiography, pseudo-obstruction, 579
Radioligand binding techniques, 80
Radiology, 165–182
  defaecatory disorders, 459
  GORD, 506–508
  limitations of, 165
  oesophagus, 337
  techniques, 165
  UOS, 359–360
Radionuclide ejection fraction, 234
Radionuclides, 228
Radio-opaque bolus, 176
Radio-opaque markers, 181–182
Radiopharmaceuticals, 233
Radiopills see Radiotelemetry,
    radiocapsules
Radioscintigraphy, 228–241
  antral emptying, 231–232
  biliary dynamics, 232–235

colonic transit, 235–237
data acquisition, 231, 235
data analysis, 231, 235–237
dosimetry, 228–229
enterogastric reflux, 232–233
fundal emptying, 231–232
gastric emptying, 230–232
gastro-oesophageal reflux, 230
oesophageal transit, 229
radiation risks, 229
Radiotelemetry, 200, 211–227
  aerial detecting system, 214
  ambulatory subjects, 215, 216, 222–
      223
  applications, 215–225
  colonic pressure measurement, 217–
      219
  data collection and storage
      equipment, 214
  data handling and analysis, 215
  digital data storage, 215
  free-fall applications of pH capsules,
      222–223
  gastric pressure, 217
  history, 211
  implantation of pH sensors, 223–224
  implantation of radiocapsules, 216
  inductance type pressure-sensitive
      radiocapsules, 212–213
  miscellaneous uses, 219–221
  pH sensing applications, 221–225
  pH-sensitive capsules, 213
  portable recording systems, 215
  pressure-sensing applications, 216–
      221
  pressure-sensitive capsules, 212–213
  principles, 211
  radiocapsules, 211–213
    general applications, 211
    types available, 211
  receiving and recording systems,
      213–215
  rectal pressure measurement, 217–
      219
  redox potential, 213
  small intestinal pressure, 217
  system requirements, 213
  temperature detection, 213
  transit measurement, 225
Ranitidine, 530
Rapid eye movement (REM) sleep, 95
Rapid phasic contraction frequency,
    542–543
Re-anastomosis, motor consequences
    of, 697–700
Rectal compliance, 456
Rectal function assessment, 458
Rectal motor complexes (RMCs), 98
Rectal pressure, 453
Rectal prolapse, 659–660, 661
Rectal sensation
  impairment of, 657–658
  in constipation, 627–630
Recto-anal inhibitory reflex (RAIR),
    453–454, 458, 658, 667

Recto-anal tract, examination of, 170
Rectocele, 171, 660
Rectosigmoid junction, 7
Rectosphincteric dyssynergia, 604
Rectosphincteric reflex, 676
Rectum, 8, 449
  herniation of, 662
  innervation, 450–451
  intussusception of, 661
  pressure measurement, 217–219
Redox potential, 213
Reduced rectal compliance, 664–665
Reflex control of gastric emptying, 19
Reflex motor responses, 19
Reflex oesophageal peristalsis, 19
Reflex relaxation
  of internal anal sphincter, 19
  of stomach, 19
Reflux oesophagitis, 176
  Savary-Miller classification, 508
REM sleep, 98, 101
REM–non-REM sleep, effect of late
    meal, 100
Repetitive bursts of action potentials
    (RBAPs), 258
Resin casting techniques, biliary tract,
    393
Resistivity of various body parts, 280
Respiratory inversion point (RIP), 368
Retrograde motor activity, 176
Reversed segments, 706–707
Rotavirus, 522
Roux gastrectomy, 192
Roux jejunal limb, 681
Roux-en-Y reconstructions, 304
Roux-en-Y syndrome, 258
Roux-limb reconstruction, 681

Sacral reflex function, 631
Sampling reflex, 453
Sarcoplasmic reticulum, 38, 48
Satiety sensation, 75
Schabadasch's plexus, 18, 19
Scintigraphic defaecography
  data analysis, 238–239
  defaecation, 237–239
  protocol, 238
Scintigraphy
  gallbladder, 539
  oesophageal motor function, 491–
      492
  pseudo-obstruction, 579
  scleroderma, 485
Scintiscanning, oesophagus, 338
Scleroderma, 204, 205, 483–485
  manometry, 485
  myopathy, 571
  scintigraphy, 485
Secondary plexus, 13
Secretin, 134, 406
Segmenting stationary contractions,
    170–173
Serosal patching, 707
Serotonin, 25

Sexual abuse and constipation, 604, 632
Short-chain (or volatile) fatty acid (SCFA) solution, 418
Short spike bursts (SSBs), 434–436
Shunt fascicle, 21
Silver impregnation, 28
Single firer EMG, 458
Sleep, 95–103
  aims of measuring gastrointestinal motor activity during, 102
  and gastrointestinal motility, 95
  and IBS, 101–102
  clustered motor hyperactivity during, 206
  normal MMC during, 203
Sleeve catheters, 458
Slow waves, 290, 292, 410–411, 451
  colonic smooth muscle, 430
  surgical intervention, 693
Small bowel, 410–426
  motility patterns, 201
  peristalsis, 175
  resection and bypass, 684–686
  stress, 108–109
  transection, 676, 684
Small bowel disease, 684
Small intensely fluorescent (SIF) cells, 27
Small intestine, 5–7
  altered motility in, 119
  digestive status, 130–131
  electromyography, 266–268
  feedback inhibition, 388
  in IBS, 585
  intramural nerves, 17–18
  motility in disease, 423–425
  motor activity, 57
  pH measurement, 222
  postoperative-ileus, 548–550
  pressure measurement, 217
  stages of motor development, 58
Smooth muscle, 569
  electrical activity recording, 256–257
  from inflamed gut, 120–121
  function in inflamed intestine, 121–123
  infiltration, 571
  motor control, 51–52
  oesophageal body disorders, 475–485
  structure of, 32–48
Smooth muscle cells, 33, 43, 51, 120, 145, 569, 570, 691, 692
Solitary rectal ulcer syndrome, 659–660
Somatic nervous system, 451
Somatostatin, 53, 88–89, 141, 159, 401, 402
  peptide structure, precursors and localization, 89
  sites and mechanisms of enteric actions, 89
Spastic colitis, 127
Spectral analysis, 328

Sphincter of Oddi, 393
  cholescintigraphy, 542
  dysfunction, 540–545
    endoscopic sphincterotomy (ES), 545
  dyskinesia, 542–544, 545
  electromyography, 397
  investigations, 540–541
  manometry, 394–397, 403–406, 542–544
  morphology, 399–401
  motility, 406
  stenosis, 542, 545
  treatment, 545
  ultrasonography, 398–399, 541
Sphincter substitutes, 703–706
Sphincteric mechanism, 457
Spike potentials, 290–291
Spinal cord, 145
Sporadic hollow visceral myopathy, 192
Stach's plexus, 19
Steady burst neurons, single-spike pattern, 25
Stomach, 4–5
  abnormal electrogastrographic rhythms, 296–305
  anatomical regions, 4
  computed tomography image, 5
  contractility of, 287
  digestion and dispersion of food, 381–382
  digestive status, 130
  electromyography, 265
  extrinsic denervation, 676
  extrinsic innervation, 378–379
  extrinsic vs intrinsic control of gastric motility, 379
  functional morphology, 373–374
  intramural nerves, 17
  intrinsic innervation, 377
  motility disorders, 522–537
  motor activity, 56–57
  muscle layers, 373–374
  musculature, 32–33
  myoelectrical activity, 265, 290–291
  neuromuscular anatomy, 373–374
  normal electrogastrographic activity, 294–296
  normal motility, 379
  normal motor functions, 673
  parasympathetic nerve supply, 5
  peristalsis, 173
  postoperative ileus, 548
  reflex relaxation of, 19
  reservoir function, 380–381
  schematic diagram, 373
  segmenting contractions, 170
  sensory innervation, 379
  small capacity, 680
  stress, 104–107
  transit of digesta, 133
Stool consistency, 595
Stool frequency, 595–598
Stool weight, 595

Strain gauge catheter, 207
Strain gauges, 213, 322
Stress, 104–117
  and disease, 113–115
  and functional disorders, 104
  animal studies, 104–105, 108, 109
  as physiological response, 112
  concepts of, 112
  environmental, 112–113
  experimental investigations, 104–112
  human studies, 105–107, 109–112
  large bowel, 109–112
  maladaption, 113–115
  oesophagus, 104
  reaction stereotypes, 113–115
  research perspectives, 115
  small bowel, 108–109
  stomach, 104–107
Striated muscle activity, in achalasia, 479
Striated muscle disorders, 473–475
Striated sphincter dysfunction, 660–663
Stroma, 40–43
Submucosa, 44
Submucosal neurons, 48
Submucous plexus, 13, 15
Substance K, 159
Substance P, 25, 84, 120, 123, 158, 159, 401, 402, 406
Sucking activity
  after birth, 54–55
  in utero, 53–55
  mechanism of, 54–55
  oesophageal phase, 55
  oropharyngeal phase, 55
Sufentanyl, 157
Sulphasalazine in mouth–caecum transit measurement, 317
Supravital methylene blue, 28
Surgical procedures, 192
  animal studies, 674–676
  clinical outcome, 678–688
  for malignant neoplasms, 683
  historical perspectives, 678–680
  increasing effective absorptive area, 707–709
  motility effects, 674–676
  physiological basis for effects of, 691
  restorative, 703–709
Suspensor duodeni, 43
Swallowing activity
  after birth, 54–55
  defects in neural control of, 474
  difficulties in, 474
  in utero, 53–55
  mechanism of, 54–55
  motility after, 345–355
  motor programme of, 75
  oesophageal phase, 55
  oropharyngeal phase, 55
Sympatholytics, 556
Synaptic transmission, in intramural enteric nerves, 25
Systemic lupus erythematosus, 484

Tachy Oddia, 542–544
Tachyarrhythmias, 304
Tachygastrias, 298–304
Tachykinins, 84–85, 159
　endogenous, 85
　peptide structure, precursors,
　　localization, receptor subtypes,
　　84
　sites and mechanisms of action, 84–85
Taenia coli, 34, 35, 37, 38, 41
Taeniae, 7
T-cell function, 122
Temperature detection,
　radiotelemetry, 213
Tertiary plexus, 13
Tetrodotoxin, 144
Thiopentone, 556
Thoracolumbar pathways, 11–12
　entering into craniosacral pathways,
　　11–12
Thyrotropin-releasing hormone, 137
Tissue resistivities, 280
T-lymphocytes, 122, 123
Total gastrectomy, 304
Tracer studies, pseudo-obstruction,
　579–580
Transcutaneous gastric electrical
　activity, 286–287
Transection
　bowel wall, 676
　motor consequences of, 697–700
Transit
　chemical detection, 308–318
　principle of, 308
　colonic, radioscintigraphy, 235–237
Transit measurement, radiotelemetry,
　225
Transit rate, 176–182
Transit slowering surgical procedures,
　703–707
Transitional zone, 9
Transmitter substances of enteric
　neurons, 25
Traumatic spinal cord transection, 526
Trazodone, 492
Trichinella infection, 121–127
Trichinella spiralis, 123, 126
Trifluperidol, 556
Trimebutine, 645
Trimethaphan, 153
Trinitrobenzene sulphonic acid
　(TNB), 126

Trituration, 381–382
Truncal vagotomy, 679
Trypanosoma cruzi, 481
Tumor necrosis factor α (TNFα), 124
Tyramine, 154

U-50488, 157
Ulcerative colitis, 120, 127
Ultrasound, 242–255
　advantages, 254
　antral contraction characteristics, 248
　antral filling and emptying, 247
　antral motor functions, 246–247
　antral peristaltic rhythmicity, 247
　antroduodenal coordination, 250–
　　251
　apparatus, 243–245
　application, 243
　biliary duct, 398–399
　clinical applications, 253
　development of, 242–243
　duration of study, 252
　future applications, 252–254
　gallbladder, 398
　gastric emptying, 247
　gastroduodenal reflux, 250–251
　history, 242
　inter- and intra-observer variability,
　　251
　lateral movement of antrum after
　　feeding, 251–252
　limitations, 254
　luminal flow, 250–251
　machine description, 243–245
　measurements, 245–247
　pancreatic duct, 398–399
　pharmacological considerations, 253
　physiological considerations, 253
　plotting and measurement of region
　　of interest, 244
　real-time, 242
　real-time, high-resolution, 242
　recording and storage of images, 244
　reliability of measurements, 251–252
　reproducibility and subject
　　variability, 251
　reproducibility between different
　　laboratories, 251
　sphincter of Oddi, 398–399, 541
　technique, 245
　test meal selection, 244

Upper anal canal (UAC), 450
Upper gastrointestinal pressure profile,
　192–193
Upper gastrointestinal tract, pH
　sensing applications, 221–225
Upper oesophageal sphincter (UOS),
　337, 473, 474
　achalasia, 360
　anatomy, 357
　'at rest' motility, 339
　manometry, 360–361
　motility after swallowing, 345–347
　physiology, 358–359
　radiology, 359–360
　responsiveness, 364
　spasm, 360

Vagi
　motor functions, 27
　sensory functions, 27
Vagotomy, 71
Vagovagal arc, 70, 72
Vagovagal reflexes, 27–28
Varicella zoster, 522
Vasoactive intestinal polypeptide
　(VIP), 27, 53, 79, 85–86, 121,
　377, 401, 402, 406, 443, 700
Vasopressin, 491
Ventromedial nucleus of the
　hypothalamus (VMH), 138
Villi, 6
Viral infection, 522
Visceral musculature
　development of, 44–45
　hypertrophy of, 45–48
Visceral myopathies, 571
Visceral neuropathies, 571, 572–577
Volume measurements, 332
Vomiting, 192

Wall movements, 170–176
Wallenberg syndrome, 474
Weaning, 53

Zenker's diverticulum, 475
Zollinger–Ellison syndrome, 679, 683